Pediatric Radiation Oncology
Third Edition

Pediatric Radiation Oncology
Third Edition

Edward C. Halperin, M.D.
The Leonard R. Prosnitz Professor and Chairman
Department of Radiation Oncology
Professor, Department of Pediatrics
Duke University Medical Center
Durham, North Carolina

Louis S. Constine, M.D.
Professor of Radiation Oncology and Pediatrics
Section Chief, Pediatric Radiation Oncology
University of Rochester Medical Center
Rochester, New York

Nancy J. Tarbell, M.D.
Head, Pediatric Radiation Oncology Unit
Director, Office for Women's Affairs
Massachusetts General Hospital
Harvard Medical School
Boston, Massachusetts

Larry E. Kun, M.D.
Chairman, Department of Radiation Oncology
St. Jude Children's Research Hospital
Director, Section of Radiation Oncology
University of Tennessee College of Medicine
Memphis, Tennessee

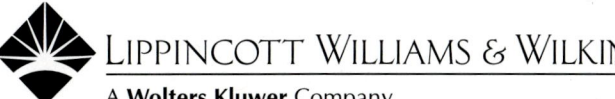

LIPPINCOTT WILLIAMS & WILKINS
A **Wolters Kluwer** Company
Philadelphia • Baltimore • New York • London
Buenos Aires • Hong Kong • Sydney • Tokyo

Manufacturing Manager: Kevin Watt
Production Manager: Robert Pancotti
Production Editor: Jeff Somers
Indexer: Michael Ferreira
Compositor: Lippincott Williams & Wilkins Desktop Division
Printer: Maple Press

Printed in the United States of America

9 8 7 6 5 4 3 2 1

Library of Congress Cataloging-in-Publication Data
Pediatric radiation oncology / Edward C. Halperin ... [et al.]. — 3rd ed.
     p.   cm.
   Includes bibliographical references and index.
   ISBN-0-7817-1500-8 (alk. paper)
   1. Tumors in children—Radiotherapy. I. Halperin, Edward C.
   [DNLM: 1. Neoplasms—in infancy & childhood. 2. Neoplasms—radiotherapy.
3. Radiotherapy—in infancy & childhood. QZ 275P3713 1999]
RC281.C4P447 1999
618.92'99406402—dc21
DNLM/DLC
for Library of Congress   98-33919
                                                                CIP

For our children

Contents

Preface ix

Acknowledgments xi

1. The Cancer Problem in Children 1

2. Leukemia 10

3. Supratentorial Brain Tumors Except Ependymomas; Brain Tumors
   in Babies and Very Young Children 37

4. Tumors of the Posterior Fossa and the Spinal Canal 80

5. Retinoblastoma 126

6. Neuroblastoma 163

7. Hodgkin's Disease 203

8. Non-Hodgkin's Lymphoma 233

9. Ewing's Sarcoma 245

10. Osteosarcoma 267

11. Rhabdomyosarcoma 289

12. Soft-Tissue Sarcomas Other Than Rhabdomyosarcoma; Desmoid Tumor . . . 320

13. Wilms' Tumor 343

14. Tumors of the Liver and Biliary Tree 373

15. Germ and Stromal Cell Tumors of the Gonads and Extragonadal
    Germ Cell Tumors 386

16. Endocrine, Aerodigestive Tract, and Breast Tumors 395

17. Langerhans' Cell Histiocytosis 422

18. Skin Cancer, Hemangioma, and Lymphangioma 446

19. Late Effects of Cancer Treatment 457

20. Secondary Tumors 538

21. Anesthesia for External-Beam Radiotherapy
    (In collaboration with Scott Schulman) 563

22. Stabilization and Immobilization Devices 576

Subject Index 587

Preface

In 1986, we conceived the idea of a new textbook of pediatric radiation oncology. There was no shortage of general textbooks in radiation oncology at that time. There were, in fact, several in existence and many more to come. There was not, however, a textbook specifically devoted to the use of radiation therapy for the treatment of childhood cancer. The texts that were available in the marketplace of the mid-1980's were largely devoted to adult cancer. We believed that there was a need for a focused text in pediatric radiation oncology and we set out to write it.

Most clinical oncology textbooks are hefty tomes, edited by several physicians, with each chapter assigned to individual authors so that the book is written by one to three dozen experts. For the reader to do justice to any individual chapter, several hours of study are required. From its inception, our concept for *Pediatric Radiation Oncology* was at variance with this common textbook practice. We believed that a text was needed wherein each section, individually devoted to a specific tumor type, could be read at one sitting. We imagined the need of a house officer or practitioner, confronted with a case of childhood cancer at the end of a busy clinical day, and preparing to present the case the next day at morning rounds: time did not allow for a long trip to the library, the copying of multiple articles from the primary literature, their synthesis, and the formulation of a case management plan by morning. We felt that we could and should write a book wherein this hypothetical clinician could find enough background information to understand the disease he or she faced, what was called for in diagnostic and staging studies, what the treatment strategy ought to be, and when and how to employ radiation therapy. By morning rounds the physicians could not presume themselves to be experts—but could present themselves as informed, competent, and ready to explore the topic in more depth.

As we conceived this book, we felt that it would be best written by a team. The chapters should reflect controversies in management. All major sides of an issue should be presented so that the reader may form their own opinion. We did not, and do not, shirk from offering our opinion on many topics of controversy, but we have striven to be fair to alternative views. This book is intentionally not a practice of pediatric radiation oncology book, i.e., a formulaic book that represents the treatment philosophy of one institution. We have tried to write all the chapters with a common voice, avoiding repetition and maintaining reasonable uniformity of style. We have included tables and illustrations that might be classified as historical. We believe that it is instructive and humbling to see how much was known about childhood cancer by our forebears in this discipline.

The response to our vision, as expressed in the first two editions of *Pediatric Radiation Oncology*, has been gratifying. We believe that the book has found a niche in the medical literature. We have been honored by supportive reviews and gracious praise and have benefited from the many helpful suggestions we have received from readers over the years. The selection of the book for the Association of Residents in Radiation Oncology (ARRO)'s "you should have" list was particularly appreciated. Buoyed by the medical community's support of the first two editions, and persuaded that new knowledge in the specialty warranted a thoroughly updated text, we undertook this Third Edition.

It's hard to believe that over a decade has passed since we began the first edition of this book. It is gratifying to have witnessed how far our discipline has come, and daunting to realize how far we have to go. We hope that the three editions of this text have contributed to an improved understanding of the benefits and risks of radiotherapy for children. We trust that the dissemination of knowledge about pediatric radiation oncology will improve the quality and quantity of life for children afflicted with cancer.

Edward C. Halperin, M.D.
Louis S. Constine, M.D.
Nancy J. Tarbell, M.D.
Larry E. Kun, M.D.

Acknowledgments

For all those children who have taught us about life, bravery, pain, and serenity; as well as for what they have taught us about clinical pediatric radiation oncology, we are grateful beyond words. We pray that *Pediatric Radiation Oncology* will serve, in the ultimate measure of our days, as some small repayment for what our patients have given to us.

The manuscript for the Third Edition was prepared by Ruth Aultman. Were it not for the skilled and devoted work of Ms. Aultman, the book would never have been completed. Additional manuscript preparation was done by Patricia Bray (Memphis), Ann G. Muhs (Rochester), and Carole Obst (Memphis). Stuart Freeman, David Dritsas, Jeffrey Somers, and the staff of Lippincott Williams & Wilkins were, at all times, courteous and helpful.

We are indebted to our teachers: J. Robert Cassady, Juan A. del Regato, Sarah Donaldson, Samuel Hellman, Henry Kaplan, Rita M. Linggood, Leon Rosenberg, Philip Rubin, Stephen Sallan, Herman D. Suit, Samuel O. Thier, and John Truman.

The love of our families has been a source of constant strength to us.

Pediatric Radiation Oncology
Third Edition

1

The Cancer Problem in Children

THE EXTENT OF THE PROBLEM

In 1900, cancer trailed typhoid fever, malaria, smallpox, measles, scarlet fever, whooping cough, diphtheria, croup, influenza, dysentery, erysipelas, tuberculosis, venereal disease, meningitis, acute bronchitis, pneumonia, accidents, birth injuries, and violence as a cause of death in children in the United States (1,2). Cancer mortality per 100,000 persons in the United States and Canada from 1911 to 1916 was 3.7 for 1- to 4-year-olds, 1.4 for 5- to 9-year-olds, 1.3 for 10- to 14-year-olds, and 2.8 for 15- to 19-year-olds. Death from cancer, as a percentage of mortality from all causes, constituted only 0.43% for these same age groups (1).

At the end of the twentieth century, in economically developed countries, cancer in children has become a significant problem in comparison to other causes of childhood mortality (3). There are 7,500 to 8,000 new cases of cancer per year among children in the United States and approximately 1700 cancer deaths (4–6). This later statistic places cancer as the second leading cause of childhood death in the United States among 1- to 14-year-olds—following accidents and preceding congenital anomalies and homicide (6,7). For the youngest children, however, cancer is not a major cause of mortality. Cancer does not even appear on the list of the ten leading causes of infant death in the United States (8). The leading causes of death in infants are congenital anomalies, disorders relating to short gestation and low birth weight, and sudden infant death syndrome.

The incidence of cancer is lowest for 5- to 14-year-olds (10–13 new cases per 100,000 per year) and highest for 0- to 4-year-olds and 15- to 19-year-olds (19–21 new cases/100,000 per year) (Table 1) (9). The mortality rate from cancer for children is approximately 3 deaths per 100,000 population per year (5,10). The most recent *Vital Statistics of the United States* reports approximately 100 cancer deaths per year in 0- to 1-year-olds, 500 in 1- to 4-year-olds, and 1,100 in 5- to 14-year-olds (11,12).

Although cancer is a major cause of childhood death in developed countries, it continues to trail infections as a cause of mortality in developing countries (6,13–15). In many parts of the world, nutritional standards, housing, climate, and sanitation conditions create relative childhood mortality statistics such as those reported in the industrialized countries earlier in this century. It is likely, however, that future improvements in the standard of living, the success of immunization programs, and dissemination of medical services will

TABLE 1. *US and Canada age-specific cancer incidence rate per 1,000,000 by age and sex*

	US		Canada	
Age (y)	Male	Female	Male	Female
<1			26.9	24.7
0–4	20.7	18.9		
1–4			24.1	19.2
5–9	12.5	9.7	13.0	10.4
10–14	12.6	11.2	12.3	10.8
15–19	21.3	20.6	20.0	19.6

From refs. 5 and 10 with permission.

1

make inroads against infectious disease and thereby make childhood cancer a major cause of death in developing nations. Finally, there is almost certainly some variation in childhood cancer rates between countries because of differing abilities to ascertain and treat cases in different parts of the world.

THE RELATIVE FREQUENCY OF THE VARIOUS TYPES OF CHILDHOOD CANCER

The relative frequency of the various types of childhood cancer is influenced by whether we are examining incidence or mortality and by how we stratify by age, sex, or nation. Among the most commonly used data are those of the Surveillance, Epidemiology, and End Results (SEER) program. SEER is a continuing project of the Biometry Branch of the United States National Cancer Institute

(NCI). The program draws data from several population-based cancer reporting systems covering approximately 10% of the total population of the United States (5,16). The adjusted relative frequency of the common forms of childhood cancer from SEER is shown in Table 2. Leukemias, brain and spinal tumors, lymphomas, sympathetic nervous system tumors (neuroblastoma), kidney (Wilms') tumors, and soft tissue and bone sarcomas are the most frequent childhood cancers. The common epithelial tumors of adults are rare in children.

Childhood cancer deaths for the United States are shown in Table 3. In general, approximately one-third of childhood cancer deaths are caused by leukemia, and about one-fifth of these deaths are by brain tumors (5,11,17,18). The relative frequency of cancer types varies as a function of age groups. The most common tumors of neonates (≤28 days

TABLE 2. *Childhood cancer in the US: percent distribution by histology, SEER data 1973–1987*

Leukemias	31.4%	
Acute lymphocytic leukemia		23.6%
Acute nonlymphocytic leukemia		4.7%
Chronic myeloid leukemia		0.7%
Lymphomas	12.4%	
Hodgkin's disease		5.1%
Non-Hodgkin's lymphoma		3.8%
Burkitt's lymphoma		1.5%
Central nervous system	17.6%	
Ependymoma		1.7%
Astrocytoma		9.6%
Medulloblastoma		4.2%
Sympathetic nervous system, i.e., neuroblastoma and ganglioneuroblastoma	8.1%	
Retinoblastoma	2.9%	
Wilms' tumor	6.3%	
Hepatic tumors	1.3%	
Hepatoblastoma		0.9%
Hepatic carcinoma		0.4%
Bone	5%	
Osteosarcoma		2.6%
Ewing's sarcoma		2.0%
Soft-tissue sarcoma	7.1%	
Rhabdomyosarcoma, embryonal sarcoma, and soft-tissue Ewing's tumor		3.6%
Fibrosarcoma, neurofibrosarcoma and other fibromatous neoplasms		1.7%
Other soft-tissue sarcomas		1.8%
Germ cell, trophoblastic other gonadal neoplasms	3.2%	
Carcinoma and other malignant epithelial neoplasms	4.0%	
Thyroid		
Nasopharyngeal		
Melanoma		

From ref. 4, with permission.

TABLE 3. *Reported yearly US cancer deaths for the five leading cancer sites, by gender, for individuals <15 years of age*

Male		Female	
All cancer	978	All cancer	721
Leukemia	359	Leukemia	238
Brain and CNS	255	Brain and CNS	205
Endocrine	113	Endocrine	74
Non-Hodgkin's lymphoma	63	Bones and joints	44
Soft tissue	47	Soft tissue	37

From ref. 18, with permission.

of age), for example, are teratomas, retinoblastoma, rhabdomyosarcoma, and neuroblastoma (19). In 15- to 20-year-olds, the list is headed by lymphoma (25%), epithelial tumors (18%), bone malignancies (15%), followed by leukemia, central nervous system (CNS) tumors, and gonadal/germ cell tumors (10% each) (20).

Reviews of the incidence and mortality of childhood cancer are available from national and political subdivision registries throughout the world (16,21–25). Table 4 demonstrates the similar childhood cancer incidence rates in Australia, the United Kingdom, and the United States. While the absolute frequency of certain tumors is reported to be higher in developing countries than in industrialized states, there is likely to be variation in reporting standards, diagnostic techniques, and

TABLE 4. *Cancer incidence rates for the most common childhood malignancies, per 100,000 individuals ≤14 years in Australia, US, and UK*

	Australia	UK	US
Acute lymphoblastic leukemia	4.0	3.0	3.1
Hodgkin's disease	0.4	0.4	0.7
Non-Hodgkin's lymphoma	0.6	0.6	0.8
CNS tumors	3.0	2.5	2.9
Neuroblastoma	1.0	0.7	0.9
Retinoblastoma	0.4	0.4	0.4
Wilms' tumor	0.8	0.7	0.8
Osteosarcoma	0.2	0.3	0.4
Ewing's tumor	0.3	0.2	0.3
Rhabdomyosarcoma	0.5	0.4	0.5
Nonrhabdomyosarcoma soft-tissue sarcoma	0.4	0.2	0.2

From refs. 5, 17, and 54, with permission.

histopathologic review (24,26). In Cuba, the most frequent childhood tumor is leukemia (31%), followed by lymphoma (18%), CNS tumors (15%), sympathetic nervous system tumors (7%), soft-tissue sarcomas (6%), and renal tumors (5%) (13). In Thailand, leukemias are most frequent (40%), followed by CNS tumors (14%), lymphoma (12%), bone tumors (4%), and soft-tissue sarcomas (4%) (27).

TRENDS IN CHILDHOOD CANCER MORTALITY RATES

Table 5 demonstrates that from 1950 to 1992 the mortality rate from childhood cancer has fallen dramatically in the United States. This finding is additionally illustrated in Table 6. In 1960 to 1963, the 5-year cancer survival rate for children was 28%. This rate had risen to 71% by 1986 to 1992. Particularly impressive gains have been posted for acute lymphocytic leukemia, bone tumors (predominantly osteosarcoma and Ewing's sarcoma), Hodgkin's disease, non-Hodgkin's lymphoma, soft-tissue sarcomas (including rhabdomyosarcoma and nonrhabdomyosarcoma soft-tissue sarcomas), and Wilms' tumor. While gains have also been achieved for acute myelocytic leukemia, neuroblastoma, and brain tumors, the improvements have either been less dramatic or confined to certain subgroups or stages. In general, however, the diagnosis and treatment of childhood cancer has been one of the success stories of modern medicine.

It is clear that when compared to adult cancer, childhood cancer is a vanishingly rare event. For example, in 1991 there were

TABLE 5. *43-Year trends in US childhood cancer mortality rates*

Age group (y)	1950	1975	1992
0–4	11.0	5.1	2.9
5–14	6.6	4.7	3.0

Age-adjusted to the 1970 US standard population; rates per 100,000 population.
From ref. 5, with permission.

TABLE 6. *Trends in 5-year cancer survival rates for US children <15 years of age, 1960–1992*

Site	1960–1963	1970–1973	1974–1976	1977–1979	1980–1982	1983–1985	1986–1992
All sites[a]	28%	45%	56%	61%	65%	68%	71%
Acute lymphocytic leukemia	4	34	53	67	70	70	79
Acute myeloid leukemia	3	5	14	26	21[b]	32[b]	33
Bones and joints	20[b]	30[b]	54[b]	52[b]	54[b]	58[b]	65
Brain and other nervous system	35	45	54	57	55	62	61
Hodgkin's disease	52[b]	90	79	83	91	91	92
Neuroblastoma	25	40	52	53	53	54	63
Non-Hodgkin's lymphoma	18	26	45	51	62	70	71
Soft tissue	38[b]	60[b]	60	69	65	78	72
Wilms' tumor	33[b]	70[b]	74	77	86	86	93

Year at diagnosis

[a]Excludes basal and squamous cell skin cancer and *in situ* carcinomas except bladder.
[b]The standard error of the survival rates is between 5–10%.
From refs. 6 and 18, with permission.

143,758 reported deaths *from lung cancer alone* in the United States (5,6). The comparative infrequency of childhood cancer is highlighted by the fact that more people in the United States die of lung cancer in 1 week than children die of all forms of cancer in 1 year. Looking at the impact of cancer solely in this manner, however, obscures the issue. If one looks at a death from cancer in terms of *potential years of life lost* then one readily appreciates that the consequences of the death of an 8-year-old from acute lymphocytic leukemia will have greater statistical weight than the death of an 82-year-old from small cell carcinoma of the lung. Therefore, the success of medical treatment of childhood cancer has a significant public health impact when considered in terms of the person-years of potential life saved or lifetime earnings. There is a lifetime saved for every child cured of cancer (9).

IS THE INCIDENCE OF CHILDHOOD CANCER INCREASING?

SEER, the Manchester Children's Tumor Registry in Northwestern England, a registry for Queensland, Australia, the Greater Delaware Valley Pediatric Tumor Registry, and a study from Canada indicate an increase in cancer incidence in children of approximately 1% per year in the 1970s and 1980s

(28–30). While a study in Denmark did not find a rising incidence, overall the evidence supports an increase in childhood cancer incidence (21).

The data concerning changes in the incidence of acute leukemia in childhood is somewhat conflicting. Some reports indicate it is rising and some show it to be stable. Improvements in diagnosis have decreased the number of children labeled as "leukemia, not otherwise specified" and increased the number of children given a specific leukemia type as a diagnosis. Most studies, however, indicate an increase in the incidence of childhood brain tumors and lymphoma (28,29).

If we accept the premise that the overall incidence of childhood cancer is rising, then we must bear in mind several potential confounding factors. To wit: (a) The frequency of childhood cancer is so low that it takes only a few cases, in registries covering a small population base, to suggest a change in incidence (31); (b) As the diagnostic tools of modern medicine improve, more children will be correctly diagnosed with cancer as opposed to another diagnosis. This may be particularly important for brain tumors (28). It has been suggested that exposure to magnetic fields emanating from electric transmission and distribution lines and certain electrical household appliances may be associated with some childhood tumors. The available studies are contradictory (30). In summary, an explanation for the increase in childhood cancer incidence is, as yet, not established.

WHAT DOES "CURE" MEAN IN PEDIATRIC ONCOLOGY?

The English word "cure" is derived from the Latin term *cura* and the Old French term *cure*—both meaning *care*. The generally accepted definition in medicine for cure is "successful medical treatment; the action or process of healing a wound, a disease, or a sick person; restoration to health" (32). There are several mathematical and statistical definitions of cure. Cure may be defined as that state where "the expectation of life of a group of patients free of disease become similar to that of the general population of the same sex and age constitution" (33). One way of expressing this type of probability of survival is a "relative" survival rate. The relative survival rate is the ratio of the observed percentage of survival to the percentage expected on the basis of general population experience, adjusted for age, sex, race, and calendar year. Utilizing this definition, a population of patients would be cured when a graph plotting relative survival rate showed a horizontal line (34).

Pinkel (35) has summarized the criteria of biologic cure as (a) completion of all cancer treatment, (b) continuous freedom from cancer relapse, and (c) minimal or no risk of subsequent relapse. It is important to consider the continuous cancer-free survival (other commonly used terms are relapse-free survival and event-free survival) and the overall survival in the construction of survival curves. Overall survival rates will reflect factors other than biologic curability, including: (a) death due to complications of treatment; and (b) subjective factors such as the will of the patient to continue living with cancer or its repeated relapses, the determination of the physician to keep the patient alive, and the technical and financial resources available to the physician and the patient (35).

Collins (36) provided a definition of cure, concerning Wilms' tumor, which is worth noting because it is of historical interest as well as of some practical use:

> If one accepts the prenatal origin of this tumor as occurring within a fixed period of embryonic development, then the time of recognition and diagnosis would depend upon the rate of growth....If the rate of growth was characteristic of an individual tumor, then this would not only govern the time of first appearance of the primary tumor but would also place limits upon the length of time in which a recurrence might be expected to develop. A tumor present at birth had to develop to clinically recognizable size in a period of 9 months or less. If it were to recur following surgical removal, then this should require no longer than an additional 9 months. A tumor first recognized at the age of 5 years and incompletely removed should again reach the size of clinical recognition either as a recurrence at the primary site or as a distant metastasis in a period not to exceed 5 years plus 9 months.

There is no biologic evidence that the "prenatal origin" of childhood tumors necessarily implies that tumor doubling times are correlated with the patient's age at the time of diagnosis.

Collins' hypothesis, however, has generally agreed with the observed rates of recurrence in Wilms' tumor and medulloblastoma. Because it is in agreement with clinical data, even though there is no modern biologic rationale to support it, Collins' hypothesis is of some use in determining that point in time beyond which a child treated for Wilms' tumor or medulloblastoma is unlikely to relapse.

The reported cure rates in pediatric cancer may be affected by artifacts of data acquisition and analysis. The "zero-time shift" or "lead-time bias" will extend the statistical length of survival without prolonging life. This phenomenon occurs when a new screening test or imaging study leads to the detection of a previously unknown tumor. Even if therapy is ineffectual, survival is increased by the interval provided by the earlier detection of the cancer. The "Will Rogers effect" occurs when there are improved techniques for detection of cancer metastases. These new data allow patients to migrate from lower stages of cancer to higher. Such migration improves survival in lower stages by eliminating those with metastatic disease. Survival also improves in higher stages because of the addition of people with minimal metastatic disease. Survival improves in each stage while overall survival for the cancer is unaffected. This phenomenon is named after the American humorist Will Rogers, who is reputed to have remarked during the economic depression of the 1930s that "when the Okies left Oklahoma and moved to California, they raised the average intelligence in both states" (37).

With improving cure rates in childhood cancer, it is apparent that we must move beyond the statistical definition of cure (20,38). Cure means more than "the absence of disease." It is important to provide the child with a "functional" cure, regaining or retaining the ability to conduct oneself in society without major handicaps and by minimizing the need for significant support. Planning for adequate limb function, ambulation, and activities of daily living are crucial in planning a course of treatment. Rehabilitation including physical, occupational, and recreational therapy plays an important part in follow-up care. A comprehensive pediatric cancer rehabilitation program requires individuals with expertise in prosthetics, orthoses, ostomy care, gait training, and pain management (22,39–42). Attention to the child's emotional status is also important. This includes the preservation and nurturing of a sense of well-being on the part of the child and their family. The family should be given every measure of support in dealing with illness and restoration of health. The diagnosis and treatment of cancer will generate severe emotional and financial strains on a family.

Parental separation and divorce, sibling behavior problems, and the weight of family responsibilities during adversity complicate the treatment and rehabilitation of the pediatric cancer patient (43,44). The pediatric radiation oncologist should ensure an ongoing relationship with the child and family after treatment to contribute to the rehabilitative process. As the survival rates for pediatric cancers im-

prove, we will have an increasing population of young adults who are cancer survivors. These individuals will pose new problems for medicine and society: What will be appropriate medical surveillance for late effects of treatment, including secondary malignancy? How shall these patients be counseled concerning reproduction? What special needs will such individuals have concerning employment, disability and health insurance, and psychological support (41)? The pediatric radiation oncologist will play an important role in understanding these issues and implementing solutions (45). Fortunately, there is an evolving body of literature addressing these questions, including a recommended monograph (46).

QUANTITATIVE MEASUREMENT OF THE QUALITY OF LIFE

As emphasized in the previous section, the goals of therapy for the child with cancer should include not only the cure but restoration of function. Adult oncologists have long recognized the value of qualitative measurements of functional status of patients. By giving a numerical value to the patient's functional status, one can track performance of a single patient over time and, in clinical trials, assess the performance of a large number of individuals. Among the most popular scales for the assessment of adult functional status is the one promulgated by David Karnofsky: the Karnofsky performance scale (KPS) (47). The KPS assigns a value of 0% to 100% to a patient based on the degree of impairment. The KPS has been used in the assessment of children with cancer, but it is not entirely appropriate. The KPS emphasizes the ability to care for oneself, the need for assistance, and the ability to carry on with normal activity. In addition, the KPS score is usually assigned by the treating clinician. The "work" of children is play, and the person best able to judge the child's play is an observant parent. In pediatric oncology, therefore, the Lansky Play–Performance Scale is more suitable because it is designed

TABLE 7. *The Lansky play–performance scale*

A parent is asked to select the description that best describes the child's play during the past week, averaging out good and bad days.

100%	Fully active
90%	Minor restrictions in physical strenuous play
80%	Restricted in physically strenuous play (i.e., chasing games); may tire more easily but otherwise active
70%	Both greater restriction of, and less time spent in, active play
60%	Ambulatory 50% of time; limited active play with adult assistance, supervision
50%	Considerable adult assistance required for any active play; fully able to engage in quiet play (set up games, turn on TV, etc.)
40%	Able to initiate most quiet games
30%	Needs considerable assistance even for quiet activities
20%	Play entirely limited to very passive activities initiated by others (i.e., watching television)
10%	Completely disabled, no play
0%	Unresponsive

Modified from ref. 48.

to quantitate the degree to which cancer has disrupted the child's play (48). The parent is asked to select the description that best describes the child's play during the previous week, averaging good and bad days. A value from 0% to 100% is selected, just as in the KPS (Table 7).

THE SITE OF CARE AND THE PEDIATRIC CANCER TEAM

The effective use of combined modality therapy has been a rewarding approach to pediatric cancer management. A coordinated group of medical and surgical specialists with expertise and interests in the clinical care of children with cancer, as well as in basic and clinical research, best directs the child's care. The complete pediatric cancer center will be staffed by a pediatric medical oncologist, specially trained nurses, a pediatric diagnostic radiologist, surgeons with expertise in pediatric oncology, anesthesiologists, psychiatrists, physiotherapists, physicians' assistants, and skilled social workers. The group must also include a radiation oncologist committed to pediatric care and with experience in radiotherapy for children (3,45) (Table 8).

TABLE 8. *Requirements for a pediatric cancer center*

I. The **medical staff** should include a qualified pediatric hematologist/oncologist; pediatric radiation oncologist; pediatric general surgeon; surgeons with pediatric expertise in neurosurgery, urology, and orthopedic surgery; a pathologist with expertise in the pathology of tumors of children and adolescents; and pediatric subspecialists in anesthesiology, diagnostic radiology, intensive care, infectious disease, cardiology, endocrinology, nephrology, and neurology.

II. The **allied health staff** should include pediatric nurses, social workers, pharmacists, psychologists, child life specialists, recreational therapists, physical and occupational therapists, and chaplains with expertise in childhood cancer.

III. The **physical plant** of the hospital/medical center should include an appropriate in-patient unit for the care of children with cancer, ambulatory clinic for treatment and monitoring of children with cancer, pediatric intensive care unit, hematopathology laboratory capable of performing cell phenotype analysis, clinical chemistry laboratory able to monitor antibiotic and antineoplastic drug levels, blood bank, pharmacy capable of preparation and dispensing of antineoplastic agents as well as total parenteral nutrition, diagnostic radiology suite, and radiation oncology department.

IV. The **institution** should conduct a regularly scheduled multidisciplinary pediatric tumor board and offer access to ongoing clinical protocols via one of the pediatric cancer treatment groups.

Based on Section on Hematology/Oncology Guidelines for the pediatric cancer center and role of such centers in diagnosis and treatment. *Pediatrics* 1997; 99:139–141.

There is evidence that the diagnosis and treatment of some pediatric malignancies, particularly those dependent on complex radiotherapy, is better conducted at university-affiliated medical centers. In an analysis of children with brain tumors, survival was compared for those children who received all or part of their treatment at university cancer centers versus those who received all or part of their treatment at community hospitals (49). For children with medulloblastoma, the 5-year survival rate was $2\frac{1}{2}$ times greater for children treated at university hospitals compared to those treated at community hospitals. For brain stem gliomas there was also a greater probability of survival for those children treated at university hospitals. The 5-year projected survival rates for cerebellar astrocytoma, Grade I and II supratentorial astrocytoma, ependymoma, and glioblastoma multiforme (where survival is arguably less dependent on irradiation) for university-treated patients were similar to those for community hospital-treated patients.

In another analysis, the survival rates of Wilms' tumor patients were studied. Children treated in a coordinated university and cancer center treatment program, in an upstate New York county, were compared with those treated in smaller counties without large treatment centers (17). From 1950 to 1959, an era in which there was relatively poor treatment for Wilms' tumor, there was no significant difference in survival between these two groups. However, from 1967 to 1972, there was a significant improvement in survival for those children treated in the county with the coordinated university and cancer treatment program.

Another study addressed the influence of place of treatment on diagnosis, treatment, and survival in Wilms' tumor, rhabdomyosarcoma, and medulloblastoma in the Delaware Valley area (50). There was an improved probability of survival in children treated for medulloblastoma and rhabdomyosarcoma at cancer centers when compared to that of children treated in noncancer centers. For Wilms' tumor, however, there were no major differences in management strategy or survival between cancer centers and noncancer centers. A study from the Children's Cancer Group indicated improved survival for children with acute leukemia treated at pediatric institutions (20,38).

The available data suggest that there is a benefit to treatment at a university-based or regional cancer center in situations where the treatment is rapidly evolving and where success requires complex treatment approaches with technically difficult surgery and/or radiotherapy. However, it appears that the site of treatment does not alter survival rates for those patients in whom a cure may be achieved with surgical intervention alone, tumors for which there is no significant curative treatment, and tumors requiring multimodality therapy where the acquisition of the most up-to-date protocol information as well as the services of a consulting expert are available in the community hospital (51–53).

REFERENCES

References particularly recommended for further reading are indicated by an asterisk.

1. Dublin LI. Mortality statistics of insured wage-earners and their families. New York: Metropolitan Life Insurance Company, 1919.
2. North SND, Director, Bureau of the Census, Department of Commerce and Labor. *Special reports: mortality statistics 1900–1904.* Washington, DC: US Government Printing Office, 1906:76–89.
3. American Academy of Pediatrics. Guidelines for the pediatric cancer center and role of such centers in diagnosis and treatment. *Pediatrics* 1986;77:916–917.
4. Miller RW, Young Jr JL, Navakovic B. Childhood Cancer. *Cancer* 1994;75(Supp):395–405.
5. *SEER cancer statistics review, 1973–1992. Tables and graphs.* Bethesda: US Department of Health and Human Services (NIH Pub. No. 96-2789), 1995:57.
6. Wingo PA, Tang T, Bolden S. Cancer statistics 1995. *CA Cancer J Clin* 1995;45:8.
7. Pediatric oncology group. Progress against childhood cancer: the pediatric oncology group experience. *Pediatrics* 1992;89:597–600.
8. Ventura SJ, Peters KD, Martin JA, Maurer JD. Births and deaths: United States, 1996. *Mon Vital Stat Rep* 1997;46:29–34.
9. Bleyer WA. The impact of childhood cancer on the United States and the world. *Cancer J Clin* 1990;40: 355–367.
10. *Canadian cancer incidence atlas, volume 1: Canadian cancer incidence.* Ottowa: Minister of National Health and Welfare, 1995:138–139.
11. Dorgan CA, ed. *Statistical record of health & medicine.* New York: Gale Research Inc., 1995:49.
12. US Department of Commerce. *116th Edition, statistical abstract of the United States 1996.* Washington, DC: US Department of Commerce, 1996:94–95.
13. Martin AA, Alpert JA, Reno JS, Lonchong M, Grueiro S. Incidence of childhood cancer in Cuba (1986–1990). *Cancer* 1997;72:551–555.
14. Nkanza NK. Paediatric solid malignant tumors in Zimbabwe. *Cent Afr J Med* 1989;35:496–501.
15. Panda BK, Dandapat MC, Parida N. Patterns of paediatric solid malignant tumours in southern Orissa. *J Indian Med Assoc* 1989;87:136–137.
16. Parkin DM, Stiller CA, Draper GJ, Bieber CA, Terracini B, Young JD, eds. *International incidence of childhood cancer.* Lyon: World Health Organization, International Agency for Research on Cancer, 1988:101–107.
17. Gurney JG, Davis S, Severson RK, Fang J-Y, Ross JA, Robison LL. Trends in cancer incidence among children in the US. *Cancer* 1996;78:532–541.

18. Parker SL, Tong T, Bolden S, Wingo PA. Cancer statistics 1997. *CA Cancer J Clin* 1997;47:5–27.

19. Plaschkes J. Epidemiology of neonatal tumours. In: Puri P, ed. *Neonatal tumours.* London: Springer-Verlag, 1996:1–1a.

20. Lewis IJ. Cancer in adolescence. *Br Med J* 1996;52: 887–897.

21. DeNully Brown P, Hertz H, Olsen JH, Yssing M, Scheibel E, Jensen OM. Incidence of childhood cancer in Denmark 1943–1984. *Int J Epidemiol* 1989;18: 546–555.

22. Goodman MT, Yoshizawa CN, Kolonel LN. Ethnic patterns of childhood cancer in Hawaii between 1960 and 1984. *Cancer* 1989;64:1758–1763.

23. Groves FD, Craig JF, Chen VW, Fontham ETH, Zavala DE, Correa P. Pediatric cancer in New Orleans. *J La State Med Soc* 1990;142:27–30.

24. McWhirter WR, Petroeschevsky AL. Childhood cancer incidence in Queensland, 1979–1988. *Int J Cancer* 1990;45:1002–1005.

25. Savitz DA, Zuckerman DL. Childhood cancer in the Denver metropolitan area 1976–1983. *Cancer* 1987;59: 1539–1542.

26. Merrill RM, Feuer EJ. Risk-adjusted cancer—incidence rates (United States) *Cancer Causes Control* 1996;7: 544–552.

27. Sriamporn S, Vatansapt V, Martin N, et al. Incidence of childhood cancer in Thailand 1988–1991. *Paediatr Perinat Epidemiol* 1996;10:73–85.

*28. Bunin GR, Feurer EJ, Witman PA, Meadows AT. Increasing incidence of childhood cancer: report of 20 years experience from the Greater Delaware Valley Pediatric Tumor Registry. *Paediatr Perinat Epidemiol* 1996;10:319–338.

29. Cushman Jr JH. U.S. reshaping cancer strategy as incidence in children rises. *NY Times* 1997 Sept. 29:1.

30. Kraut A, Tate R, Tran N. Residential electric consumption and childhood cancer in Canada (1971–1986). *Arch Environ Health* 1994;3(49):156–159.

31. Walter SD. Letter to the editor. *Arch Environ Health* 1996;51(6):467.

32. *Compact edition of the Oxford English dictionary.* Oxford: Oxford University Press, 1985.

33. Easson EC, Russell MH. The cure of Hodgkin's disease. *Br Med J* 1963;1:1704–1707.

34. Frei E, Gehan EA. Definition of cure for Hodgkin's disease. *Cancer Res* 1971;31:1828–1833.

35. Pinkel D. Cure of the child with cancer—definition and perspective. In: *American Cancer Society: proceedings of the national conference on the care of the child with cancer.* New York: American Cancer Society, Inc. 1979:191–200.

36. Collins VP. Wilms' tumor: its behavior and prognosis. *J La State Med Soc* 1955;107:474–480.

*37. Feinstein AR, Sasin DM, Wells CK. The Will Rogers phenomenon: stage migration and new diagnostic techniques as a source of misleading statistics for survival in cancer. *N Engl J Med* 1985;312:1604–1608.

38. Nachman J, Sather HN, Buckley JD, et al. Young adults 16–21 years of age at diagnosis entered on Children's Cancer Group acute lymphoblastic leukaemia and acute myeloblastic leukaemia protocols. *Cancer* 1993; 71:3377–3385.

39. Gerber LH, Binder H. Rehabilitation of the child with cancer. In: Pizzo PA, Poplack DG, eds. *Principles and practice of pediatric oncology.* Philadelphia: JB Lippincott, 1993:1079–1090.

40. Hammond D. Progress in the study, treatment and cure of the cancers of children. In: Burchenal JH, Oehgen HF, eds. *Cancer achievement, challenges, and prospects for the 1980's.* New York: Grune & Stratton, 1981:171–190.

41. Hays DM, Landsverk J, Ruccione K, Schoonover D, Zilber SL, Siegel SE. Employment problems and workplace experience of childhood cancer survivors. In: Green DM, D'Angio GJ, eds. *Late effects of treatment for childhood cancer.* New York: Wiley-Liss, 1992:171–178.

42. Meyer WH. Principles of total care: rehabilitation. In: Fernbach DJ, Vietti TJ, eds. *Clinical pediatric oncology.* St. Louis: CV Mosby, 1991:285–294.

43. Craft AW, Pearson ADJ. Three decades of chemotherapy for childhood cancer: from cure "at any cost" to "cure at least cost." *Cancer Surv* 1989;8:605–629.

44. Dickens M. *Miracles of courage.* New York: Dodd, Mead & Co., 1985.

45. Constine LS, Donaldson SS. Pediatric radiation oncology—subspecialty training? *Int J Radiat Oncol Biol Phys* 1992;24:881–884.

*46. Schwartz CL, Hobbie WL, Constine LS, Ruccione KS. *Survivors of childhood cancer: assessment and management.* St. Louis: Mosby, 1994.

47. Karnofsky DA, Burchenal JH. The clinical evaluation of chemotherapeutic agents in cancer. In: MacLeod CM, ed. *Evaluation of chemotherapeutic agents.* New York: Columbia University Press, 1949:191–205.

48. Lansky LL, List MA, Lansky SB, Cohen ME, Sinks LF. Toward the development of a play performance scale for children (PPSC). *Cancer* 1985;56:1837–1840.

49. Duffner PK, Cohen ME, Flannery JT. Referral patterns of childhood brain tumors in the state of Connecticut. *Cancer* 1982;50:1636–1640.

50. Kramer S, Meadows AT, Pastore G, Jarrett P, Bruce D. Influence of place of treatment on diagnosis, treatment, and survival in 3 pediatric solid tumors. *J Clin Oncol* 1984;2:917–923.

51. Cohen ME, Duffner PK, Kun LE, D'Souza B. The argument for a combined cancer consortium research data base. *Cancer* 1985;56:1897–1901.

52. Lennox EL, Stiller CA, Morris-Jones P, Kinnier-Wilson LM. Nephroblastoma: treatment during 1970–1973 and the effect of inclusion in the first Medical Research Council trial. *Br Med J* 1979;2:567–569.

53. Stiller CA, Draper GJ. Treatment, centre size, trial entry and survival in acute lymphoblastic leukaemia. *Arch Dis Child* 1989;64:798–807.

2

Leukemia

Bone Marrow Transplantation for Leukemia and Anemia

Leukemia is the most common form of childhood cancer. It represents about 31% of all pediatric cancers in the United States. The relative frequency of leukemia is similar throughout the world. It constitutes 40% of all childhood cancer in Thailand and 31% in Cuba (1,2). Approximately 2,500 new cases are diagnosed annually in the United States representing an incidence of 3.1 per 100,000 children under the age of 14 years (3). Acute lymphoblastic leukemia (ALL) is the dominant type, accounting for 75% to 80% of childhood leukemias. Acute non-lymphoblastic leukemias (ANLLs), most often acute myelogenous leukemia (AML, 16%), comprises the remaining 20% to 25%. Chronic forms of leukemia are rare in children (3%) (4,5).

The frequency of ALL is increased in certain genetic disorders, including syndromes associated with chromosome fragility and impaired DNA repair mechanisms (Fanconi's anemia, Bloom syndrome), Down syndrome (trisomy 21) and inherited immunodeficiencies (e.g., Wiskott-Aldrich syndrome) (5–9). Exposure to ionizing radiation *in utero* has been linked to an excess incidence of ALL in childhood (10,11). The occurrence of AML has been well documented in survivors of other forms of childhood cancer. The development of AML is related to exposure to alkylating agents and topoisomerase-2 in-hibitors, especially the epipodphyllo-toxins. This later form of AML is associated with chromosome 11q23 translocations (4).

ACUTE LYMPHOBLASTIC LEUKEMIA

ALL presents most often in children between 2- and 10-years-old. Five percent of cases occur in infants (less than 2 years of age), and approximately 20% occur in adolescents (12). The median age at diagnosis is 4 years. Boys are affected more commonly, with a sex ratio of 1.3:1 (6). The incidence is significantly higher in US whites than in US blacks.

ALL is a clonal expansion of dysregulated, immature lymphoid cells (13). It is a regulatory disorder of cellular development in which proliferation and differentiation are uncoupled (14). The morphology is characterized by the blast form. Blast cells can be characterized by cytochemistry, immunologic surface markers, and chromosome and receptor gene rearrangements. The immunophenotype is indicative of the stage of lymphoid differentiation at which malignant transformation has occurred (15).

Approximately 80% to 85% of ALL cases are of B-cell lineage (16). B cells are bone marrow-derived lymphocytes at the final stage of antigen-independent differentiation

(17). Committed precursors within the developmental lineage of B lymphocytes may be identified as the malignant cell line in most children. Of the B-cell lineage ALL cases, 2% to 3% are mature B-cell immunophenotypes that express surface membrane immunoglobulin (sIg⁺). About 20% to 25% of patients have pre–B-cell ALL. The pre–B-cell lineage is identified by the absence of surface immunoglobulin (sIg⁻) but the presence of immunoglobulin heavy chains within the cytoplasm (cIg⁺). About 90% of these cases express CD10, the common ALL antigen, on the cell surface [common ALL antigen positive (CALLA⁺)]. The majority of ALL (55% to 60% of cases) appear to be derived from clonal growth of early pre–B-lymphocyte lines, signified only by cell surface expression of B-cell differentiation antigens without surface or cytoplasmic immunoglobulin (CD10⁺, CD19⁺, cIg⁻, sIg⁻). A transitional pre–B-cell ALL (1% of cases) has been recognized (18,19).

B-precursor ALL may be separated into prognostic groups as a guide to therapy. Patients 1 to 10 years old with a white blood cell (WBC) count at presentation of <50,000 are *standard risk*. Patients ≥10 years old with a WBC count ≥50,000 are *high risk* (20). Not all cooperative groups select a WBC count of 50,000 as the cut-off point (Table 1). Some authorities also define an *intermediate risk* group (i.e., WBC count of 10–25,000 to 50–75,000) and/or incorporate cytogenetic findings in the grouping system (21). Ploidy also appears to be useful in predicting outcome in B-lineage ALL. A modal chromosome number >50 or DNA Index >1.16 (hy-

perdiploidy) is associated with a 4-year event-free survival of >90% (22).

T cells also originate in the bone marrow, subsequently "centering" in the thymus for maturation and differentiation. T-cell leukemia accounts for 15% to 20% of childhood ALL, occurring more often in adolescents. T cells are identified by the expression of surface antigens recognized by monoclonal T-cell antibodies (23). Clinical correlations with T-cell ALL include older age, male sex, significant elevation of WBC count, mediastinal mass, and palpable peripheral nodes. The majority of T-cell ALL cases are considered high-risk because of high WBC count, older age, and/or bulk disease (large mediastinal mass, massive splenomegaly, lymphadenopathy >3 cm) (21). Although felt to be a "continuum" of the more distinctly identified T-cell mediastinal lymphoblastic malignant lymphoma, T-cell ALL is signified by a striking degree of overt systemic involvement. T-cell ALL has been shown to relate to an earlier progenitor of T lymphocytes than seen in T-lymphoblastic malignant lymphomas (23). Compared to the pre–B-cell types of ALL, T-cell ALL is more frequently associated with extramedullary disease both at diagnosis and as a pattern of relapse (24).

Chromosomal translocations have been documented in the bone marrow of up to 75% of children with ALL (25) (Table 2). B-cell ALL is associated with the same t(9;14) abnormality noted in B-cell malignant lymphomas of childhood. The Philadelphia chromosome, or t(9;22), is present in 3% of childhood ALL and correlates with a high risk of treatment failure (26,27). The event-free survival for t(9;22) ALL is also poor (22). Significant elevation of the WBC count has been correlated with the t(4;11) alteration in B-lineage leukemias. In T-cell ALL, 25% of children show the distinctive t(11;14) marker (28). The t(1;19) translocation is associated with a high WBC count. Survival has been increased from 50 to 80% with more intensive therapy (22). The t(8;14) translocation is, however, a relatively favorable prognostic sign (21).

TABLE 1. *Relationship between age (≥1 year old), white blood count at presentation, and survival in B-precursor ALL*

White blood cell count		Age	
		1–9 y	>10 y
<50,000	4-year EFS	80%	66%
>50,000	4-year EFS	67%	41%

EFS, event-free survival; y, years of age.
Modified from refs. 20 and 21.

TABLE 2. *Clinically relevant genetic subgroups of childhood acute lymphoblastic leukemia*

Chromosome abnormality	Associated with cell type	Frequency	Mechanism	Estimated 5-year event-free survival
t(12;21)	B	21–24%	Chimeric transcription factor	85–90%
t(1;19)	B	5–6%	Chimeric transcription factor	70–80%
t(4;11) and other 11q23 translocations	B	4–8%	Chimeric transcription factor	20–30%
t(9;22)	B	3–4%	Tyrosine kinase over expression	25–35%
t(1;14)	T	3%	Enhanced gene expression	60–70%
t(8;14)	B	2%	Enhanced gene expression	70–80%
t(11;14)	T	1%	Enhanced gene expression	60%
dic(9;12)	B	1%	—	90%
Hyperdiploid (>50 chromosomes)	B	27%	—	80–90%
Hypodiploid (<45 chromosomes) and near haploid	B	1%	—	20–30%

Modified from refs. 22 and 39.

Clinical Presentation

The pathophysiology of the symptoms and signs of ALL are explicable on the basis of the proliferation of abnormal lymphoblasts. Replacement of normal bone marrow elements by leukemic cells results in neutropenia (with frequent or recurrent infections), thrombocytopenia (with bruising or bleeding), and anemia (with generalized malaise). Direct signs of leukemic infiltration occur as peripheral lymphadenopathy, mediastinal lymph node enlargement, hepatosplenomegaly, and retroperitoneal adenopathy. Bone pain is common due to leukemic periosteal infiltration. The diagnosis of ALL is based on bone marrow aspiration. A chest radiograph is important to identify mediastinal disease.

The WBC count is below 10,000 at diagnosis in about 50% of cases, between 10,000 and 50,000 in 30%, above 50,000 to 100,000 in 10% of cases, and higher than 100,000 in another 10% of cases. The correlation between presenting WBC count and prognosis has been found to be strong in multivariate analyses. The small proportion of cases with "hyperleukocytosis" (WBC count >200,000) present specific management problems, including fluid and electrolyte balance during rapid cell lysis, potential leukostasis, and intracerebral microinfarcts and hemorrhage (29).

Central nervous system (CNS) involvement is clinically apparent in 5% of children at diagnosis, with initial CNS leukemia more frequent among infants (30). The international definition of CNS involvement is ≥5 WBC/ul in the cerebrospinal fluid (CSF) with blast cells in the CSF by cytologic analysis or cranial nerve palsy/palsies (21). There have been attempts to subtype the extent of CSF involvement. In a St. Jude Children's Research Hospital (SJCRH) series, children were grouped as CNS 1 (negative cytology), CNS 2 (positive cytology, WBC count < 5 WBC/ul), and CNS 3 (positive cytology, WBC count ≥5 WBU/ul) (31,32). It is not clear if CNS 2 disease has a worse prognosis than CNS1—the data is conflicting (21).

Asymptomatic CSF pleocytosis is the most common presentation of CNS ALL. These children may also present with one or more cranial nerve deficits, usually involving the facial nerve (VII). In rare instances, VIIth nerve palsy may occur with negative CSF cytology, presumably implying nerve root infiltration at the base of the skull (33). Extradural spinal cord compression, rarely documented at diagnosis, is likely related to focal extradural extension from involved vertebrae.

Ophthalmic manifestations of leukemia can be seen in more than 30% of all newly diagnosed patients (34). Retinal hemorrhages are felt to be related to thrombocytopenia or anemia; however, retinal leukemic infiltrates are uncommon. The optic discs may be directly involved by leukemic infiltration through advanced subarachnoid extension, usually in association with meningeal involvement (35).

Treatment

In 1948, Farber et al. (36) demonstrated the efficacy of chemotherapy by the introduction of short-lived clinical remissions in ALL using aminopterin, an analogue of methotrexate. Frei and Freireich (37) explored the ability of methotrexate (MTX), 6-mercaptopurine (6-MP), and steroids to induce and maintain remissions. Subsequently, investigators at SJCRH developed a curative approach for ALL in a seminal series "total therapy" protocols.

There are four basic therapeutic elements of ALL therapy: *initial remission induction, intensification-consolidation therapy designed to eliminate residual blast cells, prevention of overt CNS disease, and continuation therapy*. Therapy usually lasts from 2.5 to 3 years. For high-risk ALL, intermittent *intensification* or *reinduction* is an important component of therapy (38).

Induction treatment typically includes prednisone or dexamethasone, vincristine, and L-asparaginase. Maintenance therapy utilized 6-MP and systemic MTX. Intensification may include high-dose intravenous methotrexate, VM-16, and L-asparaginase (21,39).

Many investigations have sought to improve results in ALL by overcoming the development of drug resistance (30,40–43). Efforts to overcome drug resistance have focused on more intensive induction therapy with early intensification to immediately decrease the leukemic population liable to develop drug resistance. The induction/intensification regimen of the Berlin–Frankfurt–Munster (BFM) group includes vincristine, prednisone, asparaginase, cyclophosphamide, cytosine arabinoside, 6-MP, and intrathecal (IT) MTX. The regimen has achieved a long-term continuous complete remission rate of 75% (43). The results in the BFM studies have also been impressive in improving continuous complete remission rates for patients with high-risk ALL. In fact, the early BFM intensification and repeated reintensification for those with classic high-risk factors, eliminated the negative impact of high WBC count in their studies (44). Similar data, indicating a benefit from early intensive therapy, have been reported from the Dana–Farber Cancer Institute (DFCI); researchers at DFCI have added high-dose systemic MTX to the induction regimen, followed by early intensification with repeated high-dose asparaginase (41,45). In some "front-ended" treatment programs reinduction or intensive consolidation regimens follow the initial induction/intensification therapy, especially for children with high-risk features.

The duration of chemotherapy has gradually been shortened, from initial regimens of 36 to 60 months to current studies of 18 to 30 months. The use of continuous 6-MP and weekly MTX has been varied to include intermittent "reinduction," alternating drug pairs, or interrupted, intensive continuation therapy (40) (Fig. 1).

Role of Radiation Therapy

Preventive CNS Therapy

The pathogenesis of CNS involvement in ALL has been elegantly described by Price and Johnson (15). Perivascular infiltrates originate along the fine subpial vessels, extending into the subarachnoid space and, with advanced disease, directly into the brain parenchyma. Tumoricidal concentrations of chemotherapeutic agents are difficult to achieve systematically due to limited drug penetration through the blood–brain barrier. IT drug administration results in adequate, if often non-uniform, exposure of the superficial meninges; tumoricidal concentrations are limited to the surface cell layers. Theoretically, differences in the apparent efficacy of prolonged IT preventive therapy for low-risk

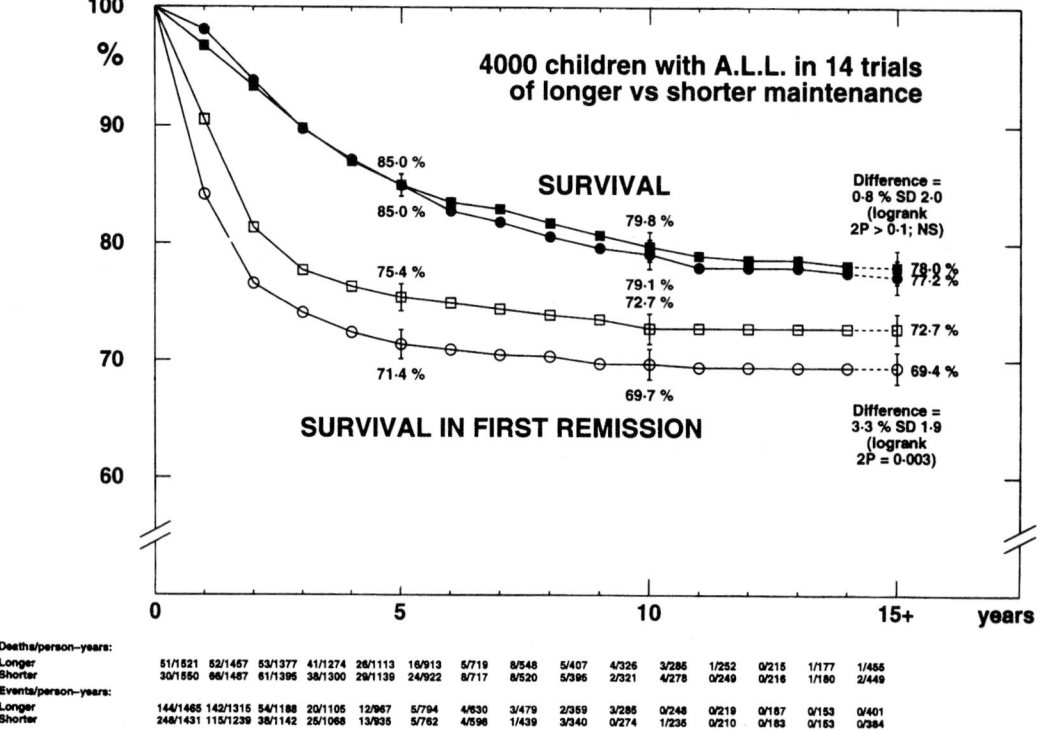

FIG. 1. The Childhood Acute Lymphoblastic Leukemia Collaborative Group conducted an overview of 42 clinical trials involving 12,000 randomized children. The data in this figure is derived from 4,000 children in 14 clinical trials of longer vs. shorter maintenance therapy. This figure conveys the generally excellent overall survival rate achievable in childhood ALL ($\approx$ 77% at 15 years), the equally good survival in first remission ($\approx$ 71%), as well as the suggestion that longer and more intense maintenance chemotherapy improves survival. The upper pair of lines describes survival, the lower pair of lines (open symbols) show survival in first remission from the time of randomization. Both pairs of data derive from stratified analyses. The squares and circles denote longer maintenance therapy vs. shorter therapy respectively (This figure is reproduced with permission of The Lancet and the Childhood ALL Cooperative Group secretariat. *Lancet* 1996;347:1783–1788.)

ALL and the apparent inadequacy for high-risk presentations may reflect quantitative differences in the extent of subclinical meningeal infiltrates, with thicker cell layers in high-risk presentations limiting control due to the physical characteristics of drug penetration (46).

The initial trials between 1962 and 1967, achieved improved rates of remission (>80%); however, they showed only 15% long-term survival (38,47,48). Clinical trials at SJCRH established the efficacy of "preventative" or "prophylactic" irradiation given early in the course of therapy (49). Study V

utilized craniospinal irradiation (CSI; 24 Gy/15–16 fractions) soon after obtaining hematologic remission. Fifty percent of the 35 patients remain alive in long-term follow-up. This represented the first cohort of ALL survivors, indicating the potential for curative treatment (47). Study VI randomly assigned children to receive CSI (24 Gy/15 fractions) or no specific CNS preventive therapy. The rate of isolated CNS relapse without directed CNS therapy was 67%; following preventive CSI, meningeal involvement occurred in only 4% (50). The incidence of CNS relapse without CSI was similar regardless of the WBC count at diagnosis (11). Earlier studies had shown no preventive effect using CSI at a dose level of only 12 Gy (50).

Subsequent trials confirmed the equivalence of CSI and cranial irradiation (CrI) combined with concurrent IT-MTX, while the latter approach significantly reduced the degree of hematosuppression, immunologic compromise, and concern regarding later spinal growth attendant to full neuraxis irradiation (48,51,52). Protocol regimens using CrI (at dose levels of 24 Gy) and IT-MTX repeated intermittently throughout continuation therapy have reported rates of initial CNS relapse below 5%. The high continuous complete remission rates achieved in the BFM and DFCI regimens include systematic use of CrI, confirming the low risk of meningeal relapse rate after CrI/IT-MTX (43,53). It is against such data, with isolated CNS relapse at or below a 5% to 7% incidence, that all trials seeking alternative CNS treatment must be measured.

Although late effects can be seen without CrI, concerns regarding late effects of CrI in a population with a median age of only 4 years have led to numerous trials testing alternative strategies for CNS therapy (9,54). The optimal CNS treatment is still controversial, and the number of patients who receive CrI varies greatly between cooperative groups and institutions (43,55–59).

The use of IT-MTX alone early in the course of consolidative therapy has been ineffective. The Children's Cancer Study Group (CCSG) reported a 38% incidence of subsequent isolated CNS failure (60). Pediatric Oncology Group (POG) tested "triple IT" chemotherapy (MTX, cytosine arabinoside, prednisone) given repeatedly throughout continuation therapy versus CrI plus limited-duration IT-MTX. At 4 years, the incidence of primary CNS relapse was identical at 4% with either form of therapy (61). The latter study has been criticized for lack of adequate follow-up or subsequent reporting and a relatively low rate of absolute survival and continuous complete remission, potentially masking a benefit from CrI in any of the prognostic groups.

Attempts to improve the efficacy of CNS preventive therapy without irradiation have involved combinations of systemic MTX and IT therapy. Administration of high doses of intravenous (IV) MTX combined with IT-MTX produces higher levels of CSF MTX than does either route alone (32). Initial studies explored the effectiveness of two cycles of intermediate-dose IV-MTX and concurrent IT-MTX compared to CrI with IT-MTX. For children with standard-risk ALL (WBC count <30,000; age 2–8 years), overall survival was similar, although the IV-MTX group experienced a statistically higher rate of isolated CNS relapse, which was directly compensated by superior hematologic remission. The difference in preventive CNS therapy was more pronounced in the subset with high-risk ALL; isolated CNS relapse occurred in 40% following IV-MTX, as compared with 10% after CrI. The impact of effective CNS preventive therapy was masked by poor systemic control in both arms of the study (62). Of interest, the IV-MTX group experienced significantly fewer episodes of extraneural, extramedullary relapse (in particular, testicular relapse).

Building on the apparent efficacy of systemic MTX in prolonging hematologic remission and preventing extramedullary relapse outside the CNS, a prospective study of IV/IT-MTX versus CrI/IT-MTX in "favorable-risk ALL" was pursued at SJCRH between 1979 and 1983. A total of 360 children were randomized to IV/IT-MTX repeated at 6-week intervals for 18 months versus CrI (18 Gy/12 fractions) soon after hematologic remission with concurrent IT-MTX. In both groups, IT-MTX was repeated throughout continuation therapy. In a liberally defined favorable-risk ALL population with WBC count <100,000, disease-free survival at 4 years favored the IV/IT-MTX group: 67% versus 56%. Improved survival in the former group reflects hematologic and testicular control; the rate of isolated CNS relapse was 10% with IV/IT-MTX and 4% following CrI (63).

Although confirming the efficacy of a regimen combining high-dose IV-MTX and IT chemotherapy, additional analysis of the SJCRH study indicates a substantial impact of CNS therapy in those who might be categorized as "intermediate risk" (WBC count 25,000–100,000). These patients experienced a significantly higher rate of isolated CNS relapse following IV/IT-MTX: 30% at 4 years compared to 2% following CrI ($p < 0.001$) (55). Within the better-risk subset with WBC count <25,000, there was no statistically significant difference in CNS relapse in this study.

The 1997 report of the Cancer and Leukemia Group B (CALGB) 7611 study, compared intermediate dose IV-MTX plus IT-MTX versus 24 Gy CrI plus IT-MTX. Hematologic relapse-free survival favored intermediate dose IV-MTX (73% vs. 57%), CNS relapse-free survival favored CrI (72% vs. 92%), and 12-year continuous remission was equivalent (40%, adequate for a 1976 study) (64).

The trials just summarized appear to show relative equivalence in CNS preventive therapy for patients with low-risk ALL, defined as WBC count <25,000. Treatment regimens repeatedly incorporating intensive systemic chemotherapy with IT drugs during the course of maintenance, achieve high rates of sustained overall and hematologic remission with adequate CNS control. Such results have been achieved without the added concerns of combining high-dose MTX and CrI producing neurologic toxicity (65). Additional follow-up of patients will be needed to ensure that results are truly equivalent for standard-risk children.

One study suggests that IT chemotherapy and more intensive systemic chemotherapy is equivalent to CrI plus IT chemotherapy in intermediate risk ALL. The Associazione Italiana di Ematologia ed Oncologic Pediatrica (AIEOP) achieved an 78% 6-year event-free survival and a <1% isolated CNS relapse rate in intermediate risk ALL without CrI (66).

For patients with high-risk ALL (defined as WBC count >25,000), T-cell disease, or CNS involvement at diagnosis, there is a significantly higher likelihood of controlling occult meningeal leukemia with the addition of CrI (40,43,45,55). The issue of sequencing systemic chemotherapy and CrI has led to delayed irradiation in most current protocols, incorporating an interval of intensive chemotherapy with or without high-dose MTX before initiating CrI. Preliminary data confirm the efficacy and rationale of the latter approach, with excellent early CNS control rates and little suggestion of added neurologic toxicity (30,67). We are aware of a report of 21 children with high-risk ALL treated without CrI with no subsequent CNS relapses (68). Such an assertion will require wider confirmation.

What are the indications for prophylactic cranial irradiation in contemporary practice? There is, at least, partial consensus among the major pediatric institutions and cooperative groups. Most agree that CrI is indicated for T-cell ALL with an initial WBC count >50,000. Some also favor CrI for B-precursor ALL with a high WBC count—although there is wide variation in the definition of "high." Other relative indications for CrI are Philadelphia chromosome positive ALL, ALL with lymphomatous features, and/or t(1;19) or t(11;14) disease (21).

In an attempt to keep the excellent CNS control rates while decreasing late effects, the DFCI conducted a randomized trial of two irradiation regimens (69). High-risk patients (defined at the DFCI as age <2 or >9 years, WBC count >20,000, or T-cell disease) were randomized to either a hyperfractionated regimen of 90 cGy given twice daily to 1800 cGy or to conventional irradiation of 180 cGy once daily over 10 treatments to the same total dose (1800 cGy). In a 1992 report covering the period between November 1987 and July 1991, 200 children with high-risk ALL were randomized. With a median follow-up of 29 months, there had been only one CNS relapse in the conventionally treated group. Neuropsychological testing and assessment of differences in growth effects were ongoing. There have been no subsequent published reports. It is our understanding (S.E. Sallan, *personal communication*, March 1998) that both radiation programs have approximately a 99% CNS event-free survival. The type of CNS prophylaxis does not appear to affect overall survival. Growth appears uninfluenced by q.d. versus b.i.d. irradiation—although irradiated children grow less well than unirradiated children.

Importance of CNS Therapy

Effective CNS therapy has increased the number of long-term, disease-free survivors of childhood ALL (70). Nesbit et al. (51,52) suggested that CNS relapse should be avoided to limit the toxicities of meningeal leukemia and additional therapy, noting no apparent difference in survival with or without effective preventive therapy for subclinical disease. Subsequent analyses have shown a benefit in long-term survival related to effective CNS preventive therapy (36,71,72). Following an isolated CNS relapse, there is an increase in subsequent hematologic relapse and death in addition to repeated episodes of meningeal leukemia, along with added neurologic toxicities. George et al. (71) reported that the disease-free survival following CNS failure in the SJCRH experience was only 17%. Ortega et al. (72) noted an identical 16% secondary relapse-free survival in the CCSG study. The CCSG data do indicate better survival following CNS relapse in the group who initially received inadequate preventive therapy. The 21% survival in the group relapsing without prior CrI, contrasts with the 8% survival in those failing in the meninges following CrI. However, the ultimate "salvage rate" remains unacceptably low after an "isolated" CNS relapse (53,72). The risk of hematologic relapse in the SJCRH series was 74% after CNS failure compared to 46% without CNS failure (71). Of the 31 patients with a CNS relapse after intensive chemotherapy and CrI from the DFCI, only four patients were alive without disease at 25 to 71 months (53). The impact of effective CNS preventive therapy seems obvious. The impact of CNS relapse on the quality of survival has been analyzed by Ochs et al. (67), describing a significantly greater incidence of seizures, neurologic dysfunction, and intellectual delays among those patients surviving CNS relapse.

Overt CNS Leukemia

The management of overt CNS leukemia is somewhat less controversial than the choice of appropriate preventive therapy. Although CNS remission can be achieved with IT, systemic, or intraventricular chemotherapy, durable control of meningeal disease has only been documented following the addition of CNS irradiation (46,72). In patients with cranial nerve palsies, limited-volume irradiation to the base of skull region may facilitate nerve recovery (33). Such therapy (approximately 10–15 Gy at 150 cGy/fraction) is discounted in plans for later definitive therapy: delayed CrI in conjunction with intermittent IT chemotherapy repeatedly through the course of consolidation therapy.

CNS leukemia at diagnosis is present in 3% to 5% of children with ALL. The 1996 report of CCSG patients with CNS disease at diagnosis, entering treatment between 1983 and 1989, described a variety of types of chemotherapy (typically vincristine, prednisone, L-aspariginase $\pm$ daunorubicin and/or cyclophosphamide induction; consolidation with 6-MP or 6 thioguanine, MTX with cytosine arabinoside (ara-c), cyclophosphamide, and other drugs, and delayed intensification and maintenance chemotherapy, along with IT chemotherapy and craniospinal irradiation. The 5-year event-free survival was 69% for 53 patients with CNS disease at diagnosis. The cranial irradiation dose was 24 Gy. The spinal dose was 12 Gy but was decreased to 6 Gy in 1989 to limit hematopoietic toxicity. There was a 90% freedom from isolated CNS relapse at 5 years. To the spine, 6 Gy seemed equivalent to 12 Gy (73). The role of CSI versus CrI for CNS leukemia at diagnosis deserves study. If 6 Gy to the spine is adequate, perhaps protocols eliminating spinal irradiation would be reasonable. One might also investigate cranial doses <24 Gy (74).

Effective treatment for overt CNS relapse includes coordination of chemotherapy and neuraxis irradiation or consideration of bone marrow transplantation (75,76). CSI alone was evaluated for meningeal leukemia in the late 1960s. Although achieving clearance of CSF cytology and symptomatology, CSI at 20 to 24 Gy (150- to 200-cGy fractions) was associated with a 40% incidence of second CNS relapse (50,72,77). In SJCRH Study IV, 33 of 49 patients randomized to no preventive CNS therapy experienced isolated CNS relapse in 33 instances. Following CSI, 13 (39%) had a second CNS relapse (50). Other studies indicated comparable rates of recurrent CNS disease after "secondary remission" following CSI (72,77).

By comparison, treatment approaches utilizing systemic chemotherapy plus initial IT chemotherapy to clear CSF cytology followed by CSI have resulted in almost uniform control of established meningeal leukemia. In a series of 14 patients, Kun et al. (76) systematically obtained control of CNS disease; however, only five children remained in secondary continuous complete remission for over 6 years after CSI (76). In a larger POG trial, children treated with CSI after achieving remission with IT triple chemotherapy maintained CNS control in 35 of 36 cases at a median 2-year interval (78). The dose of CSI must be adequate to be effective in controlling CNS disease. In a report using IT-MTX and IT-Ara-C, followed by ineffectively low-dose CSI (6–9 Gy/4–6 fractions) and maintenance intraventricular MTX, the projected rate of CNS control was only 40% (61).

Another POG trial achieved 46% disease-free survival following CNS relapse treated with CrI and IT chemotherapy and only an 11% frequency of second CNS relapse (79). Most other series indicating systematic control of meningeal disease and a proportion of durable secondary complete remissions treat with full neuraxis irradiation (67,78,80). In the POG trial reported in 1985 there was superior CNS control (97% with CSI vs. 69% with CrI) and secondary continuous complete remission (CCR) (44% vs. 7%, respectively)

following CSI (78). Forty-five of 100 cases with CNS relapse in the 1987 report of the CCSG trial experienced repeated episodes of meningeal leukemia, indicating the difficulty in controlling established or overt meningeal disease in comparison to the high rate of effective "prevention" with treatment regimens incorporating CrI (72). Reinduction chemotherapy and CSI achieved a 70% 5-year disease-free survival and a 5% secondary CNS relapse in a 1983 to 1989 SJCRH study (74).

The limited proportion of children enjoying long-term secondary disease control after meningeal leukemia reflects the high proportion of hematologic relapse following overt CNS disease (71,72). Bone marrow relapse occurs in 50% to 75% of cases in the literature, although more intensive systemic reinduction therapy combined with CSI indicates apparent improvement in short-term studies (81,82). Therefore, some institutions recommend bone marrow transplantation after CNS relapse, especially for those children who received CrI during primary treatment. Early results of 19 patients undergoing autologous bone marrow transplantation (ABMT) following CNS relapse compare favorably with studies utilizing CSI; 12 of the 19 children remain in CCR after ABMT, with a median follow-up of 39 months (83).

Leukostasis

Leukostasis may develop in cerebral blood vessels in patients who present with extremely high WBC counts. Thrombi may lead to infarction and intracranial hemorrhage. Such patients are usually managed with chemotherapy, allopurinol, hydration, and alkalization. Some radiotherapists feel that a brief course of CrI (1.5–2 Gy/2–4 fractions) is helpful, but this is almost always unnecessary.

Radiotherapeutic Management

Volume

For preventive CNS therapy, the target volume for CrI includes the entire intracranial subarachnoid space. The caudal margin of the field extends to the bottom of the second cervical vertebra. Although intraocular relapse has generally been associated with advanced meningeal leukemia or hematogenous seeding, standard guidelines for preventive CrI include the posterior retina and orbital apex, encompassing the extension of the subarachnoid space along the optic nerves (Fig. 2).

Proper attention to volume for preventive CrI is imperative. The margins at the base of the skull have often been closely or inadequately covered, with confusion largely regarding the region of the cribriform plate and lower limit of the temporal fossa. Anatomic limits are illustrated in Fig. 3, indicating the proximity of the cribriform plate to the upper aspect of the orbit and the relatively inferior limit of the temporal fossa on a lateral skull radiograph. Analyses of the position of the cribiform plate relative to the orbital roofs, utilizing computed tomography, indicate that the relative positions can vary with age and that the cribiform plate can be quite low. In order to cover the cribiform plate with a lateral beam it will be necessary, in most children, to encompass part of the superior retina.

To adequately encompass the CSF bearing area around the optic nerve where it joins the posterior aspect of the retina and orbit, while

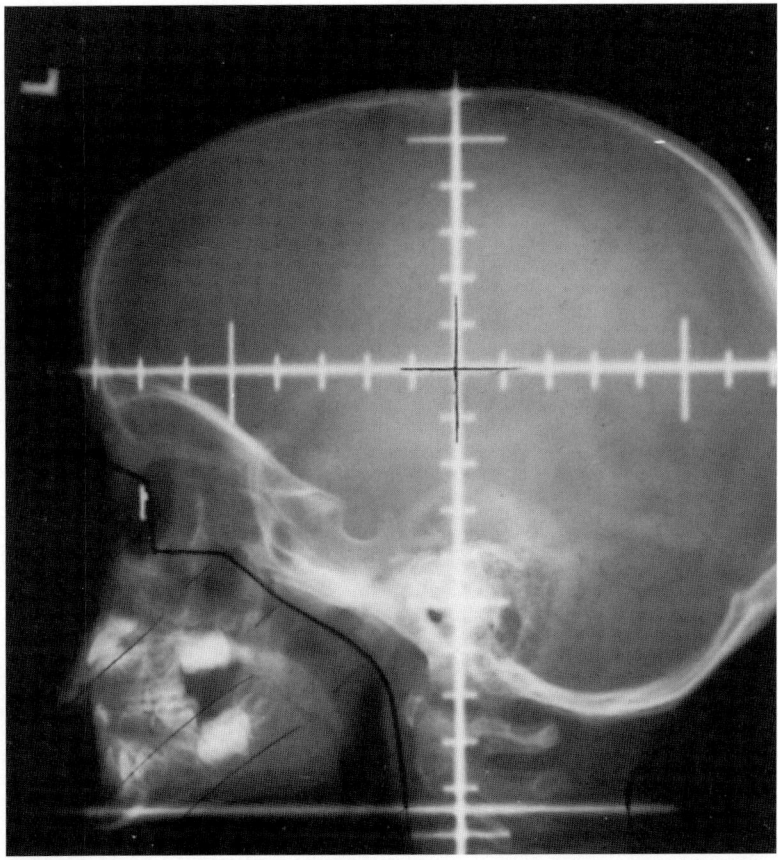

FIG. 2. Cranial irradiation field, outlining treatment that encompasses the entire cranial subarachnoid space, extending down to the second cervical vertebrae. Margins at the cribiform plate and temporal fossa are derived from anatomy as demonstrated in Fig. 3. The lead markers outline the bony orbital rims, with inclusion of the posterior aspects of the orbit within the irradiated volume.

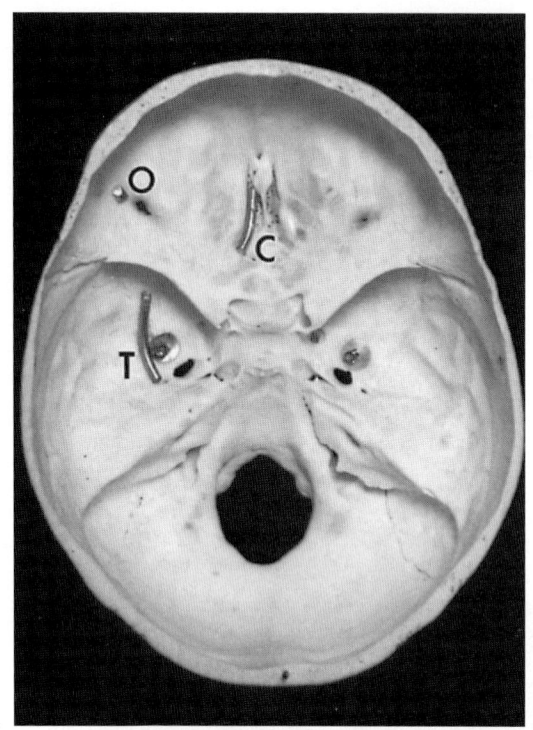

A

FIG. 3. Skull views outlining anatomic limits of the base of skull for inclusion of the intracranial subarachnoid space. **A:** Lead markers have been placed in the subfrontal region at the level of the cribriform plate (c), in contrast to the lateral subfrontal region representing the roof of the orbit (o); the inferior limits of the temporal fossa are outlined (T). **B:** The projection of the cribriform plate (c) and the temporal fossa (T) are indicated on the lateral radiograph of the skull.

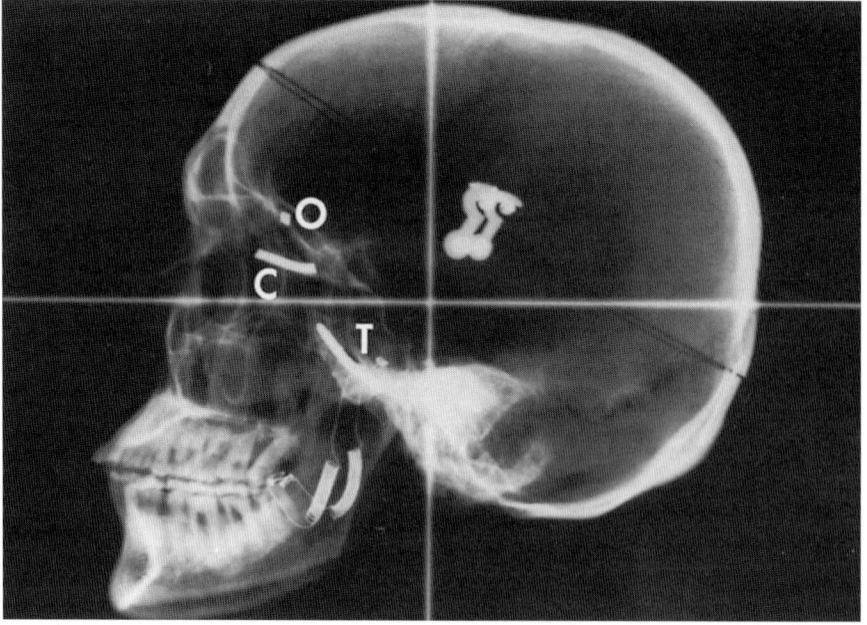

B

sparing the anterior half of the globe and lens, specific geometric techniques and/or blocking must be utilized.

Use of a 4 degree to 5 degree gantry angle to correct for divergence at the level of the orbital rim is quite simple and reproducible (Fig. 4) (84). The amount of "flash" beyond the scalp does not appear to be critical for linear accelerator beams. For cobalt-60 teletherapy, "flash" of 1 cm or more beyond the skull has been recommended (71). Some clinicians choose to deal with the question of divergence by placing the central axis of the beam near the eye and using a "half-beam block."

For CSI, the target volume includes the subarachnoid space within the cranial volume and the spine. Recommendations for the cranial field are identical to those noted previously for preventive cranial irradiation; the caudal margin is generally lower than C2 to appropriately adjoin a posterior spinal field. The caudal margin of the spinal field must extend below the lower limit of the thecal sac, which is determined by sagittal MRI. Ideal homogeneity and reproducibility of daily setup require correction for divergence in three dimensions, illustrated in the technique for CSI in Fig. 1, Chapter 4. Lateral craniocervical fields require correction for divergence, at the orbits and at the lower field margin where the posterior spinal field adjoins the cervical component of the lateral treatment fields. Correction at the orbits is achieved by gantry angle similar to that noted for cranial irradiation; in addition, the field is angled about the horizontal axis to achieve parallelism with the superior divergence of the posterior spinal field. Caudal divergence of the lateral craniocervical fields can be corrected by calculating the angle of divergence based on the height of the craniocervical field and appropriately angling the pedestal of the treatment couch. (Also see discussion of the technique of CSI in Chapter 4.)

Despite detailed attention to the correction for potential inhomogeneity at the junction, it is good practice to change the junction by 1 to 2 cm at least one or two times during the course of CSI. Although the technique for neuraxis therapy can be successfully implemented in a supine position by specific modifications of the treatment couch, the daily setup, reproducibility, and immobilization are significantly simpler and more accurate when using a prone position. A customized cast can be fabricated prior to simulation. (See the discussion of stabilization devices in Chapter 22.)

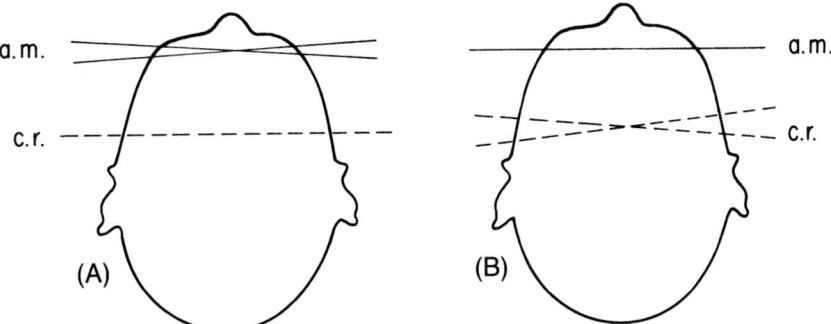

FIG. 4. Illustration of a simple means of achieving parallelism at the level of the anterior margin of the orbital rims (a.m.) for cranial irradiation. **A:** Parallel opposed fields result in divergent beams at the orbital rims, resulting in irradiation of the anterior aspect of the contralateral eye. **B:** A 4-degree to 5-degree gantry angle achieves a nonopposed field pair at the central ray (c.r.) while resulting in a parallel anterior margin (a.m.). (From ref. 153, with permission.)

Dose

The standard dose for preventive CrI is 18 Gy. Historical studies of SJCRH clearly showed that a dose level of 12 Gy/8 fractions without added IT chemotherapy was inadequate. The efficacy of 24 Gy (given at 150–160 cGy/fraction once daily) had been confirmed (65). Sequential studies by the CCSG indicated the apparent equivalence of 18 Gy/9–12 fractions and 24 Gy/12–20 fractions for patients with standard risk factors (defined largely as WBC count <50,000) (51,52). Although marked by the difficulty of sequential rather than prospective comparisons, patients with a high WBC count (>50,000) showed a suggestive, but statistically insignificant, difference in control of subclinical CNS disease favoring 24 Gy (40–99,100). Studies in the BFM group have utilized doses of irradiation between 12 and 24 Gy, dependent on the risk factors at diagnosis (43). Most current studies in the United States utilizing preventive CrI for high-risk ALL incorporate a 1- to 12-month interval of intensive systemic and IT MTX prior to CrI. A dose of 18 Gy in 10–12 fractions appears to be adequate in this group (30,59). It may be that improvements in chemotherapy have allowed a decrease in the effective total dose of CrI that is required for initial CNS treatment of leukemia.

For CrI to control overt meningeal leukemia following CNS remission induction, dose levels for the cranial fields have ranged from 24 to 30 Gy (at 150 cGy/fraction), whereas those for the spinal fields have ranged from 15 to 24 Gy. Data from POG, CCSG, and SJCRH indicate excellent early CNS control with doses of 24 Gy into the cranial vault and 6–14 Gy into the spine (30,73,78). The SJCRH study reflects therapeutic CSI in a population including children with relapsed ALL who were previously irradiated with 18- or 24-Gy primary treatment (81,82). Low dose protracted CSI 6 Gy in 4 days followed by monthly CSI to 18 Gy (total) has also been described (85).

Equipment Factors

The precision of linear accelerator irradiation suggests the advantage of this technique over cobalt-60 teletherapy for CrI and, in particular, CSI. Photon energies in excess of 6 MV are not recommended for CrI, due to depth dose differences suggesting the advantage of maximal ionization closer to the surface for meninges immediately beneath the calvarium (86). Although spinal techniques have been reported using an electron beam, conventional CSI utilizes low-energy photons to homogeneously irradiate the spinal canal (87). While theoretically sparing exit dose through the viscera (including the thyroid and abdominal organs), electron beam irradiation is not likely to achieve significant advantages for bone growth and invites questions regarding homogeneity of dose within the spinal canal at divergent depths along the axis of the vertebral column.

Testicular Leukemia

In the past, there was a debate as to whether the testes was, just as the CNS, a sanctuary site wherein leukemic cells were relatively protected from chemotherapy (a "blood–testes barrier" analogous to a "blood–brain barrier") or whether testicular leukemia is simply a barometer of extramedullarly leukemia, foretelling a general recurrence (88). The evidence indicates that the later concept is far more likely to be true. The compelling arguments include: (a) sufficiently high doses of systemic methotrexate substantially reduce the risk of testicular leukemia, indicating the ability of the drug to reach the target organ (63). It has been shown, in the rat, that methotrexate easily reaches the testicular interstitum (89). (b) Boys with testicular recurrence, treated with only local irradiation, generally develop a bone marrow recurrence within a few months. (c) Patients with apparently isolated testicular recurrence of ALL have been shown to have abdominal lymph node involvement on exploratory laparotomy (75,90).

Reports of ALL treatments in the 1970s indicated a clinical risk of testicular involvement in 5% to 16% of boys. At necropsy the incidence was 64% to 92% (91,92). The incidence of testicular involvement had been higher in adolescents and in T-cell ALL. The incidence of testicular relapse indicated a possible role for testicular biopsy at completion of continuation therapy to detect subclinical disease (93). In a trial reported in 1980, prophylactic testicular irradiation significantly reduced the incidence of testicular relapse but did not influence survival (91). With the evolution of more intensive systemic chemotherapy, several series indicate virtual elimination of testicular relapse (41,63). In the current era, the value of testicular biopsy on completion of therapy appears to have been successfully negated by more adequate systemic chemotherapy (44,94).

Currently, overt testicular disease is present at diagnosis in approximately 2% of boys with ALL (95). It appears to respond adequately to systemic chemotherapy, without requiring subsequent testicular irradiation. A matched-pair analysis from SJCRH indicates that boys with testicular disease at diagnosis have a poorer event-free survival and overall survival than those without this finding (95).

It is likely that testicular relapse occurring during continuation therapy signifies resistance to systemic therapy. Bowman et al. (96) and others (91) have found that testicular disease during chemotherapy is almost uniformly bilateral and has systematically been associated with hematologic relapse within 3 to 6 months. The rare instances of late testicular relapse, occurring 6 or more months following cessation of chemotherapy, have often been clinically unilateral. Although biopsies have failed to confirm subclinical disease in the contralateral testis in up to 75% of such cases, there is no clinical series documenting efficacy of unilateral orchiectomy or unilateral testicular irradiation without addressing the presumed microscopic involvement of the contralateral testis (96). Recently, five patients have been described who suffered a testicular relapse between 8 and 71 months following conclusion of chemotherapy (88). All were treated with chemotherapy and radiotherapy was omitted. No additional leukemic relapses were observed with 1 to 15 years of follow-up. This single series raises the possibility that some boys with testicular relapse

may be treated without radiotherapy. This idea would require confirmation by others before being adopted over the longstanding use of local irradiation.

Treatment of testicular infiltration occurring during or after continuation therapy includes reinduction systemic drug therapy plus local irradiation. The target volume for radiation therapy includes the entire scrotal region, encompassing the testes and epididymis bilaterally. Dose levels of 24–25 Gy at 150–200 cGy/fraction have been successful in controlling most instances of testicular relapse (50). Some have argued for a higher dose because of in-field failures at 21–26 Gy (97). Treatment techniques may incorporate either appropriate-energy electron beam or low-energy photon irradiation, the latter often requiring bolus to ensure buildup for younger children. Attention to patient position to ensure adequate testicular descent into the scrotum is critical during treatment. One wishes to avoid exit irradiation into the pelvis or penile shaft, if at all possible. For many cases an anterior oblique photon beam with the penile shaft taped onto the abdomen of a child in a supine "frog-leg" position works well.

ACUTE MYELOGENOUS LEUKEMIA

Approximately 20% of children with leukemia present with AML, with approximately 500 newly diagnosed cases in the United States each year (98). AML subtypes are most commonly defined by the French–American–British (FAB) morphology (Table 3). Chromosomal abnormalities are frequent in AML. The most common abnormalities are trisomy 8, t(8;21), t(15;17), t(9;11), or t(10;11), and inv 16 (4,39,99). Patients with t(8;21) have a relatively favorable prognosis when treated with high-dose cytarabine. Acute promyelocytic leukemia is frequently associated with t(15;17). There is a high rate of complete remission in these patients when treated with all-*trans*-retinoic acid with anthracycline-based chemotherapy (100).

Despite the fact that AML generally occurs at an older median age than ALL (approximately 9–10 years), if leukemia occurs in the

TABLE 3. *The French–American–British (FAB) classification of acute myelogeneous leukemia*

Fab type	Percentage of total	Prominent feature(s)
MO	2	Large and agranular blasts with minimal myeloid diffeeantiation
M1	10–18	Poorly differentiated myeloblasts
M2	27–29	Myelocytic
M3	5–10	Promyelocytic, associated with t(15;17)
M4	16–25	Myelomonocytic, associated with chromasome 11 translocations
M5	13–22	Monocytic, associated with chromosome 11 translocations
M6	1–3	Erythroleukemia
M7	4–8	Megakarkyocytic

From refs. 4, 151, and 152, with permission.

first 4 weeks of life it is usually AML. Extreme elevation of the WBC count (>100,000) complicates initial management in about 20% of cases, contributing significantly to early deaths due to hemorrhage and leukocytosis in the brain or lungs. Most children present with pallor, fatigue, bleeding, or fever. The more typical WBC count is <50,000.

Current drug regimens incorporating cytosine arabinoside and an anthracycline (most often daunomycin) have achieved remission rates of 70% to 85%. This is a substantial improvement over past rates (101–104). Median duration of remission, however, has infrequently exceeded 18 to 24 months; relapse in 40% to 50% of cases and deaths in remission (5% or greater) limit the ultimate rate of continuous remission to 40% to 45% (102,104).

The overall incidence of CNS involvement in AML was similar to the high rates seen in ALL without adequate preventive therapy. CNS involvement at diagnosis, in fact, has been reported in a higher proportion of patients than noted in ALL: 5% to 15% of children (4,103,105). CNS disease is more common with an initial WBC count over 25,000 and in infants <2 years of age at diagnosis (106).

The long-term survival rate for childhood AML, historically, was about 10%. It is now about 40% (4). Initial therapy addresses life-threatening presenting symptoms such as infection, hemorrhage, leukostasis, or tumor lysis syndrome. Initial chemotherapy is high-dose cytosine arabinoside and daunorubicin. Many programs also include 6-TG and etoposide. Intrathecal chemotherapy (cytosine arabinoside and/or MTX) and CrI has substantially reduced the occurrence of isolated CNS relapses (102,107). Specific presentations, including inversion of chromosome 16 in M4 myelomonocytic leukemia, are associated with higher rates of CNS failure, possibly justifying preventive CrI (108).

CNS involvement in AML presents typically with CSF pleocytosis. Cranial nerve palsies are infrequent. A small proportion of children present with intracerebral masses more compatible with "chloromas." The word *chloroma* derives from chlorine (chlor) and tumor (oma). Chlorine is invoked because the green color of chlorine gas is reminiscent of the tumor's color (106). Treatment with IT chemotherapy and delayed CrI (24 Gy at 150 cGy/fraction) has been successful in achieving long-term remissions free of subsequent CNS failure in a small subset of cases following meningeal relapse. There are some data that appear to indicate adequate control of meningeal disease using systemic and IT chemotherapy alone (102,106).

BONE MARROW TRANSPLANTATION

Bone marrow transplantation is a modification of cancer therapy developed to overcome the hematologic limitations of antineoplastic agents. Protocols incorporating bone marrow transplantation permit "supralethal" doses of hematosuppressive total-body irradiation (TBI) and chemotherapy, relying on reconstitution of normal bone marrow function following infusion of exogenous marrow elements. By eliminating the dose-limiting concerns of hematologic toxicity, bone marrow transplantation allows substantial dose escalation of agents limited by marrow toxicity in the conventional setting. Bone marrow transplantation, thereby, achieves greater dose-related tumor cell kill by irradiation and chemotherapy. In addition, the immunologic activity of infused lymphocytes from donor marrow has an antitumor effect (109,110) (Table 4).

Bone marrow transplantation includes a conditioning or preparative regimen (usually TBI and either cyclophosphamide or cytosine arabinoside or VP-16 or chemotherapy alone) followed by marrow infusion, intensive supportive care, and some degree of immunosuppression to avoid or limit graft-versus-host-disease (GVHD) (111,112).

Early studies with bone marrow transplantation established the ability of TBI to provide sufficient immunosuppression to permit marrow engraftment. The addition of cyclophosphamide was necessary to achieve a greater degree of tumor cell kill, limiting the frequency of leukemic relapse (112). Initial trials of bone marrow transplantation for ALL and ANLL in relapse indicated some efficacy, with ultimate survival in 10% of otherwise incurable cases. Subsequent studies by Thomas and co-workers (113,114), using high-dose cyclophosphamide plus TBI showed continued improvements in survival. Failure was due to recurrent ALL (60% of those failing therapy) and death from opportunistic infection or sequelae of acute GVHD.

Bone Marrow Transplantation for Childhood AML

The currently available chemotherapy programs for AML induce initial remission in approximately 75% of children. Long-term survival is achieved in about 40% (4,115). The relatively poor survival of children with AML has given impetus to the use of bone marrow transplantation. Some favor transplantation in first remission if there is a suitable family donor. Others believe transplantation should be reserved for second or subsequent remissions. Several single-institution studies have demonstrated that in the 25% of children with

TABLE 4. *Glossary of terms related to bone marrow transplantation*

Allogeneic transplantation—Harvesting of suitable bone marrow from an individual other than the patient (Greek *allos* = other) for transplantation into the patient. Suitability is determined by HLA matching (See "Histocompatibility complex.") The donor may be a relation or someone identified by a donor registry system.
Autologous transplantation—Removal of a patient's own marrow when a complete remission has been induced. This is followed by ablative treatment of the patient with the hope of destruction of any residual tumor and rescue with the patient's own bone marrow. (See "Marrow purging.")
Graft-versus-host disease—A disease in which immunologically competent donor cells react against antigens in a immunologically depressed recipient. It is characterized by fever, exfoliative dermatitis, hepatitis, diarrhea, and abdominal pain, which may progress to ileus. The severity of graft-versus-host disease is described by a standardized grading system. (See *Bone Marrow Trans* 1995;15:825–828.)
Graft-versus-leukemia effect—There are antineoplastic effects mediated by the graft. Leukemic relapse tends to occur less frequently in patients in whom graft-versus-host disease develops compared to those in whom it does not.
Histocompatibility complex—The word "histocompatibility" refers to the ability of cells to survive without immunological interference. The ability of the human immune system to differentiate "self" from "nonself" is determined by the products (the antigens) of the major histocompatibility complex whose genes are located on the short arm of chromosome 6. There are six major types of these antigens. They are: Class I HLA consists of HLA A, B, and C. Class II HLA consists of HLA DP, DR, and DQ. It is common to refer to the degree of compatibility between donor and recipient marrow in allogeneic transplant in terms of these six HLA antigens, i.e., "a five out of six match" or a "six out of six match."
Marrow purging—Treatment of the autologous marrow in an attempt to minimize the effects of the infusion of a significant number of malignant cells.
Syngeneic transplantation—Transplantation of bone marrow between identical twins. Donor–host cell incompatibility should be eliminated.

Definitions were derived, in part, from Thomas CL, ed. *Taber's cyclopedic medical dictionary, 13th edition.* Philadelphia: F.A. Davis Company, 1977; Berkow R, ed. *Sixteenth edition. The Merck manual of diagnosis and therapy.* Rahway: Merck Research Laboratories, 1992; Forman SJ, Blume KG, Thomas ED, eds. *Bone marrow transplantation.* Boston: Blackwell Scientific Publications, 1994.

AML who have a suitably matched famiy member (HLA-matched sibling or closely matched family member), and who are transplanted in the first remission, the survival rate is 40% to 60%— apparently better than with chemotherapy alone (115,116). For the 75% of children without a related donor, one must consider treatment with chemotherapy alone versus a transplant with either autologous, purged marrow, an unrelated donor, or umbilical cord blood. Single-institution studies with autologous transplant have achieved survivals of 17% to 40%, approximately the same as with chemotherapy alone (115,117).

Two pediatric randomized trials have evaluated autologous versus allogeneic transplantation versus chemotherapy for AML. An Italian cooperative study compared outcome in children with AML in first remission who received allogeneic transplants from HLA-compatible donors following cyclophosphamide/TBI preparation (18 patients) versus bone marrow transplantation with autologous unpurged marrow with chemotherapy alone preparation (32 patients) versus conventional chemotherapy without bone marrow transplantation (32 patients). There was not an intention-to-treat analysis and 16 patients (17%) were unevaluable because of protocol or randomization violations. The 2-year disease-free survival was: allogeneic transplantation (76%), autologous transplantation (31%), and chemotherapy alone (12%) (118).

POG Study 8821 randomized children to ABMT versus intensive consolidation chemotherapy. Children with suitable donors underwent allogeneic transplantation. Event-free survival 3 years after randomization by intention-to-treat analysis was: allogeneic transplantation (52%), autologous transplantation (38%, $p = 0.01$ vs. allogeneic), and chemotherapy alone (36%, $p = 0.2$ vs. autologous, $p = 0.07$ vs. allogeneic) (119).

Bone Marrow Transplantation for ALL

Modern treatment programs for ALL achieve disease-free survival rates in excess of 70%. Those children who relapse, however, have a poor outcome. Conventional chemotherapy for salvage results in less than 30% disease-free survival (120). Fortunately, survival following bone marrow transplantation for ALL is quite good.

In 1957, E. Donnall Thomas, M.D., following extensive animal experimentation, performed a bone marrow transplant on a young girl with ALL utilizing her identical twin as a donor. The patient received approximately 800 cGy of TBI as a midline dose. The patient survived for 6 months before her leukemia relapsed. She ultimately died. In 1977, Thomas published a series of patients with ALL who were transplanted: 22 in second, third, and fourth remission, and 20 in relapse. About one-half of the patients were less than 18 years of age and the long-term survival rate was about 30% (121). In recognition of his work, Thomas shared the 1990 Nobel Prize in Medicine or Physiology.

A team from Memorial Sloan-Kettering achieved a 5-year actuarial survival of 69% with sibling donors for transplantation of ALL in second remission (46). Similar results, with survival rates on the order of 40% to 58%, have been achieved with sibling donors in a German Cooperative Study, at the University of Minnesota, the University of Washington, Seattle, and Case Western Reserve University (120,122–124). Most programs use TBI/Cyclosphamide for preparation. The largest study, with the longest follow-up, is from Seattle with a 40% Kaplan-Meier disease-free survival at 10 years (123,125).

The success of bone marrow transplantation for relapsed disease has given encouragement to the early employment of this procedure for poor prognosis ALL. Therefore, some patients will be referred for transplantation in first remission because of unfavorable clinical or cytogenetic factors (i.e., Philadelphia chromosome positive ALL in first remission) (109,126–128). Limited data in the treatment of ALL following initial hematologic relapse suggest that a subset of patients, primarily those failing more than 18 months after achieving initial remission, may obtain long-term secondary disease control without bone marrow transplantation (81,82).

Bone Marrow Transplantation for Fanconi's Anemia

Fanconi's anemia is an autosomal recessive disorder characterized by progressive pancytopenia, thumb and radial abnormalities, growth retardation, abnormal skin pigmentation with cafe au lait spots, kidney or urinary tract abnormalities, micropthalmia, small face, and cardiac malformations. The phenotype is variable (129–132). Fanconi's anemia cells are hypersensitive to random chromatid breakage when stressed by DNA cross-linking agents. The diagnosis can be confirmed by demonstration of spontaneous chromatid breaks in preparations of phytohemagglutinin-stimulated peripheral blood lymphocytes. Greater than 90% of Fanconi's anemia patients develop full-blown aplastic anemia. With supportive care and androgens, about 50% of patients die by age 20 years and close to 100% are dead by 50 years of age (129). There is a tendency to develop malignancies, including leukemia.

The only cure for Fanconi's anemia is bone marrow transplantation. Cells from Fanconi's patients are unusally sensitive to irradiation (131). For this reason, the radiation dose and volume are restrained in preparative programs for bone marrow transplantation. The best established program is thorocoacbominal irradiation (TAI) to 5 Gy in a single fraction at approximately 10 cGy/min in conjunction with cyclophosphamide (Fig. 5).

Bone Marrow Transplantation for Aplastic Anemia

Aplastic anemia is a disease characterized by pancytopenia and a hypocellular bone marrow. It has been associated with a variety of infectious and chemical causes, but in most patients no cause is identified. Mortality in

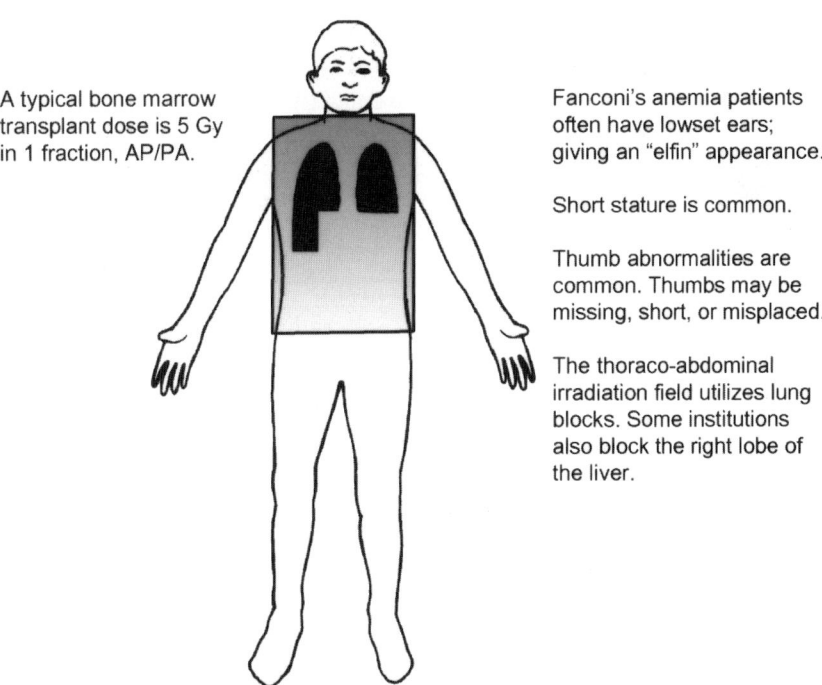

A typical bone marrow transplant dose is 5 Gy in 1 fraction, AP/PA.

Fanconi's anemia patients often have lowset ears; giving an "elfin" appearance.

Short stature is common.

Thumb abnormalities are common. Thumbs may be missing, short, or misplaced.

The thoraco-abdominal irradiation field utilizes lung blocks. Some institutions also block the right lobe of the liver.

FIG. 5. Thoracoabdominal irradiation is often used to prepare a child for bone marrow transplantation for Fanconi's anemia. The lungs are blocked. At some institutions it is also customary to block the right lobe of the liver.

severe aplastic anemia is extremely high. A bone marrow transplantation may be curative.

Graft failure is a well-recognized complication following bone marrow transplantation for aplastic anemia, particularly in heavily transfused patients. Radiotherapy is generally used to prepare the recipient and appears to improve the probability of engraftment compared to cyclophosphamide alone. The techniques used include cyclophosphamide plus either total lymphoid irradiation (TLI, 7.5 Gy × 1), TLI (3 Gy × 1), TLI (1 Gy × 6, t.i.d. = 6 Gy), or TAI (6 Gy × 1). One should be able to achieve a 70% to 80% long-term survival with a graft failure rate of <10%. The available data favors TLI (7.5 Gy × 1) or TAI (6 Gy × 1) (133,134).

Placental Blood Transplantation

Allogeneic bone marrow transplantation can cure some hematological malignancies, bone marrow failure syndromes, immunodeficiency disorders, and inborn errors of metabolism. The success of allogeneic transplantation, of course, depends on the identification of a suitable matched donor and the avoidance of GVHD. In recent years, *placental blood from a sibling donor* has been used as a source of hematopoietic stem cells for allogeneic transplantation. The feasibility of using *banked placental blood from unrelated donors* has recently been established (135). With banked placental blood, it appears that engraftment can regularly be achieved with partial HLA incompatibility and with relatively mild GVHD. Banked placental blood has several potential advantages: it can be obtained more quickly than the time typically needed to find an unrelated bone marrow donor via computerized registries, the time required to prepare the patient for transplantation is relatively short, and the possibilities for transplantation are increased—particularly for African-American children where there is a relative paucity of suitable donors available via computerized adult registries. As far as is known, when TBI or thoraco-abdominal irradiation are used for an umbilical cord

blood transplant, the same radiation dose, dose rate, and fractionation parameters are used as for conventional allogeneic transplantation (135).

Is TBI Necessary for Bone Marrow Transplantation for Leukemia?

TBI, usually with cyclophosphamide, has been used as preparation for bone marrow transplantation since the inception of the procedure. With the introduction of fractionated programs, TBI has been proven effective and the morbidity of the technique has been reduced. There has been, however, considerable impetus to identify alternative, nonradiation programs for bone marrow transplant preparation (134a). In pediatrics, of course, this desire has been driven by the hope of reducing late effects of radiation (136). The most popular alternative to TBI/Cyclophosphamide (TBI/CY) is Busulfan/Cyclophosphamide (BU/CY).

A study by the Societe Francaise de Greffe de Moelle of allogeneic bone marrow transplantation for children with AML in first remission compared, in a nonrandomized fashion, TBI/CY versus Bu/200 mg per kg[+] CY versus BU/120 mg per kg[+] CY (137). The relapse rate was 10% for TBI/CY versus 13% for high dose CY/BU versus 54% for lower dose CY/BU. Event-free survival was 82% for TBI/CY versus 80% for higher dose CY/BU versus 46% for lower dose CY/BU (137).

A randomized study, largely of adults with AML in first remission receiving allogeneic transplants, by the Groupe d'Etudes de la Greffe de Moelle Osseuse compared TBI/CY to BU/CY. At 2 years, the disease-free survival was 72% for TBI/CY versus 47% for BU/CY. Overall survival was 75% for TBI/CY versus 51% for BU/CY. Relapse rate was 14% for TBI/CY versus 34% for BU/CY (138).

A retrospective review from the Japanese Bone Marrow Transplant Registry also demonstrated significantly better overall survival and relapse rates for patients who had a TBI containing program compared to chemotherapy alone programs (139). A randomized trial of TBI/CY versus BU/CY in adults and children with AML in first or greater remission receiving autologus bone marrow transplant treatment at the University of Minnesota found similar disease-free survival at 2-years for patients in first remission (TBI/CY 67% vs. BU/CY 50%). For patients in greater than first remission there was a strong trend toward improved disease-free survival with TBI/CY (42% vs. BU/CY 9%, $p = 0.06$) (140,141). An adult Southwest Oncology Group Study found no significant difference between TBI/Etoposide and BU/CY for patients with acute leukemia or CML (142).

The Nordic Bone Marrow Transplant Group conducted a randomized trial of 167 patients, mostly adults, with allogeneic transplants for AML, ALL, and CML. When patients of all stages were lumped together the 3-year relapse-free survival favored TBI/CY (67%) versus BU/CY (56%, $p = 0.07$). For patients beyond first remission, the TBI/CY seemed clearly superior (61% vs. 18%, $p = 0.005$). The TBI containing program was associated with less venoocclusive disease and hemorrhagic cystitis than the chemotherapy alone program (143).

TBI/CY is either equivalent or superior to BU/CY and should be utilized prior to bone marrow transplantation for AML or ALL—with the possible exception of infants. There has also been concern raised that busulfan is unpredictably absorbed from the gastrointestinal tract in children (140).

Radiotherapeutic Management of Bone Marrow Transplantation with TBI

TBI is fundamental in bone marrow transplantation preparative regimens for most malignant diseases. The target volume includes the entire body; especially in leukemia, it is important not to completely block any area that might harbor circulating blast cells. These variables make comparisons between techniques difficult.

There are many physical factors that can be varied in TBI for bone marrow transplantation. The *fractionation* may be single (usually 10 Gy) or multiple. If the fractionation is multiple it may be given b.i.d. or t.i.d. The *total fractions*, therefore, may range from 1 to 11 or 12 over 1 to 4 to 5 days. The *dose per fraction* may be 1.25 to 10 Gy. A variety of *dose rates* have been utilized ranging from <5 cGy/min to 30–40 cGy/min. Some institutions use *partial or full attenuation blocks* of the lung or liver for all or part of the course of TBI. Many institutions use *attenuators* or tissue equivalent bolus to deal with variations in tissue thickness. As discussed later in the chapter, *boost fields* may be directed to the testes or to the marrow of the ribs, which are shielded by lung blocks. The *patient position* may be standing, seated, or supine and the *beam arrangement* may be laterals, anterior/posterior or obliques. Institutions vary in the *beam energy* selected and the use, at higher energies, of beam spoilers (144,145). Some common set-ups are shown schematically in Figs. 6 and 7. Among the more common dose and fractionation schemes are 1.5 Gy b.i.d. × 9 = 13.5 Gy, 125 Gy t.i.d. × 12 = 15 Gy, 2 Gy b.i.d. × 6 = 12 Gy, 225 Gy q.i.d. × 5 = 1125 Gy (56,60,126,145,146). With multiple-fraction-day treatment the normal tissue sparing effect of low-dose rate is less noticeable and 10 to 30 cGy/min is frequently used. With more limited fractionation, lower dose rates are used (147–149).

There are conflicting reports about the benefit of single-fraction versus fractionated regimens in nonrandomized series, although most reports (including a randomized study from Seattle) favor the fractionated group (112). Fractionation clearly improves normal tissue tolerance and, therefore, reduces late effects. This has been most clearly demonstrated in the decrease in cataracts seen after fractionated TBI (150). In young children, fractionation is clearly superior to single fraction regimens to decrease late effects such as growth impairment.

Most experiences with bone marrow transplantation and refractory ALL have shown a significant incidence of testicular failure. Of boys surviving more than 5 months after TBI, 25% developed primary testicular relapse in

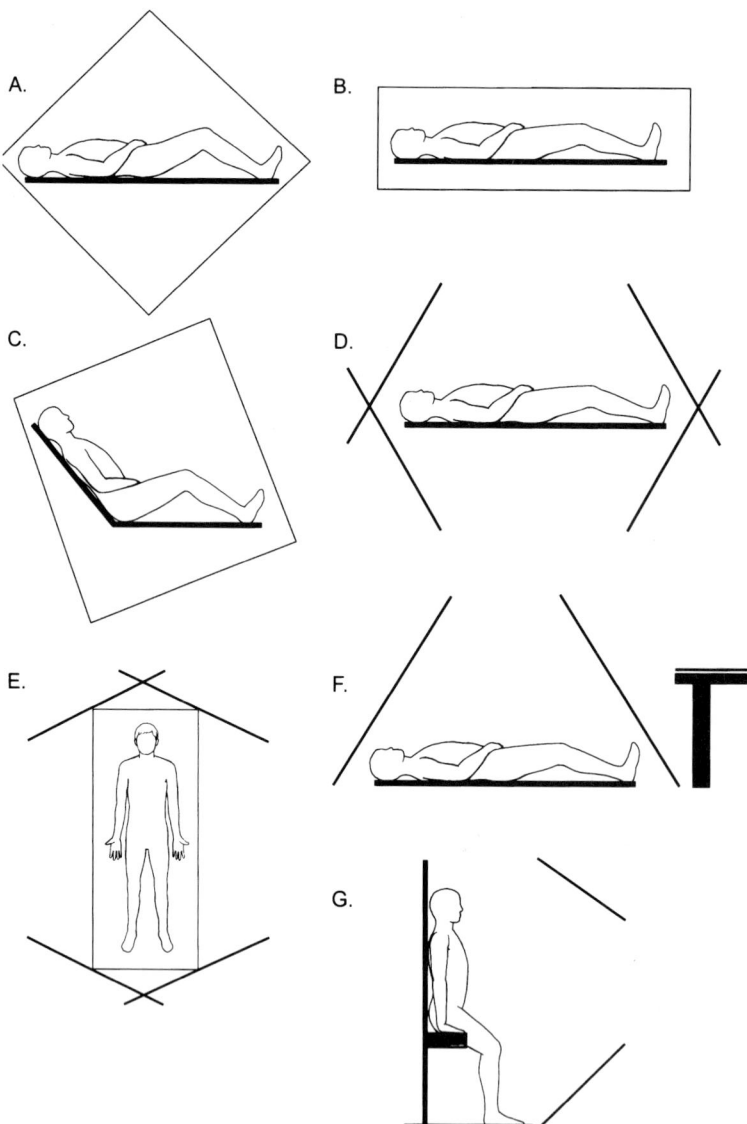

FIG. 6. There are a large variety of techniques available for the administration of total body irradiation. The techniques include: **(A)** a lateral approach with the patient supine and the collimator of the treatment machine rotated to fit the patient in the beam; **(B)** a lateral approach with the patient supine and the use of a very extended distance from the treatment machine to the patient so that a rectangular beam may be used; **(C)** a lateral approach with the patient in a semi-recumbent position and the collimator of the treatment machine rotated to fit the patient in the beam; **(D)** a specially prepared total body irradiation suite with one treatment machine mounted in the ceiling and one in the floor—the patient is placed on a treatment couch between the units; **(E)** a specially prepared total body irradiation suite with two machines mounted at opposite ends of the room—the patient is irradiated in the lateral position while on a treatment couch between the units; **(F)** a conventional treatment unit is used with the patient on the floor of the treatment room, instead of on the treatment couch, to obtain the necessary extended distance; **(G)** the patient is seated on a specially constructed seat to allow anterior/posterior treatment—some institutions use lung shielding during the photon treatment and then "boost" the ribs with electron beams.

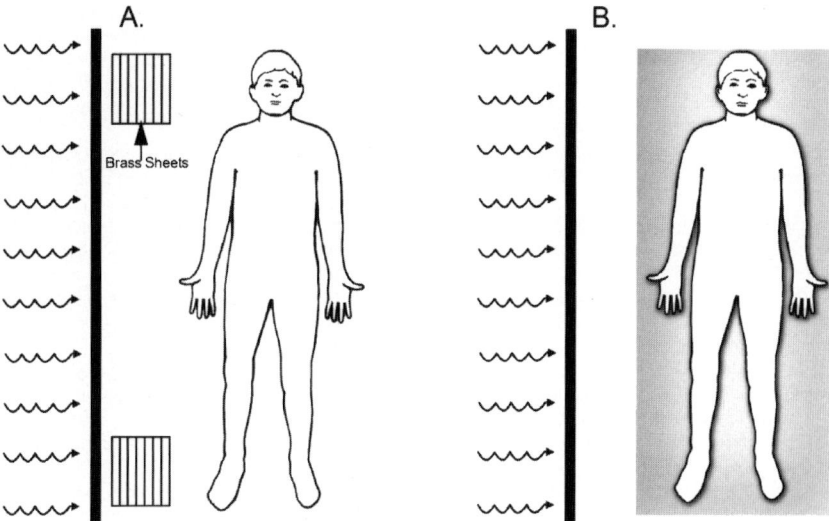

FIG. 7. The human body has an irregular surface contour and varies in internal density. In an attempt to achieve homogenous dose during total body irradiation, some institutions interpose brass plates in the radiation beam **(A)** to attenuate the dose to the thinner parts of the body such as the head and neck, and the distal lower extremities. This technique may also be used in an attempt to reduce the dose to the lungs. Others try to deal with the problem of irregular contour by using tissue equivalent material, packed around the body **(B)**, to create a more uniform contour.

the Seattle trials (124). Memorial Sloan-Kettering Cancer Center has used a 400 cGy/1–2 fraction to "boost" the testes, with no subsequent testicular relapses (122).

COMPLICATIONS

Complications of radiotherapy in the treatment of leukemia are reviewed in Chapter 19.

REFERENCES

References particularly recommended for further reading are indicated by an asterisk.

1. Martin AA, Alert JA, Reno JS, Lonchong M, Grueiros. Incidence of childhood cancer in Cuba (1986–1990) *Int J Cancer* 1997;72a:551–555.
2. Sriamporn S, Vatanasapt V, Martin N, et al. Incidence of childhood cancer in Thailand 1988–1991. *Paediatr Perinat Epidemiol* 1996;10:73–85.
3. Young JL, Percy CL, Asire AJ, eds. Surveillance, epidemiology, and end results: incidence and mortality data, 1973–77. *Natl Cancer Inst Monogr* 1981;57: 98–101.
*4. Ebb DH, Weinstein HJ. Diagnosis and treatment of childhood acute myelogenous leukemia. *Pediatr Clin North Am* 1997;44:847–862.
5. Miller RW, Young Jr JL, Navakovic B. Childhood cancer. *Cancer* 1994;75:395.
6. Hanson MR, Mulvihill JJ. Epidemiology of childhood cancer. In: Levine AS, ed. *Cancer in the young.* New York: Masson, 1980:3–12.
7. Miller RW. Relation between cancer and congenital defects: an epidemiologic evaluation. *J Natl Cancer Inst* 1968;40:1079–1085.
8. Miller RW. Neoplasia and Down's syndrome. *Ann NY Acad Sci* 1970;171:637–644.
9. Mulhern RK, Wasserman AL, Fairclough D, et al. Memory function in disease-free survivors of childhood acute lymphoblastic leukemia given CNS prophlylaxis with or without 1,800cGy cranial irradiation. *J Clin Oncol* 1988;6:3315–3320.
10. Bross IDJ, Natarajan N. Leukemia from low-level radiation: identification of susceptible children. *N Engl J Med* 1972;287:107–110.
11. Gibson RW, Bross IDJ, Grahma S, et al. Leukemia in children exposed to multiple risk factors. *N Engl J Med* 1968;219:906–909.
12. Reaman G, Zelter P, Bleyer WA, Amendola B, Level C, Sather H, Hammond D. Acute lymphoblastic leukemia in infants less than one year of age: a cumulative experience of the Children's Cancer Study Group. *J Clin Oncol* 1985;3:1513–1521.
*13. Kun LE. Acute lymphoblastic leukemia. *Semin Radiat Oncol* 1997;7:185–194.

14. Greaves M. A natural history for pediatric acute leukemia. *Blood* 1993;82:1043–1051.
15. Price RA, Johnson WW. The central nervous system and childhood leukemia. I. The arachnoid. *Cancer* 1973;31:530–533.
16. Pui C-H, Behm F, Crist W. Clinical and biologic relevance of immunologic marker studies in childhood acute lymphoblastic leukemia. *Blood* 1993;82: 343–362.
17. Korsmeyer SJ. Antigen receptor genes as molecular markers of lymphoid neoplasms. *J Clin Invest* 1987; 79:1291–1295.
*18. Crist WM, Grossi CE, Pullen J, Cooper MD. Immunologic markers in childhood acute lymphocytic leukemia. *Semin Oncol* 1985;12:105–121.
19. Crist WM, Boyett J, Jackson J, et al. Prognostic importance of the pre-B-cell immunophenotype and other presenting features in B-lineage childhood acute lymphoblastic leukemia: a Pediatric Oncology Group study. *Blood* 1989;74:1252–1259.
20. Smith M, Arthur D, Camitta B, et al. Uniform approach to risk classification and treatment assignment for children with acute lymphoblastic leukemia. *J Clin Oncol* 1996;14:18–24.
*21. Kun LE. Acute lymphoblastic leukemia. *Semin Oncol* 1997; 7:185–194.
*22. Rubinitz JE, Crist WM. Molecular genetics of childhood cancer: implications for pathogenesis, diagnosis and treatment. *Pediatrics* 1997;100:101–107.
23. Roper M, Crist WM, Metzgar R, et al. Monoclonal antibody characterization of surface antigens in childhood T-cell lymphoid malignancies. *Blood* 1983; 61:830–837.
24. Crist W, Pullen J, Boyett J, et al. Acute lymphoid leukemia in adolescents: clinical and biologic features predict a poor prognosis—a Pediatric Oncology Group study. *J Clin Oncol* 1988;6:34–43.
25. Pui C-H, Crist WM, Look AT. Biology and clinical significance of cytogenetic abnormalities in childhood acute lymphoblastic leukemia. *Blood* 1990;76: 1449–1463.
26. Fletcher JA, Lynch EA, Kimball VM, Donnelly M, Tantravahi R, Sallan SE. Translocation (9;22) is associated with extremely poor prognosis in intensively treated children with acute lymphoblastic leukemia. *Blood* 1991;77:435–439.
27. Ribeiro RC, Abromowitch M, Raimondi SC, Murphy SB, Behm F, Williams DL. Clinical and biologic hallmarks of the Philadelphia chromosome in childhood acute lymphoblastic leukemia. *Blood* 1987;70: 948–953.
28. Look TA. The emerging genetics of acute lymphoblastic leukemia: clinical and biologic implications. *Semin Oncol* 1985;12:92–104.
29. Maurer HS, Steinherz PG, Graynon PS, et al. The effect of initial management of hyperleukocytosis on early complications and outcome of children with acute lymphoblastic leukemia. *J Clin Oncol* 1988;6: 1425–1432.
30. Rivera GK, Mauer AM. Controversies in the management of childhood acute lymphoblastic leukemia: treatment intensification, CNS leukemia and prognostic factors. *Semin Hematol* 1987;24:12–26.
*31. Mahmoud HH, Rivera GK, Hancock ML, et al. Low leukocyte counts with blast cells in cerebrospinal fluid

of children with newly diagnosed acute lymphoblastic leukemia. *N Engl J Med* 1993;329:314–319.
32. Shapiro WR, Young DF, Mehta BM. Methotrexate: distribution in cerebrospinal fluid after intravenous, ventricular and lumbar injections. *N Engl J Med* 1975;293:161–166.
33. Paryani SB, Donaldson SS, Amylon MD, Link MP. Cranial nerve involvement in children with leukemia and lymphoma. *J Clin Oncol* 1983;1:542–545.
34. Schachat AP, Markowitz JA. Ophthalmic manifestations of leukemia *Arch Ophthalmol* 1989;107: 697–700.
35. Schwartz CL, Miller NR. The optic nerve as the site of initial relapses in childhood ALL. *Cancer* 1989; 63:1616–1620.
*36. Farber S, Diamond LK, Mercer RD, Sylvester RF, Wolff JA. Temporary remission in acute leukemia in children produced by folic acid antagonist, 4-amino pteroylglutamic acid (aminopterin). *N Engl J Med* 1948;238:787.
37. Freireich EJ. The road to the cure of acute lymphoblastic leukemia: a personal perspective. *Oncology* 1997;54:265–269.
*38. Pinkel D. Curing children with leukemia. *Cancer* 1986;59:1683–1691.
*39. Pui C-H. Acute lyphoblastic leukemia. *Pediatr Clin North Am* 1997;44:831–846.
40. Niemeyer CM, Hitchcock-Bryan S, Sallan SE. Comparative analysis of treatment programs for childhood acute lymphoblastic leukemia. *Semin Oncol* 1985;12: 122–130.
41. Niemeyer CM, Gelber RD, Tarbell NJ, et al. Low dose versus high dose methotrexate during remission induction in childhood acute lymphoblastic leukemia. *Blood* 1991;78(10):2514–2519.
42. Gustafson G, Lie SO. Acute leukemias. In: Voute PA, Kalifa C, Barrett A, eds. *Cancer in Children: clinical management.* Oxford: Oxford University Press, 1998: 99–118.
*43. Riehm H, Gadner H, Hente G, et al. Results and significance of six randomized trials in four consecutive ALL-BFM studies. *Haematology and blood transfusion* 1990;33:439–450.
44. Pui C-H, Dahl GV, Bowman WP, et al. Lack of clinical utility of elective testicular biopsy performed during chemotherapy for childhood leukemia. *Lancet* 1985;2:410–412.
45. Clavell LA, Gelber RD, Cohen HJ, et al. Four-agent induction and intensive asparaginase therapy for treatment of childhood acute lymphoblastic leukemia. *N Engl J Med* 1986;315:657.
46. Bleyer WA, Poplack DG. Intraventricular versus intralumbar methotrexate for central-nervous-system leukemia. *Med Pediatr Oncol* 1979;6:207–213.
47. Aur RJA, Hustu HO, Verzosa MS, Wood A, Simone JV. Comparison of two methods of preventing central nervous system leukemia. *Blood* 1973;42:349.
48. Aur RJA, Simone JV, Hustu HO, Verzosa M, Pinkel D. Cessation of therapy during complete remission of childhood acute lymphocytic leukemia. *N Engl J Med* 1974;291:1230.
49. Dahl GV, Simone JV, Hustu HO, Mason C. Preventive central nervous system irradiation in children with acute non-lymphocytic leukemia. *Cancer* 1978;42: 2187–2192.

50. Hustu HO, Aur RJA. Extramedullary leukemia. *Clin Haematol* 1978;7:313–337.

*51. Nesbit ME Jr, Robinson LL, Littman PS, et al. Presymptomatic central nervous system therapy in previously untreated childhood acute lymphoblastic leukaemia: comparison of 1800 rad and 2400 rad: a report for Children's Cancer Study Group. *Lancet* 1981;1:461–466.143.

52. Nesbit ME Jr, Sather HN, Ortega J, et al. Effect of isolated central nervous system leukaemia on bone marrow remission and survival in childhood acute lymphoblastic leukaemia. A report for Children's Cancer Study Group. *Lancet* 1981;2:1386–1389.

*53. Gelber R, Sallan SE, Cohen HJ, et al. Central nervous system treatment in childhood acute lymphoblastic leukemia: long-term followup for patients diagnosed 1973–1985. *Cancer* 1993;72:261–270.

54. Bleyer WA. Neurologic sequelae of methotrexate and ionizing radiation. A new classification. *Cancer Treat Rep* 1981;65:89–98.

55. Abromowitch M, Ochs J, Pui C-H, Fairclough D, Murphy SB, Rivera GK. Efficacy of high-dose methotrexate in childhood acute lymphocytic leukemia: analysis by contemporary risk classifications. *Blood* 1988;71:866–869.

56. Poplack DG, Reaman GH. Successful prevention of CNS leukemia without cranial irradiation. *Am J Clin Oncol* 1989;8:213.

57. Pui C-H, Behm FG, Raimondi SC, et al. Secondary acute myeloid leukemia in children treated for acute myeloid leukemia. *N Engl J Med* 1989;321:136–142.

58. Pullen J, Boyett J, Frankel L, et al. Extended triple intrathecal (T.I.T.) chemotherapy provides efficient central nervous system (CNS) prophylaxis for both good and poor prognosis patients with non-T, non-B, acute lymphoblastic leukemia (ALL); substitution of intermediate dose methotrexate (IDM) for T.I.T. after consolidation provides less effective protection for the CNS. *Proc Am Soc Clin Oncol* 1988;7:176.

59. Tarbell NJ, Gelber RD, Barr R, et al. Efficacy of hyperfractionated cranial irradiation in childhood ALL. *Blood* 1992;80[Suppl 1]:207A.

60. Nesbit ME, Sather HN, Robinson LL, et al. Sanctuary therapy: a randomized trial of 724 children with previously untreated acute lymphoblastic leukemia. *Cancer Res* 1982;42:674–680.

61. Sullivan MP, Humphrey GB, Vietti TJ, et al. Superiority of conventional intrathecal methotrexate therapy with maintenance over intensive intrathecal methotrexate therapy, unmaintained, or radiotherapy (2000–25000 rads tumor dose) in treatment for meningeal leukemia. *Cancer* 1975;35:1066–1073.

*62. Freeman AI, Weinberg V, Brecher ML, et al. Comparison of intermediate-dose methotrexate with cranial irradiation for the post-induction treatment of acute lymphocytic leukemia in children. *N Engl J Med* 1983;308:477–484.

63. Abromowitch M, Och I, Pui CH, et al. High-dose methotrexate improves clinical outcome in children with ALL: St. Jude Total Therapy Study X. *Med Pediatr Oncol* 1988;16:297–203.

64. Freeman AI, Boyett JM, Glicksman AS, et al. Intermediate-dose methotrexate versus cranial irradiation in childhood acute lymphoblastic leukemia: a ten-year follow-up. *Med Pediatr Oncol* 1997; 28:98–107.

*65. Bleyer WA, Poplack DG. Prophylaxis and treatment of leukemia in the central nervous system and other sanctuaries. *Semin Oncol* 1985;12:131–148.

*66. Conter V, et al. Extended intrathecal methotrexate may replace cranial irradiation for prevention of CNS relapse in children with intermediate-risk acute lymphoblastic leukemia treated with Berlin-Frankfurt-Munster based intensive chemotherapy. *J Clin Oncol* 1995;13:2497–2502.

67. Ochs JJ, Rivera G, Aur RJ, Hustu HO, Berg R, Simone JV. Central nervous system morbidity following an initial isolated central nervous system relapse and its subsequent therapy in childhood acute lymphoblastic leukemia. *J Clin Oncol* 1985;3:622–626.

*68. Hasle H, Helgestad J, Christensen JK, Jacobsen BB, Kamper J. Prolonged intrathecal chemotherapy replacing cranial irradiation in high-risk acute lymphatic leukaemia: long-term follow-up with cerebral computed tomography scans and endocrinological studies. *Eur J Pediatr* 1995;154:24–29.

*69. Tarbell NJ, Amato DA, Down JD, Mauch P, Hellman S. Fractionation and dose rate effects in mice: a model for bone marrow transplantation in man. *Int J Radiat Oncol Biol Phys* 1987;13:1065–1069.

70. Editorial. Leukemia and the central nervous system. *Lancet* 1985;i:1196.

71. George SL, Ochs JJ, Mauer AM, Simone JV. The importance of an isolated central nervous system relapse in children with acute lymphoblastic leukemia. *J Clin Oncol* 1985;3:776–781.

72. Ortega JA, Nesbit ME, Sather HN, Robinson LL, D'Angio GJ, Hammond GD. Long-term evaluation of a CNS prophylaxis trial—treatment comparisons and outcome after CNS relapse in childhood ALL: a report from the Children's Cancer Study Group. *J Clin Oncol* 1987;5:1646–1654.

*73. Cherlow JM, Sather H, Steinherz P, et al. Craniospinal irradiation for acute lymphoblastic leukemia with CNS disease at diagnosis—a report from the Children's Cancer Group. *Int J Radiat Oncol Biol Phys* 1996;36:19–27.

*74. Kun LE. CNS disease at diagnosis: a continuing challenge in childhood lymphoblastic leukemia. *Int J Radiat Oncol Biol Phys* 1996;36:257–259.

75. Baum E, Heyn R, Nesbit M, Tilford D, Nachman J. Occult abdominal involvement with apparently isolated testicular relapse in children with acute lymphocytic leukemia. *Am J Pediatr Hematol Oncol* 1984;6:343–346.

76. Kun LE, Camitta BM, Mulhern RK, et al. Treatment of meningeal relapse in childhood acute lymphoblastic leukemia. I. Results of craniospinal irradiation. *J Clin Oncol* 1984;2:359–364.

77. Castro JR, Sullivan MP. Cerebrospinal axis radiation therapy for meningeal leukemia with tumor dose levels in the range of 2000 rad. *Radiology* 1972;104:543.

78. Land VJ, Thomas PRM, Boyett JM, et al. Comparisons of maintenance treatment regimens for first central nervous system relapse in children with acute lymphocytic leukemia: a Pediatric Oncology Group study. *Cancer* 1985;56:81–87.

79. Winnick NJ, et al. Treatment of CNS relapse in children with acute lymphoblastic leukemia: a Pediatric Oncology Group study. *J Clin Oncol* 1993;11:271–278.

80. Willoughby MCN. Treatment of CNS leukemia. In:

Mastrangelio A, Poplak DG, Riccardi R, eds. *Central nervous system leukemia: prevention and treatment.* Boston: Martinus Nijhoff, 1983:113.

81. Rivera GK, Buchanan G, Boyett JM, et al. Intensive retreatment of childhood acute lymphoblastic leukemia in first bone marrow relapse: a Pediatric Oncology Group study. *N Engl J Med* 1986;315: 273–278.

82. Rivera GK, Ochs J, Roberson PK, et al. Intensive salvage therapy for isolated initial CNS relapses in childhood ALL. *Blood* 1986;68:231(abst).

83. Weisdorf DJ, Billett AL, Hannan P, Ritz J, Sallan SE, Steinbuch M, Ramsay NK. Autologous versus unrelated donor allogeneic marrow transplantation for acute lymphoblastic leukemia. *Blood* 1997;90(8): 2962–2968.

84. Kline RW, Gillin MT, Kun LE. Cranial irradiation in acute leukemia: dose estimate in the lens. *Int J Radiat Oncol Biol Phys* 1979;5:117–121.

85. Belasco J, Goldwein J, Lange B, et al. Monthly low-dose cranio-spinal (C-S) radiotherapy (RT) to 18 Gy after CNS relapse in children with acute lymphoblastic leukemia (ALL). *Proc ASCO* 1996;15:368.

86. Gillin MT, Kline RW, Kun LE. Cranial dose distribution. *Int J Radiat Oncol Biol Phys* 1979;5:1903–1906.

87. Maor MH, Fields RS, Hogstrom KR, van Eys J. Improving the therapeutic ratio of craniospinal irradiation in medulloblastoma. *Int J Radiat Oncol Biol Phys* 1985;11:687–697.

88. van den aBerg H, Langeveld NE, Veenhof CHN, Behrendt H. Treatment of isolated testicular recurrence of acute lymphoblastic leukemia without radiotherapy: a report from the Dutch late effects study group. *Cancer* 1997;79:2257–2262.

89. Riccardi R, Vigersky RA, Barnes S, Bleyer WA, Poplack DG. Methotrexate levels in the interstitial space and seminiferous tubule of rat testis. *Cancer Res* 1982;42:1617–1619.

90. Kuo TT, Tschange TP, Chu JY. Testicular relapse in childhood acute lymphocytic leukemia during bone marrow remission. *Cancer* 1976; 2604–2612.

91. Medical Research Council. Testicular disease in acute lymphoblastic leukæmia in childhood. *Br Med J* 1978;1:334–338.

92. Nesbit Jr ME, Robinson LL, Ortega JA, Sather HN, Donaldson M, Hammond D. Testicular relapse in childhood acute lymphoblastic leukemia: association with pretreatment patient characteristics and treatment. A report for Children's Cancer Study Group. *Cancer* 1980;45:2009–2016.

93. Ortega JJ, Javier G, Toran N. Testicular infiltrates in children with acute lymphoblastic leukemia: a prospective study. *Med Pediatr Oncol* 12:386–393.

94. Hudson MM, Frankel LS, Mullins J, Swanson DA. Diagnostic value of surgical testicular biopsy after therapy for acute lymphocytic leukemia. *J Pediatr* 1985;107:50–53.

95. Gaijar A, Ribeiro RC, Mahmoud HH, et al. Overt testicular disease at diagnosis is associated with high risk features and a poor prognosis in patients with childhood acute lymphoblastic leukemia. *Cancer* 1996;78: 2437–2442.

96. Bowman WP, Aur RJA, Hustu HO, Rivera G. Isolated testicular relapse in acute lymphocytic leukemia of childhood: categories and influence on survival. *J Clin Oncol* 1984;2:924–929.

97. Blatt J, Sherins RJ, Niebrugge D, Bleyer WA, Poplack DG. Leydig cell function in boys following treatment for testicular relapse of acute lymphoblastic leukemia. *J Clin Oncol* 1985;3:1227–1231.

98. Li FP, Bader JL. Epidemiology of cancer in childhood. In: Nathan DG, Oski FA, eds. *Hematology of infancy and childhood.* Philadelphia: WB Saunders, 1987:918–941.

99. D'Angio GJ, Littman P, Nesbit M, et al. Evaluation of radiation therapy factors in prophylactic central nervous system irradiation for childhood leukemia: a report from the Children's Cancer Study Group. *Int J Radiat Oncol Biol Phys* 1981;7:1031–1038.

100. Tallman MS. Differentiating therapy with all-trans retinoic acid in acute myeloid leukemia. *Leukemia* 1996;10(Suppl 1):S12–15.

101. Creutzig U, Ritter J, Riehm H, et al. Improved treatment results in childhood acute myelogenous leukemia: a report of the German cooperative study AML-BFM-78. *Blood* 1985;65:298–304.

102. Creutzig U, Ritter J, Budde M, Jurgens H, Riehm H, Schellong G. Treatment results in childhood AML, with special reference to the German studies BFM-78 and BFM-83. *Hamatologie und Bluttransfusion* 1987; 31:30–34.

103. Lampkin BC, Woods W, Strauss R, et al. Current status of the biology and treatment of acute non-lymphocytic leukemia in children. (Report from the ANLL strategy group of the Children's Cancer Study Group). *Blood* 1983;61:215–228.

104. Weinstein H, Grier H, Gelber R, et al. Post remission induction intensive sequential chemotherapy for children with AML—treatment results and prognostic factors. In: Buchner T, Schellong G, Hiddemann W, et al., eds. *Haematology and blood transfusion, vol 30: Acute leukemias.* New York: Springer-Verlag, 1987:88–92.

105. Kay HEM. Development of CNS leukemia in acute myeloid leukemia in childhood. *Arch Dis Child* 1976; 51:73–74.

106. Pui C-H, Dahl GV, Kalwinsky DK, Look AT, Mirro J, Dodge RK, Simone JV. Central nervous system leukemia in children with acute nonlymphoblastic leukemia. *Blood* 1985;66:1062–1067.

107. Dahl GV, Kalwinsky DK, Murphy S, et al. Cytokinetically based induction chemotherapy and splenectomy for childhood acute nonlymphocytic leukemia. *Blood* 1982;60:856–863.

108. Holmes R, Keating MJ, Cork A, et al. A unique pattern of central nervous system leukemia in acute myelomonocytic leukemia associated with inv(16) (p13q22). *Blood* 1985;65:1071–1078.

109. Champlin R, Gale RP. Bone marrow transplantation for acute leukemia: recent advances and comparison with alternative therapies. *Semin Hematol* 1987;24: 55–67.

110. Cheson BD, Lacerna L, Leyland-Jones B, Sarosy G, Wittes RE. Autologous bone marrow transplantation. Current status and future directions. *Ann Intern Med* 1989;110:51–65.

111. Blume KG, Forman SJ, O'Donnell MR, et al. Total body irradiation and high dose etoposide: a new

preparatory regimen for bone marrow transplantation of patients with advanced hematologic malignancy. *Blood* 1987;69:1015–1020.

*112. Thomas ED, Clift RA, Hersman J, et al. Marrow transplantation for acute nonlymphoblastic leukemia in first remission using fractionated or single-dose irradiation. *Int J Radiat Oncol Biol Phys* 1982;8: 817–821.

113. Johnson FL, Thomas ED, Clark BS, Chard RL, Hartmann JR, Storb R. A comparison of marrow transplantation with chemotherapy for children with acute lymphoblastic leukemia in second or subsequent remission. *N Engl J Med* 1981;305:846–851.

114. Thompson CB, Sanders JE, Flournoy N, Buckner CD, Thomas ED. The risks of central nervous system relapse and leukoencephalopathy in patients receiving marrow transplants for acute leukemia. *Blood* 1986;67:195–199.

115. Sanders JE, Flournoy N, Thomas ED, et al. Marrow transplant experience in children with acute lymphoblastic leukemia: an analysis of factors associated with survival, relapse, and graft-versus-host disease. *Med Pediatr Oncol* 1985;13:165–172.

116. Long GD, Blume KG. Allogeneic bone marrow transplantation for acute myeloid leukemia. In: Forman SJ, Blume KG, Thomas ED, eds. *Bone marrow transplantation*. Boston: Blackwell Scientific Publications, 1994:607–617.

117. Yeager AM. Autologous bone marrow transplantation for acute myeloid leukemia. In: Forman SJ, Blume KG, Thomas ED, eds. *Bone marrow transplantation*. Boston: Blackwell Scientific Publications, 1994: 709–730.

118. Arcese W, Amadori S, Testi AM, et al. Allogeneic vs. autologous BMT v. intensive chemotherapy in childhood ANLL during first complete remission: AIEOP experience. *Bone Marrow Trans* 1991;7[Suppl 3]: 71–74.

*119. Ravindranath Y, Yeager AM, Chang MN, et al. Autologous bone marrow transplanation versus intensive consolidation chemotherapy for acute myeloid leukemia in childhood. *N Engl J Med* 1996;334: 1428–1434.

*120. Sanders JE. Bone marrow transplantation for pediatric malignancies. *Pediatr Clin North Am* 1997;44: 1005–1020.

121. Thomas ED. ALL and beyond: implications for other hematologic malignancies. *Leukemia* 1997;11[Suppl 4]:S43–45.

122. Brochstein JA, Kernan NA, Groshen S, et al. Allogeneic bone marrow transplantation after hyperfractionated total body irradiation and cyclophosphamide in children with acute leukemia. *N Engl J Med* 1987; 317:1618–1624.

123. Chao NJ, Forman SJ. Allogeneic bone marrow transplantation for acute lymphoblastic leukemia. In: Forman SJ, Blume KG, Thomas ED, eds. *Bone marrow transplantation*. Boston: Blackwell Scientific Publications, 1994:618–628.

124. Sanders JE, Thomas ED, Buckner CD, et al. Marrow transplantation for children in first remission of acute nonlymphoblastic leukemia: an update. *Blood* 1985; 66:460–462.

125. Sanders JE, Thomas ED, Buckner CD, Doney K, et

al. Marrow transplantation for children with acute lymphoblastic leukemia in second remission. *Blood* 1987;70:324–326.

126. Butturini A, Rivera GK, Bortin MM, Gale RP. Which treatment for childhood acute lymphoblastic leukemia in second remission? *Lancet* 1987;1:429–432.

127. Fletcher JA, Kimball VM, Lynch E, et al. Prognostic implications of cytogenic studies in an intensively treated group of children with ALL. *Blood* 1989;74: 2130–2135.

128. Forman SJ, O'Donnell MR, Nademanee AP, et al. Bone marrow transplantation of patients with Philadelphia chromosome-positive acute lymphoblastic leukemia. *Blood* 1987;70:587–588.

129. Alter BP. Fanconi's anemia: current concepts. *Am J Pediatr Hematol Oncol* 1992; 14:170–176.

130. DeBaun MR, Wall DA, Watson MS. Microcephaly with short stature, macrocytosis, and pancytopenia. *Am J Pediatr Hematol Oncol* 1993; 15:356–360.

131. Gluckman E, Hows J. "Bone marrow transplantation in Fanconi's anemia." In: Forman SJ, Blume KG, Thomas ED, eds. *Bone marrow transplantation*. Boston: Blackwell Scientific Publications, 1994: 902–909.

132. Strathdee CA, Buchwaldl M. Molecular and cellular biology of Fanconi anemia. *Am J Pediatr Hematol Oncol* 1992;14:177–185.

133. Castro-Malaspina H, Childs B, Laver J, et al. Hyperfractionated total lymphoid irradiation and cyclophosphamide for preparation of previously transfused patients under going HLA-identical marrow transplantation for severe aplastic anemia. *Int J Rad Oncol Biol Phys* 1994;29:847–854.

*134. McGlave PB, Haake R, Miller W, Kim T, Kersey J, Ramsay NK. Therapy of severe aplastic anemia in young adults and children with allogeneic bone marrow transplantation. *Blood* 1987;70:1325–1330.

*135. Kurtzberg J, Laughlin M, Graham ML, et al. Placental blood as a source of hematopoietic stem cells for transplantation into unrelated recipients. *N Engl J Med* 1996;335:157–166.

136. *Seer Cancer Statistics Review 1973–1992. Tables and Graphs*. Bethesda: U.S. Depart of Health and Human Services (NIH Pub. No. 96-1789), 1995:463.

*137. Michel G, Gluckman E, Esperou-Bourdeau H, et al. Allogeneic bone marrow transplantations for children with acute myeloblastic leukemia in first complete remission: impact of conditioning regimen without total-body irradiation—a report from the Societe Francaise de Greffe de Moelle. *J Clin Oncol* 1994;12: 1217–1222.

138. Blaise D, Maraninchi D, Archimbaud E, et al. Allogeneic bone marrow transplantation for acute myeloid leukemia in first remission: a randomized trial of busulfan-cytoxan versus cytoxan-total body irradiation as preparative regimen. *Blood* 1992;79:2578–2582.

139. Inoue T, Ikeda H, Yamazaki H, et al. Role of total body irradiation as based on the comparision of preparation regimens for allogeneic bone marrow transplantation for acute leukemia in first complete remission. *Strahlenther Onkol* 1993;169:250–255.

140. Dusenbery KE, Woods WG. In response to B. Shank. *Int J Radiat Oncol Biol Phys* 1995;31:202–203.

*141. Dusenbery KE, Daniels KA, McClure JS, et al. Randomized comparision of cyclophosphamide-total body irradiation vs. busulfan-cyclophosphamide conditioning in autologous bone marrow transplantation for acute myeloid leukemia. *Int J Radiat Oncol Biol Phys* 1995;31:119–128.

142. Blume KG, Kopecky KJ, Henslee-Downey JP, et al. A prospective randomized comparison of total body iradiation etoposide versus busulfan-cyclophosphamide as preparatory regimens for bone marrow transplantation in patients with leukemia who were not in first remission. *Blood* 1993;81:2187–2193.

*143. Ringden O, Ruutu T, Remberger M, et al. A randomized trial comparing busulfan with total body irradiation as conditioning in allogeneic marrow transplant recipients with leukemia; a report from the Nordic Bone Marrow Transplant Group. *Blood* 1994;894:2723–2730.

144. Planskay B, Bedford AM, Davis FM, Tapper PD, Loverock LT. Physical aspects of total-body irradiation at the Middlesex Hospital (UCL group of hospitals), London 1988–1993: I. Phantom measurements and planning methods. *Phys Med Biol* 1996;41:2307–2326.

145. Planskaky B, Tapper PD, Bedford AM, Davis FM. Physical aspects of total-body irradiation at the Middlesex Hospital (UCL group of hospitals), London 1988–1993:II. *In vivo* planning and dosimetry. *Phys Med Biol* 1996;41:2327–2343.

146. Peters LJ, Withers HR, Cundiff JH, Dicke KA. Radiobiological considerations in the use of total-body irradiation for bone-marrow transplantation. *Radiology* 1979;13:243–247.

147. Broerse JJ, Dutriex A, Noordijk EM, eds. Physical, biological and clinical aspects of TBI. *Radiother Oncol* 1990;18(Suppl 1):11–162.

148. Obcemea CH, Rice RK, Mijnheer BJ, et al. Three-dimensional dose distribution of total body irradiation by a dual source total body irradiator. *Int J Radiat Oncol Biol Phys* 1992;24:789–793.

149. Shank B, Chu FCH, Dinsmore R, et al. Hyperfractionated total body irradiation for bone marrow transplantation. Results in seventy leukemia patients with allogeneic transplants. *Int J Radiat Oncol Biol Phys* 1983;9:1607–1611.

*150. Deeg JD, Flournoy N, Sullivan KM. Cataracts after total body irradiation and marrow transplantation: a sparing effect of dose fractionation. *Int J Radiat Oncol Biol Phys* 1984;10:957–964.

3

Supratentorial Brain Tumors Except Ependymomas; Brain Tumors in Babies and Very Young Children

Nearly 20% of all neoplasms in children arise within the central nervous system (CNS). The incidence of CNS tumors in children has increased over the past 2 to 3 decades (1). The frequency of brain tumors by site and histology is indicated in Table 1. The current World Health Organization (WHO) classification of CNS neoplasms is summarized in Table 2 (2,3).

Nearly one-half of pediatric CNS tumors are supratentorial tumors. Anatomically, the supratentorial cranial compartment (Fig. 1) includes the cerebral hemispheres (i.e., the frontal, parietal, temporal, and occipital lobes), the diencephalon (i.e., the hypothalamus, optic chiasm, and thalamic/caudate nucleus/putamen structures, the latter generally considered together as the "thalamic region"), and the pineal region (i.e., the pineal gland and posterior third ventricular region). Tumors are commonly categorized by regions that correlate with specific clinical findings and histologic types: suprasellar lesions (including glial tumors of the optic chiasm and adjacent hypothalamic area, craniopharyngiomas, and germ cell tumors of the anterior third ventricular region), central or deep-seated lesions (gliomas of the thalamic region plus pineal region tumors including germ cell, embryonal, and glial neoplasms), and peripheral lesions (gliomas, ependymo-

mas, and embryonal tumors of the cerebral hemispheres).

Advances in neuroimaging have greatly improved the accuracy of diagnosis and staging of CNS tumors. Magnetic resonance imaging (MRI) is often the only imaging tool sensitive enough to identify small hemispheric tumors presenting with seizures. Although MRI provides unique and often diagnostic information in suprasellar and pineal region lesions, computerized tomography (CT) better delineates calcification (typically seen in craniopharyngiomas and malignant germ cell tumors). Positron emission tomography (PET), single photon emission tomography (SPECT), and magnetic resonance spectroscopy (MRS) are of potential value in assessing tumor viability or differentiating posttherapy changes from tumor progression; correlations between MRS and tumor grade or type have also been noted (4–8).

Modern neurosurgical techniques have virtually eliminated the necessity to consider radiation therapy and/or chemotherapy without a histologic diagnosis in supratentorial tumors (9). There is no apparent advantage to the patient or radiation oncologist in considering therapy based on imaging alone (10). Exceptions include (a) the infrequent malignant pineal or suprasellar germ cell tumors diag-

TABLE 1. *Relative incidence of common brain tumors in children*

Supratentorial tumors	(45–50%)	Infratentorial tumors	(50–55%)
Astrocytoma	23%	Medulloblastoma	20%
Malignant gliomas (anaplastic	6%	Astrocytoma	15%
astrocytoma, glioblastoma multiforme)		Brainstem glioma	10%
Craniopharyngioma	6%	Ependymoma	6%
Embryonal tumors (PNET and others)	4%		
Pineal region tumors/intracranial germ			
cell tumors	4%		
Ependymoma	3%		
Oligodendroglioma	2%		
Other (meningioma, ganglioma, choroid			
plexus tumors, others)	2%		

From refs 2, 146, and 150, with permission.

nosed by elevated levels of α-fetoprotein (AFP) or β-human chorionic gonadotropin (β-HCG); and (b) optic pathway tumors that involve the optic nerve alone or the chiasm in conjunction with adjacent optic pathway structures, particularly in the setting of neu-rofibromatosis (11). For craniopharyngiomas, the imaging diagnosis can frequently be confirmed by simple cyst aspiration, documenting the presence of diagnostic squamous cells and/or cholesterol crystals in the cyst fluid (12).

TABLE 2. *Histopathologic classification of CNS tumors—WHO classification 1994*

1. Tumors of neuroepithelial tissue
   astrocytic tumors (astrocytoma, anaplastic astrocytoma, glioblastoma, pilocytic astrocytoma, pleomorphic
      xanthoastrocytoma, subependymal giant cell astrocytoma)
   oligodendroglial tumors (oligodendroglioma, anaplastic oligodendroglioma)
   ependymal tumors (ependymoma, anaplastic ependymoma, myxopapillary ependymoma)
   mixed gliomas (oligodendroglioma, others)
   choroid plexus tumors
   neuronal tumors (gangliocytoma, ganglioglioma, desmoplastic infantile neuroepithelioma,
      dysembryoplastic neuroepithelial tumor)
   pineal tumors (pineocytoma, pineoblastoma)
2. Embryonal tumors
   medulloepithelioma
   neuroblastoma
   ependymoblastoma
   primitive neuroectodermal tumors (PNETs)
      medulloblastoma (posterior fossa, cerebellar)
      cerebral or spinal PNETs
3. Tumors of meningothelial cells
   meningioma
   malignant meningioma
4. Tumors of the uncertain histogenesis
   hemangioblastoma
5. Germ cell tumors
   germinoma
   embryonal carcinoma
   endodermal sinus tumor
   choriocarcinoma
   teratoma
   mixed germ cell tumors
   ependymoblastoma
5. Tumors of the sellar region
   pituitary adenoma
   craniopharyngioma

From refs. 3 and 188, with permission.

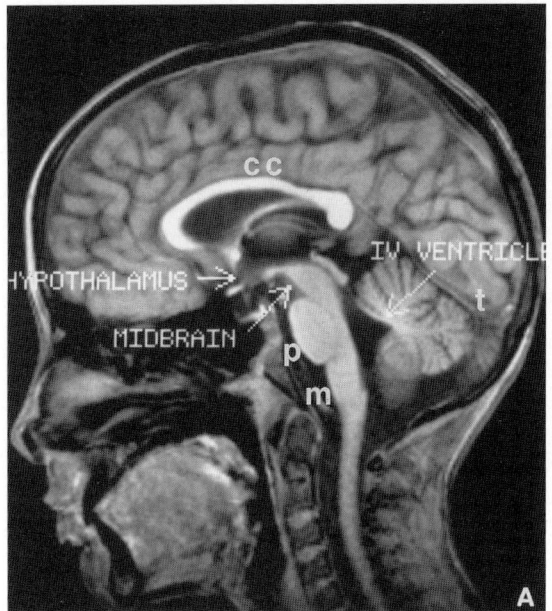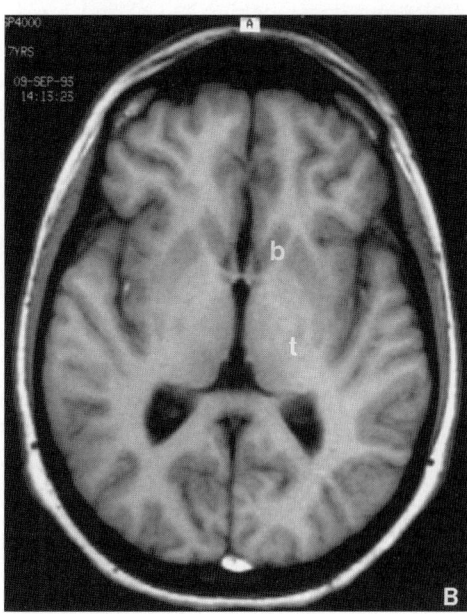

FIG. 1. Sagittal **(A)** and axial **(B)** MRI of the normal brain. Note tentorium *(t)* separating supratentorial volume from infratentorial or posterior fossa region **(A)**. The supratentorial compartment includes the cerebral hemispheres, basal ganglia *(b)* and thalamic nuclei *(t)*, and the lateral ventricles **(B)**, the hypothalamus and corpus callosum *(cc)* **(A)**. The posterior fossa **(A)** includes the cerebellum and the brainstem (midbrain, pons-P, medulla-M); the fourth ventricle is central within the posterior fossa **(A)**.

ETIOLOGY

Although brain tumors are mostly sporadic, a number of pediatric brain tumor presentations are associated with recognized neurocutaneous or other genetic syndromes (13).

Neurofibromatosis is a relatively common congenital disorder associated with CNS tumors (14). Clinical criteria for type I neurofibromatosis (NF1) include six or more café au lait spots and/or peripheral neurofibromas. NF1 is an autosomal dominant syndrome linked to a 17q chromosomal defect (15). Fully 15% to 20% of children with NF ultimately present with CNS neoplasms, usually gliomas of the visual pathways or low-grade tumors of the diencephalon, cerebral hemispheres, or posterior fossa (16). Low-grade gliomas associated with NF1 may be biologically less aggressive than similar gliomas in the general population (17,18).

The extremely indolent subependymal giant cell astrocytoma occurs in children with tuberosclerosis, a hereditary disorder signified also by cutaneous acneiform lesions and angiofibromas, mental retardation, and renal insufficiency; CNS findings include hamartomatous periventricular lesions known as "tubers."

The Li-Fraumeni familial tumor syndrome includes brain tumors and sarcomas in children in association with breast cancer, sarcomas, and brain tumors in related young adults (19). The syndrome is associated with p53 deletion abnormalities and a relatively high incidence of secondary, treatment-related neoplasms (20).

Radiation-induced meningiomas have long been recognized. Reports indicate a disturbing incidence of secondary gliomas, most often malignant or high grade, in long-term survivors of childhood acute lymphoblastic leukemia (ALL) (21–23). The estimated risk is 1% to 3% following routine preventive cranial irradiation; a dose-response relationship has been suggested, with minimal incidence following doses below 20 Gy and a risk approximating 10% following cumulative doses in excess of 30 Gy (generally in children with repeated courses of cranial irradiation in association with CNS relapse).

CLINICAL PRESENTATION

Supratentorial tumors generally present with localizing neurologic symptoms. Seizures are the most common symptom in cerebral hemispheric lesions, especially in those arising in the temporal lobe. Lateralizing neurologic signs (motor and/or sensory) occur in thalamic region tumors, often associated with symptoms of increased intracranial pressure. Suprasellar tumors typically occlude the foramen of Monro, resulting in symptoms of increased intracranial pressure. Visual signs (e.g., visual field cuts and/or decreased acuity) and endocrine abnormalities (e.g., diminished growth hormone, cortisol, and/or thyroid stimulating hormone, and/or signs of delayed or precocious puberty) are frequently apparent with the midline suprasellar lesions. Youngsters with suprasellar tumors may show features of the diencephalic syndrome signified by hyperactivity and asthenia, the latter in spite of normal or increased food intake. Pineal region tumors produce hydrocephalus by compressing the aqueduct of Sylvius; specific ocular signs (e.g., Parinaud's syndrome) are classically noted as subsequently discussed (24).

LOW-GRADE HEMISPHERIC AND DIENCEPHALIC ASTROCYTOMAS

Low-grade supratentorial astrocytomas of childhood occur predominantly in the central regions of the diencephalon, including the hypothalamic-optic chiasmatic region and the thalamus. Cerebral hemispheric astrocytomas account for 40% of the supratentorial lesions, occurring primarily in the temporal and frontal lobes (25,26).

The astrocytic neoplasms are classified histologically by the dominant cell type (3,27, 28).

Fibrillary astrocytomas are comprised of long, thin cells highlighted by a crisscrossing background matrix of neuroglial fibrils. The tumors are often circumscribed in the diencephalon, but may be diffuse or poorly marginated in the cerebral hemispheres. *Gemistocytic* astrocytomas are a relatively uncommon variant that present as benign-appearing, often circumscribed lesions with a high rate of recurrence; these tumors frequently demonstrate malignant degeneration within several years after initial presentation (29). *Protoplasmic* astrocytomas are characterized by large, rounded astrocytes with abundant cytoplasm and a background virtually devoid of fibrils (30).

The fibrillary, gemistocytic, and protoplasmic astrocytomas may be grouped together with "astrocytomas, not otherwise specified, (NOS)" as *ordinary astrocytomas* to distinguish them from the common *juvenile pilocytic astrocytoma (JPA)* (27,31). The ordinary astrocytomas may show malignant degeneration, accruing successive genetic abnormalities that result in a more malignant phenotype in up to 40% of recurrent, uncontrolled lesions (26,32–34). Whether the genotypical progression documented in adult malignant gliomas occurs in children is yet unclear (35,36).

The classic Kernohan system for grading ordinary astrocytomas (cytologically identifying astrocytomas as Grades I, II, III, or IV) has largely been replaced by a histologic system advanced by Burger et al. (27,37), the WHO (3), and others (28,31). The WHO system categorizes JPAs as grade 1, other differentiated astrocytomas as grade 2, anaplastic (malignant) astrocytoma as grade 3, and glioblastoma multiforme (GBM) as grade 4 (3).

JPAs are low-grade neoplasms histologically signified by elongated bipolar astrocytes organized in a parallel array of glial fibers giving a "hairlike" or piloid appearance (28). The sparsely cellular tumors are signified by microcysts and Rosenthal's fibers (amorphous eosinophilic material formed by plump, degenerating astrocytes) (38). Macro-

scopically, visible cystic components are often present, sometimes with much less prominent solid tumor components. The tumors may be circumscribed or may extend along white matter tracks, dependent on location (28) (Fig. 2). JPA is the most common tumor in the diencephalic region and comprises 25% of hemispheric astrocytomas (9,25,38,39). JPA is unique in retaining low-grade characteristics even when uncontrolled or recurrent. The tumor is typically relatively nonaggressive, although rapid progression and dissemination (or multifocal presentations, see subsequent text) certainly occur (40–43).

Less common astrocytic tumors include the following tumors.

Pleomorphic xanthoastrocytomas are benign astrocytic tumors presenting in children as large, peripherally located hemispheric lesions, often involving the leptomeninges (44). The tumor appears aggressive histologically, with cellular pleomorphism and numerous mitoses, but is biologically benign; there are few reports of recurrence or malignant degeneration after surgery alone (45).

Subependymal giant cell astrocytomas are sharply marginated tumors that occur along the linings of the lateral ventricles. The tumors are benign, nearly hamartomatous lesions requiring therapy (most often surgery alone) only if progressive or symptomatic.

Uncommonly, low-grade gliomas present as diffusely infiltrating tumors involving two or more cerebral lobes. The latter tumors are often nonenhancing on CT and MRI, and in children they may show relatively little mass effect. These diffuse lesions appear to represent an uncommon entity, usually referred to as *gliomatosis cerebri* (46). Surgery is limited to biopsy; early response to irradiation is almost always followed by recurrence within 1 year. Low-grade gliomas involving both right and left thalamic regions (i.e., bithalamic tumors) are noted in up to 25% of pediatric thalamic region astrocytomas and seem to have an aggressive course similar to

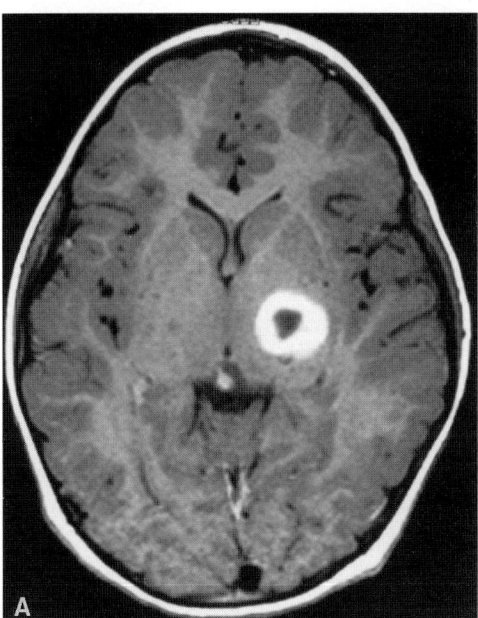 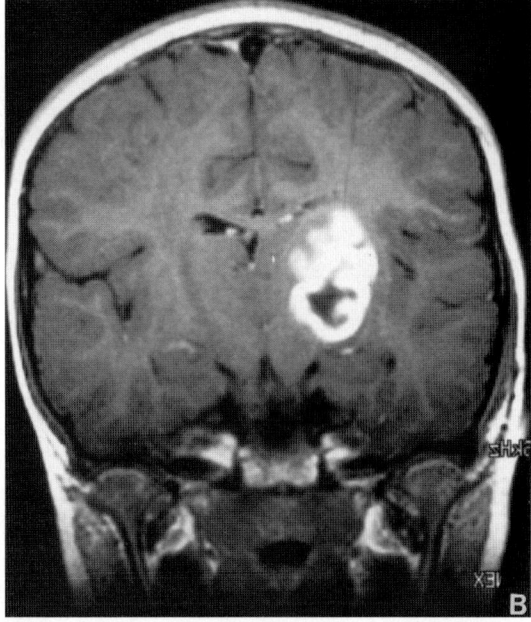

FIG. 2. (A, B) Juvenile pilocytic astrocytoma of left thalamus, a localized, well-circumscribed lesion occurring in a 7-year-old boy. This type of lesion can be approached surgically, but is also an excellent target for three-dimensional conformal irradiation (Fig. 4) or stereotactic radiotherapy (fractionated radiosurgery).

that of the more diffuse gliomatosis cerebri (47).

Therapy

Surgery

Management of low-grade gliomas is generally determined by the site of origin. Tumors arising in the cerebral hemispheres are often resectable. Pediatric reports indicate total removal in up to 90% of cerebral hemispheric astrocytomas and mixed oligoastrocytomas (25,42,48). Low recurrence rates are reported both for JPA and for ordinary astrocytomas following total resection (25,33,42, 48–52). Tumors involving the dominant medial temporal lobe, motor strip region, or Broca's speech cortex may be unresectable due to the neurologic deficits attendant to surgery.

Neurosurgical resection has only recently been reported in the central thalamic and hypothalamic astrocytomas (53–55). The surgical series are selected by tumor size and anatomic location; resection is potentially applicable in fewer than one-third of children with diencephalic gliomas. Series by Bernstein et al. (53) and by Kelly (56) document relative safety in resecting selected tumors, with serious morbidity limited to less than 5% to 10% of cases. Short-term follow-up indicates freedom from recurrence in a majority of children following resection, although long-term results are pending (53,56). For most diencephalic presentations, surgery is limited to stereotactic biopsy, cyst decompression, and ventriculoperitoneal (VP) shunt as required.

Radiation Therapy

Radiation therapy is clearly effective in low-grade gliomas, achieving tumor response and durable disease control in a significant proportion of pediatric cases (26,50–52, 57–59). The indications for radiation therapy and timing relative to surgery and, more recently, chemotherapy remain controversial

(17,48,60) *(Table 3)*. A classic review of low-grade astrocytomas, by Leibel et al. (50), showed a survival advantage at 10 years following irradiation for incompletely resected astrocytomas: 35% versus 11% with surgery alone. In supratentorial ordinary astrocytomas, 10-year survival following surgery and irradiation was statistically superior to surgery alone in reports by Shaw et al. (51) and Shibamoto et al. (52): 39% versus 19% and 41% versus 11%, respectively. The latter series address children and adults; although superior outcome was reported in younger patients, numbers limit significance both in children and in adults less than 30-years old. A more recent analysis from Pollack et al. (26), shows a 10-year benefit for postoperative irradiation following incomplete resection of cerebral hemispheric astroctyomas: 82% progression-free survival versus 42%; a significant benefit in overall survival was not apparent. Identically impressive progression-free results following incomplete resection and irradiation have been noted in series from the University of California, San Francisco (UCSF) and Mayo Clinic: 81% and 87%, respectively, at 10 years (51,61). Pediatric Oncology Group (POG) and Children's Cancer Study Group (CCG) initiated a prospective study to test the impact of immediate versus delayed irradiation in children with intracranial astrocytomas: children lacking tumor-related neurologic symptoms following *incomplete* resection were randomized to observation versus irradiation. Unfortunately, an insufficient number of cases eligible for randomization were accrued, and the trial was discontinued.

JPAs predominate in diencephalic childhood gliomas (51,62). Prolonged progression-free survival following irradiation alone for hypothalamic tumors likely reflects both the nature of tumors in this site and the efficacy of irradiation (61–64). Survival exceeding 70% at 10-years postirradiation is common for these tumors (12,61–63). In thalamic astrocytomas, pilocytic histology is less prevalent; 10-year survival results range from 33% to 60% after therapy (9,12,47). The efficacy

TABLE 3. *Decision making in supratentorial low grade gliomas—cooperative outcome data*

| Tumor type | Modality | Selection | Outcome | | Other | Series/Ref. |
			5-yr PFS	5-yr OS		
Cerebral hemisphere	Complete resection	95% GTR	95%	95%	78% PFS (12 yr)	Paris (25)
		47% GTR	89%	95%		SJCRH (48)
		20% GTR	100%	100%	10 y data	U.Pitts (26)
	Incomplete resection + irradiation	49% incomplete resection + irradiation	83%	90%	10 y data	U.Pitts (26)
Diencephalic thalamic	Surgery ± irradiation	32% incomplete resection		50%		Toronto (53)
		69% resection	69%			Mayo (56)
	Irradiation			38%		R.Marsden (12)
Diencephalic hypothalamic/ optic chiasm	Surgery —chiasm/ exophytic ± irradiation	Selected 53% resected			69% FFP <1–4 y	NYU (55)
					79% "well"	Toronto (54)
	Irradiation —hypothalamic			76%	64% 10y OS	Marsden (92)
			70%	93%		U.Cinn (63)
	—optic chiasm		89%	84%	84% 10y PFS	Marsden (92)
			80%	94%	73% 10y PFS	Toronto (17)
				89%	100% 10y data	Boston (59)
	CT —optic chiasm/ hypothalamic (CBCDA/VCR)		@3 yrs	77%		Packer (60)

GTR, gross total resection; PFS, progression-free survival; OS, overall survival; FFP, freedom from progression; CBCDA, carboplatin; VCR, vincristine.

of radiation therapy for diencephalic astrocytomas can be additionally documented by measuring tumor response using clinical and imaging parameters (9,57,59,63,64) (Fig. 3).

In managing astrocytomas in children, one must balance the often indolent natural history, the relative effectiveness of total resection versus that of irradiation, and the potential morbidities, early and late, of surgery and irradiation. One of the few reports of observation alone (no surgery or radiotherapy) in cerebral hemispheric astrocytomas tracked adults presenting primarily with seizures. Nearly 60% showed increase in tumor size or neurologic deficit requiring therapy at a median of 29 months after diagnosis. Survival, however, did not differ from a contemporaneous group of initially operated cases (65). Observation has been recommended for children below 3 to 5 years of age with diencephalic or tectal plate (midbrain) tumors (66,67). It is important to recognize that durable disease control is achievable with radiation therapy in a substantial proportion of symptomatic or progressive astrocytomas. "Expectant" surveillance in controlled settings may be appropriate, for example, in young children with limited hypothalamic tumors, or following incomplete resection of central or hemispheric astrocytomas, particularly JPA. Inherent in such an approach is the commitment to intervene appropriately with documented disease progression, including use of primary radiation therapy or additional surgery, as indicated.

The potential risks of delayed intervention include irreversible neurologic impairment attendant to tumor growth, malignant degeneration, and the increased potential for late morbidities if delayed irradiation results in a larger target volume (33,61,68,69). The impetus toward delayed irradiation is based on potential reduction in radiation-related neurotoxicities (especially neuropsychologic and

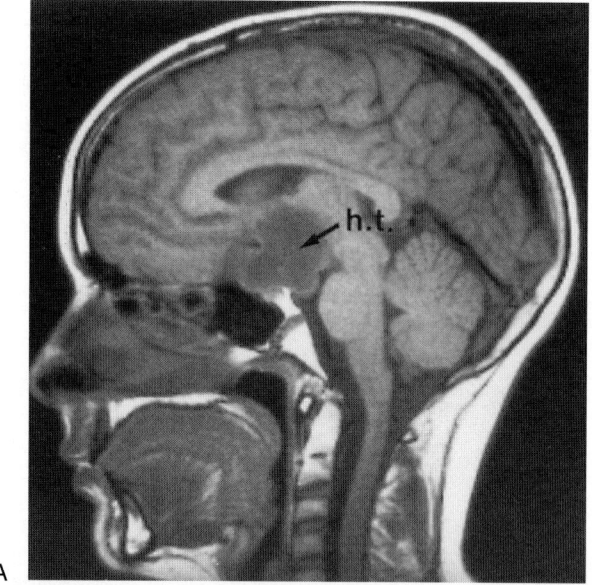

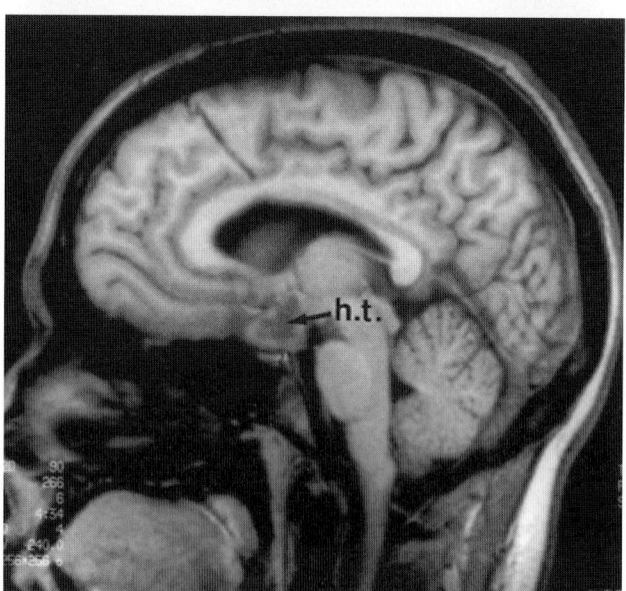

FIG. 3. Tumors of the optic chiasm and hypothalamic region: a well-delineated lesion involving the posterior aspect of the chiasm and adjacent hypothalamus **(A)**; appearance 5 years following local irradiation **(B)**. Current treatment approach is highlighted in Fig. 4. Approximately 10% to 20% of these lesions demonstrate multifocal or metastatic tumor at diagnosis **(C)**, a presentation that may be compatible with long-term response or stabilization.

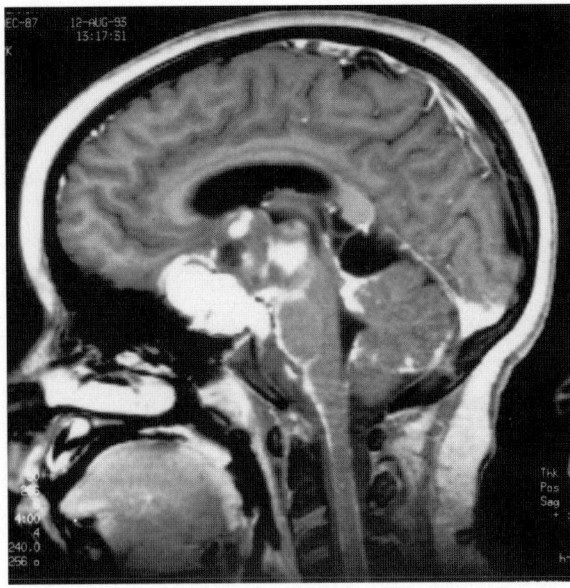

C

FIG. 3. *Continued.*

neuroendocrine changes) associated with treatment below ages 3 to 5 years or, perhaps, before puberty. Precision volume radiation techniques, including three-dimensional conformal irradiation, fractionated radiosurgery, proton beam therapy, or highly selected use of single-fraction radiosurgery, may offer advantages that alter the risk-benefit ratio in favor of earlier radiation therapy in central gliomas (70–75).

Chemotherapy

The use of initial chemotherapy for low-grade gliomas has been studied primarily in hypothalamic/chiasmatic tumors (see subsequent text). Follow-up studies suggest similar response and disease control rates for astrocytomas and other low-grade sites (60,76). Although chemotherapy has been associated with only a modest objective response rate, data does indicate a prolonged disease stabilization interval in progressive low-grade gliomas, approximating 3 years (60). The goal of delayed irradiation for such an interval may be worthwhile, especially in young children. Use of carboplatin, alone or combined with vincristine,

has been relatively effective and to date associated with few serious late toxicities (60,76,77).

Radiotherapeutic Management

Volume

The target volume for low-grade astrocytomas is usually localized to the imaging-defined tumor with limited margin. JPAs are usually well-circumscribed lesions; 95% isodose coverage with dosimetric margins of 1 cm or less, including the tumor and cyst wall (if present), appears to be adequate. The target is usually defined by contrast-enhanced T1 sequence on MRI. Similar guidelines are appropriate for the well-delineated ordinary astrocytomas, using 1- to 2-cm margins. For the occasional JPA or more common ordinary astrocytomas without uniform enhancement, the T1 image is generally adequate; proton density or flare sequences sometimes highlight the lesion more adequately. It is unusual to see more extensive changes on T2 sequence for low-grade lesions.

For diffusely infiltrating or poorly circumscribed ordinary astrocytomas, a margin of 2 to 3 cm is recommended, based on both T1 and T2 sequences on MRI (78). Anatomic routes of potential extension, particularly along the white matter tracks, should be considered in outlining the target volume. Gemistocytic astrocytomas are treated as malignant gliomas, with 3-cm margins defining the 95% volume.

Cases with multifocal presentations or subarachnoid seeding are generally treated with craniospinal irradiation, although the require-ment for coverage of the entire neuraxis is unproven (40,41).

Dose

Dose-response data indicate improved disease control beyond 45 to 50 Gy (9). Shaw et al. (51,78), showed an advantage with radia-

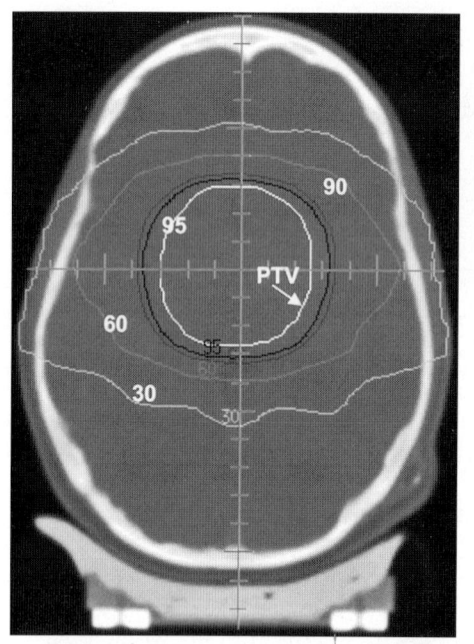

A

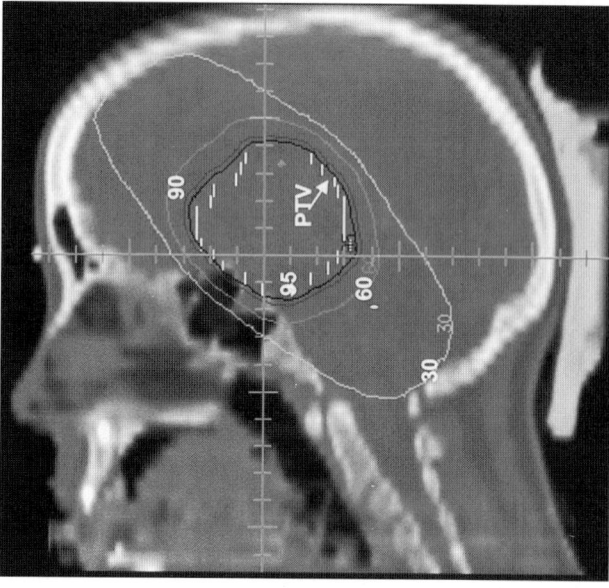

B

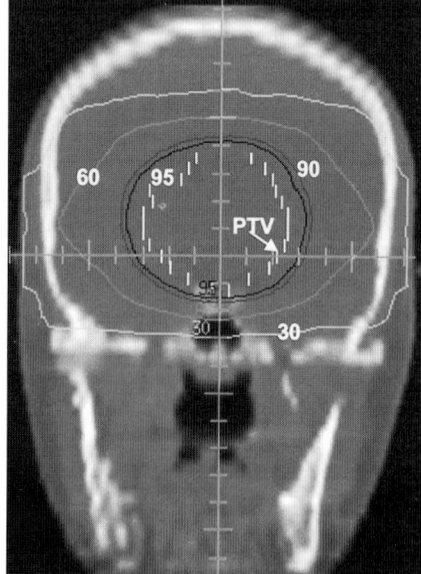

C

FIG. 4. **(A, B, C)** Three-dimensional conformal planning for central diencephalic astrocytoma, an approach that achieves conformation of dose (here 54 Gy) to the lesion through six noncoplanar fields.

tion therapy only at doses greater than 53 Gy. For children under 5 years of age, we recommend 50 to 55 Gy using 150 to 180 cGy per fraction. For children under 2 years of age, one generally tries to delay irradiation; when such therapy is required, a dose of 45 to 50 Gy to small volumes is appropriate. In children at least 5-years old, the traditional dose of 54 to 55 Gy is recommended at 150 to 180 cGy per fraction.

Technique

Ideal techniques achieve close conformation of the high-dose irradiated volume to a well-defined local target volume. Multiple fields, based on single-plane or noncoplanar techniques as available, are utilized to a dose distribution maximally conformed to the tumor volume (Fig. 4). For relatively spherical central lesions up to 3 or 4 cm in diameter, stereotactic radiotherapy or fractionated radiosurgery may be appropriate (79,80). In developing treatment techniques, maximal sparing of the temporal lobes and pituitary-hypothalamic region is sought to diminish some of the more common neuropsychologic and neuroendocrine effects of therapy. There is limited experience with single-fraction radiosurgery for small, circumscribed astrocytomas, including those located in the diencephalic region; long-term disease control and toxicities appear to be acceptable in highly selected cases (70,74).

Results

Long-term disease-free survival has been reported in up to 90% of children following complete resection of cerebral hemispheric tumors; for similarly managed thalamic tumors, small series report 60% to 90% disease control (26,48,53,81). Incomplete resection and adjuvant irradiation have resulted in 80% progression-free survival in hemispheric astrocytomas at 10 years (26). For thalamic tumors treated with postbiopsy irradiation, 40% to 50% survive free of progression (9,12,47, 82). Hypothalamic tumors have a more favorable outcome following primary irradiation,

with 10-year progression-free survival rates approximating 70% (9,12,63,83).

OPTIC PATHWAY TUMORS

Optic pathway tumors (OPTs) represent 4% to 6% of childhood brain tumors. OPTs may involve the optic nerves alone (approximately 25% of cases) or the optic chiasm alone or in combination with optic nerve involvement in 20% to 40% of children; in 33% to 60% of cases, the tumors involve the hypothalamus, often with additional extension to the optic tracts (17,84,85) (Fig. 5). OPTs occur predominately in young children; 25% present before 12 to 18 months of age, and 50% present before 4 to 5 years (84–86).

Between 25% and 40% of childhood OPTs are associated with neurofibromatosis. Conversely, of children with neurofibromatosis, up to 5% to 10% are found to have tumors of the optic pathways either on screening evaluation or during follow-up (87). Children with NF1 may have a more indolent disease course (83).

Clinical presentation is most often with diminished vision. In young children, increased pressure endocrinopathies, and diencephalic syndrome may predominate. Histologically, 80% to 90% of cases are low-grade astrocytomas, frequently gliomas and gangliogliomas. Mixed JPA, or malignant gliomas, account for 10% to 20% (17,55,83,88).

The nature of OPTs has been debated. Hoyt and Baghdassarian (89) and Imes and Hoyt (90) have argued that OPTs are usually associated with clinical progression or death in fewer than 25% of cases (89,90). Most pediatric oncologists differ with this view (11, 18,84,85). While acknowledging the sometimes indolent nature of OPTs, serial observations in major pediatric clinics indicate progression in up to 75% of children, most often within 1 to 2 years of initial presentation (17,83). Other signs of aggressive behavior include frequent extension to or invasion of the adjacent hypothalamus and/or other aspects of the optic pathways and, infrequently, involvement of the subarachnoid space or

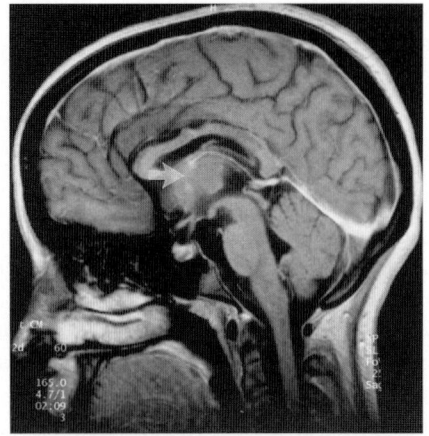

A

FIG. 5. Optic chiasm gliomas present as localized lesion **(A)**, **(B)**, or as tumors that extend along the optic tracts **(C)**; especially with tumors may extend to involve the optic nerves and may extend posteriorly to the lateral geniculate body. Note the tracking of the middle cerebral arteries (m.c.a.) through the tumor.

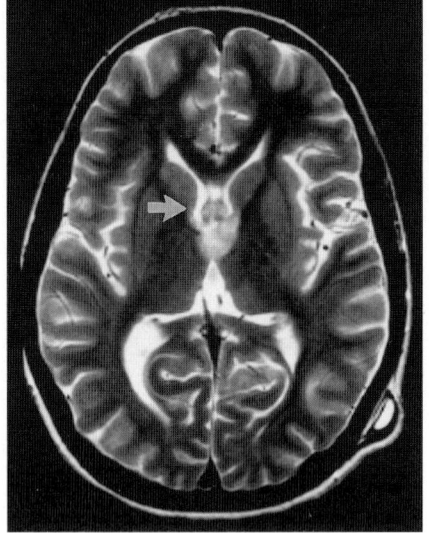

B

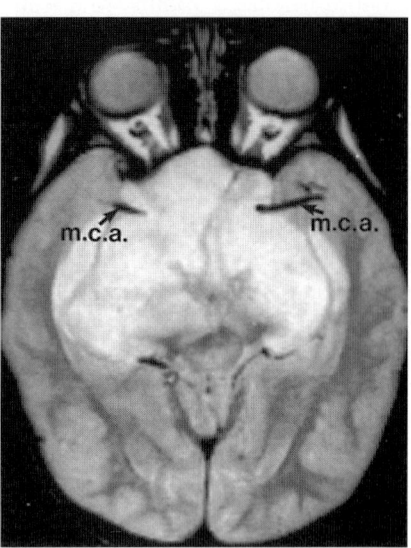

C

other sites within the CNS (40–43). Mortality within 10 years of diagnosis is uncommon, although ultimate disease-related mortality has been documented in up to 40% of cases (12, 17,59,84).

Several series identify the typical optic pathway tumors as optic pathway/hypothalamic gliomas, indicating the difficulty differentiating the origin from hypothalamic (57, 72). Although lesions extending to or originating within the hypothalamus may be somewhat more aggressive than lesions confined to the visual pathways, up to 25% to 50% of selected, asymptomatic children have been free of progression for 5 years or longer without therapeutic intervention. Preliminary data suggest adequate "retrieval" with secondary therapy at the time of progression during observation (17,83).

Therapy

Surgery

Surgery has classically been the preferred treatment for unilateral tumors of the optic nerve (17,84,88). Observation may be selected, especially if there is residual vision associated with a lesion confined to the intraorbital-optic nerve. Alvord and Lofton (84) reported progression in 70% of children with untreated lesions within 6 years of diagnosis, although it was rarely associated with tumor-related mortality. Most series indicate more indolent, perhaps truly hamartomatous, behavior in children with neurofibromatosis (17,88).

For lesions involving the optic pathways, there is limited data suggesting a role for surgical resection. Decompression or limited resection may be successful in restoring vision (91). Series from Hospital for Sick Children, Toronto, and New York University suggest a somewhat broader role for local excision in selected presentations. The latter authors indicate removal of lesions of partially infiltrating low-grade optic pathway astrocytomas with surprisingly little added visual compromise; long-term follow-up data is yet unavailable (54,55,88).

Typical lesions involving components of the visual pathways beyond the optic chiasm/hypothalamic region (i.e., with imaging extension to the optic nerves, optic tracts, or into the optic radiation) may be managed without biopsy confirmation. The vast majority of these tumors are low-grade astrocytomas and most often, can be managed based on the clinical and imaging diagnosis. Globular tumors that involve the chiasm and hypothalamus are best biopsied; a small but important percentage of these lesions may be germ cell tumors or more aggressive gliomas histologically (91).

Radiation Therapy

Treatment is indicated for (a) significant visual and/or neurologic deficits at presentation; or (b) documented progression, by clinical evaluation and/or neuroimaging (17,60, 84,86). Radiation therapy is highly effective for chiasmal gliomas: 10-year *progression-free* survival rates (i.e., disease control) exceed 70% to 80% (17,59,92,93). Although overall survival at 10 years is unaffected by the initial therapeutic approach (i.e., observation, resection, chemotherapy, or irradiation), progression-free survival rates at 5 and 10

years are substantially higher following radiation therapy (11,12,17,60,93). Efficacy is also apparent in reports documenting measurable tumor reduction in approximately 50% of children, often apparent over several years post-therapy (57,59). Visual improvement is reported in 25% to 35% of children following irradiation (59,83,86,93). Visual deterioration is reported in 10% to 20% of children postirradiation, largely related to cystic degeneration (and consequent increased mass effect at the chiasm) or unrecognized increased intracranial pressure (17,59,83,92,93).

Balancing the indications for radiation therapy and, in particular, the timing, is appropriate concern regarding sometimes unique late radiation-related toxicities. The young age at diagnosis, central location and often extensive optic pathway involvement, and associated genetic syndromes (NF1) are all factors associated with significant neurocognitive deficits; this is especially true for young children (59,83,86,93). The frequency of late vascular events in children with brain tumors is highest among those with OPTs, especially in children presenting before 2 to 3 years of age (86,94–96). Moyamoya syndrome is signified by total obliteration of the major vessels at the circle of Willis; incomplete brain perfusion is provided by peripheral meningeal vessels. The syndrome has been noted following irradiation, perhaps related to cicatricial constriction of vessels tracking through chiasmal/hypothalamic gliomas. An incidence approaching 18% has been reported, especially noted among young children (less than 1- to 2-years old) with NF1 (94). The Toronto group has related a 10% incidence of second malignant neoplasms following irradiation in OPTs; of interest, a series from Children's Hospital of Los Angeles shows the same rate of anaplastic degeneration in JPA following surgery alone (17,32, 81).

Chemotherapy

Mostly because of the radiation-associated toxicities in young children, Packer et al. (97)

initially explored primary chemotherapy in children less than 5-years old with primary optic pathway gliomas. Initial experience with Actinomycin D (dactinomycin) and vincristine resulted in stabilization in a majority of children and objective tumor reduction in approximately 25%. Although more than 60% of children required irradiation by 5-years postdiagnosis, the approach resulted in a potentially significant delay in initiating radiation therapy interval in view of the age of the study population—the median time to progression was 3 years (97). Subsequent experience with an 18-month regimen of carboplatin and vincristine has shown a significant rate of objective tumor reduction (reporting greater than 50% tumor reduction in one-third of patients), early progression in only 10%, and a 3-year progression-free survival rate of 77% (60). The results with chemotherapy appear to be independent of age, presence of NF1, histology, or disease extent (60). Early experience suggests favorable outcome with secondary irradiation following progression during or after chemotherapy, although the duration of follow-up is yet limited (17,60, 83). Toxicity with carboplatin and vincristine has been limited, and early data suggests continued intellectual development during chemotherapy (11,97). There is a balance between duration of disease control (clearly superior with radiation therapy) and moderate-term control apparently absent some of the toxicities associated with irradiation in this age group (17,83). Current protocols address initial chemotherapy in a variably defined set of eligible age groups in up to 5, 10, or 15 years chronologically or until completion of puberty. Additional experience and follow-up will yet determine the "appropriate" age thresholds for initial chemotherapy or irradiation in those requiring treatment.

Radiotherapeutic Management

Volume and Technique

Local volumes are utilized, often confined to the suprasellar region for lesions that are limited to the chiasm with or without hypothalamic involvement. The central lesions are often ideal for three-dimensional conformal or stereotactic radiotherapeutic (i.e., fractionated radiosurgery) approaches, limiting the dose to the surrounding cerebral hemispheres (79,80). The use of proton beam therapy will be prospectively explored over the next several years (72). For lesions extending along the optic tracts or beyond (occasionally to involve the optic radiation, toward or to the occipital lobes), there may be only limited gain from the use of three-dimensional conformal approaches, the large target volumes sometimes requiring wide opposed lateral field configurations. Caution is urged in defining true "neoplastic extension" versus NF1-type changes on MRI.

Dose

Dose-response analyses suggest improvement with doses approximating 50 to 54 Gy at 150 to 180 cGy per fraction (85). Reduction to 45 Gy at 150 cGy daily is appropriate in youngsters less than 3-years old (93).

OLIGODENDROGLIOMA

Oligodendrogliomas represent 2% of supratentorial tumors in children. The generally circumscribed tumors occur most often in the cerebral hemispheres. Data specific for pediatric oligodendrogliomas are limited; treatment recommendations are largely based on adult experience.

Total surgical resection is the treatment of choice for accessible lesions. Gross total resection has been documented in 20% to 25% of all cases, although apparently more frequently in children and adolescents (98,99). Survival rates at 10 years following total excision is reported to be 60% in the Mayo Clinic series; among six children, five survived (78, 99).

For incompletely resected oligodendrogliomas, a short-term benefit for radiation therapy has been documented. Shaw et al. (99) reported 5-year survival of 25% followiing subtotal resection compared to 62% with the addition of radiation doses in excess of 50 Gy; by 10 years, the survival rates were similar with (31%) and without (25%) irradiation. A long-term benefit was apparent in a retrospective review from UCSF: 56% 10-year survival with postoperative irradiation compared to 18% following incomplete surgery alone (100). In contrast, other series have failed to show a benefit from irradiation (98,101). Histologic grade has increasingly been cited as a prognostic indicator in oligodendrogliomas (99,102). Because oligodendrogliomas represent a spectrum of aggressiveness, it is difficult to be dogmatic concerning radiotherapy's role based on the retrospective clinical literature. If an initial approach similar to that with astrocytomas is adopted, one would generally intervene with irradiation only for tumors that show progression or recurrence after initial surgery. Radiation parameters are similar to those noted for astrocytomas. Anaplastic oligodendrogliomas are managed similarly to other malignant supratentorial gliomas in children, although the outcome tends to be superior to anaplastic astrocytoma and glioblastoma (103,104).

Information regarding chemotherapy indicates objective responses to alkylating agents, platinum compounds, and multidrug regimens (105). The PCV regimen (procarbazine, CCNU (lomustine), vincristine) has been notedly effective in anaplastic oligodendrogliomas in adults (106). Combined radiation therapy and PCV has been associated with excellent disease control, including patients with anaplastic oligodendoglioma (107). Limited chemotherapy has been associated with sufficient tumor reduction to permit delayed gross total resection in tumors initially felt to be unresectable (105,108).

The "benign" nature of oligodendrogliomas is open to question, with few reports documenting survival rates in excess of 25% beyond 15 years (99,100,109,110). Long-term results following contemporary surgery and irradiation are limited in the literature (99).

RARE LOW-GRADE NEOPLASMS

Gangliogliomas are biologically benign neoplasms containing neuronal (ganglion cells) and glial (astrocytes) elements (28, 111). The tumors occur primarily in children. Gangliogliomas arise throughout the CNS, most often within the cerebral hemispheres, especially in the temporal lobes (112–114). The tumors are usually well-circumscribed and often resectable; recurrence is uncommon (111,113). Malignant transformation is rare in these tumors; when documented, it has generally been the glial elements that have been identified as anaplastic or malignant (28). There are few indications for radiation therapy in children. Progressive, unresectable lesions may respond to irradiation with treatment factors similar to those used for low-grade astrocytomas (113).

Neurocytomas are clinically indolent tumors that present as intraventricular lesions, usually in the third ventricle. Neurocytomas are composed of small neuronal cells thought to represent a benign neoplasm derived from cells midway in the maturation process of neuronal differentiation (28,38,62). The lesion is generally resectable. Rare hemispheric neurocytomas seem to require only local excision (62).

Dysembryoplastic neuroepithelial tumors (DNT or DNET) are biologically indolent, often sizable cerebral cortical tumors typically presenting with a longstanding seizure history (115,116). The tumors may be considered "quasi-hamartomatous," requiring surgery alone (38,115,116).

MALIGNANT GLIOMAS

Supratentorial malignant gliomas represent approximately 6% of brain tumors in children. Children seem to present a continuum of the adult data, suggesting more favorable histology and outcome inversely related to age. Children have an increased proportion of anaplastic astrocytomas among the malignant gliomas and have arguably longer survival intervals (117–119). Histologic grading is most often by the three-tiered system of astrocytoma, anaplastic (or malignant) astrocytoma, and GBM (37).

Supratentorial malignant gliomas arise primarily as cerebral hemispheric tumors; 20% to 30% present primarily in the thalamus or basal ganglia (104,117,118). Imaging characteristics are similar to those in adults, with often poorly marginated, peripherally enhancing lesions on MRI or CT associated with surrounding white matter changes ("edema") and often central necrosis. Adult studies have shown infiltration of the small, round anaplastic cells well into the perilesional low-density areas on CT or areas of abnormal signal on T2 MRI (120–122). The infiltrative characteristics of high-grade gliomas indicate some caution in aggressive surgery and high-dose local radiation techniques; the histologic studies are at odds with clinical data substantiating a direct relationship between tumor control and (a) degree of resection, and (b) high-dose focal radiation therapy (104,117, 121,123–128) It is yet unclear whether treatment modifications resulting in improved survival beyond 2 to 3 years may be associated with late marginal or distant tumor recurrence. Although primarily a local disease process, leptomeningel dissemination is present in 10% to 15% of children at diagnosis; the pattern of failure remains predominantly local, although several pediatric studies have shown a frequency of leptomeningeal dissemination approaching 30% (104,118).

Therapy

Surgery

Surgical resection has often been limited in extent due to the poorly circumscribed nature of the tumor and the attendant lack of aggressive neurosurgical intent. Recent series indicate a rate of gross total resection approximating 25% in cerebral malignant gliomas in this age group; complete resection is less common in the central thalamic lesions (104,117,123). There does appear to be a significant correlation between degree of resec-

tion (especially gross total vs. incomplete removal and survival); survival rates in three pediatric series exceed 60% at 3 to 5 years, among those children with imaging-confirmed gross total resection; correlation with disease extent and histologic grade is important in interpreting such results (104,117,123,129).

Radiation Therapy

Radiation therapy is a primary component of initial management of pediatric malignant gliomas. Adult studies have documented the impact of adequate radiation therapy on survival, although survival beyond 2 years is almost entirely among those with anaplastic astrocytoma rather than GBM. Two decades of cooperative group studies have shown (a) equivalent results with wide local fields versus whole-brain irradiation, (b) a dose response suggesting treatment to at least the 55- to 60-Gy level with conventional fractionation, and (c) no clear benefit to hyperfractionation to dose levels of 72 Gy and little gain from conventional or hyperfractionated doses beyond 72 Gy (124,125,130,131).

Pediatric experience with interstitial brain implants suggests increased survival in the highly selected subset of children eligible for stereotactic brachytherapy, similar to that apparent in adults (127,132–134). Experience from Heidelberg, UCSF, and St. Jude Children's Research Hospital (SJCRH) indicates reasonable tolerance for high-activity, removable 125I implants even in children under 4 to 5 years of age (135–137). Outcome in 11 children treated at SJCRH suggests a marginal benefit in survival in comparison to conventionally treated children (103,104,135). The frequency of treatment-related intralesional necrosis is at least comparable to that in adults; extensive posttreatment white matter changes and functional deficits have limited enthusiasm for this approach (103,138) (Fig. 6).

Stereotactic radiosurgery for pediatric brain tumors parallels the broader experience in adults (79,139). Preliminary experience shows no unique complications in the

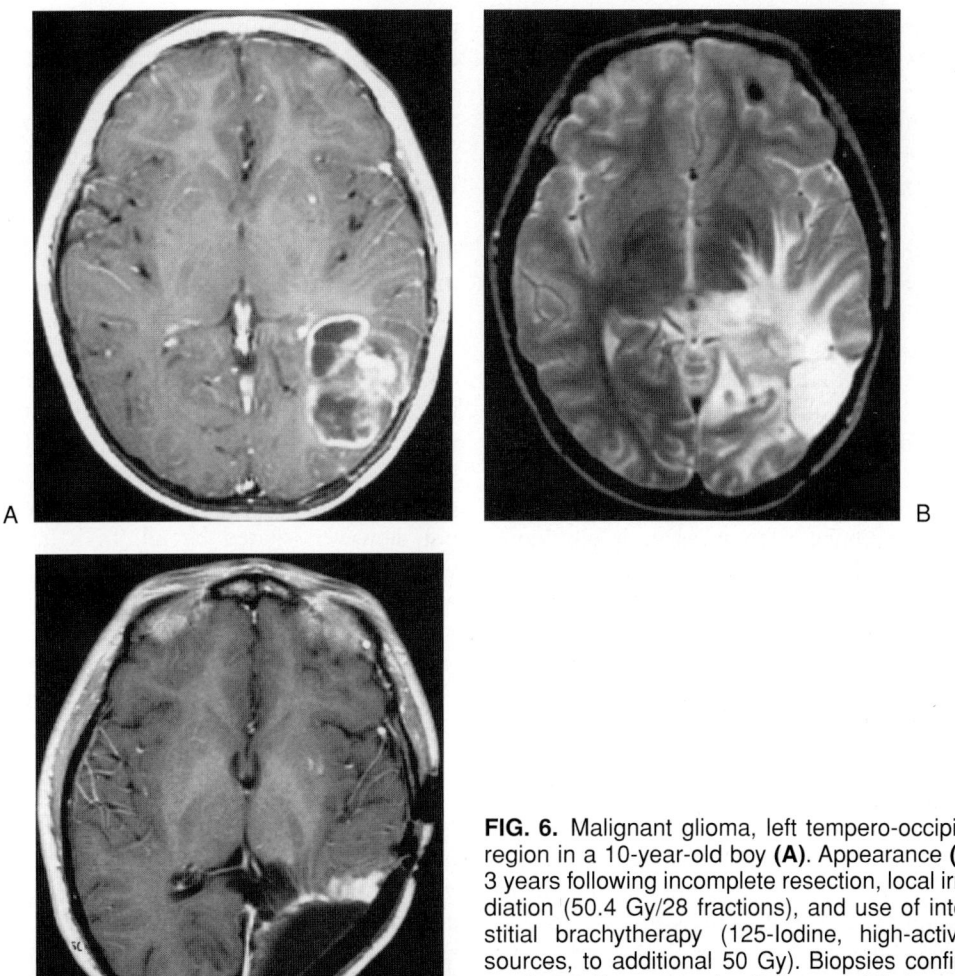

FIG. 6. Malignant glioma, left tempero-occipital region in a 10-year-old boy **(A)**. Appearance **(B)** 3 years following incomplete resection, local irradiation (50.4 Gy/28 fractions), and use of interstitial brachytherapy (125-Iodine, high-activity sources, to additional 50 Gy). Biopsies confirm postirradiation necrosis. Follow-up **(C)** 8-years posttreatment and 5 years after resection of necrotic site.

younger age group. The suggested decrease in post-therapy necrosis requiring resection in comparison to interstitial implants may indicate a potential advantage for radiosurgery as a more homogeneous "local intensive boost," which may be technically superior to interstitial implants in the pediatric age group (126).

Chemotherapy

Chemotherapy for adult malignant gliomas has consistently shown a statistically significant, if clinically marginal, gain in time to progression and survival (58,140). The increased benefit in adults less than 40-years old and with anaplastic astrocytomas (versus GBM) leads one to anticipate increased benefit in children. The first significant prospective trial addressing chemotherapy (vincristine, CCNU, and prednisone) and irradiation showed an apparently significant benefit in the cohort treated with combined modality therapy: Sposto et al. (142), reported 5-year event-free survival approaching 45% versus 17% for those who received radiation therapy alone, postoperatively. The report is problematic: it indicated a benefit only among those with GBM, involved a relatively small number of patients, and reported only three long-term survivors in the combined modality arm (142). Follow-up data, in fact, indicates a significant number of cases misinterpreted as malignant gliomas, and a subsequent trial showed survival at 5 years in only 25% of children with reviewed malignant gliomas treated on the same "standard" regimen. The "8-in-1" regimen tested by CCG achieved no advantage in disease control (123).

Interest in overcoming the theoretical blood–brain barrier and the potential advantage of dose intensification have stimulated investigation of high-dose chemotherapy with autologous bone marrow rescue in childhood malignant gliomas. Finlay et al. (143) initially described four complete responses in ten children treated with high-dose thiotepa/VP-16 with or without BCNU (carmustine), including durable responses in two children. Subsequent studies in single institutions, and by the CCG, support the finding of a small but significant number of complete responses with this technique (103,143). Balanced against the enthusiasm for high-dose chemotherapy is the frequency of significant morbidity, including fatal acute toxicities in 20% to 25% as experienced by Finlay et al. (143,144). Ongoing trials in single institutions and the cooperative groups should establish the efficacy and ultimate toxicities with this approach.

Radiotherapeutic Management

Volume and Technique

The target volume is best defined by the enhancing lesion and surrounding low-density change (on CT) or signal abnormality (on T2 MRI). A detailed review of imaging and histologic extent in untreated patients with malignant gliomas suggests that a 3-cm margin around the target volume as defined provides adequate coverage, avoiding full brain irradiation in most presentations (121,122).

What is the correct definition of target volume? Is it contrast-enhancing tumor or tumor plus edema? The clinician's uncertainty is related to the question of whether the area of the brain, adjacent to tumor, that is referred to as "edematous" by the neuroradiologist, contains normal neural tissue plus water or, in addition, is infiltrated in total or in part by tumor. If that area referred to as "edematous" is truly that, then the radiotherapy field margin is defined in relation to the contrast-enhancing tumor edge. If the "edema" contains tumor, then the clinician might elect to irradiate tumor plus edema plus a margin around the edema. In most supratentorial malignant gliomas cases, the "edema" contains tumor cells (121). For this reason, some clinicians select target volumes that include the "edema." This view is not, however, shared by all. In a tumor in which the survival and local tumor control are poor, it will be difficult to establish the superiority of one radiotherapy field design policy over another.

The use of three-dimensional conformal irradiation has a theoretical advantage in significantly limiting the volume of normal brain exposed to high-dose levels (71). Such therapy is generally advantageous for localized, unilateral tumors. Tumors that arise centrally often show infiltration within or across the corpus callosum to the contralateral hemisphere, suggesting broad coverage (with limited benefit from conformal approaches) for central tumors.

Dose

The conventional dose-volume relationships indicate levels of 45 to 54 Gy to the wide local volume (3 cm beyond tumor extent as described previously), with subsequent "boost," often defined as a 1-cm margin around the enhancing lesion, to a cumulative dose of 55 to 60 Gy (124,128). Hyperfractionated irradiation to the 72-Gy level (utilizing 1.2 Gy b.i.d. with interfraction interval of 6 to 8 hours) has been utilized but has not been shown to be superior in adult studies; whether this offers an advantage in tumor control or diminished neurotoxicity has yet to be adequately assessed in pediatrics (130).

Use of interstitial brain implants has largely focused on removable high-activity 125I implants. Doses of 50 Gy focally in combination with wide-field external beam irradiation mimics the broader experience available in adults (127,133,134). Comparable data for a stereotactic radiosurgical boost suggest that a dose of 15 Gy delivered in one fraction may be as effective as an interstitial implant (126).

Results

Median survival times for pediatric malignant gliomas approximate 18 to 24 months in all recent series (104,117,123). Event-free survival is as high as 60% among the minority of patients in whom a gross total resection is apparent, confirmed by post-operative neuroimaging (104,117,123). Among those with identifiable residual after surgery, representing over 75% of childhood cases, the progression-free survival rate at 3 to 5 years is only 15% to 20%, slightly higher among the anaplastic astrocytomas than the glioblastomas (104,123).

BRAIN TUMORS IN INFANTS AND YOUNG CHILDREN

Children less than 2-years old account for 10% to 15% of pediatric CNS neoplasms (12,145–147). Symptoms in this age group usually include increased head size, lethargy, and vomiting. Tumors are predominantly supratentorial; in comparison to older children, lesions are more often histologically malignant and overtly metastatic within the neuraxis (145,148–150). The most common tumor types include the embryonal neoplasms (medulloblastoma and the supratentorial embryonal tumors [including the primitive neuroectodermal tumors (PNETs) and pineoblastomas]), astrocytomas (particularly optic chiasmatic/hypothalamic lesions), ependymomas, and malignant gliomas. Unique to this age group are the *atypical teratoid/rhabdoid tumors*, often confused with medulloblastoma in the very young; this embryonal tumor is discussed in the section on embryonal tumors.

Intracranial teratomas and choroid plexus tumors occur most often in this age group. Choroid plexus tumors include papillomas and carcinomas, typically arising in the lateral ventricles, but occurring in third or fourth ventricles as well. Histology can be uncertain in predicting benign or malignant behavior; outcome correlates with the degree of brain invasiveness as a sign of malignant biology (27,28,151,152). The infantile desmoplastic neuroepithelial tumors (or desmoplastic infantile gangliogliomas and astrocytomas) also arise predominantly in the very young, often signified by sizable, peripherally located lesions that may appear aggressive at first histologic inspection, but generally represent low-grade neoplasms rarely recurring after primary resection (38,116,153).

Most pediatric series indicate lower survival rates for brain tumors presenting in children less than 2- to 4-years old (12,146,147, 154). In addition to the unfavorable tumor characteristics noted, the therapeutic ratio for surgery and radiation therapy is less favorable (46,155). Operative morbidity and mortality rates are higher in infants than in older children, in part related to incomplete myelinization and diminished plasticity of the brain; mortality rates approaching 5% to 10% have been documented (148,155,156). Following radiation therapy, cognitive dysfunction, somatic alterations, endocrine deficits, and neurotoxicity are more pronounced than in older children (145,157–160).

Conventional surgery and irradiation have resulted in 5-year survival rates of 40% to 50% or less in infants with brain tumors (12,154,161,162). Outcome in medulloblastoma is significantly poorer in young children: 32% to 48% versus 50% to 71% for those over 2- to 5-years old in three major institutional and cooperative group studies (163–165). A similar difference is apparent in ependymomas; Sutton et al. (166) reported a 26% 5-year survival rate in children 1- to 3-years old compared to 51% in older children. In malignant gliomas, there has been relatively little age-related difference in outcome amongst children (118,123). Overall, 10-year survival in infants with malignant brain tumors has been recorded at 25% to 30% in reports from the Children's Hospital of Philadelphia and a combined Children's Hospital of Alabama-Rainbow Babies and Children's Hospital in Cleveland-Duke University analysis; survival rates for low-grade or benign tumors approach 75% to 85% in this age group (145,148).

Therapy

For low-grade neoplasms, the approach in infants and younger children is similar to that in older children, but with greater reliance on surgery or initial chemotherapy for central lesions as one generally prefers to delay or defer irradiation. For malignant lesions, most of the cooperative group studies in North America and Europe since the mid-1980s have explored the use of primary postoperative chemotherapy, using delayed, diminished, or no irradiation depending on the goals and philosophy of the respective group or institution (145,149,167–170) (Table 4). The experience has allowed unparalleled assessment of the frequency and durability of response in malignant CNS tumors using prolonged or high-dose, multiagent chemotherapy. Specific results are subsequently detailed; one can summarize the several large series as documenting (a) a high rate of chemoresponsiveness; (b) durable disease control without irradiation in only a small minority of cases, primarily those with localized disease amenable to complete resection at diagnosis; (c) disease control rates disappointingly similar to those achieved with surgery and irradiation in older series, still well below the 30% to 50% level following initial, prolonged chemotherapy and irradiation; (d) small amounts of data suggesting a role for additional exploration of altered radiation parameters (i.e., limited dose and volume) in selected, protocol settings, and (e) an overall rate of disease control (approximating 25% to 40%) that challenges additional evolution in techniques for this age group, now stimulating a third generation of studies that will study dose-intensive chemotherapy and may reintroduce irradiation at an earlier interval (46,145,149,167–174).

Surgery

Contemporary neurosurgical techniques allow primary resection of low-grade cerebral hemispheric gliomas and selected small, localized hypothalamic and thalamic lesions with seemingly acceptable rates of significant morbidity (55,88,145,148,175). Long-term outcome following radical resection of diencephalic tumors is yet unavailable with reference to ultimate pituitary-hypothalamic function and intellectual development (54,55, 88).

TABLE 4. *Malignant tumors in infants (<3 yr)—initial postoperative chemotherapy*

Tumor type	Chemotherapy	Consolidative	@ 1 yr PFS OS	@ 2 yr PFS OS	@ 5 yr PFS OS	Series/Ref
Medulloblastoma	Cy, V, CD, VP	All	42%	34%		POG (149)
	8-in-1	0	60%	35%	20%	CCG (168)
	MOPP	PD only			46% 72%	MDACC (167)
Supratentorial PNET[a]	Cy, V, CD, VP	All		19%		POG (149)
	8-in-1	0		23%		CCG (168)
Ependymoma	Cy, V, CD, VP	All		42%		POG (149)
	8-in-1	0		38%	18%	CCG (168)

[a]includes pineoblastomas.

Cy, cyclophosphamide; V, vincristine; CD, cisplatin; VP, etoposide; 8-in-1, V, CCNU, procarbazine, hydroxyurea, CD, cytarabine, prednisone, and Cy; PFS, progression-free survival; OS, overall survival; POG, Pediatric Oncology Group; CCG, Children's Cancer Group; MDACC, M.D. Anderson Cancer Center; RT, radiation therapy.

For malignant tumors, gross total resection is often feasible despite extensive local involvement in posterior fossa tumors (medulloblastomas and ependymomas); supratentorial lesions (primarily malignant gliomas and embryonal tumors) tend to be more extensive and often less amenable to complete resection (11,161,166,176,177,178). Delayed definitive surgery following initial chemotherapy may result in sufficient tumor reduction to allow judicious resection of macroscopic disease, potentially limiting the target volume for radiation therapy and, in specific settings, the required radiation dose for "microscopic disease residual" (113,149,179).

Radiation Therapy

Radiation therapy is an option for low-grade gliomas in this age group, generally reserved for tumors that have documented progression following surgery and chemotherapy. (See section on Radiation Therapy for Optic Pathway Tumors.) It is important to recognize the indications for radiation therapy and to intervene when imaging or clinical signs indicate tumor progression (17,83,154).

The majority of children with malignant tumors treated "on study" with initial chemotherapy ultimately require irradiation (145, 149,180). The earlier data from the POG infant study was based on systematic irradiation at planned completion of 12 to 24 months of chemotherapy (149). More recent studies have utilized a "primary chemotherapy approach," generally requiring irradiation only for disease that is progressive during or after chemotherapy, or residual on completion of planned chemotherapy. Irradiation seems to add significantly to disease control on completion of chemotherapy in ependymomas, and is effective in achieving secondary disease control among children with medulloblastoma treated at the time of disease progression or residual (172,173).

The number of children ultimately controlled without irradiation is estimated at only 10% to 20% (149,168,170,178). Attendant to clinical investigations in this age group using initial, often prolonged chemotherapy is the commitment to seriously consider full-dose or modified radiation therapy for children with progressive or residual disease during or after chemotherapy. Even among those with neuraxis dissemination, full-dose irradiation for children older than 18 to 36 months has achieved durable secondary disease control in 25% to 40% of cases resistant to chemotherapy (145,173,181). A decision to forgo irradiation should be based on disease-free status for malignant tumors and progression-free status for low-grade tumors following initial surgery and chemotherapy. Whether one can safely omit irradiation in those with neuraxis dissemination at presentation regardless of chemotherapy response is uncertain (145,149, 168,170,181,182).

Chemotherapy

The initial study of primary MOPP chemotherapy at M.D. Anderson Cancer Center showed long-term survival in 8 of 11 infants with medulloblastoma; 6 of 8 survivors had not received radiation therapy (167).

Duffner et al. (149) reported the first POG trial with initial postoperative chemotherapy in 1993. The regimen included cycles of cyclophosphamide/vincristine and cisiplatin/VP-16. Progression-free survival at 2 years was 42% for ependymomas, 54% for malignant gliomas, 19% for supratentorial PNETs, and 34% for medulloblastomas (Fig. 7). As in other infant trials, failures beyond 2 years have been uncommon with the "malignant" histiotypes (i.e., medulloblastoma, malignant gliomas/brainstem gliomas, supratentorial PNETs); notably, ependymomas have continued to fail at and beyond 5 years posttherapy (145,149,167,172).

A more recent CCG trial in medulloblastoma and PNETs utilized the "8-in-1" chemotherapy approach alone . There was little adherence to the suggested use of local or neuraxis irradiation. In a series largely reflecting chemotherapy disease control, Geyer et al. (168) reported 3-year disease control in only 22% of children. A similar regimen in

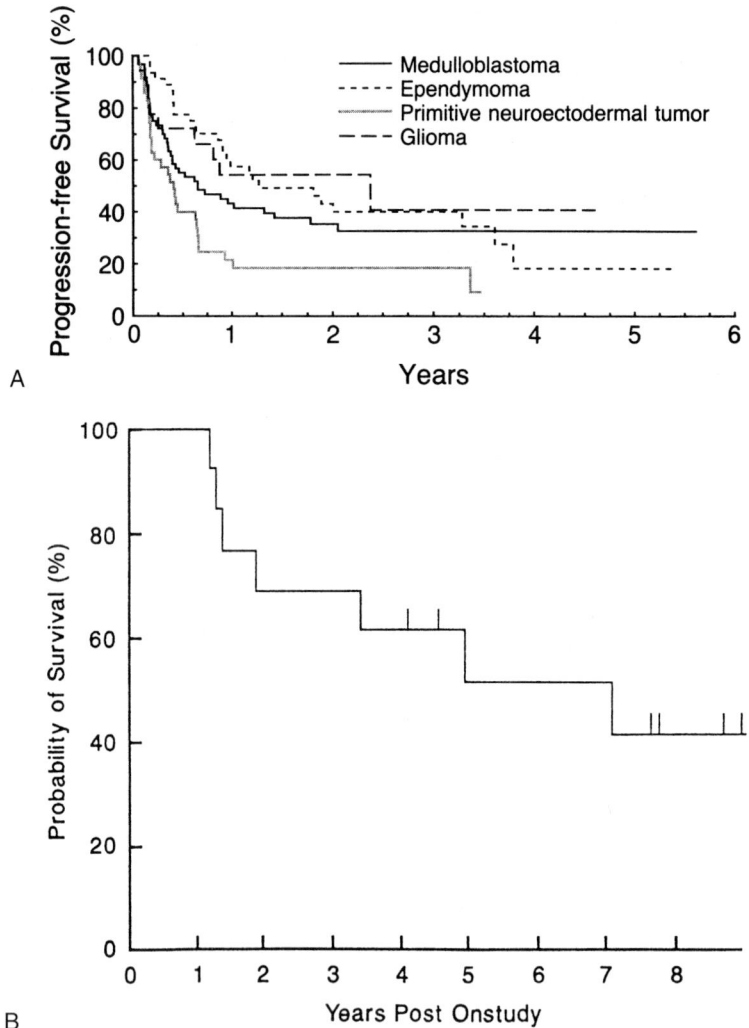

FIG. 7. Outcome in infants with malignant brain tumors following initial postoperative chemotherapy and delayed postoperative consolidative irradiation: progression-free survival by histologic type (**A**, based on POG 8633) (149) and long-term survival following retrieval for medulloblastoma, progressive during chemotherapy or persistent on completion of chemotherapy (**B**, based on St. Jude Children's Research Hospital experience) (105,181).

malignant gliomas showed disease control in 44% with anaplastic astrocytoma and 0% with GBM (178).

The "Headstart" program popularized by Mason and colleagues has utilized "induction" chemotherapy followed by a high-dose regimen (busulphan, VP-16, thiotepa) and autologous marrow rescue (170). Long-term disease control is not significantly different from the experience reported by Geyer; only among the subset successfully proceeding through the high-dose regimen does a subset analysis show disease control approaching 50% (170).

Although limited in number, the series reported by Dupuis-Girod and colleagues (182), showed a 75% objective response rate to high-dose busulfan/thiotepa in medulloblastoma progressive after a traditional infant chemotherapy regimen. Among 13 patients with only local tumor progression treated with consolidative posterior fossa irradiation, the freedom from progression rate at 3 years is 70%; by comparison, none of the 9 cases with M$^+$ disease achieved durable disease control despite craniospinal irradiation (182).

Radiotherapeutic Management

Volume and Technique

Radiation parameters are similar to those in older children; most protocols require craniospinal irradiation for localized medulloblastoma and supratentorial PNETs, pineoblastomas, choroid plexus carcinomas, and any histologic type associated with overt leptomeningeal dissemination. Infants with low-grade or malignant gliomas or localized ependymomas (regardless of degree of differentiation or anaplasia) require only local radiation therapy. For low-grade gliomas, the target volume should include the primary tumor with a 1-cm margin for the majority of lesions that are discrete and circumscribed on imaging; for those that appear more infiltrating or extending along white matter tracks, the target volume should include all areas of known extension (being careful to differentiate tumor involvement from imaging changes more typically associated with NF1 in such patients). Those with malignant or aggressive histologic types require 2- to 3-cm margins as described for older children. Three-dimensional conformal irradiation offers a considerable potential advantage in targeting and delivering the intended dose with greater sparing of the critical, adjacent normal brain for supratentorial tumors, posterior fossa boost volumes, and localized infratentorial lesions (e.g., dorsally exophytic brainstem gliomas and, investigationally, ependymomas) (183). For centrally located tumors with spherical configuration, trials of fractionated stereotactic radiosurgery (or stereotactic radiotherapy) suggest a similar or greater advantage in disease control and an idealized tumor:normal tissue therapeutic ratio (74,79,184).

The use of more limited volumes, including irradiation limited to the posterior fossa for medulloblastoma in infants achieving a complete response to intensive chemotherapy or treatment limited to only the tumor bed in ependymomas, is supported by some of the early data regarding high-dose chemotherapy and patterns of disease relapse (170,172,182). Such restriction of radiation volume must be considered highly investigational, appropriate only in the setting of an approved therapeutic trial.

Dose

The recommended dose to the neuraxis is 30 to 32 Gy for children under 2-years old and 35 to 36 Gy for children over 2- to 3-years old with residual or recurrent disease or with neuraxis dissemination at diagnosis or at the time of initiating radiation therapy. Reduced dose irradiation has been successful in children with M0 disease: the initial POG study used only 24 Gy for children in "complete response" with M0 disease at diagnosis, and Goldwein et al. (185) reports disease control of 70% in a small series of similar children who received only 18 Gy to the neuraxis. The dose to the primary target volume is 50 Gy (for those less than 2-years old) to 54 Gy (for those over 2-years old). With response to chemotherapy, "consolidative" doses have been reported at 48 to 50 Gy (149). The French series that combined high-dose chemotherapy and local posterior fossa consolidation for progressive medulloblastoma used only 36 Gy (182). Doses for low-grade gliomas (45–50 Gy for those less than 1-year old and 50 Gy for those 1- to 2-years old) are raised to 50 to 54 Gy in children over 2- to 3-years old. Data reported for malignant gliomas has been based on dose levels of 50 to 54 Gy in this age group (171).

Results

Overall results in children with malignant histiotypes approximate 20% to 35% disease control at 3 years. Five-year data is similar to the earlier time frame for medulloblastoma, supratentorial PNETs, and malignant gliomas; for ependymomas, there has been a steady falloff in progression-free survival toward the 20% to 25% range at 5 years (12, 149,168,172,178). Pineoblastomas and atypical teratoid/rhabdoid tumors in this age group have done notoriously poorly, with few if any survivors beyond 1 year (149,186). Outcome in young children with low-grade gliomas is more favorable, with disease control rates approaching 80% following surgery, initial chemotherapy, or initial/delayed use of irradiation (9,12,17,26,48,53,93,145,161,162,187).

EMBRYONAL CNS TUMORS (PRIMITIVE NEUROECTODERMAL TUMORS OR PNETS AND ATYPICAL TERATOID/RHABDOID TUMORS)

The 1993 WHO classification of embryonal CNS tumors seeks to clarify the controversies regarding the PNET "concept" (3,188,189). The supratentorial primitive neuroectodermal tumor (PNET) was initially reported by Hart and Earle in 1973 as an aggressive cerebral tumor occurring predominantly in young children (190). The tumor is comprised of undifferentiated neuroepithelial cells with focal areas of divergent differentiation toward glial, neuronal, and mesenchymal lines and unique molecular markings (189–192). In 1983, Rorke (193) introduced the "PNET" as a unifying concept grouping together the cellular "small blue cell" CNS tumors with or without focal or uniform differentiation. Included among PNETs were the supratentorial neuroblastomas, ependymoblastomas, pineoblastomas, medulloepitheliomas, and the undifferentiated PNETs identified by Hart and Earle; in addition, medulloblastomas were included as "posterior fossa PNET"(193). The tumors share relatively similar histologic appearances, a tendency to seed along the cerebrospinal fluid (CSF) pathways, and relative responsiveness to irradiation and chemotherapy. Those skeptical of the broad PNET designation have argued that malignant transformation could oc-

cur not only at the level of the primitive multipotential neuroepithelial cell precursor as suggested by the "PNET concept," but also within the committed neuronal and glial cell lines at later stages of differentiation (27,188, 194).

The clinical outcome of medulloblastoma and the supratentorial embryonal tumors continues to differ; even the several supratentorial entities show different survival rates in different series (i.e., ependymoblastoma vs. pineoblastoma vs. neuroblastoma vs. medulloblastoma, etc.) (168,174,176,188,189,195, 196).

Table 2 shows the WHO classification of embryonal CNS tumors, maintaining the distinct clinical entities (i.e., the primitive medulloepithelioma, pineoblastoma, ependymoblastoma, and neuroblastoma). The category of "primitive neuroectodermal tumors" is specifically distinguished for medulloblastoma ("posterior fossa PNET") and the primitive supratentorial lesion with little or multiple divergent lines of differentiation identified as supratentorial PNET (3,188).

The embryonal tumors occur predominantly in young children. In the POG infant malignant CNS tumor study, 18% of cases were grouped as embryonal supratentorial tumors; one-half of these can be classified as PNET, lacking a recognizable dominant line of differentiation, and the other one-half can be classified as one of the specific embryonal tumor types (149).

Medulloepithelioma is the most primitive embryonal tumor, histologically showing features of primitive medullary epithelium and primitive tubular structures. Focal differentiation toward glial, neuronal, and/or mesenchymal lines are often present (196). *Primitive polar spongioblastoma* is a rare cerebral tumor thought to be derived from migrating glial precursor cells and characterized by immature unipolar glial cells with or without focal differentiation toward astrocytic or oligodendroglial elements (194).

Ependymoblastoma is a poorly differentiated embryonal tumor including ependymal differentiation signified by multilayered rosettes similar to those seen in retinoblastoma (Flexner-Wintersteiner rosettes) (28). The tumor is felt to be a specific embryonal neoplasm, different from the differentiated and anaplastic ependymomas (discussed in Chapter 4) that occur both in the posterior fossa and supratentorially (38,188,194).

The *cerebral neuroblastoma* ranges histologically from an undifferentiated tumor similar to the extra-CNS childhood neuroblastoma often including unilayered Homer Wright rosettes, to lesions demonstrating considerable ganglionic differentiation (194, 197).

The tumor most often confused with medulloblastoma histologically and by contiguous anatomic location is the *pineoblastoma* (Fig. 8). The tumor is believed to arise from pineal parenchymal cells, histologically signified by undifferentiated small round cells, usually including scattered Homer Wright rosettes. The tumor may mimic

retinoblastoma, including fleurettes and Flexner-Wintersteiner rosettes (186,198).

The embryonal tumors present as solid or partially cystic lesions (Fig. 8). Although the undifferentiated classic PNET and cerebral neuroblastoma may present as well-demarcated lesions, the embryonal tumors are generally invasive (162,189,190,194). Leptomeningeal dissemination is apparent at the time of diagnosis or at the time of initial tumor recurrence/progression in approximately one-third of children with pineoblastoma, ependymoblastoma, and undifferentiated supratentorial PNET (149,162,176,199). Although some question has been raised regarding the frequency of CSF failure in localized cerebral neuroblastoma, most reports indicate a frequency of CNS dissemination similar to that noted previously (195,197,200). Also controversial is the frequency of extra-CNS and peritoneal metastases associated with ventricular peritoneal shunts (201,202). There

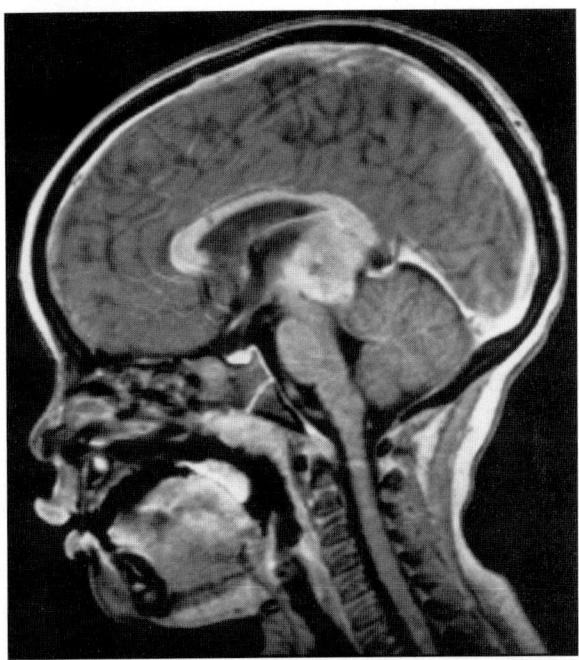
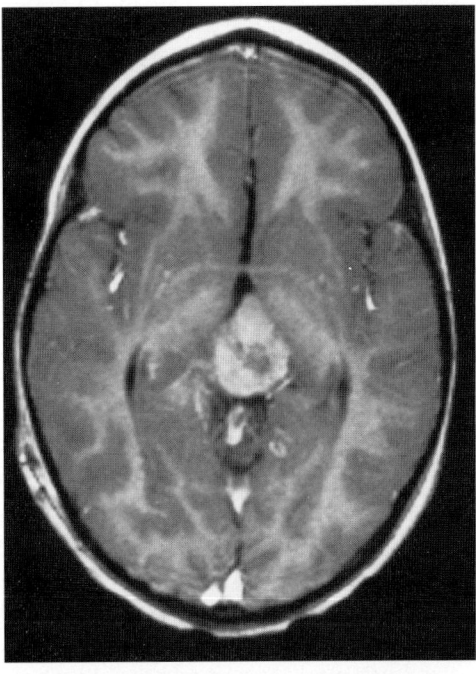

A   B

FIG. 8. Pineoblastoma presenting in a 2-year-old girl, a sizable central lesion that often responds promptly to chemotherapy and/or irradiation; experience in this age group shows few if any long-term survivals despite aggressive intervention.

are occasional children who develop peritoneal seeding of tumor concentrated around the shunt tip following a ventriculoperitoneal shunt. In the absence of any other tumor relapse, these nodules are considered shunt-borne metastases. It is not clear, however, if there is a statistically significant increased risk of systemic dissemination of CNS tumors in shunted children.

Separate from the PNETs are the immature, highly aggressive tumors identified as *atypical teratoid/rhabdoid* tumors (187,203). The tumors are of uncertain histogenesis and occur almost exclusively in young children as posterior fossa or supratentorial lesions (187). Rorke et al. (187) reports that up to 20% to 25% of infant medulloblastomas are, on review, actually atypical teratoid/rhabdoid tumors. The lesions are associated with a chromosome 22 abnormality, and although often responsive to chemotherapy (especially carboplatin-containing regimens) and irradiation, the disease course is almost always signified by rapid recurrence and neuraxis dissemination (187). Survival beyond 1 to 2 years has been only anecdotal (187,204).

Therapy

The basic principle of surgical resection is limited by disease extent and site. Undifferentiated supratentorial PNET, cerebral neuroblastoma, and ependymoblastoma may be resectable in up to 25% to 50% of cases, more often in tumors that are grossly cystic (149,168,176,189,190,195). Pineoblastomas are generally approached by stereotactic biopsy or limited resection (10,162,186).

Postoperative irradiation is indicated for the embryonal CNS tumors. Classic studies indicate disease control in less than 25% of cases with supratentorial PNET and pineoblastoma (10,189,205,206). The addition of chemotherapy to often limited surgery and craniospinal irradiation has been associated with a 60% survival rate in pineoblastomas in children more than 18-months old (186). Similar rates are preliminarily reported following similar chemotherapy (vincristine, CCNU,

prednisone or the 8-in-1 regimen) (174). In relatively small series, outcome following surgery and irradiation for cerebral neuroblastoma has approached 60% survival beyond 2 to 5 years (195,197).

Radiotherapeutic Management

Volume and Technique

Most series documenting more favorable outcome in the literature have included full neuraxis irradiation for the embryonal CNS tumors (174,176,186,199,205). The exception is a single report documenting disease control in six children with localized cystic cerebral neuroblastoma following surgery and limited volume irradiation (195). The technique for craniospinal irradiation is discussed in Chapter 4. The local "boost" is confined to the preoperative tumor volume, corrected for tissue shifts that occur during resection of often sizable lesions; in practice, the preoperative volume is diminished to the tumor bed and residual neoplasm. Margins of 2 to 3 cm are indicated for all but the most circumscribed tumors, often followed by a more limited field with 1-cm dosimetric margins for a final "boost." As in other supratentorial lesions, the use of three-dimensional conformal irradiation offers potential advantage in coverage and limiting the dose of adjacent normal brain volumes.

Dose

The dose of craniospinal irradiation is comparable to that used in medulloblastoma, with full neuraxis doses of 35 to 36 Gy in children beyond 3 to 5 years of age (176,186). There has been little experience, to date, documenting outcome after reduced neuraxis irradiation (similar to the 23.4 Gy level utilized in favorable or low-stage medulloblastoma, see Chapter 4) in conjunction with chemotherapy (207). Ongoing trials will address this issue as a potentially valid alternative. Treatment to the primary tumor volume is generally to a cumulative dose of 54 to 55 Gy, often incorporating an additional reduction in target volume after 50 Gy.

CRANIOPHARYNGIOMA

Craniopharyngiomas are benign tumors of epithelial origin believed to arise from remnants of Rathke's pouch in the suprasellar region. The typical adamantinous craniopharyngioma is a calcified, cystic tumor derived from embryonic cell rests of enamel organs located adjacent to the tuber cinereum along the pituitary stalk (28,208). The less common squamous cell craniopharyngioma occurs almost exclusively in adults; the latter type is rarely calcified and often presents as a solid lesion without cyst formation. The adamantinous craniopharyngioma seen in children and adolescents includes solid components and often large, complex cysts filled with fluid containing high lipid content and cholesterol granules, typically described as "crankcase oil."

Craniopharyngiomas are well-circumscribed, encapsulated extra-axial lesions. The argument for surgical resection is based on the marginated nature of the tumor. Confounding, however, is the location of the tumor, often found adherent to the optic nerves or chiasm, the major vessels at the circle of Willis, the tuber cinereum, and the hypothalamus. Infiltration into the tuber cinereum and the presence of small tumor islets within the adjacent hypothalamus have been noted, indicating locally invasive potential (208, 209).

Anatomically, 70% of childhood craniopharyngiomas are retrochiasmatic in location, usually extending superiorly into the third ventricle and along the hypothalamus (Fig. 9). The multicystic lesion may include cystic extension into the basal cisterns and even into the posterior fossa. In 30% of cases, the tumor is prechiasmatic, occurring between the optic nerves and pushing the chiasm posteriorly (209–211). The latter tumors are more accessible and less adherent to vital suprasellar structures.

Children present with visual disturbances (most often visual field deficits, less likely decreased acuity) and symptoms of increased intracranial pressure. Endocrine deficits at diagnosis are apparent in 50% to 90% of children studied, most often including diminished growth hormone, diabetes insipidus (noted in only 10% to 15% of cases preoperatively), and decreased gonadotropin, thyroid-stimulating hormone (TSH), and/or adrenocorticotropic hormone (ACTH). Changes in personality and altered cognitive function have been noted in up to 50% of children at presentation (208,212–215).

Therapy

The treatment of craniopharyngiomas is controversial. Total resection is often curative in this technically "benign" neoplasm. Matson's classic 1969 neurosurgical text (216), described complete resection in 44 of 57 children preceding the modern era of the operating microscope; 10 of the 44 had required more than one surgical procedure to effect gross total removal. Numerous contemporary series reporting primary surgical intent note attempted total resection in 50% to 80% of children (209,210,215–218). A review of treatment strategies in academic pediatric neurosurgical centers in North America indicated a vast majority of programs are oriented toward surgical resection as the treatment of choice in most childhood craniopharyngiomas (217). Postoperative imaging indicates residual calcification, consistent with residual tumor, in 15% to 50% of "totally resected" cases (210,214,215,219). The rate of clinical recurrence following total resection is 10% to 30% and clearly linked to the presence of postoperative residual, including the small "calcified flecks" that signal tumor residual (210,211,214,215,217,219–221).

Balanced against the low-failure rate following aggressive surgery are risks of mortality (3%) and major postoperative morbidity (defined as significant visual loss or neurologic dysfunction, 10%) (209,210,215,217). Most important is the skill and experience of the surgeon—tumor control and morbidity rates correlate strongly with the number of cases per-

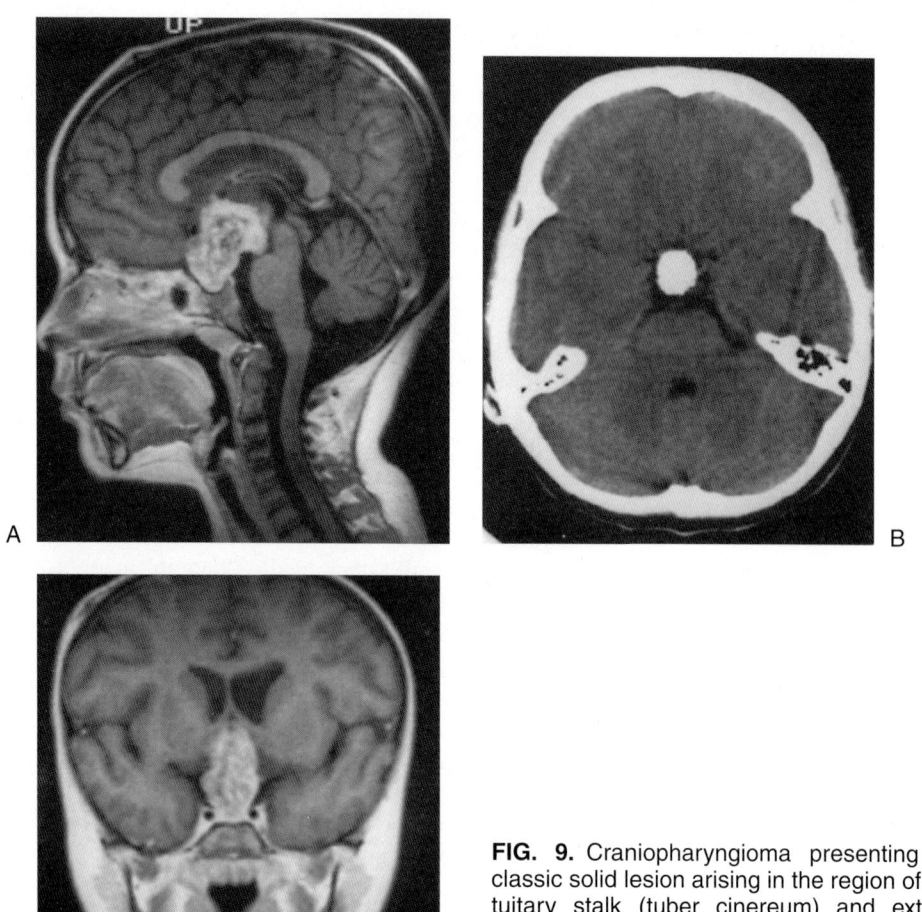

A

B

C

FIG. 9. Craniopharyngioma presenting as a classic solid lesion arising in the region of the pituitary stalk (tuber cinereum) and extending cephalad into the third ventricular region with a significant cystic component. With irradiation alone or following planned limited resection, a three-dimensional conformal or stereotactic radiotherapy approach is ideal for most of these lesions.

formed annually in the treating center (217, 222). Dissection is associated with fusiform dilatation of the internal carotid artery in up to 15% of cases (96). Tumor recurrence and operative morbidity/mortality are more frequent in the more common retrochiasmatic craniopharyngiomas (209,210,214). Among the most common operative sequelae is an 80 to 90% incidence of diabetes insipidus, one of the most difficult endocrinopathies to manage in long-term survivors, and an incidence of morbid hypothalamic obesity as high as 50% (208–210, 214,220,221,223,224).

Kramer and colleagues (225) first reported the efficacy of limited surgical decompression and primary irradiation for craniopharyngiomas from London's Royal Marsden Hospital in 1961. A 15-year update indicated progression-free survival in all six children (226). Subsequent experience at the Royal Marsden Hospital has documented survival rates at 10 and 15 years of 84% and 79%, respectively, in patients treated between 1950 and 1981 by simple cyst aspiration or limited decompression followed by irradiation (12). Among 27 children treated by modern supervoltage techniques between 1970 and 1981, survival at 5, 10, and 15 years is reported at 100%, 96%, and 96%, respectively; these results are equal to or better than the best radical resection series (12,213). An additional experience at Jefferson (227), also demonstrates 80% 20-year disease control following limited surgery and irradiation.

There is considerable literature confirming long-term disease control in 80% to 95% of children with varying degrees of less than radical surgery combined with irradiation (214,217–219,221,227–230) (Table 5). Although acute reactions are quite infrequent, one anticipates late endocrine changes after irradiation (including growth hormone deficiency, less frequent accelerated or delayed sexual development, and diminished TSH and/or ACTH secretion). Radiation-related diabetes insipidus is distinctly uncommon (221, 224,229). Late vascular events are reported, if infrequently, as a cause of neurologic toxicity after irradiation; Kramer et al.'s later Jefferson experience (227), documented late vascular and neurologic events in 10% of long-term survivors, correlated to a subset of children treated at dose levels (greater than 61 Gy) beyond those utilized in current practice.

The option of incomplete resection and observation, delaying irradiation until later progression, is unattractive. Despite the low-grade histology of craniopharyngiomas, clinically detectable tumor progression is apparent in 70% of incompletely removed cases within 2 to 3 years (209,210,214). There may be a role for limited radiosurgery if tumor residual is limited in size and anatomically positioned remote from the chiasm and hypo-thalamus (231). Second surgery is associated with diminished efficacy and greatly increased surgical morbidities (210,215,217). Results of delayed irradiation at the time of recurrent disease are inferior to those achieved with planned postoperative irradiation: 25% versus 78% (227). It should be noted that some patients who have cyst enlargement in the first few months following radiotherapy may not have truly progressive tumor. A majority of children will ultimately have stabilization and ultimate regression of the cyst, or require simple cyst aspiration for associated neurologic symptoms (226,232). It appears that the cells composing cranio-pharyngiomas may continue, for a period of time, to secrete fluid despite having sustained a lethal radiation injury (232). In some instances, progressive but isolated cystic enlargement may require intracystic irradiation using ^{32}P or other pure beta emitters (201, 233).

Primary total resection and limited surgery with planned primary irradiation achieve excellent disease control. The controversy regarding primary treatment includes the balance of relatively high rates of immediate postsurgical sequelae (endocrinopathies including diabetes insipidus, visual deterioration in up to 25% of cases, and major neurologic complications) versus recognized rates of late postirradiation sequelae (growth hormone and other endocrinopathies, late vascular events, secondary carcinogenesis) (217, 218). Comparative reports of neurocognitive and overall functional levels favor children treated by limited surgery and irradiation (213,218,221,228,229).

TABLE 5. *Outcome in craniopharyngioma*

Primary modality	Series total no.	% Complete resection[a]	PFS	10 y Survival	Series/Ref
Surgery	31	61%	63%		CHOP (214)
	50	90%	66%		Toronto (210)
	27	78%	85%		Child. Mem (209)
Limited surgery + primary RT	77 (1950–86)			83%	Marsden (12)
	27 (1970–81)			96%	Marsden (213)
	37 (1970–90)			86%	Boston (221)

[a]By operative impression.
CHOP, Children's Hospital of Philadelphia.

Radiotherapeutic Management

Volume and Technique

The volume of irradiation is limited to the well-marginated tumor, including its cystic components. It is important to accurately map out the cystic areas; cystic extensions posteriorly or inferiorly may be obscured by the basal cisterns. Following decompression, one can target the reduced cystic volume. Following partial resection, it is prudent to limit irradiation to the postoperative extent only if one is assured that the cyst wall was removed in toto. Conventional techniques include coronal arcs utilizing head position to avoid exit through the thyroid, three-field coronal or four-field axial obliqued configurations (avoiding exit through the eyes and, preferably, the neck and torso), or opposed lateral high-energy beams when required by disease extent. Stereotactic or three-dimensional conformal techniques should replace most other approaches except in extraordinarily large tumors requiring conformal lateral field arrangements (234). These techniques decrease the volume of normal tissue irradiated and offer the promise of reduced neuropsychological sequelae of irradiation (184,235). Experience with single-fraction radiosurgery has been reported; the number of cases appropriately managed by such an approach is limited, largely to those with small foci of post-surgery residual that can be easily targeted when remote from the chiasm, major vessels, and hypothalamus (231).

Intracavitary radionuclide insertion is a valid approach for tumors that are largely cystic, either in an effort to delay primary surgery or external irradiation (e.g., in children below 3 to 4 years of age) or with residual or recurrent cyst formation following definitive surgery or radiation therapy. A catheter is passed into the cyst at craniotomy or by stereotactic guidance. Based on the cyst volume, an appropriate dose of isotope in diluent is instilled into the cavity. Most contemporary experience is with beta emitters such as ^{32}P and ^{90}Yt, delivering a high dose (i.e., 200 Gy) to the cyst wall (39,233,236). Centers using intracystic brachytherapy as primary management report high rates of uncomplicated disease control in a majority of tumor presentations (233,236).

Dose

An external beam dose response has been documented up to 54 to 55 Gy using 180 cGy fractions daily (12,213,227). There is no evidence that doses more than 55 Gy add to disease control in pediatric craniopharyngioma; late complications, including chiasmal injury, are increased with dose levels above 60 Gy (12,213,227).

Results

Long-term disease control rates for craniopharyngioma should approximate 80% to 90%, with a definite plateau on both disease-free and overall survival beyond 5 to 10 years. Such results are achievable among those selected for surgery who have successfully undergone gross total resection (210,211,214, 215,217,219–221). Similar data is available following limited surgery and irradiation (12, 127,213,218,227,229,230,237).

PINEAL REGION TUMORS/INTRACRANIAL GERM CELL TUMORS

Pineal region tumors include a unique spectrum of neoplasms presenting in the posterior third ventricular region (Table 6). Approximately 80% of the pineal region tumors in children and adolescents are *germ cell tumors* (representing 60% to 70%) or *pineal parenchymal tumors* (i.e., pineoblastomas and less common pineocytomas, representing 10% to 20%). Other types include glial tumors (astrocytomas, ependymomas) and arachnoid cysts. With MRI, gliomas occurring in the pineal region are now often identified as neoplasms primary in the adjacent tectal plate or midbrain. Low-grade and malignant astrocytomas have been reported as pineal region tumors (10,238).

TABLE 6. *Pineal region tumors—relative incidence*

Tumor type	Relative frequency (%)	Characteristics
Germinoma	40–60%	Predominately adolescent males, (–) AFP; may have isolated (+) BHCG (typically to <15–75 units)
Malignant germ cell tumors endodermal sinus tumor choriocarcinoma malignant teratoma immature teratoma	20–25%	(+++) AFP (+++) HCG; frequent intralesional hemorrhage
Pineal parenchymal tumor pineoblastoma pineocytoma	14%	Predominately in young children Uncommon in children/adolescent
Glioma astrocytoma ependymoma	15%	

Intracranial *germ cell tumors* occur within the diencephalic structures, almost exclusively as midline third ventricular lesions, located in the pineal region in 50% to 60% of presentations and in the anterior third ventricular or suprasellar region in 30% to 35% of cases. Uncommonly, primary intracranial germ cell tumors originate in the basal ganglia or thalamic nuclei (24,239–243). Germ cell tumors are rare in North America and Europe, representing fewer than 1% to 3% of pediatric CNS neoplasms; in Japan and Taiwan they are reported to represent up to 5% to 9% of childhood brain tumors (24,240). The full range of germ cell histiotypes present intracranially: *germinomas* (60% to 70%), "more malignant germ cell types" (i.e., *embryonal carcinomas* or *endodermal sinus tumors* or *choriocarciomas*, collectively accounting for 15% to 20%), and *teratomas* (benign, immature, and malignant types accounting for 15% to 20%) (24,238,240,244, 245). [*Malignant teratomas* are admixtures of benign teratomatous lesions with one or more malignant germ cell lines such as embryonal carcinoma, endodermal sinus tumor, or choriocarcinoma, or malignant elements of rhabdomyosarcoma, neuroblastoma, or epithelial carcinoma (238).]

Pineal region germinomas occur most often in adolescent males. Suprasellar germ cell tumors occur throughout the first two decades; there is no gender predilection (10,24,239). In very young children, the most common pineal region tumors are pineoblastomas.

Pineoblastomas are embryonal CNS tumors believed to originate from pineal parenchymal cells (see previous section on embryonal CNS tumors). *Pineocytomas* are "mature" parenchymal cell neoplasms, which are quite rare lesions in children, clinically benign in adolescents, and potentially malignant in young children (246–248).

Pineal region tumors present most often with increased intracranial pressure due to compression of the adjacent Sylvian aqueduct. Ocular signs are classically noted, including features of *Parinaud's syndrome*: decreased upward gaze, abnormal pupillary responses described as near-light dissociation (i.e., limited constriction to light but retained pupillary response to accommodation), and diminished convergence (24,249).

In suprasellar germ cell tumors, the "classic triad" includes diabetes insipidus, precocious or delayed sexual development, and visual deficits (242,250). In adolescent males, one may find symptoms of suprasellar involvement associated with primary pineal tumors, occasionally in the absence of imaging evidence of suprasellar involvement. Concurrent pineal and suprasellar germinomas is recognized as ("*multiple midline germinomas*"), accounting for 5% to 10% of intracranial ger minomas; the phenomenon appears to represent multicentric tumor development or subependymal laminar infiltration around the third ventricle, rather than subarachnoid or CSF pathway metastasis (6,24,202,239,251, 252).

Alpha-fetoprotein may be present in serum or CSF in embryonal carcinoma, endodermal sinus tumor, or malignant teratoma; elevated levels are diagnostic of a malignant germ cell histiotype and exclude the diagnosis of a pure germinoma (244,245). Beta-HCG is elevated in a subset of germinomas (10% to 20% of pure germinomas show levels above 5 to 10 IU, up to 50 to 70 IU; higher levels are in "germinomas with syncytiotrophoblastic giant cells"); significant elevation (typically above 1000 IU) is associated with choriocarcinoma (24,244,245,253–256).

Therapy

Treatment of pineal region and CNS germ cell tumors is rather controversial, from the decision to establish histology to the role of surgery, radiation parameters, and the appropriate role for chemotherapy. Although excellent disease control has been reported in series based on clinical/imaging diagnosis (i.e., without histologic confirmation), identifying specific radiation, chemotherapy, and surgery is dependent on a histologic diagnosis. Most North American investigators routinely rec-

ommend histologic confirmation for pineal region and suprasellar tumors, except in those uncommon presentations where tumor markers establish a diagnosis. Radiation therapy is the standard treatment and "control arm" for alternative investigations in germinomas; it is a significant component of therapy for the malignant germ cell types (253,257–260). Intracranial germ cell tumors are chemoresponsive; the use of combined chemotherapy and limited-volume or limited-dose irradiation has been reported as a potentially attractive treatment approach (253,261–265) (Table 7). The use of chemotherapy alone has been associated with higher rates of recurrence and mortality than one would consider acceptable (254,255).

Surgery

Earlier data documented rates of operative mortality (10% to 33%) and major morbidity (over 25%) that discouraged surgical intervention beyond often necessary ventriculoperitoneal shunt insertion (10,199). Contemporary surgical techniques permit stereotactic or open biopsy for pineal region tumors with low rates of mortality (less than 1% to 3%) and morbidity (10,199,253,261, 266). A prior suggestion that biopsy predisposed the patient to a higher risk of subarachnoid dissemination has not been confirmed (266–269). The wide variation in tumor his-

TABLE 7. *Outcome in intracranial germinoma*

Primary management	RT volume/1° dose[a] (chemotherapy)	No.	5-yr Survival	Series/Ref
RT	CSI/50–55 Gy	22	85%	Kyoto (257)
	<CSI	38	86%	
	CSI/45–55 Gy	22	86%	Boston (202)
	<CSI/40–50 Gy	48	87%	European (263)
	<CSI/44 Gy	25	90%	Mayo (252)
CT + reduced RT	<CSI/30 Gy[b] (cyclo)	11	91%	Allen (253,261)
CT + reduced RT	<CSI/24 Gy[b] (CDDP, VP-16)	10	100%[c]	Hokkaido (264)
CT	(CD, VP, B)	45	84%[d]	"International" (255)

[a]RT volume (CSI = craniospinal component; <CSI = cranial, ventricles, or wide local volumes *without* full CSI).
[b]series utilized CSI only for M+.
[c]2-yr progression-free survival
[d]2-yr event-free survival is 42%
CD, cisplatin; VP, VP16; B, bleomycin; RT, radiation therapy; CT, chemotherapy.

tiotypes in the anterior third ventricular region (e.g., astrocytomas of the hypothalamic/chiasmatic area, craniopharyngiomas, and hamartomas as well as germinomas or other germ cell tumors) and relative surgical accessibility have long indicated biopsy for suprasellar presentations.

A nonoperative approach for pineal region tumors had been to assume the relative dominance of *germinoma* cell type, especially among adolescent boys, and initiate locate irradiation as a "histologic test." Prompt tumor reduction (by 20 to 25 Gy) was interpreted to be "diagnostic" of germinoma. Subsequent therapy included primary irradiation based on institutional policies (local, cranial, or craniospinal fields) (202,257,259, 267). If a tumor showed limited early response to the "test" dose, then surgical intervention and/or radiation volume/dose are based on the presumption of a benign (e.g., teratoma, glioma) or malignant (e.g., malignant germ cell histiotype) tumor (12,202, 267). Although the "radiation test dose" is neither reliable nor recommended by the authors, analyses show differences in outcome that only marginally favor histologic series (256,259,260,267).

Potentially resectable gliomas or teratomas can be successfully approached; malignant teratomas or more aggressive germ cell types, known to experience higher failure rates following irradiation with or without chemotherapy, have been operated on with varying reports of success (10,156, 261). The potential role of stereotactic radiosurgery to "boost" local disease, which persists after conventional radiotherapy or chemotherapy is under investigation in children with malignant intracranial germ cell tumors (270). Significant deterioration in postshunt or postbiopsy functional status can be noted in pineal region tumors, often associated with malignant germ cell histiotypes or noted tumor progression; patients with dramatic neurologic impairment may respond to radiotherapeutic intervention, warranting intensive supportive care early in the course of urgent irradiation.

Radiation Therapy

Radiation therapy has been the major curative modality for pineal region and suprasellar germinomas. Long-term disease control rates range from 60% to over 90% (202,242,256, 259,260,266–268,271).

Chemotherapy

Intracranial germ cell tumors are chemosensitive, with excellent objective response rates documented for cyclophosphamide, carboplatin, cisplatin/VP-16, ICE (ifosfamide/carboplatin/VP-16), and CDDP/VP-16/bleomycin (253–255,261–265). Objective response rates approach 100% for germinomas (254,255,261,264,265).

There is now information regarding long-term follow-up in two moderate-sized series using preirradiation chemotherapy [carboplatin in a trial by Allen et al. (261), CDDP/VP-16 for localized/marker negative germinoma and added bleomycin for "higher risk" germinoma in the series by Sawamura et al. (264)] and limited irradiation (24 to 30 Gy locally, with 0 to 21 Gy to the neuraxis); excellent survival (100%), disease control (more than 95%), and outcome characteristics have been described (253,261,262,264). The approach is under prospective study in POG, testing serial reductions of local irradiation dose in conjunction with chemotherapy.

The use of chemotherapy alone has been tested in an "international protocol." Serial reports of the first drug regimen (CDDP/VP-16/bleomycin) indicate high initial response rates, but disease progression or recurrence in 50% of patients. Treatment-related mortality approximates 15% (254,255). Disease control has been notably difficult amongst children with elevated β-HCG, despite pure germinoma histology (255). Salvage has been achieved with "reinduction" cyclophosphamide and craniospinal irradiation among children documenting progression during or after the chemotherapy protocol. For the more malignant germ cell types, added chemotherapy is indicated, using a CDDP- or carbo-platin-based regimen (254,255,265,267).

Radiotherapy Management

Volume and Technique

There has been continuing debate regarding the necessity for full cranial or craniospinal radiation volumes in pineal region or suprasellar germinomas. The majority of recent publications favor limiting the radiation volume to the primary tumor (alone) or including a proportion of the ventricular system (i.e., third ventricle region or the entire intracranial ventricular volume) or an initial whole brain field followed by whole ventricles followed by a primary tumor boost. The size and maturity of a 1978 report by Sung et al. (250) provided the major support for those favoring craniospinal irradiation (CSI) for germinomas. The pre-CT era experience showed a greater than 10% risk of subarachnoid dissemination in pineal region tumors; among biopsied suprasellar germinomas, neuraxis dissemination occurred in 43% (250).

Evidence of disease beyond the primary site is apparent in 10% to 30% of intracranial germinomas at diagnosis. Third ventricular disease is apparent as multiple midline presentations, classically involving the pineal and suprasellar recess areas, but sometimes showing multiple nodules along the linings of the ventricle (202,251,257,268,271). CSF involvement has been documented in less than 15% of cases in North American series, but up to 60% of cases in Japan (59,252,253,267). Overt spinal seeding, however, is rarely demonstrable by imaging (257,271). The implication of CSF cytology is unclear; Shibamoto et al. (257) described disease-free survival in 6 of 6 children with positive CSF cytology following irradiation limited to the third ventricular volume (259).

A large proportion of clinical series reporting disease control rates in excess of 90% over the past two decades have been based on low-dose craniospinal irradiation as a component of therapy (199,241,257,263,266,267,

269). More recent analyses favor local radiation volumes, several centers reporting similar disease control rates with far more restricted radiation volumes (256,257,266,268, 272). The incidence of spinal failure, specifically, has been reported to be 0% to 10% following irradiation limited to the cranium (257,259,260,268,272). Less than full cranial irradiation has been associated, by some, with an incidence of intracranial recurrence of 15% (252,266,271). In light of the preceding evidence, CSI has a marginal benefit for intracranial germinomas treated by irradiation alone. The potential 10% to 15% gain is not uniformly recognized and must be judgementally weighed against the potential added toxicities of 24 to 25 Gy to the neuraxis. For older teenagers, the use of CSI is considered "appropriate therapy," albeit not required; the more common recommendation is for wide local radiation fields. For younger children, one would argue that the putative gain from CSI may not exceed even the low likelihood of significant functional toxicities.

Local radiation volumes include the primary tumor only, using a 1- to 2-cm dosimetric margin. Localized midline lesions in the pineal or suprasellar regions may be ideal for stereotactic radiotherapy techniques (i.e., fractionated radiosurgery); three-dimensional conformal approaches may be equally advantageous. When using local irradiation after induction chemotherapy, the initial target volume should include the anatomic extent of the tumor at diagnosis; the subsequent boost volume may be restricted to the postchemotherapy region or the pineal region as reconfigured after tumor reduction. For tumors with third ventricular involvement, the initial treatment volume should include the entire third ventricular structure (at a minimum); some would argue to include the entire intracranial ventricular system, a volume only slightly smaller than the full cranium. Advocates of full cranial fields recommend initial coverage to the broader volume, followed typically by a boost to the local tumor. A commitment to local irradiation restricts indications for CSI to those with overt imaging evidence of dissemination (242,248,252,257,266,268,270,271,273).

For malignant germ cell histiotypes, incorporation of a final stereotactic radiosurgical "boost" to the local tumor site may be an appropriate escalation of standard approaches.

Dose

Dose-response data for intracranial germinomas is classically at the 50-Gy level (202, 242,266,267,271). More recent analyses suggest a dose level of 45 Gy may be more appropriate (252,259,273).

The elective dose to the neuraxis (i.e., for M0 disease) is 24 to 25 Gy; in patients with positive cytology, neuraxis levels of 24 to 30 Gy have been used successfully. Similarly, in patients requiring full cranial irradiation or large ventricular volumes, the dose to the initial volume is typically 24 to 30 Gy. The ventricular system then received about 10 Gy. Boost volumes (local or third ventricular) are treated to the same 45 to 50 Gy level, as noted previously.

Successful salvage (for patients with progressive or recurrent disease during or after primary chemotherapy) has been reported with similar doses to the neuraxis (30 Gy) and local tumor region (50 Gy) (183).

Results

Five-year disease-free survival is documented at or above 80% to 90% in reports for pineal region germinomas. Comparable control rates are now reported for suprasellar germinomas (10,242,258,259,266,267,271,273). Short-term results are similar with induction chemotherapy and more limited irradiation (253,261,264). It is important to recognize a 10% to 15% incidence of late failure (202, 252,271). Disease control with primary irradiation seems to be independent of β-HCG elevation among intracranial germinomas; patients with significantly elevated levels (greater than 50 to 70 IU) and pure germinoma do poorly with primary chemotherapy (254,256).

For the aggressive malignant germ cell tumors (i.e., other than germinomas), survival rates at 5 years have been limited to 0% to 33% following irradiation (24,141,199,261, 267,274,275).

REFERENCES

References particularly recommended for further reading are indicated with an asterisk.

1. Gurney JG, Davis S, Severson RK, et al. Trends in cancer incidence among children in the U.S. *Cancer* 1996;78:532–541.
2. Childhood Brain Tumor Consortium. A study of childhood brain tumors based on surgical biopsies from ten North American institutions: sample description. *J Neurooncol* 1988;6:9–23.
*3. Kleihues P, Burger PC, Scheithauer BW. The new WHO classification of brain tumours. *Brain Pathol* 1993;3:255–268.
4. Alger JR, Frank JA, Bizzi A, et al. Metabolism of human gliomas: assessment with H-1 MR spectroscopy and F-18 fluorodeoxyglucose PET1. *Radiology* 1990; 177:633–641.
5. Broniscer A, Gajjar A, Bhargava R, et al. Brain stem involvement in children with neurofibromatosis Type 1: Role of magnetic resonance imaging and spectroscopy in the distinction from diffuse pontine gliomas. *Neurosurgery* 1997;40:331–338.
6. Kollias SS, Barkovich AJ, Edwards MSB. Magnetic resonance analysis of suprasellar tumors of childhood. *Pediatr Neurosurg* 1991–1992;17:284–303.
7. Sutton LN, Wang ZJ, Wehrli SL, et al. Proton spectroscopy of suprasellar tumors in pediatric patients. *Neurosurgery* 1997;41:388–395.
8. Tzika AA, Vigneron DB, Ball WS Jr., et al. Localized proton MR spectroscopy of the brain in children. *J Magn Reson Imaging* 1993;3:719–729.
9. Albright AL, Price RA, Guthkelch AN. Diencephalic gliomas of children: a clinicopathologic study. *Cancer* 1985;55:2789–2793.
10. Edwards MSB, Hudgins RJ, Wilson CB, et al. Pineal region tumors in children. *J Neurosurg* 1988;68: 689–697.
11. Sutton LN, Molloy PT, Sernyak H, et al. Long-term outcome of hypothalamic/chiasmatic astrocytomas in children treated with conservative surgery. *J Neurosurg* 1995;83:583–589.
*12. Bloom HJG, Glees J, Bell J. The treatment of long-term prognosis of children with intracranial tumors: a study of 610 cases, 1950–1981. *Int J Radiat Oncol Biol Phys* 1990;18:723–745.
13. Mulvihill JJ. Clinical ecogenetics: cancer in families. *N Engl J Med* 1985;312:1569.
14. Riccardi VM. Neurofibromatosis: past, present and future. *N Engl J Med* 1991;324:1283–1285.
15. Shearer P, Parham D, Kovnar, et al. Neurofibromatosis type I and malignancy: review of 32 pediatric cases treated at a single institution. *Med Pediatr Oncol* 1994;22:78–83.
16. Lewis RA, Gerson LP, Axelson KA, et al. Von Reck-

linghausen neurofibromatosis. II. Incidence of optic gliomata. *Ophthalmology* 1984;91:929–935.

*17. Jenkin D, Anygalfi S, Becker L, et al. Optic glioma in children: surveillance, resection, or irradiation? *Int J Radiat Oncol Biol Phys* 1993;25:215–225.

18. Listernick R, Darling C, Greenwald MJ, et al. Optic pathway tumors in children: the effect of neurofibromatosis type 1 on clinical manifestations and natural history. *J Pediatr* 1995;127:718-722.

19. Li FP, Fraumeni JF Jr. Soft tissue sarcomas, breast cancer, and other neoplasms: a familial syndrome? *Ann Intern Med* 1969;71:747.

20. Birch JM, Hartley AL, Tricker KJ, et al. Prevalence and diversity of constitutional mutations in the P53 gene among 21 Li-Fraumeni families. *Cancer Res* 1994;54:1298.

21. Neglia JP, Meadows AT, Robinson LL, et al. Second neoplasms after acute lymphoblastic leukemia in chldhood. *N Engl J Med* 1991;325:1330–1336.

22. Rimm IJ, Li FC, Tarbell NJ, et al. Brain tumors after cranial irradiation for childhood acute lymphoblastic leukemia. *Cancer* 1987;59:1506–1508.

23. Walter A, Ochs J, Hudson M, et al. Secondary brain tumors in children treated for ALL on St. Jude Children's Research Hospital. *J Clin Oncol*, 1998. (in press).

24. Jennings MT, Gelman R, Hochberg F. Intracranial germ-cell tumors: natural history and pathogenesis. *J Neurosurg* 1985;63:155–167.

25. Hirsch J-F, Rose CS, Pierre-Kahn A, et al. Benign astrocytic and oligodendrogcytic tumors of the cerebral hemispheres in children. *J Neurosurg* 1989;70: 568–572.

26. Pollack IF, Claassen D, Al-Shboul Q, et al. Low grade gliomas of the cerebral hemispheres in children: an analysis of 71 cases. *J Neurosurg* 1995;82:536–547.

*27. Burger PC, Scheithauer BE, Vogel FS, eds. *Surgical pathology of the nervous system and its coverings*, 3rd ed. New York: Churchill Livingstone, 1991.

28. Russell DS, Rubinstein LJ, eds. *Pathology of tumors of the nervous system.* Baltimore: Williams & Wilkins, 1989.

29. Krouwer HG, Davis RL, Silver P, et al. Gemistocytic astrocytomas: a reappraisal. *J Neurosurg* 1991;74: 399–406.

30. Prayson RA, Estes ML. Protoplasmic astrocytoma. A clinicopathologic study of 16 tumors. *Am J Clin Pathol* 1995;103:705–709.

31. Daumas-Duport C, Scheithauer B, O'Fallon J, et al. Grading of astrocytomas. A simple and reproducible method. *Cancer* 1988;62:2152–2165.

32. Dirks PB, Jay V, Becker LE, et al. Development of anaplastic changes in low-grade astrocytomas of childhood. *Neurosurgery* 1994;34:68–78.

33. Laws ER, Taylor WF, Clifton MB, et al. Neurosurgical management of low-grade astrocytoma of the cerebral hemispheres. *J Neurosurg* 1984;61:665–673.

34. Linskey ME, Gilbert MR. Glial differentiation: a review with implications for new directions in neurooncology. *Neurosurgery* 1995;36:1–22.

35. Furnari FB, Huang H-JS, Cavenee WK. Molecular biology of malignant degeneration of astrocytoma. *Pediatr Neurosurg* 1996;24:41–49.

36. Litofsky NS, Hinton D, Raffel C. The lack of a role for p53 in astrocytomas in pediatric patients. *Neurosurgery* 1994;34:967–973.

*37. Burger PC, Vogel FS, Green SB, et al. Glioblastoma multiforme and anaplastic astrocytoma: pathologic criteria and prognostic implications. *Cancer* 1985;56: 1106–1111.

38. Burger PC, Fuller GN. Pathology trends and pitfalls in histologic diagnosis, immunopathology, and applications of oncogene research. *Neurol Clin* 1991;9: 249–271.

39. Pollack IF, Lunsford LD, Slamovits TL, et al. Stereotactic intracavitary irradiation for cystic craniopharyngiomas. *J Neurosurg* 1988;68:227–233.

40. Gajjar A, Bhargava R, Jenkins JJ, et al. Low-grade astrocytoma with neuraxis dissemination at diagnosis. *J Neurosurg* 1995;83:67–71.

41. Mamelak AN, Prados MD, Obana WG, et al. Treatment options and prognosis for multicentric juvenile pilocytic astrocytoma. *J Neurosurg* 1994;81:24–30.

42. Pollack IF, Hurtt M, Pang D, et al. Dissemination of low grade astrocytomas in children. *Cancer* 1994;73: 2869–2878.

43. Prados M, Mamelak AN. Metastasizing low grade gliomas in children. Redefining an old disease. *Cancer* 1994;73:2671–2673.

44. Kepes JJ, Rubinstein LJ, Eng LF. Pleomorphic xanthoastrocytoma: a distinctive meningocerebral glioma of young subjects with relatively favorable prognosis: a study of 12 cases. *Cancer* 1979;44:1839–1852.

45. Whittle IR, Gordon A, Misra BK, et al. Pleomorphic xanthoastrocytoma—report of four cases. *J Neurosurg* 1989;70:463–468.

46. Zeltzer PM. Toward a cure for infants with brain tumors: the challenge for the 1990's. *Br J Cancer* 1992;66:41–49.

47. Reardon D, Gajjar A, Walter A, et al. Pediatric thalamic gliomas: 10 year St. Jude Children's Research Hospital experience. *J Neurooncol* 1997;33:285.

48. Gajjar A, Sanford RA, Heideman R, et al. Low-grade astrocytoma: a decade of experience at St. Jude Children's Research Hospital. *J Clin Oncol* 1997;15: 2792–2799.

49. Forsyth PA, Shaw EG, Scheithauer BW, et al. Supratentorial pilocytic astrocytomas. *Cancer* 1993;72: 1335–1342.

50. Leibel SA, Sheline GE, Wara WM, et al. The role of radiation therapy in the treatment of astrocytomas. *Cancer* 1975;35:1551–1557.

51. Shaw EG, Daumas-Duport C, Scheithauer BW, et al. Radiation therapy in the management of low-grade supratentorial astrocytomas. *J Neurosurg* 1989;70: 853–861.

52. Shibamoto Y, Kitakubu Y, Takahashi M, et al. Supratentorial low-grade astrocytoma: correlation of computed tomography findings with effect of radiation therapy and prognostic variables. *Cancer* 1993;72: 190–195.

53. Bernstein M, Hoffman HJ, Halliday WC, et al. Thalamic tumors in children: long-term followup and treatment guidelines. *J Neurosurg* 1984;61:649–656.

54. Hoffman HJ, Soloniuk DS, Humphreys RP, et al. Management and outcome of low-grade astrocytomas of the midline in children: a retrospective review. *Neurosurgery* 1993;33:964–971.

55. Wisoff JH, Abbott R, Epstein F. Surgical management of exophytic chiasmatic-hypothalamic tumors of childhood. *J Neurosurg* 1990;73:661–667.

56. Kelly PJ. Stereotactic biopsy and resection of thalamic astrocytomas. *Neurosurgery* 1989;25:185–195.

57. Fletcher WA, Imes RK, Hoyt WF. Chiasmal gliomas: appearance and long-term changes demonstrated by computerized tomography. *J Neurosurg* 1986;65: 154–159.

58. Levin VA, Silver P, Hannigan J. Superiority of post-radiotherapy adjuvant chemotherapy with CCNU, procarbazine, and vincristine (PCV) over BCNU for anaplastic gliomas: NCOG 6G61 final report. *Int J Radiat Oncol Biol Phys* 1990;18:321–324.

59. Tao ML, Barnes PD, Billett AL, et al. Childhood optic chiasm gliomas: radiographic response following radiotherapy and long-term clinical outcome. *Int J Radiat Oncol Biol Phys* 1997;39:579–587.

60. Packer RJ, Ater J, Allen J, et al. Carboplatin and vincristine chemotherapy for children with newly diagnosed progressive low-grade gliomas. *J Neurosurg* 1997;86:747–754.

61. Wallner KE, Gonzales M, Sheline GE. Treatment results of juvenile pilocytic astrocytoma. *J Neurosurg* 1988;69:171–176.

62. Nishio S, Takeshita K, Fujii K, et al. Supratentorial astrocytic tumours of childhood: a clinicopathologic study of 41 cases. *Acta Neurochir* 1989;101:3–8.

63. McLaurin RL, Breneman J, Aron B. Hypothalamic gliomas: review of 18 cases. *Pediatr Neurosurg* 1987;7:19.

64. Woo SY, Donaldson SS, Cox RS. Astrocytoma in children: 14 years' experience at Stanford University Medical Center. *J Clin Oncol* 1988;6:1001–1007.

65. Recht LK, Lew R, Smith TW. Suspected low grade glioma: is deferring treatment safe? *Ann Neurol* 1992; 31:431–436.

66. Boydston WR, Sanford RA, Muhlbauer MS, et al. Gliomas of the tectum and periaqueductal region of the mesencephalon. *Pediatr Neurosurg* 1991;17: 234–238.

67. Morantz RA. Radiation therapy in the treatment of cerebral astrocytoma. *Neurosurgery* 1987;20: 975–982.

68. Leibel SA, Sheline GE. Review article: radiation therapy for neoplasms of the brain. *J Neurosurg* 1987;66:1–22.

69. Muller W, Schroder R. Supratentorial recurrences of gliomas: morphological studies in relation to time intervals with astrocytomas. *Acta Neurochir (Wien)* 1977;37:75–91.

70. Grabb PA, Lunsford LD, Albright AL, et al. Stereotactic radiosurgery for glial neoplasms of childhood. *Neurosurgery* 1996;38:696–702.

71. Leibel SA, Kutcher GJ, Mohan R, et al. Three-dimensional conformal radiation therapy at the Memorial Sloan-Kettering Cancer Center. *Semin Radiat Oncol* 1992;2:274–289.

72. Loeffler JS, Smith AR, Suit HD. The potential role of proton beams in radiation oncology. *Semin Oncol* 1997;24:686–695.

73. Schwade JG, Houkek PV, Landy HJ, et al. Small-field stereotactic external-beam radiation therapy of intracranial lesions: fractionated treatment with a fixed

halo immobilization device. *Radiology* 1990;176: 563–565.

74. Somaza SC, Kondziolka D, Lunsford LD, et al. Early outcomes after stereotactic radiosurgery for growing pilocytic astrocytomas in children. *Pediatr Neurosurg* 1996;25:109–115.

75. Souhami L, Olivier A, Podgorsak EB, et al. Fractionated stereotactic radiation therapy for intracranial tumors. *Cancer* 1991;68:2101–2108.

76. Friedman HS, Krischer JP, Burger P, et al. Treatment of children with progressive or recurrent brain tumors with carboplatin or iproplatin: a Pediatric Oncology Group randomized phase II study. *J Clin Oncol* 1992;10:249–256.

77. Packer RJ, Lange B, Ater J, et al. Carboplatin and vincristine for recurrent and newly diagnosed low grade gliomas of childhood. *J Clin Oncol* 1993;11:850–856.

78. Shaw EG, Scheithauer BW, O'Fallon JR. Management of supratentorial low-grade gliomas. *Oncology* 1993;7:97–107.

79. Dunbar SF, Tarbell NJ, Kooy HM, et al. Stereotactic radiotherapy for pediatric and adult brain tumors: preliminary report. *Int J Radiat Oncol Biol Phys* 1994;30:531–539.

80. Landy HJ, Schwade JG, Houdek PV, et al. Long-term follow-up of gliomas treated with fractionated stereotactic irradiation. *Acta Neurochir* 1994;62:67–71.

81. Krieger MD, Gonzalez-Gomez I, Levy ML, et al. Recurrence patterns and anaplastic change in a long-term study of pilocytic astrocytomas. *Pediatr Neurosurg* 1997;27:1–11.

82. Krouwer HGJ, Prados MD. Infiltrative astrocytomas of the thalamus. *J Neurosurg* 1995;82:548-557.

83. Janss AJ, Grundy R, Cnaan A, et al. Optic pathway and hypothalamic/ chiasmatic gliomas in children younger than age 5 years with a 6-year follow-up. *Cancer* 1995;75:1051–1059.

84. Alvord EC, Lofton S. Gliomas of the optic nerve or chiasm: outcome by patients' age, tumor site, and treatment. *J Neurosurg* 1988;68:85–98.

85. Wong JYC, Wara W, Sheline GE. Optic gliomas: a reanalysis of the University of California, San Francisco, experience. *Cancer* 1987;60:1847–1855.

86. Packer RJ, Savino PJ, Bilaniuk LT, et al. Chiasmatic gliomas of childhood: a reappraisal of natural history and effectiveness of cranial irradiation. *Child's Brain* 1983;10:393–403.

87. Listernick R, Louis DN, Packer RJ, et al. Optic pathway gliomas in children with neurofibromatosis 1: consensus statement from the NF1 Optic Pathway Glioma Task Force. *Ann Neurol* 1997;41:143–149.

88. Hoffman HJ, Humphreys RP, Drake JM, et al. Optic pathway/hypothalamic gliomas: a dilemma in management. *Pediatr Neurosurg* 1993;19:186–195.

89. Hoyt WF, Baghdassarian SA. Optic glioma of childhood: natural history and rationale for conservative management. *Br J Ophthalmol* 1969;53:793–798.

*90. Imes RK, Hoyt WF. Childhood chiasmal gliomas: update on the fate of patients in the 1969 San Francisco study. *Br J Ophthalmol* 1986;70:179–182.

91. Medlock MD, Scott RM. Optic chiasm astrocytomas of childhood. 2. Surgical management. *Pediatr Neurosurg* 1997;27:129–136.

92. Bataini JP, Delanian S, Ponvert D. Chiasmal gliomas:

results of irradiation management in 57 patients and review of literature. *Int J Radiat Oncol Biol Phys* 1991;21:615–623.

93. Horwich A, Bloom HJG. Optic gliomas: radiation therapy and prognosis. *Int J Radiat Oncol Biol Phys* 1985;11:1067.

94. Kestle JRW, Hoffman HJ, Mock AR. Moyamoya phenomenon after radiation for optic glioma. *J Neurosurg* 1993;79:32–35.

95. Rudoltz MS, Regine WF, Langston JW, Kovnar EH, Sanford RA, Kun LE. Multiple causes of cerebrovascular events in children with tumors of the parasellar region. *J Neurooncol* 1998;37:251–261.

96. Sutton LN. Vascular complications of surgery for craniopharyngioma and hypothalamic glioma. *Pediatr Neurosurg* 1994;21:124–128.

97. Packer RJ, Sutton LN, Bilaniuk LT, et al. Treatment of chiasmatic/hypothalamic gliomas of childhood with chemotherapy: an update. *Ann Neurol* 1988;23:79–85.

98. Reedy PD, Bay JW, Hahn JF. Role of radiation therapy in the treatment of cerebral oligodendroglioma: an analysis of 57 cases and a literature review. *Neurosurgery* 1983;67:224-230.

99. Shaw EG, Scheithauer BW, O'Fallon JR, et al. Oligodendrogliomas: the Mayo Clinic experience. *J Neurosurg* 1992;76:428–434.

100. Wallner K, Gonzales M, Sheline GE. Treatment of oligodendrogliomas with or without postoperative radiation. *J Neurosurg* 1988;68:684–688.

101. Dorhman GJ, et al. Oligodendrogliomas in children. *Surg Neurol* 1978;10:21–25.

102. Burger PC, Rawlings CE, Cox, EB, et al. Clinocopathologic correlations in the oligodendroglioma. *Cancer* 1987;59:1345–1352.

103. Heideman RL, Douglass EC, Krance RA, et al. High dose chemotherapy and autologous bone marrow rescue followed by interstitial and external beam radiotherapy in newly diagnosed pediatric malignant gliomas. *J Clin Oncol* 1993;11:1458–1465.

104. Heideman RL, Kuttesch J Jr, Gajjar AJ, et al. Supratentorial malignant gliomas in childhood: a single institution perspective. *Neurosurgery* 1997;80:497–504.

105. Gajjar A, Heideman RL, Kovnar EH, et al. Response of pediatric low grade gliomas to chemotherapy. *Pediatr Neurosurg* 1993;19:113–120.

106. Cairncross JG, MacDonald DR. Successful chemotherapy for recurrent malignant oligodendroglioma. *Ann Neurol* 1988;23:460–464.

107. Allison RR, Schulsinger A, Vongtama V, et al. Radiation and chemotherapy improve outcome in oligodendroglioma. *Int J Radiat Oncol Biol Phys* 1997;37: 399–403.

108. Sanford RA, Kun LE, Langston JW, et al. Pitfalls in the management of low grade gliomas. *Pediatr Neurosurg* 1991;11:133–149.

109. Mork SJ, Lindegaard K-F, Halvorsen TB, et al. Oligodendroglioma: incidence and biological behavior in a defined population. *J Neurosurg* 1985;63:881–889.

110. Shaw EG, Scheithauer BW, Gilbertson DT, et al. Postoperative radiotherapy of supratentorial low grade gliomas. *Int J Radiat Oncol Biol Phys* 1989;16: 663–668.

111. Johnson JH, Hariharan S, Berman J, et al. Clinical outcome of pediatric gangliogliomas: ninety-nine cases over 20 years. *Pediatr Neurosurg* 1997;27:203–207.

112. Garrido E, Becker LF, Hoffman HJ, et al. Gangliogliomas in children: a clinicopathologic study. *Child's Brain* 1978;4:339–346.

113. Mickle JP. Ganglioma in children. A review of 32 cases at the University of Florida. *Pediatr Neurosurg* 1992;18:310–314.

114. Sutton LN, Packer RJ, Rorke LB, et al. Cerebral gangliomas during childhood. *Neurosurgery* 1983;13: 124–128.

115. Daumas-Duport C, Scheithauer BW, Chodkiewicz J-P, et al. Dysembryoblastic neuroepithelial tumors of young patients with intractable partial seizures: report of thirty-nine cases. *Neurosurgery* 1988;23: 545–556.

116. Van den Berg SR, May EE, Rubinstein LJ, et al. Desmoplastic supratentorial neuroepithelial tumors of infancy with divergent differentiation potential ("desmoplastic infantile gangliogliomas"). *J Neurosurg* 1987;66:58–71.

117. Campbell JW, Pollack IF, Martinez AJ, et al. High-grade astrocytomas in children: Radiologically complete resection is associated with an excellent long-term prognosis. *Neurosurgery* 1996;38:258–264.

118. Dropcho EJ, Wisoff JH, Walker RW, et al. Supratentorial malignant gliomas in childhood: a review of 50 cases. *Ann Neurol* 1987;22:355–364.

119. Prados M, Levin V. Malignant supratentorial gliomas in childhood. *Pediatr Neurosci* 1987;13:144–151.

120. Burger PC, Heinz ER, Shibata T, et al. Topographic anatomy and CT correlations in the untreated glioblastoma multiforme. *J Neurosurg* 1988;68:698–704.

121. Halperin EC, Bentel G, Heinz ER, et al. Radiation therapy treatment planning in supratentorial glioblastoma multiforme: an analysis based on post mortem topographic anatomy with CT correlations. *Int J Radiat Oncol Biol Phys* 1989;17:1347–1350.

122. Kelly PJ, Daumas-Duport C, Scheithauer BW, et al. Stereotactic histologic correlations of computed tomography—and magnetic resonance imaging-defined abnormalities in patients with glial neoplasms. *Mayo Clinic Proc* 1987;62:450–459.

123. Finlay JL, Boyett JM, Yates AJ, et al. Randomized phase III trial in childhood high-grade astrocytoma comparing vincristine, lomustine, and prednisone with the eight-drugs-in-1 day regimen. *J Clin Oncol* 1995;13:112–123.

124. Garden AS, Maor MH, Yung WKA, et al. Outcome and patterns of failure following limited-volume irradiation for malignant astrocytomas. *Radiother Oncol* 1991;20:99–110.

125. Liang BC, Thornton AF Jr, Sandler HM, et al. Malignant astrocytomas: focal tumor recurrence after focal external beam radiation therapy. *J Neurosurg* 1991; 75:559–563.

126. Loeffler JS, Alexander E III, Shea WM, et al. Radiosurgery as part of the initial management of patients with malignant gliomas. *J Clin Oncol* 1992;10: 1379–1385.

127. Scharfen CO, Sneed PK, Wara WM, et al. High activity iodine-125 interstitial implant for gliomas. *Int J Radiat Oncol Biol Phys* 1992;24:583–591.

128. Wallner KE, Galicich JH, Krol G, et al. Patterns of failure following treatment for glioblastoma multiforme and anaplastic astrocytoma. *Int J Radiat Oncol Biol Phys* 1989;16:1405–1409.

129. Boyett JM, Yates AJ, Gilles FH, et al. When is a high-grade astrocytoma (HGA) not a HGA? Results of a central review of 226 cases of anaplastic astrocytoma (AA), glioblastoma multiforme (GBM), and other-HGA (Oth-HGA) by five neuropathologists. To be presented at 34th annual ASCO meeting in Los Angeles, 15–18 May, 1998 (abst).

130. Nelson DF, Curran WJ Jr, Scott C, et al. Hyperfractionated radiation therapy and bis-chlorethyl nitrosourea in the treatment of malignant glioma: Possible advantage observed at 72.0 Gy in 1.2 b.i.d. fractions. Report of the Radiation Therapy Oncology Group protocol 8302. *Int J Radiat Oncol Biol Phys* 1993;25:193–207.

*131. Walker MD, Strike TA, Sheline GE. An analysis of dose—effect relationship in the radiotherapy of malignant gliomas. *Int J Radiat Oncol Biol Phys* 1979; 5:1725.

132. Florell RC, Macdonald DR, Irish WD, et al. Selection bias, survival, and brachytherapy for glioma. *J Neurosurg* 1992;76:179–183.

133. Loeffler JS, Alexander E, Wen PJ, et al. Results of stereotactic brachytherapy used in the initial management of patients with glioblastoma. *J Natl Cancer Inst* 1990;82:1918–1921.

134. Prados MD, Gutin PH, Phillips TL, et al. Interstitial brachytherapy for newly diagnosed patients with malignant gliomas: the UCSF experience. *Int J Radiat Oncol Biol Phys* 1992;24:593–597.

135. Fontanesi J, Muhlbauer M, Heideman RL, et al. High activity 125I interstitial irradiation in the treatment of pediatric central nervous system tumors: a pilot study. *Pediatr Neurosurg* 1995;22:289–298.

136. Gutin PH, Edwards MSB, Wara WM, et al. Preliminary experience with 125I-brachytherapy of pediatric brain tumors. *Pediatr Neurosurg* 1985;5:187–206.

137. Voges J, Sturm V, Berthold F, et al. Interstitial irradiation of cerebral gliomas in childhood by permanently implanted 125 iodine–preliminary results. *Klin Padiatr* 1990;202:270–274.

138. Taylor JS, Langston JW, Reddick WE, et al. Clinical value of proton magnetic resonance spectroscopy for differentiating recurrent or residual brain tumor from delayed cerebral necrosis. *Int J Radiat Oncol Biol Phys* 1996;36:1251–1261.

139. Loeffler JS, Rossitch E Jr, Siddon R, et al. Role of stereotactic radiosurgery with a linear accelerator in treatment of intracranial arteriovenous malformations and tumors in children. *Pediatrics* 1990;85: 774–782.

*140. Fine HA, Dear KB, Loeffler JS, Black PM, Canellos GP. Meta-analysis of radiation therapy with and without adjuvant chemotherapy for malignant gliomas in adults. *Cancer* 1993;71:2585–2597.

141. Patel SR, Buckner JC, Smithson WA, et al. Cisplatin-based chemotherapy in primary central nervous system germ cell tumors. *J Neurooncol* 1992;12:47–52.

142. Sposto R, Ertel IJ, Jenkin RDT, et al. The effectiveness of chemotherapy for treatment of high grade astrocytoma in children: results of a randomized trial. *J Neurooncol* 1989;7:165–177.

143. Finlay JL, August C, Packer R, et al. High-dose multi-agent chemotherapy followed by bone marrow "rescue" for malignant astrocytomas of childhood and adolescence. *J Neurooncol* 1990;9:239–248.

144. Garvin J, Finlay J, Walker R, et al. High dose chemotherapy and autologous bone marrow rescue for high-risk central nervous system (CNS) tumors in children under six years of age. *Proc ASCO* 1992;11(abstr).

145. Cohen BH, Packer RJ, Siegel KR, et al. Brain tumors in children under 2 years: treatment, survival and long-term prognosis. *Pediatr Neurosurg* 1993;19: 171–179.

*146. Duffner PK, Cohen ME, Myers MH, et al. Survival of children with brain tumors: SEER program, 1973–1980. *Neurology* 1986;36:597–601.

147. Stiller CA, Bunch KJ. Brain and spinal tumors in children aged under two years: incidence and survival in Britain, 1971–85. *Br J Cancer* 1992;66:S50–S53.

148. Brown K, Mapstone TB, Oakes WJ. A modern analysis of intracranial tumors of infancy. *Pediatr Neurosurg* 1997;26:25–32.

*149. Duffner PK, Horowitz ME, Krischer JP, et al. Postoperative chemotherapy and delayed radiation in children less than three years of age with malignant brain tumors. *N Engl J Med* 1993;328:1725–1731.

150. Gilles FH, Sobel EL, Tavare CJ, et al. Age-related changes in diagnoses, histological features, and survival in children with brain tumors: 1930–1979. *Neurosurgery* 1995;37:1056–1068.

151. Duffner PK, Kun LE, Burger PC, et al. Postoperative chemotherapy and delayed radiation in infants and very young children with choroid plexus carcinomas. *Pediatr Neurosurg* 1995;22:189–196.

152. Pancalet P, Sainte-Rose C, Lellough-Tubiana A, et al. Papillomas and carcinomas of the choroid plexus in children. *J Neurosurg* 1998;88:521–528.

153. Taratuto AL, Monges J, Lylyk P, et al. Superficial cerebral astrocytoma attached to dura: Report of six cases in infants. *Cancer* 1984;54:2505–2512.

154. Jenkin D, Greenberg M, Hoffman H, et al. Brain tumors in children: long-term survival after radiation therapy. *Int J Radiat Oncol Biol Phys* 1995;31: 445–451.

155. Albright AL, Wisoff JH, Zeltzer PM, et al. Current neurosurgical treatment or medulloblastoma in children. *Pediatr Neurosurg* 1989;177:633–641.

156. Stein BM. Surgical therapy of benign pineal tumors. In: Neuwelt EA, ed. *Diagnosis and treatment of pineal region tumors.* Baltimore: Williams & Wilkins, 1984:254–272.

157. Jannoun L, Bloom HJG. Long-term psychological effects in children treated for intracranial tumors. *Int J Radiat Oncol Biol Phys* 1990;18:747–753.

158. Johnson DL, McCabe MA, Nicholson HS, et al. Quality of long-term survival in young children with medulloblastoma. *J Neurosurg* 1994;80:1004–1010.

159. Mulhern RK, Hancock J, Fairclough D, et al. Neuropsychological status of children treated for brain tumors: a critical review and integrative analysis. *Med Pediatr Oncol* 1992;20:181–191.

160. Shalat S, Beardwell C, Pearson D, et al. The effect of varying doses of cerebral irradiation on growth hormone production in children. *J Endocrinol* 1976;8: 287–290.

161. Deutsch M. Radiotherapy for primary brain tumors in very young children. *Cancer* 1982;50:2785–2789.

162. Jooma R, Hayward RD, Grant DN. Intracranial neoplasms during the first year of life: analysis of 100 consecutive cases. *Neurosurgery* 1984;14:31–41.

163. Evans AE, Jenkin RDT, Sposto R, et al. The treatment of medulloblastoma. Results of a prospective randomized trial of radiation therapy with and without CCNU, vincristine, and prednisone. *J Neurosurg* 1990;72:572–582.

164. Hughes EN, Shillioto J, Sallan SE, et al. Medulloblastoma at the Joint Center for Radiation Therapy between 1968–1984. The influence of radiation dose on the patterns of failure and survival. *Cancer* 1988;61:1992–1998.

165. Tait DM, Thornton-James H, Bloom HCG, et al. Adjuvant chemotherapy for medulloblastoma: the first multicentre control trial of the International Society of Pediatric Oncology (ISOP I). *Eur J Cancer* 1990;26:464–469.

166. Sutton LN, Goldwein J, Perilongo G, et al. Prognostic factors in childhood ependymomas. *Pediatr Neurosurg* 1990–1991;16:57-65.

*167. Ater JL, van Eys J, Woo SY, et al. MOPP chemotherapy without irradiation as primary postsurgical therapy for brain tumors in infants and young children. *J Neurooncol* 1997;32:243–252.

168. Geyer JR, Zeltzer PM, Boyett JM, et al. Survival of infants with primitive neuroectodermal tumors or malignant ependymomas of the CNS treated with eight drugs in 1 day: a report from the Children's Cancer Group. *J Clin Oncol* 1994;12:1607–1615.

169. Kuhl J, Beck J, Bode U, et al. Delayed radiation therapy (RT) after postoperative chemotherapy (PCH) in children less than 3 years of age with medulloblastoma. Results of the trial HIT-SKK'87, and preliminary results of the pilot trial HIT-SKK'92. *Med Pediatr Oncol* 1995;25:250.

170. Mason WP, Grovas A, Halpern S, et al. Intensive chemotherapy and bone marrow rescue for young children with newly diagnosed malignant brain tumors. *J Clin Oncol* 1998;16:210–221.

*171. Duffner PK, Krischer JP, Burger PC, et al. Treatment of infants with malignant gliomas: The Pediatric Oncology Group experience. *J Neurooncol* 1996;28:245–256.

172. Duffner PK, Krischer JP, Sanford RA, et al. Prognostic factors in infants and very young children with intracranial ependymomas. Pediatric Neurosurgery '98 (Proceedings from Ependymoma meeting, New York, 21–23 Nov '97. (*In press*, 1998).

173. Gajjar A, Mulhern RK, Heideman RL, et al. Medulloblastoma in very young children: outcome of definitive craniospinal irradiation following incomplete response to chemotherapy. *J Clin Oncol* 1994;12:1212–1216.

174. Zeltzer P, Boyett J, Finlay J, et al. Prognostic factors for survival in high risk primitive neuroectodermal tumors (PNET)s in children: report from the Children's Cancer Group CCG-921. *Proc ASCO* 1993;12:415.

175. Tomita T, McLone DG, et al. Brain tumors during the first twenty-four months of life. *Neurosurgery* 1985;17:913–919.

176. Albright AL, Wisoff JH, Zeltzer P, et al. Prognostic factors in children with supratentorial (nonpineal) primitive neuroectodermal tumors. A neurosurgical perspective from the Children's Cancer Group. *Pediatr Neurosurg* 1995;22:1–7.

177. Albright AL, Wisoff JH, Zeltzer PM, et al. Effects of medulloblastoma resections on outcome in children:

a report from the Children's Cancer Group. *Neurosurgery* 1996;38:265–271.

178. Geyer JR, Finlay JL, Boyett JM, et al. Survival of infants with malignant astrocytomas. A report from the Children's Cancer Group. *Cancer* 1995;75:1045–1050.

179. Horowitz ME, Mulhern RK, Kun LE, et al. Brain tumors in the very young child. Postoperative chemotherapy in combined-modality treatment. *Cancer* 1988;61:428–434.

180. Packer RJ, Sutton LN, Atkins TE, et al. A prospective study of cognitive function in children receiving whole-brain radiotherapy and chemotherapy: 2-year results. *J Neurosurg* 1989;70:707–713.

181. Walter A, Gajjar A, Heideman R, et al. Survival of young children with medulloblastoma at St. Jude Children's Research Hospital. To be presented at American Society of Clinical Oncology 34th Annual Meeting, Los Angeles, CA, 16–19 May, 1998. (abstr).

182. Dupuis-Girod S, Hartmann O, Benhamou E, et al. Will high dose chemotherapy followed by autologous bone marrow transplantation supplant cranio-spinal irradiation in young children treated for medulloblastoma? *J Neurooncol* 1996;27:87–98.

183. Merchant TE, David BJ, Sheldon JM, et al. Radiation therapy for relapsed CNS germinoma after primary chemotherapy. *J Clin Oncol* 1998;16:204–209.

184. Shrieve DC, Tarbell NJ, Alexander E, et al. Stereotactic radiotherapy; a technique for dose optimization and escalation for intracranial tumors. *Acta Neurochir* 1994;62:118–123.

185. Goldwein JW, Radcliffe J, Packer RJ, et al. Results of a pilot study of low-dose craniospinal radiation therapy plus chemotherapy for children younger than 5 years with primitive neuroectodermal tumors. *Cancer* 1993;71:2647–2652.

186. Jakacki RI, Zeltzer PM, Boyett JM, et al. Survival and prognostic factors following radiation and/or chemotherapy for primitive neuroectodermal tumors of the pineal region in infants and children: a report of the Children's Cancer Group. *J Clin Oncol* 1995;13:1377–1383.

187. Rorke LB, Packer RJ, Biegel JA, et al. Central nervous system atypical teratoid/rhabdoid tumors of infancy and childhood: definition of an entity. *J Neurosurg* 1996;85:56–65.

188. Kleihues P. Neuroepithelial tumours. In: Kleihues P, Burger PC, Scheithauer BW, eds. *Histological typing of tumours of the central nervous system.* New York: Springer-Verlag, 1994.

189. Pigott TJ, Punt JAG, Lowe JS, et al. The clinical, radiological and histopathological features of cerebral primitive neuroectodermal tumours. *Br J Neurosurg* 1990;4:287–298.

*190. Hart MN, Earle KM. Primitive neuroectodermal tumors of the brain in children. *Cancer* 1973;32:890–897.

191. Cruz-Sanchez FF, Rossi ML, Hughes JT, et al. Differentiation in embryonal neuroepithelial tumors of the central nervous system. *Cancer* 1991;67:965–976.

192. Raffel C, Gilles FE, Weinberg KI. Reduction of homozygosity and gene amplification in central nervous system primitive neuroectodermal tumors of childhood. *Cancer Res* 1990;50:587–591.

*193. Rorke LB. The cerebellar medulloblastoma and its relationship to primitive neuroectodermal tumors (presidential address). *J Neuropathol Exp Neurol* 1983;42:1–15.

194. Rubinstein LJ. Embryonal central neuroepithelial tumors and their differentiating potential [review article]. *J Neurosurg* 1985;62:795–805.

*195. Berger MS, Edwards MSB, Wara WM, et al. Primary cerebral neuroblastoma: long-term followup review and therapeutic guidelines. *J Neurosurg* 1983;59: 418–423.

196. Molloy PT, Yachnis AT, Rorke LB, et al. Central nervous system medulloepithelioma: A series of eight cases including two arising in the pons. *J Neurosurg* 1996;84:430–436.

197. Bennett JP, Rubinstein LJ. The biological behavior of primary cerebral neuroblastoma: a reappraisal of the clinical course in a series of 70 cases. *Ann Neurol* 1984;16:21–27.

198. Herrick MK, Rubinstein LJ. The cytological differentiating potential of pineal parenchymal neoplasms (true pinealomas), a clinicopathological study of 28 tumours. *Brain* 1979;102:280–320.

199. Linggood RM, Chapman PH. Pineal tumors. *J Neurooncol* 1992;12:85–91.

200. Horten BC, Rubinstein LJ. Primary cerebral neuroblastoma: a clinicopathological study of 35 cases. *Brain* 1976;99:735–736.

201. Gururangan S, Heideman RL, Kovnar EH, et al. Peritoneal metastases in two patients with pineoblastoma and ventriculoperitoneal shunts. *Med Pediatr Oncol* 1994;22:417–420.

202. Rich TA, Cassady Jr, Strand RD, et al. Radiation therapy for pineal and suprasellar germ cell tumors. *Cancer* 1985;55:932–940.

203. Hanna SL, Langston JW, Parham DM, et al. Primary malignant rhabdoid tumor of the brain: clinical, imaging, and pathologic findings. *J Neuroradiol* 1993; 14:107–115.

204. Olson TA, Bayar E, Kosnik E, et al. Successful treatment of disseminated central nervous system malignant rhabdoid tumor. *J Pediatr Hematol Oncol* 1995; 17:71–75.

205. Gaffney CC, Sloane JP, Bradley NJ, et al. Primitive neuroectodermal tumours of the cerebrum: pathology and treatment. *J Neurooncol* 1985;3:23–33.

206. Kosnik EJ, Boesel CP, Bay J, et al. Primitive neuroectodermal tumors of the central nervous system in children. *J Neurosurg* 1978;48:741–746.

207. Packer RJ, et al. Early results of reduced-dose radiotherapy plus chemotherapy for children with nondisseminated medulloblastoma (MB): a Children's Cancer Group Study. *Pediatr Neurosurg* 1995;55: 518.

208. Adamson TE, Wiestler OD, Kleihues P, et al. Correlation of clinical and pathological features in surgically treated craniopharyngiomas. *J Neurosurg* 1990; 73:12–17.

209. Tomita T, McLone DG. Radical resections of childhood craniopharyngiomas. *Pediatr Neurosurg* 1993; 19:6–14.

210. Hoffman HJ, De Silva M, Humphreys RP, et al. Aggressive surgical management of craniopharyngiomas in children. *J Neurosurg* 1992;76:47–52.

211. Hoffman HJ. Surgical management of craniopharyngioma. *Pediatr Neurosurg* 1994;21:44–49.

212. Anderson CA, Wilkening GN, Filley CM, et al. Neurobehavioral outcome in pediatric craniopharyngioma. *Pediatr Neurosurg* 1997;26:255–260.

213. Rajan B, Ashley S, Gorman C, et al. Craniopharyngioma–long term results following limited surgery and radiotherapy. *Radiother Oncol* 1993;26:1–10.

214. Weiss M, Sutton L, Marcial V, et al. The role of radiation therapy in the management of childhood craniopharyngioma. *Int J Radiat Oncol Biol Phys* 1989; 17:1313–1321.

215. Yarsargil MG, Curcic M, Kis S, et al. Total removal of craniopharyngiomas. Approaches and long-term results in 144 patients. *J Neurosurg* 1990;73:3–11.

216. Matson DD. Craniopharyngiomas. *Neurosurgery of infancy and childhood.* Springfield, IL: Charles C. Thomas, 1969:544–574.

217. Sanford RA. Craniopharyngioma: results of survey of the American Society of Pediatric Neurosurgery. *Pediatr Neurosurg* 1994;21:39–43.

218. Scott RM, Hetelekidis S, Barnes PD, Goumnerova L, Tarbell NJ. Surgery, radiation, and combination therapy in the treatment of childhood cranio-pharyngioma—a 20-year experience. *Pediatr Neurosurg* 1994;21:75–81.

219. Wen B-C, Hussey DH, Staples J, et al. A comparison of the roles of surgery and radiation therapy in the management of craniopharyngiomas. *Int J Radiat Oncol Biol Phys* 1989;16:17–24.

220. DeVile CJ, Grant DB, Kendall BE, et al. Management of childhood craniopharyngioma: can the morbidity of radical surgery be predicted? *J Neurosurg* 1996;85:73–81.

*221. Hetelikidis S, Barnes PD, Tao ML, et al. Twenty year experience in childhood craniopharyngioma. *Int J Radiat Oncol Biol Phys* 1993;27:189–195.

222. Sweet WH. History of surgery for craniopharyngiomas. *Pediatr Neurosurg* 1994;21:28–38.

223. Curtis J, Daneman D, Hoffman HJ, et al. The endocrine outcome after surgical removal of craniopharyngiomas. *Pediatr Neurosurg* 1994;21:24–27.

224. Sklar CA. Craniopharyngioma: endocrine sequelae of treatment. *Pediatr Neurosurg* 1994;21:120–123.

225. Kramer S, McKissock W, Concannon JP. Craniopharyngiomas: treatment by combined surgery and radiation therapy. *J Neurosurg* 1961;18:217–226.

226. Kramer S, Southard M, Mansfield CM. Radiotherapy in the management of craniopharyngiomas: further experience and late results. *Am J Roentgenol Radium Ther Nucl Med* 1968;103:44–52.

227. Regine WF, Kramer S. Pediatric craniopharyngiomas: long-term results of combined treatment with surgery and radiation. *Int J Radiat Oncol Biol Phys* 1992;24:611–617.

228. Brada M, Thomas DGT. Craniopharyngioma revisited. *Int J Radiat Oncol Biol Phys* 1993;27:471–475.

229. Fischer EG, Welch K, Shillito J Jr, et al. Craniopharyngiomas in children. Long-term effects of conservative surgical procedures combined with radiation therapy. *J Neurosurg* 1990;73:534–540.

230. Laws ER. Conservative surgery and radiation for childhood craniopharyngiomas. *J Neurosurg* 1991; 74:1025.

231. Lunsford LD, Pollack BE, Kondziolka DS, et al. Stereotactic options in the management of craniopharyngioma. *Pediatr Neurosurg* 1994;21:90–97.

232. Constine L, Randall SH, Rubin P, McDonald J. Craniopharyngiomas: fluctuation in size following surgery and radiation therapy. *Neurosurgery* 1989;24: 53–59.

233. Backlund E-O, Axelsson B, Bergstrand C-G, et al. Treatment of craniopharyngiomas—the stereotactic approach in a ten to twenty-three years' perspective. I. Surgical, radiological and ophthalmological aspects. *Acta Neurochir* 1989;99:11–19.

234. Kooy HM, van Herk M, Barnes PD, et al. Image fusion for stereotactic radiotherapy and radiosurgery treatment planning. *Int J Radiat Oncol Biol Phys* 1994;28:1229-1234.

235. Stephanian E, Lunsford LD, Coffey RJ, Bissonette DJ, Flickinger JC. Gamma knife surgery for sellar and suprasellar tumors. *Neurosurg Clin N Am* 1992; 3:207–212.

236. Van den Berge JH, Blaauw G, Breeman WAP, et al. Intracavitary brachytherapy of cystic craniopharyngiomas. *J Neurosurg* 1992;77:545–550.

237. Flickinger JC, Lunsford LD, Singer J, et al. Megavoltage external beam irradiation of craniopharyngiomas: analysis of tumor control and morbidity. *Int J Radiat Oncol Biol Phys* 1990;19:117–122.

238. Herrick MK. Pathology of pineal tumors. In: Neuwelt EA, ed. *Diagnosis and treatment of pineal region tumors.* Baltimore: Williams & Wilkins, 1984:31–60.

239. Glenn OA, Barkovich AJ. Intracranial germ cell tumors: a comprehensive review of proposed embryonic derivation. *Pediatr Neurosurg* 1996;24:242–251.

240. Ho DM, Lieu H-C. Primary intracranial germ cell tumor. Pathologic study of 51 patients. *Cancer* 1992; 70:1577–1584.

241. Huh SJ, Shin KH, Kim H, et al. Radiotheray of intracranial germinomas. *Radiother Oncol* 1996;38: 19–23.

242. Legido A, Packer RJ, Sutton LN, et al. Suprasellar germinomas in childhood. A reappraisal. *Cancer* 1989;63:340–344.

243. Yasue M, Tanaka H, Nakajima M, et al. Germ cell tumors of the basal ganglia and thalamus. *Pediatr Neurosurg* 1993;19:121–126.

244. Bjornsson J, Scheithauer BW, Okazaki H, et al. Intracranial germ cell tumors: pathological and immunohistochemical aspects of 70 cases. *J Neuropathol Exp Neurol* 1985;44:32–46.

245. Felix I, Becker LE. Intracranial germ cell tumors in children: an immunohistochemical and electron microscopic study. *Pediatr Neurosurg* 1990–1991;16: 156–162.

246. Borit A, Blackwood W, Mair WGP. The separation of pineocytoma from pineoblastoma. *Cancer* 1980;45: 1408–1418.

247. DiSclafani A, Hudgins RJ, Edwards MSB, et al. Pineocytomas. *Cancer* 1989;63:302–304.

248. Schild SE, Scheithauer BW, Schomberg PJ, et al. Pineal parenchymal tumors. Clinical, pathologic, and therapeutic aspects. *Cancer* 1993;72:870–880.

249. Erlich SS, Apuzzo MLJ. The pineal gland: anatomy, physiology, and clinical significance. *J Neurosurg* 1985;63:321–341.

250. Sung D, Harisiadis L, Chang CG. Midline pineal tumors and suprasellar germinomas: highly curable by irradiation. *Radiology* 1978;128:745–751.

251. Dayan AD, Marshall AHE, Miller AA, et al. Atypical teratomas of the pineal and hypothalamus. *J Pathol Bacteriol* 1966;92:1–28.

*252. Haddock MG, Schild SE, Scheithauer BW, et al. Radiation therapy for histologically confirmed primary central nervous system germinoma. *Int J Radiat Oncol Biol Phys* 1997;38:915–923.

253. Allen JC. Controversies in the management of intracranial germ cell tumors. *Neurol Clin* 1991;9:441–452.

254. Balmaceda C, Diez B, Villablanca J, et al. Chemotherapy only strategy in primary central nervous system germ cell tumors (CNS GCT): results of an international study. *J Neurooncol* 1993;15:S3.

255. Balmaceda C, Heller G, Rosenblum M, et al. Chemotherapy without irradiation: a novel approach for newly-diagnosed central nervous system (CNS) germ cell tumors (GCT): results of an international cooperative trial. *J Clin Oncol* 1996;14:2908–2915.

256. Shibamoto Y, Takahashi M, Sasai K. Prognosis of intracranial germinoma with syncytiotrophoblastic giant cells treated by radiation therapy. *Int J Radiat Oncol Biol Phys* 1997;37:505-510.

257. Shibamoto Y, Abe M, Yamashita J, et al. Treatment results of intracranial germinoma as a function of the irradiation volume. *Int J Radiat Oncol Biol Phys* 1988;15:285–290.

258. Shibamoto Y, Takahashi M, Abe M. Reduction of the radiation dose for intracranial germinoma: A prospective study. *Br J Cancer* 1994;70:984–989.

*259. Shirato H, Nishio M, Sawamura Y, et al. Analysis of long-term treatment of intracranial germinoma. *Int J Radiat Oncol Biol Phys* 1997;37:511–515.

*260. Wolden SL, Wara WM, Larson DA, et al. Radiation therapy for primary intracranial germ-cell tumors. *Int J Radiat Oncol Biol Phys* 1995;32:943–949.

261. Allen JC, Kim JH, Packer RJ. Neoadjuvant chemotherapy for newly diagnosed germ-cell tumors of the central nervous system. *J Neurosurg* 1987;67:65–70.

262. Allen JC, DaRosso RC, Donahue B. A phase II trial of preirradiation carboplatin in newly diagnosed germinoma of the central nervous system. *Cancer* 1994; 74:940–944.

263. Calaminus G, Bamberg M, Baranzelli MC, et al. Intracranial germ cell tumors: a comprehensive update of the European data. *Neuropediatrics* 1994;25:26–32.

264. Sawamura Y, Shirato H, Ikeda, et al. Induction chemotherapy followed by reduced-volume radiation therapy for newly diagnosed central nervous system germinoma. *J Neurosurg* 1998;88:66–72.

265. Yoshida J, Sugita K, Kobayashi T, et al. Prognosis of intracranial germ cell tumors: Effectiveness of chemotherapy with cisplatin and etoposide (CDDP and VP16). *Acta Neurochir* 1993;120:111–117.

266. Jenkin D, Berry M, Chan H, et al. Pineal region germinomas in childhood: treatment considerations. *Int J Radiat Oncol Biol Phys* 1990;18:541–545.

267. Dearnaley DP, A'Hern RP, Whittaker S, et al. Pineal and CNS germ cell tumors: Royal Marsden Hospital experience 1962–1987. *Int J Radiat Oncol Biol Phys* 1990;18:773–781.

*268. Linstadt D, Wara WM, Edwards MSB, et al. Radiotherapy of primary intracranial germinomas: the case against routine craniospinal irradiation. *Int J Radiat Oncol Biol Phys* 1988;15:291–297.

269. Wara WM, Jenkin RDT, Evans A, et al. Tumors of the pineal and suprasellar region: Children's Cancer

Study Group treatment results 1960–1975. A report from Children's Cancer Study Group. *Cancer* 1979; 43:698–701.

270. Dempsey PK, Lunsford LD. Stereotactic radiosurgery for pineal regional tumors. *Neurosurg Clin N Am* 1992;3:245–253.

271. Glanzmann C, Seelentag W. Radiotherapy for tumours of the pineal region and suprasellar germinomas. *Radiother Oncol* 1989;15:31–40.

*272. Dattoli MJ, Newall J. Radiation therapy for intracranial germinoma: the case for limited volume treatment. *Int J Radiat Oncol Biol Phys* 1991;19:429–433.

273. Shibamoto Y, Oda Y, Yamashita J, et al. The role of cerebrospinal fluid cytology in radiotherapy planning for intracranial germinoma. *Int J Radiat Oncol Biol Phys* 1994;29:1089–1094.

274. Graziano SL, Paolozzi FP, Rudolph AR, et al. Mixed germ-cell tumor of the pineal region. *J Neurosurg* 1987;66:300–304.

275. Kobayashi T, Yoshida J, Ishyama J, et al. Combination chemotherapy with cisplatin and etoposide for malignant intracranial germ-cell tumors. An experimental and clinical study. *J Neurosurg* 1989;70: 676–681.

Tumors of the Posterior Fossa
and the Spinal Canal

The posterior fossa occupies the lower one-half of the posterior aspect of the cranium, bounded *anteriorly* by the clivus and posterior clinoid and *posteriorly* by the calvarium, at and below the level of the inion (Fig. 1). Inferiorly, the posterior fossa is bordered by the occipital bone; laterally, it is bordered by portions of the temporal, occipital, and parietal bones. Superiorly, the margin is defined by the tentorium cerebellae, i.e., portion of the dura mater extending from the basisphenoid adjacent to the posterior clinoid, rising to cover the cerebellum, and extending posteriorly and inferiorly to insert at the level of the inion. The cerebellum and brainstem are contained within the posterior fossa. Over one-half of all childhood brain tumors arise in the posterior fossa. The most common types are medulloblastoma, low-grade astrocytomas of the cerebellum, brainstem tumors, and ependymomas (1,2) (see Table 1, Chapter 3). In this chapter, we address the more common posterior fossa tumors and the relatively uncommon spinal cord tumors in children.

MEDULLOBLASTOMA

Medulloblastoma is a primitive cerebellar tumor of neuroectodermal origin. The tumor accounts for 20% of pediatric brain tumors, or approximately 400 cases per year in the United States (1). Medulloblastoma was first identified in Bailey and Cushing's 1925 classification of central nervous system (CNS) tumors (3,4). The classic description defined medulloblastoma as a primitive or embryonal tumor of the cerebellum, theoretically derived from the progenitor medulloblast located in the external granular layer of the cerebellum.

In 1983, Rorke proposed a broader "umbrella" concept of primitive neuroectodermal tumors (PNETs), including medulloblastoma as one of a group of related "small, round, blue cell" embryonal tumors occurring throughout the CNS (5). Tumors categorized as PNETs also include those classically identified as medulloepithelioma, ependymoblastoma, cerebral neuroblastoma, and pineoblastoma, all typically comprised of immature small, round, blue cells and sharing a tendency toward subarachnoid dissemination. Included are tumors that show little differentiation or show multiple, divergent lines of differentiation (i.e., without a dominant component) and have been classically characterized by location, e.g., medulloblastoma in the posterior fossa, pineoblastoma in the pineal region, supratentorial (cerebral hemispheric) PNET, as described by Hart and Earle (5,6). The PNETs share relative responsiveness to chemotherapy and irradiation (5). The concept has not been uniformly accepted; several prominent neuropathologists have strongly favored retaining the nomenclature for specific histiotypes based on unique differences in histology, site-specific behavior, and outcome (7–9). There has also been confusion with the peripheral or extraneural PNETs (e.g., extra-

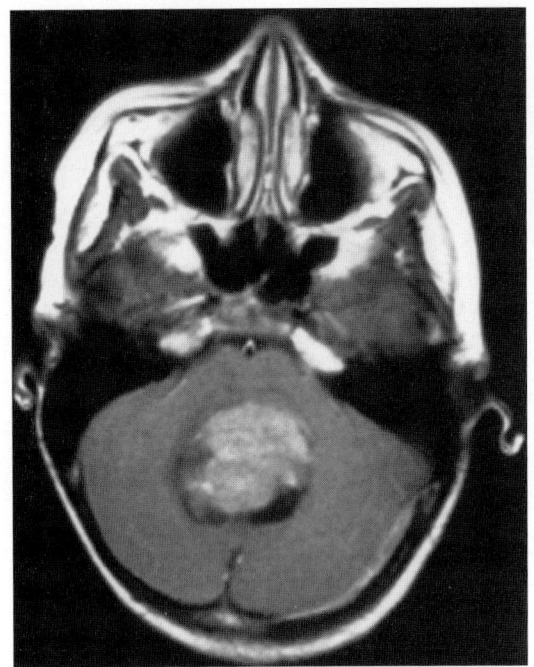

A

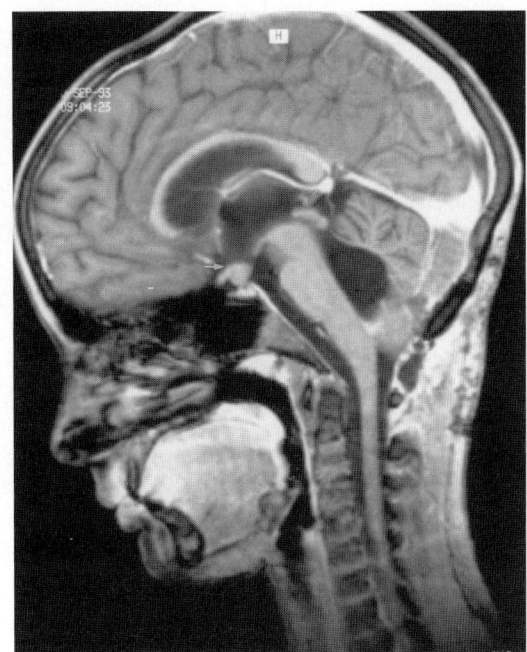

B

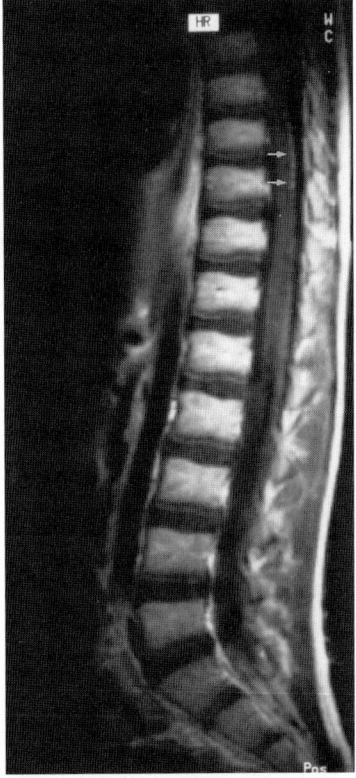

C

FIG. 1. Medulloblastoma, originating classically in the cerebellar vermis **(A)** and **(B)**, with signs of subarachnoid spread in the hypothalamic region **(B)** and along the spine **(C)**.

osseous Ewing's sarcoma or peripheral neuroepithelioma), tumors that are not related to the so-called PNETs arising within the CNS.

The 1993 World Health Organization (WHO) classification of CNS neoplasms attempts to rationalize the PNET concept, grouping most of the primitive tumors as "embryonal neoplasms" and retaining the specific identity of those tumors with specific lines of differentiation (e.g., ependymoblastoma, neuroblastoma) (8,10) (see Table 2, Chapter 3). Pineoblastomas are listed separately by anatomic site, categorized amongst pineal region tumors. The WHO classification recognizes embryonal tumors of divergent or little differentiation as PNETs; those occurring in the posterior fossa retain the designation of medulloblastoma (8,10). Histologically similar supratentorial tumors that lack specific or dominant lines of differentiation are coded as "supratentorial PNETs."

Histologically, medulloblastoma is a densely cellular neoplasm comprised predominantly of small, round, blue cells. The putative "medulloblast" had been theorized as a primitive cell of the cerebellar external granular layer active during embryogenesis. The origin has now been identified from the actively replicating cells of the subependymal matrix zone located in the external granular layer of the posterior medullary velum (11,12). Differentiation may be apparent toward neuronal and/or glial (astrocytic, oligodendroglial, and, less commonly, ependymal) lines; differentiation along mesenchymal lines (primary muscular) may be present as a variant termed medullomyoblastoma (12,13). Recent data suggests that tumors with cytochemical evidence of glial or neuronal differentiation are associated with relatively unfavorable outcome (14). Cytogenetic findings include loss of 17p, 10q, 16q, or chromosome 11 in 30% to 40% of cases; in addition, excess of 17q or chromosome 7 has been noted in nearly 20% of cases (15–17).

The median age at diagnosis is 5- to 6-years old. Approximately 20% of medulloblastomas present in infants less than 2-years old; the tumor occurs uncommonly in adults. Boys are affected more often than girls (18). In the Duke University Medical Center medulloblastoma series, the four most common presenting symptoms were vomiting (67% of patients), headache (60%), ataxia (40%), and nausea (39%) (19). Increased intracranial pressure results from tumor obstructing cerebrospinal fluid (CSF) flow through the Sylvian aqueduct and fourth ventricle. Between 50% and 75% of patients present to medical attention with less than or approximately 3 months of symptoms. It appears that a short duration of symptoms is associated with the diagnosis of more advanced medulloblastoma (20). Increased intracranial pressure results from tumor obstructing CSF flow through the Sylvian aqueduct and fourth ventricle. The most common signs are papilledema and truncal ataxia; cranial nerve abnormalities (especially the fifth) are less common. The tumor may arise laterally within the cerebellar hemispheres, particularly in adolescents.

Medulloblastomas arise most often in the midline cerebellar vermis. The tumor characteristically grows into the fourth ventricle, obstructing CSF. Infiltration around the fourth ventricle is common, often involving the brachium pontis and extending onto the ventricular floor (i.e., the brainstem). Cranial magnetic resonance imaging (MRI) is the definitive diagnostic study (21). Medulloblastomas are relatively well-defined, typically solid lesions with uniform or, less often, nonhomogeneous contrast enhancement. By computerized tomography (CT) scan, the tumor is often hyperdense, reflecting high cellularity.

Medulloblastoma is the classic CNS tumor associated with CSF seeding or metastasis. Subarachnoid dissemination is reported at diagnosis in 10% to 30% of children at diagnosis (22,23). Tumor deposits are documented by gadolinium-enhanced spinal or cranial MRI in 10% to 20% of cases; lumbar CSF cytology is positive less often (less than 5% to 10% as an isolated finding, 10% with concurrent imaging evidence of metastasis) (24). Neuraxis disease typically involves the spinal subarachnoid space; intracranial metastasis is less frequent, often noted in the region of the basal or suprasellar cisterns (Figs. 1–2). Postoperative staging requires: (a) imaging of the brain to assess degree of resection and potential subarachnoid metastasis (ideally within 24 hours, but acceptable up to 72 hours postsurgery); (b) spinal MRI (gadolinium-enhanced study approximately 10 to 14 days postsurgery to assess potential overt metastasis); and (c) lumbar CSF cytology (best obtained immediately after spinal imaging).

The Chang staging system has been used for staging medulloblastoma (25). The system was developed in the pre-CT era and is based on the size and invasiveness of the primary tumor at surgery and evidence of spread outside the posterior fossa (Table 1). Tumors are considered "early T-stage" with T1 to T3a lesions (i.e., tumors involving the fourth ventricular region without brainstem involvement); "high T-stage" tumors include those with infiltration of the brainstem (T3b) or extension beyond the posterior fossa (T4). Imaging diagnosis of brainstem invasion is not as reliable as surgical observation. "M" stage is based on subarachnoid metastasis, progressively coding abnormal CSF cytology (M1) or imaging evidence of noncontiguous tumor within the cranium (M2) or spine (M3). Extraneural disease (most often confined to the bone marrow) is present in less than 1% to 2% of cases at presentation, coded as M4. There is little data to substantiate any current role for "T" stage as an independent parameter predicting outcome or defining therapy (24,26–28). A comparison of otherwise "early medulloblas-

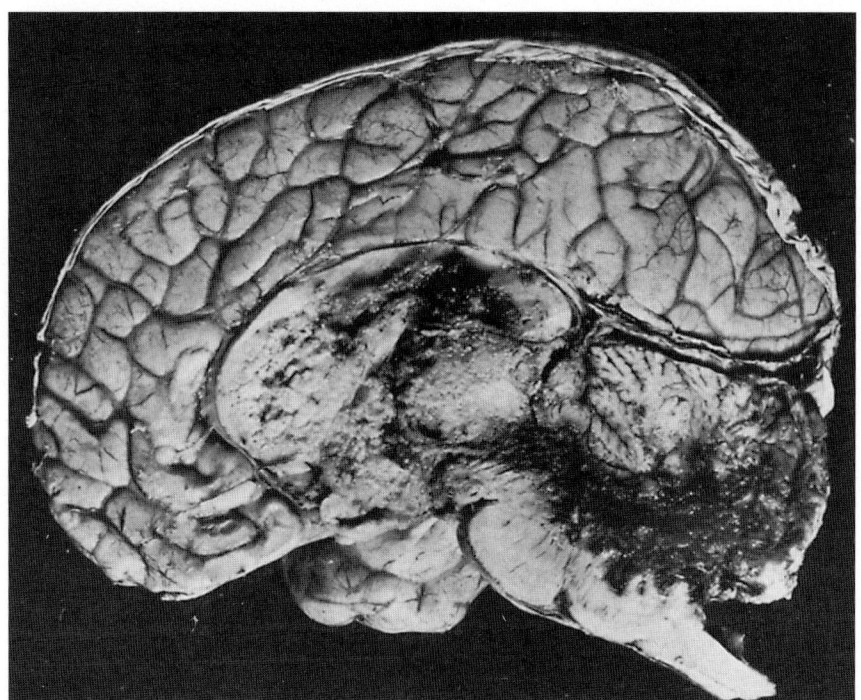

FIG. 2. In Harvey Cushing's 1932 work, *Intracranial Tumors*, he described the brain section taken from a patient who was "thoroughly radiated. Note invasion of the medulla and massive obliteration of the cerebral ventricles by tumor." Cushing stated that "I believe that its [medulloblastoma] thorough local removal by dissection or by suction is the proper procedure...Radiation should subsequently be begun as early as possible and it should be distributed over the entire cerebrospinal axis. By this combination of radical extirpation and radiation a complete subsidence of all symptoms for a year and sometimes longer may be anticipated." (Reprinted with permission of C. C. Thomas, Publishers; Springfield, Illinois and the assistance of the Rare Book Room, Duke Medical School Library.)

TABLE 1. *Chang staging for medulloblastoma*[a]

T_1	Tumor <3 cm in diameter	M_0	No evidence of subarachnoid or hematogenous metastasis
T_2	Tumor ≥3 cm in diameter	M_1	Tumor cells found in cerebrospinal fluid
T_{3a}	Tumor >3 cm in diameter with extension	M_2	Intracranial tumor beyond primary site (e.g., into the aqueduct of Sylvius and/or into the subarachnoid space or in the third or foramen of Luschka or lateral ventricles)
T_{3b}[b]	Tumor >3 cm in diameter with unequivocal extension into the brain stem	M_3	Gross nodular seeding in spinal subarachnoid space
T_4	Tumor >3 cm in diameter with extension up past the aqueduct of Sylvius and/or down past the foramen magnum (i.e., beyond the posterior fossa)	M_4	Metastasis outside the cerebrospinal axis (esp. bone marrow, bone)

[a]A pre-CT era system described by Chang (25), modified by J. Langston (*personal communication,* 1988).
[b]T_{3b} is generally defined by *intraoperative* demonstration of tumor extension into the brainstem.

toma" (defined as M0 with complete or near total resection, *v.i.*), for example, shows equivalent outcome among those with brainstem invasion (T3b) versus without such (T1–T3) (29). "M" stage, however, is a highly significant prognostic factor; intensity of therapy in current protocols and outcome are strongly related to the presence or absence of metastatic disease (23,26,28,30).

Therapy

Surgery

Harvey Cushing's classic 1930 report of his experience with medulloblastoma (4), demonstrated the inability of surgery alone to cure this tumor; only 1 of 61 patients survived 3 years following surgery with ($n = 33$) or without ($n = 29$) limited irradiation.

The importance of *maximal, judicious* surgical resection is apparent in most contemporary series (26,30–34). *Gross total resection* (i.e., no evidence of residual tumor seen at surgery and negative postoperative imaging) or *near total resection* (best defined as minimal residual: more than 90% resection estimated by the surgeon and less than 1.5 cm² residual on postoperative imaging) are associated with superior outcome in comparison to *subtotal* (51% to 90% resection) or *partial resection* (11% to 50% removal) and *biopsy*

only (less than 10% removal) (26). Table 2 summarizes data from series documenting the influence of degree of surgical resection on survival. A correlation between degree of resection and local tumor extent (i.e., infiltration into the brainstem or cerebellopontine peduncle limiting complete removal) can be inferred. Data from the Children's Cancer Study Group (CCG) indicates gross total or near total resection in approximately 90% of children. Survival appears to correlate more significantly with amount of tumor residual (i.e., the surgical result as documented on immediate postoperative imaging) than with the surgeon's impression of degree of resection; data confirming the value of minimal residual disease is most apparent among children with M0 disease (26,35). For tumors adherent to or invading the brainstem, a report from St. Jude Children's Research Hospital (36) shows no advantage to pursuing gross total resection compared to near total removal; morbidity appears to be greater with the more aggressive surgical approach.

Operative mortality has been reduced to 2% or less in pediatric neurosurgical centers. Aggressive surgery may, however, be associated with significant morbidity (26,37,38). The "posterior fossa syndrome" has been described in up to 10% to 15% of children following posterior fossa craniotomy. The syndrome is signified by difficulty swallowing,

TABLE 2. *Degree of surgical resection and outcome in medulloblastoma*

				Disease-free survival at 5 yr					
Interval	First author (ref)	Number of patients	Percent with total resection	Survival of patients with total resection	Percent of patients with near total resection	Survival of patients with near total resection	Percent of patients with limited resection	Survival of patients with limited resection	Significant difference?
1977–1987	Jenkin (33)	72	39	93%	30	41%	30	48%	Yes
1968–1984	Hughes (32)	60	30		48	69% (total + near total resection)	22	40%	Yes
1984–1989	Bailey (30)	122	NA		53	61%	47	54%	No
1985–1988	Gentet (31)	61	82	58%	18	61%	NA		No
1986–1990	Albright (41)	93	NA		73	72% (total + near total resection)	25	56%	0.06

as well as truncal ataxia, "mutism," and, less often, respiratory failure; symptoms and signs are typically noted after a 12- to 24-hour period of initially uneventful postoperative recovery (24,37,38). Disabling neurologic signs often improve dramatically, sometimes over many months after surgery. It is important to maintain an aggressive, curative approach (including radiation therapy) in children with this syndrome, anticipating significant neurologic recovery, which may not be apparent early in the course of irradiation.

The routine use of ventriculoperitoneal (VP) shunts to reduce intracranial pressure prior to posterior fossa craniotomy resulted in significant improvement in operative morbidity and mortality when introduced 40 years ago. The risk of shunt-borne metastases is minimal (39,40). There have been several reports implicating shunts in the dissemintation of medulloblastoma. There are other studies that find no increased incidence of medulloblastoma dissemination in the presence of a shunt. It is not clear, therefore, if the presence of CSF shunts leads to an increased incidence of extraneural metastases. We may conclude that while shunt-borne metastases do occur, the event is so infrequent as to not require a change in tumor management policy as a result of the presence of a shunt. Children with VP shunts typically become shunt dependent (39,41). Shunt failure or infection may com-

plicate long-term survival, requiring revision or replacement in nearly 25% of children measured at 5-years postinsertion. In many academic pediatric neurosurgical centers, it is standard procedure to place a ventricular drain, as needed, at the time of surgery. The surgeon can often document reestablishment of CSF flow following fourth ventricular tumor resection. Later shunt insertion may be required in up to 25% of children (24). Such an approach provides physiologic CSF dynamics for the majority of children, avoiding potential late events related to an indwelling VP shunt.

Radiation Therapy

The efficacy of radiation therapy in medulloblastoma was reported within a decade of Cushing's initial description of the tumor. Cutler et al. (42) reported the radiation responsiveness of medulloblastoma and the value of "preventive irradiation" of the entire neuraxis based on Cushing's clinical series. The seminal report documenting cure of medulloblastoma with craniospinal irradiation (CSI) was published by Bloom in 1969 (43), documenting 32% survival at 5 years and 25% disease-free survival at 10 years. Numerous subsequent reports confirm increasing rates of disease control with modern radiation techniques (24,29,30,32,33,45).

Modifications of radiation volume, dose, and fractionation have been explored. Data confirm the value of standard full neuraxis irradiation rather than more limited treatment volumes (with the possible exception of very young children; *v.i.*); established neuraxis dose levels are superior to reduced dose CSI when postoperative therapy is restricted to radiation therapy (11, 20, 41, 76, 181) Reduction in craniospinal dose in conjunction with contemporary chemotherapy may be appropriate for a subset of children treated in an investigational protocol setting (28).

Chemotherapy

Phase II trials have documented the chemoresponsiveness of medulloblastoma. Modern series indicate efficacy for alkylating agents (cyclophosphamide), platinum compounds (cisplatinum, carboplatinum), etoposide (administered orally), and multidrug regimens (including MOPP, cisplatinum/VP-16, cyclophosphamide/vincristine, cyclophosphamide/melphalan) (46–51).

Single-institution data have suggested a benefit for combined modality treatment, in-

cluding adjuvant chemotherapy, in selected cases of medulloblastoma (52,53). Randomized trials in both CCG and International Society for Pediatric Oncology (SIOP) between 1978 and 1981 tested surgery and standard postoperative irradiation with versus without adjuvant CCNU/vincristine (with added prednisone in the CCG study). There was no overall benefit with such chemotherapy: survival and disease-free survival were not statistically improved (27,54) (Table 3). A parallel Pediatric Oncology Group (POG) study (1979 to 1986) suggested an overall survival benefit in randomizing children to receive adjuvant MOPP chemotherapy: 5-year survival 74% versus 56% ($p = 0.06$) with postoperative irradiation alone (55).

The CCG-941 and SIOP-1 studies did document significant improvement with chemotherapy in "high-risk" patients, variably identified in the two cooperative group studies to include those with metastatic disease, incomplete resection, age less than 2 years, high "T" stage, and/or brainstem involvement (27,54) (Table 3). The efficacy of adjuvant chemotherapy has been most convincingly shown in Packer's studies of chemoradiation, using

TABLE 3. *Adjuvant chemotherapy for medulloblastoma*

Schema	CSI dose	Subset	Chemo	Outcome @ 5 yr PFS	Outcome @ 5 yr OS	Group/Ref
(RT + V) ± CCNU/pred/V[a]	36 Gy	All	0	50%	65%	CCG (27)
		All	+	59%	65%	
		High-risk[b]	0		0	
		High-risk	+		46%	
(RT + V) ± CCNU/V	36 Gy	All	0	42%		SIOP (54)
		All	+	55%		
		High-risk[c]	0	25–35%		
		High-risk	+	48–58%		
S ± MTX + RT	36 Gy	All	0	60%		SIOP-2 (30)
		All	+	75%		
	24 Gy	All	0	69%		
		All	+	41%		
(RT + V) + CDDP/CCNU/V	36 Gy	High-risk[d]	+	85%		Packer (28)
		(M_0)[e]	+	90%		
		(M_+)[e]	+	67%		
	23.4 Gy	Low stage	+	82%		CCG 9892 (69)

[a]V, vincristine; MTX, methotrexate; CDDP, cisplatin
[b]high-risk, M_{1-3}/T_{2-4} ($n = 30$ total)
[c]high-risk, T_{3-4} or partial resection
[d]high-risk, incomplete resection; brainstem involvement, ± M_+
[e]M_0, localized; M_+, subarachnoid dissemination

postoperative irradiation and concurrent vincristine, followed by eight courses of CCNU/cisplatinum/vincristine (28). In negatively selected high-risk patients (defined as T3b or brainstem invasion, and/or significant local residual tumor, and/or metastatic disease), disease-free and overall survival at 5 years have been reported at 85% and 83%, respectively (28). Although one would no longer identify T3bM0/resected patients as high risk, the outcome in the entire cohort reported by Packer et al. is, nevertheless, superior to published results with irradiation alone (Table 3), even when selected as "favorable" (i.e., T1–3aM0 cases status/postresection). For M0 patients, Packer et al. (28) reported 90% 5-year disease-free survival in a five institution trial. For patients with metastatic involvement, Packer et al. (28) report 67% 5-year disease-free survival, a substantial improvement over other published series. Cooperative group studies are ongoing in Europe and North America to prospectively confirm the outcome attributed to the platinum/CCNU/vincristine regimen.

Trials of "upfront," often phase II, chemotherapy for patients with measurable residual disease (incomplete resection and/or neuraxis dissemination) have shown excellent response rates to cisplatinum/VP-16, carboplatinum, carboplatinum/VP-16, high-dose methotrexate, and cyclophosphamide/cisplatinum/vincristine (49–51). The studies have established high rates of objective response (generally more than 50% to 75%); theoretically, radiation control may be facilitated by the reduction in tumor burden associated with response to chemotherapy. Problematic is a low but recognized rate of disease progression, even during a "brief" 12- to 16-week schema of preirradiation chemotherapy (49,56). The potential facilitation of radiation control must also be balanced against the potential induction of radiation resistance or accelerated repopulation, events that may theoretically occur during preirradiation chemotherapy and may diminish ultimate disease control with irradiation. In a report from Mosijczuk et al. (57), 23% of patients progressed prior to irradiation, of

more concern though was that another 25% failed to begin or complete intended irradiation (57). POG has just completed a randomized trial of pre- versus postirradiation CDDP/VP-16 for high-risk disease; preliminary analysis favors the radiation therapy-chemotherapy sequence, although final reporting is yet incomplete.

Current management for medulloblastoma incorporates chemotherapy for most presentations, combined with standard or modified radiation therapy. North American drug regimens incorporate cisplatinum (or, less commonly, carboplatinum), CCNU or cyclophosphamide, and vincristine and/or VP-16. Pending additional data, postoperative irradiation followed by chemotherapy appears to be the preferable schema.

For disease recurrent after radiation therapy (with or without chemotherapy), demonstration of chemotherapy responsiveness and subsequent high-dose chemotherapy with autologous bone marrow or peripheral stem cell rescue has resulted in a small proportion of durable secondary disease control (58).

Radiotherapeutic Management

Volume

Medulloblastoma is the seminal tumor identified with subarachnoid dissemination. The requirement for full CSI has been recognized for over 5 decades. In reviewing serial treatment regimens in Sweden, Landberg et al. (59) noted serial improvements in survival rates with increasing radiation volume: 5% 10-year survival following limited posterior fossa irradiation, 15% following irradiation to the posterior fossa and spinal canal, and 53% after CSI. Reported failures in the subfrontal region additionally document the necessity to completely encompass the cranial and spinal subarachnoid space; such failures clearly represent inadequate dose to the subfrontal area, a potential site of geographic miss or underdosage that requires particular attention in CSI planning and delivery (60,61).

A French cooperative trial of limited-volume irradiation (including the posterior fossa and spinal axis only) in conjunction with aggressive chemotherapy also confirms the importance of "comprehensive" CSI. The notably poor outcome and unique predominance of early neuraxis failures (largely supratentorial and spinal in location) associated with reduced-volume therapy led to early closure of the study (62). All available data is based on "boost" volumes defined by the anatomic limits of the posterior fossa (*v.i.*). There is rationale for *investigating* the use of three-dimensionally defined target volumes based on the initial tumor bed, at least for a component of the dose now utilized to boost the entire posterior fossa (63). Similarly, there is interest in additionally studying limited radiation volumes (restricting irradiation to the posterior fossa only) in conjunction with high-dose chemotherapy in well-controlled trials of selected infants with limited stage disease. It will be several years before sufficient data is available to know whether such modifications are safe (i.e., equally effective) and result in reduced radiation-related morbidities.

Dose

Medulloblastoma is a relatively radiosensitive tumor. *In vitro* studies by Fertil and Malaise (64) demonstrated a favorable surviving fraction at 2 Gy (SF2Gy = 28%), comparable to most other embryonal pediatric tumors and notably different from the clinically less responsive malignant gliomas. There is considerable data indicating a correlation between dose to the posterior fossa primary site and outcome; local disease control and survival have been related to posterior fossa doses of 50 to 55 Gy using conventional fractionation at 160 to 180 cGy per fraction (32, 33,65).

The proper neuraxis radiation dose to the full brain and spinal canal is more difficult to define. Most of the recent data documenting disease-free survival rates beyond 50% are based on cranial doses of 35 to 40 Gy and spinal doses of 30 to 35 Gy (32,33,44,66).

The "standard" for CSI for M0 disease in children more than 2- to 3-years old has been accepted at 35 to 36 Gy over the past 2 decades. In children with overt meningeal seeding at diagnosis, CSI is continued to a slightly higher total (38 to 40 Gy), with local boost volumes (i.e., overt, nodular sites of intracranial or spinal leptomeningeal disease) to cumulative levels of 45 to 50 Gy.

Tomita and McLane's 1986 report of excellent disease control in selected totally resected lesions treated with only 25 Gy CSI, prompted a national trial of reduced neuraxis dose irradiation (67). POG and CCG jointly studied favorably selected children more than 3-years old with limited stage tumors (T1-3aM0 using the Chang system) following near total or total resection (with less than 1.5 cm³ residual on postoperative neuroimaging). Patients were randomized between 1986 and 1990 to conventional CSI (36 Gy at 180 cGy per fraction) versus reduced dose CSI (23.4 Gy at 180 cGy per fraction); all cases received standard dose to the posterior fossa (54 Gy). The study was closed prior to planned completion of accrual due to an excess of isolated neuraxis failures in the experimental, reduced dose arm (68). Formal analysis of the study at a minimum 5-years posttherapy (median follow-up interval of 7 years) shows a marginal benefit to standard dose CSI: 63% 5-year disease-free survival versus 54% following reduced dose CSI ($p = 0.058$); the incidence of isolated neuraxis failure remains higher in the lower dose arm (29).

This study provides a new easily recognized standard for surgery and modern irradiation, resulting in 63% disease-free survival at 5 years in relatively favorable medulloblastoma (29). The established efficacy of cisplatinum-containing chemotherapy and the narrowing differences between 36 Gy CSI versus 23.4 Gy with added follow-up have encouraged additional explorations of reduced neuraxis irradiation. A joint POG/CCG trial randomizing standard dose CSI (36 Gy) versus reduced dose CSI (23.4 Gy) *plus* chemotherapy (vincristine/CCNU/cisplatinum) represented the ideal test of relative efficacy and comparative toxicities for children with "favorable, low stage" medulloblastoma. Unfortunately, the biases of clinical investigators and difficulty in the perceived "equivalence" of the two arms during parental interviews for informed consent prevented sufficient accrual, and the study was closed due to inadequate numbers after just 18 months. In the interim, a CCG "pilot" study utilizing the experimental arm (reduced dose CSI plus chemotherapy) for children between 1.5 and 10 years of age accrued over 70 cases. Preliminary analysis shows greater than 80% progression-free survival at 3 years, results at least comparable to those with standard dose irradiation alone in the earlier low stage POG/CCG study (69).

The current intergroup POG/CCG study accepts the presumed benefit of combined reduced dose CSI plus chemotherapy for children more than 3-years old with "standard risk" medulloblastoma. The trial accessions patients with limited residual (less than 1.5 cm^2) M0 disease to CSI (23.4 Gy) with concurrent vincristine, followed by cisplatinum and vincristine with either CCNU ("control arm") or cyclophosphamide ("experimental arm"). Perhaps the most important goal of the study is to confirm disease control at or above the 75% to 80% level for "favorable" medulloblastoma using reduced dose CSI and effective chemotherapy. The randomization to CCNU versus cyclophosphamide may identify a new regimen permitting additional dose escalation or diminished hematologic toxicities.

Trials of hyperfractionated CSI include neuraxis doses of 30 to 48.4 Gy at 100 to 110 cGy per fraction b.i.d., with greater than 6-hour interfraction interval; cumulative doses for the posterior fossa have been 66 to 72 Gy with similar fractionation (70–73). It is premature to assess the added efficacy and/or reduced late toxicities that might accompany altered fractionation studies.

Technique

The goal of achieving uniform dose throughout the subarachnoid space, encompassing the entire intracranial vault and spinal canal, represents one of the most technically demanding aspects of radiation oncology. There are several techniques appropriate for the administration of CSI (74). Fundamental is the use of opposed lateral fields including the cranium and upper cervical spinal canal, matching a posterior spinal field including the full spinal subarachnoid space or, in larger children, the upper one-half of the spinal canal (with a separate, matched lower posterior spinal field) (75).

It is important to establish immobilization and reproducibility of setup. Prone positioning is generally preferable as it allows greater extension of the chin (minimizing potential bone growth changes due to the exit of the posterior spinal field) and simplifies technical maneuvers at the critical junction between the lateral craniocervical fields and the posterior spinal field. Immobilization can be achieved through a customized plaster cast, use of the Alpha Cradle system, or a Vac-Loc (76). (Discussed in Chapter 22.) Supine techniques may be appropriate for very young children requiring sedation or anesthesia; detailed attention to the junction area is required when adapting the more familiar prone geometry to supine CSI use.

In planning CSI, it is simpler to first simulate the spinal field(s); establishing the length of the spinal field defines the collimator angle necessary for homogeneity with the craniocervical fields. The lower border of the spinal field is set at the bottom of S-2 or the lowest level of the thecal sac as determined by MRI, whichever is lower (45). The upper portion of the spinal field is set in the area of C-5 to C-7. In small children the entire spine can be encompassed with one field; in children older than 4 to 5 years, however, two adjacent spinal fields are usually required. If two fields are necessary, lateral radiographs are taken to include the isocenter and junctional margin of each spinal field to establish the spinal cord depth for dose prescription and calculation of the gap at the surface to provide relative uniformity at the spinal depth. Whenever two spinal fields are required, it is important to change the level of the junction concurrently when "feathering" the craniocervical junction. The width of the spinal field should be sufficient to dosimetrically encompass the full width of the spinal canal. There has been debate whether a "spade" configuration is necessary to allow adequate lateral coverage at the lower sacral margin. Halperin's anatomic study (77), documents the importance of covering the sacral foramina, often requiring some blocking of the superior component of the spinal volume (Fig. 3).

The brain and upper cervical spine are treated with lateral fields. The collimators for the lateral fields are angled to match the divergence of the posterior spinal field (Fig. 4).

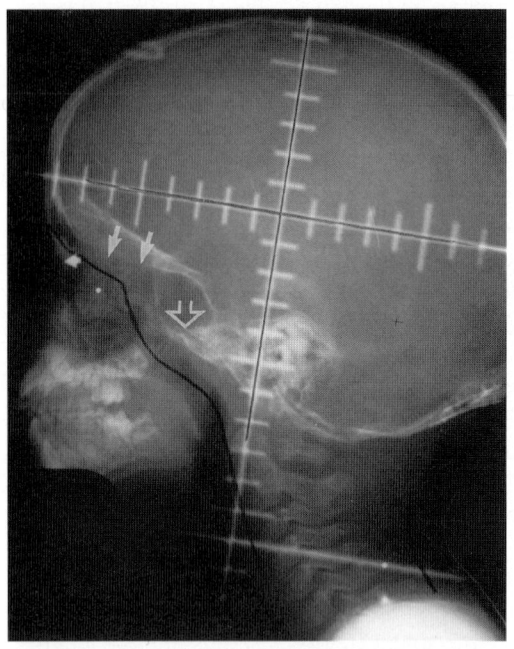

A

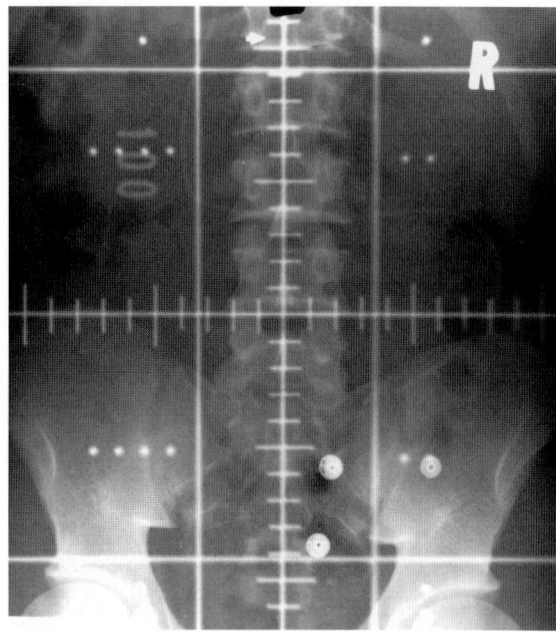

B

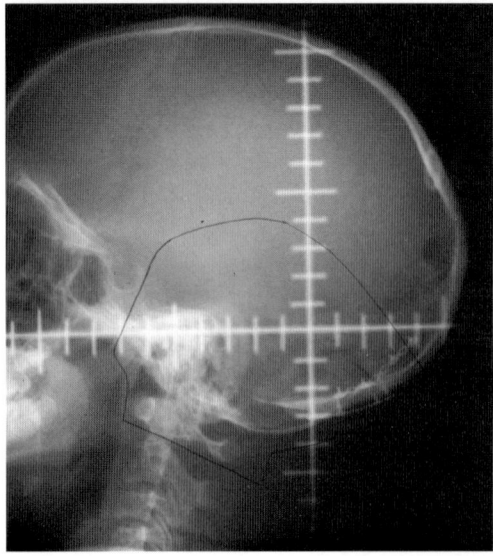

C

FIG. 3. Cranial **(A)** and spinal **(B)** fields utilized for medulloblastoma or other CNS tumors requiring CSI. Note the highlighted cribriform plate *(solid arrows)* and base of the temporal lobe/middle cranial fossa *(open arrow,* **A**). A classic posterior fossa boost field is pictured **(C)**. Many centers utilize a three-dimensional conformal approach to relatively spare the cochlea and pituitary-hypothalamic region during the posterior fossa component of therapy (Fig. 6).

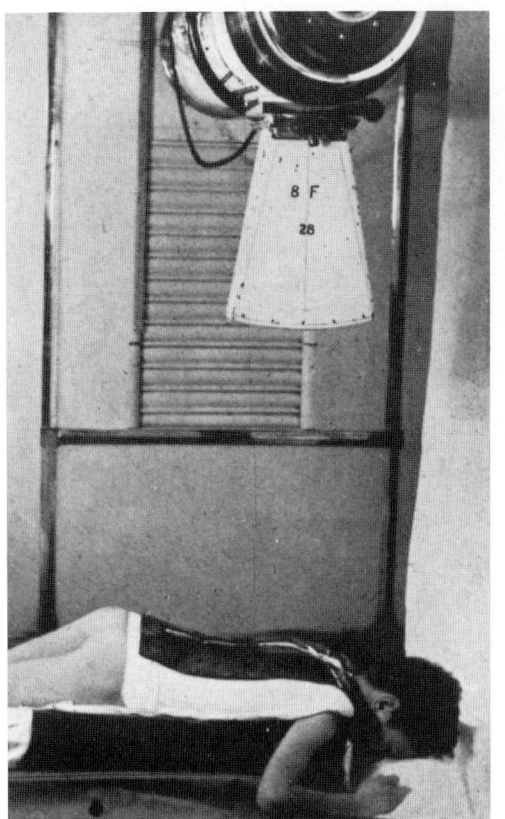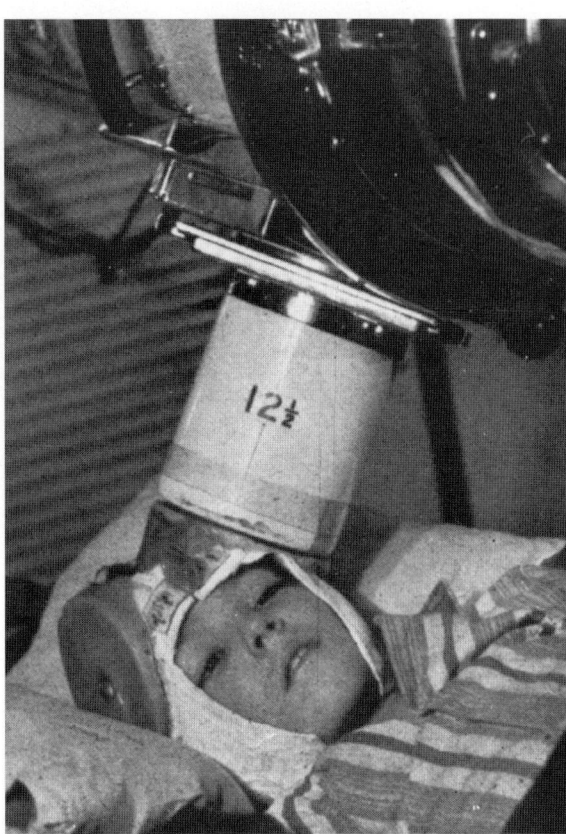

A   B

FIG. 4. A: The famous English radiation oncologist Ralston Paterson illustrated, in 1948, his method of treating the "whole C.N.S. in continuity" with 200–250 KV x-rays. Note the posterior field intended to encompass the whole spine exposed via a narrow spinal slit in the lead jacket as well as the whole head(s). **B:** The anterior brain was treated with oblique head fields, apparently wedged and with a head stabilization device. (Reproduced with permission from Paterson R. The treatment of malignant disease by radium and x-rays being a practice of radiotherapy. London: Edward Arnold & Co., 1948.)

The cranial fields need to accommodate serial decreases in length to "feather" the junction zone; if asymmetric collimators are not available to allow diminution of the caudal portion of the lateral fields while maintaining the isocenter, the length of the craniocervical fields needs to be sufficient to permit ultimate symmetric shrinkage by 6 to 10 cm. A table angle is generally used to correct for caudal divergence of the craniocervical fields (Fig. 5). Although detailed analysis shows only minimal inhomogeneity if a correcting table angle is not used (74), full three-dimensional attention at the junction zone permits more confident abutting of the lateral craniocervi-cal and posterior spinal fields. Eliminating a "gap" actually simplifies daily setup; with proper attention to technique and "feathering" to anatomically distribute any potential inhomogeneity, a three-dimensional junction with abutting fields provides maximal homogeneity within the spinal canal. As an alternative, asymmetric jaws can be used to avoid divergence at this junction; the technique creates somewhat greater divergence in blocking the eyes at the critical cribriform plate region and limits the spinal length, requiring a spinal junction even with younger children. Even with the "ideal" craniocervical match using asymmetric jaws, it is important to feather all

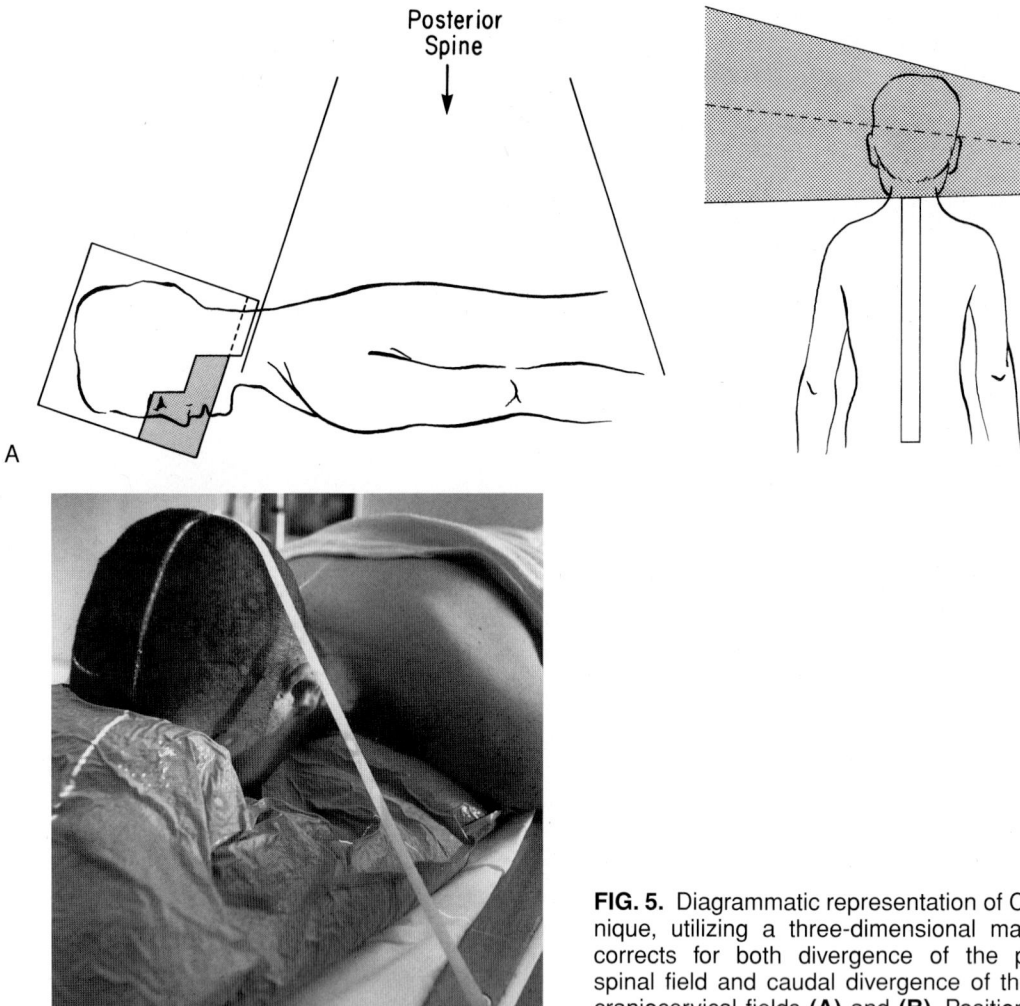

FIG. 5. Diagrammatic representation of CSI technique, utilizing a three-dimensional match that corrects for both divergence of the posterior spinal field and caudal divergence of the lateral craniocervical fields **(A)** and **(B)**. Positioning and immobilization device for the patient for CSI **(C)**.

junctional zones, shifting the anatomic junction site by at least 5 to 10 mm every 8 to 9 Gy, effectively once a week.

The cranial fields require exquisite attention to include the entire intracranial subarachnoid space. The most difficult area is at the level of the cribriform plate, where there is often little margin to allow one to block the eyes and dosimetrically encompass the critical subfrontal cribriform site. Reports of subfrontal recurrences have been noted even by highly respected institutions, documenting the particular technical difficulty in achieving

adequate coverage at this site (60,61,77–79). For older children, the pneumatized frontal sinuses allow sufficient margin to obviate concern with adequate attention to the cribriform anatomy (Fig. 3). In younger children, the margin above the eye may be extremely close, but should permit coverage of the subfrontal area without resorting to an anterior electron boost, aimed between the eyes, or other inhomogeneous techniques suggested in the past (79).

The posterior fossa boost is delivered by parallel opposed lateral fields. The anterior border of the posterior fossa is, on a lateral radiograph, at the posterior clinoid. The superior border of the tentorium is best identified on postoperative sagittal MRI scan; if unavailable, one can estimate the superior margin as 1 cm higher than the midpoint between the foramen magnum and the vertex. To cover the inferior and posterior borders, one sets field edges beyond the calvarium with a lower border typically at the lower border of C-1. Current investigations to restrict the boost volume to the tumor bed (rather than the anatomic posterior fossa), at least at dose levels above 36 Gy, require at least 5-years follow-up before such can be adopted beyond strictly controlled investigational settings. The goal of three-dimensional conformal irradiation, targeting the tumor bed, is to relatively diminish the dose to the cochlea (especially important with combined irradiation and cisplatin) and the hypothalamic-pituitary region (Fig. 6).

The use of spinal electron irradiation has been explored to minimize the exit dose through the length of the body (80). Theoretically, one can reduce potential late effects on the lungs and heart, as well as the absorbed dose in the childhood thyroid. Detailed dosimetry has been performed in phantoms for the use of electron fields in CSI (80). Whether inhomogeneity across the vertebral bodies will result in accentuated kyphoscolosis is yet unclear. The clinical outcome of this technique has been summarized by Gaspar et al. (81), noting no apparent difference in late complications comparing children treated with electron versus photon spinal irradiation.

Delivery

CSI results in predictable, if quantitatively variable, acute changes in the peripheral blood counts. Monitoring for neutropenia and/or thrombocytopenia, most often noted during or after the third week of CSI without preceding chemotherapy, is critically important. Traditionally, CSI is interrupted if the neutrophil count falls below 500 to 1,000 cells per mL, especially if the child is febrile.

When necessary to permit completion of neuraxis irradiation, granulocyte colony stimulating factor (G-CSF) may be used to correct neutropenia; thrombocytopenia may require platelet transfusion (126). In most settings, radiation therapy for medulloblastoma begins with CSI. If blood counts require CSI to be interrupted for more than 2 or 3 consecutive days, initiation of posterior fossa irradiation will provide continuity and limit unnecessary interruption in irradiation at the primary site. One should return to CSI as soon as hematologic status permits. In settings where CSI follows chemotherapy, extended hematosuppression delaying initiation of CSI may favor beginning with posterior fossa irradiation to allow earlier radiation therapy and delay neuraxis therapy until hematologically feasible.

Nausea and vomiting are generally more pronounced in older children. Use of antiemetics is important in preventing "anticipatory" vomiting that may be more difficult to control. Phenothiazines or, more recently, ondansatron, is usually successful. Rarely, corticosteroids may be necessary at low dose levels, particularly early in the postoperative period.

Results

Long-term disease-free survival following surgery and irradiation approximates 60% for medulloblastoma (Fig. 7, Table 4). The data showing improvement to the 80% range with the addition of cisplatinum-containing chemotherapy has short follow-up (28). Factors associated with more favorable outcome include age more than 2 to 3 years, localized presentations (i.e., M0), and tumors amenable to near total or total resection. Biologic factors that may impact on survival include DNA index (with conflicting data in the literature), immunochemical documentation of neuronal and/or glial differentiation, and the presence of specific cytogenetic or chromosomal abnormalities (14,16,83,84). Investigations to additionally improve outcome seek improvement in disease control and reduction in functional limitations attendant to therapy.

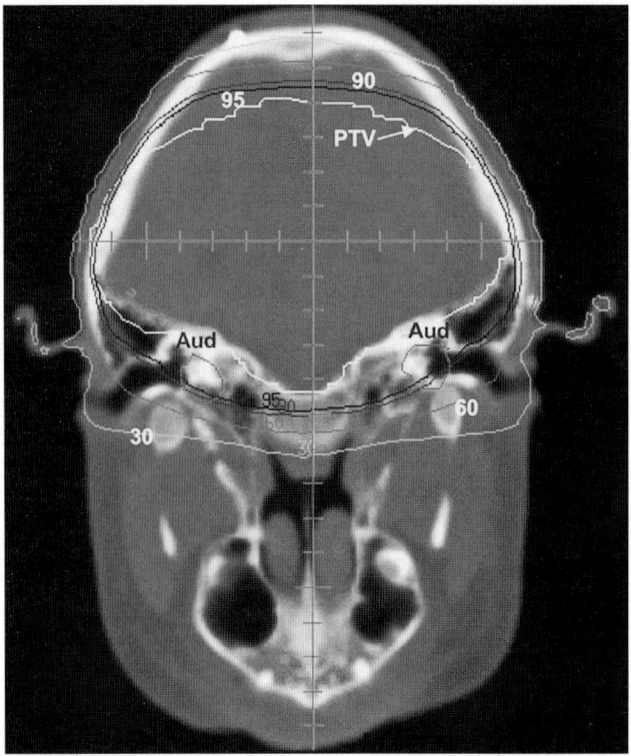

A

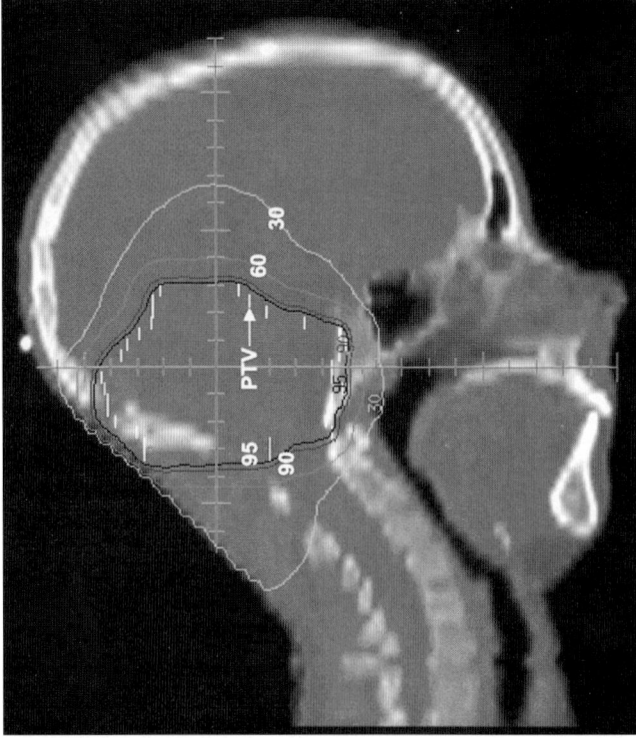

B

FIG. 6. (A, B) Three-dimensional conformal approach to encompass the posterior fossa, utilizing four noncoplanar fields; note the dose distribution in the region of the hearing apparatus is relatively diminished for this component of therapy.

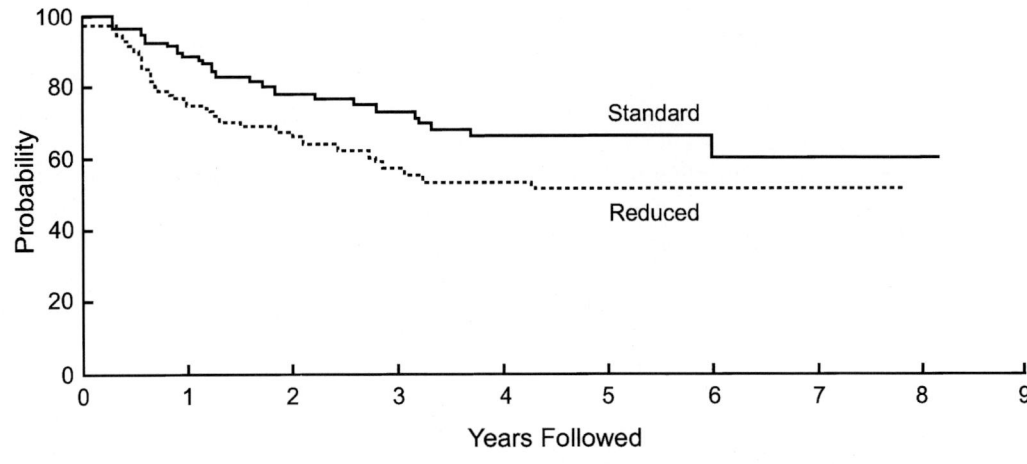

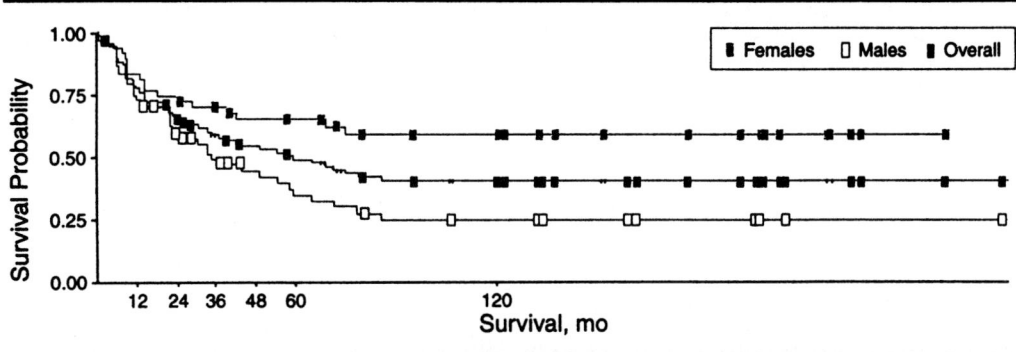

FIG. 7. A: Outcome following surgery and irradiation for favorable medulloblastoma (selected by localized disease following gross total or near total resection with less than 1.5 cm^2 residual and no apparent evidence of brainstem invasion): survival and disease-free survival in the POG 8631/CCG 923 study (1986–1990, *n* = 123) (29). **B:** Kaplan-Meier analysis for overall survival and survival according to sex for patients with medulloblastoma, 21 years of age or younger, treated with surgery and postoperative radiotherapy at the University of California, San Francisco, between 1970 and 1995. There were 62 males and 47 females in the study group. Survival was significantly better for females (*p* = 0.01). The median for overall survival was 59 months. (Reprinted with permission from Weil MD, Lamborn K, Edwards MSB, Wara WM. Influence of a child's sex on medulloblastoma outcome. *JAMA* 1998;279:1474–1476.)

TABLE 4. *Outcome in medulloblastoma—contemporary series*

Patient population	No.	Surgery	RT	Chemotherapy	5-yr PFS	5-yr OS	10-yr OS	Series/Ref
All (1968–1984)	60	All	CSI 36Gy	0	68%		44%	JCRT (32)
All (1977–1987)	72	All	CSI 36Gy	few	64%	71%	63%	Toronto (33)
Low stage (1986–1990)[a]	63	Complete, near total	CSI 36Gy	0	63%			POG/CCG (29)
High risk (1983–1991)[b]	63	Variable	CSI 36Gy	CDDP/CCNU/V	85%			Packer (28)

[a]low stage, near or total resection, no brainstem invasion, M_0
[b]high stage, incomplete resection ± brainstem invasion ± M_+

BRAINSTEM GLIOMAS

The brainstem is the connecting structure that joins the "long tracts" from the cerebral hemispheres and midline diencephalic nuclei with the cerebellar tracks, forming the spinal cord as the tracks exit through foramen magnum. Within the brainstem are the nuclei of the cranial nerves, the reticular activating system, and vital functional centers (e.g., respiratory). The brainstem includes three anatomic segments: the midbrain rostrally, the pons, and the medulla caudally. Brainstem tumors are a heterogeneous group of tumors that share common astrocytic histologies but evidence divergent clinical behavior related to the anatomic region of involvement and the pattern of growth. The tumor types are identified by their apparent anatomic segment of origin and the macroscopic appearance, defined as *diffuse* or *focal* lesions. Focal lesions are generally limited to tumors that are circumscribed on imaging and involve less than 50% of just one segment of the brainstem (85).

As a group, brainstem gliomas constitute approximately 10% of intracranial tumors in children. The peak incidence occurs between the ages of 5 and 9 years; males are affected more commonly than females. The most common presenting symptoms include diplopia, motor weakness, and difficulty with speech, swallowing, and walking. Neurologic signs include ataxia, cranial nerve palsies (most frequent are the pontine nerves, VI and VII, followed by the medullary nerves, IX, X, XI, and XII, and, less often, the midbrain nerves, III, IV, and V) and long tract signs (motor weakness, most often hemiparesis) (86,87). A review of the anatomy of the brainstem readily demonstrates why this constellation of signs occurs (Fig. 8). The most common type of brainstem glioma is the *diffusely infiltrating pontine glioma*, comprising 70% of brainstem tumors. Tumors of the *midbrain* and *medulla* may be diffuse or focal; even diffuse tumors typically show considerably less infiltration and expansion of the brainstem than seen with the pontine gliomas. Focal intrinsic tumors do occur within the pons, as do dorsally exophytic tumors; both types enjoy considerably more favorable outcome than the more typical infiltrating pontine tumors (85–90).

The duration of symptoms correlates with the type of brainstem glioma. Children with pontine gliomas typically relate a brief history

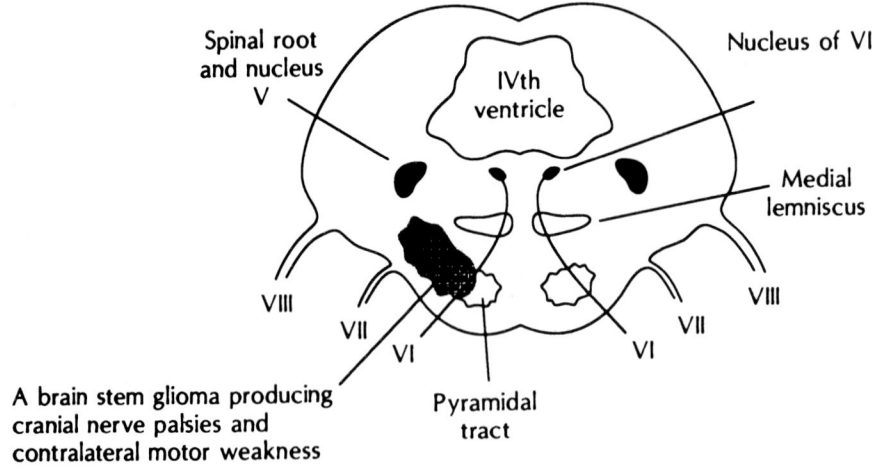

FIG. 8. A lower pontine glioma interferes with motor function on one side of the body and with contralateral function of cranial nerves VI and VII. These two cranial nerves are most commonly affected by brainstem tumors. Ataxia can result from involvement of the fibers of the middle cerebellar peduncle.

of neurologic symptoms; for classic pontine gliomas, protocol eligibility requires the duration of symptoms to be less than 6 months. Neurologic signs required for pontine glioma protocols include at least 2 of 3 major categories of neurologic signs (i.e., cranial nerve deficits, long tract signs, ataxia) are present (91–93). Increased intracranial pressure (secondary to obstructive hydrocephalus) is not common among pontine gliomas. Midbrain tumors and dorsally exophytic tumors of the pons or pontomedullary junction often present with obstruction at the aqueduct of Sylvius or the fourth ventricle, respectively. The more focal, less aggressive brainstem tumors are often associated with prolonged symptoms, typically confined to cranial nerve abnormalities alone, ataxia, or gradual onset of increased intracranial pressure (94–96).

MRI is the definitive test for diagnosis and delineation of tumor extent and type (Figs. 9–10). The typical diffusely infiltrating pontine glioma is homogeneous or hypodense on T1 imaging, but readily appreciated on T2 sequence. The tumor expands the pons, often showing exophytic growth, as well, in the ventral, dorsal, or lateral projections. The disease infiltrates into the other brainstem segments, sometimes as far rostrally as into the thalamus, and frequently extends into the cerebellopontine peduncle (brachium pontis) toward or into the cerebellum. There is often little enhancement, although inhomogeneous areas of focal enhancement or signs of intralesional hemorrhage or necrosis may be noted (21,85).

Biopsy of the classic, diffusely infiltrating pontine glioma is unnecessary (26,97,98). Histologic series show roughly equal proportions of low-grade (fibrillary astroctyoma or WHO Grade II astrocytoma) and malignant (anaplastic astroctyoma or glioblastoma multiforme) types (87,99). There is no consistent correlation between histology and outcome; all *diffusely infiltrating* pontine tumors show extremely poor duration of response to irradiation and median survival of less than 1 year (89,93,100,101). It is of interest that the vast majority of such tumors show malignant astrocytoma at autopsy; even tumors showing

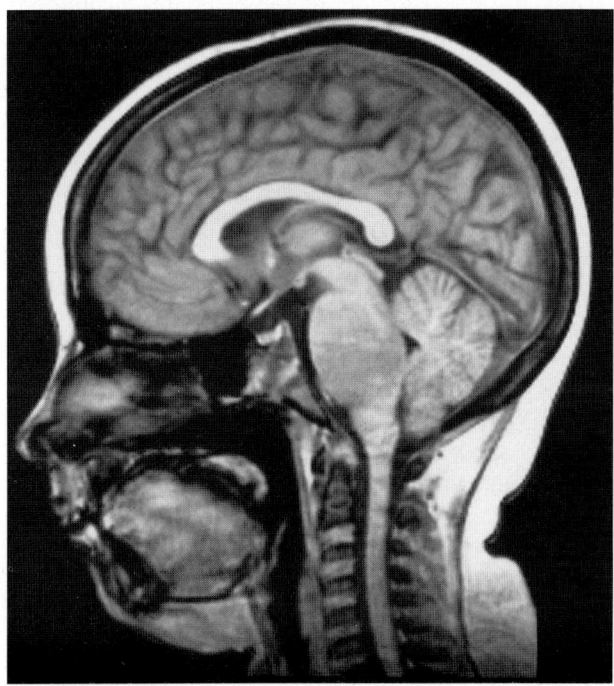

FIG. 9. Brainstem gliomas: classic and most common diffusely infiltrating pontine glioma.

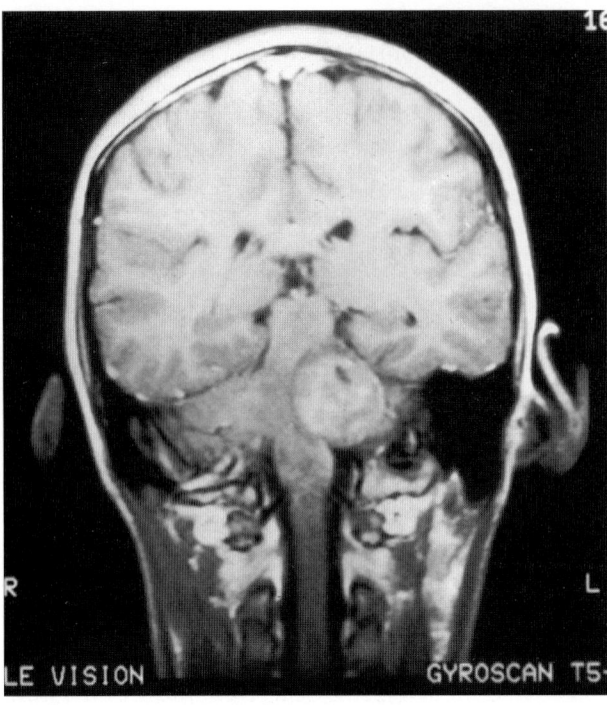

FIG. 10. An 11-year-old girl presented to medical attention with a 1 month history of diplopia, dizziness, and progressive headache. Physical examination showed mild left VI and VII cranial nerve dysfunction with poor finger to nose testing. The MRI demonstrated a large left brainstem mass. Taken to the operating room at a community hospital, a subtotal resection of a tumor invading the brainstem was performed. The pathology showed glioblastoma multiforme. The tumor location, short duration of symptoms, and aggressive histology all portend a poor prognosis. The roles of biopsy and surgical resection in primary brainstem tumors of childhood are controversial. Surgical resection is indicated in selected cases. The risks of surgery in this location are, however, considerable. These issues are discussed in detail in the text.

low-grade histology at biopsy are often malignant when analyzed at autopsy less than 1 to 2 years after diagnosis (102,103). Lacking evidence that low-grade tumors require a less aggressive approach or demonstrate superior outcome, there is no apparent benefit derived from a biopsy procedure when the imaging and clinical picture are indicative of a typical diffusely infiltrating, expansile pontine glioma (64,87,98).

Hoffman et al. (95) identified a less common, highly specific brainstem tumor now recognized as a dorsally exophytic "benign" brainstem tumor. This tumor type represents approximately 15% of brainstem lesions (96,104). The lesion characteristically fills the fourth ventricle, presenting with symptoms and signs of increased intracranial pressure. In most cases, the tumor enhances briskly with gadolinium (Fig. 11). The origin from the floor of the fourth ventricle (the dorsal surface of the pons or medulla; the tumor often arising at the pontomedullary junction) may be suggested by MRI, but is usually apparent only at the time of surgery. These tu-

mors are almost systematically juvenile pilocytic astrocytomas (JPAs); the prognosis has been quite favorable (95,96,104).

Focal tumors of the pons are uncommon. One specific presentation includes isolated facial nerve palsy or similar, limited neurologic dysfunction associated with a small, enhancing intrapontine lesion (94). Such tumors are low grade (often juvenile pilocytic astrocytoma or WHO Grade I) and enjoy a favorable prognosis.

Tumors of the midbrain may involve the tegmentum or the tectal plate. *Tegmental* tumors are usually fibrillary astrocytomas (WHO Grade II). The tumors may involve the tegmentum focally or may infiltrate through much of the midbrain. Lesions may show uniform enhancement or little contrast enhancement. Presenting signs include extraocular muscle palsy and/or long track involvement. Biopsy is preferred, especially for lesions contiguous with the pineal region. *Tectal plate* tumors are usually quite small and well demarcated, confined to the tectal plate and best visualized on MRI.

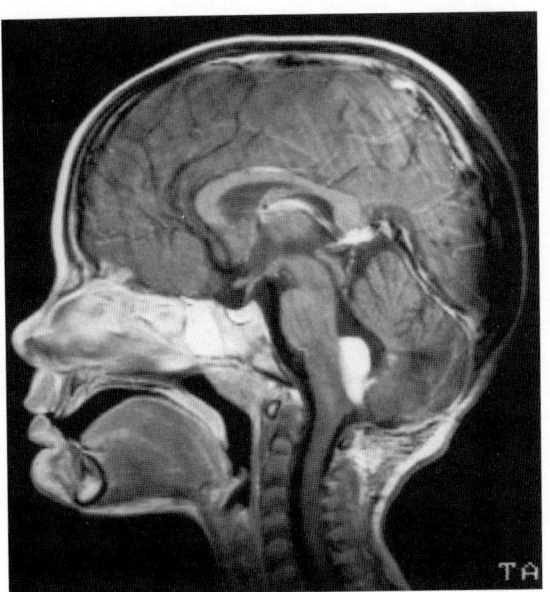
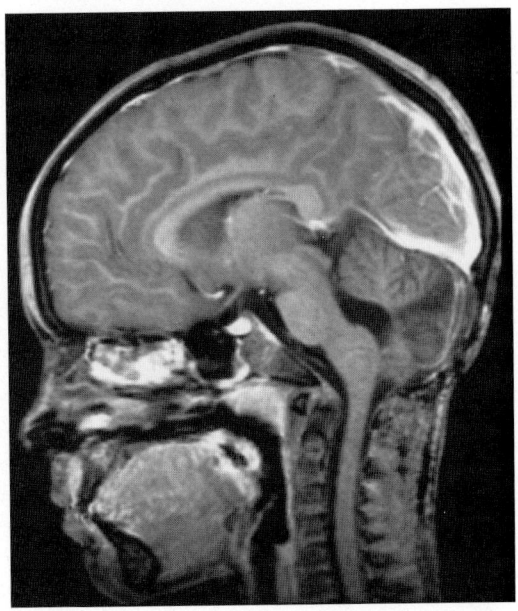

FIG. 11. Brainstem astrocytomas: dorsally exophytic brainstem juvenile pilocytic astrocytoma (JPA) (**A**) presents as a sizable lesion filling the IVth ventricle, but is attached only along the floor at the level of the pontomedullary junction (**B**, postoperative); appearance 4 years after irradiation for documented post-surgical progression shows decreased mass effect and lack of enhancement.

Many such tumors likely comprised the former diagnosis of "idiopathic obstructive hydrocephalus," small mass lesions obstructing the aqueduct often not demonstrable on CT scan. Ventriculoperitoneal shunt is usually required. MRI shows the focal nature of tectal lesions, most frequently signified by brisk enhancement; biopsy generally confirms juvenile pilocytic histology (WHO Grade I). These tumors are typically indolent; observation alone is usually the treatment of choice (105). Somewhat controversial is the timing of biopsy. If the tumor is anatomically confined to the tectum and stable over an initial 3- to 6-month period of observation, biopsy may be deferred until or if there is evidence of tumor progression requiring therapy. Lesions that are atypical (e.g., cystic) or where there is some question whether the lesion has originated in the adjacent pineal region may require biopsy at diagnosis; if confirmed as a low-grade astrocytoma, subsequent observation is appropriate.

Therapy

Surgery

The role of surgery in classic pontine gliomas is quite limited. Routine biopsy is not recommended. A small proportion of tumors that are otherwise characteristic of diffusely infiltrating gliomas present with large cysts or focal areas of hemorrhage or necrosis within the pons. When such components are peripheral in location and can be approached safely, an initial surgical procedure to "decompress" the lesion may be helpful (86,87,98,106).

For dorsally exophytic tumors, partial resection will establish the diagnosis (by surgical observation of the origin from the brainstem and histology) and reduce the obstructing mass within the fourth ventricular region. There appears to be no advantage to aggressive surgery in which the limits of resection within the brainstem may be difficult to identify and associated with unnecessary morbidity. Partial resection alone is associated with greater than 60% to 70% freedom from progression at 5 to 10 years (95,96,99, 104). Small focal lesions intrinsic to the pons may be biopsied if safely approachable; one cannot insist on biopsy if the differential is limited and the biopsy-associated morbidity is high.

Lesions within the tegmentum should be biopsied, although the potential morbidity of stereotactic biopsy is recognized due to the proximity of the central veins. Occasional resection has been reported for midbrain tumors (90). Tumors of the lower medulla or cervicomedullary region are similar to low-grade astrocytomas of the spinal cord. Biopsy or attempted gross total resection have been reported; results following surgery alone have been impressive if limited to a small number of neurosurgical centers (90,97,107). Histology is usually low-grade astrocytoma (WHO Grade II); malignant gliomas have been noted (87,97).

Radiation Therapy

Children with diffusely infiltrating pontine gliomas often initially respond impressively to irradiation; approximately 70% show improvement in neurologic symptoms and signs over a several week interval during and after irradiation (92,108). Improvement in MRI has been reported in 30% to 70% of children (92,100). Objective response is almost always followed by signs of progressive disease within 8 to 12 months (92,100).

Clinical response has also been noted in tegmental midbrain lesions and tumors of the medulla, where radiation therapy is more likely to achieve long-term disease control (88,89). For tectal plate or dorsally exophytic pontomedullary astrocytomas, irradiation is safely deferred until signs of disease progression are apparent on imaging (96,99, 104). Once progression has been documented on serial imaging (noted in up to 25% of dorsally exophytic tumors), there has been almost uniform disease control measured out to more than 5 years following local irradiation (96,99,104). Intrinsic focal

pontine lesions often require irradiation at diagnosis due to attendant neurologic signs (94). With the availability of precision volume techniques (i.e., three-dimensional conformal irradiation or fractionated radiosurgery), the risk:benefit ratio may favor earlier radiation intervention in localized, low-grade brainstem lesions.

Chemotherapy

There has been little evidence of efficacy for chemotherapy in brainstem tumors. An earlier prospective, randomized trial of CCNU/vincristine/prednisone showed no benefit in these tumors despite purported efficacy in supratentorial high-grade gliomas (109). For the classic pontine gliomas, preirradiation chemotherapy has shown some responsiveness: a small series testing high-dose cyclophosphamide demonstrated objective response in four children with brainstem gliomas; a POG study revealed objective response (by imaging criteria) in 3 of 32 patients (110,111). It is difficult to measure objective response in this tumor system; the POG series, for example, showed few imaging measurable responders, and the majority of cases required radiotherapeutic intervention prior to the planned completion of four cycles of cisplatin and cyclophosphamide (111). Although anecdotal responses have been documented following oral VP-16 in pontine gliomas, there have been no durable responders reported in the several phase II studies that have included children with brainstem gliomas (112).

For focal, low-grade gliomas, the use of chemotherapy prior to irradiation is an extrapolation from diencephalic low-grade tumors, which may be rational in selected settings. For the majority of children, even those at or below 3 to 4 years of age, symptomatic or progressive dorsally exophytic or focal pontine lesions can be effectively treated with focal radiation techniques. It is difficult to anticipate any significant advantage in delaying definitive therapy with intervening chemotherapy.

Radiotherapeutic Management

Volume

MRI and autopsy studies document contiguous extension of pontine gliomas (a) linearly through the adjacent medulla and/or midbrain, and (b) axially into the brachium pontis, the cerebellopontine angle, and adjacent portions of the cerebellar hemispheres (85,113). Leptomeningeal involvement has been noted in up to 10% to 15% of children with diffusely infiltrating pontine lesions, most often involving the subarachnoid space about the brainstem, the basal cistern, or the upper cervical cord; spinal canal involvement has also been documented (93,114). A small proportion of focal, low-grade brainstem lesions (often JPAs) are associated with neuraxis dissemination, most often noted at diagnosis (94,115,116).

The pattern of failure for pontine gliomas is generally one of local recurrence. Wide local irradiation is indicated, with target volumes subtending both the pons and the adjacent midbrain, medulla, and anterior cerebellum. Diffuse, infiltrating pontine gliomas are often incompletely or nonenhancing lesions; the greatest tumor extent on T1 or T2 images should define the local treatment volume. For infiltrating tumors of the midbrain and medulla, margins of 1 to 2 cm beyond the imaging evident lesion are appropriate. Focal lesions of the tectum can be treated with limited target volumes; the discrete lesions generally require only the identifiable tumor with a dosimetric margin. Fractionated stereotactic radiosurgery (or "stereotactic radiotherapy") may provide ideal coverage for the latter tumor types (117). For dorsally exophytic tumors, the volume can conform to the disease process based on MRI; the anterior margin at the brainstem should encompass at least 5 to 10 mm of apparently normal brainstem ventral to the tumor as documented on MRI. A multifield of three-dimensional conformal approach can relatively spare the temporal lobes, potentially important in this young age group.

Dose

Conventional irradiation using single daily fractions (180 to 200 cGy per fraction) to total doses of 50 to 55 Gy has been associated with 5-year survival rates of 30% to 40% in classic single institution reports from the 1960s through the 1980s (118,119). These studies include patients with all subsets of brainstem tumors, most diagnosed in the pre-CT era. Despite the anticipated predominance of diffusely infiltrating pontine gliomas, the "classic" series include an undetermined proportion of children with relatively favorable brainstem lesions and often extend the definition of such tumors to include the more favorable thalamic gliomas (88,113,119). When limited to classic diffusely infiltrating pontine gliomas, selected by modern imaging and clinical criteria as summarized previously, a recent POG study using conventionally fractionated radiation therapy has resulted in less than 10% progression-free survival at 2 years (120).

A decade-long series of trials has evaluated the impact of high-dose, hyperfractionated irradiation for brainstem gliomas. The initial experience with hyperfractionated delivery was reported from the Univesity of California at San Francisco (UCSF), suggesting improved outcome following 100 cGy b.i.d. to 72 Gy (91,121). The rationale is similar to other trials in CNS tumors, based on the relative sparing of dose-limiting late CNS effects using smaller fraction sizes, permitting dose escalation of potential benefit regarding tumor control (122,123). Using the early results of the UCSF trial and mathematical models of the alpha/beta ratios for normal CNS and tumor characteristics, the clinical cooperative groups serially tested escalating doses of hyperfractionated irradiation. Table 5 summarizes outcome for selected, unfavorable brainstem gliomas, progressively limited to the more aggressive diffusely infiltrating pontine gliomas as eligibility criteria became more stringent during the course of the past decade (93). One can appreciate a suggested, but statistically marginal, benefit in 2-year and long-

TABLE 5. *Multiple-fraction-per day radiotherapy for children with brainstem tumors*

Institution or group (ref.)	No.	Cranial nerve palsy (%)	Long tract signs (%)	Median duration of symptoms	Pretreatment biopsy (%)	Dose/fraction (Gy)	Total dose (Gy)	Median survival time (mo)	Survival (%)		
									1 yr	2 yr	3 yr
POG (92,93, 118,125)	34	79	56	2	35	1.1	66	11	48	6	3
POG (92,93, 118,125)	57	93	60	1	40	1.17	70.2	10	40	23	20
POG (92,93, 118,125)	39	92	66	1	21	1.26	75.6	10	40	22	
CHOP (100, 108,114,101, 127)	15	100	27	1	27	1.2	64.8	11	48		
CHOP (100, 108,114,101, 127)	35	91	43	1	20	1	72	NS	30	28	28
UCSF (85,88, 89,121,196)	39	NS	NS	a	53	1	66–78	10.8[b]			36[b]
Duke University (124)	11	82	38	1	9	1.1–1.17	60.5–71.5	11	54	0	
New York University (197)	18	NS	NS	<6	44	1	72	14	—	—	28

POG, Pediatric Oncology Group; CHOP, Children's Hospital of Philadelphia; UCSF, University of California at San Francisco; NS, not stated.
[a]Duration of symptoms influenced survival.
[b]Includes some patients with thalamic tumors.
Modified and updated from reference 85.

term survival at dose levels of 70.2 Gy (POG study at 117 cGy b.i.d.) or 72 Gy (CCG and multiinstitutional experience at 100 cGy b.i.d.) compared to the initial dose levels of 66 Gy (100 to 110 cGy per fraction, felt to be "isoeffective" with 54 Gy at 180 cGy fractions once daily), and the dose-escalated level of 75.6 Gy (POG at 126 cGy/fraction b.i.d.) or 78 Gy (CCG at 100 cGy/fraction b.i.d.) (92,93,100,101).

The experience with hyperfractionated irradiation has, perhaps, been most important as it provided enthusiastic support for neurosurgeons, pediatric neurologists, and pediatric oncologists to focus on brain tumor trials and develop some understanding of radiation parameters (124). Later data from the initial UCSF trial confirmed the mixture of brainstem tumor types, with positive outcome limited to the focal tumors often outside the pons (88,89,91). The number of long-term survivors with diffusely infiltrating pontine gliomas remains quite limited; a late update of the POG study, including all three serially escalating dose arms studied between 1984

and 1990, shows only 9 survivors of 130 enrolled (125).

A prospective, randomized trial of hyperfractionated versus conventionally fractionated irradiation had been felt to be unsupportable in the mid-1980s when the "control" arm promised survival rates below 10%. A single-arm study of hyperfractionated irradiation with concurrent cisplatinum as a potential radiosensitizer was completed in POG without apparent undue toxicity (126). A subsequent trial prospectively compared conventional to hyperfractionated radiation delivery, incorporating concurrent cisplatinum in both arms to provide the potential for improving outcome. The radiotherapy arms were either hyperfractionated delivery (70.2 Gy at 117 cGy b.i.d.) or conventional fractionation (54 Gy at 180 cGy q.i.d.). Median survival time in both arms is a disappointing 8 months using now standard criteria for high-risk pontine gliomas; the survival curves are coincident, with 2-year survival of 10% in both arms (120).

More recent studies have refocused investigational management on combined chemoradiation (using concurrent etoposide), biologic response modifiers (with concurrent interferon or tamoxifen), and radiosensitizers (testing estramustine) (127,128). Most trials have reverted to conventionally fractionated irradiation (124). The most recent POG trial suggests that conventionally fractionated irradiation to 54 to 55.8 Gy (at 180 cGy daily fractions) is, again, the "standard" regimen for diffusely infiltrating pontine lesions (120). For the low-grade, focal brainstem tumors, dose levels of 50 to 54 Gy are used; particularly with three-dimensional planning/delivery, focal radiation techniques permit utilization of the higher dose level even in very young children.

Technique

Diffusely infiltrating pontine gliomas were typically irradiated with parallel opposed lateral fields intended to encompass the tumor volume with a margin of 2 to 3 cm (92). At some insitutions three-dimensional treatment planning is used to treat with two lateral and a vertex field. The use of higher energy linear accelerators (e.g., 10 to 18 MV or greater) results in a more favorable dose distribution than can be achieved with lower energies. The lower border of the radiation volume typically extends to C-1 or C-2 to allow a margin below disease extending into the medulla; because of narrower separation at this level, one should follow off-axis dosimetry. With high-dose regimens, it is appropriate to block the C1–2 volume as it approaches the intended cumulative dose level. New developments in three-dimensional tumor reconstruction and computer-aided simulation allow more localized dose delivery, potentially important in the infiltrating pontine tumors treated with concurrent cytotoxic chemotherapy or radiation modifiers.

For focal brainstem gliomas (including tectal plate lesions, dorsally exophytic pontomedullary tumors, and focal intrinsic lesions of the midbrain, pons, or medulla), tumor size and configuration often define the best approach using conventional delivery (including coronal arcs or 3-, 4-field approaches) or three-dimensional planning and delivery (conformal irradiation or fractionated stereotactic radiosurgery).

Delivery

Children with diffusely infiltrating brainstem gliomas usually require corticosteroids at diagnosis to hasten control of neurologic symptoms. For those not receiving corticosteroids at the initiation of radiation therapy, one should consider initiating a low-dose regimen (e.g., dexamethasone at 2 to 4 mg b.i.d.) for children with large primary lesions. Children with rapidly deteriorating neurologic signs may require high-dose corticosteroids and use of mannitol to control local edema and mass effect prior to initiating irradiation.

Irradiation is generally well tolerated. Acute reactions include radioepidermitis, most pronounced in the external auditory canal and the retroauricular region when using parallel opposed lateral fields; such reactions may be more pronounced with hyperfractionated delivery (92,100,101).

A significant proportion of patients with brainstem tumors demonstrate clinical and imaging evidence of apparent "progressive tumor" within 1 to 4 months of completing radiation therapy (91–93,101,114). Following high-dose hyperfractionated irradiation, 10% to 40% of patients may require reinstitution of corticosteroids or remain corticosteroid-dependent for several months after therapy (91–93,100,101). Patients should not immediately be considered therapeutic failures; a majority of children will stabilize or improve following a 3- to 12-week interval. Imaging changes during this interval include focal enhancement (often in a previously nonenhancing lesion), cyst formation (or cystic degeneration), or intralesional hemorrhage/necrosis (114). Differentiating such subacute phenomena from tumor progression may be extremely difficult, often apparent only with time to observe the clinical course. Positron emission tomography using fluordeoxyglucose (FDG-PET) has been of purported value in selected series; conversion of a "hot" lesion to a "cold" one following irradiation may be more compatible with subacute radiation changes than tumor progression (129). Preliminary data has also suggested that magnetic resonance spectroscopy may provide differential information in this setting (130).

Results

Approximately 60% to 70% of patients with classic pontine gliomas will have a stabilization or improvement of their functional status following irradiation. Time to progression may be difficult to document in this tumor system; cooperative group studies report median time to progression approximating 6 to 8 months. Median survival intervals are only 8 to 12 months in patients selected for high-risk pontine glioma studies (92,93,100, 101). There appears to be no difference for hyperfractionated versus conventionally fractionated irradiation in this setting (120).

Children with focal, intrinsic tumors of the midbrain or medulla show long-term survival after irradiation estimated at 50% to 70% (21,85,94). Survival at 10 years following surgery with or without necessary irradiation for dorsally exophytic brainstem gliomas approaches 75% (95,96,99,104). Similar rates are quoted for the focal pontine lesions of limited size after localized irradiation (94).

EPENDYMOMAS

Intracranial ependymomas represent 3% to 6% of intracranial neoplasms in children; two-thirds occur as primary infratentorial tumors. Posterior fossa or fourth ventricular ependymomas arise along the linings of the fourth ventricle, most often as midline lesions filling the fourth ventricle. The tumors generally originate from the ventricular floor where attachment is commonly noted at the level of the obex (the caudal-most aspect of the fourth ventricle along the posterior surface of the medulla, where the fourth ventricle ends and the central spinal canal begins). The tumors frequently extend into the foramina of Lushka, growing toward the cerebellopontine angle and extending caudally along the upper cervical spine (131,132) (Figs. 12–13). Particularly in young children, ependymomas may originate at the cerebellopontine angle, presenting as lateral rather than midline lesions (133). The less common supratentorial lesions occur as intracerebral tumors, often adjacent to the third or lateral ventricular regions (132,134).

Ependymomas are histologically comprised of polygonal cells with large vesicular nuclei and cytoplasmic granules. Characteristic are ependymal rosettes, formed by tumor cells oriented radially around a central lumen; cells also have a tendency to orient themselves around blood vessels, forming perivascular pseudorosettes (11,102). The origin is from the ependymal central neuroepithelial cells during embryogenesis or as malignant degeneration of mature ependymal cells in the ventricular linings or the subependymal zones of cellular proliferation. Supratentorial ependymomas may be remote from the ventricular system; such tumors theoretically arise from ependymal cell rests.

There is uncertainty with regard to histologic classification or grading of ependymomas (11,102,135). The tumor categories include:

- differentiated, or ordinary, ependymomas (herein identified as "ependymoma");
- anaplastic ependymomas (identified by focal or diffuse areas of increased cellular density and/or cytologic evidence of cellular anaplasia); anaplastic characteristics are more common within supratentorial than fourth ventricular lesions;
- myxopapillary ependymomas: well-differentiated, papillary-like tumors occurring most often as primary spinal cord lesions, typically at the level of the cauda equina; or
- ependymoblastoma, an extremely rare, highly malignant form of primitive embryonal supratentorial tumor occurring in infants with embryonal cell types and ependymal characteristics (see Chapter 3). Ependymoblastomas are excluded from ad-

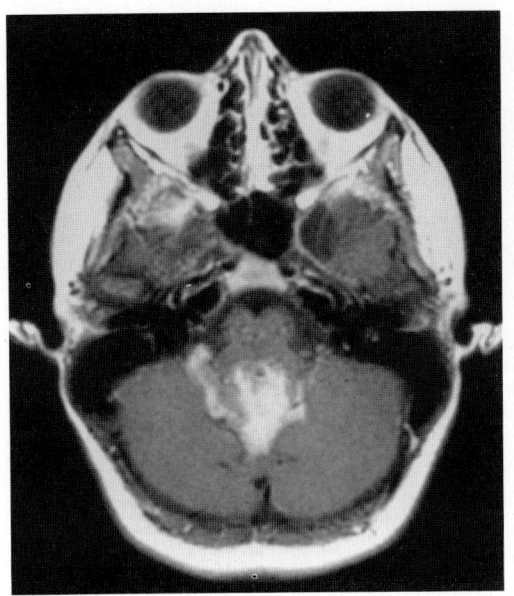
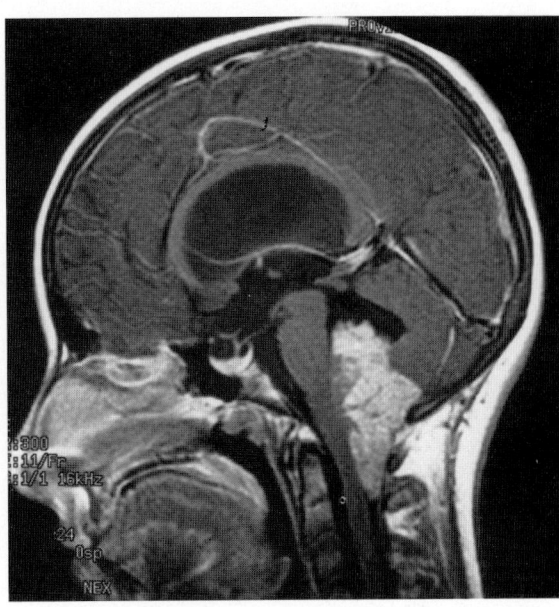

A   B

FIG. 12. Posterior fossa ependymoma, typically extending from the region of the IVth ventricle, through the foramen of Luschka **(A)** and caudally beyond the cerebellopontine angle along the cervicomedullary junction **(B)**.

ditional discussion relative to fourth ventricular ependymomas.

There are conflicting reports with respect to the correlation between tumor grade (i.e., ependymoma versus anaplastic ependymoma) and survival. Although a majority of radiation oncology-related series indicate superior survival for differentiated ependymomas compared to anaplastic forms, the neuropathology literature expresses caution regarding modifications of treatment based on histologic "grade" as clinicohistologic correlations are unproven (135–137). If one reviews recent series reporting outcome, one finds data indicating: equivalent results for ependymoma and anaplastic ependymoma, superior survival for ependymomas, or superior survival for anaplastic ependymomas (138–141). One major series suggests a unique classification system based on a specific feature (focal areas of hypercellularity) to identify a statistically significant histologic predictor (131). There is no consistent data supporting a higher rate of local recurrence or neuraxis dis-

semination amongst anaplastic ependymomas when compared to differentiated histologic types (131,140–143).

There is a male sex predilection, although young children show equal gender distribution or even a slight female predominance. The median age at diagnosis is 3 to 4 years; younger children (less than 3- to 5-years old) have less favorable outcome, particularly in posterior fossa ependymomas (131,142).

Symptoms are usually nonspecific, related to fourth ventricular obstruction with attendant headaches and vomiting; ataxia is also common. Children with disease involving the cerebellopontine (CP) angle, with or without tumor growing into the upper cervical spine, will frequently show torticollis and/or CP angle cranial nerve signs (especially unilateral hearing loss) (132,133). MRI often shows a nonhomogeneously enhancing lesion, diagnostic when there is characteristic involvement through the foramen of Lushka, to or from the CP angle, or extension along the upper cervical spine. Approximately 50% of children show tumor extension into the cervi-

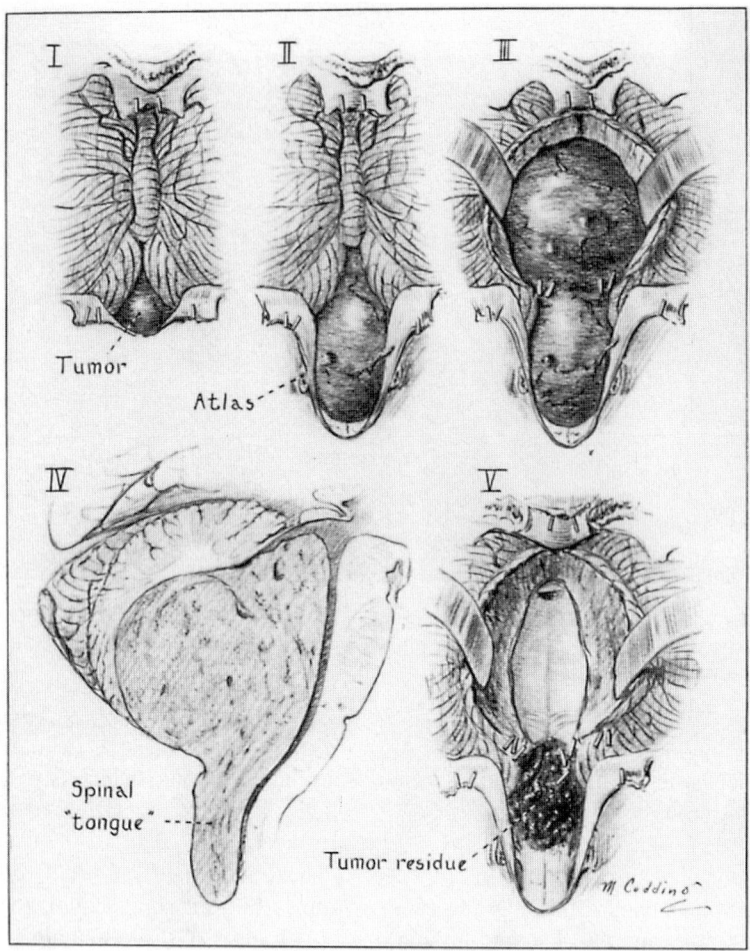

FIG. 13. In 1929, Harvey Cushing operated on a man with a cerebellar ependymoma and described a characteristic finding of this tumor—its tendency to extend into the cervical spine: "a tongue of tumor was disclosed projecting downward into the spinal canal...for its proper exposure it was necessary to laminectomize the atlas...." The illustration demonstrates the stages of operative exposure and subtotal resection. (Reprinted from Cushing's 1932 edition of *Intracranial Tumors* with permission of C. C. Thomas, Publishers: Springfield, Illinois and the assistance of the Rare Book Room, Duke Medical School Library.)

cal spinal canal; tumor growth frequently extends to the C-2 area and has been documented to the C-5 level (131,141).

Therapy

Surgery

Surgical resection is often incomplete in posterior fossa ependymoma. Fourth ventricular lesions are usually adherent along the brainstem, especially at the level of the obex where surgical damage can result in significant cardiorespiratory compromise (132,144). Total resection is limited in tumors involving the CP angle, where dissection amongst the cranial nerves is technically difficult (131–133). Tumors extending to the anterior aspect of the medulla challenge surgical exposure and are often attached along the basilar artery or focally along the ventral brainstem. Experience indicates complete resection (based on surgical impression and postoperative imaging) in approximately 30% to 50% of cases. There is a significant relationship between degree of resection and outcome in most reports of childhood ependymomas. Tomita (144) noted 5-year progression-free survival only among the subset of children with gross total resection: 33% versus 0% for those with incomplete surgery. A review from the Children's Hospital Medical Center in Boston similarly noted 0% 10-year freedom from progression when postoperative imaging indicated residual tumor, compared to 75% for patients with imaging-confirmed complete resection ($p = 0.03$) (145). Table 6 summarizes the correlation between degree of resection and outcome in major reports.

Operative morbidity in pediatric neurosurgery is often most apparent in posterior fossa ependymomas. Operative mortality has diminished from 15% to 20% to levels below 3% to 5% (131,132,144). The incidence of new postoperative neurologic deficits has approached 30% in the literature; temporary mutism, ataxia, and/or respiratory complications requiring tracheostomy are amongst the more serious occurrences (38,131,144).

Radiation Therapy

Radiation therapy has been a routine component of therapy for ependymomas since the 1950s (Fig. 4). The relatively favorable results summarized previously following surgical resection are almost systematically based on the addition of postoperative irradiation (44,131,

141,144–146,183). Two series confirm the contribution of radiation therapy: Pollack et al. (146) recorded overall 5-year survival of 45% with surgery and irradiation compared to 13% with surgery alone; Rousseau et al. (141) noted similar results: 63% survival at 5-years postirradiation versus 23% without irradiation. Although long-term progression-free survival in children with residual ependymoma treated with radiation therapy averages less than 30%, the ability to achieve durable disease control has been documented (Table 5). The excellent results with complete resection and postoperative irradiation continue to support early, systematic use of radiation therapy especially for posterior fossa lesions. The impact of irradiation on disease control has also been suggested in infants managed by primary postoperative chemotherapy. The first POG infant brain tumor study included a group who received systematic irradiation after 1 year of chemotherapy and a younger subset scheduled to receive irradiation after 2 years of chemotherapy. Long-term disease control has been significantly higher in the former group with earlier irradiation (147). Among the most controversial unresolved questions for the radiation oncologist is the appropriate target volume, recommendations ranging from full CSI to treatment limited to the imaging defined region of tumor residual (44,139,141–143,148,149).

Chemotherapy

Ependymomas are relatively chemosensitive tumors, with objective responses demon-

TABLE 6. *Impact of surgical resection in combined surgery–radiation therapy for pediatric ependymomas*

| Interval | Outcome measure | Surgical resection | | Incomplete(n) | Series/Ref |
		Gross total (n)	"Radical" (n)		
1975–1989	5-yr PFS (all sites)	80% (10)	60% (23)	21% (18)	CHOP (132)
1970–1987	5-yr PFS (post fossa)	100% (5)		19% (21)	H.SickChild (131)
1985–1990	5-yr PFS (all sites)	82% (29)		35% (27)	POG (155)
1975–1989	5-yr PFS (all sites)	51% (38)		26% (42)	I-GusRoussy (191)
1975–1993	5-yr PFS (all sites)	68% (23)	(imaging –,+)	9% (14)	Pitts.Child (146)

PFS, profession-free survival

strated following cisplatinum or carboplatinum and alkylating agents in phase II trials (48). The only prospective, randomized trial tested adjuvant chemotherapy (CCNU, vincristine, prednisone) following surgery and irradiation (150). Disease-free survival was no different with CSI alone (5/14) than CSI plus chemotherapy (10/22). Disease-free survival for the entire group was 42% with a medial follow-up of 88 months. Multiagent regimens have shown tumor response in the preirradiation setting, including cyclophosphamide/VP-16, cyclophosphamide/vincristine, and MOPP (47). Trials continue to test preirradiation chemotherapy responsiveness (e.g., topotecan in POG). There is no data suggesting a role for routine, adjuvant chemotherapy.

Radiotherapeutic Management

Volume

The selection of treatment volume for ependymomas has been an issue of considerable controversy. Posterior fossa ependymomas are known to have the ability to extend in continuity up to the aqueduct and down to the high cervical spine (131,132). Ependymomas also have the ability to seed the craniospinal axis via the CSF. The incidence of neuraxis dissemination varies in the literature; several review articles summarize the frequency at approximately 12% (139,140,143,151–153). Bloom (151) initially reported relatively frequent seeding among high-grade posterior

fossa ependymomas, recommending CSI for such presentations. Several series questioned the necessity to use full neuraxis therapy, noting a predominantly local pattern of failure and a significant incidence of dissemination largely as a secondary event following one or more local recurrences (139,141–143,148, 154) (Tables 7 and 8). Late follow-up of Bloom's Royal Marsden experience, in fact, reported neuraxis dissemination in only 2 of 33 children with local posterior fossa tumor control, in addition noting no difference between children who had received CSI and those treated with only local volumes. There was no difference between ependymomas (5% total incidence of CSF dissemination) or anaplastic ependymomas (8.7% incidence) (143). A prospective study, only preliminarily reported by POG, has shown neuraxis disease at diagnosis in only 1 of 37 children with posterior fossa differentiated ependymomas; following local irradiation, CSF metastasis has been reported in only one of these children at 7 years posttherapy (155). The latter study required CSI for anaplastic infratentiorial ependymomas; following CSI, 3 of 10 have failed concurrently at the primary site and in the neuraxis (155). Paradoxically, preliminary analysis of a follow-up POG trial testing local, posterior fossa hyperfractionated irradiation has shown neuraxis involvement at the time of initial failure in 5 of 35 cases (156).

The broad body of current data regarding posterior fossa ependymomas favors local irradiation: the incidence of isolated primary

TABLE 7. *Intracranial ependymoma—neuraxis involvement at diagnosis*

Site	Tumor Histology	No.	M_1	$M_{2-3}M_+$	Total	Series/Ref
IT	Ependy.	27	0	1	1	CHOP (142)
	Anaplastic	13	2	0	2	
IT	Anaplastic	14	0	1	1	MSKCC (149)
ST	Anaplastic	14	1	0	1	
All	All	45	3	1	4	IGR (141)
IT	All	25	5	3	7	U.Pitts (146)
ST	All	12			1	
IT	All	43	2	0	2	POG (155)
ST	All	10	1	0	1	

ST, Supratentorial; IT, Infratentorial; Ependy, classic ependymoma; Anaplastic, anaplastic ependymoma.

TABLE 8. *Infratentorial ependymomas—subarachnoid dissemination at first failure*

No. of patients with radiation volume		Total no. of patients	M$_+$ at initial failure	Series/Ref
Post. Fossa	CSI			
4	13	17	0	Child Mem (144)
6	29	35	1	HSC/PMH (131)
27	6	33	3	CHOP (142, 148)
33	10	43	5	POG (155)

Post. Fossa, posterior fossa; CSI, craniospinal irradiation; HSC/PMH, Hospital for Sick Children/Princess Margaret Hospital; CHOP, Children's Hospital of Philadelphia; POG, Pediatric Oncology Group.

neuraxis failure following resection and local irradiation seems to be at or below the 10% level; to date, there has been no evidence that "preventive" CNS irradiation improves the outcome of differentiated or anaplastic ependymomas (131,139,141–143,148,149, 155). "Local" irradiation traditionally implies treatment encompassing the entire posterior fossa, extending inferiorly to the C-2 level (or lower to allow 2 to 3 cm below disease when there is extension below the foramen magnum). Increasing observations note that local failures often involve sites of initially identifiable residual disease or areas of attachment identified at surgery. Reduction of the target volume to cover only the initial tumor bed rather than the entire posterior fossa is currently under investigation. There is an evolving experience with stereotactic radiotherapy (or fractionated radiosurgery), targeting only the bed on postoperative imaging or identified by the surgeon (117). Use of stereotactic radiosurgery as a single-fraction boost has also been successful in a limited trial reported from St. Jude (157). Outside the study setting, the target volume for differentiated and anaplastic posterior fossa ependymomas remains the posterior fossa, covering sites of initial or potential disease involvement.

Dose

Dose-response data for ependymoma is relatively rare. Reports confirm greater radiation efficacy with dose levels above 45 or 50 Gy (139,142,148,149,158). In series limited to anaplastic ependymomas, Children's Hospital of Philadelphia reported 3-year survival of 55% following more than 45 Gy to the primary volume, compared to 0 for those with dose levels below 45 Gy; Memorial/Sloan Kettering similarly noted a correlation between dose to the primary lesion and outcome (142,149).

Technique

The standard technique for posterior fossa irradiation is parallel opposed lateral fields; for ependymomas (with little tendency to infiltrate diffusely or metastasize within the posterior fossa), opposed high energy beams may be appropriate. Current three-dimensional conformal approaches have targeted the tumor bed (rather than the entire posterior fossa) or only the site(s) of residual disease (Fig. 14). It is too early to estimate the frequency and pattern of failure.

Delivery

Standard immobilization techniques are utilized, particularly when three-dimensional conformal techniques define rather narrow margins. Significant acute treatment-related toxicities are largely limited to cutaneous reactions. For most children treated after complete or near total resection, it is unnecessary to utilize corticosteroids during irradiation.

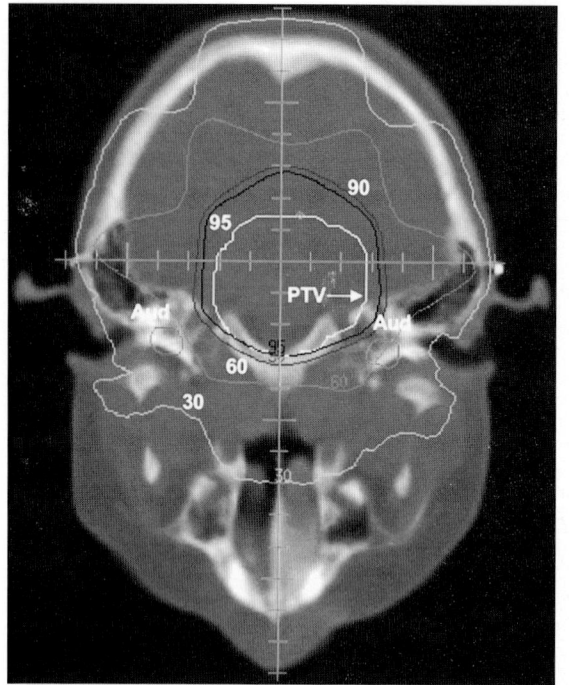

A

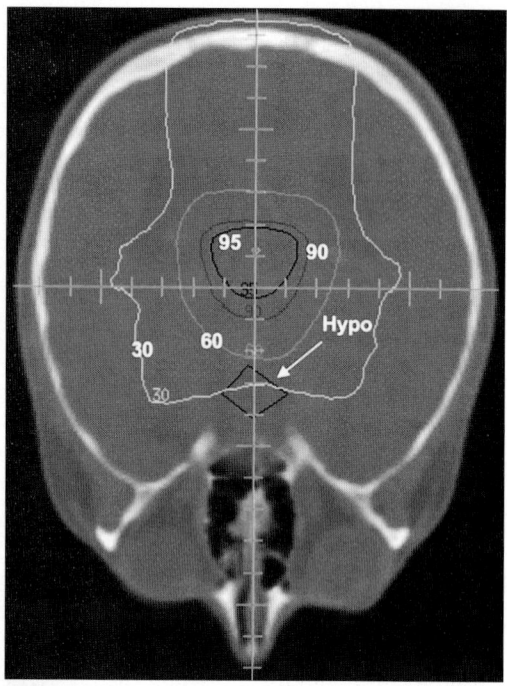

B

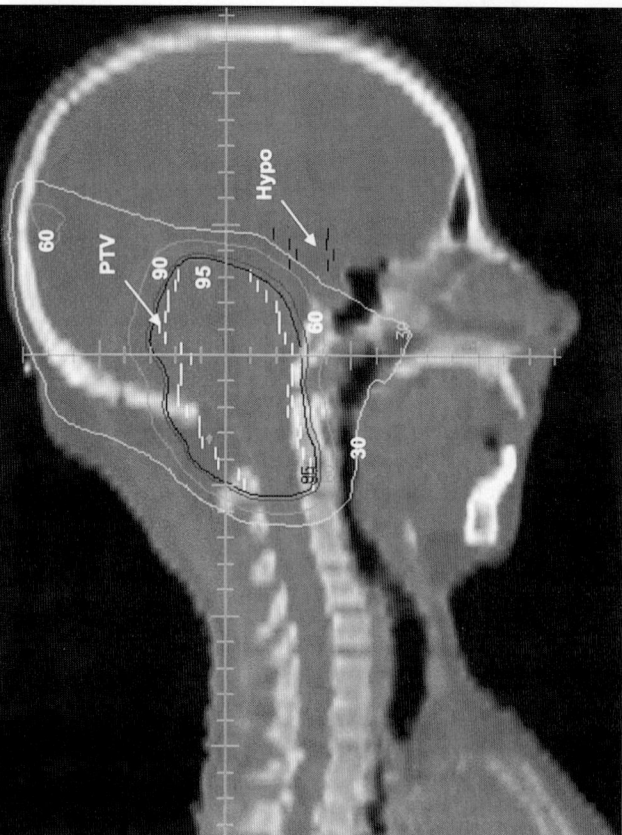

C

FIG. 14. Three-dimensional conformal approach for treating ependymoma following near total resection, targeting the tumor bed with a 1.5 cm margin (defining the somewhat broader PTV). The 3-field noncoplanar approach achieves relative dose conformation and relatively spares the hearing apparatus (Aud), as well as the pituitary-hypothalamic region (Hypo).

Results

Overall results in various series indicate 5-year survival rates approximating 45% to 65% for children over 2- to 4-years old (Table 5). Progression-free survival rates approach 40% to 50%. For children with gross total resection followed by irradiation, disease-free survival at 5 years ranges from 60% to 80%. Following incomplete resection and irradiation, progression-free survival averages only 20% to 30% at 5 years (131,139,141–143, 146).

CEREBELLAR ASTROCYTOMAS

Cerebellar astrocytomas comprise 15% of childhood brain tumors. The tumors are typically well-circumscribed, slowly growing lesions with prominent cyst formation (159,160). The classic cystic cerebellar astrocytoma presents as a unilocular cyst with a prominent mural nodule. Cushing was the first to describe the entity in 1931 (161), commenting on the "benign" nature of cerebellar astrocytomas, associated with low morbidity and mortality. Initially, Cushing failed to recognize that the mural nodule represented the active neoplastic portion of cystic cerebellar astrocytomas. Without removal of the nodule, the cyst was likely to recur. Once the neoplastic nature of the nodule was recognized and the nodule was removed at surgery, results improved dramatically (162).

Cerebellar astrocytomas are divided histologically into JPAs (noted in 75% to 85% of cases) or diffuse astrocytomas (15% to 20%) (11,163). The JPA consists of bipolar (piloid) astrocytes intermixed with Rosenthal fibers and areas of microcystic, loose-textured astrocytes (11,163). Diffuse astrocytomas are identified as fibrillary astrocytomas or astrocytomas NOS; uncommonly, such tumors are oligoastroctyomas. It is controversial whether malignant gliomas occur in the cerebellum in children. Shinoda et al. (164) described five children with histologic signs of anaplastic astrocytoma or glioblastoma among 19 cerebellar astrocytomas; the clinical course in each of the children was certainly consistent with a malignant glioma. Standard neuropathology texts debate whether true malignant astrocytomas can arise in the cerebellum, especially among young children (11,102). The occurrence is most uncommon.

The median age at diagnosis is 5 to 6 years. Although 20% occur in young children (less than 2 to 3 years), it is rarely found in infants in the first year of life (159,165,166). Presenting symptoms are often confined to those associated with increased intracranial pressure (headaches, vomiting, less often diplopia), altered cerebellar function (poor coordination, dyspraxic speech, ataxia), or cranial nerve deficits, which occur less frequently.

The majority of tumors arise in the cerebellar hemispheres; approximately one-third are primary vermis lesions. The most characteristic appearance on CT or MRI is a large, well-circumscribed tumor with prominent cysts (unilocular or multilocular). The nodular or solid portion of the tumor characteristically enhances briskly. In 40% to 60% of cases, the cyst wall does not enhance; in such cases, the cyst is technically a reactive structure without tumor cells in the cyst wall (165). The remaining ± 40% of tumors are either "false cysts," signified by focal or diffuse cyst wall enhancement (in which case the cyst wall is a part of the neoplastic process) or diffuse (solid) tumors. The latter are more likely to show direct extension to the cerebellopontine peduncle or the brainstem (159,160,166). Cerebellar JPAs have been associated with multifocal CNS involvement, representing either neuraxis dissemination or multifocal tumorigenesis. Although less frequent than noted in diencephalic tumors of the same histology, "metastatic" disease has been documented in up to 5 to 10% of cases, most often at the time of diagnosis (167–169). The incidence of remote disease has only recently become apparent; in general, evaluation of the spinal axis (i.e., spinal MRI) is reserved for cerebellar astrocytomas with disease apparent beyond the primary site on cranial MRI.

Therapy

Surgery

Surgical resection is the treatment of choice for cerebellar astrocytomas. Long-term disease control, even in the presence of known postoperative residual, has been well documented since Cushing's initial operative series (161). For classic cystic cerebellar astrocytomas, gross total resection has been reported in 70% to 90% of cases (162,163,170). A review from Children's Hospital of Los Angeles (160), indicated imaging evidence of residual tumor in 11 of 18 cases coded surgically as "total resection." The clinical behavior of these tumors remains quite indolent, often noting long-term disease stabilization despite documented tumor residual. Among cases coded largely by surgical impression, Garcia et al. (170) noted recurrence in only 1 of 40 children after gross total resection, between 1928 and 1980, with a median follow-up approaching 50 years. A review of 112 cases over a similar timeframe similarly indicated freedom from progression in 95% of cases after total resection (162). Following incomplete resection, disease progression (or recurrence) has been noted in 30% to 60% of cases at 5 to 10 years or more; importantly, long-term survival remains at or above the 60% level (160,162,170). Despite the "indolent" nature of these tumors, the median time to recurrence approximates 2 years (160,162). A recently completed CCG/POG trial addressing astrocytomas in children should soon provide prospective data addressing the frequency of gross total resection, based on central review of operative records and postoperative imaging, and the incidence of recurrence or progression after gross total or incomplete resection.

Radiation Therapy

There is no established role for radiation therapy in the primary management of cerebellar astrocytomas. The sentinel issue revolves around the question of prognostic factors that may predict recurrence after surgery alone. Most series indicate increased risk of recurrence in solid (versus cystic) tumors and in diffuse (versus juvenile pilocytic) histologic types. In a sizable Mayo Clinic series combining children and adults treated between 1960 and 1984, 10-year survival was 81% with JPA compared to 7% for diffuse histologies; most of the latter cases occurred in adults over 20-years old (163). Analyses restricted to children have shown similar, if less dramatic, differences: the majority of series correlate solid tumors with diffuse histologies, both solid tumors and diffuse histologies with brainstem involvement and with incomplete resection (159,160,166,171).

Indications for radiation therapy have included incompletely resected tumors or those with diffuse or unfavorable histologies (171, 172). There is no data substantiating improvement in disease control with postoperative irradiation (166,170,173). Series that have suggested efficacy in selected settings (residual cystic cerebellar astrocytoma, incomplete resection regardless of histology, or solid tumor types) include numbers that remain statistically nonsignificant (162,170,172). There is interest in testing stereotactic radiosurgery (either as a single fraction or with fractionated stereotactic radiotherapy) to focal sites of disease residual; enthusiasm will be based on a documented rate of progression after incomplete surgery from the cooperative group study as well as the apparent efficacy and toxicities of such intervention in controlled settings (117).

Chemotherapy

There is no substantial data addressing the impact of chemotherapy in cerebellar astrocytomas to date.

Radiotherapeutic Management

Indications for radiation therapy are generally limited to children with documented progressive or recurrent disease who have undergone a second, incomplete resection or who are felt to be unresectable at the time of progression/recurrence (173). In such cases, standard techniques include local irradiation (to the tumor bed with a 1-cm margin) to dose levels of 50 to 54 Gy.

The treatment of high-grade cerebellar astrocytomas is controversial. As in adults, there has been debate regarding the necessity to irradiate the entire neuraxis. Anecdotal cases indicate an incidence of CSF seeding from cerebellar malignant gliomas that has ranged from 3 of 4 to 0 of 4 (174,175). UCSF has reported 5-year survival in 4 of 6 children following full cranial or local posterior fossa irradiation (176). The indications for CSI are generally limited to children with documented subarachnoid metastasis or multifocal disease, regardless of histology. The implications for malignant cerebellar astrocytomas are largely theoretical. Long-term survival has been documented in children with the rare multifocal/metastatic low-grade astrocytomas (167–169).

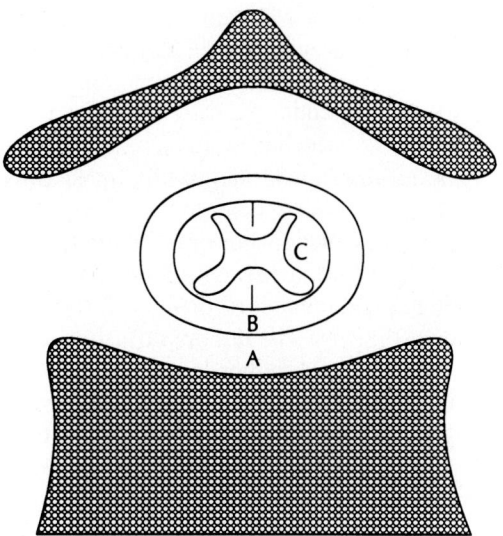

FIG. 15. Classification of spinal tumors. **A:** Extramedullary, extradural. **B:** Extramedullary, intradural. **C:** Intramedullary, intradural.

Results

Overall survival rates in childhood cerebellar astroctyomas are 80% to 90% at over 10 years (159,160,165,166). Survival rates are highest among those with JPA histology and gross total resection. For incompletely resected diffuse astrocytomas, long-term survival rates of 45% to 60% have been reported (159,162,163,166).

SPINAL CORD NEOPLASMS

Spinal cord neoplasms are uncommon in children. Tumors involving the spinal canal are classified as *intradural* when (a) confined to the spinal canal (termed *intramedullary*) or (b) arising from the cauda equina or intradural components of the nerve roots (*extramedullary*). *Extradural* tumors are extraneural neoplasms that arise outside the nervous system (Fig. 15). The extradural lesions extend into the canal by direct growth (from osseous tumors of the vertebrae or adjacent soft-tissue lesions) or by insinuation through the spinal foramina. Tumors that grow through a spinal foramen (or adjacent foramina) extend linearly beyond the cord segment of entry, accounting for the so-called "dumbbell" description; such presentations are most common in neuroblastomas, paravertebral soft-tissue tumors of the "Ewing's family" (i.e., peripheral PNET), or neurofibromas. Management of extradural presentations is discussed in chapters related to the primary tumor type. Nervous system tumors arising in the spinal cord and cauda equina are discussed in this section.

Primary spinal cord neoplasms account for approximately 5% of central nervous system neoplasms in the pediatric age group. It is difficult to extrapolate adult data regarding spinal cord tumors to children; spinal cord tumors represent a greater proportion of CNS neoplasms in adults, and the relative histologic and anatomic frequencies are almost mirror image presentations compared to those in children (177,178). Astrocytomas are the most common spinal cord tumors in children, accounting for 60% of primary neoplasms. Ependymomas account for 30%; other gliomas (gangliogliomas, oligodendrogliomas) and neurilemommas (neurofibromas usually associated with neurofibromatosis type I) comprise the remaining 10% (178).

Over 80% of pediatric spinal cord *astrocytomas* are low-grade neoplasms, most often fibrillary and less commonly pilocytic in type. Astrocytomas occur primarily in the cervical and thoracic regions of the cord, presenting as circumscribed or more infiltrating lesions (Fig. 16). The tumors diffusely widen the involved cord; tumor length averages six spinal cord segments (179). Over 30% to 40% are associated with sizable intraspinal cysts (107,178,180). The cysts typically extend in cephalad and caudal directions from the solid tumor, representing fluid-filled components that may more than double the overall length of the lesion. The cyst wall is usually not a part of the tumor process (178,180,181). Malignant gliomas (*high-grade astrocytomas*: anaplastic astrocytoma and glioblastoma multiforme) account for less than 10% to 20% of astrocytic lesions of the cord. The spinal malignant gliomas are clinically aggressive lesions; there is suggestion in the literature that such tumors are relatively more frequent in infants (177,178,180).

Holocord astrocytomas extend over much of the length of the cervicothoracic cord. Holocord lesions have been described in up to 60% of primary astroctyomas of the spine; more recent data shows that the majority represent lengthy cystic extensions of more localized lesions, although the solid tumor components may involve a significant length of the spinal cord (181,182). Tumors of the *cervicomedullary junction* seem to represent an anatomic extension into the lower brainstem of astrocytic neoplasms histologically and clinically similar to those occurring within the cervical spinal cord (107).

The less common glial tumors include *oligodendrogliomas* and *gangliogliomas*. These tumors are usually discrete, well-circumscribed intraspinal lesions that occur within the cervical, thoracic, or cervicomedullary junction regions; presenting

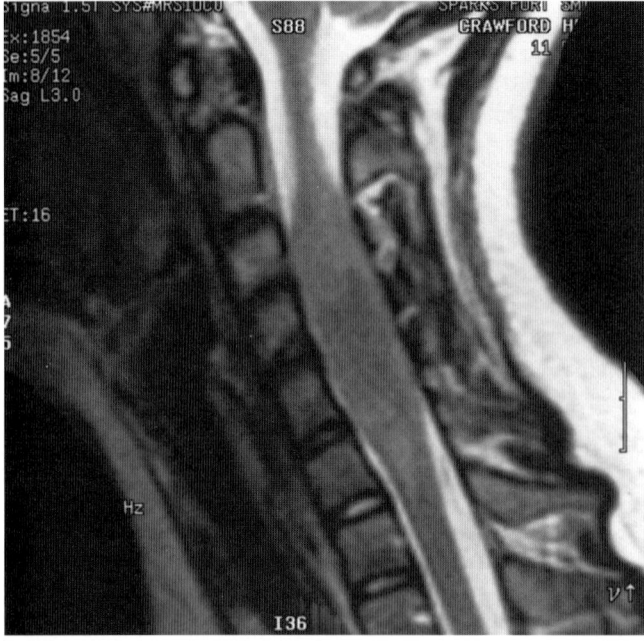
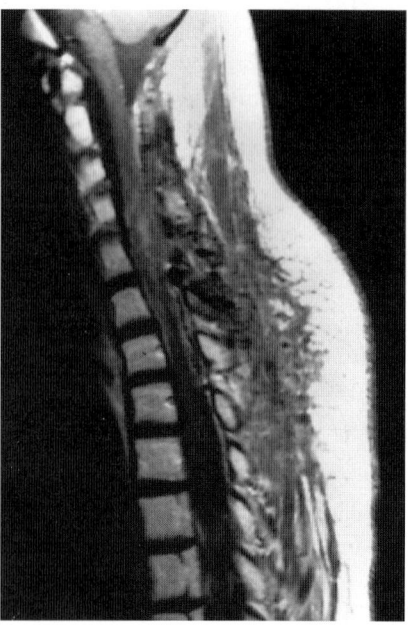

FIG. 16. Intramedullary spinal cord astrocytoma: lesion involving the cervico-thoracic cord **(A)**; child is free of disease following subtotal resection **(B)** and irradiation.

characteristics are similar to the astrocytomas (183).

Spinal cord *ependymomas* predominate amongst intamedullary tumors in adults, but comprise only a third of primary spinal neoplasms in children. The spinal cord primaries represent no more than 5% of all ependymomas in children (177,178). The majority arise in the low thoracic-lumbar region, involving the conus medullaris or the cauda equina. Ependymomas tend to be discrete, focal tumors when presenting as intramedullary lesions of the cervial or thoracic cord; tumor length averages 3 to 5 spinal segments (184). Most such ependymal lesions are histologically differentiated ependymomas. The more common pediatric tumor is the myxopapillary ependymoma. The latter tumors are low-grade, "indolent" lesions signified histologically by papillary growth and mucin formation; these tumors have been described as "recapitulating" the structure of the filum terminale (185). Two-thirds occur in the cauda equina, presumably arising from the filum; 30% present as tumors of the conus medullaris, and 5% as atypical myxopapillary tumors of the cervical or thoracic cord (Fig. 17). Rarely, myxopapillary ependymomas present as subcutaneous tumors connected to a sacrococcygeal sinus tract. Presumably arising from an embryonic rest, the sacrococcygeal lesions occur in infants without contiguity with the spinal cord of filum terminale (186).

Spinal cord tumors usually present with slowly progressive symptomatology; the average duration of symptoms in children was 2 years in a review from the Mayo Clinic (178). The most frequent symptoms include long tract signs, most apparent as subtle, gradually progressive changes in gait. Spinal pain is commonly noted, usually limited to the thoracic or cervical region of origin. Pain is classically increased at night when the child is recumbent (182,183). It is not rare to see lower thoracic cord pain evaluated as intraabdominal symptomatology, including laparotomy for suspected appendicitis. Radicular pain is relatively less common. Numbness or sphincter dysfunction occur in 10% of cases

(178,181,182). Children with cervical or cervicomedullary tumors often present with torticollis or head tilt. Spinal changes are less frequent with cervicothoracic lesions, presenting as kyphoscoliosis at the involved spinal level (183). Symptoms and signs of increased intracranial pressure may be noted at diagnosis of a primary, localized spinal cord tumor. The pathophysiology is incompletely understood, but is theoretically related to increased cerebrospinal fluid protein and/or altered CSF flow, resulting in ventriculomegaly and classic associated symptoms absent any discernible intracranial pathology (187).

MRI provides ideal evaluation of spinal cord neoplasms. One can usually distinguish intramedullary from extramedullary lesions. Tumor extent is generally well appreciated on MRI (Fig. 16). It is sometimes difficult to discern subtle cystic changes from solid tumor extension; intraoperative ultrasound can be a more sensitive tool in this regard. Low-grade astrocytomas and gangliogliomas are usually nonenhancing tumors, best delineated on T-2 or proton spin density sequences. Pilocytic astrocytomas enhance uniformly; ependymomas are typically enhancing lesions. In evaluating spinal cord tumors, it is important to image the entire length of the spinal canal; one can see "skip" intramedullary involvement uncommonly in astrocytomas. In ependymomas, it is standard to image the entire neuraxis. Rarely, intracranial ependymomas can masquerade as a primary intraspinal or cauda equina tumor, with an occult intracranial primary and symptoms due to spinal metastasis. Subarachnoid dissemination does occur in malignant gliomas and ependymomas, although involvement at diagnosis is rare; staging is appropriate prior to consideration of postoperative management (180,184).

Therapy

Surgery

The primary management for most intradural spinal tumors is surgery. While radi-

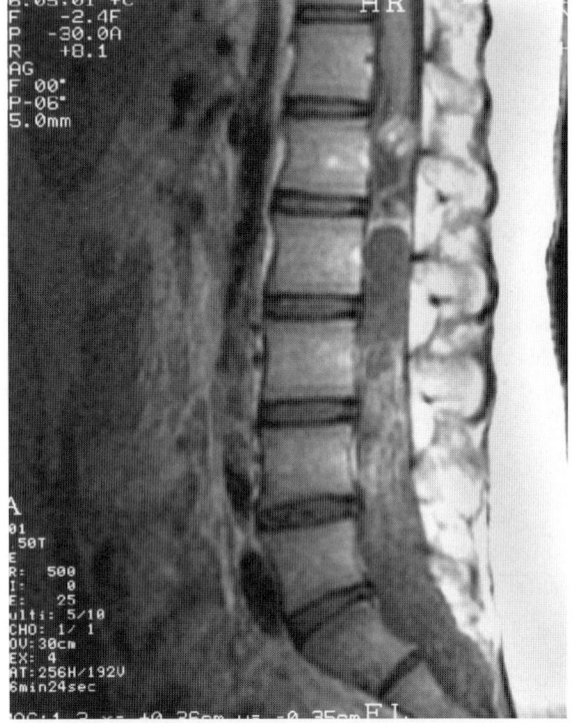

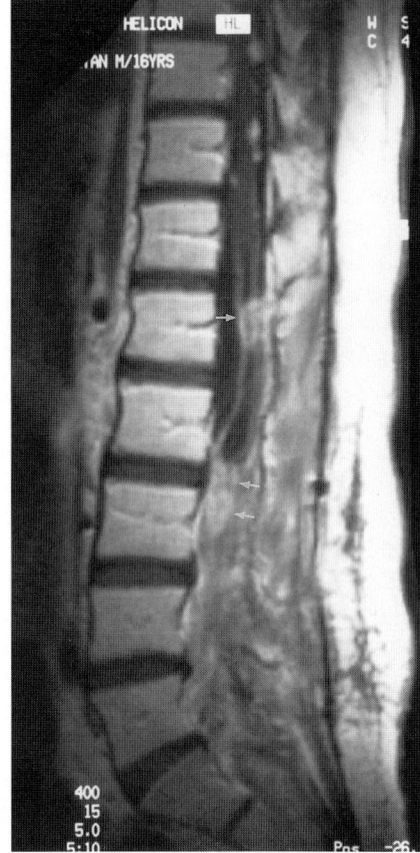

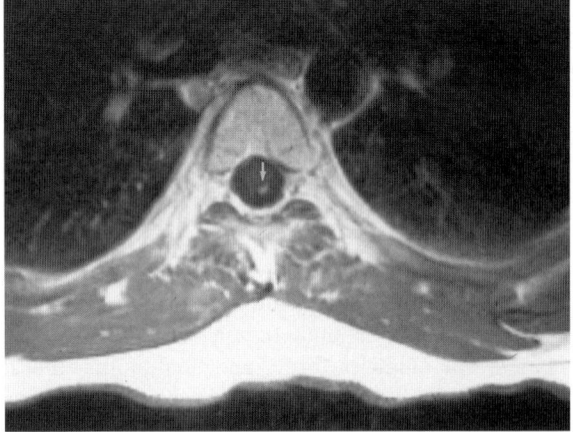

FIG. 17. Myxopapillary ependymoma of the cauda equina, documenting extensive disease that involves the cauda and nerve roots **(A)**; postoperative imaging shows residual and subarachnoid deposits **(B)** and **(C)**. Disease controlled at 5 years following surgery and CSI.

cal intramedullary resection had been infrequent, improved technology and extensive experience with intramedullary lesions has greatly facilitated the radical or gross total resection of a large percentage of pediatric intraspinal neoplasms. The use of midline myelotomy and ultrasonic dissection has allowed discrete dissection of intraspinal gliomas; the leading pediatric neurosurgeons relate less long-term morbidity following judicious complete resection, often technically approached from just outside the tumor margin, than from biopsy with attendant intralesional swelling or potential hemorrhage (181,188). Laminectomy and myelotomy are typically limited to the region of solid tumor involvement, guided intraoperatively by diagnostic ultrasound. Spinal evoked potentials guide the surgical procedure, allowing intra-operative monitoring for preservation of long track function (181). Postoperative morbidity, defined as increased neurologic deficit, is generally limited and ultimately resolving for tumors above the T-9 level; intraspinal astro-cytomas at the T9-12 level are reported to have the most significant operative-related morbidity (181).

Summary data from ten reported series combining pediatric and adult experience largely prior to the last decade, indicated total excision in 16% of low-grade spinal *gliomas* (primarily *astrocytoma*) (180). The 20-year re-view of pediatric spinal astrocytomas from the Mayo Clinic related radical excision in 2 of 32 children (178). The latter series noted im-proved outcome following total or subtotal re-section compared to decompressive laminec-tomy and biopsy alone: 100% survival at 5 years (with or without irradiation) versus 53% (178). Epstein (181) has serially presented a sizable experience with radical resection of spinal cord astrocytomas, relating excellent functional outcome and nearly uniform dis-ease control amongst children with low-grade astrocytomas managed by primary, aggressive resection. In reporting 152 children resected over a 4-year interval (1982 to 1986), he sug-gests little long-term operative morbidity and, with incomplete follow-up information, few instances of disease recurrence following pri-mary radical operation (181). For low-grade histologies, updated data indicates progres-sion-free survival after surgery alone exceed-ing 90% at over 5 years in spinal cord and cer-vicomedullary junction tumors (189). Other series, each including only a small number of children with radical resection, confirm high rates of disease control following gross total resection (177,178,180). The high rates of dis-ease control following radical resection and acceptable morbidity for spinal surgery sug-gest primary surgical management for low-grade astrocytomas. Outcome amongst malig-nant gliomas has been systematically poor, with only anecdotal survival beyond 3 to 5 years for anaplastic astrocytomas or glioblas-tomas (178,180).

For spinal *ependymomas*, gross total resec-tion has been documented in 25% to 100% of cases in series often combining pediatric and adult experience (184,185,190). The more common myxopapillary ependymomas in children are amenable to gross total resection, especially when involving the cauda equina. Although detailed dissection is often neces-sary for lesions that adhere to numerous nerve roots comprising the cauda, data from the Royal Marsden Hospital (1950 to 1987) indi-cates total resection in 42% of 24 cases of cauda equina tumors, with 92% progression-free survival at 5 years (184). For lesions of the conus medullaris, the latter series indi-cated resection in only 2 of 14 cases (184). Documenting the change in neurosurgical technique and outcome, Whitaker et al. (184) noted no instances of gross total resection among 20 cervicothoracic intraspinal ependy-momas; more recent experience from Mc-Cormick et al. (190) (1976 to 1988), indicated resection in all 23 children and adults with in-tramedullary tumors, only one of whom had experienced recurrence. Surgery alone has been associated with survival rates at 5 years of 86% to 100% (184,191). Among 25 chil-dren with spinal ependymomas, Epstein noted no recurrences (189).

Epstein describes almost equal facility in dissecting cervicomedullary lesions, defining such tumors as "upward extension" of spinal cord tumors based on tumor type, pattern of growth, the ability of surgery to achieve tu-mor resection comparable to that described for spinal tumors, and favorable outcome fol-lowing gross total resection alone (107,189).

Radiation Therapy

The use of postoperative irradiation for spinal cord tumors has been controversial and, largely, inconsistent. With improved neuro-surgical methodology, there is no clear bene-fit from systematic radiation therapy in child-hood gliomas or ependymomas.

The literature readily documents 50% to 60% survival rates at 5 years following surgery and irradiation for spinal *astrocy-*

tomas; in general, irradiation has been utilized after incomplete resection (170,178,180, 192,193). Lacking comparative data, a rational approach includes maximal surgical resection. For incompletely resected tumors, one can support observation for low-grade gliomas (especially pilocytic histologies and for prepubertal children in whom the risk:benefit ratio may favor delaying radiation intervention). Although long-term freedom from progression has been documented after incomplete surgery alone, postoperative radiation therapy is generally indicated with (a) imaging evidence of disease residual, and (b) disease unlikely to be amenable to later, more complete resection (170,178,192,194). If one adopts a policy of observation, it is important to commit to later second surgery (when feasible) and irradiation (unless the second surgery results in imaging-confirmed total resection).

For spinal cord *ependymomas*, there is more convincing evidence supporting surgery alone for intramedullary and cauda equina tumors (190,193). The indolent nature of myxopapillary tumors of the cauda equina favors observations in the settings of total resection or minimal disease residual (180,184,194). In the review from Whitaker et al. of the Royal Marsden experience with spinal ependymomas (intramedullary and cauda equina), gross total resection had been achieved in only 15 of 58 cases (28%). Thirty of 33 incompletely resected and all 11 biopsied cases received postoperative irradiation, with progression-free survival at 5 years estimated at 60% (184). By comparison, the 15 admittedly selected cases managed by surgery alone showed 92% free of progression at 10 years (184). Curran et al. (180) compiled 127 children and adults with spinal ependymomas, documenting 80% progression-free outcome at 4 years: 90% for cauda equina presentations and 63% for intramedullary lesions. In smaller single institution reports, long-term outcome at 10 years has varied from 43% to 63% and as high as 89% progression-free following incomplete surgery and irradiation (184,192–194). Although the impact of histo-

logic grade in ependymomas remains controversial, the radiotherapy literature indicates less favorable outcome for high-grade or anaplastic ependymomas, with fairly uniform recommendation that such cases receive systematic postoperative irradiation (177,184, 192).

Radiotherapeutic Management

Volume

Local irradiation is utilized for most spinal cord tumors. Localized intramedullary astrocytomas and ependymomas are generally treated to the tumor bed, based on pre- and postoperative MRI; a margin of 3 to 5 cm is recommended. For *astrocytomas*, one typically sees decompression or obliteration of the rostral and caudal cystic components after resection of the solid tumor; in such instances, it appears that radiation therapy can be limited to the "bed" of the solid component (180,181,184,188). For spinal *ependymomas*, Garrett et al. (195) found no benefit to full spinal (or craniospinal) treatment volumes compared to local irradiation alone. Whitaker et al. (184) reported use of CSI in 40% of irradiated cases; there was no difference in outcome suggesting a benefit to wider field irradiation. For cauda equina tumors, one generally includes the proximal sacral nerve roots with the local radiation volume.

Neuraxis dissemination has been rare amongst spinal cord tumors. Local failure has predominated in astrocytomas; dissemination has accompanied local failure anecdotally in malignant gliomas or high-grade astrocytomas. A similar predominance of local failure has been documented for spinal ependymomas. Among eight failures in the series by Whitaker et al. (184), six were localized to the primary tumor site and two recurred as intracranial lesions. Although likely to underestimate the "true" rate of neuraxis failure, Curran et al. (180) found a frequency of 2% among 127 cases compiled from the literature; Whitaker et al. (184) estimated the incidence of intracranial failure at 5.8% among

259 reported cases. Although supporting the use of "neuraxis staging" procedures at diagnosis and failure, the outcome data and pattern of failure analyses support the use of local volumes for all localized spinal cord tumors, including high-grade lesions based on available data.

Dose

The local radiation dose for spinal cord gliomas has been fairly consistently reported at the 50-Gy level. The dose is based at least as much on estimated cord tolerance as documentation of tumoricidal dose levels; single institution and collected series indicate no apparent dose-response relationship beyond 50 Gy (at 200 cGy per fraction) or 50 to 54 Gy (at 180 cGy per fraction) for *astroctyomas* (177,180). For ependymomas, similar analyses indicate a dose-response at the 45- to 50-Gy level, most authors favoring a dose at or below 50 Gy (typically at 180 cGy per fraction) (170,177,180,195).

Technique

Primary spinal cord tumors are typically treated with a single posterior photon field. The use of compensators should be considered if there is significant variation in depth across the height of the spinal field. A posterior wedge pair is favored in settings where exiting beams will not exceed conservative tolerance limits for the kidneys, lung, or heart. Electrons may be used to treat spinal cord tumors if one accounts for inhomogeneous absorption of electrons in vertebral bone as well as variation in depth.

Results

Overall survival in spinal cord *astrocytomas* is estimated at 80% at 5 years and 55% at 10 years (178,180). Prognosis is affected by histologic grade and, more recently, by the extent of surgical resection. For ependymomas, overall survival is comparable, with recent figures indicating 70% 5-year survival and

more than 60% 10-year survival. Outcome is dependent on site of origin (with long-term survival rates exceeding 90% for cauda equina tumors versus 60% for intramedullary tumors or those arising in the conus medullaris) (184,194). Children, differentiated ependymomas (versus anaplastic or high grade), and patients with radical or complete resection appear to enjoy relatively favorable outcome (180,184).

REFERENCES

References particularly recommended for further reading are indicated by an asterisk.

1. Gurney JG, Davis S, Severson RK, et al. Trends in cancer incidence among children in the U.S. *Cancer* 1996;78:532–541.
2. Walker AE, Robins M, Weinfeld FD. Epidemiology of brain tumors: The national survey of intracranial neoplasms. *Neurology* 1985;35:219–226.
3. Bailey J, Cushing H. Medulloblastoma cerebelli, common type of mid-cerebellar glioma of childhood. *Arch Neurol Psychiatry* 1925;14:192–224.
4. Cushing H. Experiences with the cerebellar medulloblastomas: a critical review. *Acta Pathol Microbiol Scand* 1930;1:1–86.
5. Rorke LB. The cerebellar medulloblastoma in its relationship to primitive neuroectodermal tumors: presidential address. *J Neuropathol Exp Neurol* 1983;42:1–15.
*6. Hart MN, Earle KM. Primitive neuroectodermal tumors of the brain in children. *Cancer* 1973;32:890–897.
7. Fields WS, ed. *Primary brain tumors, a review of histologic classification.* New York: Springer-Verlag, 1989.
8. Kleihues P, Burger PC, Scheithauer BW. The new WHO classification of brain tumours. *Brain Pathol* 1993;3:255–268.
9. Rubinstein LJ. Embryonal central neuroepithelial tumors and their differentiating potential. *J Neurosurg* 1985;62:795–805.
10. Kleihues P, Burger PC, Scheithauer BW, eds. *Histological typing of tumours of the central nervous system.* Berlin: Springer-Verlag, 1994.
11. Russell DS, Rubinstein LJ. *Pathology of tumours of the nervous system.* London: Edward Arnold, Baltimore: Williams and Wilkins, 1989.
12. Trojanowski JQ, Fung K-M, Rorke LB, et al. In vivo and in vitro models of medulloblastomas and other primitive neuroectodermal brain tumors of childhood. *Mol Chem Neuropathol* 1994;21:219–239.
13. Burger PC, Grahmann FC, Bliestele A, et al. Differentiation in the medulloblastoma. A histological and immunohistochemical study. *Acta Neuropathol* 1987;73:115–123.
14. Janss AJ, Yachnis AT, Silber JH, et al. Glial differentiation predicts poor clinical outcome in primitive

neuroectodermal brain tumors. *Ann Neurol* 1996;39: 481–489.

15. Batra SK, McLendon RE, Koo JS, et al. Prognostic implication of chromosome 17p delections in human medulloblastomas. *J Neurooncol* 1995;24:39–45.

16. Reardon DA, Michalkiewicz E, Boyett JM, et al. Extensive genomic abnormalities in childhood medulloblastoma by comparative genomic hybridization. *Cancer Res* 1997;57:4042–4047.

17. Thomas GA, Raffel C. Loss of heterozygosity on 6q, 16q, and 17p in human central nervous system primitive neuroectodermal tumors. *Cancer Res* 1991;51: 639–643.

18. Roberts RO, Lynch CF, Jones P, et al. Medulloblastoma: a population-based study of 532 cases. *J Neuropathol Exp Neurol* 1991;50:134–144.

19. Halperin EC, Friedman HS. Is there a correlation between duration of presenting symptoms and stage of medulloblastoma at the time of diagnosis? *Cancer* 1996;78(4):874–880.

20. Halperin EC. Concerning the inferior portion of the spinal radiotherapy field for malignancies that disseminate via the cerebrospinal fluid. *Int J Radiat Oncol Biol Phys* 1993;26:357–362.

21. Barkovich AJ. *Pediatric neuroimaging*, 2nd ed. New York: Raven Press, 1995:321–437.

22. Deutsch M. Medulloblastoma: staging and treatment outcome. *Int J Radiat Oncol Biol Phys* 1988;14: 1103–1107.

23. Boyett J, Zeltzer P, Finlay J, et al. Progression-free survival (PFS) and risk factors for primitive neuroectodermal tumors (PNET) of the posterior fossa (PF) [Medulloblastoma] in children: report of the Children's Cancer Group (CCG) randomized trial, CCG-921. *Proc ASCO* 1995;14:147.

24. David KM, Casey ATH, Hayward RD, et al. Medulloblastoma: is the 5-year survival rate improving? *J Neurosurg* 1997;86:13–21.

25. Chang CH, Housepian EM, Herbert C Jr. An operative staging system and a megavoltage radiotherapeutic technic for cerebellar medulloblastoma. *Radiology* 1969;93:1351–1359.

26. Albright AL, Wisoff JH, Zeltzer PM, et al. Effects of medulloblastoma resections on outcome in children: a report from the Children's Cancer Group. *Neurosurgery* 1996;38:265–271.

*27. Evans AE, Jenkin RDT, Sposto R, et al. The treatment of medulloblastoma: results of a prospective randomized trial of radiation therapy with and without CCNU, vincristine, and prednisone. *J Neurosurg* 1990;72:572–582.

28. Packer RJ, Sutton LN, Elterman R, et al. Outcome for children with medulloblastoma treated with radiation and cisplatin, CCNU, and vincristine chemotherapy. *J Neurosurg* 1994;81:690–698.

29. Thomas PRM, Deutsch M, Mulhern, et al. Reduced dose vs. standard dose neuraxis irradiation in low stage medulloblastoma: The POG and CCG Study. SIOP XXVII Meeting-Abstracts. *Med Pediatr Oncol* 1995;25:277.

30. Bailey CC, Gnekow A, Wellek S, et al. Prospective randomized trial of chemotherapy given before radiotherapy in childhood medulloblastoma. International Society of Paediatric Oncology (SIOP) and the (German) Society of Paediatric Oncology (GPO): SIOP II. *Med Pediatr Oncol* 1995;25:166–178.

31. Gentet JC, Bouffet E, Doz F, et al. Preirradiation chemotherapy including "eight drugs in 1 day" regimen and high-dose methotrexate in childhood medulloblastoma: results of the M7 French Cooperative Study. *J Neurosurg* 1995;82:608–614.

32. Hughes EN, Shillito J, Sallan SE, et al. Medulloblastoma at the Joint Center for Radiation Therapy between 1968 and 1984. *Cancer* 1988;61:1992–1998.

33. Jenkin D, Goddard K, Armstrong D, et al. Posterior fossa medulloblastoma in childhood: treatment results and a proposal for a new staging system. *Int J Radiat Oncol Biol Phys* 1990;19:265–274.

34. Jenkin D, Greenberg M, Hoffman H, et al. Brain tumors in children: long-term survival after radiation treatment. *Int J Radiat Oncol Biol Phys* 1995; 31(3): 445–451.

35. Bourne JP, Geyer R, Berger M, et al. The prognostic significance of postoperative residual contrast enhancement on C7 scan in pediatric patients with medulloblastoma. *J Neurooncol* 1992;14:263–270.

36. Gajjar A, Sanford RA, Bhargava R, et al. Medulloblastoma with brain stem involvement: the impact of gross total resection on outcome. *Pediatr Neurosurg* 1996;25:182–187.

37. Aguiar PH, Plese JP, Ciquini O, et al. Transient mutism following a posterior fossa approach to cerebellar tumors in children: a critical review of the literature. *Childs Nerv Syst* 1995;11:306–310.

38. Cochrane DD, Gustavsson B, Poskitt KP, et al. The surgical and natural morbidity of aggressive resection for posterior fossa tumors in childhood. *Pediatr Neurosurg* 1994;20:19–29.

39. Berger MS, Baumeister B, Geyer JR, et al. The risk of metastases from shunting in children with primary central nervous system tumors. *J Neurosurg* 1991;73: 872–877.

40. Halperin EC, Samulski T, Oakes WJ, Friedman HS. Fabrication and testing of a device capable of reducing the incidence of ventricular shunt promoted metastases. *J Neurooncol* 1996;27:39–46.

41. Albright AL, Wisoff JH, Zeltzer PM, et al. Current neurosurgical treatment of medulloblastomas in children. *Pediatr Neurosci* 1989;15:276–282.

42. Cutler EC, Sosman MC, Vaughan WW. Place of radiation in treatment of cerebellar medulloblastoma: report of 20 cases. *Am J Roentgenol Radium Ther Nucl Med* 1936;35:429–453.

43. Bloom HJG, Glees J, Bell J. The treatment and prognosis of medulloblastoma in children. *AJR* 1969;105: 43–62.

*44. Bloom HJG, Glees J, Bell J. The treatment of long-term prognosis of children with intracranial tumors: a study of 610 cases, 1950–1981. *Int J Radiat Oncol Biol Phys* 1991;18:723–745.

45. Dunbar S, Barnes P, Tarbell NJ. Radiographic determination of the caudal border of the spinal field in craniospinal irradiation. *Int J Radiat Oncol Biol Phys* 1993;26:669–673.

46. Ashley DM, Meier L, Kerby T, et al. Response of recurrent medulloblastoma to low-dose oral etoposide. *J Clin Oncol* 1996;14:1922–1927.

47. Duffner PK, Horowitz ME, Krischer JP, et al. Postoperative chemotherapy and delayed radiation in children less than 3 years of age with malignant brain tumors. *N Engl J Med* 1993;328:1725–1731.

48. Friedman HS, Oakes WJ. The chemotherapy of pos-

terior fossa tumors in childhood. *J Neurooncol* 1987; 5:217–229.

49. Heideman RL, Kovnar EH, Kellie SJ, et al. Preirradiation chemotherapy with carboplatin and etoposide in newly diagnosed embryonal pediatric CNS tumors. *J Clin Oncol* 1995;13:2247–2254.

50. Kovnar EH, Kellie SJ, Horowitz ME, et al. Pre-irradiation cisplatin and etoposide in the treatment of high-risk medulloblastoma and other malignant embryonal tumors of the central nervous system: a phase II study. *J Clin Oncol* 1990;8:330–336.

51. Mastrangelo R, Lasorella A, Riccardi R, et al. Carboplatin in childhood medulloblastoma/PNET: feasibility of an in vivo sensitivity test in an "up-front" study. *Med Pediatr Oncol* 1995;24:188–196.

52. Packer RJ, Sutton LN, Goldwein JW, et al. Improved survival with the use of adjuvant chemotherapy in the treatment of medulloblastoma. *J Neurosurg* 1991;74: 433–440.

53. Tarbell NJ, Loeffler JS, Silver B, et al. The change in patterns of relapse in medulloblastoma. *Cancer* 1991; 68:1600–1604.

*54. Tait DM, Thornton-Jones H, Bloom HJG, et al. Adjuvant chemotherapy for medulloblastoma: the first multi-centre controlled trial of the International Society of Paediatric Oncology (SIOP1). *Eur J Cancer* 1990;26:464–469.

*55. Krischer JP, Ragab AH, Kun L, et al. Nitrogen mustard, vincristine, procarbazine, and prednisone as adjuvant chemotherapy in the treatment of medulloblastoma. A Pediatric Oncology Group study. *J Neurosurg* 1991;74:905–909.

56. Hartsell WF, Gajjar A, Heideman RL, et al. Patterns of failure in children with medulloblastoma: effects of preirradiation chemotherapy. *Int J Radiat Oncol Biol Phys* 1997;39:15–24.

57. Mosijczuk AD, Nigro MA, Thomas PRM, et al. Preradiation chemotherapy in advanced medulloblastoma: A Pediatric Oncology Group pilot study. *Cancer* 1993;72:2755–2762.

58. Mahoney DH, Strother D, Camitta B, et al. High-dose melphalan and cyclo-phosphamide with autologous bone marrow rescue for recurrent/progressive malignant brain tumors in children: a pilot Pediatric Oncology Group study. *J Clin Oncol* 1996;14: 382–388.

59. Landberg TG, Lindgren ML, Cavallin-Stahl EK, et al. Improvements in the radiotherapy of medulloblastoma 1946–1975. *Cancer* 1980;45:670–678.

60. Jereb B, Reid A, Ahuja RK. Patterns of failure in patients with medulloblastoma. *Cancer* 1982;50: 2941–2947.

61. Wara WM, Le Q-T X, Sneed PK, et al. Pattern of recurrence of medulloblastoma after low-dose craniospinal radiotherapy. *Int J Radiat Oncol Biol Phys* 1994;30:551–556.

62. Bouffet E, Bernard JL, Frappaz D, et al. M4 protocol for cerebellar medulloblastoma: supratentorial radiotherapy may not be avoided. *Int J Radiat Oncol Biol Phys* 1992;24:79–85.

63. Merchant TE, Happersett L, Finlay JL, et al. Conformal radiation therapy for medulloblastoma. *J Neurooncol* 1998 (*in press*).

64. Fertil B, Malaise EP. Intrinsic radiosensitivity of human cell lines is correlated with radioresponsiveness of human tumors: analysis of 101 published survival curves. *Int J Radiat Oncol Biol Phys* 1985;11: 1699–1707.

65. Silverman CL, Simpson JR. Cerebellar medulloblastoma: the importance of posterior fossa dose to survival and patterns of failure. *Int J Radiat Oncol Biol Phys* 1982;8:1869–1876.

66. Merchant TE, Wang M-H, Haida T, et al. Medulloblastoma: long-term results for patients treated with definitive radiation therapy during the computed tomography era. *Int J Radiat Oncol Biol Phys* 1996; 36:29–35.

67. Tomita T, McLane DG. Medulloblastoma in childhood: results of radical resection and low dose neuroaxis radiation therapy. *J Neurosurg* 1986;64: 238–242.

*68. Deutsch M, Thomas PRM, Krischer J, et al. Results of a prospective randomized trial comparing standard dose neuraxis irradiation (3,600 cGy/20) with reduced neuraxis irradiation (2,340 cGy/13) in patients with low-stage medulloblastoma: a combined Children's Cancer Group-Pediatric Oncology Group study. *Pediatr Neurosurg* 1996;24:167–177.

69. Packer RJ. Early results of reduced-dose radiotherapy plus chemotherapy for children with non-disseminated medulloblastoma (MB): A Children's Cancer Group Study. *Pediatr Neurosurg* 1995;55:518.

70. Allen JC, Nirenberg A, Donahue B. Hyperfractionated radiotherapy and adjuvant chemotherapy for high risk PNET. *J Neurooncol* 1992;12:263.

71. Hudes RS, Gajjar A, Heideman RL, et al. High dose hyperfractionated craniospinal irradiation (HF-CSI): feasibility, acute toxicity, outcome and late sequelae. (abst '98)

72. Prados M, Edwards M, Wara W, et al. Hyperfractionated radiotherapy in the management of patients with medulloblastoma. *J Neurooncol* 1992;12:263.

73. Prados M, Wara WM, Edwards MSB, et al. Hyperfractionated craniospinal radiation therapy for primitive neuroectodermal tumors: early results of a pilot study. *Int J Radiat Oncol Biol Phys* 1993;28: 431–438.

*74. Tatcher M, Glicksman AS. Field matching considerations in craniospinal irradiation. *Int J Radiat Oncol Biol Phys* 1989;17:865–869.

75. Holupka EJ, Humm JL, Tarbell NJ, et al. Effect of set-up error on the dose across the junction of matching cranial-spinal fields in the treatment of medulloblastoma. *Int J Radiat Oncol Biol Phys* 1993;27: 345–352.

76. Goldschmidt EJ, Holst RJ. Medulloblastoma immobilization and treatment considerations. *Med Dosim* 1990;15:7–11.

77. Halperin EC. Impact of radiation technique upon the outcome of treatment for medulloblastoma. *Int J Radiat Oncol Biol Phys* 1996;36:233–239.

78. Donnal J, Halperin EC, Friedman HS, Boyko CB. Subfrontal recurrence of medulloblastoma. *Am J Neuroradiol* 1992;13:1617–1618.

79. Jereb B, Krishnaswami S, Reid A, et al. Radiation for medulloblastoma adjusted to prevent recurrences to the cribriform plate region. *Cancer* 1984;54:602–604.

80. Maor MH, Fields RS, Hogstrom KR, et al. Improving the therapeutic ratio of craniospinal irradiation in medulloblastoma. *Int J Radiat Oncol Biol Phys* 1985; 11:687–697.

81. Gaspar LE, Dawson DJ, Tilley-Guilliford SA, et al.

Medulloblastoma. Long-term follow-up of patients treated with electron irradiation of the spinal field. *Radiology* 1991;180:867–870.

82. Marks LB, Halperin EC. The use of G-CSF during craniospinal irradiation. *Int J Radiat Oncol Biol Phys* 1993;26:905–906.

83. Gajjar AJ, Heideman RL, Douglass EC, et al. Relation of tumor-cell ploidy to survival in children with medulloblastoma. *J Clin Oncol* 1993;11:2211–2217.

84. Zerbini C, Gelber RD, Weinberg D, et al. Prognostic factors in medulloblastoma including DNA ploidy. *J Clin Oncol* 1993;11:616–622.

85. Barkovich AJ, Krischer J, Kun LE, et al. Brainstem gliomas: a classification system based on magnetic resonance imaging. *Pediatr Neurosurg* 1990;16: 73–83.

86. Albright AL, Price RA, Guthkelch AN. Brain stem gliomas of children. A clinicopathological study. *Cancer* 1983;52:2313–2319.

87. Albright AL, Guthkelch AN, Packer RJ, et al. Prognostic factors in pediatric brain-stem gliomas. *J Neurosurg* 1986;65:751–755.

88. Prados MD, Wara WM, Edwards MSB, et al. The treatment of brain stem and thalamic gliomas with 78 Gy of hyperfractionated radiation therapy. *Int J Radiat Oncol Biol Phys* 1995;32:85–91.

89. Shrieve DC, Wara WM, Edwards MSB, et al. Hyperfractionated radiation therapy for gliomas of the brainstem in children and adults. *Int J Radiat Oncol Biol Phys* 1992;24:599–610.

90. Vandertop WP, Hoffman HJ, Drake JM, et al. Focal midbrain tumors in children. *Neurosurgery* 1992;31: 186–194.

91. Edwards MSB, Wara WM, Urtasum RC, et al. Hyperfractionated radiation therapy for brainstem glioma: a Phase I-II trial. *J Neurosurg* 1989;70: 691–700.

92. Freeman CR, Krischer JP, Sanford RA, et al. Final results of a study of escalating doses of hyperfractionated radiotherapy in brain stem tumors in children. *Int J Radiat Oncol Biol Phys* 1993;27:197–206.

*93. Freeman CR. Hyperfractionated radiotherapy for diffuse intrinsic brain stem tumors in children. *Pediatr Neurosurg* 1996;24:103–110.

94. Edwards MSB, Wara WM, Ciricillo SF, et al. Focal brain-stem astrocytomas causing symptoms of involvement of the facial nerve nucleus: long-term survival in six pediatric cases. *J Neurosurg* 1994;80: 20–25.

95. Hoffman HJ, Becker L, Craven MA. A clinically and pathologically distinct group of benign brain stem gliomas. *Neurosurgery* 1980;7:243–248.

96. Pollack IF, Hoffman HJ, Humphreys RP, et al. The long-term outcome after surgical treatment of dorsally exophytic brain-stem gliomas. *J Neurosurg* 1993;78:859–863.

97. Epstein F, McCleary EL. Intrinsic brain-stem tumors of childhood: surgical indications. *J Neurosurg* 1986; 64:11–15.

98. Pierre-Kahn A, Hirsch J-F, Vinchon M, et al. Surgical management of brain-stem tumors in children: results and statistical analysis of 75 cases. *J Neurosurg* 1993; 79:845–852.

99. Stroink AR, Hoffman HJ, Henrick EB, et al. Diagno-

sis and management of pediatric brain stem gliomas. *J Neurosurg* 1986;65:745–750.

100. Packer RJ, Boyett JM, Zimmerman RA, et al. Hyperfractionated radiation therapy (72 Gy) for children with brain stem gliomas. A Children's Cancer Group Phase I/II trial. *Cancer* 1993;72:1414–1421.

101. Packer RJ, Boyett JM, Zimmerman RA, et al. Outcome of children with brain stem gliomas after treatment with 7800 cGy of hyperfractionated radiotherapy. A Children's Cancer Group Phase I/II trial. *Cancer* 1994;74:1827–1834.

102. Burger PC, Scheithauer BW, Vogel FS, eds. *Surgical pathology of the nervous system and its coverings*, 3rd ed. New York: Churchill Livingstone, 1991.

103. Mantravadi RVP, Phatak R, Bellur S, et al. Brain stem gliomas: an autopsy study of 25 cases. *Cancer* 1982; 49:1294–1296.

104. Khatib ZA, et al. Predominance of pilocytic histology in dorsally exophytic brain stem tumors. *Pediatr Neurosurg* 1994; 20:2–10.

105. Boydston WR, Sanford RA, Muhlbauer MS, et al. Gliomas of the tectum and periaqueductal region of the mesencephalon. *Pediatr Neurosurg* 1991–1992; 17:234–238.

106. Hibi T, Shitara N, Genka S, et al. Radiotherapy for pediatric brain stem glioma: radiation dose, response, and survival. *Neurosurgery* 1992;31:643–651.

107. Epstein F, Wisoff J. Intra-axial tumors of the cervicomedullary junction. *J Neurosurg* 1987;67:483–487.

108. Packer RJ, Nicholson HS, Johnson DL, et al. Dilemmas in the management of childhood brain tumors: brainstem gliomas. *Pediatr Neurosurg* 1991–1992; 17:37–43.

109. Jenkin RDT, Boesel C, Ertel I, et al. Brain–stem tumors in childhood: a prospective randomized trial of irradiation with and without adjuvant CCNU, VCR, and prednisone. *J Neurosurg* 1987;66:227–233.

110. Allen JC, Helson L, Jereb B. Preradiation chemotherapy for newly diagnosed childhood brain tumors: a modified phase II trial. *Cancer* 1983;52:2001–2006.

111. Kretschmar CS, Tarbell NJ, Barnes PD, et al. Pre-irradiation chemotherapy and hyperfractionated radiation therapy 66 Gy for children with brain stem tumors. *Cancer* 1993; 72:1404–1413.

112. Allen JC, Siffert J. Contemporary chemotherapy issues for children with brainstem gliomas. *Pediatr Neurosurg* 1996;24:98–102.

113. Halperin EC. Pediatric brain stem tumors: patterns of treatment failure and their implications for radiotherapy. *Int J Radiat Oncol Biol Phys* 1985;11: 1293–1298.

114. Packer RJ, Zimmerman RA, Kaplan A, et al. Early cystic/necrotic changes after hyperfractionated radiation therapy in children with brain stem gliomas. Data from the Children's Cancer Group. *Cancer* 1993;71:2666–2674.

115. Gajjar A, Bhargava R, Jenkins JJ, et al. Low-grade astrocytoma with neuraxis dissemination at diagnosis. *J Neurosurg* 1995;83:67–71.

116. Gajjar A, Sanford RA, Heideman R, et al. Low-grade astrocytoma: A decade of experience at St. Jude Children's Research Hospital. *J Clin Oncol* 1997;15: 2792–2795.

117. Dunbar SF, Tarbell NJ, Kooy HM, et al. Stereotactic

radiotherapy for pediatric and adult brain tumors: preliminary report. *Int J Radiat Oncol Biol Phys* 1994;30(3):531–539.

118. Freeman CR, Suissa S. Brain stem tumors in children: results of a survey of 62 patients treated with radiotherapy. *Int J Radiat Oncol Biol Phys* 1986;12: 1823–1828.

119. Kim TH, Chin HW, Pollan S, et al. Radiotherapy of primary brain stem tumors. *Int J Radiat Oncol Biol Phys* 1980; 6:51–57.

*120. Mandell L, Kadota R, Douglass EC, et al. It is time to rethink the role of hyperfractionated radiotherapy in the management of children with newly diagnosed brainstem glioma? Results of a Pediatric Oncology Group Phase III trial comparing conventional versus hyperfractionated radiotherapy. *Int J Radiat Oncol Biol Phys* 1997;39[Suppl 2]:143.

121. Edwards MSB, Levin V, Wara W. Hyperfractionation radiation therapy for brain stem glioma in children. *J Neurooncol* 1987;5:170.

122. Thames HD Jr, Peters LJ, Withers HR, et al. Accelerated fractionation vs. hyperfractionation: rationales for several treatments per day. *Int J Radiat Oncol Biol Phys* 1983;9:127–138.

123. Withers HR, Peters LJ, Thomas HD, et al. Hyperfractionation. *Int J Radiat Oncol Biol Phys* 1982;8: 1007–1009.

*124. Hebert ME, Halperin EC, Oakes WJ, et al. Multiple-fraction-per-day radiotherapy for patients with brain stem tumors. *J Neurooncol* 1993;17:131–138.

125. Freeman CR, Bourgouin PM, Sanford RA, et al. Long term survivors of childhood brain stem gliomas treated with hyperfractionated radiotherapy, clinical characteristics and treatment related toxicities. *Cancer* 1996;77:555–562.

126. Kadota RP, Mandell LR, Fontanesi J, et al. Hyperfractionated irradiation and concurrent cisplatin in brain stem tumors: a Pediatric Oncology Group pilot study (9139). *Pediatr Neurosurg* 1994; 20: 221–225.

127. Packer RJ, Prados M, Phillips P, et al. Treatment of children with newly diagnosed brain stem gliomas with intravenous recombinant b-interferon and hyperfractionated radiation therapy. A Children's Cancer Group Phase I/II Study. *Cancer* 1996;77: 2150–2156.

128. Walter AW, Gajjar A, Ochs J. Carboplatin and etoposide with hyperfractionated radiation therapy in children with newly diagnosed pontine gliomas: a phase I/II study. *Med Pediatr Oncol* 1998;30:28–33.

129. Griebel M, Friedman HS, Halperin EC, et al. Reversible neurotoxicity following hyperfractionated radiation therapy of brain stem glioma. *Med Pediatr Oncol* 1991;19:182–186.

130. Taylor JS, Langston JW, Reddick WE, et al. Clinical value of proton magnetic resonance spectroscopy for differentiating recurrent or residual brain tumor from delayed cerebral necrosis. *Int J Radiat Oncol Biol Phys* 1996;36:1251–1261.

131. Nazar GB, Hoffman HJ, Becker LE, et al. Infratentorial ependymomas in childhood: prognostic factors and treatment. *J Neurosurg* 1990;72:408–417.

132. Sutton LN, Goldwein J, Perilongo G, et al. Prognostic factors in childhood ependymomas. *Pediatr Neurosurg* 1990–1991;16:57–65.

133. Sanford RA, Kun LE, Heideman RL, et al. Cerebellar pontine angle ependymoma in infants. *Pediatr Neurosurg* 1997;27:84–91.

134. Centeno RS, Lee AA, Winter J, et al. Supratentorial ependymomas. Neuroimaging and clinicopathological correlation. *J Neurosurg* 1986;64:209–215.

135. Rawlings CE III, Giangaspero F, Burger PC, et al. Ependymomas: a clinicopathologic study. *Surg Neurol* 1988;29:271–281.

136. Rorke LB. Relationship of morphology of ependymoma in children to prognosis. *Prog Exp Tumor Res* 1987;30:170–174.

137. Ross GW, Rubinstein LJ. Lack of histopathological correlation of malignant ependymomas with postoperative survival. *J Neurosurg* 1989;70:31–36.

138. Carrie C, Mottolese C, Bouffet E, et al. Non-metastatic childhood ependymomas. *Radiother Oncol* 1995; 36:101–106.

139. Kovalic JJ, Flaris N, Grigsby, Pirkowski M, Simpson JR, Roth KA. Intracranial ependymoma long term outcome, patterns of failure. *J Neurooncol* 1993;15: 125–131.

140. Rezai AR, Woo HH, Lee M, Cohen H, Zagzag D, Epstein FJ. Disseminated ependymomas of the central nervous system. *J Neurosurg* 1996;85:618–624.

141. Rousseau P, Habrand JL, Sarrazin D, et al. Treatment of intracranial ependymomas of children: review of a 15-year experience. *Int J Radiat Oncol Biol Phys* 1994;28:381–386.

142. Goldwein JW, Leahy JM, Packer RJ, et al. Intracranial ependymomas in children. *Int J Radiat Oncol Biol Phys* 1990;19:1497–1502.

143. Vanuystel LJ, Bessell EM, Ashley SE, et al. Intracranial ependymoma: long-term results of a policy of surgery and radiotherapy. *Int J Radiat Oncol Biol Phys* 1992;23:313–319.

144. Tomita T, McLone DJ, Das L, et al. Benign ependymomas of the posterior fossa in children. *Pediatr Neurosci* 1988; 14–277.

145. Healey EA, Braners PD, Kupsky WJ, et al. The prognostic significance of postoperative residual tumor in ependymoma. *Neurosurgery* 1991;28:666–672.

146. Pollack IF, Gerszten PC, Martinez AJ, et al. Intracranial ependymomas of childhood: Long-term outcome and prognostic factors. *Neurosurgery* 1995;37: 655–667.

147. Duffner PK, Krischer JP, Sanford RA, et al. Prognostic factors in infants and very young children with intracranial ependymomas. *Pediatr Neurosurg* 1998; 28:215–222.

*148. Goldwein JW, Corn BW, Finlay JL, et al. Is craniospinal irradiation required to cure children with malignant (anaplastic) intracranial ependymomas? *Cancer* 1991;67:2766–2771.

149. Merchant TE, Haida T, Wang M-H, et al. Anaplastic ependymoma: treatment of pediatric patients with or without craniospinal radiation therapy. *J Neurosurg* 1997;86:943–949.

150. Lefkowitz I, Evana A, Splosto R, et al. Adjuvant chemotherapy of childhood posterior fossa (PF) ependymoma: craniospinal irradiation with or without CCNU, vincristine (VCR) and prednisone (P). *Proc Am Soc Clin Oncol* 1989;8:87.

*151. Bloom HJG. Intracranial tumors: response and resistance to therapeutic endeavors, 1970–1980. *Int J Radiat Oncol Biol Phys* 1982;8:1083–1113.

152. Kun LE, Kovnar EH, Sanford RA. Ependymomas in children. *Pediatr Neurosci* 1988;14:57.

153. Salazar OM. A better understanding of CNS seeding and brighter outlook for postoperatively irradiated patients with ependymomas. *Int J Radiat Oncol Biol Phys* 1983;9:1231–1234.

154. Goldwein JW, Glauser TA, Packer RJ, et al. Recurrent intracranial ependymomas in children: survival, patterns of failure, and prognostic factors. *Cancer* 1990; 66:557–563.

155. Kun LE, Kovnar E, Kepner J, et al. Ependymomas in children—A prospective study of post-operative radiation therapy. *Pediatr Neurosurg* 1998 (*in press*).

156. Kovnar EH, Curran W, Tomita T, et al. Hyperfractionated irradiation for childhood ependymoma: improved local control in subtotally resected tumors. Presented at the 8th Int'l Symposium on Pediatric Neuro-Oncology, Rome, Italy, 1998, May 6–9 (abstr).

157. Aggarwal R, Yeung D, Muhlbauer M, et al. Efficacy and feasiblility of stereotactic radiosurgery in the primary management of unfavorable pediatric ependymoma. *Radiother Oncol* 1997;43:269–273.

158. Marks JE, Adler SJ. A comparative study of ependymomas by site of origin. *Int J Radiat Oncol Biol Phys* 1982;8:37–43.

159. Ilgren EB, Stiller CA. Cerebellar astrocytomas: Clinical characteristics and prognostic indices. *J Neurooncol* 1987;4:293–308.

160. Schneider JH Jr, Raffel C, McComb JG. Benign cerebellar astrocytomas of childhood. *Neurosurgery* 1992;30:58–63.

161. Cushing H. Experiences with the cerebellar astrocytomas: a critical review of 76 cases. *Surg Gynecol Obstet* 1931;52:129–191.

162. Ilgren EB, Stiller CA. Cerebellar astrocytomas: therapeutic management. *Acta Neurochir* 1986;81:11–26.

163. Hayostek CJ, Shaw EG, Scheithauer B, et al. Astrocytomas of the cerebellum. A comparative clinicopathologic study of pilocytic and diffuse astrocytomas. *Cancer* 1993;72:856–869.

164. Shinoda J, Yamada H, Sakai N, et al. Malignant cerebellar astrocytic tumours in children. *Acta Neurochir* 1989;98:1–8.

165. Lapras C, Patet JD, Lapras CH Jr., et al. Cerebellar astrocytomas in childhood. *Childs Nerv Syst* 1986;2: 55–59.

166. Sgouros S, Fineron PW, Hockley AD. Cerebellar astrocytoma of childhood: long-term follow-up. *Childs Nerv Syst* 1995;11:89–96.

167. Mamelak AN, Prados MD, Obana WG, et al. Treatment options and prognosis for multicentric juvenile pilocytic astrocytoma. *J Neurosurg* 1994;81:24–30.

168. Pollack IF, Hurtt M, Pang D, et al. Dissemination of low grade intracranial astro-cytomas in children. *Cancer* 1994;73:2869–2878.

169. Prados M, Mamelak AN. Metastasizing low grade gliomas in children. Redefining an old disease. *Cancer* 1994;73:2671–2673.

170. Garcia DM, Marks JE, Latifi HR, et al. Childhood cerebellar astrocytomas: is there a role for postoperative irradiation? *Int J Radiat Oncol Biol Phys* 1990; 18:815–818.

171. Gjerris F, Klinken L. Long-term prognosis in children with benign cerebellar astrocytoma. *J Neurosurg* 1978;49:179–184.

172. Conway PD, Oechler HW, Kun LE, et al. Importance of histologic condition and treatment of pediatric cerebellar astrocytoma. *Cancer* 1991;67:2772–2775.

173. Larson DA, Wara WM, Edwards MSB. Management of childhood cerebellar astrocytoma. *Int J Radiat Oncol Biol Phys* 1990;18:971–973.

174. Kopelson G, Linggood RM. Infratentorial glioblastoma: the role of neuroaxis irradiation. *Int J Radiat Oncol Biol Phys* 1982;8:999–1003.

175. Kopelson G. Critique of "primary malignant cerebellar astrocytomas in children: a signal for postoperative craniospinal irradiation" [Letter]. *Int J Radiat Oncol Biol Phys* 1982;8:1818–1819.

176. Chamberlain MC, Silber P, Levin VA. Poorly differentiated gliomas of the cerebellum: a study of 18 patients. *Cancer* 1990;65:337–340.

177. Kopelson G, Linggood RM, Kleinman GM, et al. Management of intramedullary spinal cord tumors. *Radiology* 1980;135:473–479.

178. Reimer R, Onofrio BM. Astrocytomas of the spinal cord in children and adolescents. *J Neurosurg* 1985; 63:669–675.

179. DeSousa AL, Kalsbeck JE, Mealey J, et al. Intraspinal tumors in children. A review of 81 cases. *J Neurosurg* 1979;51:437–445.

180. Curran WJ Jr, D'Angio GJ. Nonsurgical management of spinal tumors. In: Ashley DG, Curran WJ Jr, D'Angio GJ, et al., eds. *Spinal tumors in children and adolescents, the international review of child neurology.* New York: Raven Press, 1990:71–84.

181. Epstein F. Spinal cord astrocytomas of childhood. *Prog Exp Tumor Res* 1987;30:135–153.

182. Epstein F, Epstein N. Surgical management of holocord intramedullary spinal astrocytomas in children. *J Neurosurg* 1981;54:829–832.

183. Pascual-Castroviejo I, ed. *Spinal cord tumors in children and adolescents.* New York: Raven Press, 1990.

184. Whitaker SJ, Bessell EM, Ashley SE, et al. Postoperative radiotherapy in the management of spinal cord ependymoma. *J Neurosurg* 1991;74:720–728.

185. Sonneland PRL, Scheithauer BW, Onofrio BM. Myxopapillary ependymoma. A clinicopathologic and immunocytochemical study of 77 cases. *Cancer* 1985; 56:883–893.

186. Ciraldo AV, Platt MS, Agamanolis DP, et al. Sacrococcygeal myxopapillary ependymomas and ependymal rests in infants and children. *J Pediatr Surg* 1986;21:49–52.

187. Rifkinson-Mann J, Wisoff JH, Epstein F. The association of hydrocephalus with intramedullary spinal cord tumors: a series of 25 patients. *Neurosurgery* 1990;27:749–754.

188. Epstein F, Epstein N. Surgical treatment of spinal cord astrocytomas of childhood. A series of 19 patients. *J Neurosurg* 1982;57:685–689.

189. Epstein F. Intraaxial tumors of the cervicomedullary junction in children. *Pediatr Neurosurg* 1987;7:117.

190. McCormick PC, Torres R, Post KD, et al. Intramedullary ependymoma of the spinal cord. *J Neurosurg* 1990;72:523–532.

191. Schiffer D, Chio A, Girodana MT, et al. Histologic prognostic factors in ependymoma. *Childs Nerv Syst* 1991;7:177–182.

192. Lindstadt DE, Wara WM, Leibel SA, et al. Postoperative radiotherapy of spinal cord tumors. *Int J Radiat Oncol Biol Phys* 1989;16:1397–1403.

193. O'Sullivan C, Jenkin RD, Dohery MA, et al. Spinal cord tumors in children: long-term results of combined surgical and radiation treatment. *J Neurosurg* 1994;81:507–512.

194. Chun HC, Schmidt-Ultrich RK, Wolfson A, et al. External beam radiotherapy for primary spinal cord tumors. *J Neurooncol* 1990;9:211–217.

195. Garrett PG, Simpson WJK. Ependymomas: results of radiation treatment. *Int J Radiat Oncol Biol Phys* 1983;9:1121–1124.

196. Wara WM, Linstadt DE, Larson DA: management of primary brain stem gliomas and spinal cord gliomas. *Semin Rad Oncol* 1991;1:50–53.

197. Donahue B, Allen J, Siffert J, Rosovsky M, Pinto R, et al. Patterns of recurrence in brain stem gliomas: evidence for craniospinal dissemination. *Int J Rad Oncol Biol Phys* 1998;40:677–680.

Retinoblastoma

HISTOLOGY AND PATTERNS OF GROWTH

Retinoblastoma (RB) is the most common malignant intraocular tumor of childhood. The tumor is of neuroepithelial origin and arises from the nucleated layers of one or both eyes (1). RB consists of undifferentiated small anaplastic cells, which may be round or polygonal. Scant cytoplasm surrounds the large nuclei, which characteristically stain deeply with hematoxylin. Calcification commonly occurs in necrotic areas (2,3). Both Flexner and Wintersteiner described the arrangement of the more differentiated malignant cells of RB in neuroepithelial rosettes. These Flexner-Wintersteiner rosettes appear to represent an attempt to differentiate into photoreceptor cells (4) (Fig. 1).

As an RB grows, it may cause a retinal detachment secondary to a solid or multifocal mass (endophytic type of growth) (Fig. 2). Endophytic tumors may break through the inner layers of the retina to the vitreous. The tumor may also form a pedunculated mass (exophytic type of growth). Both patterns of growth may occur in the same eye, and neither one is of prognostic significance (5). It is not unusual for RB to seed the vitreous. These vitreous seeds may grow even though they lack a blood supply (2).

INCIDENCE

The reported incidence of RB ranges from 1 in 14,000 live births to 1 in 34,000 (4,6). There are approximately 200 to 350 new cases per year in the United States and 50 in the United Kingdom (2,4–8). The tumor may be more frequent in Latin America (9).

RB shows no predilection for sex, race, or the right or left eye. Between 65% and 80% of the cases are unilateral, and 20% to 35% are bilateral (2,4,10–14). The frequency of bilateral tumors will be higher at institutions serving as referral centers for more complicated cases. Bilaterality may be ascertained concurrently or sequentially.

The diagnosis may be made from shortly after birth until 5 to 7 years of age. The mean age of detection is 2 to 4 months, and the vast majority of cases are discovered before 3 years of age (2,4,15,16). Unilateral RB patients are, in general, diagnosed at an older age than are bilateral disease patients. In the Mayo Clinic series the median ages at diagnosis were 4.5 months for bilateral disease and 22 months for unilateral—an observation supported by others (5,8,17).

THE GENETICS AND MOLECULAR BIOLOGY OF RETINOBLASTOMA

In 1972, Alfred G. Knudson, Jr. proposed a simple genetic model to explain the origins of RB. He sought to understand how the disease might have a familial (i.e., hereditary) form and a sporadic (i.e., nonhereditary) form. In a retrospective statistical analysis, he plotted the logarithm of the proportion of cases not yet diagnosed against age for bilateral (i.e., hereditary) and unilateral (largely nonhereditary) forms of RB (18,19). The graph for the bilateral type generated a straight line, whereas the unilateral type cre-

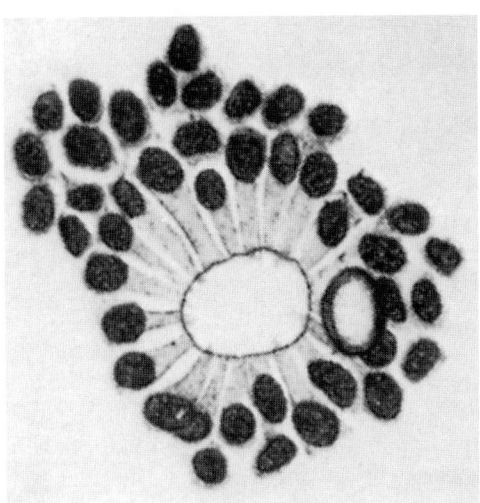

FIG. 1. A rosette characteristic of differentiated retinoblastoma—after a drawing by Wintersteiner. Note the cylindrical nuclei and fine protoplasm extensions toward the lumen. (From ref. 38, with permission.)

ated a curved line with second-order kinetics. Knudson inferred that the bilateral type was explicable by a single random somatic event acting in the presence of an existing germ-line mutation, whereas the unilateral form resulted from two somatic events. He also analyzed the number of tumors in patients with bilateral RB. He found that the mean number was three and that the distribution of the number of tumors followed the Poisson equation. The tumor events were, he concluded, random and independent (14,18, 19).

In its simplest statement, Knudson's model suggests that children with sporadic RB are genetically normal at conception. During embryonic development, two somatic mutations (also called two genetic "hits") occur in the cell line leading to the retinal photoreceptors. The resulting doubly mutated primordial retinal cell proliferates into RB tumors. In famil-

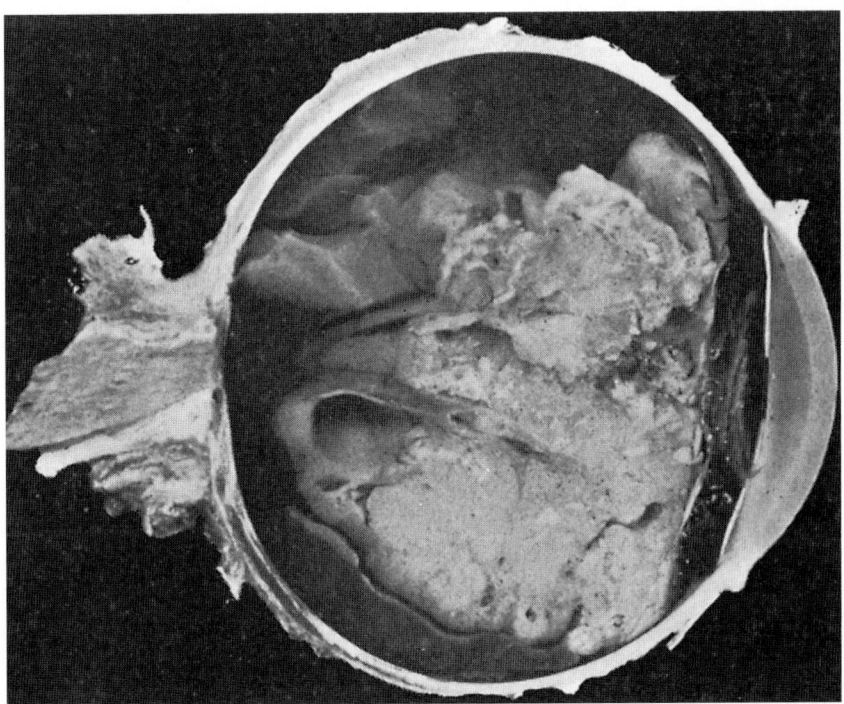

FIG. 2. The renowned pathologist James Ewing, in the 1919 edition of his textbook of tumor pathology, recognized the "glioma of the retina" as being composed of "small round-cells...arranged in small alveoli or rosettes after the manner of neuro-epithelial rosettes...[occurring] almost exclusively in infants...The congenital character is most remarkable." (Ewing J. *Neoplastic diseases: a text-book on tumors.* Philadelphia: W.B. Saunders, 1919.)

ial RB, the fertilized egg already carries one copy of the mutant gene (one "hit"). All the descendants of this cell carry the mutation. If any cell sustains a somatic mutation (a second "hit") to reach the doubly mutated state required for tumor induction, RB develops. The "two-hit hypothesis," as proposed, had the potential to explain both forms of RB (14, 18–21) (Fig. 3).

Knudson's hypothesis explained neither the precise gene affected nor the nature of the mutation or gene product, which caused the malignancy (21). A few years after Knudson's seminal paper, however, cytogenetic studies disclosed that some RB had a deletion on the long arm (called the "q" arm) of chromosome 13. The deletion included the number 14 band on the chromosome and is conventionally abbreviated 13q14. This deletion is homozygous in tumor cells. Homozygosity, or the loss of heterozygosity, appears to be the predicted two "hits." The RB gene was isolated by mo-

lecular cloning in 1986 and is 200 kb in length (21–24).

What protein is normally produced by the deleted 13q14 RB gene? How does it regulate cell growth? Why does its absence lead to malignancy? The search for the answers to these questions is at the heart of the burgeoning field of molecular cancer biology. In general, we may think of tumor formation as the possible result of mutations in two classes of genes: proto-oncogenes and tumor suppressor genes. When mutations occur in proto-oncogenes, which result in a gain of function and unbridled cell growth, they are referred to as oncogenes. Proto-oncogenes participate in cell growth and proliferation via several mechanisms: the elaboration of cellular growth factors; the production and deployment of membrane growth factor receptors; intracellular signal transducers, which conduct growth-promoting signals from the membrane deep into the interior of

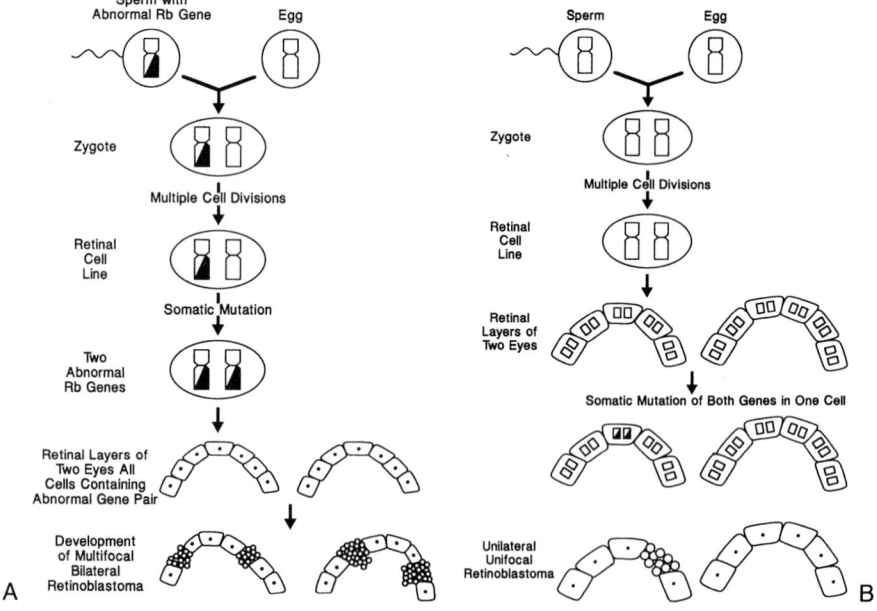

FIG. 3. A: In heritable bilateral retinoblastoma a gamete carrying a defective Rb gene (the "first hit") forms a zygote heterozygous at the Rb locus. A later somatic mutation inactivates the other Rb gene (the "second hit"), allowing bilateral multifocal tumors. **B:** In nonheritable retinoblastoma, inactivation of both genes in a retinal cell ("two hits") by somatic mutations leads to the development of unilateral unifocal disease. (Modified from ref. 74.)

the cell; and transcription factors that promote the ultimate production of proteins, which lead to cell proliferation. It is clear that proto-oncogenes have desirable physiologic functions in fetal development, normal childhood growth, wound healing, and desirable cell proliferation such as occurs in the aero-digestive tract, gut, and bone marrow. When, however, proto-oncogenes go awry and become oncogenes, then the persistent cell growth that results, without appropriate restraints of time and space, leads to cancer.

Tumor suppressor genes, in contrast, provide signals that constrain cell proliferation. Mutations in the tumor suppressor genes behave in a recessive manner at the molecular level. Consistent with Knudson's hypothesis, when mutations occur in both alleles (two "hits") then the suppressive behavior of the gene is fully lost, i.e., only when both copies of the gene are inactivated by mutations does an abnormal phenotype, malignant transformation, occur in a cell. A child born with one defective copy of a tumor suppressor gene has a predisposition to cancer. If the second copy of the gene is rendered inactive by a mutation, then the carcinogenic potential is realized. However, a child with two defective tumor suppressor genes has fully lost a constraint on cell growth and cancer will ensue.

The retinoblastoma protein, abbreviated as pRB, is intimately involved in control of the cell cycle. There is a transcription factor that helps drive the cell through the cell cycle to mitosis named E2F (the name comes from its initial identification as being involved in the adenovirus E2 promoter). When pRB binds E2F, then E2F is not free to activate promoters of DNA synthesis. In addition, the pRB-E2F complex downregulates the expression of many G_1 exit-promoting genes such as c-*myc* and c-*myb*. In this way, pRB inhibits the cell from duplicating itself. If pRB is phosphorylated, the phosphorus groups displace the E2F from its binding site. Then the E2F launches into action and promotes cell division. If the pRB is absent or defective, then the factors leading to cell proliferation have no countervailing force.

To use a metaphor, consider cell growth as being similar to sitting in the driver's seat of an automobile. To move the car forward, the driver pushes down on the accelerator pedal. To stop the car, the driver moves their foot to the brake pedal. Oncogenes are similar to pushing down on the accelerator, a gain of function leads to motion. Tumor suppressor genes, however, press on the cell's brakes. When tumor suppressor genes fail to exercise their normal restraint, then the metaphorical foot is removed from the brake and the car (or cell) moves forward into a proliferative stage (20,21,25–27).

A generation of pediatric radiation oncologists were taught that RB has an autosomal dominant inheritance pattern with an 80% to 90% penetrance (1,8). This is now known to not be precisely correct. RB is the result of an autosomal recessive—only in the presence of damage to two alleles (two "hits") will cancer develop. It must be the case that, in the presence of an inherited single defective allele, the occurrence of a mutation in the second allele is frequent—this gives the impression of dominant inheritance.

RB may be inherited from an affected parent or may be the result of sporadic mutations (28). While most cases of RB are sporadic, between 25% and 40% are familial (inherited from an affected parent who survived RB, a nonaffected gene carrier parent who has no clinical signs of having RB, or a parent with a new germ-line mutation). Hereditary cases are usually bilateral and multifocal; they occur at a young age compared to sporadic cases, which are, in comparison, more often unifocal and unilateral and occur at an older age. Of all new RB patients, about 10% will have a positive family history and, almost always, bilateral disease. Of the 90% with no family history, 20% to 30% will be found to have bilateral disease and be hereditary. The remaining 65% to 80% are unilateral. Of these unilateral cases, about 10% prove to be hereditary and 90% nonhereditary (14) (Fig. 4).

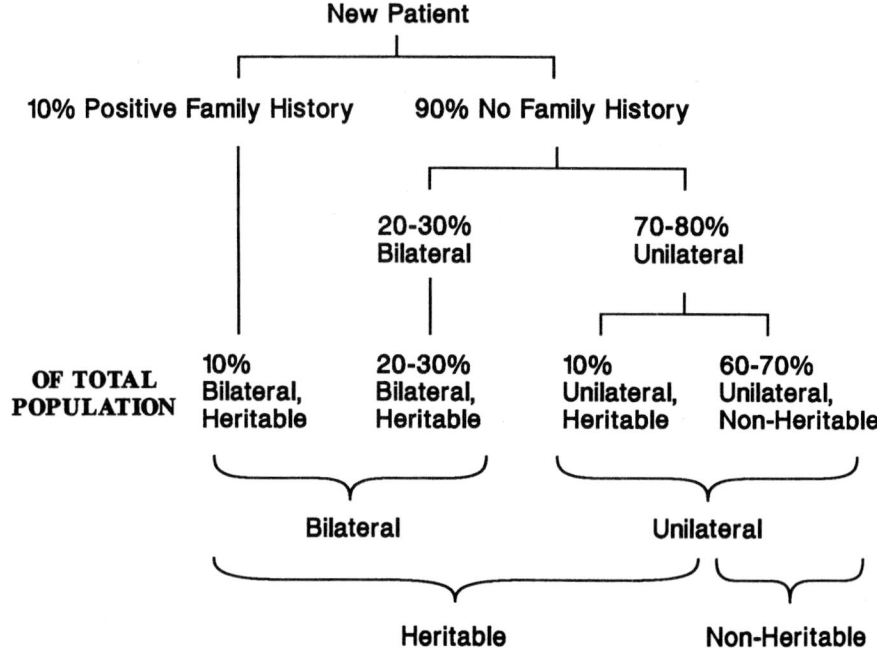

FIG. 4. The distribution of unilateral and bilateral, as well as heritable and nonheritable, cases of retinoblastoma. (Modified from ref. 1.)

WORKUP

RB commonly presents with a white pupillary light reflex (termed *leukocoria*) (5,11, 29). The parents may note this abnormal appearance in a flash photograph (Fig. 5), because photographic flash bounces light through the pupil and conjunctiva to produce a red appearance in a color snapshot. However, large RB, or a RB producing retinal detachment, will produce the white reflex when the flash bounces off it. This effect can also be seen with a handheld ophthalmoscope. RB may also be discovered by a pediatrician or ophthalmologist while doing a surveillance examination of a child with a positive family history or during the course of a routine examination.

On physical examination one notes a raised white, white-yellow, or white-pink mass (2). Tortuous vessels may be seen feeding the tumor. Cells may break off from the main tumor mass and grow as small vitreous seeds (5). Because RB may be multifocal, it is vital to examine the entire retinal surface, with the examination performed generally under anesthesia.

When RB presents as a mass, the differential diagnosis includes astrocytic hamartoma, *Toxocara canis* granuloma, the infected emboli of subacute bacterial endocarditis or toxoplasmosis, and other types of severe uveitis. When RB causes retinal detachment, the differential diagnosis includes Coats' disease, retrolental fibroplasia, and persistent hyperplastic vitreous (2,4–6,8). Biopsy of a suspected RB or vitreous aspiration for enzyme studies are generally felt to be contraindicated because of the risk of choroidal seeding (5). The consequences of intraocular procedures in RB patients are discussed later in this chapter.

Retinal drawings and photographs, along with a written description, are used to record if single or multifocal tumors are present (Fig. 6). Ultrasound is also useful for documenting tumor location and size. (Fig. 7) The cornea–back of the lens distance can also be mea-

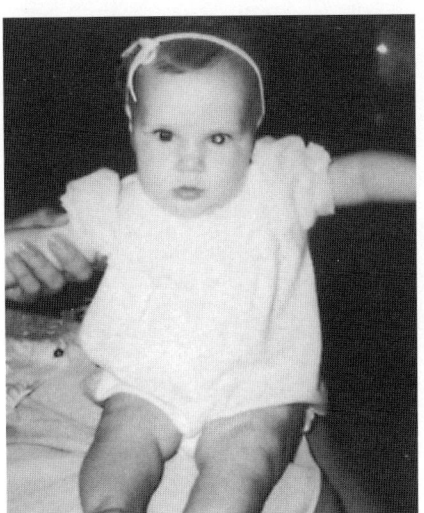
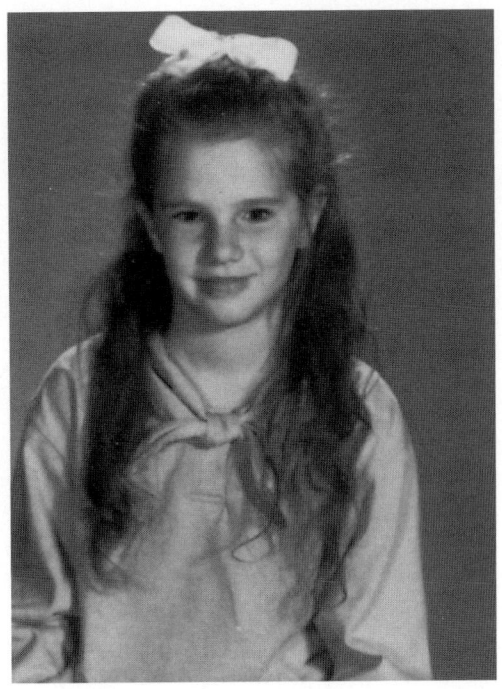

A B

FIG. 5. A,B: Leukocoria in a flash photograph of a 6-month-old child with retinoblastoma. Irradiated with 43.6 Gy, she retains excellent vision at 10-year follow-up. (Reproduced with permission of the child's parents.)

sured with ultrasound to aid in lateral field radiotherapy planning. Computerized tomography (CT) scan is an effective way of demonstrating tumor calcification. A cranial CT scan may accompany the orbital study to assess the presence of intracranial extension of the primary tumor and the possibility of a synchronous pineal tumor.

Among the tests used for the determination of metastatic disease are a lumbar puncture with cerebrospinal fluid (CSF) cytology and a bone marrow biopsy and aspirate (30). Pratt et al. (31) reported no positive CSF cytologies or bone marrow aspirates in 109 children with RB confined to the globe. The only positive studies were in patients with extraocular tumor extension (i.e., through the sclera or beyond the cut end of the optic nerve) or with bone, distant soft tissue, or brain metastases. In Pratt et al. (31), data is supported by a 1997 study from Riyadh, Saudia Arabia. In children

with disease confined to the eye who were treated with external beam irradiation, 0 of 49 had a positive CSF, 0 of 50 had a positive bone marrow biopsy/aspirate, 0 of 54 had a positive bone scan. In children with more advanced disease requiring enucleation and orbital irradiation, the frequency of positive staging studies was: CSF cytology 0 of 27, bone marrow examination 0 of 28, and bone scan 0 of 26. In the patients presenting with locally advanced and/or metastatic disease there were some positive staging studies: CSF cytology positive in 7 of 31 (23%) and bone scan positive in 5 of 27 (19%) (32). In modern practice, routine lumbar puncture and bone marrow aspiration are not justified for RB confined to the retina without optic nerve involvement or other suggestion of extraocular extension. In the presence of symptoms suggestive of metastatic disease, a bone scan and plain bone films are indicated.

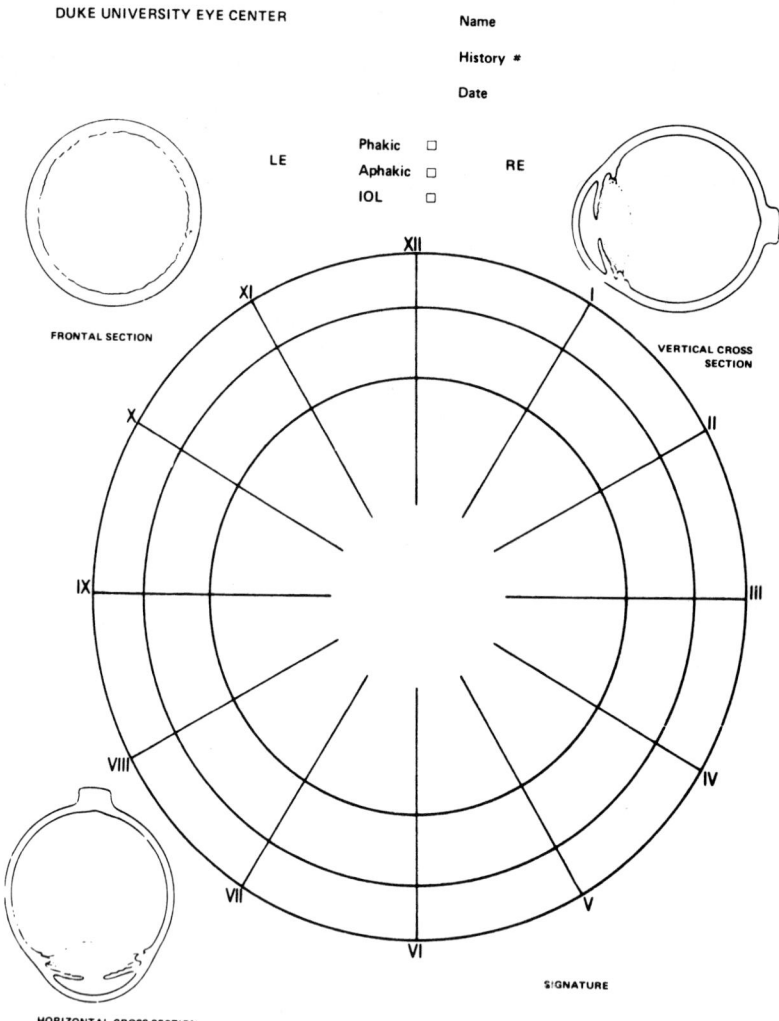

FIG. 6. A standard retinal drawing used to localize intraocular tumors. The drawing represents the inner curved surface of the eye. The space between the outermost circle and the middle circle represents the pars plana. The middle circle is the ora serrata—the anterior termination of the retina. The most inner circle is the geometric equator of the globe. The macula, the yellow spot in the center of the retina, is indicated by the central area of the drawing. The macula contains a pit, the fovea centralis, where closely packed cones function as the area of most acute vision. The optic nerve's exit (the optic nerve "head" or "disc") is 2-mm medial to the macula. The disk is approximately 1.5 mm in diameter and is often used as a ruler to describe tumor dimensions (i.e., so many "disc diameters" in width).

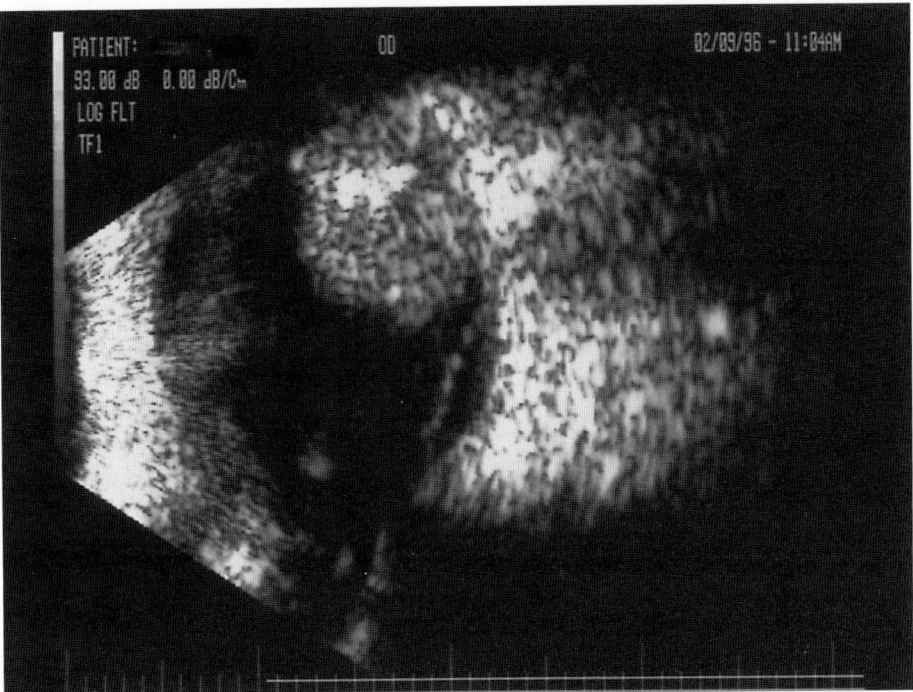

FIG. 7. Ultrasonography may be of considerable assistance to the pediatric radiation oncologist in the diagnosis and treatment of retinoblastoma. This 18-month-old child had unilateral retinoblastoma. The circular globe is clearly seen in the image with the lens on the left. The tumor mass with internal calcification is seen in the upper right portion of the image of the globe. (The tumor was located superiortemporal in the patient.) Adjacent to the tumor an area of retinal detachment is clearly seen. Preservation and restoration of vision was dependent on the ability to control the tumor as well as the re-attachment of the detached retina. The ultrasound was also used to determine the distance between the front of the cornea and the back of the lens to direct the use of the Schipper device (see Fig. 14).

PROGNOSTIC FACTORS AND STAGING

The staging system for RB must fulfill at least two requirements. First, it must predict the likelihood of cure—a requirement placed on all staging systems for malignancy. An important emphasis of RB treatment, however, is not only cure but preservation of sight in the affected eye. To this end, some eyes are treated with chemotherapy, cryotherapy, laser photocoagulation, hyperthermia, radioactive plaque, and external beam radiotherapy as an alternative to enucleation. The secondary requirement for staging, therefore, is to predict the likelihood of visual preservation.

The most widely used grouping system for RB was proposed by Algernon Reese (6) and Robert Ellsworth (33) (Table 1). This system does not do well discriminating survival probability. It does, however, serve as guide to the chance of visual preservation with conservative therapy. There are at least two staging systems published that attempt to predict prognosis for survival and include information on disease extension beyond the globe (9,31). Of these systems the St. Jude Children's Research Hospital (SJCRH) is somewhat more frequently used (Table 2).

Histologic evaluation of an enucleated eye is a useful tool to ascertain prognosis. Invasion of the choroid has usually been considered a poor prognostic sign. It is almost certainly true that hematogenous spread of RB does occur via choroidal vessels. Choroidal invasion, however, is not rare: It occurs in up to 62% of

TABLE 1. *The Reese–Ellsworth system of classifying retinoblastoma*[a]

Group I: Very favorable
A. Solitary tumors, <4 DD[b] in size, at or behind the equator.
B. Multiple tumors, none larger than 4 DD in size, all at or behind the equator.
Group II: Favorable
A. Solitary tumors, 4–10 DD in size, at or behind the equator.
B. Multiple tumors, 4–10 DD in size, all at or behind the equator.
Group III: Doubtful
A. Any lesion anterior to the equator.
B. Solitary tumors, larger than 10 DD in size, behind the equator.
Group IV: Unfavorable
A. Multiple tumors, some larger than 10 DD.
B. Any lesion extending anterior to the ora serrata.
Group V: Very Unfavorable
A. Massive tumors involving more than half of the retina.
B. Vitreous seeding.

[a]See refs. 2, 33, 15, and 6.
[b]The optic nerve's exit (the optic nerve "head" or "disc") is approximately 1.5 mm in diameter. The disc diameter (DD) is often used as a ruler to describe tumor dimensions (i.e., so many DD in size).

cases. Distant metastases are rare. It seems that the prognostic correlation is less with choroidal invasion alone than with the *volume* of choroidal invasion and its correlation with other risk factors. Involvement of the optic nerve beyond the lamina cribosa is a risk factor

TABLE 2. *The St. Jude Children's Research Hospital staging system of retinoblastoma*

I. Intraocular diseases
  Ia. Retinal tumor, single or multiple
  Ib. Extension to lamina cribosa
  Ic. Uveal extension
II. Orbital disease
  IIa. Orbital tumor
    IIa1. Scattered episcleral cells
    IIa2. Orbital invasion
  IIb. Optic nerve
    IIb1. Invasion of optic nerve to cut end
    IIb2. Invasion of optic nerve beyond the cut end
III. Intracranial metastases
  IIa. Positive CSF
  IIb. Mass lesion in the CNS
IV. Hematogenous metastasis
  IVa. Positive bone marrow
  IVb. Facial bone lesions ± positive marrow
  IVc. Other organ involvement

From refs. 9 and 110, with permission.

for orbital recurrence and central nervous system (CNS) dissemination. Even worse is the involvement of the distal cut end of the optic nerve with tumor (3). Tumor involvement of the scleral emisseric veins and episcleral tissues also forebodes a poor prognosis. Multivariate analysis of data from 330 children at St. Bartholomew's and Moorefield's Eye Hospitals showed that the deleterious effect of extensive choroidal invasion as a prognostic factor was lost in the absence of either retrolaminar (behind lamina cribosa) or cut end of the optic nerve invasion. Two patient groups had a particularly poor prognosis: retrolaminar extension and extensive choroidal invasion (5-year survival 31%) and extensive choroidal invasion and cut end of optic nerve invasion (5-year survival 25%) (5). In 62 children only one death was attributable to metastatic disease from choroidal invasion alone (34,35). There is no clear correlation between tumor differentiation and prognosis (36). The clinical implications of histologic evaluation of the enucleated eye are considered later in this chapter.

SELECTION OF THERAPY

The primary goal of RB therapy is cure. Because RB infrequently metastasizes, the chance of cure is excellent. The actuarial overall 5-year survival rate for 731 children with RB seen at St. Bartholomew's and Moorefield's Eye Hospitals from 1960 to 1988 was 87% (5). The 50-month actuarial overall survival of 52 SJCRH patients with initial intraocular disease was 97% (9). Therefore, it is appropriate to assert that a secondary goal of treatment is preservation of vision in the affected eye. Enucleation is recommended only in a blind eye or an eye, which does not have a reasonable expectation of sight after cryotherapy, phototherapy, or radiotherapy. Every effort should be made to *preserve vision* in a *sighted* eye. This rule pertains to both bilateral and unilateral disease. Generally, however, children with unilateral disease have locally advanced tumors with little hope of vision, and, therefore, these patients generally undergo enucleation. In bilateral disease, enucleation of the more severely affected eye is

indicated only if this eye is blind. *If both eyes are sighted, then an effort should be made to preserve both eyes.*

Enucleation

In an enucleation for RB, anterior traction is placed on the globe after severing the rectus muscles. The optic nerve is then cut near its exit from the socket. Obtaining a long segment of nerve is important in the event the tumor is within the nerve. In young children, orbital growth is reduced after enucleation. As the child grows, the orbit appears relatively small. This may be ameliorated by a properly fitting orbital prosthesis.

A review of the New York Hospital experience showed that primary enucleation was performed in 97% of eyes in unilateral cases seen from 1951 to 1965 and 87% from 1966 to 1980. Enucleation was used in 67% of eyes in bilateral cases treated from 1951 to 1965 and 58% in 1966 to 1980 (37). Similarly, Shields et al. (38,39) reported a reduction in the proportion of children having an eye removed for RB from 96% in 1974 to 1978 to 75% for 1984 to 1988.

Enucleation is indicated in unilateral RB, where the eye is blind. In bilateral RB, when both eyes are blind a bilateral enucleation is done. If one eye is blind a unilateral enucleation is done. Enucleation is also indicated in unilateral or bilateral tumor, when glaucoma follows rubeosis iridis with visual loss. It is also recommended when local recurrence of tumor can no longer be controlled with more conservative measures (15,40).

Exenteration

An exenteration is the removal of the globe, extraocular muscles, lids, nerves, and orbital fat. Blood loss may be significant. In the opinion of some ophthalmologists the indications for exenteration in RB include: (a) extensive local tumor breaching the globe (exenteration in this situation will generally be followed by postoperative radiotherapy and chemotherapy), and (b) recurrence of tumor

in the socket after enucleation. Some cases of local recurrence, however, may be locally managed with external beam radiotherapy, a radioactive implant or a radioactive mold, and chemotherapy (*vide infra*).

Local Therapy

The four local therapies for RB are cryotherapy, photocoagulation, laser hyperthermia, and radioactive plaque applications.

Until recently, in children at high risk for multicentric disease, local therapy was thought only to be appropriate when there could be serial follow-up with repeated local therapy or with external beam radiotherapy when necessary. In children with bilateral disease, an average of five foci of tumors are randomly distributed (2,41). These foci may not appear simultaneously but may occur months after successful local treatment of the sentinel lesion. In children with multifocal disease or in those at high risk of developing multifocal disease, as well as in children with large tumors, local therapy, the old argument concluded, should generally not be used.

Modern thinking concerning local therapy is now far different. With the increase in use of systemic chemotherapy, local therapy is now used in multifocal disease. Local therapy may be interspersed with chemotherapy or follow it. Programs using focal therapy in this way are reviewed in the chemotherapy section of this chapter.

Photocoagulation

The technique of photocoagulation is based on obliteration of the retinal vessels. With the child under anesthesia a white retinal burn is created, surrounding the tumor by 1 mm, by "painting" with the laser beam. Special attention is directed to closing feeding vessels (42). The tumor is encircled by the burn and regression depends on interruption of blood supply. Direct photocoagulation of RB should be avoided because small explosions can release viable tumor cells into the vitreous and lead to tumor recurrence (5). In primary therapy, photocoagulation may be used for tumors less than or equal to 4.5 mm at the base and less than or equal to 2.5 mm thick, provided that they are not close to the macula or disc where retinal damage would generate large scotoma. Vitreous seeding is a contraindication (12,40). Photocoagulation may be used for small tumor recurrences after prior irradiation in order to avoid the risks of reirradiation. With proper case selection photocoagulation has a local tumor control probability of about 70% (42).

Laser Hyperthermia

Laser hyperthermia is generated by a diode laser (810 nm) on continuous mode. A single spot, 0.8 to 2.0 mm, is placed on the center of the tumor using the aiming beam. An output of 300 to 700 mW is selected based on the tumor size. Tumors are heated for 10 to 30 minutes per session. It is estimated that a central tumor temperature of about 46°C is reached. As the heat disperses throughout the tumor the temperature decreases about 2°C for each millimeter outside the treatment spot. In this technique the heat is used principally to enhance the binding and cytotoxicity of platinum drugs— an assertion supported by experiments utilizing rabbit ocular melanoma (43). Whole eye hyperthermia in combination with external beam irradiation has been shown to be effective in controlling murine transgenic RB but has not, to our knowledge, been used in humans (44).

Cryotherapy

With cryotherapy a tumor is localized and indented, transsclerally, with a nitrous oxide cryoprobe. The freeze (−80°C) is then applied until the tumor is completely covered with a frozen vitreous. The freeze–thaw cycle is then repeated at least three times (45,46). Cryotherapy is indicated for the primary therapy of RB in the following situations: (a) small tumors anterior to the equator, without vitreous seeding, which can be reached with the cryoprobe (posterior tumors are difficult to reach, and the risks of freezing the macula or nerve increase); (b) local recurrence or tumor

persistence following irradiation; (c) in conjunction with chemotherapy. Only 1% of 575 patients seen from 1951 to 1965 received cryotherapy at New York Hospital whereas 23% of patients seen from 1966 to 1980 did (37).

Cryotherapy can induce acute retinal edema and accumulation of subretinal fluid. To avoid retinal detachment, some opthalmologists use the laser to create a retinal barrier to fluid leakage. Disruption of the retina by cryotherapy may increase intravitreal penetration of systemic carboplatin (46).

Radioactive Plaque Application

Plaques are used for solitary 2- to 16-mm basal diameter unilateral lesions located greater than 3 mm from the optic disc or fovea, generally with a thickness less than 10 mm, for two lesions that are small enough or close enough to be covered by one plaque, and for local failure following other therapy (Fig. 8). Plaques can be used if there is a small amount of vitreous seeding over the tumor apex (11,29,47–50).

Prior to the operative procedure, the tumor's dimensions are ascertained by physical examination and ultrasonography. One derives a maximum basal diameter of the tumor and a maximum height. In treatment planning, it is customary to allow 1 mm for scleral thickness—although there is some normal variation in this measurement (51,52). The operative procedure begins with a careful eye examination using magnifying lenses. After confirming the tumor anatomy, the surgeon opens the conjunctiva around the periphery of the limbus (a periotomy). Muscle hooks are used to snare rectus muscles and rotate the eye. Traction sutures are sometimes used. It may be necessary to disinsert a muscle in order to visualize the tumor. With the room darkened, a transilluminator is placed over the pupil. The shadow, cast by the tumor, is marked on the sclera with a marking pen or with electrocautery. Tumors that cannot be transilluminated are located by ultrasound. A clear dummy plaque is then brought into the

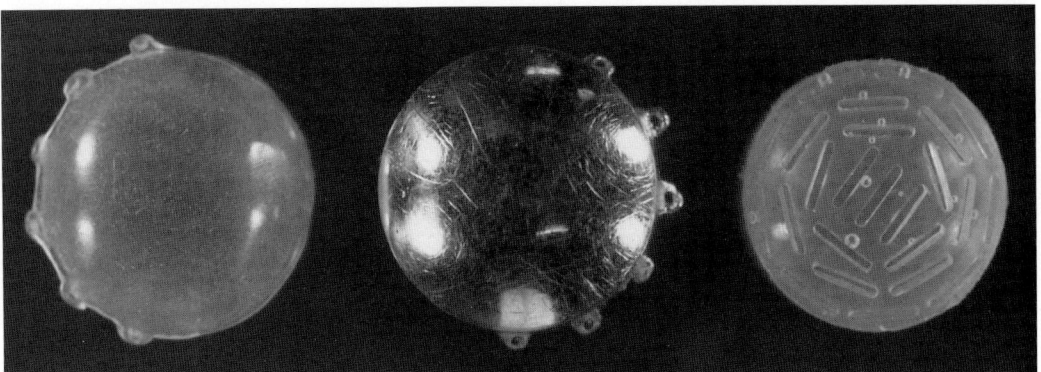

FIG. 8. Equipment for I 125 ocular plaque construction and placement includes, from left to right, a dummy plaque to aid in the placement of the necessary retention sutures, a gold backing with lug holes for sutures and a plastic insert to hold the radioactive I 125 seeds.

operative field. We allow 1.5 to 2 mm of margin on either side of the basal diameter; that is, an 8.5-mm tumor is plaqued with a 12- to 14-mm device. The dummy is utilized to place the two sutures through the lug holes and into the sclera. The dummy is then removed and replaced with the radioactive plaque. The retention sutures are tied, and the eye is rotated back into place. The conjunctiva is then closed. The patient generally remains hospitalized for the duration of the application. The plaque is then removed (53).

There are several types of plaques available. The ^{60}Co plaque (1.17 and 1.33 MeV, half-life 5.2 years) may be purchased in a circular or crescenteric configuration to fit around the optic nerve (54). The ^{60}Co ball applicator is a platinum-coated 6-mm sphere attached to a ring (16). The ^{125}I plaque (27 to 35 keV, half-life 60 days) with lip consists of ^{125}I seeds glued in a carrier within a gold shield. These plaques are available in circular or notched configuration. ^{192}Ir (295 to 612 keV, half-life 74.5 days) and ^{109}Ru (beta emitter) plaques are also available (55,56).

The four available plaques (^{60}Co, ^{125}I, ^{192}Ir, ^{109}Ru) each have advantages and disadvantages. ^{60}Co plaques may be purchased and assembled in standard sizes. The relatively long half-life means that the plaque may be used for several years before the treatment times become unacceptably long. The high-

energy ^{60}Co and the breadth of the high-dose isodose curves mean that thick and infiltrative tumors can be treated. Shielding of periocular normal tissues behind the plaque is, however, impossible. Effective shielding on the back of the plaque is achievable with ^{125}I and ^{109}Ru. Shielding from the gold lip on the ^{125}I plaque requires expert placement lest tumor be missed. ^{125}I plaques must be assembled for each case; while this involves extra work, it does allow individualization of the plaque. Hospital personnel exposure is minimal with ^{125}I or ^{109}Ru. A shielded ^{125}I plaque with a lead eye patch will allow the child's parent to provide care with appropriate and acceptable radiation safety precautions (11, 29,47–50).

Using ^{60}Co plaques, Stallard (57) administered 40 Gy to the tumor apex in 1 week. Sixty-three of 69 children with tumor involving one-fourth of the retinal area or less were successfully treated with a plaque. When the tumor involved one-fourth to one-half of the retinal area, success was achieved in 8 of 10 instances. Among the best characterized clinical series of plaque brachytherapy for RB is that of the Wills Eye Hospital of Philadelphia (11,29,48–50,53,58). Over 90 children have been treated with plaque brachytherapy for recurrent RB or residual RB and over 35 patients have been treated primarily with a plaque (48–50,58). The median tumor apex dose administered was 40 Gy. I^{125} was the most commonly used isotope followed by Co^{60}, Ir^{191}, and Ru^{106}. In general, the clinical results from Wills have been excellent. In recurrent or relapsed RB cases, regression occurred in 89%. Recurrences developed in 11% during a mean follow-up of 52 months. Vision greater than or equal to 20/400 was obtained in 62% (48–50).

In the past, it was reported that for large tumors with vitreous seeds, multiple sequential plaques (rotating plaques) could be used. In this technique, two plaques are applied in one operation to opposite quadrants of the eye. In a second operation these two plaques are rotated to the remaining quadrants. In a third operation the plaques are removed. This technique gives about 40 Gy to midvitreous and 160 Gy to the sclera. Initial reports indicated that useful vision was retained in 14 of 16 patients treated with plaques as the single irradiation modality. Useful vision was retained in 22 of 36 cases plaqued after failure of some other treatment (11,29,48). Later reports showed a significant incidence of radiation retinopathy with this technique and it is now rarely used (53).

In carefully selected patients with small primary RB or for recurrent tumors after other treatment, a radioactive single plaque application of 40 Gy to tumor apex is reasonable therapy. With growth in the use of chemotherapy as primary treatment for RB, plaque therapy has joined photocoagulation laser treatment, and cryotherapy as an adjuvant focal treatment following or interspersed with chemotherapy. When a plaque is used in a child who has also received chemotherapy, some ophthalmologists feel that 40 Gy as an apical dose is too high. The occurrence of a few cases of post brachytherapy retinitis has lead to a dose reduction to 25 to 30 Gy to the tumor apex (43) (C. Shields, *personal communication,* 1997). Plaques have little chance of producing orbital bone hypoplasia and should not contribute to the risk of orbital bone sarcoma. Conventional plaques rarely will be associated with cataracts, retinopathy, or hemorrhage (11,29,48).

External Beam Radiotherapy

When RB is multifocal and/or close to the macula or optic nerve with preservation of vision, it has been found that cryotherapy, photocoagulation, or plaque therapy by themselves will not be adequate and that enucleation is too drastic. In such situations, which are quite common, external beam irradiation or chemotherapy, plus focal therapy are used. These types of therapy are also indicated for large tumors and vitreous seeding. Hilgartner (59) reported treatment of a case of bilateral retinoblastoma with x-rays in 1910. Verhoeff cured a case of retinoblastoma with x-ray treatment in 1918. The patient died in 1972 with tumor controlled (60). The Reese-Ellsworth grouping system may be used to predict the probability of success for external beam irradiation (Table 3). Large lesions have a proclivity to fail after teletherapy. Some say that anterior lesions are also more likely to fail after teletherapy, but the reader is cautioned that the risk of failure of anterior lesions is probably related to the practice, by some radiotherapists, of treating with a lateral beam with the anterior field edge at the rim of the bony orbit. This technique will underdose the anterior globe (8,12,61–64). Technical factors play a large role in the probability of success of external beam therapy and the frequency of complications.

Technique

The goals of conventional external beam radiotherapy are to provide a homogeneous and tumoricidal dose to the retinal anlage and vitreous and to respect tolerance of normal tissue structures. At least five arguments have been put forward in support of this expansive view of treatment volume: (a) RB represents, in many cases, a "field change" where all retinal cells have a genetic neoplastic potential. The entire retina must, therefore, be treated. (b) Vitreous seeding can occur. (c) Multiple tumors may arise from a primary RB. (d) Tumor may spread via the subretinal space. (e) Retinal differentiation progresses from posterior to anterior and from superior to inferior.

TABLE 3. *Visual preservation in retinoblastoma with external beam irradiation as a function of initial Reese–Ellsworth group[a]*

Group	I	II	III	IV	V
Columbia 1969 (12)[b]	84% (43)	67% (45)	69% (33)	30% (37)	15% (66)
Stanford 1987 (13)[b]	88% (8)	60% (5)	67% (8)	0% (2)	33% (15)
Cornell 1983, children <6 months old (55)[c,d]	89%	82%	80%	56%	10%
Utrecht 1985 (73)	100% (14)	100% (9)	83% (10)	79% (14)	0% (5)
Norwegian Radium Hospital 1986 (117)[b]	100% (5)	100% (5)	100% (1)	100% (1)	
Curie Institute 1987 (114)[e]	0% (1)	100% (2)	0% (1)	50% (2)	38% (13)
Cornell 1988 (62,63)[b,d,f]		100% (31)			60% (14)
Mayo 1989[b] (17)	100% (1)	100% (1)	85% (13)	50% (14)	83% (6)
Arhus 1989 (119)[g]			61% (46)		
Wills Eye Hospital 1990 (11)[g]	100% (2)	83%	100% (6)	67% (3)	50% (5)
Duke 1992 (70)[b,h]			100% (8)	100% (8)	100% (4)
U. of Washington/ S. Florida 1994 (64a)[e,h,i,j]		83%/100% (6)	71%/71% (7)		
St. Jude Children's Research Hospital 1995, >1 yr old (67)	100% (1)	67%/67% (6)	67%/100% (3)	100% (1)	57%/100% (7)
St. Bartholomew's Hospital 1995 (65), whole eye technique	88%/100% (16)	56%/84% (55)	59%/82% (68)	14%/43% (7)	45%/66% (29)
St. Bartholomew's Hospital 1995 (74), lens sparing technique	78%/100% (18)	67%/88% (33)	64%/91% (11)	100% (5)	
St. Jude Children's Research Hospital, 1996 <1 yr old (80)	75%/100% (20)	100% (6)	50%/100% (6)	100% (2)	43%/57% (7)
Memorial Sloan-Kettering and the New York Hospital-Cornell 1996 (61)	67%/88% (96)	67%/88% (96)	67%/88% (96)	44%/60% (84)	44%/60% (84)
Duke 1996 (71)	86% (15)	86% (15)	86% (15)	86% (15)	
Hahneman University and Wills Eye Hospital 1996 (83)	79% (4)	79% (10)	20% (7)	20% (2)	20% (11)
King Faisal Specialist Hospital & Research Center 1997 (32)[e,b]	86% (7)	100% (6)	50% (8)	67% (15)	54% (28)

[a]The numbers within the body of the table, in parentheses, are the number of eyes per group.

[b]Patients were treated with external beam radiotherapy, but cryotherapy, plaques, or laser therapy may have been used for salvage. In some series the need for additional treatment, following radiotherapy, approaches 50%.

[c]Patients were treated with a variety of primary therapies.

[d]Series which probably share some patients.

[e]These patients also received chemotherapy.

[f]Modifed lateral beam technique.

[g]Primary therapy includes external beam treatment and/or plaque.

[h]These series principally contain macular tumors.

[i]Lateral field only.

[j]First number is control with radiotherapy alone. Second number is eye preservation including focal salvage therapy.

Subclinical disease may exist in the immature retina and must be included in the treatment (17). The argument in favor of a more restrictive tumor volume is that selected cases will be unilateral and unifocal and, therefore, amenable to more focal irradiation—such as might be delivered to a fixed target with protons.

The dimensions of the eye of young children have been well-characterized (Fig. 9).

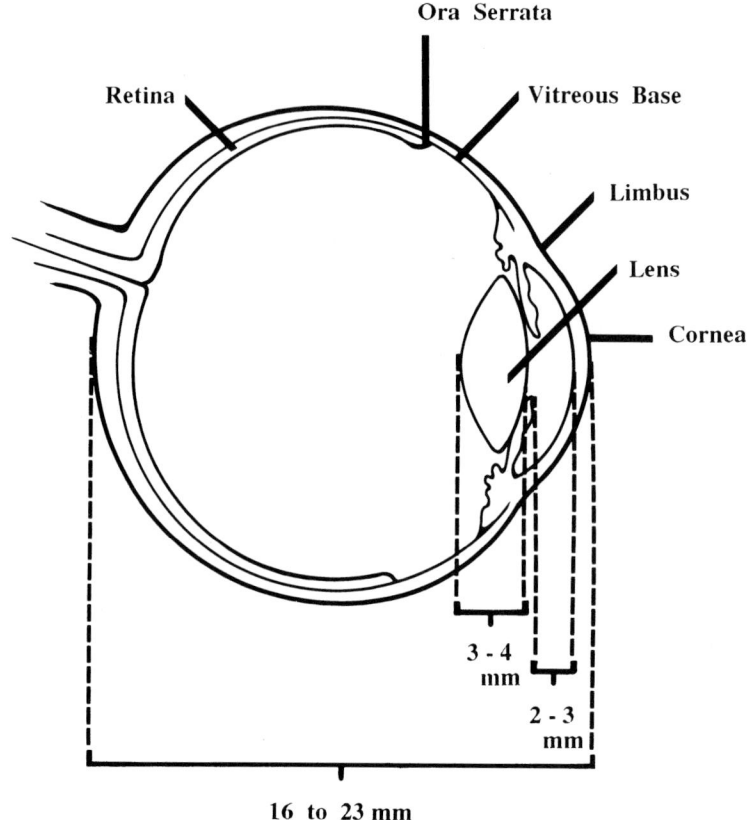

FIG. 9. The range of measurements of relevant dimensions of a young child's eye. In any individual case, measurements may be made by ultrasound.

The outer sagittal diameter of the eye varies from 16 to 17 mm at birth and increases rapidly to an average of 22.5 to 23 mm at 3 years of age (51,52). In any individual patient the axial intraocular dimensions may be measured by ultrasonic biometry and ocular CT.

One of the earliest techniques for the external beam irradiation of RB was developed by Algernon Reese in the 1930s. Using an orthovoltage unit, treatment was delivered through temporal and nasal portals. The technique attempted to avoid the lens by having the nasal portal angled 24 to 30 degrees (Fig. 10). A high bone dose was given by the orthovoltage apparatus. A "saddle nose" deformity developed in long-term survivors along with depression of the temporal bone (7).

In modern pediatric radiation oncology patient immobilization is recognized as crucial to precision irradiation of the designated treatment volume with minimization of radiation to normal tissue. In RB treatment anesthesia is generally required. Immobilization and anesthesia for pediatric radiotherapy are fully discussed in Chapters 21 and 22. Two special points are, however, warranted in this discussion. When a plaster or thermoplastic head holder is prepared for treatment, and the anesthesia gas mask is placed, care must be taken to allow an unobstructed view of the eye(s) so that the fields may be correctly set. Second, ketamine anesthesia produces lateral nystagmus. If a blocking technique is used that relies on the eye being a stable target, then ketamine will generally be unacceptable as the anesthetic agent.

The contemporary radiotherapist may choose among a large number of techniques:

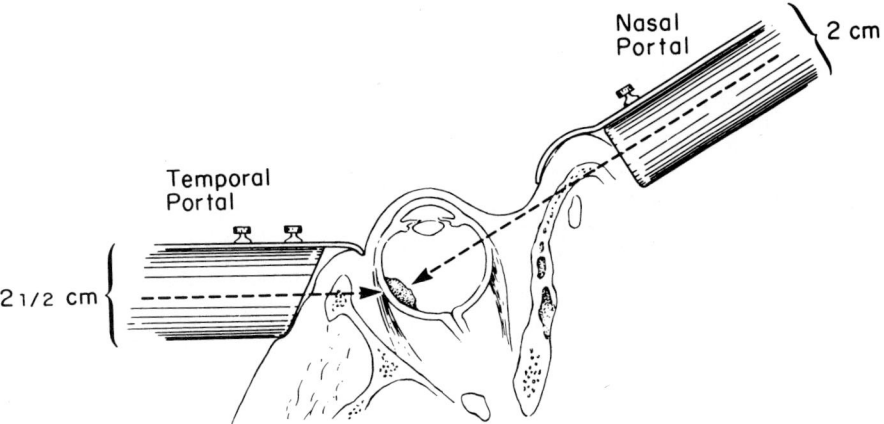

FIG. 10. In the 1930s, Reese utilized orthovoltage beams to externally irradiate retinoblastoma while attempting to spare the lens. The high bone dose produced cosmetic deformities. (From ref. 7, with permission.)

1. A lateral-beam megavoltage technique with the anterior field border set at the lateral bony orbit has been used. A direct lateral field is used following enucleation in the contralateral side. When the contralateral globe is in place, the beam is slightly angled posteriorly to avoid exit dose into the lens of the fellow eye (Fig. 11) (64). The distance from the back of the lens to the ora serrata is 1 to 1.5 mm, making techniques that endeavor to treat the entire retina from a lateral approach, yet miss the posterior part of the lens, highly impractical (64). Utilization of only a lateral beam may result in tumor recurrence at or near the ora serrata (7,12,64). However, small anterior failures can be treated with cryotherapy and, therefore, if there is no gross disease near the ora serrata, this technique may be adequate (7).

2. A direct anterior ^{60}Co or linear accelerator field treats the entire eye and spares the opposite eye. There is no sparing of the lens, cataract formation is almost certain, the lacrimal gland is fully irradiated (thereby potentially impairing tear production), and dose exits through the brain. However, the single anterior field is easy to set up, is reproducible, and homogeneously irradiates the entire vitreous and retina (7,15,33,61–63,65). Because the cataract will take time to develop, mitigating the problem of disuse amblyopia, and may

be treated surgically, advocates of the anterior field are assuaged (66–68).

3. A half-beam blocked lateral field has been used to sharpen the beam edge. Field sizes ranging from 3 × 6 cm to 5 × 10 cm are typically used for a 3 × 3-cm to 5 × 5-cm treatment area. The field edge may be set at the bony orbit or between the bone and the limbus. A field anterior edge about halfway between the limbus and edge of the bony orbit will cover the ora serrata. Treatment may be given with a lateral beam with photons alone or with mixed photon/electron straight lateral and lateral oblique beams (7,33,61–63,69).

For children with unilateral disease, straight lateral fields are replaced, by many clinicians, with oblique fields. Superior and inferior oblique fields will miss the uninvolved eye. The price of an inferior oblique field, of course, is exit dose into the frontal lobe of the brain. A superior oblique field will exit into the maxillary sinus and mouth (Fig. 12).

4. A two-field technique using a lateral field and an anterior field with a hanging lens block is an attempt to achieve a homogeneous retinal dose yet spare the lens (7,26) (Fig. 13). This is probably the most widely used approach (8,67,68,70,71). The fields are weighted 75% to 80% from the lateral and 20% to 25% from the anterior. There are two alternative tech-

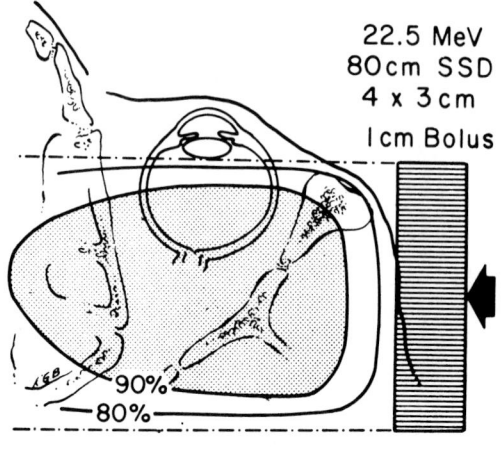

22.5 MeV
80 cm SSD
4 x 3 cm
1 cm Bolus

90%
80%

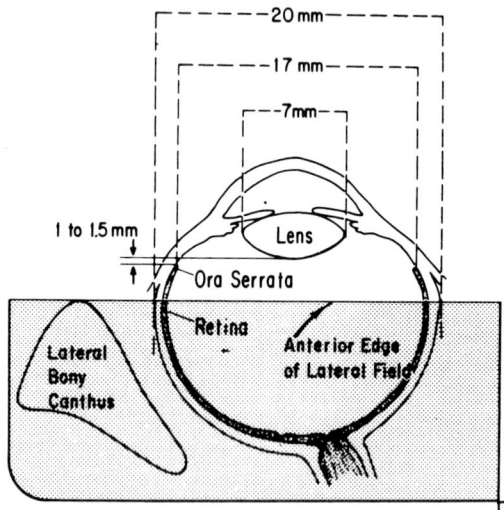

20 mm
17 mm
7mm

1 to 1.5 mm

Lens

Ora Serrata

Retina

Lateral
Bony
Canthus

Anterior Edge
of Lateral Field

FIG. 11. A direct lateral supervoltage field with anterior border set at the bony orbit. (From ref. 12, with permission.)

niques. One continues to use the lateral field but uses an anterior electron field with a contact lens mounted lead block for the lens. Small displacements of the contact lens will significantly affect the dose from the anterior field (7,33,61–63). A second modification uses anterior photons without the hanging eye block when it is feared that the hanging block will shield posterior pole tumor (71).

5. Schipper (72,73) has described a precision lateral technique which calls for a specially devised machine-mounted device which, by way of a scale, sets the anterior field edge just behind the lens (Fig. 14). Measurement of the lens depth in each patient is necessary for proper beam alignment (69,72,73). This elegant technique is particularly appropriate for posterior pole lesions (5). Schipper's technique uses a linear accelerator, modified with a beam splitting and extended collimation system, to produce a nondivergent and almost penumbra-free anterior beam edge. The depth of the posterior margin of the lens is measured by ultrasound. A contact lens or plumbob with an attached rod and scale measuring system allows placement of the beam behind the lens. Either a straight or angled lateral beam is used—depending on whether the clinician wishes to avoid exit dose to the other eye (74).

6. A superior dose distribution for RB treatment might be achieved with a proton beam. With a lateral approach the patient with unilateral RB would benefit from sparing of the other eye because of the stopping characteristics of the protons related to deposition of energy via the Bragg peak. Even in bilateral cases the possibility of sparing some normal tissue is held out as a benefit to reduce the risks of radiation-induced malignancy. Nine patients have been treated with protons for RB at the Harvard Cyclotron Laboratory; preliminary results are encouraging (J. Munzenrider, *personal communication*, 1993). Photon irradiation using sterotactic techniques in a fractionated schema are also available (75).

With most techniques using a lateral beam, blocking is used. This blocking spares the pituitary and some of the tooth buds. This generally produces a "D"-shaped field.

Which is the *best* technique for external beam treatment of RB? In a retrospective review from Riyadh, Saudi Arabia, Pradhan et al. (32) compared eye survival in 26 children treated with external beam radiotherapy with lateral fields to 38 children in which anterior fields were used for part or all of the treatment. Forty-four of the total population of 64 children (84%) had Group IV or V disease. No difference in eye survival was found between the two groups (32). Foote et al. (17) from the Mayo Clinic, however, did report a benefit to

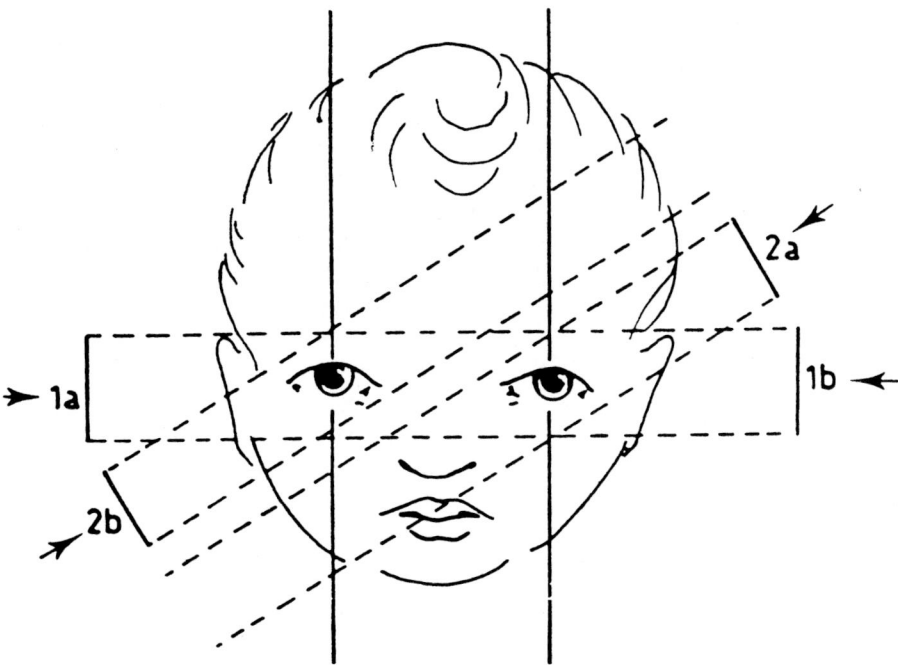

FIG. 12. In this schematic fields 1a and 1b demonstrate simultaneous irradiation of bilateral disease with opposed fields. Fields 2a and 2b illustrate the use of oblique fields in unilateral disease intended to spare the opposite eye. (Reproduced with permission from Dr. Jan Schipper, *Thesis retinoblastoma*, 1980, illustrated in *Opthalmology* 1996;103:263–268.)

whole eye irradiation using anterior fields versus a lateral lens-sparing technique. The tumor control rate with the former was stated to be superior (7 of 11, 64% versus 29%) but the overall ocular survival was comparable between the two techniques (whole eye 82% versus lens sparing 79%) (17). An excellent retrospective comparison of lens sparing versus whole eye irradiation for Groups I to III disease from St. Bartholomew's Hospital, London, included 201 children. The eye preservation rate was 85% following whole eye and 92% after lens sparing radiotherapy (*p* = 0.55) (65,74). Blach et al. (76,77) has updated a series by McCormick et al. (62,63), which indicated, in a retrospective review, that a lateral-beam technique with the beam edge set 2 to 3 mm behind the limbus is preferred to a technique utilizing a more posteriorly set lateral beam and an anterior electron field with lens-sparing block. The more posterior field arrangement was associated with anterior fail-

ures. Many other series confirm anterior failures when anterior-segment-sparing techniques are used (61–63) (Fig. 15). Twenty patients with large macular RB were treated at Duke with a lateral 4-MV photon half-blocked beam set halfway between the limbus and bony orbit and an anterior field (sometimes using a hanging eye block, weighted lateral to anterior 4 or 5:1). With 1 to 8 years follow-up, there are no local failures and four clinically significant cataracts (70).

Inspection of Table 4 shows that, in general, control of Groups I to III disease with lens-sparing external beam irradiation alone is fairly good in contemporary series, i.e., 40% to 80%. The addition of photocoagulation, cryotherapy, and plaque therapy results in an ultimate eye preservation rate of 67% to 100% for Groups I to III disease. When new tumors develop in patients treated with lens-sparing external beam techniques, the majority of the recurrences are located anterior in

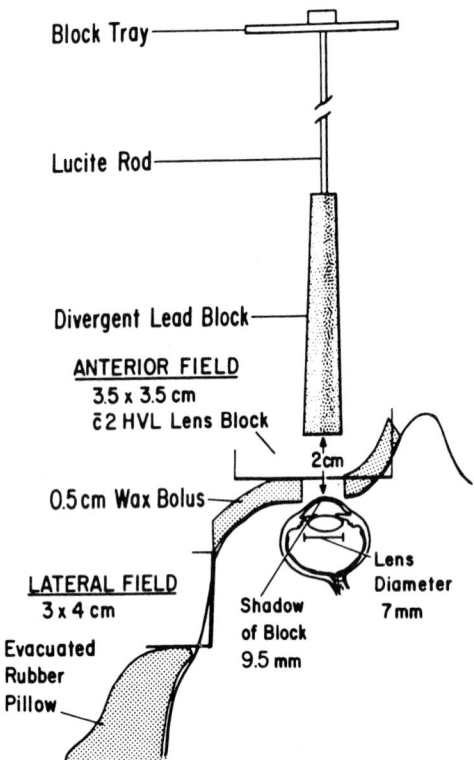

Block Tray

Lucite Rod

Divergent Lead Block

ANTERIOR FIELD
3.5 x 3.5 cm
c̄ 2 HVL Lens Block

2 cm

0.5 cm Wax Bolus

LATERAL FIELD
3 x 4 cm

Shadow
of Block
9.5 mm

Lens
Diameter
7 mm

Evacuated
Rubber
Pillow

FIG. 13. A two-field technique using a lateral field with an anterior field and a hanging eye block. If the contralateral eye is in place, the lateral field is angled posteriorly. (From ref. 64, with permission.)

the eye (74). Clearly, failure to irradiate the anterior retina in a tumor in which the entire retinal surface is at risk for tumor will lead to recurrence. Even when careful placement of the anterior beam edge is done with a half-beam blocked lateral field, or a Schipper device, it is almost impossible to perfectly irradiate the most anterior retina and reproducibly miss the lens. It is for this reason that many radiation oncologists supplement a lateral beam with some dose from an anterior field (with an 80%:20% lateral:anterior weighting) to bring up the dose anteriorly. The overall eye preservation rate in patients with anterior failures following lateral beam alone treatment remains quite good. This is due to the frequent success of focal salvage therapies such as cryotherapy, laser, or plaque (74).

Lateral techniques which utilize a sufficiently anterior placed field border (with or without a lightly weighted anterior beam) or a single anterior field are the best techniques to avoid anterior failures. Defenders of the former technique cite the possibility of reducing the risk of injury to anterior structures and brain, whereas supporters of the latter invoke ease of setup and the alleged manageable nature of complications (5,8,17,61–63).

Any external beam RB technique should (a) encompass the entire retinal anlage, (b) avoid the fellow eye if uninvolved, and (c) limit the dose to normal tissue. Individual radiotherapists must adopt a technique that fulfills the aforementioned criteria within the context of their own equipment and expertise while respecting the circumstances of the individual patient.

Dose

Is there a radiation dose-reponse relationship for external beam therapy for RB?

Stallard (57) performed serial sections of RB treated with brachytherapy and concluded that 35 Gy was the appropriate dose delivered in 7 days. A large number of dose/fraction schemes have been proposed for external beam treatment, ranging from 2 to 3.8 Gy per fraction to a total dose of 30 to 60 Gy (2,12,33,61–65,67,69,72–74,78–81). Objective data which speak to the establishment of an optimum tumor dose include (a) a 1969 report by Cassady et al. (12) that 32 to 35 Gy was no less effective than 40 to 45 Gy, and (b) the observation that late ill effects of irradiation on the retina (i.e., chorioretinitis) are infrequent at doses of 50 Gy or less (12,62,63). In 1972, Thompson et al. (82) published an analysis of treatment time and total dose suggesting improved local control at higher doses. These authors recommend 2.5 Gy per fraction, four fractions per week, to 50 Gy.

In 1985, Abramson (7), reviewing the Cornell and Columbia experience, reported no influence of the size of tumor on the control rate with radiotherapy. Tumors less than 3 DD in size were cured as often as those 3 to 10 DD in size or larger. Abramson did, however, observe

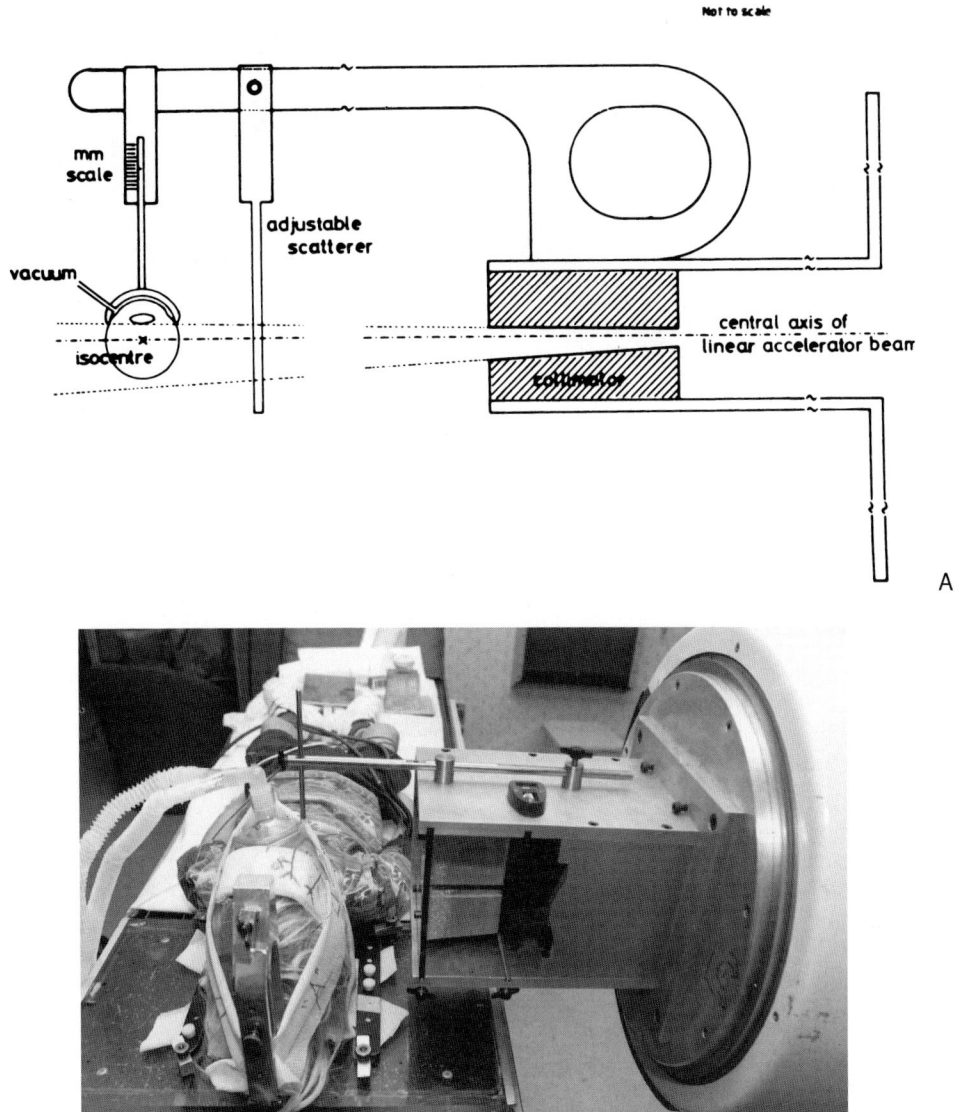

FIG. 14. A: A special retinoblastoma treatment applicator designed to set the treatment beam just at the posterior pole of the lens. The position is adjusted with the scale and contact lens assembly. (From ref. 69, with permission.) **B:** A modification of such a device in operation.

a dose-response relationship as a result of dose inhomogeneities from lateral-beam treatment. This is shown in Fig. 15. A review of the Mayo Clinic experience by Foote et al. (17) in 1989 found no dose-response relationship over the 45- to 50-Gy dose range in 4 to 5 1/2 weeks for tumors less than 4 DD in size, tumors 4 to 10 DD in size, or Reese-Ellsworth Group III

cases. Based on a small number of patients, local control was thought to be associated with higher doses in Group V cases and in tumors greater than 10 DD in size. In 1996, a group from Wills Eye Hospital in Philadelphia, however, found an inverse relationship between tumor control and tumor size following external beam irradiation. Tumor control with radiation

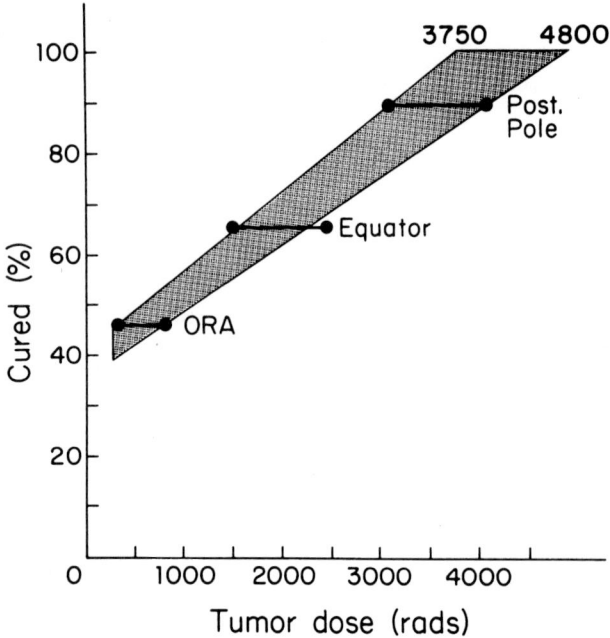

FIG. 15. With a single lateral photon technique for the treatment of retinoblastoma, particularly if the beam is not half-beam blocked, the dose across the retinal anlage is quite inhomogeneous. Abramson has observed that if the beam's anterior edge is not set sufficiently close to the limbus, then the ora serrata may receive only 10% to 30% of the prescribed dose, the equator 50%, and the posterior pole 90% to 100%. He plotted the local tumor control of tumors as a function of their ocular location. The more posterior the tumor, the higher the rate of local control. By relating the dose which was likely administered to the eye at the ora, equator, and posterior pole and plotting it against the local control rate, a dose-response curve is generated. While the observation is of considerable interest, it only argues in favor of a dose at least in excess of 37.5 Gy. This analysis does not provide guidance as to what is the best dose in the 37.5- to 50-Gy range that can be administered homogeneously with multiple field technique. (From ref. 7, with permission.)

TABLE 4. *Reported eye preservation rates following lens sparing external beam radiation therapy*

Author (ref.)	Year of report	Number of eyes irradiated	Groups I–V		Groups I–III	
			RT	RT + salvage	RT	RT + salvage
Cassady (12)	1969	223	49%	69%		73%
Egbert (13)	1978	38		58%		80%
Schipper (73)	1985	54	41%	81%	54%	94%
Foote (17)	1989	25	29%	79%	40%	80%
Fontanesi (67,80)	1995, 1996	7[a]	71%	71%	67%	67%
		13[b]	67%	76%	60%	100%
Toma (74)	1995	67	72%	93%	69%	92%
Blach (61)	1996	67[c]	38%	71%	37%	81%
		113[d]	65%	78%	84%	94%

[a]>1 yr of age
[b]<1 y of age
[c]Anterior lens-sparing technique or modified lateral beam technique
[d]Modified lateral beam technique

alone as a function of maximum basal tumor diameter was 88% (less than 5 mm), 93% (5.1–10 mm), 72% (10.2–15 mm), and 50% (greater than 15 mm) (83).

A review of the St. Bartholomew's Hospital, London, data described the using of varying dose and fraction schemes over the period 1970 to 1985. Tumor control was minimally better with 40 to 44 Gy in 20 fractions than 35 to 36 Gy in 9 to 12 fractions but little can be concluded from this retrospective review with multiple uncontrolled variables (65). Messmer et al. (84) from Germany reported a higher tumor recurrence rate with a mean dose of 40 Gy versus 50 Gy (49% versus 22%). Fontanesi et al. (67,80), however, found the reverse in a small number of patients: control with less than 36 Gy (71%) was superior to that obtained with greater than 36 Gy (50%).

What may we conclude? (a) High dose per fraction radiotherapy is associated with an increasing risk of late effects. Data from Lausanne, Switzerland, demonstrates an increase in retinopathy at greater than or equal to 2.5 Gy/fraction (32); (b) with improvements in anesthesia technique, it is not plausible to argue in favor of high dose per fraction irradiation with three fractions per week "because the anesthesia is too difficult." It is not. RB patients should be treated 5 days per week at less than or equal to 2 Gy per fraction. (c) In view of the somewhat contradictory data, most clinicians will choose a dose based on the tolerance of normal tissue rather than on an unfounded belief in unassailable dose-response information. Daily doses of 1.8 to 2.0 Gy, 5 days per week, to a total dose of 40 to 45 Gy is most commonly selected. For large tumors and/or vitreous seeding, some will treat to 48 to 50 Gy.

Chemotherapy

A multiinstitutional study conducted under the auspices of the Pediatric Oncology Group (POG) and the Children's Cancer Study Group (CCSG) and reported in 1981 evaluated chemotherapy (cyclophosphamide 30 mg/kg and vincristine 0.05 mg/kg) every 3 weeks for 37 weeks in 88 children with Group V disease following enucleation. No overall or disease-free survival advantage was shown over enucleation alone (5,7,8,86). In 1969, Cassady et al. (12) found no advantage to intracarotid triethylenemamine in conjunction with radiotherapy when compared to radiotherapy alone in terms of local control or survival for advanced intraocular disease.

Few quarrel with the use of chemotherapy in metastatic RB. Traditionally, the most active agent in metastatic disease was said to be cyclophosphamide (5,8). Some clinicians now favor cisplatinum or carboplatinum and vincristine plus etoposide. In metastatic disease as well as in orbital recurrence or trilateral RB, as discussed elsewhere in this chapter, chemotherapy has produced responses and may prolong survival. The value of drugs in this situation is, however, debatable. A case may be made that certain factors (i.e., sublaminar tumor extension, massive choroidal invasion, or tumor in the cut end of the optic nerve) help predict orbital or systemic relapse. Proponents argue that adjuvant chemotherapy may favorably impact that risk of relapse (9).

In 1995 to 1998, a series of publications in refereed journals and meeting abstracts, as well as platform presentations and word-of-mouth began to describe attempts to treat intraocular RB primarily with chemotherapy (87). Because the control of advanced retinoblastoma is relatively poor with external beam irradiation alone, and because external beam irradiation is associated with orbital and midfacial bone deformity, lacrimal gland dysfunction, and an increased risk of second malignant neoplasms (all discussed subsequently in this chapter), it is not unreasonable to seek alternatives. Few chemotherapy programs rely on drugs alone to cure. Most, instead, combine chemotherapy with interspersed vigorous focal therapy (cryotherapy, laser photocoagulation, laser hyperthermia, or plaque therapy) and/or external beam irradiation.

Less than 125 patients, treated with programs that rely on chemotherapy, have been described in any detail (Table 5) These pa-

TABLE 5. *1994–1997 Published reports of treatment of intraocular retinoblastoma with primary chemotherapy with or without including focal therapy or external beam radiotherapy, as primary treatment*

Institution (Ref.)	Number of Patients	Number of Eyes	Reese–Ellsworth grouping	Treatment program	Follow-up (yr)	Primary therapy relapse-free survival	Comments
Tata Memorial Hospital, Bombay (111)	1	2	NS	CAPE	1.4 yr	1/1 (100%)	
Hospital for Sick Children, Toronto (23,88)	21	28	Ia 4 Ib 2 IIa 1 IIb IIIa 3 IIIb 1 IVa 1 IVb Va 4 Vb 8	CVT + CSA Cryo + laser	0.1–4.8 yr	89% overall 7/8 for Vb(87%) of patients	1 therapy-related death 1 remission sustained with I-125 plaque
Relapsed patients	9	12	Ia 3 Ib 0 IIa 2 IIb 0 IIIa 0 IIIb 0 IVa 1 IVb 0 Va 1 Vb 5	VT ≠ C + CSA + Cryo + laser	0.1	67% of patients	1 patient cured by external beam irradiation
Children's Memorial Hospital, Chicago (45)	6	11	IIb IIIa 3 IIIb 0 IVa 1 IVb 0 Va 2 Vb 4	Carbo E + Cryo + laser hyperthermia + plaque	<2.24 yr	4/11 eyes (36%) 1/6 patients (16%)	4 eyes salvaged by external beam irradiation

Institution (ref)	No. patients	No. eyes	b V at relapse	Chemotherapy	Follow-up	Response	Comments
Saga Prefectural Hospital (115)	1	1		CAP MCHU Carbo	>3 yr	1/1 (100%)	
St. Bartholomew's Hospital, London (116)	14	24	a13 V, b11 V	VE Carbo + EBRT	median 5 yr	17/24 (71%) of eyes, 7/14 (50%) of patients	1 eye salvaged; 2 deaths: 1 from RB, one from SMN
Children's Hospital, Los Angeles (43)		38	15 I, 9 II, 4 III, 0 IV, a0 V, b10 V	Carbo + laser hyperthermia		24/38 (63%) of eyes	Some eyes were salvaged by additional chemotherapy or EBRT
		35	3 I, 7 II, 0 III, 4 IV, a3 V, b18 V	Carbo + E + V + EBR and/or Cryo and/or laser and/or laser hyperthermia and/or plaque		10/35 (29%) of eyes	Carbo + laser hyperthermia controlled 0/10 Vb eyes. 10/14 (71%) of Groups I–IV controlled. 0/21 of Group V
Wills Eye Hospital, Philadelphia (118)	20	31	a2 I, b0 I, a2 II, b1 II, a1 III, b2 III, a1 IV, b0 V, a6 V, b16 V	Carbo VE ± EBRT ± laser ± Cryo ± laser hyperthermia ± plaque	Mean 0.54 (2–13 m)	31/31 eyes, 20/20 patients (100%)	
NY Hospital, New York (113[a])	7	11	NS	Carbo	NS	NS	Tumor (not eye) complete + partial response rate: 12/22 (55%)
King Faisal Specialist Hospital, Riyadh (32)	28	31	I–III 9, IV–V 22	VAC + EBRT	Mean 48.5 m	78% of group I–III eyes, ~28% of Group IV–V eyes	Nonrandomized study: no benefit to the addition of chemotherapy

C, cyclophosphamide; A, adriamycin; P, cisplatin; E, etoposide; V, vincristine; T, teniposide; Csa, cyclosporine A; Cryo, cryotherapy; Carbo, carboplatin; MCNU, ramusine; EBRT, external beam radiation therapy; NS, not specified.

tients include a mix of Reese-Ellsworth groups, *de novo* treatment and relapsed patients, a variety of drugs (often varying in type, dose, or sequencing within one series), often minimal follow-up, ascribing of complete and partial responses to drugs by allowing the results of adjuvant focal therapy to be included (radiotherapy series generally score patients receiving additional focal therapy as failures), and a lack of uniform reporting with results described by eyes, patients, or even, in some series, individual tumors within eyes.

What is the critical reader to make of this data? In Table 5 the results from nine institutions are shown. It seems without dispute that there are many children who will initially respond to chemotherapy. In addition, there appear to be some patients cured and spared enucleation or external beam radiotherapy. In many patients, however, chemotherapy has failed to achieve the desired end, particularly in the difficult Group V cases. Vigorous advocates of institutional data will argue that one may identify superior chemotherapy programs from the crowded field of choices (i.e., Wills Eye Hospital or Hospital for Sick Children, Toronto). It is, in our view, not appropriate to render such pronouncements with so few patients and such limited follow-up.

The use of cyclosporine A in the Toronto series is premised on the notion that the activity of the multiple drug resistance (MDR) gene is correlated with chemotherapy-resistance by RB. The MDR gene product is a transmembrane pump that abets the efflux of many chemotherapy drugs from cells (88,89). Cyclosporine A blocks the MDR pump and should, the argument concludes, increase cell kill by foiling this tumor cell defense mechanism. The importance of MDR in human tumors, and the efficacy of cyclosporine A, are both open questions. MDR has been shown to be of no prognostic importance in RB, of questionable importance in neuroblastoma, and the data for retinoblastoma is conflicting.

Plans are afoot for an international retinoblastoma cooperative group trial to test the role of chemotherapy. Drafts of the protocol, in circulation in the fall of 1998, included a trial of carboplatin, vincristine, and etoposide with focal therapy for bilateral retinoblastoma where at least one eye is Group Vb or harbors tumor greater than 13 mm or with substantial retinal detachment or substantial retinal tumor seeding. The study is particularly aimed at eyes in which would have been enucleated or received external beam irradiation. The study question is whether the addition of cyclosporine A is beneficial. Patients will be randomized to receive or not receive this drug. A second study will be open to children with bilateral retinoblastoma with at least one eye with Reese-Ellsworth Groups II to IV disease that would normally require enucleation or external beam irradiation. Patients will receive carboplatin, etoposide, and vincristine and focal therapy. There is no randomization. Guidelines for the using of adjuvant plaque therapy and salvage external beam irradiation are under development.

SPECIAL SITUATIONS

Trilateral Disease

Trilateral RB is a rare but well-recognized entity consisting of bilateral RB associated with ectopic RB of the pineal or suprasellar region. A forme fruste of trilateral RB has been described in which unilateral RB is associated with intracranial tumor (90). The intracranial lesion can cause signs of raised intracranial pressure (anorexia, ataxia, lethargy, vomiting) or, when the lesion is suprasellar, diabetes insipidus (5,91).

Since the publication of the second edition of this textbook, at least four estimates of the incidence of trilateral RB have appeared in the literature from the United Kingdom and the United States (Table 6). Most cases appear in children with biateral RB. The frequency of trilateral RB has led some authorities to argue in favor of "screening" cranial CT or MRI to make the diagnosis. The population at prime risk are children with bilateral RB within the first 3 to 4 years after diagnosis (90,91). It seems reasonable to perform intracranial imaging at the diagnosis of all cases of RB (when many clinicians do CT of the orbits

TABLE 6. *Incidence of midline intracranial tumors (trilatral disease) in retinoblastoma*

	Overall	Bilateral familial RB	Bilateral sporadic RB
West Midlands Regional Children's Tumour Research Group (90)	3%	5%	12.5%
Wills Eye Hospital (112)	4%	8%	5%
NY Hospital/Memorial Sloan-Kettering Cancer Center (91)	5%	10%	6%
St. Bartholomew's Hospital (94a)	—	—	—

RB, retinoblastoma.

anyway) and every 3 to 6 months thereafter for 3 to 4 years in bilateral RB. If a pineal/suprasellar mass is found, a decision must be made concerning biopsy.

For some clinicians the presence of a calcified, discrete midline mass of the pineal or suprasellar regions in the setting of heritable bilateral RB is sufficient to make the diagnosis of trilateral disease (5). Other oncologists, however, feel more comfortable with a biopsy of the intracranial lesion.

The treatment of trilateral disease with surgery alone or in combination with radiotherapy resulted in no long-term survivors (5,90–94). Six cases of trilateral RB were reported in 1994 from Memorial Sloan-Kettering Cancer Center. Three were treated with craniospinal irradiation (CSI) plus chemotherapy, two with chemotherapy alone, and one with no treatment. All patients died from tumor in 2 to 12 months (91). Five patients with trilateral RB seen in the West Midland's Health Authority, U.K., and reported in 1996, died at 1 to 31 months following diagnosis (90). In 1986, the pediatric neurooncology group at Duke reported that cyclophosphamide and vincristine were active in patients with recurrent trilateral RB (92). Subsequently, the same group has described three children with newly diagnosed trilateral RB treated with systemic (cyclophosphamide, vinscristine) and intrathecal (methotrexate, hydrocortisone, cytarabine) chemotherapy along with orbital irradiation and, in two cases, CSI. Two patients are alive without evidence of disease 3 and 8 years following diagnosis. One is alive with persistent disease 2 years after diagnosis (94).

The use of radiotherapy in trilateral RB poses an interesting challenge to the radiotherapist. The orbital disease is usually irradiated first, accompanied and followed by chemotherapy, with CSI given last in the sequence. Knowing this, the radiotherapist must set up the orbital fields with the understanding that they will be called on to partially overlap and then match-on the CSI fields. Particular attention is paid to the optic chiasm dose in this situation. It is possible, utilizing rigid patient immobilization and three-dimensional treatment planning, to administer CSI and a boost to the intracranial tumor with reasonable safety even at some time removed from ocular irradiation (93).

Re-treatment

Among the most difficult problems to confront the pediatric radiation oncologist is the selection of therapy in a child who has suffered recurrent RB in an eye previously externally irradiated to full dose. If the recurrent lesion is small and favorably located, it may be treated with photocoagulation, cryotherapy, or a radioactive plaque—often with success. Amendola and co-workers (11,29,48) plaqued 29 eyes, 28 with Group V disease, for recurrent tumor. Tumor progression in 14 eyes ultimately required enucleation. The remaining 15 eyes (52%) have preservation of vision.

In some situations, the clinician will be faced with the choice of enucleation or re-irradiation with external beam. Abramson reported re-treatment of 15 eyes that, at the time of tumor recurrence, could be classified as Groups I to III. Twelve (80%) of these eyes survived. Of the 89 eyes that, at the time of tumor recurrence, were Group IV or V, only two (2.2%) survived. Nine of the 14 salvaged eyes had useful vision. The overwhelming cause of enucleation was progressive tumor, not radiation damage. There appears to be no increase in secondary nonocular tumors in children receiving two courses of radiotherapy (78).

Metastases

As previously discussed, RB may gain access to the brain and spinal cord in its advanced stages. CNS or systemic dissemination of RB has a grave prognosis. The eyes are treated as dictated by the individual stage. Cranial irradiation or CSI are given if chemotherapy holds disease in check until the child reaches a more advanced age where radiation's ill effects may be muted. Such a therapeutic plan is analogous to that used in children less than 3 years of age with brain tumors (see Chapter 3).

For bony metastases causing pain, palliative radiotherapy is appropriate. We generally use doses of 20 to 40 Gy, similar to those for metastatic neuroblastoma (8) (see Chapter 6).

Choroidal Invasion, Extraocular Extension, and Orbital Recurrence

In developed countries, cases of extraocular extension or orbital recurrence following initial treatment of RT are rare. At academic centers, such cases will often be referred from institutions where the initial treatment was given by physicians who thought, at first, that they were dealing with another diagnosis. By making the best possible use of the available data and by relying on sound clinical reasoning, the pediatric radiation oncologist can try to make the best of vexing cases.

Earlier in this chapter, we pointed out that histologic evaluation of the enucleated eye can, to some extent, predict prognosis (34,95). Extensive involvement of the choroid along with either retrolaminar extension of tumor or, even worse, involvement of the cut end of

the optic nerve predict a poor outcome. Patients with these problems are subject to either local recurrence of tumor in the orbit, CNS disease, or systemic tumor. It is reasonable to consider more aggressive adjuvant treatment in these cases in an attempt to improve the outcome.

Another important prognostic factor is the performance of a prior intraocular procedure in RB patients. RB may initially be misdiagnosed. The increase in the availability of technology in vitreous surgery has, as an unforeseen consequence, resulted in more children undergoing intraocular surgery in an attempt to confirm an inflammatory cause for visual loss or in an attempt to improve vision (96). The surgeon will be surprised and dismayed to find that RB is the true diagnosis. RB may, by such procedures, be seeded by breach of the scleral or corneal barrier. One of the authors has seen a patient with tumor growing directly through the previous incision. Children who have undergone a prior intraocular operative procedure before definitive enucleation are at risk for orbital recurrence of tumor and nodal and hematogenous dissemination.

Recurrence of RB in the orbit following enucleation has, historically, carried an extremely poor prognosis for survival. Only 1 of 16 children with orbital recurrence was a long-term survivor in the St. Bartholomew's and Moorefield Eye Hospital's 1987 report (80). Children succumbed to CNS tumor, systemic disease, and uncontrolled orbital tumor. More recently, long-term survivors have been reported following local excision of the tumor, orbital external beam, and, in one case, intracavitary irradiation and chemotherapy (32,77,97).

Based on the available data, we recommend postoperative external beam irradiation to the orbit for children with invasion of the cut end of the optic nerve, extrascleral extension, and/or a prior intraocular operative procedure. At the time of enucleation, the residual optic nerve may retract back into the optic foramen. The radiotherapist must use sufficiently large fields to encompass this area of persistent disease. Depending upon whether the residual disease is minimal or extensive, a dose of 45 to 60 Gy is given (5,7,16,63,96–98). Usually an anterior and lateral oblique wedge pair of fields are used. An intracavitary brachytherapy boost may be utilized (97). Full cranial irradiation is probably not necessary. This view must be tempered, however, by the fact that CNS metastasis occasionally occur in this patient population (9,32). Local orbital recurrence of RB should be treated with tumor excision and local orbital irradiation. Some patients with local orbital recurrence of RB die of tumor extension into the CNS. There may be situations when the orbital irradiation will need to be combined with cranial irradiation or CSI (5). Systemic chemotherapy is generally given for orbital tumor relapse, for retrolaminar and cut end of optic nerve invasion, or if there has been a prior intraocular surgical procedure. Some pediatric medical oncologists favor the addition of intrathecal chemotherapy because of concerns over CNS tumor in these situations (99). If intrathecal chemotherapy is used, we have been restrained in using "prophylactic" cranial irradiation or CSI in these young patients.

Clinical data to defend the views presented is now available. From 1985 to 1993, 11 children with major choroidal invasion and retrolaminar optic nerve tumor invasion received chemotherapy at St. Bartholomew's Hospital, London. Children with positive optic nerve margins received orbital irradiation. With a minimum of 1 year of follow-up, there have been no deaths (35). Twenty-five children at SJCRH with Stage IIb1–IIb2 disease were treated with chemotherapy plus orbital irradiation. Twenty-two are survivors (88%); deaths occurred from CNS relapse, CNS plus bone marrow relapse, and second malignant neoplasm (9). From Saudia Arabia, 28 children with risk factors following enucleation such as retrolaminar tumor extension, a positive cut optic nerve end, and/or extrascleral involvement received orbital irradiation and, in 19 of 28 cases, vincristine, actinomycin-D, and cyclophosphamide. Local control was achieved in 71%, and disease-free survival appears to

be on the order of 60%. Relapses occurred distantly, or in the socket or brain (32).

LATE EFFECTS

Secondary Nonocular Tumors

The evidence is persuasive that the 13q-14 deletion of heritable RB produces a malignant diathesis. The relative risk (RR) for death from a second tumor is much higher among patients with bilateral RB (RR = 60) than among those with unilateral disease (RR = 3.8). The obviously first manifests itself in the development of the index case of RB. In long-term survivors of heritable RB, there is an extremely high incidence of secondary nonocular tumors. The most common secondary malignant neoplasms (SMNs) occurring within the radiation field in survivors of heritable RB are osteosarcoma, fibrosarcoma, and other spindle cell sarcomas. SMNs developing out of the radiotherapy field also include osteosarcoma and the soft tissue sarcomas. This list needs to be broadened, however, to include malignant melanoma and thyroid carcinoma. In addition, there is a long list of less common SMNs, which have developed in long-term survivors of heritable RB (7,25, 100,101).

In children treated with hereditary RB, the incidence of SMNs increases with time. The median latency period is 15 years (102,103). At 10 years, the incidence of SMNs is about 10%, at 20 years it is about 20%, at 30 years it is estimated to be about 25%, and at 50 years, 51% (34,89,103). Initially, Abramson et al. (7,10), described even higher risks: 20% at 10 years, 50% at 20 years, and 90% at 30 years. A comprehensive evaluation of SMNs in RB by Eng et al. (100) is based on a large number of RB patients, including patients from New York and Boston. In a 1993 report, at 40 years of follow-up, the cumulative mortality for all second tumors was 26% for bilateral RB and 1.5% for unilateral RB. The Eng study includes those previously reported by Abramson and, therefore, superseded those reports (Fig. 16).

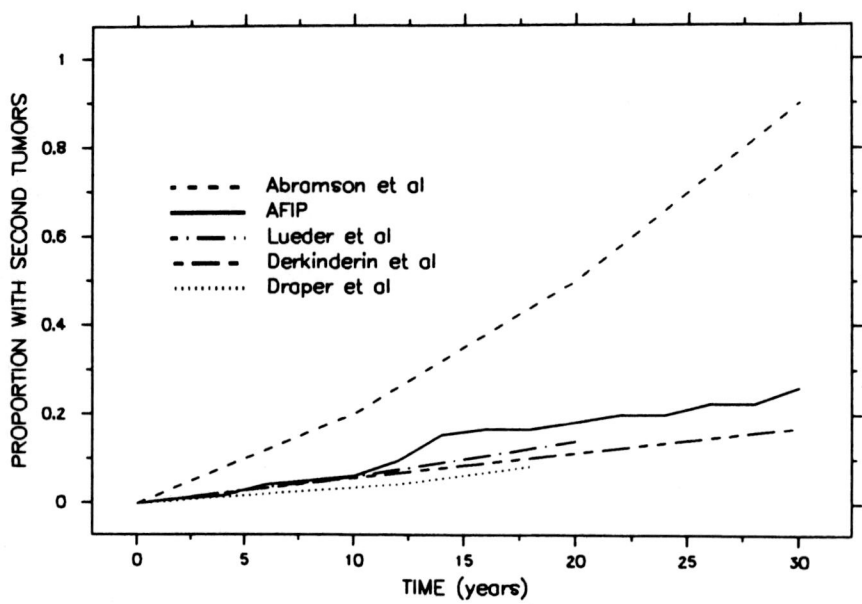

FIG. 16. The risk of secondary nonocular tumors for children with bilateral retinoblastoma from several published studies described in the text. (From ref. 101, with permission.)

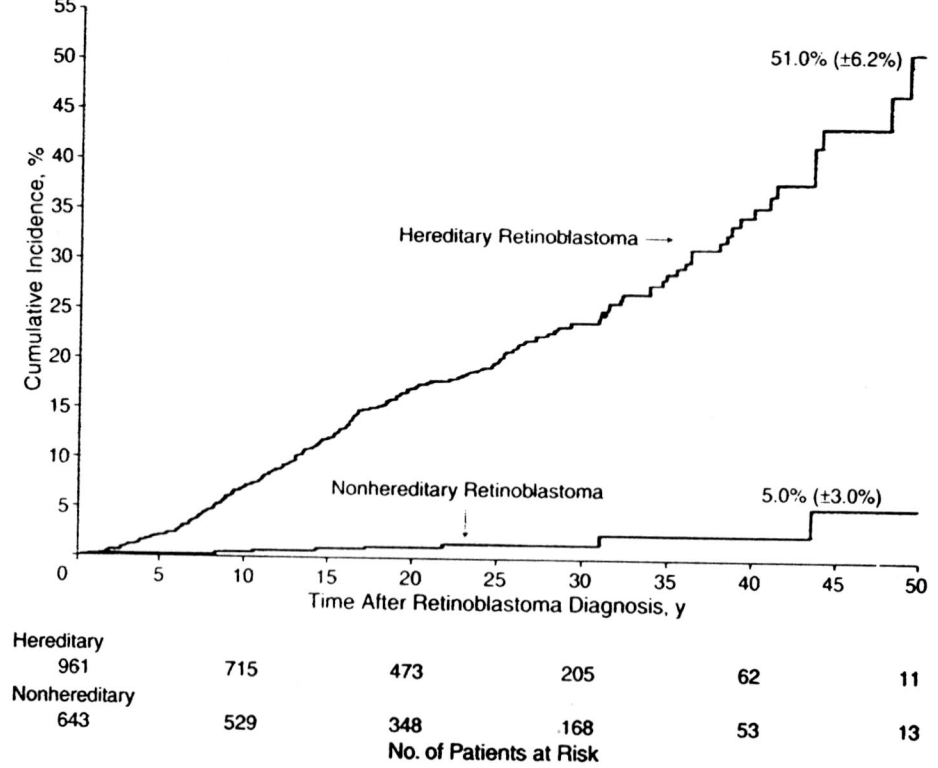

FIG. 17. Cumulative incidence (± standard error) of second cancers following the diagnosis of retinoblastoma in 961 patients with hereditary disease and 643 patients with nonhereditary disease. (From ref. 103, with permission.)

In a 1997 report, the cumulative incidence of second cancer at 50 years after diagnosis was 51% (103). All the major studies agree that the risk of SMN is greater in heritable RB survivors who received radiotherapy than in those patients who did not. Roarty et al. (101), for example, found a 30-year SMN incidence rate of 29% within the field of radiation for 137 patients who received radiotherapy. The incidence of 8% outside the field of irradiation was similar to the 6% rate for the 78 patients who did not receive radiation. Abramson et al. (7,10), also found a significant reduction in the incidence of SMN outside the field of radiation or in patients never irradiated. Among bilateral RB patients, Eng et al. (100) found that cumulative mortality from second neoplasms at 40 years follow-up was 30% for irradiated patients and 6% for those who did not receive irradiation. Wong et al. found that, at 50 years, the cumulative incidence of second cancers was 58% in irradiated heritable retinoblastoma patients versus 27% in nonirradiated patients (Fig. 17). Dosimetry data, collected for patients with secondary bone and soft tissue sarcoma, showed a stepwise increase in secondary tumor relative risk with increasing dose (103) (Fig. 18). In an analysis confined to bilateral cases the incidence of second tumors at 30 years was 34% for children irradiated at less than 12 months of age, 22% for children irradiated at greater than 12 months of age, and 18% for those not irradiated (102).

Draper et al. (104), have developed some evidence to implicate cyclophosphamide as a risk factor for SMN in heritable RB. In an extensive review of heritable RB, they found that the estimated incidence rate 12 years after diagnosis for tumors in the field of radiation was 4.2% for patients given chemotherapy and 2.9% for patients not given chemo-

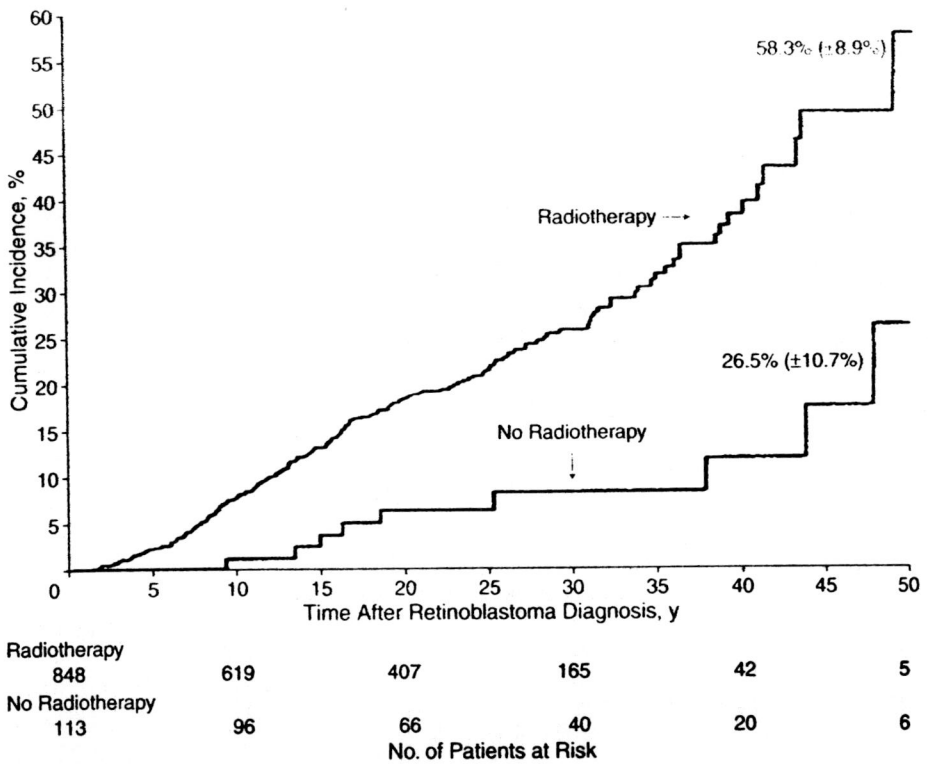

FIG. 18. Cumulative incidence (± standard error) of second cancers following diagnosis of retinoblastoma in patients with hereditary disease, by presence or absence of radiation treatment. (From ref. 103, with permission.)

therapy. The rates for tumors outside the radiation field (including patients not irradiated) was 4.6% for those receiving chemotherapy and 1% for those not receiving it.

Children with heritable RB have a field change rendering them subject to malignant transformation. Radiotherapy, and perhaps chemotherapy, adds an additional insult. Radiotherapy shortens the latent period for SMN, increases the incidence of SMN, and affects the distribution of SMN (102). In summary, for heritable retinoblastoma radiotherapy compounds the risk of SMN upon a background of high risk.

CATARACTS

Fontanesi et al. (80) noted that clinically significant posterior pole cataracts developed in 23 of 27 eyes (85%) treated with anterior fields. The Mayo Clinic reported 4 of 14 (28%) posterior cataracts using a lens sparing technique (17). In seven eyes followed for more than 36 months, Hernandez et al. (83), generally using lateral plus anterior fields, observed lens changes in all cases—three requiring lens extraction. Radiation-induced cataracts following radiotherapy of RB can be removed successfully and vision can be corrected (1). Shields and colleagues (66) removed cataracts in 38 RB patients (42 eyes) from 1973 to 1989. Nineteen eyes (45%) had final visual acuities of 20/20 to 20/50. Twelve eyes (29%) had macular tumors with postoperative visual acuities of 20/80 to counting fingers. Buckley and Heath (70) extracted cataracts from three eyes with macular tumors and observed near vision acuities of 20/60, 10/200, and localizing 2-mm beads at 13 inches. The risks of cataract removal after RB treatment include amblyopia, retinal detachment, and the risk of tumor dissemination if RB was not controlled by irradiation (66).

ORBITAL DEVELOPMENT

Children treated with radiotherapy or enucleation for RB are at significant risk for orbital and midfacial growth retardation insofar as their orbital bones are growing during treatment. In long-term survivors of RB, these orbital growth injuries may be apparent. In recent years investigators have sought to quantify the changes in orbital development wrought by treatment.

Imhof et al. (105,106) examined children treated at Utrecht University Hospital in the Netherlands and followed for a mean of approximately 8 years. Direct measurements were made of the orbital width and height and the orbital-tragus distance. In general, high dose per fraction external beam irradiation had been used (3 Gy/fraction × 15 = 45 Gy 8 MV photons). The mean orbital width, height, and distance between the tragus and outer orbital edge were significantly shorter in irradiated versus nonirradiated orbits in patients with unilateral RB as well as versus control eyes. External Beam Radiation Therapy (EBRT) given to children less than 6 months of age was more injurious than when it was used in older children. Enucleation plus EBRT was not worse than EBRT alone.

Findings by Imhof et al. are supported by a slightly less detailed study from Essen, Germany, by Messmer et al. (107). The German researchers evaluated 99 patients, diagnosed at the median age of 10 months, and at a median age at last follow-up of 16 years. In those children and adolescents with anophthalmic sockets, there was a significantly less satisfactory cosmetic and functional outcome in those patients who received EBRT before or after enucleation (Fig. 19). Midfacial hypoplasia was also clearly related to the using of enucleation and/or irradiation (Fig. 20).

Fontanesi and his collaborators at SJCRH have evaluated the orbital development in long-term survivors of RB using a CT scan obtained at a median age of 13 years. Because the orbital interior is roughly conical, the orbital volume was assessed with a scan slice at the level of the optic nerve using the equation for the volume of a cone ($v = \pi r^3 h/3$). In patients with unilateral RB the orbit on the enucleated side was smaller in 20 of 24 cases and larger in 4 cases. The median orbital volume difference was 1.5 cm^3. This relatively small

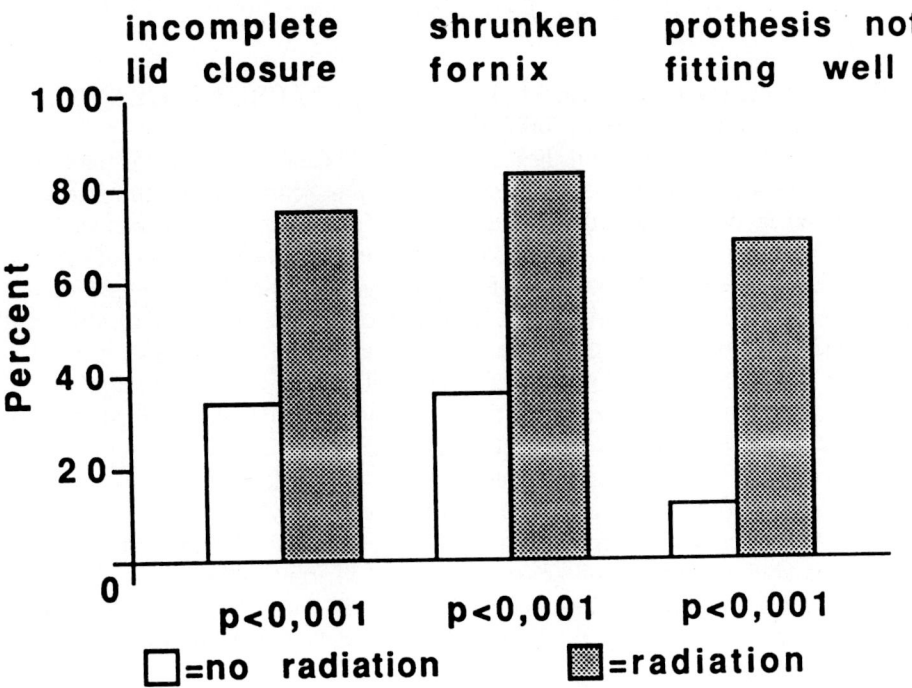

FIG. 19. Radiation plus enucleation can produce significant orbital problems. In anopthalmic children deformities were heightened by the addition of radiation. (From ref. 107, with permission.)

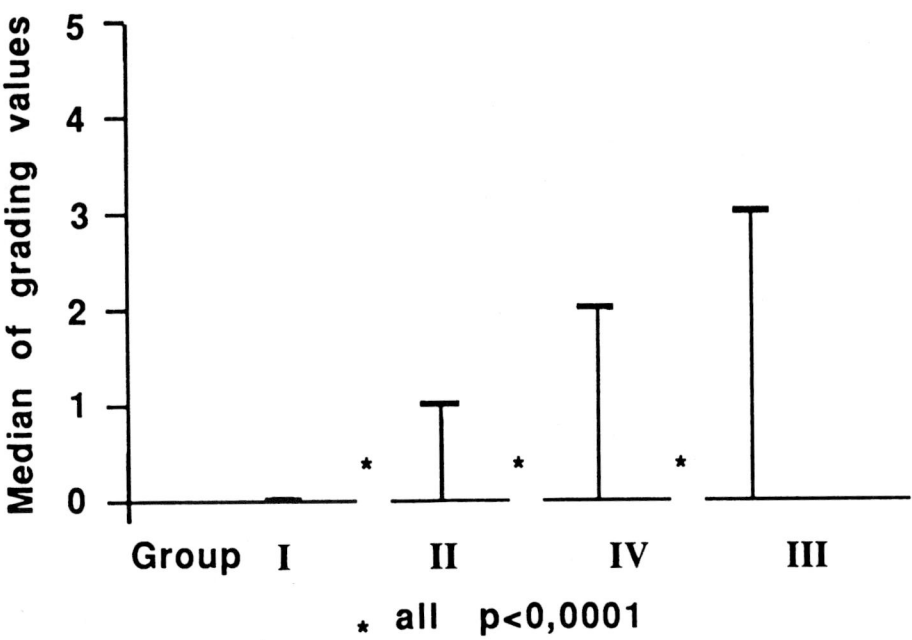

FIG. 20. Utilizing a clinical grading system, Messmer et al. did subjective grading of deformity of mid-facial structures following treatment for retinoblastoma. Midfacial hypoplasia correlated with therapy. Group 1 consists of patients treated with photocoagulation or cryotherapy only; group 2 is patients treated with enucleation without irradiation; group 3 is patients treated with enucleation with radiation; and group 4 includes children treated with radiation without enucleation. (From ref. 107, with permission.)

difference may be the result of the use of orbital prostheses that stimulate bony orbital
growth. In 18 children with bilateral disease
treated with enucleation on one side and irradiation on the other, the enucleated side had
the smaller volume in six cases, the irradiated
side was smaller in ten, and there was no difference in two (54).

The available literature confirms the impression of senior clinicians caring for children
with RB: radiation and, to some extent, enucleation without a properly fitting prosthesis can
lead to retardation of bony and soft tissue
growth of the midface (orbits, ethmoid bones,
nasal bridge). Hypo-telorism, enophthalmos,
depressed temporal bones, atrophy of the tem-
poralis muscle, narrow and deep orbits, and a
depressed nasion can be the result (108). These
effects are accentuated if radiotherapy is used
in the very young (less than 6 months of age)
and at doses greater than 35 Gy (54,106).

LACRIMAL GLAND

In 1955 Cogan, Fink, and Donaldson (109),
of the Massachusetts Eye and Ear Infirmary,
did a series of experiments concerning the irradiation of the orbital glands of rabbits. Rabbits have two orbital glands opening onto the
conjunctiva. One, a sebaceous gland, called a
Harderian gland and the other a true lacrimal
gland. They irradiated rabbit orbits to varying
doses and excised and weighed the glands at
45 days or later. The results, shown in Fig. 21,
demonstrate a definite decrease in gland size
with increasing dose.

Imhof et al. studied lacrimal function in 45
eyes of 34 irradiated patients who underwent
tear function tests a mean of 86 months following irradiation (106). Irradiated eyes had a
significant lessening of tear production as well
as a significant reduction in tear protein production when compared with a control group

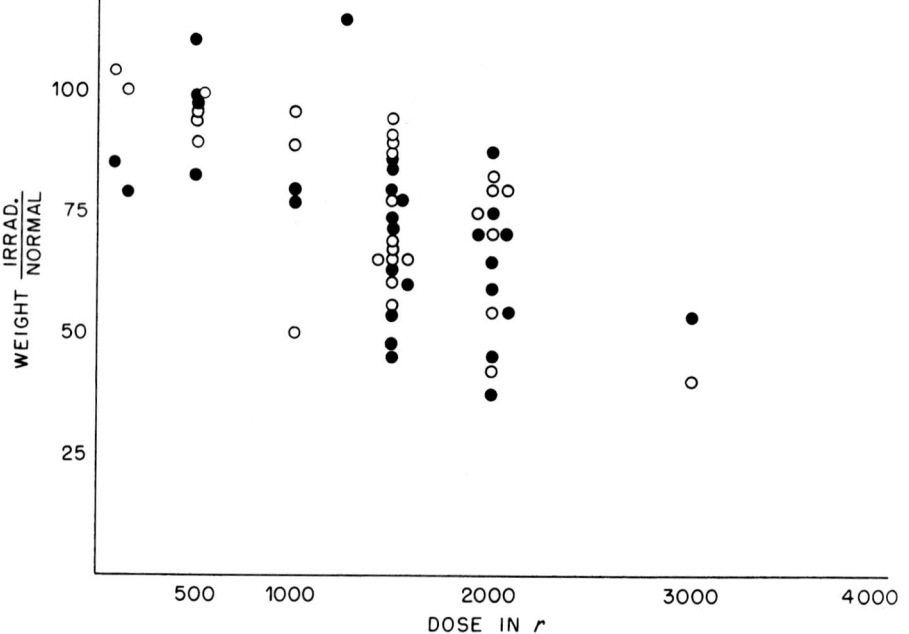

FIG. 21. In a study by Cogan et al., the weight of the two orbital glands of the rabbit were evaluated
following irradiation. The Harderian gland is the sebaceous gland. Rabbits also have a true lacrimal
gland. The relative weights of the irradiated and normal Harderian gland (*open circles*) are compared
to the weights of the irradiated and normal lacrimal glands (*closed circles*). Although there is great
individual variation, there is clearly a decrease in gland size with increasing doses of irradiation.
(From ref. 109, with permission.)

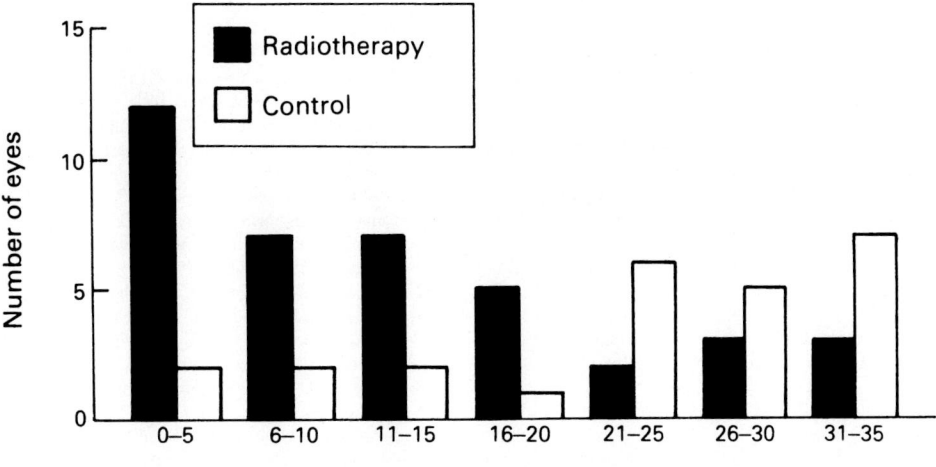

FIG. 22. The Schirmer test may be used for quantifying the effects of retinoblastoma irradiation on lacrimal function. A small piece of filter paper is inserted into the lower conjunctival fornix folded at right angles over the ciliary body of the lid, where it is left in position. Normal secretion ought to moisten at least 1.5 cm of the strip as measured from the fold in 5 min. The test, while crude, provides an indication of excessive larcrimation or of marked hyposecretion or the absence of tears. In this study, from researchers in Amsterdam and Utrech, children irradiated with a lateral beam for retinoblastoma are shown, on average, to have less tear production than unirradiated controls. (From ref. 105, with permission.)

(Fig. 22). Although many radiation oncologists attempt to shield the lacrimal gland, some long-term survivors of RB will have diminished tears and diminished stability of the tear film. Such children may be prone to keratopathies. Keratitis as a side-effect of irradiation for RB has been reported with varying frequency: 28% by Imhof et al., 3 of 30 (10%) of patients treated at less than 1 year of age, and 2 of 15 patients (13%) treated at greater than 1 year of age by Fontanesi et al. (67,80,106).

REFERENCES

*References particularly recommended for further reading are indicated by an asterisk.

1. Cowell JK, Hungerford J, Jay M, Rutland P. Retinoblastoma—clinical and genetic aspects: a review. *J R Soc Med* 1987;81:220–223.
2. Abramson DH. Retinoblastoma: diagnosis and management. *CA Cancer J Clin* 1982;32:130–140.
3. Redler LD, Ellsworth RM. Prognostic importance of choroidal invasion in retinoblastoma. *Arch Ophthalmol* 1973;90:294–296.
4. Duke-Elder S, Darbree JH, eds. Diseases of the retina. *System of ophthalmology*, vol X. St. Louis: CV Mosby, 1957:671–727.
5. Kingston JE, Hungerford JL. Retinoblastoma. In: Plowman PN, Pinkerton CR, eds. *Paediatric oncology: clinical practice and controversies*. London: Chapman & Hall Medical, 1992:268–290.
6. Reese AB. *Tumors of the eye,* 3rd ed. Hagerstown, MD: Harper & Row, 1976:90–122.
*7. Abramson DH. Treatment of retinoblastoma. In: Blodi FC, ed. *Contemporary issues in ophthalmology, vol 2: Retinoblastoma.* New York: Churchill Livingstone, 1985:63–93.
8. Donaldson SS, Egbert PR, Lee W-H. Retinoblastoma. In: Pizzo PA, Poplack DG, eds. *Principles and practice of pediatric oncology.* Philadelphia: JB Lippincott, 1993:683–696.
9. Schvartzman E, Chantado G, Fandino A, deDavila MT, Raslawski E, Manzitti J. Results of a stage-based protocol for the treatment of retinoblastoma. *J Clin Oncol* 1996;14:1532–1536.
10. Abramson DH, Ellsworth RM, Kitchin FD, Tung G. Second nonocular tumors in the retinoblastoma survivors: are they radiation-induced? *Ophthalmology* 1984;91:1351–1355.
11. Amendola BE, Lamm FR, Markae AM, et al. Radiotherapy of retinoblastoma: a review of 63 children treated with different irradiation techniques. *Cancer* 1990;66:21–26.
*12. Cassady JR, Sagerman RH, Tretter P, Ellsworth RM.

Radiation therapy in retinoblastoma. *Radiology* 1969;93:405–409.

13. Egbert PR, Donaldson SS, Moazed K, Rosenthal AR. Visual results and ocular complications following radiotherapy for retinoblastoma. *Arch Ophthalmol* 1978;96:1826–1830.

14. Hart P. The role of the retinoblastoma gene in tumour pathogenesis. *Clin Oncol* 1992;4:125–129.

15. Bedford MA, Bedotta C, MacFaul PA. Retinoblastoma: a study of 139 cases. *Br J Ophthalmol* 1971; 55:19–27.

16. Gaitan-Yanguas M. Retinoblastoma: analysis of 235 cases. *Int J Radiat Oncol Biol Phys* 1978;4:359–365.

*17. Foote RL, Garretson BR, Schamberg PJ, et al. External beam irradiation for retinoblastoma: patterns of failure and dose-response analysis. *Int J Radiat Oncol Biol Phys* 1989;116:823–830.

18. Knudson AG. Hereditary cancer, oncogenes, and antioncogenes. *Cancer Res* 1985;45:1437–1443.

*19. Knudson AG, Strong LC. Mutation and cancer: a model for Wilms' tumor of the kidney. *J Nat Cancer Inst* 1972;48:313–324.

*20. Varmus H, Weinberg RA. *Genes and the biology of cancer.* New York: Scientific American Library, 1993.

21. Weinberg RA. The retinoblastoma gene and gene product. *Cancer Surv* 1992;12:43–57.

22. Gallie BL. Gene carrier detection in retinoblastoma. *Ophthalmol* 1980;87:591–595.

23. Gallie BL, Budning A, DeBoer G, et al. Chemotherapy with focal therapy can cure intraocular retinoblastoma without radiotherapy. *Arch Ophthal* 1996; 114:1321–1328.

24. Gallie BL, Dunn JM, Chan HSL, Hamlet PA, Phillips RA. The genetics of retinoblastoma: relevance to the patient. *Pediatr Clin NA* 1991;38:299–315.

25. Druja TP, Cavanee W, White R, et al. Homozygosity of chromosome 13 in retinoblastoma. *N Engl J Med* 1984;310:550–553.

26. Leis JF, Livingston DM. Tumor suppressor genes and their mechanism of action. In: Bishop JM, Weinberg RA, eds. *Scientific American: Molecular Oncology.* New York: Scientific American, 1996:111–142.

27. Levine AJ. Tumor suppressor genes. In: Mendelsohn J, Howley PM, Israel MA, Liotta LA. *The molecular basis of cancer.* Philadelphia: WB Saunders, 1995: 86–104.

28. Cavenee WK, Hansen MF, Nordenskjold M, et al. Genetic origin of mutations predisposing to retinoblastoma. *Science* 1985;228:501–503.

29. Amendola BE, Markoe AM, Augsburger JJ, et al. Analysis of treatment results in 36 children with retinoblastoma treated by scleral plaque irradiation. *Int J Radiat Oncol Biol Phys* 1989;17:63–70.

30. MacKay CJ, Abramson DH, Ellsworth RM. Metastatic patterns of retinoblastoma. *Arch Ophthalmol* 1984;102:391–396.

*31. Pratt CB, Meyer D, Chenaille P, Crom DB. The use of bone marrow aspirations and lumbar punctures at the time of diagnosis of retinoblastoma. *J Clin Oncol* 1989;7:140–143.

32. Pradhan DG, Sandridge AL, Mullaney P, Abboud E, Karcioglu ZA, Kandil A, Mustafa MM, Gray AJ. Radiation therapy for retinoblastoma: a retrospective review of 120 patients. *Int J Rad Oncol Biol Phys* 1997; 39:3–13.

33. Abramson DH, Jereb B, Ellsworth RM. External beam radiation for retinoblastoma. *Bull NY Acad Med* 1981;57:787–803.

34. Hungerford J. Factors influencing metastasis in retinoblastoma, *Br J Ophthal* 1993;77:541.

35. Hungerford J, Kingston J, Plowman N. Orbital recurrence of retinoblastoma. *Ophthalmic Paediatr Genet* 1987;8:63–68.

36. Stannard C, Lipper S, Sealy R, Sevel D. Retinoblastoma: correlation of invasion of the optic nerve and choroid with prognosis and metastases. *Br J Ophthalmol* 1979;63:560–570.

37. Abramson DH, Niksarli K, Ellsworth RM, Servadidio CA. Changing trends in the management of retinoblastoma: 1951–1965 vs. 1966–1980. *J Pediatr Opthalmol Strabismus* 1994;31:32–37.

38. Dudgeon J. Retinoblastoma—trends in conservative management. *Br J Opthal* 1995;79:104.

39. Shields JA, Shields CL, Sivalingam V. Decreasing frequency of enucleation in patients with retinoblastoma. *Am J Opthalmol* 1989;108:185–188.

40. Abramson DH, Ellsworth RM. The surgical management of retinoblastoma. *Ophthalmic Surg Lasers* 1980;11:596–598.

41. Abramson DH, Ellsworth RM, Rozakis GW. Cryotherapy for retinoblastoma. *Arch Ophthalmol* 1982; 100:1253–1256.

42. Shields CL, Shields JA, Kiratli H, DePotter P. Treatment of retinoblastoma with indirect ophthalmoscope laser photocoagulation. *J Pediatr Opthalmol Strabismus* 1995;32:317–322.

*43. Murphree AL, Villablanca JG, Deegan WF, et al. Chemotherapy plus local treatment in the management of intraocular retinoblastoma. *Arch Opthalmol* 1996;114:1348–1356.

44. Murray TG, Roth DB, O'Brien JM, et al. Local carboplatin and radiation therapy in the treatment of murine transgenic retinoblastoma. *Arch Opthalmol* 1996;114:1385–1389.

45. Greenwald MJ, Strauss LC. Treatment of intraocular retinoblastoma with carboplatin and etoposide chemotherapy. *Ophthalmology* 1996;103: 1989–1997.

46. Wilson AH, Karr DJ, Kalina RE, Lindsley KL, Pendergrass TW. Visual outcomes of macular retinoblastoma after external beam radiation therapy. *Ophthalmology* 1994;101:1244–1249.

47. Kock E, Rosengren B, Tengrath B, Trampe E. Retinoblastoma treated with a ^{60}Co applicator. *Radiother Oncol* 1986;7:19–26.

48. Shields JA, Giblin ME, Shields CL, et al. Episcleral plaque radiotherapy for retinoblastoma. *Ophthalmology* 1989;96:530–537.

49. Shields CL, Shields JA, DePotter P, Hernandez C, Brady LW. Plaque radiotherapy for retinoblastoma. *Int Ophthalmol Clin* 1993;33:107–118.

50. Shields JA, Shields CL, DePotter P, Hernandez JC, Brady LW. Plaque radiotherapy for residual or recurrent retinoblastoma in 91 cases. *J Pediatr Opthalmol Strabismus* 1994;31:242–245.

51. Charles MW, Brown N. Dimensions of the human eye relevant to radiation protection. *Phys Med Biol* 1975; 20:202–218.

*52. Duke-Elder S, ed. The anatomy of the visual system. *System of ophthalmology,* vols. II and X. London:

Henry Kimpton, 1961:78–82 (vol. II), 1961:672–678 (vol. X).

53. Freire JE, DePotter P, Brady LW, Longton WA. Brachytherapy in primary ocular tumors. *Semin Surg Oncol* 1997;13:167–176.

54. Kaste SC, Chen G, Fontanesi J, Crom DB, Pratt CB. Orbital development in long-term survivors of retinoblastoma. *J Clin Oncol* 1997;15(3):1183–1189.

55. Abramson DH, Notterman RB, Ellsworth RM, Kitchin FD. Retinoblastoma treated in infants in the first six months of life. *Arch Ophthalmol* 1983;101:1362–1366.

56. Abramson DH, Servodidio CA, DeLillo AR, Gamell LS, Kruger EF, McCormick B. Recurrence of unilateral retinoblastoma following radiation therapy. *Ophthalmic Genetics* 1994;15:107–113.

57. Stallard HB. The treatment of retinoblastoma. *Ophthalmologica* 1966;151:214–230.

*58. Hernandez JC, Brady LW, Shields CL, Shields JA, DePotter P. Conservative treatment of retinoblastoma. The use of plaque brachytherapy. *Am J Clin Oncol* 1993;16(5):397–401.

59. Hilgartner HL. Report of a case of double glioma treated by x-rays. *Tex Med J* 1910;18:322.

60. Marcus DM, Craft JL, Albert DM. Histopathologic verification of Verhoeff's 1918 irradiation cure of retinoblastoma. *Ophthalmol* 1990;97:221–224.

*61. Blach LE, McCormick B, Abramson DH. External beam radiation therapy and retinoblastoma: long-term results in the comparision of two techniques. *Int J Radiat Oncol Biol Phys* 1996;35:45–51.

62. McCormick B, Ellsworth R, Abramson D, et al. Radiation therapy for retinoblastoma: comparison of results with lens-sparing versus lateral beam techniques. *Int J Radiat Oncol Biol Phys* 1988;15:567–574.

63. McCormick B, Ellsworth R, Abramson D, LaSasso T, Graborski E. Results of external beam radiation for children with retinoblastoma: a comparison of two techniques. *J Pediatr Ophthalmol Strabismus* 1989;26:239–243.

64. Weiss DR, Cassady JR, Peterson R. Retinoblastoma: a modification in radiation therapy technique. *Radiology* 1975;114:705–708.

64a. Weiss AH, Karr DJ, Kalina RE, Lindsley KL,Pendergrass TW. Visual outcomes of macular retinoblastoma after external beam radiation therapy. *Ophthalmology* 1994;101(7):1244–1249.

*65. Hungerford JL, Toma NMG, Plowman PN, Kingston JE. External beam radiotherapy for retinoblastoma: I whole eye technique. *Br J Ophthal* 1995;79:109–111.

66. Brooks HL Jr, Meyer D, Shields JA, Balos AG, Nelson LB, Fontanesi J. Removal of radiation-induced cataracts in patients treated for retinoblastoma. *Arch Ophthalmol* 1990;108:1701–1708.

67. Fontanesi J, Pratt CB, Hustu HO, Coffey D, Kun LE, Meyer D. Use of irradiation for therapy of retinoblastoma in children more than 1 year old: the St. Jude Children's Research Hospital experience and review of literature. *Med Pediatr Oncol* 1995;24:321–326.

68. Fontanesi J, Pratt C, Meyer D, Elverbig J, Parham D, Kaste S. Asynchronous bilateral retinoblastoma: the St. Jude Children's Research Hospital experience. *Ophthalmic Genet* 1995;16:109–112.

69. Harnett AN, Hungerford J, Lambert G, et al. Modern lateral external beam (lens sparing) radiotherapy for retinoblastoma. *Ophthalmic Paediatr Genet* 1987;8:53–61.

70. Buckley EG, Heath H. Visual acuity after successful treatment of large macular retinoblastoma. *J Pediatr Ophthalmol Strabismus* 1992;29:103–106.

71. Merrill PT, Buckley EG, Halperin EC. New and recurrent tumors in germinal retinoblastoma: is there a treatment effect? *Opthal Gen* 1996;17:115–118.

72. Schipper J. An accurate and simple method for megavoltage radiation therapy of retinoblastoma. *Radiother Oncol* 1983;1:31–41.

73. Schipper J, Tan KEWP, Van Peperzeel HA. Treatment of retinoblastoma by precision megavoltage radiation therapy. *Radiother Oncol* 1985;3:117–132.

*74. Toma NMG, Hungerford JL, Plowman PN, Kingston JE, Doughty D. External beam radiotherapy for retinoblastoma: II lens sparing technique. *Br J Opthalmol* 1995;79:112–117.

75. Loeffler JS, Alexander E III, Kooy HM, Black PMcL, Tarbell NJ. Stereotactic radiotherapy: rationale, techniques, and early results. In: DeSalles AAF, Goetsch SJ, eds. *Stereotactic Surgery and Radiosurgery.* Madison: Medical Physics Publishing, 1993:307–320.

76. Gilbert F. Retinoblastoma and recessive cells in tumorigenesis. *Nature* 1983;305:761–762.

77. Goble RR, McKenzie J, Kingston JE, Plowman PN, Hungerford JL. Orbital recurrence of retinoblastoma successfully treated by combined therapy. *Br J Ophthalmol* 1990;74:97–98.

78. Abramson DH, Ellsworth RM, Rosenblatt M, Tretter P, Jereb B, Kitchin FD. Retreatment of retinoblastoma with external beam irradiation. *Arch Ophthalmol* 1982;100:1257–1260.

79. Chatterjee B, Dulta TK, Ayyagari S, et al. Radiation schedules for advanced retinoblastoma in children. *Int J Radiol* 1977;31:100–103.

80. Fontanesi J, Pratt CB, Kun LE, Hustu HO, Coffey D, Meyer D. Treatment outcome and dose-response relationship in infants younger than 1 year treated for retinoblastoma with primary irradiation. *Med Pediatr Oncol* 1996;26:297–304.

81. Shidnia H, Hornback NB, Helveston EM, Gettlefinger T, Biglan AW. Treatment results of retinoblastoma at Indiana University Hospitals. *Cancer* 1977;40:2917–2922.

82. Thompson RW, Small RC, Stein JJ. Treatment of retinoblastoma. *AJR Am J Roentgenol* 1972;114:16–23.

*83. Hernandez JC, Brady LW, Shields JA, et al. External beam radiation for retinoblastoma: results, patterns of failure, and a proposal for treatment guidelines. *Int J Rad Oncol Bio Phys* 1996;35:125–132.

84. Messmer EP, Saverwin W, Heinrich T, et al. New and recurrent tumor foci follow local treatment as well as external beam radiation in eyes of patients with hereditary retinoblastoma. *Graefes Arch Clin Exp Ophthalmol* 1990;228:426–431.

85. Nork TM, Millecchia LL, deVenecia G, Myers FL, Vogel KA. Immunocytochemical features of retinoblastoma in an adult. *Arch Opthalmol* 1996;114:1402–1406.

86. Wolff JA, Baesel CP, Dyment PG. Treatment of retinoblastoma: a preliminary report. *Int Congress Ser* 1981;570:364–368.

*87. Ferris FL, Chew EY. A new era for the treatment of retinoblastoma. *Arch Opthalmol* 1996;114:1412.

88. Chan HSL, DeBaer G, Thiessen JJ, et al. Combining cyclosporin with chemotherapy controls intraocular retinoblastoma without requiring radiation. *Clin Cancer Res* 1996;2:1499–1508.

89. Chan HSL, deBaer G, Thorner PS, Haddad G, Gallie BL, Ling V. Multidrug resistance: clinical opportunities in diagnosis and circumvention. *Hematol Oncol Clin NA* 1994;8:383–410.

90. Amoaku WMK, Willishaw HE, Parkes SE, Shah KJ, Mann JR. Trilateral retinoblastoma: a report of five patients. *Cancer* 1996;78:858–863.

91. Blach LE, McCormick B, Abramson DH, Ellsworth RM. Trilateral retinoblastoma-incidence and outcome: a decade of experience. *Int J Radiat Oncol Biol Phys* 1994;29:729–733.

92. Malik RK, Friedman HS, Djang W, et al. Treatment of trilateral retinoblastoma with vincristine and cyclophosphamide. *Am J Ophthal* 1986;102:650–656.

93. Marks LB, Bentel G, Sherouse GW, Spencer DP, Light K. Craniospinal irradiation for trilateral retinoblastoma following ocular irradiation. *Med Dosim* 1993;18:125–128.

94. Nelson SC, Friedman HS, Oakes WJ, et al. Successful therapy for trilateral retinoblastoma. *Am J Ophthalmol* 1992;114:23–29.

94a. Kingston JE, Plowman PN, Hungerford JL. Ectopic intracranial retinoblastoma in childhood. *Br J Ophthalmol* 1985;69(10):742–748.

95. Taktikas A. Investigation of retinoblastoma with special reference to histology and prognosis. *Br J Ophthalmol* 1966;50:225–234.

96. Stevenson KE, Hungerford J, Garner A. Local extraocular extension of retinoblastoma following intraocular surgery. *Br J Ophthalmol* 1989;73:739–742.

97. Bentel G, Halperin EC, Buckley EG. Iodine-125 embedded in an orbital prosthesis for re-treatment of recurrent retinoblastoma. *Med Dosim* 1993:18:1–5.

98. Williams IG. Let there be light: the treatment of advanced retinoblastoma by external irradiation. *Proc R Soc Med* 1967;60:189–196.

99. Grzeskowiak-Melanowska J, Skorzen S, Armata J. Letter to the editor: what is the best method of prevention of therapeutic failures in CNS in high risk retinoblastoma? [Letter] *Med Pediatr Oncol* 1997;28:79.

100. Eng C, Li FP, Abramson DH, et al. Mortality from second tumors among long-term survivors of retinoblastoma. *J Natl Cancer Inst* 1993;85:1121–1128.

101. Roarty JD, McLean IW, Zimmerman LE. Incidence of second neoplasms in patients with bilateral retinoblastoma. *Ophthalmology* 1988;95:1583–1587.

102. Frank CM, Abramson DH. Second non-ocular tumors in retinoblastoma survivors: something new you need to know. *Int Symposium on Ocular Tumors*, Jerusalem, Israel. 1997:23(abstr).

103. Wong FL, Boice JD Jr, Abramson DH, et al. Cancer incidence after retinoblastoma: radiation dose and sarcoma risk. *JAMA* 1997;278:1262–1267.

104. Cavenee WK, Murphree AL, Shull MM, et al. Prediction of familial predisposition to retinoblastoma. *N Engl J Med* 1986;314:1201–1207.

105. Imhof SM, Hofman P, Tan KEWP. Quantification of lacrimal function after D-shaped field irradiation for retinoblastoma. *Br J Ophthal* 1993;77:482–484.

106. Imhof SM, Mourits MP, Hofman P, et al. Quantification of orbital and mid-facial growth retardation after megavoltage external beam irradiation in children with retinoblastoma. *Ophthalmol* 1996;103:263–268.

107. Messmer EP, Frize H, Mohr C, et al. Long-term treatment effects in patients with bilateral retinoblastoma: ocular and mid-facial findings. *Graefes Arch Clin Exp Ophthalmol* 1991;229:309–314.

108. Yue NC, Benson ML. The hourglass facial deformity as a consequence of orbital irradiation for bilateral retinoblastoma. *Pediatr Radiol* 1996;26:421–423.

109. Cogan DG, Fink R, Donaldson DD. X-ray irradiation of orbital glands of the rabbit. *Howe Laboratory of Ophthalmology* 1954;731–736.

6

Neuroblastoma

Neuroblastoma (NB) has fascinated and frustrated clinicians since its initial description (Fig. 1). Some children may be cured by minimal therapy. However, primary and metastatic NB may resist all attempts at disease eradication, relentlessly growing and causing death (1). Beyond this, NB has the broadest spectrum of clinical presentations and paraneoplastic syndromes of any childhood tumor. Progress in understanding this intriguing and distressing disease has come through an unraveling of its genetic and biologic features, which have diagnostic and prognostic value.

It is hoped that the quirky natural history sometimes displayed by NB, and the insights into its biology, may lead to more innovative treatment approaches. The complexity of NB has stimulated repeated attempts by clinicians and investigators to define and standardize staging and tumor response criteria.

EPIDEMIOLOGY AND BIOLOGY

NB constitutes 7% to 10% of all cases of childhood cancer. It is the most common malignancy of infants, accounting for one-half of infantile cancer cases (2,3). Essentially, all children with NB are diagnosed by age 10 years, 79% are younger than 4 years, and 36% are infants less than 1-year-old. The median age at diagnosis is 22 months (3–7). The annual incidence of NB is on the order of 6 to 11 per million for those under age 15 years and 28 per million for the 0- to 4-year-old subgroup. The annual mortality rate was about 5 per million for all children and 9 per million for the 0- to 4-year-old subgroup, respectively

(8–11). Approximately 15% of childhood cancer mortality is due to NB.

NB arises from primitive (fetal) adrenergic neuroblasts of neural crest tissue, which may explain its high incidence in infancy. In the embryo, continuous columns of neural crest tissue form dorsolateral to the developing neural tissue. These columns are the precursors of the spinal ganglia, the dorsal spinal nerve roots, and the chromaffin cells, which flank the abdominal aorta (12). The largest of these masses is the adrenal medulla (Fig. 2). The vast majority of cases of NB occur in an anatomical distribution consistent with the location of neural crest tissue (Fig. 3).

The frequency of neuroblastic nodules, resembling NB *in situ,* in the adrenals of autopsied infants who have died of other causes ranges from 1 in 39 to 1 in 600 autopsies (13,14). Guin et al. (14) examined the adrenal glands from 92 fetuses aborted at 17 to 20 weeks gestation and found a neuroblastic nodule in all cases. This suggests that most regress by birth. This is interpreted to mean that such nodules are embryologic adrenal remnants, as well as the cells from which adrenal medulla NB may develop. If such neuroblastic rests are not considered NB *in situ,* reserving this term for cases detected by screening infants by urinary catecholamine measurement, then the true frequency of regression is probably 2% to 5% (15). However, if lesions of borderline malignancy are included among the truly malignant NB, then the frequency of spontaneous regression may actually be higher. Additionally complicating this issue, is the observation that NB may

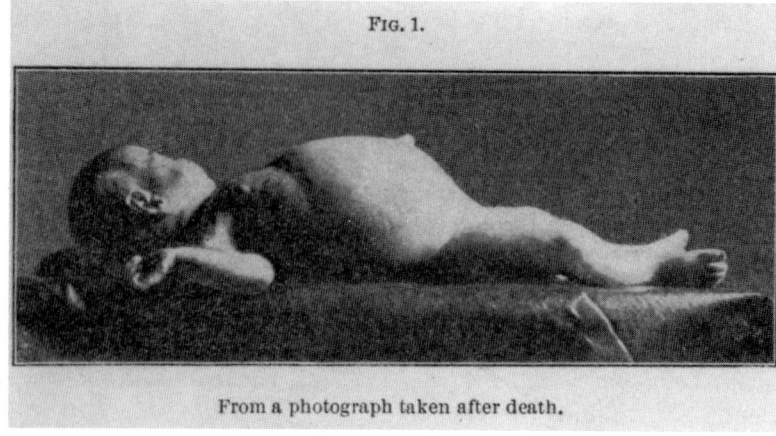

Fig. 1.

From a photograph taken after death.

A

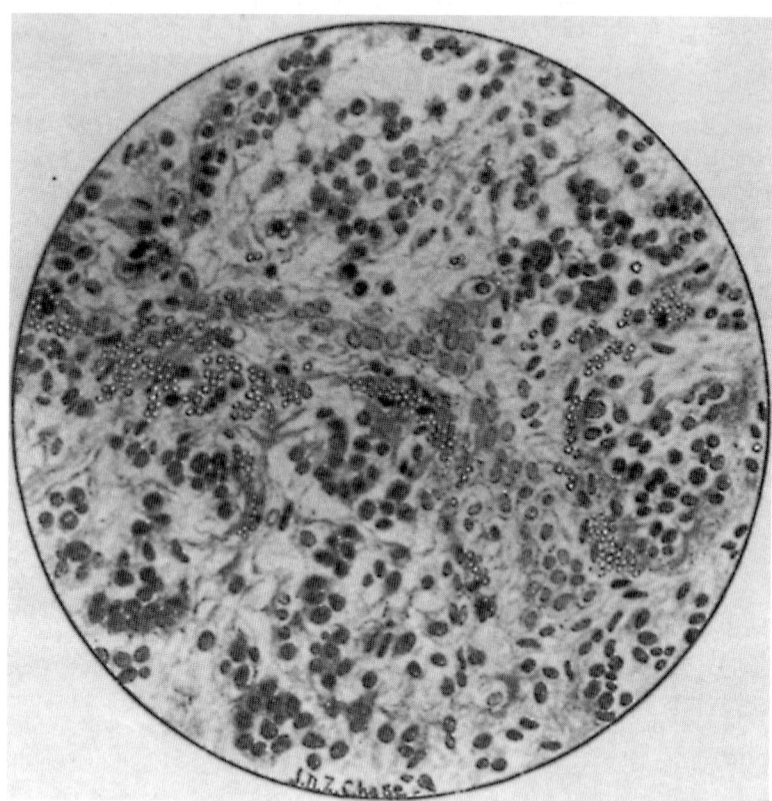

B

FIG. 1. A: William Pepper (1843–1898) described a female infant who died of "congenital sarcoma" of the adrenal gland with extensive hepatic metastasis. He was able to identify, in the literature, five similar cases. Pepper noted that "these 6 cases, besides showing such similarity to one another, have another point of interest, namely, they are so dissimilar to all other reported cases of either primary sarcoma of the supra-renals or of the liver." Pepper was a noted Philadelphia physician, medical educator, author of the fourth edition of *A Practical Treatise on the Diseases of Children* (1870), Provost of the University of Pennsylvania (1881–1894), and philanthropist. **B.** Pepper's detailed drawing of neuroblastoma infiltrating the liver. (From ref. 175, with permission.) May be compared with the modern photomicrograph, **C,** demonstrating the similar round cells with high nuclear to cytoplasm ratio.

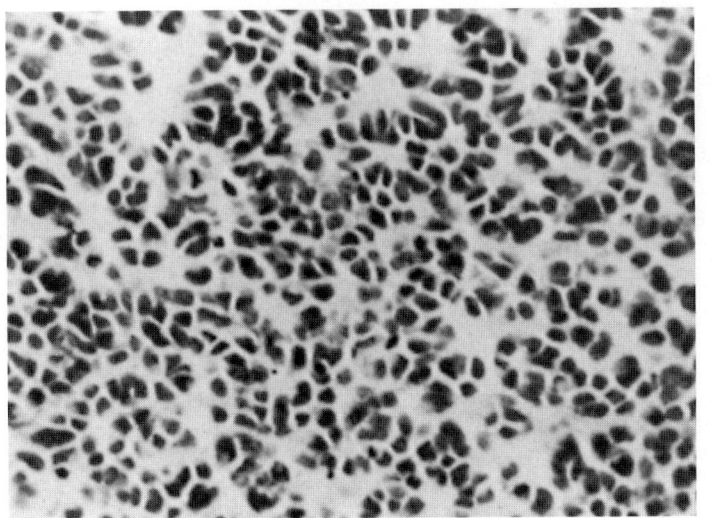

C

FIG. 1. *Continued.* Note how Pepper demonstrated the rosette formation. (Figure C is from ref. 84, with permission.) In 1910 the pathologist and microbiologist James Homer Wright, known for his development of the Wright Stain for examination of blood smears, provided a pathologic description of the tumor identified by Pepper. Wright called it a "neurocytoma or neuroblastoma, a kind of tumor not generally recognized" (195). The possibility of spontaneous regression and/or maturation of neuroblastoma was described by Cushing and Wolbach in 1927(196).

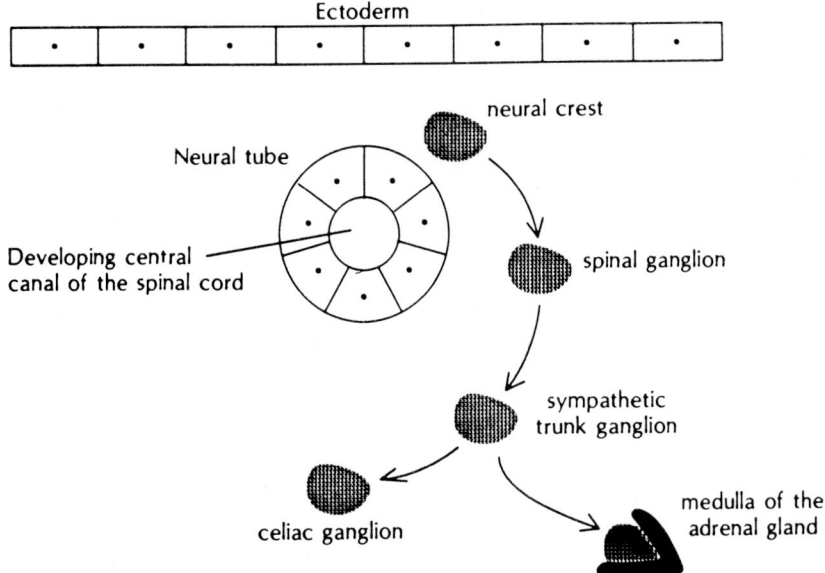

FIG. 2. Migration of the neural crest in the human embryo.

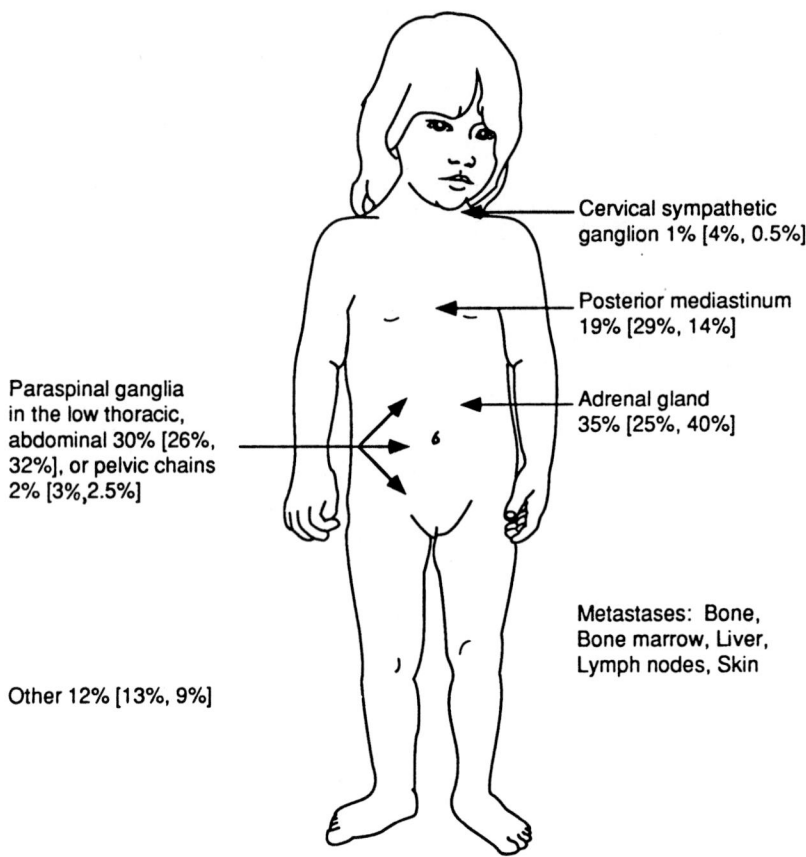

FIG. 3. Common locations of neuroblastoma. The first percentage is the overall proportion of cases at the site. The numbers in parentheses are the percentage of cases at a given site in children ≤1 year of age and >1 year of age. (Data are from ref. 5 and J. Shuster, Ph.D., Pediatric Oncology Group Statistical Office.)

show spontaneous or induced differentiation to ganglioneuroma, which suggests that the malignant transformation of these cells may relate to the inappropriate response of these cells to normal signals for morphologic differentiation. Defects in the nerve growth factor receptor (NGFR) pathway may be responsible for initiation or maintenance of the undifferentiated state of NB (5,16). Data also suggest that insulin-like growth factor II may participate in the stimulation of NB (9,10,17).

Despite these insights into the pathogenesis of NB, its etiology is unknown. Environmental exposures are unlikely to be significant. Some patients can be shown to have an autosomal dominant pattern of inheritance. Knud-

son and Strong (18) estimate that 2% to 25% of NB arises in patients with a prezygotic germinal mutation similar to the mechanisms described for familial retinoblastoma. Familial NB, bilateral, and multifocal disease is also well-described, and presents at a median age of 9 months, in contrast to 22 months for all patients (19).

Cytogenetic analysis of NB is providing new insights into its biology and natural history. A deletion or rearrangement of the short arm of chromosome 1 is found most commonly (70% of near-diploid NB) and may represent deletion (and loss of heterozygosity) of a tumor suppressor gene (5,16,20). Homogeneous staining regions (HSRs) (non-banding regions of metaphase chromosomes that stain homogeneously) and double-minute chromatin bodies (fragments of HSRs) are a manifestation of gene amplification (Fig. 4). They are derived from the distal short arms of chromosome 2, which contains the proto-oncogene N-*myc*.

Amplification of N-*myc* in primary neuroblastoma has been shown to correlate with advanced stage. Such amplification occurs in 30% to 40% of advanced-stage NB, but only in 5% to 10% of low-stage or IV-S disease and not at all in benign ganglioneuromas; it appears to be an inherent biologic property of the particular neuroblastic tumor (5,16, 20–22). Children who have N-*myc* amplification in their tumor are unlikely to respond to conventional therapy. In Children's Cancer Group protocol 3881, of 23 infants with Stage IV disease and amplified N-*myc*, 17 (74%) had progressive tumor or died. The prognostic importance of N-*myc* was confirmed in a large Italian study. Amplified N-*myc* was more frequent in children older than 1 year, with advanced stage, and elevated ferritin, neuron-specific enolase, and lactate dehydrogenase (23). A correlation between chromosome 1p deletion and N-*myc* amplification appears to exist (20).

DNA ploidy is also an important discriminator of response to chemotherapy for NB (19). In 1984, Look et al. described 23 children with unresectable NB. Of the 17 patients with hyperdiploid status, 15 were complete responders to chemotherapy and two were partial responders. None of the six patients

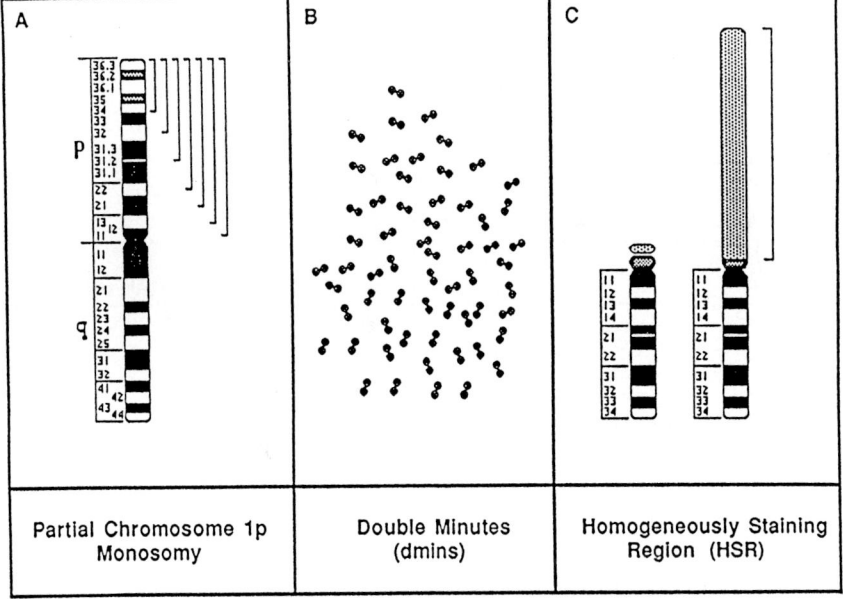

| Partial Chromosome 1p Monosomy | Double Minutes (dmins) | Homogeneously Staining Region (HSR) |

FIG. 4. Common cytogenetic abnormalities in human neuroblastomas. Shown are diagrammatic representations of the three most common cytogenetic abnormalities seen in human neuroblastomas. **A:** Deletions of the short arm of chromosome 1. The brackets indicate that the region deleted in different tumors is variable in terms of its proximal breakpoint, but the distal short arm appears to be deleted in all cases, resulting in partial 1p monosomy. **B:** Extrachromosomal double-minute chromatin bodies (dmins). These are seen in about 30% of primary neuroblastoma and are a cytogenetic manifestation of gene amplification. **C:** Homogeneously staining region (HSR). A representative HSR on the short arm of chromosome 13 is shown in this example. HSRs are a cytogenetic manifestation of gene amplification in which the amplified sequences are chromosomally integrated. (From refs. 197 and 5, with permission.)

with diploid tumors responded ($p = 0.0001$) (24). In a 1991 report, Look evaluated 298 children. In infants with Stage D disease the progression-free survival was greater than 90% for those with hyperdiploid tumors versus 0% in diploid cases. In children 12 to 24 months of age with Stage D the distinction was also striking (50% to 60% in hyperdiploid cases versus 0% in diploid, $p < 0.001$) (25). Pediatric Oncology Group Study 8743, of patients with Stages C, D, and DS, published in 1997, reported an overall 3-year survival of 94% for hyperdiploid patients versus 55% for diploid (26).

PATHOLOGY

NB is one of the small blue round cell tumors, along with non-Hodgkin's lymphoma, Ewing's sarcoma, undifferentiated soft-tissue sarcomas including rhabdomyosarcoma, and primitive neuroectodermal tumors. The classic histologic subtypes of neuroblastic tumors include NB, ganglioneuroblastoma, and ganglioneuroma (GN), reflecting a pattern of in-creasing maturation and differentiation (5, 27). The cells of NB are small and uniformly sized, with dense hyperchromatic nuclei and scant cytoplasm (Fig. 1). The cells may be densely packed, separated by thin fibrils or bundles, and necrosis and calcification can occur. Neuritic processes can be demonstrated in most cases, and pseudorosettes can be seen in 15% to 50% of cases. The other end of the spectrum, ganglioneuroma, has mature ganglion cells, neuritic processes, and Schwann cells and has more fibrillary material. Any immature cells or nuclear atypia negates this diagnosis. Patients with ganglioneuroma or ganglioneuroblastoma generally have localized tumors with favorable biologic characteristics, explaining the excellent associated prognosis.

NB has a mixture of neuroblastic and mature ganglion cells, as well as cells intermediary in their differentiation. Various immunohistochemical techniques and electron microscopy are used for diagnosis. Monoclonal antibodies will recognize neuron-specific enolase (NSE), synaptophysin, chroma-

---

TABLE 1. *Three major histopathologic classification systems for neuroblastoma*

System	Histopathologic features and age associated with prognosis
Shimada system	Favorable prognosis is associated with: 　Stroma rich, all ages, no nodular pattern 　Stroma poor, age 1.5–5 yr, differentiated, MKI < 100 　Stroma poor, age <1.5 yr, MKI < 200 Unfavorable prognosis is associated with: 　Stroma rich, all ages, nodular pattern 　Stroma poor, age >5 yr 　Stroma poor, age 1.5–5 yr, undifferentiated 　Stroma poor, age 1,5–5 yr, differentiated, MKI > 100 　Stroma poor, age <1.5 yr, MKI > 200
Joshi system	Favorable prognosis is associated with: Grade 1, all ages; Grade 2, <1 yr Unfavorable prognosis is associated with: Grade 2, age >1 yr, Grade 3, all ages
International Neuroblastoma Pathology Committee system	Classification of Neuroblastoma is based on: 　the degree of differentiation toward ganglion cells 　the amount of Schwann cell stroma present 　whether the tumor is nodular, noting particularly macronodules (which tend to be associated with a poor prognosis compared with intermixed nodules) 　the degree of calcification 　the MKI

Grade 1, Low mitotic rate (<10 mitotic figures per 10 high power fields) and calcification present; Grade 2, Either low mitotic rate or calcification present; Grade 3, Neither low mitotic rate nor calcification present; MKI, Mitosis-Karyorrhexis index (number of mitoses and karyorrhexis per 5000 cells).
Adapted from refs. 31, 32, 100, 101, 137, and 180.

granin A (CGA), and neuronal filaments (27). Electron microscopy reveals neurofilaments, neurotubules, and neurosecretory granules that contain catecholamines.

Three systems have been proposed to assess the influence of pathology on prognosis: The Shimada Classifcation, The Joshi Classification (also called the Joshi modification of the Shimada Classification), and the International Neuroblastoma Pathology Committee Classification (22,28,29). The major aspects of these three systems are summarized in Table 1. Shimada et al. (29) formulated a system based on patient age, the presence of stroma ("rich" or "poor") and nodularity, the degree of differentiation, and the mitosis-karyorrhexis index. Joshi attempted to combine conventional terminology with criteria used by Shimada and others (21,30). The terms NB and ganglioneuroblastoma are retained rather than stroma-poor and stroma-rich NB, and undifferentiated NB, poorly differentiated NB, and differentiating NB are considered distinct (based on degree of cellular density and the number of tumor cells and mitotic karyorrhectic cells per high-power field) (30). The International Neuroblastoma Pathology Committee criteria includes various histologic features designed to differentiate those NB that are embryonic and will regress from those that are neoplastic.

CLINICAL PRESENTATION AND EVALUATION

The clinical presentation of NB is dependent on the site along the sympathetic nervous system chain from which the primary tumor develops, as well as on the manifestions of metastatic disease. This varies according to patient age. The abdomen is the most common primary tumor location (50% to 80% of cases). Intraabdominal primary tumors arise in the adrenals or in a paraspinal location. The paraspinal tumors may have a "dumbbell" configuration wherein tumor extends through the neural foramina and presents with a mass lesion within the spinal canal; extradural spinal cord compression may occur. Extraab-dominal locations of the primary tumor include sympathetic ganglia in the neck (often initially thought to be lymphadenitis), posterior mediastinum, and pelvis (Fig. 3).

The earliest symptoms or signs of NB may be a palpable abdominal mass (often large, firm, irregular, and crossing the midline), a unilateral neck mass often causing Horner's syndrome, spinal cord compression, respiratory compromise due to thoracic disease or hepatic metastases placing upward pressure on the diaphragm, or bowel/bladder disturbances due to compression from a pelvic mass. About 60% of children with NB will have metastatic disease (either lymphatic or hematogenous) at the time of clinical presentation (Table 2). The symptoms in this setting are those of systemic illness: fever, weight loss, weakness, or a general failure to thrive. In some patients, the presenting symptoms are related to secretory products of the tumor. For example, intractable diarrhea (from vasoactive intestinal polypeptide) may rarely occur, usually in children with ganglioneuroblastoma or ganglioneuroma. Bone metastases present as pain, refusal to walk, skull masses, or proptosis with orbital ecchymosis. Skin metastases are common in neonates and generally have a blue tinge ("the blueberry muffin sign"). When a skin metastasis is manually compressed, one may observe blanching of the surrounding skin secondary to liberation of vasoconstrictive catecholamine. Rarely, a child with NB will present with the opsoclonus (rapid multidirectional eye movements)—myoclonus—truncal ataxia syndrome. This paraneoplastic syndrome is associated with early-stage NB,

TABLE 2. *Extent of disease at diagnosis stratified by age*

Disease extent at diagnosis	Age at diagnosis		
	≤1 year	>1 year	Total
Localized	39%	19%	26%
Regional	18%	13%	15%
Disseminated	25%	68%	52%
IV-S	18%	0%	7%

Modified from ref. 23 and courtesy of J. Shuster, Ph.D., POG Statistical Office.

and neurologic deficits may persist despite cure (31). NB may infiltrate the marrow and cause pancytopenia with resulting complications (infection, pallor, lethargy, bleeding). Intracranial metastatic disease is usually meningeal, and in infants it may cause cranial suture separation.

The diagnostic evaluation of NB includes imaging and laboratory testing with the goals of determining disease extent and prognosis, as well as identifying markers of disease activity. The primary tumor is typically imaged radiographically and with computerized tomography (CT) scan or magnetic resonance imaging (MRI). The classic radiographic sign of adrenal NB is calcification within a suprarenal soft tissue mass. The intravenous pyelogram (IVP) will show renal displacement without pelvocalyceal disruption. In the thorax, a plain radiograph will demonstrate a posterior mediastinal mass. In both abdomen and chest, CT scan and MRI are helpful in assessing possible lymph node metastases and intraspinal extension (32). Contrast vascular radiography may be requested in order to plan a surgical approach. Phosphorous magnetic resonance imaging (^{31}P MRI) has shown some promise in imaging NB and monitoring treatment response (33).

The search for distant, usually bony, metastasis includes a radionuclide bone scan and conventional radiographs. Bone metastases are most often periorbital, metaphysical, and axial in location (Fig. 5). Bone scintigraphy is more sensitive than conventional radiographs, but is sometimes difficult to interpret in infants less than 1 year old (34,35). Meta-iodobenzylguanidine (MIBG) is a guanethidine derivative of norepinephrine and epinephrine. The compound is taken up by catecholaminergic cells (7,27). It has been used in the detection of pheochromocytoma and is now frequently used in the evaluation of neuroblastoma. The MIBG is labeled with an isotope of iodine (either ^{131}I or^{123}I) and scintigraphy is performed for imaging, and, in some situations, therapy. MIBG is a sensitive and specific method (~ 90%) of assessment of the primary tumor and metastatic disease. Be-

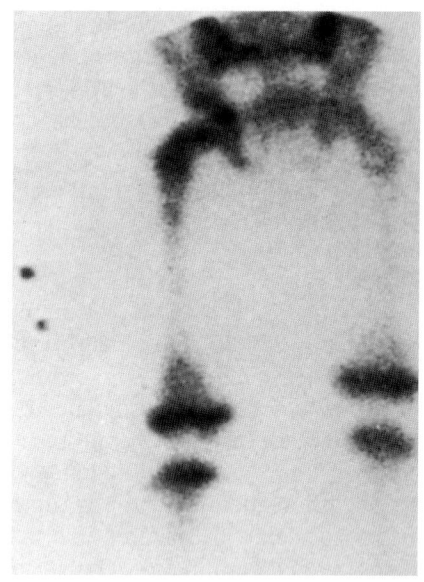

FIG. 5. Femoral metastases from neuroblastoma.

cause MIBG depends on functional uptake by tumor cells it is also useful in distinguishing residual active tumor following treatment from masses composed of scar tissue—and may be complimentary to CT scans (7,9,10, 27,36,37). ^{99m}Tc-diphosphonate bone scans continue to be used for the detection of metastatic foci in the skeleton even if MIBG studies are done. Because the MIBG scan cannot demarcate cortical bone involvement from bone-marrow infiltration, the conventional ^{99m}Tc scan remains of use to assist in making the distinction (36) (Fig. 6).

Liver involvement may be evaluated by CT, ultrasound, or radionuclide liver scan in older children because it is usually focal or nodular. In infants it may be diffuse and inapparent by imaging. For this reason, liver biopsies are recommended by some authorities for diagnostic workup of infants. This recommendation is a matter of some controversy (10). Pulmonary parenchymal metastases rarely occur in NB.

There may be extensive involvement of the bone marrow by tumor without a change in the peripheral blood counts. Bone marrow aspiration and biopsy, therefore, are performed

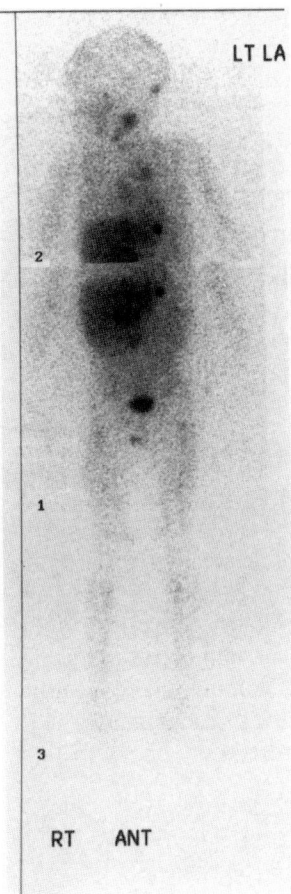
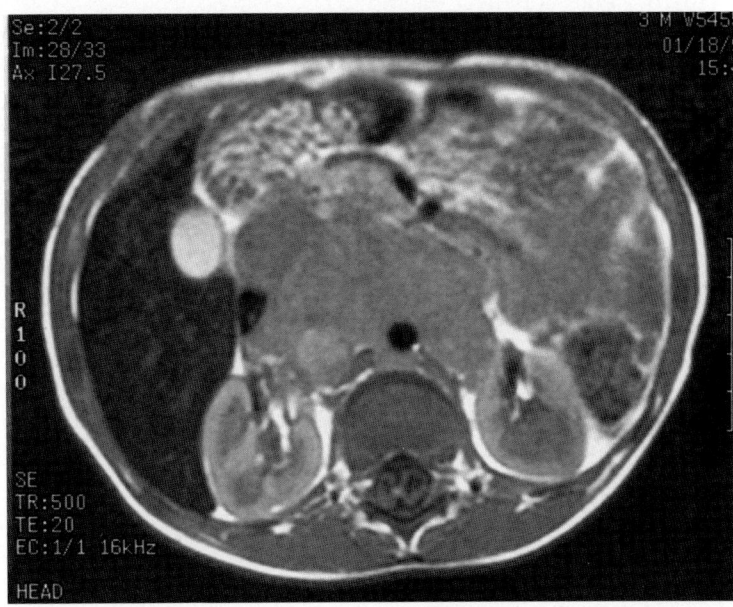

FIG. 6. A. A four year old male presented to medical attention with fever and leg pain. Chest x-ray demonstrated a posterior mediastinal mass. This MIBG scan demonstrates increased activity in the occipital region of the skull consistent with a bone metastases. There is activity in the neck which could represent either a nodal metastases or metastatic disease to the cervical spine. Activity in the left hemithorax is indeterminate as to its origin and could represent disease in the sternum, rib, or mediastinal lymph node. There is activity just below the diaphragm in the upper abdomen consistent with nodal metastasis and very slight activity in the proximal left femur. Normal findings include increased activity in the bladder as well as a bit of activity at the tip of the glans penis-almost certainly contamination from urine. **B.** This large retroperitoneal neuroblastoma encases the abdominal aorta and displaces the inferior vena cava. The tumor appears to arise from outside the kidneys. There is some retroaortic extension of tumor and the bowel is compressed anteriorly. No tumor is seen in the spinal canal. The liver and gall bladder appear to be normal.

routinely. Bilateral posterior iliac crest aspirates and core biopsies are recommended. The core biopsies should contain at least 1 cm of marrow (excluding cartilage) to be considered adequate for diagnosis. There may be extensive involvement of the bone marrow by tumor without a change in the peripheral blood counts. Small amounts of NB cells may be difficult to distinguish from hematopoietic elements. The diagnosis of NB in the bone marrow is reliably made when tumor clumps are seen in the presence of typical signs and symptoms. Recently, the use of a variety of monoclonal antibodies directed against various surface antigens for immunocytological assessment of the marrow may be used to detect tumor cells at a concentration of 1 cell per 10^6. This technology is clearly more sensitive than conventional analyses and provides prognostic information (38). It is not known, however, what level of immunocytologic bone marrow involvement warrants a change in stage. At present, tumor detected by immunocytology that is not extensive enough to be diagnosed by conventional bone marrow microscopy does not affect staging (37).

NB is associated with increased or abnormal production, secretion, and catabolism of catecholamines (or metabolites) in 90% of cases (37,39,40). Catecholamines and metabolites may be measured in the urine: norepinephrine, vanillylmandelic acid (VMA), 3methoxy-4-hydroxylphenylglycol (MHPG), and/or homovanillic acid (HVA). Dopamine may be measured in urine or serum (Fig. 7). Urinary catecholamines are typically presented as ratios to urinary creatinine. The symptoms associated with excess catecholamine production include flushing and sweating, pallor, headache, and hypertension. Diarrhea may oc-

cur and has been attributed to the excretion of vasoactive intestinal peptide (VIP). Both VIP and somatostatin can be quantified by radioimmunoassay in NB cells, and may relate to prognosis (discussed later in this chapter) (41).

STAGING AND PROGNOSTIC FACTORS

The criteria for diagnosis of NB recommended by the second INSSC are (a) unequivocal pathologic diagnosis from tumor tissue by light microscopy [with or without immunohistology, electron microscopy, increased urine or serum catecholamines or metabolites (dopamine, HVA, or VMA greater than 3.0 SD above the mean per-milligram creatinine for age)]; or (b) bone marrow aspirate or biopsy containing unequivocal tumor cells, (e.g., syncytia or immunocytologically positive clumps of cells) and increased urine or serum catecholamines or metabolites (42). A diagnosis of NB based only on compatible

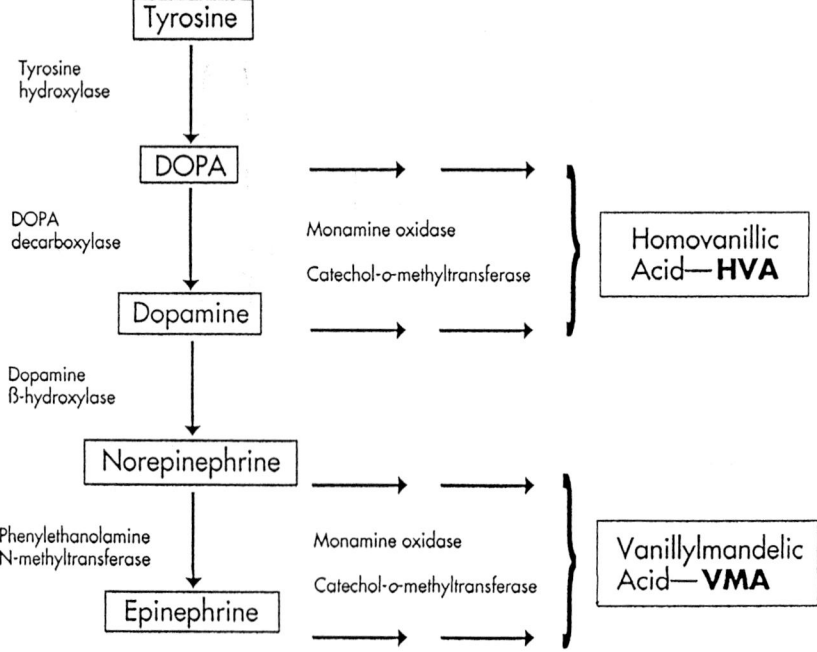

FIG. 7. A simplified diagram of catecholamine synthesis and metabolism. HVA and VMA are the urinary catecholamine metabolites that are usually measured. (From ref. 198, with permission.)

radiographic findings and elevated urinary catecholamine metabolites is insufficient because of possible confusion with ganglioneuroma or pheochromocytoma, or even other solid tumors [e.g., primitive neuroectodermal tumor (PNET), rhabdomyosarcoma], which can have false-positive urinary findings.

Staging

Three systems have been used for the staging of NB. Understanding the nuances of these systems is critical for interpreting and accurately comparing data from various reports and determining therapy (43). Evans and D'Angio (44–46) proposed a system based on the extent of the primary tumor and the presence or absence of distant metastases. A special stage (IV-S) is alloted to infants less than 1-year old with a relatively small primary tumor and metastases to the liver, skin, or bone marrow. Most children with bona fide stage 4S disease will have less than or equal to 1% tumor cells in marrow, and at most 10%. It has been speculated that the liver is a preferred site of metastases in neonates because the liver is a preferred site of blood flow in the fetus and, therefore, metastatic disease lodges in that organ (13).

The Evans-D'Angio (ED) system was criticized because its definition of stage I disease is problematic (Table 3), because primary NB arising from sympathetic ganglia are often small and not well-encapsulated. In addition, tumor resectability did not influence staging, and lymph node sampling was not required although it does influence staging (5). Hayes and colleagues (47,48) proposed an alternative staging system based on initial resectability of the primary tumor and lymph node involvement (48,49). The Pediatric Oncology Group (POG) staging system reflects this surgical evaluation for local/regional disease and regional node involvement. However, in this system the nature of the lymph node involvement is confusing (to wit: adhered to surface, within, not adhered, extracavitary, etc.). In fact, the importance of local and regional lymph node status in staging NB is uncertain. Some studies, which have prospectively sought to identify lymph node metastases, report a better survival rate in local/regional NB without nodal metastasis than with nodal disease (48,50).

Two international conferences have finalized a consensus for a new NB staging system (International Neuroblastoma Staging System or INSS). *This system is now generally accepted as the proper one for management of NB and for reporting of results.* The INSS is a postsurgical staging system with substantial reliance on the assessment of tumor resectability and surgical examination of lymph node involvement (11). The system incorporates the extent of local tumor, the degree of surgical resection, and the presence and location of involved nodes, and it maintains the special IV-S stage. In classifying tumors that cross the midline, "infiltration" (extending by contiguous invasion to/or beyond the opposite side of the vertebral bodies) was chosen to identify tumors presumably less favorable than those that are pedunculated and simply drape over the midline (Table 3) (51). The INSS uses Arabic numbers to distinguish it from the letters and Roman numerals of the other systems. The definition of stage 1 was clarified at the second INSS conference such that nodes attached to the primary (adherent to or in direct continuity with, and removed with, the primary) may be positive (42). Because gross resection of a localized tumor is associated with a favorable outcome (52,53), regardless of microscopic residual disease or involvement of attached lymph nodes, even such tumors that arise in or cross the midline may be stage 1.

Prognostic Factors

Clinical

Several clinical and biologic characteristics of NB are associated with prognosis. Various cooperative groups and investigators have attempted to select certain variables and group them to identify patients with

TABLE 3. *Neuroblastoma staging system*[a]

Evans and D'Angio (53,55)	Pediatric oncology group (86)	INSS (25,26)
Stage I	**Stage A**	**Stage 1**
Tumor confined to the organ or structure of origin.	Complete gross resection of primary tumor, with or without microscopic residual. Intracavitary lymph nodes, not adhered to and removed with primary (nodes adhered to or within tumor resection may be positive for tumor without upstaging patient to stage C), histologically free of tumor. If primary in abdomen or pelvis, liver histologically free of tumor.	Localized tumor with complete gross excision, without microscopic residual disease; representative ipsilateral lymph nodes negative for tumor microscopically (nodes attached to and removed with the primary tumor may be positive).
Stage II	**Stage B**	**Stage 2A**
Tumor extending in continuity beyond the organ or structure of origin but not crossing the midline. Regional lymph nodes on the ipsilateral side may be involved.	Grossly unresected primary tumor. Nodes and liver same as stage A.	Localized tumor with incomplete gross excision; representative ipsilateral nonadherent lymph nodes negative for tumor . microscopically
Stage III	**Stage C**	**Stage 2B**
Tumor extending in continuity beyond the midline. Regional lymph nodes may be involved bilaterally.	Complete or incomplete resection of primary. Intracavitary nodes not adhered to primary histologically positive for tumor. Liver as in stage A.	Localized tumor with or without complete gross excision, with ipsilateral nonadherent lymph nodes positive for tumor. Enlarged contralateral lymph nodes must be negative microscopically.
		Stage 3
		Unresectable unilateral tumor infiltrating across the midline,[b] with or without regional lymph node involvement; or localized unilateral tumor with contralateral regional lymph node involvement; or midline tumor with bilateral extension by infiltration (unresectable) or by lymph node involvement.
Stage IV	**Stage D**	**Stage 4**
Remote disease involving the skeleton, bone marrow, soft tissue, and distant lymph node groups, etc. (see stage IV-S).	Any dissemination of disease beyond intracavitary nodes (i.e., extracavitary nodes, liver, skin, bone marrow, bone).	Any primary tumor with dissemination to distant lymph nodes, bone, bone marrow, liver, skin and/or other organs (except as defined for stage 4S).
Stage IV-S	**Stage DS**	**Stage 4S**
Patients who would otherwise be stage I or II, but who have remote disease confined to liver, skin, or bone marrow (without radiographic evidence of bone metastases on complete skeletal survey).	Infants <1 year of age with stage IV-S disease (see Evans and D'Angio).	Localized primary tumor as defined for stage 1, 2A or 2B) with dissemination limited to skin, liver, and/or bone marrow[c] (limited to infants <1 year of age).

[a]Multifocal primary tumors (e.g., bilateral adrenal primary tumors) should be staged according to the greatest extent of disease, as defined above, and followed by a subscript letter M (e.g., 3_M).

[b]The midline is defined as the vertebral column. Tumors originating on one side and crossing the midline must infiltrate to or beyond the opposite side of the vertebral column.

[c]Marrow involvement in stage 4S should be minimal—that is, <10% of total nucleated cells identified as malignant on bone marrow biopsy or on marrow aspirate. More extensive marrow involvement would be considered to be stage 4. The MIBG scan (if performed) should be negative in the marrow.

good, intermediate, or bad prognoses. The differences in various studies likely result from differences in patient characteristics, treatment, study endpoints, and so on. As cytogenetic data is increasingly accumulated and interpreted, genetic subsets of NB that reflect clinical behavior are being identified (Tables 4 and 5).

The *stage* of disease strongly influences prognosis (Fig. 8). More than 85% of all children with POG stage A or B disease, as well as infants (less than 1 year of age) with stage C disease, survive—in contrast to approximately 60% to 80% of children older than 1 year with stage C disease, and 10% to 30% of older children with stage D disease. Implicit in the staging system is the inferior experience in treating children who have either (a) tumors that infiltrate across the midline or are unresectable, (b) contralateral or bilateral lymph node involvement, or (c) metastatic disease (54). These patients, particularly those in the latter group with cortical bone metastates, fare poorly. Stage IV-S NB was initially established in light of the observation that infants having a localized primary NB with metastases to liver, bone marrow, and/or skin had a surprisingly good prognosis and might require minimal therapy (45). Investigations into stage IV-S disease suggest, however, that subgroups may be identified with widely different prognoses (55–57). The subgrouping of Stage IV-S is discussed later in this chapter.

The *age* at diagnosis is a strong determinant of outcome, with infants less than 12 to 18 months of age faring better than older children with the same disease stage (Fig. 9). This effect is dramatic for patients with advanced stage 3 and 4 disease. Most infants with NB are long-term survivors, whereas most children diagnosed at an older age will succumb to the disease (4,6,22,28,48,49,58–65). The biologic underpinning for this is not clearly defined, but several observations can be made. Approximately 20% of infants present with stage DS (IV-S) disease, and 75% of this group (those without adverse biologic factors) survive. The DS children with favorable features might most appropriately be considered to have a disseminated neurocristopathy rather than a metastatic cancer. Older children more often present with advanced (truly metastatic) stage disease; that is, 60% to 70% of children older than 1 year present with stage D disease, compared with 25% of infants. Even with metastatic tumor at diagnosis, however, infants frequently survive. This may be related to a higher rate of spontaneous tumor regression or tumor maturation in infants. A heightened sensitivity of the immune system to NB in infants has also been postulated. Differences in the percentage of clonogenic neuroblasts and end-stage committed cells, no longer capable of tumor growth, may exist in younger patients. Carlsen et al. (58) have hypothesized that the prognosis worsens with increasing age because all NBs may be congenital. The probability of micrometastases may increase with a longer duration of exposure to tumor (age since birth) and increasing tumor burden.

TABLE 4. *Clinical and genetic subtypes of neuroblastoma*

Feature	Type 1	Type 2	Type 3
N-*myc*	Normal	Normal	Amplified
Karotype/Ploidy	Hyperdiploid	Near-diploid	Near-diploid
	Triploid	Near-tetraploid	Near-tetraploid
1p loss of heterozygosity	Absent	Present	Present
trk A expression	High	Variable or low	Low or absent
Age	<1yr	≥1 yr	1–5 yr
International Neuroblastoma Staging system stage	1,2,4S	3,4	3,4
3-yr survival	~95%	25–50%	~5%

From refs. 22, 23, with permission. (A version of this table also appears in refs. 31, 32.)

TABLE 5. *Assignment of risk group for neuroblastoma—guidelines of the Children's Cancer Group and the Pediatric Oncology Group*

International Neuroblastoma Staging System Stage	Age	N-*myc* status	Shimada histology classification	DNA ploidy	Risk group
1	0–21 yr	Any	Any	Any	Low
2A/2B	<365 d	Any	Any	Any	Low
	≥365 d–21 yr	Nonamplified	Any	NA	Low
	≥365 d–21 yr	Amplified	Favorable	NA	Low
	≥365 d–21 yr	Amplified	Unfavorable	NA	Low
3	<365 d	Nonamplified	Any	Any	Intermediate High
	<365 d	Amplified	Any	Any	Intermediate
	≥365 d–21 yr	Nonamplified	Favorable	NA	High
	≥365 d–21 yr	Nonamplified	Unfavorable	NA	High
	≥365 d–21 yr	Amplified	Any	NA	
4	<365 d	Nonamplified	Any	Any	Intermediate
	<365 d	Amplified	Any	Any	High
	≥365 d–21 yr	Any	Any	NA	High
4S	<365 d	Nonamplified	Favorable	>1	Low
	<365 d	Nonamplified	Any	= 1	Intermediate
	<365 d	Nonamplified	Unfavorable	Any	Intermediate
	<365 d	Amplified	Any	Any	High

NA, not applicable.
From refs. 23 and 33, with permission, and modified from refs. 31 and 32, as well as from Pediatric Oncology Group Protocol A3961.

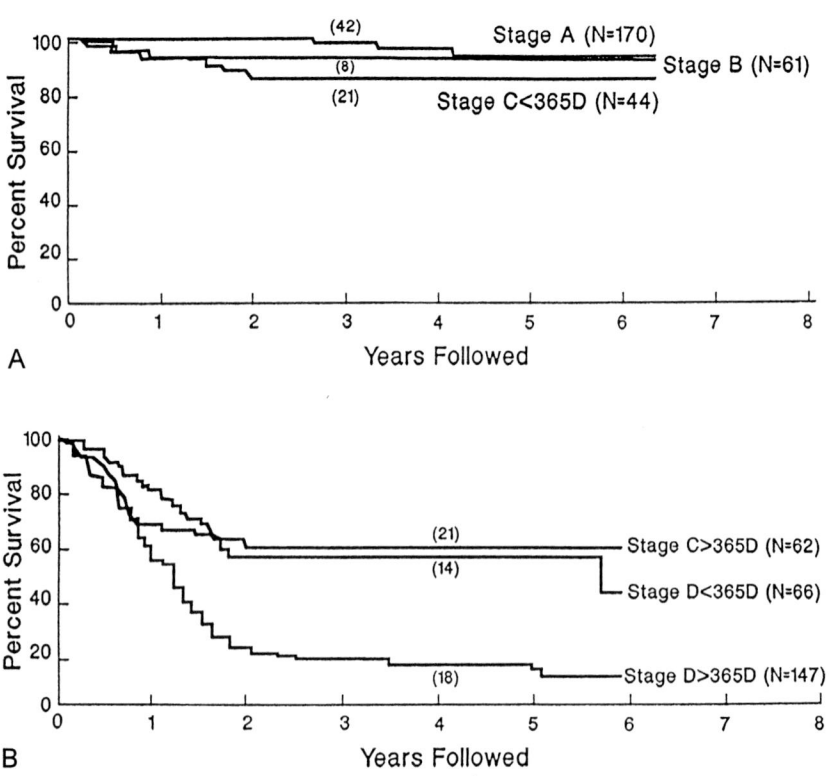

FIG. 8. Survival in 550 consecutive patients with neuroblastoma treated from 1981 to 1989 on POG protocols. Based on POG stage and age ≤ or >1 year, three prognostic groups emerged: low risk, intermediate risk, and high risk. (From ref. 5, with permission.)

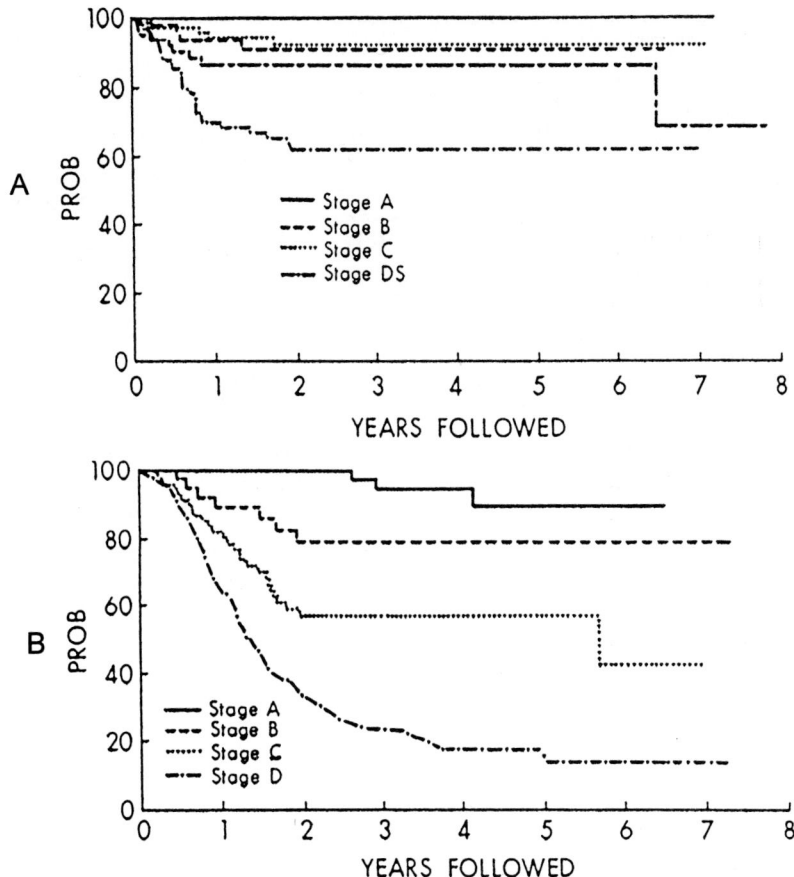

FIG. 9. Survival curves based on stage at diagnosis. Survival figures of 1001 patients with neuroblastoma treated on POG protocols from 1981 to 1989. **A:** Probability of survival of 369 infants under 1 year of age with neuroblastoma staged according to the POG staging system. **B:** Probability of survival of 632 children (≥1 year of age) with neuroblastoma according to the POG stage. (Courtesy of J. Shuster, Ph.D., POG Statistical Office and reproduced with modifications with permission from ref. 198.)

There is no difference in the survival of males versus females. While the survival of patients with thoracic primary tumors is better than those with abdominal primaries (28,62, 66,67), the tumor site is not an independent prognostic factor (58,59,67,68). Patients with thoracic primary tumors are generally younger children with lower-stage disease (69).

Biologic

Ferritin may be produced by NB cells, and thus reflects tumor burden or growth, or it may be necessary for NB cell growth (5). An elevated serum ferritin level (greater than 143 ng/mL) is found in up to half of patients with advanced stage disease, but rarely in children with localized disease. Progression-free survival is less good in children with increased levels (5,70–72).

Neuron-specific enolase is a glycolytic enzyme found in neurons. The enzyme is associated with worse survival when elevated (greater than 100 ng/mL). Elevation is more common in patients with advanced-stage disease (5,73). Neuron-specific enolase may be

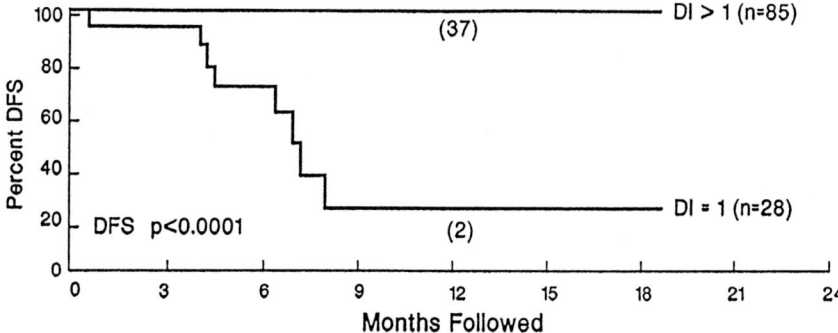

FIG. 10. Disease-free survival in 113 infants with INSS stages 2A, 2B, 3, and 4 neuroblastoma when stratified according to DNA content. DI is DNA index. (From refs. 139 and 5, with permission.)

useful for following the response to treatment.

Lactate dehydrogenase elaboration may reflect tumor cell burden or turnover, and serum elevations (greater than 1,500 IU/mL) have been found to be independently associated with a worse prognosis (62,74,75).

Certain neuropeptides (*vasoactive intestinal peptide* and *somatostatin*) have been observed to correlate with neuroblastic cellular

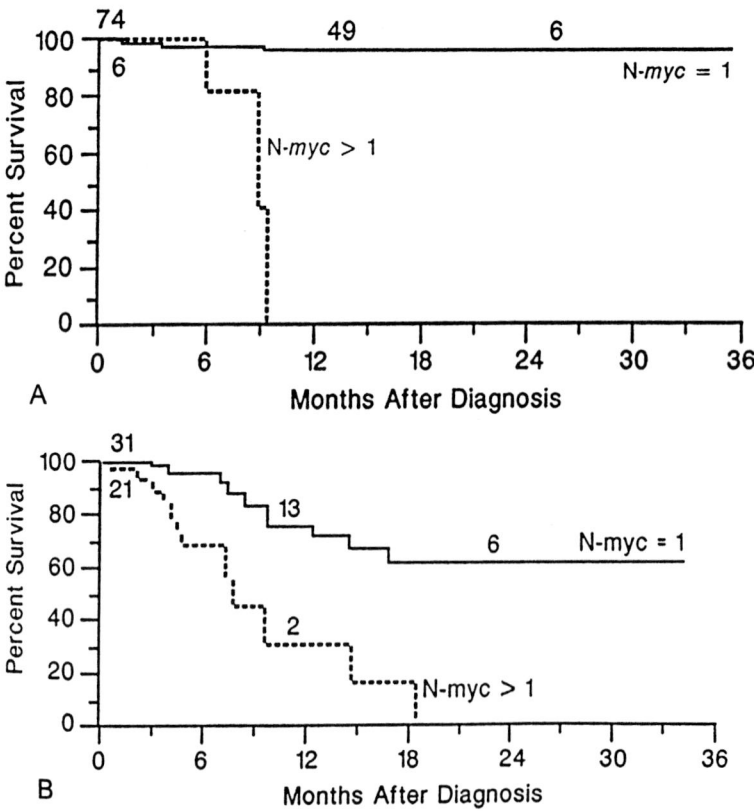

FIG. 11. Survival according to N-myc copy number. **A:** Survival according to N-myc copy number in 80 infants with POG stages B, C, D, and DS neuroblastoma. **B:** Survival according to N-myc copy number in 52 children with unresectable or metastatic neuroblastoma (POG stages C and D). (From ref. 5, with permission.)

differentiation and favorable disease stage (41).

The *MDRI* gene encodes *P-glycoprotein*, which acts as an ATP-dependent drug-efflux pump. Its expression before treatment may predict efficacy of therapy (76). This also implies that agents capable of reversing P-glycoprotein-mediated multidrug resistance may be useful in NB. Another gene that encodes for multidrug-resistance associated protein (MRP) has been reported to correlate with N-*myc* amplification and poor outcome (77). The data on this point is, however, contradictory and not all authorities agree that P-glycoprotein is of prognostic importance.

DNA index, N-myc amplification, nerve growth factor receptors, and *chromosome 1 deletion* are discussed in the section entitled "Epidemiology and Biology," (see Tables 4 and 5; Figs. 10 and 11).

High expression of the *Ha-ras p21 gene* has been correlated with lower clinical stage of tumor at diagnosis and increased patient survival; its expression was inversely associated with N-*myc* expression (77).

Ganglioside GD2 is one of the sialic acid-containing glycosphyngolipids found mainly in the cell surface membrane. Increased circulating levels may be another marker of disease activity and response to treatment (favorable prognosis level is less than 103 pmol/mL, unfavorable prognosis level is greater than 568 pmol/mL). Shed gangliosides may accelerate tumor progression, and anti-GD2 antibodies may be useful in treating NB (5,78,79).

Tables 4 and 5 categorize patients according to several clinical and biologic criteria (25,80).

SCREENING FOR NB

Because the prognosis of NB is better for younger children than older children, and because prognosis is also related to stage, it has been postulated that the tumor progresses, in an orderly manner, from early to more advanced disease. If the tumor could be diagnosed at an earlier stage in younger patients, the argument continues, then the probability of cure of NB in the overall population would be improved. This has led to the idea that with broad-based population screening of infants one might diagnose NB preclinically and achieve a vastly improved survival.

Mass screening is accomplished by parents collecting urine from their infant children by blotting filter papers against wet diapers. The filter paper is allowed to dry and is mailed to a central screening center. At the center urine is tested for the presence of excessive catecholamine metabolites (vanillymandelic and homovanillic acids). Samples are tested with techniques such as high-pressure liquid chromatography. Positive or borderline results are usually examined in more detail with gas-chromatography/mass spectrometry. Parents of children with abnormal results are contacted for confirmatory testing of the child, physical and radiographic examinations, and treatment as necessary.

The counter-argument to mass screening for NB is that it is not clear if NB does grow, in an orderly fashion, from early to more advanced disease such that it can be detected preclinically. If, in fact, advanced disease with adverse biologic factors develops without detectable step-wise progression through earlier disease with more favorable biologic characteristics, then screening may not detect tumors "before" they become more difficult to treat. Furthermore, it has already been noted that there is a fair incidence of NB *in situ* in the adrenals of infants in autopsy series—far more than the clinical incidence of NB. Perhaps NB *in situ,* or the equivalent, appears in many infants and spontaneously regresses. If so, then broad-based population screening may detect children with this entity and subject them to treatment when, in fact, the patients would have done just as well if left alone and the tumors allowed to spontaneously regress. In this sense, the counter-argument concludes, some children will be given a *diagnosis* when they never had, nor will have, a *disease.*

The costs and benefits of mass screening have now been tested in several countries and results are available for critical analysis. Consider some of the pertinent questions related to the use of mass screening for NB.

(1) *Has broad-based population screening affected the incidence of NB?*

There is no doubt that screening has produced a sharp rise in the incidence of NB. In the Quebec Neuroblastoma Screening Project, the Standardized Incidence Ratio for NB rose 2.17-fold (an increase from 54.5 expected cases of NB in the screened population to 118, $p < 0.0001$) (81). In Niigata Prefecture, Japan, screening increased the cumulative incidence of NB at 5 years of age from 10.5/100,000 live births to 18.6 (82). Screening in Saitama Prefecture, Japan, was associated with an increase in the incidence rate of NB in children less than 1 year of age from 27.9 per 10^6 population to 260.4 (83). In a large-scale study based on the Japan Children's Cancer Registry, the annual incidence rate for NB in children less than 1 year of age ranged from 23.6 to 34.13 cases per 10^6 population before screening and rose to 150.6 with screening (84,85).

(2) *Is there a difference in tumors detected by population screening and those found clinically?*

Although population-screening for NB increases the incidence of the diagnosis, the types of cases identified by screening are strikingly different from those found clinically (86,87). In the Quebec Neuroblastoma Screening Project, for example, 67% of the children diagnosed by screening had INSS stage 1, 2, or 4S disease whereas 53% of the patients diagnosed with NB who were missed by screening or were never screened had INSS stage 3 or 4 disease (81). In Miyagi Prefecture, Japan, of 18 children who had screened negative but later developed NB 12 had stage IV disease and 3 had stage III. Most had unfavorable histological features and/or amplified N-*myc* (52). There is also a higher incidence of more favorable histology in patients diagnosed at screening than those found clinically (88). Most cases diagnosed at screening have favorable biological parameters such as absence of amplification of N-*myc*, hyperdiploidy, normal serum levels of neuron specific enolase or ferritin, or absence of the chromosome 1p deletion (89–91).

Favorable NB, associated with a young age, early stage at diagnosis, and favorable biological characteristics, appears to be easily detected by screening and is associated with a favorable outcome. Unfavorable NB presents at an older age, with an advanced stage, and with unfavorable biological characteristics. Screening at or before 6 months of age does not appear to reduce the incidence of advanced stage NB in older age groups (84,85).

(3) *Does mass screening affect mortality from NB?*

The most satisfactory way to evaluate the value of screening is to document its efficacy in decreasing mortality rates (15,92). Some of the studies from Japan suggest a decrease in the mortality rate from NB associated with mass population screening (68,82,93,94). It has been suggested that other factors, including improved methods of treatment, may also influence the drop in mortality (95,96). Unfortunately, none of the studies in Canada, Europe, or Australia has yet shown any advantage of screening in terms of a decrease in mortality (91). It must be recognized, however, that most of the studies are too small to detect a small impact on survival if it exists (81,95,97,98).

(4) *If mass screening detects early tumors that are unlikely to progress to advanced, life-threatening disease, would it be possible to deal with such tumors by follow-up with imaging studies and measurements of urine catecholamines and other tumor markers instead of surgery, chemotherapy, and radiotherapy?*

In excess of 20 children, diagnosed with early stage NB by population screening, have been managed with observation alone. In most there has been a gradual decline in the level of circulating tumor markers and tumor size. Those in whom the tumor was ultimately resected because of tumor growth have generally had ganglioneuroma or ganglioneuroblastoma with scanty foci of neuroblasts (84,85,95,99,100).

(5) *Is it possible that mass screening would be useful if it were used for older children, as opposed to 6-month olds?*

In Austria screening has been performed on 7- to 12-month olds. Only a slight increase in the incidence of NB has been found in the screened group when compared to an unscreened control group. In the cases detected by screening, 13 of the 18 either had advanced stage, unfavorable histology, N-*myc* amplification, unfavorable DNA index, and/or HVA/VMA ratio greater than 1. This hints at the possibility that screening at an older age may, in fact, detect more advanced disease earlier than it would have been detected by routine clinical means (101). Whether screening repeated at a later time, such as 12 months of age, would lead to a higher rate of detection of biologically aggressive NB is unknown (92).

(6) *How will we resolve the questions concerning the value of screening for NB?*

It can be hoped that, with longer follow-up of screened populations, the full effect of screening on NB mortality in Japan, Canada, France, and the United Kingdom will be established. In addition a geographically controlled trial has been started in Germany in which 1.25 million babies will be screened and 1.25 million babies will remain unscreened. Such a large scale trial may be able to resolve some of the outstanding questions (102).

SELECTION OF THERAPY

NB is responsive to chemotherapy and radiation therapy. However, for those patients with localized disease, surgical resection alone is frequently sufficient. Other patients with localized disease have characteristics which necessitate additional treatment, including chemotherapy and possibly radiation therapy. Although those children with disseminated disease will respond to cytotoxic therapy, permanent disease eradication is infrequently achieved. It is only with intensive regimens, including bone marrow transplantation, that the cure rate of patients with advanced stage disease may be increasing. As is clear from the previous sections in this chapter, stage, age, and biologic features of each child NB must be considered in determining treatment.

Surgery

Surgery has both a diagnostic and therapeutic role. If the diagnosis has not been established by bone marrow aspirate, biochemical testing, or skin biopsy, surgery will provide histologic confirmation of malignancy. Even in the presence of a clear, nonsurgically determined diagnosis of NB, a tissue sample is important for cytogenetic analysis.

As previously stated, 20% to 40% of children present with localized disease. In children without evidence of metastatic disease, an attempt at resection is warranted if substantial morbidity (sacrifice of vital structures) can be avoided. Complete excision of the primary tumor in localized disease is associated with a very high likelihood of cure irrespective of the patient's age (103) (Table 6). For patients younger than 2 years and ED stage I or POG stage A disease, the cure rate may exceed 90% (104). If the tumor is localized but unresectable due to its intimate relationship with major blood vessels or other characteristics, the proper extent of surgery is not clear—particularly in young children, whose prognosis is excellent. Although reductive surgery prior to chemotherapy or irradiation has been advocated (105), the efficacy of such cytoreduc-

TABLE 6. *Disease-free survival in localized, totally resected, node-negative neuroblastoma (POG stage A) treated with surgery alone*

Institution or Cooperative group[a]	n	Relapse-free survival (%)
POG (145)	101	89
SJCRH (87,88)	16	94
Duke (76)	2	100
Institut Gustave-Roussy (190)	12	92
JW Riley (70)	5	100
CCSG (53)[b]	27	100
ICGN (48)	17	85
CCG Trials (124,125, 125a)		94

[a]POG, Pediatric Oncology Group; SJCRH, St. Jude Children's Research Hospital; CCG or CCSG, Children's Cancer Study Group; ICGN, Italian Cooperative Group on Neuroblastoma.
[b]Radiotherapy given at the investigator's discretion.

tion is unproven (47,49). However, even when the primary tumor is unresectable, defining its extent remains important for staging and determining optimal additional therapy.

Second-look surgical procedures are commonly used in NB. Chemotherapy and/or irradiation may produce significant interval regression of a bulky primary tumor (46,106, 107). In a POG report, 62% of children with POG stage B disease achieved a complete clinical or surgically documented response following chemotherapy (108). For patients with residual tumor, surgery may then be performed to achieve a complete response (49,106–108,109). Those children who have localized NB converted to a resectable status by interval therapy, and who undergo complete excision, have a reasonable prognosis. An intent of completely resecting the primary tumor also appears valid for patients with advanced disease (ED stage II with N-*myc* amplification, stage III, and perhaps selected patients with stage IV disease) where eventual complete excision can be accomplished in up to 60% to 65% of patients (110). In this situation, resection following chemotherapy appears to be associated with fewer complications than resection prior to chemotherapy (108). The Italian Cooperative Group for Neuroblastoma (ICGN) has reported 145 patients with localized inoperable NB or primary tumor excised with a "tumor residue more than 2 mL." Ninety-four of the 145 (65%) achieved a complete or partial response with chemotherapy, and 75 (52%) subsequently underwent complete resection.

Although the status of lymph nodes adherent to or removed with the primary tumor does not appear to predict prognosis (111), lymph nodes which are distinct (usually superior or inferior, but especially if bilateral or contralateral) from the tumor are ideally sampled. This, however, may be difficult for some patients with cervical or thoracic tumors, or infiltrative unresectable abdominal primaries. The utility of other prognostic factors suggests that aggressive attempts to acquire this information is unwarranted. Beyond this, a POG report suggests that infants with regional nodal metastases (stage C) have a favorable prognosis with limited postoperative chemotherapy, which is similar to that of infants with POG stage B NB (60). A liver biopsy should be done at the time of surgery for intraabdominal primary tumors because hepatic involvement may remain undetected by current imaging techniques (6, 48,49,112–114), although a report of children older than 1 year with POG stage C disease (INSS stage 2B and 3) questions this rationale (115). If radiotherapy is contemplated, clips should be used to mark the tumor.

The role of radical surgery in children with disseminated (stage IV) NB is uncertain (59). Some children with stage IV disease who, on clinical and radiologic grounds achieved a complete or good remission, underwent a surgical exploration in a cooperative group study (113). In 10 children no residual tumor was found, and four of these children are alive and free of tumor 3.5 to 5 years following diagnosis. Of the 62 patients in whom residual tumor was found, total resection was achieved in 34, but only six children remained free of disease. Therefore, removal of the primary tumor in stage IV disease probably does not confer a survival advantage. This experience is supported by other data, which suggest that the outcome for a patient with stage IV NB predominantly depends on the biologic aggressiveness of the tumor, not including its resectability or the actual extent of resection achieved (116). However, surgical evaluation may nevertheless be helpful in directing further therapy by identifying children with persistent and/or unresectable tumor. In addition, the increasing importance of biologic markers in the management of NB makes it important to obtain an adequate biopsy specimen to analyze molecular pathology (11).

Dumbbell tumors are, if treated surgically, dealt with by a two-stage procedure. The extraspinal component of the tumor is removed at a first operation. The extradural, intraspinal portion of the tumor is removed later. If, however, there is evidence of spinal cord compression and surgery is used, the laminectomy is performed first (117). Many institutions prefer to treat spinal cord compression with chemotherapy as discussed elsewhere in this chapter.

Infants with a small primary tumor and extensive liver metastases (stage IV-S) will, on occasion, require special surgical considerations. The enlarging liver may compromise respiratory function from upward pressure on the diaphragm, or compress the inferior vena cava or renal vein. If chemotherapy and/or local irradiation do not adequately reduce hepatic size, a Silastic sheet may be inserted in the abdominal wall to allow room for liver expansion and reduce compression of vital structures (6). Resection of the primary tumor does not influence survival in stage IV-S (56).

Radiation Therapy

Indications concerning the use of radiation therapy (RT) in children with NB continue to be refined by progress in devising effective chemotherapy and the desirability of avoiding unnecessarily aggressive treatment regimens in the young child, all on the backdrop of the recalcitrant nature of the NB in many children. NB cells in culture are generally radiosensitive (118–122), though radiation responsiveness of NB in patients is less predictable (see subsequent section entitled "Dose"). In discerning the optimal use of RT in NB, caution is necessary in interpreting reports because of the differences in staging systems used and thus the differences in patient populations treated.

LOW-RISK DISEASE

Postoperative radiotherapy is unnecessary if the primary tumor is completely excised in low-risk, localized, node-negative NB. Total surgical excision cures the majority of these children regardless of age, urinary VMA and HVA ratios, or histologic patterns (48,49,53,104,123,124). A prospective POG study of 101 children with POG stage A disease treated with surgery alone demonstrated a 2-year disease-free survival of 89% and overall survival (with salvage therapy) of 97% (104). Most recurrences were noted within one year of diagnosis, and 6 of the 9 children who relapsed were cured with chemotherapy. In Children's Cancer Group Study 3881 of ED stage I disease, the 3-year survival rate was 99% with surgery alone (53,125). Matthay et al. (53) reported outcomes in 156 patients with INSS stage 2A (ED stage II). No significant benefit was associated with the use of either chemotherapy or irradiation (53). The outcome for 75 patients treated with surgery alone was similar to that of 66 patients receiving radiotherapy (6-year progression-free survival 89% versus 94%). For the subgroup of patients with residual (postsurgical) gross or microscopic disease, survival was not influenced by the use of irradiation. Kushner et al. (126) reported 10 disease-free survivors of INSS Stage 1 NB treated with surgery alone. Six had positive margins. Some patient's tumors were diploid or N-*myc* amplified (126).

Because local control and survival rates are in excess of 90% in low-risk disease, it is unlikely that postoperative irradiation would make a positive contribution (Tables 6 and 7). The prognosis for children with localized and resected node-negative disease is excellent, and chemotherapy is indicated only in the setting of recurrence (104). The current POG/Children's Cancer Group Protocol of low-risk disease (Study P9641) treats with surgery alone. Chemotherapy is generally reserved for recurrent or progressive tumor. Radiation therapy is reserved for the vary rare instances of local recurrence in spite of surgery and chemotherapy.

TABLE 7. *Survival in Evans-D'Angio stage II and/or localized node-negative neuroblastoma and in Evans-D'Angio stage III and/or localized node-positive neuroblastoma: comparison of irradiated and nonirradiated patients*

Institution[a]	Survival	Percent	Comment	Reference
Stage II and/or localized node-negative patients				
Not irradiated				
CCSG[b]	67/75	89	E-D stage II	126
CHOP	8/10	80	E-D stage II	106
Oklahoma	6/6	100	E-D stage II, <1 year old	143
HSC	4/5	80	E-D stage II	138
SJCRH	15/15	100	SJCRH stage II	87, 88
SJCRH/POG	53/61	87	POG B (E-D stage II = 47, E-D stage III = 14) (RT in 3)	144
ICGN[c]	16/22	73	E-D stage II, unresectable	63
Irradiated				
CCSG[b]	62/66	94	E-D stage II	126
CHOP	6/10	60	E-D stage II	106
Denmark[d]	5/8	63	E-D stage II	29
Duke	6/7	86	E-D stage II	76
Florida	7/7	100	E-D stage II	99
HSC	19/24	79	E-D stage II	138
Indiana	23/31	74	E-D stage II	70
SJCRH	9/9	100	SJCRH stage IIA	87, 88
Stage III and/or localized node-positive patients				
Not irradiated				
CHOP	1/9	11	E-D stage III	106
SJCRH	11/27	41	SJCRH stage III A(N)	87, 88
ICGN[d]	11/15	73	POG stage B or C	48
POG	12/29	41	POG stage C	25
ICGN[e]	67/129	52	E-D stage III, unresectable	63
Irradiated				
Columbia	8/13	62	Regional disease, subtotal resection	114
CHOP	6/7	86	E-D stage III	106
Denmark[f]	0/3	0	E-D stage III	29
Duke	9/13	69	E-D stage III	76
	6/9	67	POG stage C	
Florida	10/14	71	E-D stage III	99
JCRT	13/16	81	E-D stage III	168, 169
JCRT	21/25[g]	84	E-D stage III	119, 120
ICGN[d]	9/14	64		48
POG	24/33	73	POG stage C	35

With the development of INSS Staging, Molecular Biological Markers, Identification of Risk Group, and more selective use of radiation therapy, these studies provide historical background and context for more recent evaluations of treatment.

[a]CHOP, Children's Hospital of Philadelphia; SJCRH, St. Jude Children's Research Hospital; ICGN, Italian Cooperative Group on Neuroblastoma; JCRT, Harvard/Joint Center for Radiation Therapy; POG, Pediatric Oncology Group, CCSG, Children's Cancer Study Group; HSC, Hospital for Sick Children, London.

[b]156 patients in total. The CCSG is reporting 6-year progression-free survival.

[c]Some of these patients may have been irradiated.

[d]Listed as tumor excision ± radiation against tumor bed, 1966–1980.

[e]Randomized prospective trial of radiotherapy versus no radiotherapy in children with minimal residual disease following surgery or with lymph node involvement. Results are relapse-free survival.

[f]A small proportion of these patients were irradiated.

[g]Failure-free local control. Radiotherapy was administered to 16/25 patients, primarily those with postchemotherapy, postsurgical residual disease.

INTERMEDIATE RISK DISEASE

In 1950, Wittenborg (127) described a beneficial effect of postoperative irradiation if gross residual tumor remained after surgery. In 1967, Perez et al. (128) reported a 41% (9/22) 5-year survival in children treated with limited surgical resection and postoperative irradiation. Only 1 of the 22 patients received adjuvant chemotherapy. The sentinel historical series supporting adjuvant irradiation is in a 1967 paper by Lingley et al. (24), showing local control in 13 of 13 children with regional disease (in retrospect, stages II to III and B to C) following incomplete resection and irradiation. Eight of 13 were long-term survivors.

For children on the more favorable end of the spectrum of localized NB, a multiplicity of studies both demonstrate and deny a survival advantage from the use of radiation therapy (Table 7). Among those which do not argue for systematic RT are the following: a prospective POG study of 61 children with POG stage B disease (E to D system: stage II = 47, stage III = 14) treated with chemotherapy followed by surgery demonstrated a 3-year disease-free survival probability of 84% (108). With censoring of three remission deaths, only 1 of 32 infants failed versus 7 of 29 children older than 1 year. Only three patients were treated with RT as a component of salvage therapy. Yet it remains possible that RT might have benefited the older children had it been given. Koop and colleagues (32,112) reported no difference in 2-year survival in ED stage II postoperatively irradiated patients (6 of 10 alive) compared to nonirradiated patients (8 of 10 alive). Thomas et al. (129) could identify no benefit for radiotherapy in 43 children with stage I to III disease. Of 34 stage II cases treated with surgery and irradiation, with or without chemotherapy, Zucker and Margulis (130) reported a 76% 5-year survival. However, 5 of 6 children treated with surgery and chemotherapy alone remained disease-free. Carlsen et al. (59) were unable to demonstrate any clear effect of therapy on long-term survival in stage I to II children; the small benefit that did exist was ascribed to chemotherapy. As previously noted, Matthay et al. (53) reviewed the records of 156 patients and found no benefit to chemotherapy and/or irradiation in stage II. Garaventa et al. (62) found no additive benefit to radiation therapy to the primary site for locally advanced disease beyond chemotherapy alone in 145 patients.

Conversely, several other studies suggest a benefit from RT for children with ED stage II disease. A retrospective review of stage II patients from Indiana University (6,131) showed 100% disease-free survival in 17 patients treated with postoperative irradiation. In four patients initially treated with surgery alone, one locally recurred and was successfully salvaged with RT. The Harvard-Joint Center for Radiation Therapy (JCRT) also systematically irradiated patients with excellent results. Data for children over 1 year of age in the Indiana and JCRT series document survival in 9 of 9 and 17 of 19, respectively (6,64,131,132). An update of the JCRT experience with 25 stage III patients over 1 year of age noted that RT was administered to 16 children, primarily for postchemotherapy, postsurgical residual disease (mean dose 23.81 ± 4.79 Gy). At a median follow-up of 85 months, there was a 72% event-free survival with failure-free local control in 21 of 25 patients (133). Overall, it would appear that RT for patients with favorable localized disease (2A in the INSS) is not warranted. This may also apply to infants with regional disease (INSS 2B/3) (134).

For children with localized NB on the less favorable end of the spectrum (i.e., advanced regional disease), several reports support a survival advantage from the use of RT (Table 7). Data identify a subgroup of patients with stage III disease who require additional treatment, namely, those older than 1 year with N-*myc* amplification. For these children the event-free survival is only 60% even with aggressive chemotherapy (135). In fact, generalizations for children with ED stage III disease are problematic because nodal sampling is not required in the ED classification system. In stage III patients, well before the period of biological staging, Koop and Johnson (112) found that postoperative irradiation improved survival (6 of 7 versus 1 of 9 patients alive with and without postoperative irradiation, respectively). It may be important to consider the influence of nodal involvement upon the effectiveness of radiation therapy within the subgroup of patients with ED stage III disease. At St. Jude Children's Research Hospital (SJCRH) where treatment generally included only surgery and chemotherapy (67), 16 of 26 (62%) children with localized, unresectable stage III lymph node-negative NB survived compared to 11 of 33 (33%) with positive nodes. In children over 1 year of age with positive nodes, survival was 17% (4 of 23). This poor outcome in node-positive patients has been confirmed by others (131a). In contrast, at Duke and the JCRT, postoperative wide-field irradiation has been used for node-positive patients (63,64,132,133,136,137). Little survival difference has been seen between node-positive and node-negative patients when RT is used. A review of the Duke experience in localized neuroblastoma, compared 21 irradiated patients (1 stage A, 11 stage B, 9 stage C; 67% more than 1-year old) to 12 patients not irradiated (4 each stages A to C, 42% more than 1-year old). All underwent initial surgery and 18 of 33 (55%) received chemotherapy. Ten-year survival of the higher risk irradiated patients was not significantly different from the unirradiated patients (70% versus 82%, $p = 0.33$). The probability of tumor relapse with a local component being part of the relapse was higher in the unirradiated patients (58% versus 5%, $p = 0.001$) (71). Survival rates at Duke and JCRT for node-positive patients are, respectively, 64% and 84%. One may speculate that the improved survival in the Duke and the JCRT node-positive patients relates to wide-field irradiation covering nodal drainage areas of the tumor bed. The impressive results of Jacobson (10 of 14 alive), also in stage III, support a recommendation for systematic irradiation in advanced local disease (138). A POG study randomized stage C patients older than 1 year to receive postoperative chemotherapy or

chemotherapy plus regional RT (24 to 30 Gy, 16 to 20 fractions) (115). Of 62 eligible patients, in the CT arm 45% and 31% achieved complete remission and remain disease-free, respectively, at a median of 35 months, and in the CT/RT arm 67% and 58% achieved complete remission and remain disease-free, respectively, at a median of 23 months. When Castleberry et al. (60) analyzed the data according to other staging systems, the RT/CT arm would appear superior for ED stage III and INSS stage 2B and 3. However, the Italian Cooperative Group of Neuroblastoma randomized children over 1 year of age with minimal residual tumor following surgery or with lymph node involvement to receive 20 to 30 Gy of irradiation versus no radiotherapy, and all the patients received Peptichemio. The relapse-free survival was the same between the two treatment groups (123).

In POG Study 8743, relying on chemotherapy (cyclophosphamide/doxorubicin and/or cisplatin/VM26) and surgery, for infants with hyperdiploid, N-*myc* nonamplified, POG stage B, INSS stage 2A disease, the 3-year disease-free-survival rate was 96% (139). In POG Study 8742 of children with stage C disease, RT was given to those patients not in complete remission following second-look surgery. Chemotherapy was cisplatin/VP-16 alternating with cyclophosphamide/doxorubicin. Retrospectively 8 patients had INSS 2A, 10 INSS 2B, and 36 INSS 3. The overall 3-year survival was 68% and N-*myc* and Shimada histology were significant predictors of outcome. The impact of RT on survival could not be determined in the study, because it was assigned nonrandomly and the majority of patients were not irradiated (140–142).

In summary, for POG stage B disease (ED stage I to III with negative lymph nodes), the value of postoperative radiotherapy is undetermined. Newer staging systems, based upon biologic markers such as oncogene amplification, may help determine which patients require adjuvant therapy (58). In ED stage III and/or with positive lymph nodes (POG stage C), there is a body of evidence that suggests that radiotherapy may increase the probability of survival and tumor local control. The most recent available trials, however, indicate that patients with N-*myc* nonamplified and favorable ploidy do reasonably well with surgery and chemotherapy. Patients with amplified N-*myc* clearly require improved methods of local and systemic control. It is a testable research question as to whether more aggressive irradiation will be of benefit to these patients. Until prospective data are available based on INSS staging, no unequivocable recommendations can be made regarding the efficacy of radiotherapy in children with intermediate risk disease.

The most recent POG/Children's Cancer Group Study for intermediate risk disease utilizes surgery to provide diagnostic material at diagnosis and to attempt maximal safe resection of the primary tumor after chemotherapy. Chemotherapy includes cyclophosphamide, doxorubicin, carboplatin, and etoposide. The duration of chemotherapy is based on the biologic risk factors. Radiation therapy is limited to situations where there is clinical deterioriation despite chemotherapy and surgery or persistent tumor after chemotherapy and second-look surgery (Children's Cancer Group/POG Protocol A3961).

HIGH-RISK DISEASE

Children older than 1 year with stage IV disease rarely survived prior to the use of aggressive multiagent chemotherapeutic regimens. Early attempts to use irradiation to cure children with advanced NB included the use of large-volume RT, either "segmental" or "sequential" fields with fractionated or single doses. Neither Sagerman (143) nor Green et al. (110) demonstrated efficacy of this technique in advanced disease. Helson et al. (144) treated eight children with stage IV NB with sequential hemibody irradiation (HBI) and combination chemotherapy. Two of the children survived free of disease at 12 and 15 months following HBI.

Fractionated total-body irradiation (TBI) has been studied by Kun et al. (145). Six stage IV patients initially achieved a complete re-mission with cyclophosphamide and adriamycin along with surgical resection of the primary tumor, local irradiation to the gross residual tumor, and adjuvant low-dose rate fractionated TBI (1 to 1.2 Gy in 10 fractions). No improvement in survival was seen. Better results were obtained by D'Angio and Evans (146) with 1 to 1.5 Gy of TBI in 50-cGy daily fractions along with each 3-week cycle of chemotherapy. A 32% actuarial survival at 24 months was reported.

With the use of aggressive, intensive chemotherapy, some older stage IV children will survive (147–150). A report from Memorial Sloan-Kettering Cancer Center described 22 children with stage IV NB who received cyclophosphamide, adriamycin, vincristine, cisplatin, VP 16, and monoclonal antibody. Surgical resection of the primary was generally done. Following chemotherapy, patients received consolidation irradiation to the primary site, based on the prechemotherapy volume, to a dose of 21 Gy at 1.5 Gy b.i.d. With a median follow-up of 18 months, 15 of 22 patients remained in remission (151). A report from Japan described a program of intensive chemotherapy and treatment of primary disease with surgery and radiation for a group of children with stage IV disease over 1 year of age—although a few patients with stage III disease and/or younger than 1 year of age were included. The 5-year event-free survival was 39% (152). The Children's Cancer Group Protocol 321P2 used a dose-intensive combination of four chemotherapeutic agents and enrolled 259 children over 1 year of age with stage IV and high-risk stage III disease. The 4 year progression-free survival was 26% (37,153).

Several attempts to cure older stage IV children have used autologous or allogeneic bone marrow transplantation, with or without TBI as a component of the preparatory regimen. Table 8 summarizes some of these recent studies. The event-free survival, for most reports, is on the order of 20% to 40%—although there is continued force of mortality as the follow-up increases. It is not clear if purging the marrow prior to reinfusion is neces-

TABLE 8. *Recent studies of bone marrow transplantation for advanced neuroblastoma (stages III–IV, C or D, or INSS 3–4)*

Reporting institution or group, year of report	Number of patients	Progression-free survival or event-free survival	Preparative regimen	Purging of the marrow?
CCSG, 1991 (176)	46	40% at 4 years	VM26, Doxo, MLP, CDDP, TBI	Yes
ENSG, 1987 (160)	32	34% at 6 years	MLP, no TBI	No
AIEOP, 1991 (49)	53	29% at 5 years	VM26, Doxo, MLP, CDDP, TBI	No
MSKCC, 1991 (111)	28	6% at 2 years	MLP, TBI	Yes
Japanese institutions, 1990 (133,173)	21	78% at 2 years, 63% at 4 years	Various regimens	Unknown
LMCE, 1991 (158)	62	40% at 2 years, 20% at 4 years, 13% at 7 years	VCR, MLP, TBI	Yes
French Multicenter Trial, 1987 (80)	33	40% at 2 years	MLP, VM26, BCNU, No TBI	Yes
POG, 1991 (65)		32% for patients transplanted in first CR, 43% in first PR	MLP, TBI	Yes
Japanese institutions, 1994[a] (132,133)	22	72% at 3 years	CDDP, MP16, THP-Doxo (in some patients), MLP, TBI (except for children <1 year of age without N-*myc* amplification)	Yes
CCG Protocol 321P3, 1996 (123,125,193)	131	37% at 6 years	VP16 or VM 26, Doxo, CDDP, TBI, L-phenylalanine mustard	Yes
Bone Marrow Transplantation Registry of AIEOP, 1996 (62)	108	31% at 8 years for those grafted in first CR, 20% in first PR, 29% in second or greater CR; 5% at 20 months for those grafted in second PR or greater	Usually vincristine, MLP, TBI	No
Three Australian Institutions, 1995 (116)	17	87% at 5 years	CDDP, VM26, Doxo, MLP, TBI	No
University of Chicago, 1995 (186)	26	39% at 5 years	TBI with either Cyclo or Cyclo/VP16 or Carboplatin/VP16 or Carboplatin/VP16/Thiotepa, CDDP/VP16/MLP, or CDDP/DTIC/VP16	Unknown: approximately one-half of the patients received allogeneic transplants
Study Group of Japan, 1995[a] (146)	31	50% at 5 years	MLP with/without VP16 or MLP/CDDP/THP-Doxo/with or without VP16; 6 of the 31 patients received TBI	Unknown; some patients received allogeneic transplants

Most series largely consist of children older than 365 days of age receiving bone marrow transplantation as primary therapy.

CCSG, Children's Cancer Study Group; ENSG, European Neuroblastoma Study Group; AIEOP, Italian Association for Pediatric Hematology-Oncology; MSKCC, Memorial Sloan-Kettering Cancer Center; LMCE, Lyons, Marseilles, Paris, East of France group; POG, Pediatric Oncology Group; Doxo, doxorubicin; THP-Doxo, Tetrahydropynyl doxorubicin; MLP, melphalan; CDDP, cisplatinum; VCR, vincristine; TBI, total-body irradiation; CR, complete remission; PR, partial remission.

[a]These three studies probably include some common patients.

sary. Some programs include marrow purging and some do not. Similarly, the necessity of TBI in the preparative program is not established and some institutions utilize it while others do not (154,155).

Although the necessity of TBI in bone marrow transplantation for neuroblastoma is not clear, there is a reasonable body of evidence supporting the use of local radiotherapy boosts to the primary site and bulky metastatic sites. Disease recurrence following bone marrow transplantation for NB is most common at previous sites of disease. Local irradiation, delivered either in preparation for the transplant or afterwards is able to significantly reduce the risk of relapse at these sites (156). In a POG study, a boost of 12 Gy in 1.2 Gy b.i.d. fractions was delivered to patients with persistent disease prior to TBI. There was an advantage in complete response rates and survival attendant to the use of the boost irradiation (157). Ikeda et al. and Kushner et al. have both reported a reduction in primary site failure rates in patients who received local boosts with radiotherapy as part of the transplant procedure (156). Sibley et al., from the University of Chicago, showed a reduction in local failures at those sites amenable to a radiotherapy boost (156). Preliminary results from a Children's Hospital of Boston/Dana–Farber Cancer Institute study of double autologous stem cell transplant using chemotherapy-based conditioning for the first transplant, melphalan/TBI for the second transplant, and selected local RT to the primary site hints at reduced local failure rates (158). The Children's Cancer Group has described 99 patients who underwent treatment with chemotherapy, surgery, and myeloablative chemotherapy plus total body irradiation. Patients with residual local disease after surgery receive local irradiation. Twenty-two of the 41 patients with recurrence developed local recurrence: 8 at the primary site alone and 14 locally plus distally. Thirty-five patients received radiotherapy to the primary site and 16 received radiotherapy to bony metastases. There was no difference in local relapse rate with or without irradiation. The two groups, however, were clearly not comparable because the irradiated patients had gross residual disease (37). Perhaps the irradiated patients seemingly equivalent local recurrence rate to the nonirradiated patients is indicative of radiotherapy's ability to improve local control in these higher risk patients (158–161).

Is intensive chemotherapy superior, inferior, or equivalent to intensive chemotherapy plus autologous bone marrow transplantation for children more than 1 year of age with advanced NB (155)? The Children's Cancer Group compared the outcome of stage IV patients treated with identical chemotherapy who then either proceeded to purged autologous bone marrow transplantation or continued on the same chemotherapy for 1 year. The decision to transplant was nonrandom and the data analysis was performed using statistical tools to measure the prognostic significance of bone marrow transplantation, rather than efficacy per se (37,162). There was an advantage for bone marrow transplantation for the group as a whole; the most significant advantage was for those children more than 2 years of age at diagnosis, those with bone or bone marrow involvement, those with N-*myc* amplification, and those who had only a partial rather than a complete response to induction chemotherapy. Another nonrandomized trial, from Japan, compared children who received intensive chemotherapy versus those who went on to transplantation. The 5-year event-free survivals were not significantly different between the two groups (152). There is also one randomized trial of the European Neuroblastoma Study Group, albeit with few patients, which favors the use of bone marrow transplantation based on 2-year survival statistics. This difference was not sustained on subsequent analysis (9,149,163). The Children's Cancer Group has accrued over 400 patients to a randomized prospective trial of autologous bone marrow transplantation versus chemotherapy. The results are not yet available (37).

METASTATIC DISEASE TREATED
WITH PALLIATIVE INTENT

Most children with NB will have metastatic disease at presentation (stage IV or POG stage D). Radiotherapy is effective in palliating symptoms secondary to bone and soft tissue metastases. A Duke study assessed the value of palliative radiotherapy for NB by retrospectively studying 40 irradiated bony sites. Pain completely or partially responded at 65% of treated sites. A subsequent recurrence of pain was seen in 23% of initially responding sites. Complete or partial palliation of soft tissue mass effect was seen in 67% of treated sites. A subsequent relapse of mass effect was seen in 28% of initially responding sites (63).

There is some preliminary data concerning palliative treatment of metastatic disease with ^{131}I-MIBG.

STAGE IV-S, INSS 4S, AND
HEPATOMEGALY

Stage IV-S NB was initially established in light of the observation that infants having a localized primary NB with metastases to liver, bone marrow, and/or skin had a surprisingly good prognosis and might require minimal therapy (45,164). Investigations into stage IV-S disease suggest, however, that subgroups may be identified with widely different prognoses. Those patients with favorable IV-S are children between the ages of 2 weeks and 12 months, regardless of the location of their metastases, as well as patients who are younger and have skin metastasis with or without associated liver or bone marrow metastases. The expected survival in this group of patients is approximately 90%. Patients having unfavorable stage IV-S disease are children 6 to 8 weeks of age or younger, particularly without skin metastases (57,165, 166). The survival in this group of patients is approximately 30%, and these patients may require more aggressive therapy. Recent investigations into stage IV-S disease suggest, however, the ability to additionally define prognostic subgroups based on N-*myc* copy number and chromosomal index (55–57). A Dutch study reported that 12% of children with stage 4S, and less than or equal to 3 copies of N-*myc* died versus 69% of those with more than 3 copies (167).

Therapeutic nihilism must not prevent therapeutic intervention when indicated in IV-S cases. A report by Stokes et al. of survival in 12 of 14 IV-S cases with radiotherapy (21 Gy) to the primary tumor and, in most cases, to the liver should be balanced against the need for such therapy and the risk of late sequelae of irradiation (142). Certainly routine radiotherapy is inappropriate in stage IV-S disease, and should only be instituted when disease progression threatens vital organ function (56). Local irradiation is a useful treatment for hepatic enlargement from stage IV-S NB (44–46,168–170). The enlarging liver may induce respiratory compromise from upward pressure on the diaphragm, produce inferior vena cava obstruction, and/or compromise renal perfusion. A 3- to 6-Gy dose of irradiation is usually required to produce a tumor response and is well within the accepted limit of hepatic irradiation tolerance. (This is additionally discussed in the "Radiotherapeutic Management" section.)

Chemotherapy

Chemotherapy is the predominant modality of treatment for most children with NB, although those with favorable, localized disease are clearly an exception. As previously discussed, children with stage I disease are cured by surgery, and the use of adjuvant chemotherapy is superfluous (Table 6). The low relapse rate in stage II disease makes it unclear if chemotherapy is appropriate. The relatively high relapse rate in localized but unresectable stage III disease (35% to 40%) and the almost uniformly fatal outcome in stage IV disease suggest that chemotherapy would be important if effective. The intensity or aggressiveness of chemotherapy generally mirrors the expected aggressiveness of the disease in the patient population under consideration (172).

Children with localized but grossly unresectable NB may have their disease controlled by induction chemotherapy and second-look surgery (60,108,115). The chemotherapy used is considered moderately aggressive and often includes cyclophosphamide, doxorubicin, cisplatin, and teniposide (5,139). A POG study of 61 children with POG stage B disease treated with cyclophosphamide/doxorubicin with crossover to cisplatin/teniposide for patients not achieving CR, and followed by surgery, demonstrated a 3-year disease-free survival probability of 84% (173). Most treatment failures occurred in children over 1 year of age. These same chemotherapeutic agents, used in a somewhat different schedule, have been successful in curing infants with POG stage C disease (3-year disease-free survival 93%) (60). The previously described POG study, which randomized stage C patients older than 1 year to receive postoperative chemotherapy versus chemotherapy/RT, used cyclophosphamide/doxorubicin, followed by these drugs alternating with cisplatin/teniposide, and then additionally administered cisplatin/teniposide for patients not achieving CR (115). Of 62 eligible patients, in the chemotherapy arm 45% and 31% achieved CR and remain disease-free, respectively, at a median of 35 months, and in the chemotherapy/RT arm 67% and 58% achieved CR and remain disease-free, respectively, at a median of 23 months. A JCRT report on 25 children with ED stage III disease treated with surgery and intensive chemotherapy used MADDOC (nitrogen mustard, doxorubicin, cisplatin, dacarbazine, vincristine, cyclophosphamide) or cisplatin and cyclophosphamide induction followed by maintenance MADDOC, followed by RT in 16 children. Event-free survival was 72% at a median of 85 months, and both N-*myc* amplification and unfavorable pathologic characteristics (Shimada system) were associated with a worse prognosis (135). The value of induction chemotherapy and second-look surgery has been observed by others (109). Infants with ED stage IV disease

treated with multiagent chemotherapy have up to a 75% 5-year actuarial event-free survival, confirming their relatively favorable prognosis (174,175).

The most frequent use of chemotherapy in NB will be for children with disseminated disease. All of the previously noted agents have been used in various combinations (32, 46,64,110,114,148,174). Vitamin B_{12}, F3TDR, and papaverine have been incorporated in some treatment programs (8,173). These agents appear to have inhibitory effects on NB cells *in vivo* and stimulate morphologic differentiation (176). Multidrug regimens can produce an initial response in up to 70% of stage IV cases (148) and may improve survival, though such gains remain modest (less than 20% survival) (58,148). POG Protocol 8104 treated children less than 1 year of age with stage D NB with induction chemotherapy plus postinduction surgery. The 5-year actuarial survival was 60% (141). Dose intensification of chemotherapy may improve outcome (177) but is associated with dose-limiting myelosuppression. Attempts to surmount this obstacle have used growth factor support or, most commonly, high-dose chemotherapy with or without TBI followed by bone marrow rescue (Table 8). As we have previously discussed, only one randomized trial of bone marrow transplantation (BMT) has been completed and another one is underway. A clear advantage to BMT versus non-BMT intensive chemotherapy has not been demonstrated (155,178). When autologous BMT is used, an advantage to purging marrow of NB cells has not been shown (155). Studies testing the effectiveness of BMT are ongoing, as are alternate methods (e.g., high-dose continuous infusion) of aggressively administering chemotherapy (69,179). Other strategies to control refractory or advanced disease, obviating severe myelosuppression, include the use of biologic response modifiers or immunotherapy, such as interleukin-2, lymphokine-activated killer cells, and [^{131}I]metaiodobenzylguanidine (180,181).

RADIOTHERAPEUTIC MANAGEMENT

Volume

The volume for irradiation of localized NB is determined by imaging studies and by the operating surgeon's description. If lymph node involvement is suspected or proven, a wide field designed to cover the primary tumor site and nodal drainage areas is appropriate. If the field must cover a portion of the vertebral body, the full width of the bone should be encompassed. This will reduce the severity of subsequent scoliosis and ensure coverage of the regional lymph nodes (63,182). Some controversy surrounds the issue of whether next-echelon lymph nodes (i.e., mediastinal lymph nodes with an upper abdominal primary tumor) need to be irradiated. Relapse in unirradiated next-echelon nodes can occur—albeit usually in conjunction with local and/or distant failure. In the Duke experience of 33 patients with stages A to C, 12 relapsed. Only 1 of the 21 irradiated patients (5%) experienced an in-field failure, whereas 7 of the 12 not receiving radiotherapy (58%) experienced an in-field failure at the time of recurrence ($p = 0.001$). Routine next-echelon nodal irradiation was not given. Five of the 12 patients who suffered a relapse had next-echelon nodal failure (NENF) as a component of relapse; only one case was an isolated NENF (137). Because extensive nodal fields may cause late morbidity as well as impair the ability to give chemotherapy, most radiotherapists cover only the primary tumor volume and immediately adjacent nodal groups. With a dumbbell-shaped tumor, careful attention must be paid to the intraspinal as well as the extravertebral components of the tumor to ensure full coverage.

As previously discussed, radiotherapy may be used for stage IV-S associated hepatomegaly. The entire liver need not be irradiated to induce tumor regression. The therapist may use portals designed to avoid the kidneys and, in girls, the ovaries. We have used two lateral fields, parallel opposed or slightly angled anteriorly, to treat the majority of the liver but spare the kidneys. This is done by placing the posterior border of the lateral field at the anterior aspect of the vertebral body. The ovaries are generally avoided by keeping the inferior border of the field at or above the superior iliac crest. Because the doses of irradiation administered for stage IV-S hepatomegaly are low, usually 3 to 6 Gy in 2 to 4 fractions, it could be argued that the kidneys are in little danger of chronic injury and that the liver could be treated with parallel opposed anterior and posterior fields. The infant kidney is, however, more sensitive to irradiation than is the kidney in older children (183,184). The child with stage IV-S disease has a high likelihood of survival and should not be subjected to a lifetime reduction of glomerular filtration rate. (See additional discussion in the section on Dose.) Stage IV NB with hepatomegaly may be treated for palliation with ports designed to cover the entire liver. The anterior/posterior parallel opposed technique is used.

NB metastases may occur in a wide variety of locations. The bone or soft-tissue site is irradiated with a moderate margin.

Dose

The D_0 for most mammalian tumor cell lines is between 1.3 and 1.5 Gy. The n is usually between 1.5 and 10. Collated data on 11 NB cell lines derived from seven patients indicate moderate cellular radiosensitivity beyond that seen for many other mammalian tumors. The median n for NB is 1.36, and the D_0 is 1.04 Gy (118,120–122,124). This low repair capacity for radiation damage implies that little sparing would result from dose fractionation. This hypothesis has been confirmed by Wheldon et al. (158), who grew human NB as multicellular tumor spheroids (MTS). There was no significant difference in the killing ability of single-dose as compared to split-dose irradiation. The absence of any substantial interfraction repair capacity of MTS may provide a radiobiologic rationale for the treatment of NB with multiple fraction-per-day irradiation. Some NB cell lines have a rapid doubling time. This would also suggest that the overall treatment time of a fractionated course of radiation should be kept short in order to prevent tumor repopulation between fractions. Deacon et al. (185), however, performed *in vitro* split-dose irradiation of a NB cell line and found a small but finite capacity for sublethal damage repair. There may be intrinsic variability in repair capabilities between NB cell lines.

Although NB is relatively radiosensitive in the laboratory, its clinical response to irradiation is variable and in-field recurrences are reported. Possible reasons for this discrepancy include the following: (a) the *in vitro* data may not be indicative of clinical NB. Cell culture techniques may select relatively radiosensitive cell lines (186). (b) NB, characterized by certain microscopic and biochemical characteristics, may actually be a spectrum of diseases. Genomic amplification of N-*myc* has been correlated with the stage and prognosis of NB, suggesting that N-myc may have a role in determining the aggressiveness of human NB (187,188) (see previous sections entitled "Epidemiology and Biology" and "Staging and Prognostic Factors"). Perhaps clinical variability in radiosensitivity is a reflection of the variation in oncogene genomic amplification in NB (186).

In 1950, Wittenborg (127) recommended a dose of 80 to 120 roentgens for gross residual NB remaining after surgery—repeated up to three times if necessary. In an attempt to identify an optimal irradiation dose for primary abdominal NB, Perez et al. (46) analyzed the 2-year survival in 27 patients receiving irradiation. There was only one survivor in five children (20%) receiving less than or equal to 10 Gy. Three of the 10 (30%) children who received 10 to 20 Gy survived, whereas 7 of 12 (58%) children who received more than 20 Gy survived. Data from this retrospective review must, however, be interpreted with great caution because the study does not control for tumor stage, tumor volume, or the patient's age, and patient numbers are small.

In a retrospective review of 20 patients with stage II or III disease receiving postoperative radiotherapy at the University of Florida (138), low doses of irradiation (9 to 20 Gy) were as effective as higher doses (30 to 40 Gy). At Duke, local control as a function of radiation dose has been analyzed in 18 patients treated postoperatively for stage II or III disease (63). All seven patients irradiated with stage II disease were locally controlled with doses of 14.8 to 26.5 Gy. Seven of 11 patients with stage III disease were locally controlled with 12 to 48.4 Gy. Four patients had true in-field recurrences. All the children with local recurrences were older than 18 months at diagnosis, and three had large treatment fields. In two of these cases, the treatment of a large volume of tumor to a dose less than 20 Gy may have contributed to the local failure. An additional retrospective analysis of the dose-response relationship for the local treatment of stage II and III NB has been conducted by Jacobson et al. (187). In children younger than 1 year of age, no local failures were seen with a dose above 12 Gy. In children between 1 and 2 years of age, no local failures were seen with doses as low as 14.4 Gy. In children over 3 years, local failures were seen at 25, 30, 39.6, and 45 Gy. Local control was achieved in 19 of 20 children less than 35 months of age and in 4 of 8 patients 36 months of age or older. A dose/local control analysis for the JCRT also suggests that higher doses are necessary for the control of NB in older patients (64). These data, therefore, suggest that older children may require more vigorous treatment for in-field control of tumor. An age-dependent dose response of NB has been hypothetically explained by a difference in the proportion of clonogenic tumor cells. An analysis of the dose-response relationship was performed at SJCRH on 53 children with POG stage C and D NB who were treated at 73 sites (188). For all disease sites, doses of greater than 25 Gy were associated with significantly improved local control.

As a basic guide, we recommend that children less than 18 months of age, receiving local field curative-intent radiotherapy for microscopic disease, receive at least 15 Gy to wide local fields with a 5- to 10-Gy cone down-boost. Older children, or those with gross disease, are given at least 15 to 20 Gy to the initial volume with a 5- to 10-Gy boost. The use of very small doses to large volumes of tumor is discouraged.

Several investigators have published recommendations for time–dose-fractionation schedules for the irradiation of metastatic NB in bone or soft tissue. The dose recommendations include daily fractions of 2 to 8.5 Gy and total doses of 4 to 32 Gy (7,109,127,128,189,190). In a retrospective evaluation of palliative radiotherapy for NB at Duke (63), there was no evidence of a dose-response relationship. All the total doses utilized in this study, however, were relatively low. The clinician is to be cautioned against selecting too low a dose for palliation of painful bony or soft-tissue lesions. Although the vast majority of children with stage IV NB will die from the malignancy, some will live for one year or more following palliative local treatment. The dose should be adequate to control the symptom for the remainder of the patient's lifetime, yet not be so high as to have a significant likelihood of complications. Fractionation depends on volume. Small fields may be treated with 16 to 20 Gy in 4 or 5 fractions, whereas large volumes are better treated with 2 to 3 Gy/fraction to 20 to 30 Gy. In the preterminal case, where timely pain control is desired with a minimum of trips to the radiotherapy department, one may administer 6 to 8 Gy once or twice with moderate success.

Palliation of hepatomegaly in stage IV-S disease can usually be accomplished by 3 to 6 Gy in 2 to 4 fractions. Regression of the liver may, however, be slow. It is occasionally necessary to repeat the dose. If possible, one should allow a 2- to 3-week interval in order to gauge response. If the dose is repeated such that the cumulative dose reaches 12 to 14 Gy, the infant's kidney should be out of the field of irradiation.

TBI prior to bone marrow transplantation will generally be given in accordance with an investigational protocol. The total doses utilized range from 7.5 to 12 Gy and are usually given in 1 to 6 fractions over 1 to 5 days (191). When local boost irradiation is administered, either before or after the preparatory regimen, the dose is dependent on whether TBI will be a component of the regimen. An appropriate total dose, including the TBI, to local sites is 20 to 30 Gy.

Techniques of Irradiation

Some abdominal and pelvic sites are best treated with parallel-opposed anterior and posterior portals. When possible, multiple fields should be used to spare normal tissues. We have often found three-dimensional reconstruction of bulky localized disease useful. A posterior mediastinal volume may be irradiated with an angled wedged posterior pair of fields. Caution should be exercised, however, in the use of a wedge pair of fields adjacent to the spinal column. The "hot spot" in such therapy may result in an inhomogeneous dose across the growth plate of the bone with a resulting spinal curvature.

RESULTS

The results of treatment by stage are denoted in Tables 6–8 and Figs. 8–12. Almost uniform survival is expected in low risk disease. The survival in intermediate risk patients is on the order of 60% to 80%. For children over 1 year of age with stage 4 disease, approximately 15% to 30% are long-term survivors, although current intensive chemotherapeutic regimens, often with marrow rescue, are encouraging for increased success (155).

COMPLICATIONS

A high incidence of spinal deformity is seen in long-term survivors of NB. Among the most common abnormalities seen are postsurgery/postirradiation kyphosis or scoliosis (182,192). The incidence of these abnormalities in 5-year survivors of NB may be as high as 76%. The factors associated with the development of spinal deformity include (a) irradiation at a very young age, (b) orthovoltage irradiation, (c) asymmetric irradiation of the spine, (d) epidural spread of tumor, and

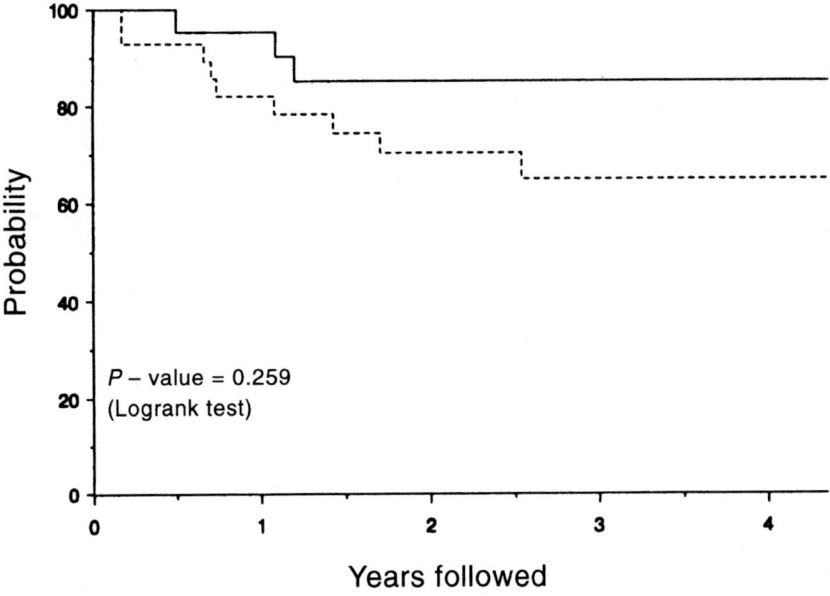

FIG. 12. Event-free survival of patients with INSS Stage 2B or 3 disease treated on Pediatric Oncology Group protocols 8742 and 9244 following complete (solid line) or incomplete (dashed line) resection of disease at diagnosis. (Reproduced from ref. 142, with permission.)

(e) laminectomy. In young children, a laminectomy may result in growth abnormality, gibbus formation, and instability of the spine. The young child with a dumbbell-shaped tumor is therefore at considerable risk for spinal deformity (63,182) (see Chapter 19).

We have observed spinal deformities in children symmetrically irradiated to the spine with a megavoltage beam. The effect of irradiation on the development of paraspinous musculature may contribute to spinal curvature. Successfully treated NB patients must be vigorously followed and observed to detect spinal deformity. Early and proper bracing may be of great benefit.

A portion of the kidney is often irradiated during NB treatment. The radiation tolerance of the adult kidney is fairly well established (20 to 25 Gy). The data for children suggest that renal tolerance is lower. Abnormalities of creatinine clearance were found by Peschel et al. (184) in three infants with stage IV-S disease who received between 12.25 and 14 Gy to one or both kidneys. It is not known if these abnormalities of creatinine clearance will be clinically significant.

FUTURE INVESTIGATIONS

Current treatment regimens for NB are risk-based; that is, the biologic characteristics of the tumor are considered together with traditional clinical prognostic factors in determining optimal therapy (Tables 4, 5, and 9). As data are accumulated, the most powerful prognostic determinants will hopefully be discerned. Areas of active investigation include (193–206):

1. Efforts to develop new chemotherapeutic agents or use old ones in novel ways (51,177,179).

2. Megatherapy (high-dose chemotherapy with or without radiotherapy) followed by marrow rescue.

3. Targeted therapy using radiolabeled metaiodobenzylguanidine (MIBG) or semi-specific monoclonal antibodies (63). Phase I and II studies of MIBG indicate a 30% to

TABLE 9. *The International Neuroblastoma Staging system's minimum recommended studies for determining the extent of disease*

Tumor site	Recommended staging tests
Primary tumor	CT and/or MRI scan with three-dimensional measurements. Ultrasound is considered suboptimal for accurate three-dimensional measurement. MIBG scan if available.
Metastatic sites[a]	
Bone marrow	Bilateral posterior iliac crest marrow aspirates and trephine (core) bone-marrow biopsies required to exclude marrow involvement. A single positive site documents marrow involvement. Core biopsies must contain at least 1 cm of marrow (excluding cartilage) to be considered adequate.
Bone	MIBG scan; ^{99m}Tc bone scan is required if MIBG scan is negative or unavailable. Plain radiographs of positive lesions are recommended.
Lymph nodes	Clinical examination (palpable nodes), confirmed histologically; CT scan for nonpalpable nodes (three-dimensional measurement).
Abdomen/liver	CT and/or MRI with three-dimensional measurements. Ultrasound is considered suboptimal for accurate three-dimensional measurement.
Chest	AP and lateral chest radiographs; Chest CT or MRI necessary only if the chest radiograph is positive, or if abdominal mass of lymph node disease extends into the chest.

[a]The MIBG scan is applicable to all sites of disease.
From refs. 25, 26, 31, and 32, with permission.

40% response rate. MIBG may also be combined with chemotherapy as consolidation therapy for bone marrow transplantation or by itself (11).

4. The use of biologic response modifiers or immunotherapy, such as interleukin-2 or lymphokine-activated killer cells (181). The retinoids, such as 13-*cis* and all *trans* retinoic acids, can cause decreased tumor cell proliferation, morphological differentiation, decreased expression of N-*myc*, and increased expression of retinoic acid in NB cell lines. Clinical studies are in progress to assess the potential benefit of these agents (11).

REFERENCES

References particularly recommended for further reading are marked with an asterisk.

1. Farber S. Neuroblastoma. *Am J Dis Child* 1940;60: 749–750(abstr).
2. Gale G, D'Angio G, Uri A, Chatten J, Koop C. Cancer in neonates: the experience at the Children's Hospital of Philadelphia, PA. *Pediatrics* 1982;70: 409–413.
3. Young JL Jr, Ries L, Silverberg E, et al. Cancer incidence, survival and mortality for children younger than 15 years. *Cancer* 1986;58:598–603.
*4. Breslow N, McCann B. Statistical estimation of prognosis of children with neuroblastoma. *Cancer Res* 1971;31:2098–2103.
*5. Brodeur G, Castleberry R. Neuroblastoma. In: Pizzo P, Poplack D, eds. *Principles and practice of pediatric oncology,* 2nd ed. Philadelphia: JB Lippincott, 1993:739–767.
6. Grosfeld JL, Baehner RL. Neuroblastoma: an analysis of 160 cases. *World J Surg* 1980;4:29–38.
7. Voute PA, Hoefnagel C, Marcuse HR, de Kraker J. Detection of neuroblastoma with [131l-meta-iodobenzylguanidine. *Prog Clin Biol Res* 1985;175:389–398.
8. Bernstein M, Leclerc J, Bunin G, et al. A population-based study of neuroblastoma incidence, survival, and mortality in North America. *J Clin Oncol* 1992; 10:323–329.
9. Castleberry RP. Neuroblastoma. *Eur J Cancer* 1997; 33:1430–1438.
10. Castleberry RP. Biology and treatment of neuroblastoma. *Pediatr Clin N Am* 1997;44:919–937.
*11. Ninane J, Pearson ADJ. Neuroblastoma. In: Pinkerton CR, Plowman PN, eds. *Paediatric oncology: clinical practice and controversies, second edition.* London: Chapman & Hall Medical, 1997:443–483.
12. Williams PL, Wendell-Smith CP, Treadgold S. *Basic human embryology.* Philadelphia: JB Lippincott, 1984:98–99.
13. Grosfeld JL. Neuroblastoma. In: Puri P, ed. *Neonatal tumours* Berlin: Springer-Verlag, 1996:29–42.
14. Guin GH, Gilbert EF, Jones B. Incidental neuroblastoma in infants. *Am J Clin Pathol* 1969;51:126–143.
*15. Carlsen N. Neuroblastoma: epidemiology and pattern of regression. Problems in interpreting results of mass screening. *Am J Pediatr Hematol Oncol* 1992; 14:103–110.
16. Brodeur G, Azar C, Brother M, et al. Neuroblastoma: effect of genetic factors on prognosis and treatment. *Cancer* 1992;70:1685–1694.
17. Israel M. Disordered differentiation as a target for novel approaches to the treatment of neuroblastoma. *Cancer* 1993;71:3310–3313.

18. Knudson A, Strong L. Mutations and cancer. Neuroblastoma and pheochromocytoma. *Am J Hum Genet* 1972;24:514–532.

19. Kushner BH, Gilbert F, Helson L. Familial neuroblastoma: case reports, literature review, and etiologic considerations. *Cancer* 1986;57:1887–1893.

20. Brodeur G, Nakagawara A. Molecular basis of clinical heterogeneity in neuroblastoma. *Am J Pediatr Hematol Oncol* 1992;14:111–116.

*21. Joshi V, Cantor A, Brodeur G, et al. Correlation between morphologic and other prognostic markers of neuroblastoma. A study of histologic grade, DNA index, N-*myc* gene copy number, and lactic dehydrogenase in patients in the Pediatric Oncology Group. *Cancer* 1993;71:3173–3181.

22. Oppedal BR, Storm-Mathisen I, Lie SA, Brandtzaeg P. Prognostic factors in neuroblastoma: clinical, histopathologic, and immunohistochemical features and DNA ploidy in relation to prognosis. *Cancer* 1988;62:772–780.

23. Tonini GP, Boni L, Pession A, et al. MYCN oncogene amplification in neuroblastoma is associated with worse prognosis, except in stage 4s: the Italian experience with 295 children. *J Clin Oncol* 1997;15:85–93.

24. Lingley JF, Sagerman RH, Santulli TV, Wolff JA. Neuroblastoma: management and survival. *N Engl J Med* 1967;277:1227–1230.

*25. Look A, Hayes F, Shuster J, et al. Clinical relevance of tumor cell ploidy and N-*myc* gene amplification in childhood neuroblastoma. A Pediatric Oncology Group study. *J Clin Oncol* 1991;9:581–591.

*26. Bowman LC, Castleberry RP, Cantor A, et al. Genetic staging of unresectable or metastatic neuroblastoma in infants: a Pediatric Oncology Group study. *JNCI* 1997;89:373–380.

27. Pochedly C, ed. *Neuroblastoma: tumor biology and therapy*. Boca Raton, FL: CRC Press, 1990.

28. Massad M, Slim MS, Mansour A, Dabbous I, Firzli S, Issa P. Neuroblastoma: report on a 21-year-experience. *J Pediatric Surg* 1986;21:388–391.

*29. Shimada H, Chatten J, Newton WA, et al. Histopathologic prognostic factors in neuroblastic tumors. Definition of subtypes of ganglioneuroblastoma and an age linked classification of neuroblastomas. *J Natl Cancer Inst* 1984;73:405–416.

*30. Joshi V, Cantor A, Altshuler G, et al. Recommendations for modification of terminology of neuroblastic tumors and prognostic significance of Shimada classification. A clinicopathologic study of 213 cases from the Pediatric Oncology Group. *Cancer* 1992;69:2183–2196.

31. Russo C, Cohn SL, Petruzzi MJ, de Alarcan PA. Long-term neurologic outcome in children with opsoclonus-myoclonus associated with neuroblastoma: a report from the Pediatric Oncology Group. *Med Pediatr Oncol* 1997;28:284–288.

32. Koop CE. Nephroblastoma and neuroblastoma. *Am J Surg* 1961;101:566–570.

33. Maris JM, Evans AE, McLaughlin AC, et al. ^{31}P Nuclear magnetic response spectroscopic investigation of human neuroblastoma *in situ*. *N Engl J Med* 1985;312:1500–1505.

34. Dauebenton JD, Fisher RM, Karabus CD, Mann MD. The relationship between prognosis and scintigraphic evidence of bone metastases in neuroblastoma. *Cancer* 1987;59:1586–1589.

35. Heisel MA, Miller HJ, Reid BS, et al. Radionuclide bone scan in neuroblastoma. *Pediatrics* 1983;71:206–209.

36. Humpl T. Neuroblastoma. *World J Urol* 1995;13:233–239.

37. Matthay K, Lukens J, Haase G, et al. Outcome and prognostic factors for 1008 children with neuroblastoma treated from 1989–1995 on Children's Cancer Group (CCG) protocols. Advances in neuroblastoma research, May 22–25, 1996, Philadelphia, PA.

38. Moss T, Reynolds C, Sather H, Romansky S, Hammond G, Seeger R. Prognostic value of immunocytologic detection of bone marrow metastases in neuroblastoma. *N Engl J Med* 1991;324:219–226.

39. LaBrosse EH, Comay E, Bohuan C, Zucker JM, Schweisguth O. Catecholamine metabolism in neuroblastoma. *J Natl Cancer Inst* 1976;57:633–643.

40. Voorhes ML, Gardner LI. Urinary excretion of norepinephrine, epinephrine, and 3-methoxy-4-hydroxymandelic acid by children with neuroblastoma. *J Clin Endocrinol Metab.* 1961;21:321–335.

41. Qualman S, O'Dorisio M, Felshman D, Shimada H, O'Dorisio T. Neuroblastoma: correlation of neuropeptide expression in tumor tissue with other prognostic factors. *Cancer* 1992;70:2005–2012.

*42. Brodeur G, Pritchard J, Berthold F, et al. Revisions of international criteria for neuroblastoma diagnosis, staging and response to treatment. *J Clin Oncol* 1993;11:1466–1477.

43. Cecchetto G, Luzzatto C, Carli M, Guglielmi M, Zanesco L. The role of surgery in non-localized neuroblastoma. Analysis of 59 cases. *Tumori* 1983;69:327–329.

44. Evans AE. Staging and treatment of neuroblastoma. *Cancer* 1980;45:1799–1802.

45. Evans AE, Baum E, Chard R. Do infants with stage IV-S neuroblastoma need treatment? *Arch Dis Child* 1981;56:271–274.

46. Evans AE, D'Angio GJ, Koop CE. Diagnosis and treatment of neuroblastoma. *Pediatr Clin North Am* 1976;23:161–170.

*47. Hayes FA, study coordinator. *Comprehensive care of the child with neuroblastoma: a stage and age oriented study.* St. Louis: Pediatric Oncology Group, 1982.

48. Hayes FA, Green A, Hustu HO, Kumar M. Surgicopathologic staging of neuroblastoma: prognostic significance of regional lymph nodes metastases. *J Pediatr* 1983; 102:59–62.

49. Hayes FA, Green AA. Neuroblastoma. *Pediatr Ann* 1983;12:366–373.

50. Ninane J, Pritchard J, Morris-Jones PH, Mann JR, Malpas JS. Stage II neuroblastoma. Adverse prognostic significance of lymph node involvement. *Arch Dis Child* 1982;57:438–442.

*51. Brodeur GM, Seeger RC, Barrett A, et al. International criteria for diagnosis, staging and response to treatment in patients with neuroblastoma. *J Clin Oncol* 1988;6:1874–1881.

52. Hata Y, Naito H, Sasaki F, et al. Fifteen years' experience of neuroblastoma: a prognostic evaluation according to the Evans and UICC staging systems. *J Pediatr Surg* 1990;25:326–329.

*53. Matthay K, Sather H, Seeger R, et al. Excellent outcome of stage II neuroblastoma is independent of residual disease and radiation therapy. *J Clin Oncol* 1989;7:236–244.

*54. Evans AE, D'Angio G, Sather H, et al. A comparison of four staging systems for localized and regional neuroblastoma: a report from the Childrens' Cancer Study Group. *J Clin Oncol* 1990;8:678–688.

55. Bourhis J, Dominici C, McDowell G, et al. N-*myc* genomic content and DNA ploidy in stage IV-S neuroblastoma. *J Clin Oncol* 1991;9:1371–1375.

56. Haas D, Ablin AR, Miller C, Zoger S, Matthay KK. Complete pathologic maturation and regression of stage IV-S neuroblastoma without treatment. *Cancer* 1988;62:818–825.

57. Wilson P, Coppes M, Solh H, et al. Neuroblastoma stage IV-S: a heterogeneous disease. *Med Pediatr Oncol* 1991;19:467–472.

58. Carlsen NLT, Christenson IBJ, Schroeder H, et al. Prognostic factors in neuroblastomas treated in Denmark from 1943–1980: a statistical estimate of prognosis based on 253 cases. *Cancer* 1986;58:2726–2735.

59. Carlsen NLT, Schroeder H, Bro PV, et al. Neuroblastoma treated at the four major child oncologic clinics in Denmark 1943–1980: an evaluation of 180 cases. *Med Pediatr Oncol* 1985;13:180–186.

60. Castleberry R, Shuster J, Altshuler G. Infants with neuroblastoma and regional lymph node metastases have a favorable outlook after limited postoperative chemotherapy: a Pediatric Oncology Group study. *J Clin Oncol* 1992;10:1299–1304.

61. Coldman AJ, Fryer CJH, Elwood JM, Sonley MJ. Neuroblastoma: influence of age at diagnosis, stage, tumor site, and sex on prognosis. *Cancer* 1980;46:1896–1901.

62. Garaventa A, DeBernardi B, Pianca C, et al. Localized but unresectable neuroblastoma: treatment and outcome of 145 cases. *J Clin Oncol* 1993;11:1770–1779.

63. Halperin EC, Cox EB. Radiation therapy in the management of neuroblastoma: the Duke University Medical Center experience 1967–1984. *Int J Radiat Oncol Biol Phys* 1986;12:1829–1837.

64. Rosen EM, Cassady JR, Frantz CN, Kretschmar C, Levey R, Sallan SE. Neuroblastoma: the Joint Center for Radiation Therapy/Dana-Farber Cancer Institute/Children's Hospital experience. *J Clin Oncol* 1984;2:719–732.

65. Simone JV. The treatment of neuroblastoma. *J Clin Oncol* 1984;2:717–718.

66. Rubie H, Hartmann O, Giron A, et al. Nonmetastatic thoracic neuroblastomas: a review of 40 cases. *Med Pediatr Oncol* 1991;19:253–257.

*67. Green AA, Casper J, Nitschke R, Smith EI, Hayes FA. The treatment of children with localized grossly unresectable (POG Stage B) neuroblastoma. *Proc ASCO* 1985;4:245.

68. Sawada T, Sugimoto T, Tanaka T, et al. Number and cure rate of neuroblastoma cases detected by the mass screening program in Japan: future aspects. *Med Pediatr Oncol* 1987;15:14–17.

69. Campbell L, Seeger R, Harris R, Villablanca J, Matthay K. Escalating dose of continuous infusion combination chemotherapy for refractory neuroblastoma. *J Clin Oncol* 1993;11:623–629.

70. Evans AE, D'Angio GJ, Propert K, Anderson J, Hann H-WL. Prognostic factors in neuroblastoma. *Cancer* 1987;59:1853–1859.

71. Hann H, Stahlhut M, Evans A. Basic and acidic isoferritins in the sera of patients with neuroblastoma. *Cancer* 1988;62:1179.

72. Silber J, Evans A, Fridman M. Models to predict outcome from childhood neuroblastoma: the role of serum ferritin and tumor histology. *Cancer Res* 1991;51:1426–1433.

73. Zeltzer PM, Marangos PJ, Evans AE, Schneider SL. Serum neuron-specific enolase in children with neuroblastoma. Relationship to stage and disease course. *Cancer* 1986;57:1230–1234.

74. Berthold F, Trechow R, Utsch S, Zieschang J. Prognostic factors in metastatic neuroblastoma: a multivariate analysis of 182 cases. *Am J Paediatr Hematol Oncol* 1992;14:107–215.

75. Shuster J, McWilliams N, Castleberry R, et al. Serum lactate dehydrogenase in childhood neuroblastoma: a Pediatric Oncology Group recursive partitioning study. *Am J Clin Oncol* 1992;15:295–303.

76. Chan H, Haddad G, Thorner P, et al. P-glycoprotein expression as a predictor of the outcome of therapy for neuroblastoma. *N Engl J Med* 1991;325:1608–1614.

77. Norris MD, Bordow SB, Marshall GM, Haber PS, Cohn SL, Haber M. Expression of the gene for multidrug-resistance-associated protein and outcome in patients with neuroblastoma. *N Engl J Med* 1996;334:231–238.

78. Castleberry R. Clinical and biologic features in the prognosis and treatment of neuroblastoma. *Curr Opin Oncol* 1992;4:116–123.

79. Valentino L, Moss T, Olson E, et al. Shed tumor gangliosides and progression of human neuroblastoma. *Blood* 1990;75:1564–1567.

80. Bourhis J, DeVathaire G, Wilson G, et al. Combined analysis of DNA ploidy index and N-*myc* genomic content in neuroblastoma. *Cancer Res* 1991;51:33–36.

81. Woods WG, Tuchman M, Robison LL, et al. A population-based study of the usefulness of screening for neuroblastoma. *Lancet* 1996;348:1682–1687.

82. Asami T, Otabe N, Wakabayashi M, Kakihara T, Uchiyama M, Asami K, et al. Screening for neuroblastoma: a 9-year birth cohort-based study in Nigata, Japan. *Acta Paediatricia* 1995;84:1173–1176.

83. Yamamoto K, Hanada R, Tanimura M, Aihara T, Hayashi Y. Natural history of neuroblastoma found by mass screening. *Lancet* 1997; 349:1102.

*84. Beesho F. Where should neuroblastoma mass screening go? *Lancet* 1996;348:1672.

85. Beesho F. Effects of mass screening on age-specific incidence of neuroblastoma. *Int J Cancer* 1996;67:520–522.

86. Kaneko Y, Kanda N, Maseki N, et al. Current urinary mass screening for catecholamine metabolites at 6 months of age may be detecting only a small portion of high-risk neuroblastomas: a chromosome and N-*myc* amplification study. *J Clin Oncol* 1990;8:2005–2013.

87. Nishi M, Miyake H, Takeda T, et al. Cases of neuroblastoma missed by the mass screening programs. *Pediatr Res* 1989;26:603–607.

88. Takeuchi LA, Hachitanda Y, Woods WG, et al. Screening for neuroblastoma in North America, pre-

liminary results of a pathology review from the Quebec project. *Cancer* 1995; 76:2363–71.

89. Ariyoshi N. Different characteristics of neuroblastomas in cases found by mass screening and nonscreening: evaluation of mass screening in neuroblastoma in Kitakyushu City. *Sangyo Ika Daigaku Zasshi* 1993;15:251–266.

90. Suita S, Zaizen Y, Sera Y, et al. Mass screening for neuroblastoma: quo vadis? A nine-year experience from the pediatric oncology study group of the Kyushu area of Japan. *J Pediatr Surg* 1996;31: 555–558.

91. Treuner J, Schilling FH. Neuroblastoma mass screening: the arguments for and against. *Eur J Cancer* 1995;31A:565–568.

*92. Murphy S, Cohn S, Craft A, et al. Consensus statement from the American Cancer Society workshop on neuroblastoma screening: do children benefit from mass screening for neuroblastoma? *CA* 1991; 41:227–230.

93. Hanawa Y, Sawada T, Tsunoda A. Decrease in childhood neuroblastoma death in Japan. *Med Pediatr Oncol* 1990;18:472–475.

94. Nishi M, Miyake H, Takeda T, Shimada M, Takasugi N, Sato Y, Hanai J. Effects of the mass screening of neuroblastoma in Sapporo City. *Cancer* 1987;60: 433–436.

95. Huddart S, Muir K, Parkes S, Mann J, Stevens M, Raafat F. Neuroblastoma: a 32-year population-based study—implications for screening. *Med Pediatr Oncol* 1993;21:96–102.

*96. Parker L. Newborn screening for neuroblastoma. *Curr Opin Pediatr* 1997;9:70–73.

97. Chauvin F, Mathieu P, Frappaz D, et al. Screening for neuroblastoma in France: methodological aspects and preliminary observations. *Med Ped Oncol* 1997; 28: 81–91.

98. Esteve J, Parker L, Roy P, et al. Is neuroblastoma screening evaluation needed and feasible? *Br J Cancer* 1995; 71:1125–31.

99. Nishihira H, Toyada Y, Ohnuma K, et al. Spontaneous regression of neuroblastoma found by mass screening. *Jpn J Pediatr Oncol* 1996;33:379.

100. Yamamoto K, Hanada R, Kikuchi A, Ichikawa M, Aihara T, Oguma E, Moritani T, Shimanuki Y, Tanimura M, Hayashi Y. Spontaneous regression of localized neuroblastoma detected by mass screening. *J Clin Oncol* 1998;16(4):1265–9.

*101. Kerbl R, Urban CE. Neuroblastoma mass screening in children. *Lancet* 1997;349:730.

*102. Parker L. Value of screening for neuroblastoma? *Lancet* 1995;346:1419.

*103. O'Reilly R, Cheung NK, Bowman L, et al. NCCN pediatric neuroblastoma practice guidelines. *Oncology* 1996; 10:1813–1822.

*104. Nitschke R, Smith EI, Schochat S, et al. Localized neuroblastoma treated by surgery—a Pediatric Oncology Group study. *J Clin Oncol* 1988;6: 1271–1279.

105. Gerson JM, Koop CE. Neuroblastoma. *Semin Oncol* 1974;1:35–46.

*106. Hasse G, O'Leary M, Ramsay N, et al. Aggressive surgery combined with intensive chemotherapy improves survival in poor-risk neuroblastoma. *J Pediatr Surg* 1991;26:1119–1123.

107. Shamberger R, Allarde-Segundo A, Kozakewich H, Grier H. Surgical management of stage III and IV neuroblastoma: resection before or after chemotherapy? *J Pediatr Surg* 1991;26:1113–1117.

*108. Nitschke R, Smith E, Altshuler G, et al. Postoperative treatment of nonmetastatic visible residual neuroblastoma: a Pediatric Oncology Group study. *J Clin Oncol* 1991; 9:1181–1188.

109. Dy V, Watson RC, Exelby PR, Hajdu SI, Helson L. Improved management of stage III neuroblastoma. *Clin Bull* 1979;9:76–81.

110. Green AA, Hustu HO, Palmer R, Pinkel D. Total-body sequential segmental irradiation and combination chemotherapy for children with disseminated neuroblastoma. *Cancer* 1976;38:2250–2257.

111. Smith I, Nitschke R, Shochat S, et al. Lack of significance of involved lymph nodes attached to localized neuroblastoma. A Pediatric Oncology Group study. *Proc Am Soc Clin Oncol* 1987;6:219(abstr).

112. Koop CE, Johnson DG. Neuroblastoma: an assessment of therapy in reference to staging. *J Pediatr Surg* 1971;6:595–600.

113. Sitarz A, Finkelstein J, Grasfeld J, et al. An evaluation of the role of surgery in disseminated neuroblastoma: a report from the Children's Cancer Study group. *J Pediatr Surg* 1983;18:147–151.

114. Wagner HP, Kaser H. The role of surgery, radio- and chemotherapy in the treatment of neuroblastoma and ganglioneuroblastoma. *Prog Pediatr Surg* 1983;16: 1–6.

*115. Castleberry R, Kun L, Shuster J, et al. Radiotherapy improves the outlook for patients older than 1 year with Pediatric Oncology Group stage C neuroblastoma. *J Clin Oncol* 1991;9:789–795; [Letter] 2076–2077.

116. Shorter N, Davidoff A, Evans A, et al. The role of surgery in the management of stage IV neuroblastoma. *Med Pediatr Oncol* 1990;18:377(abstr).

117. Shaw A. Surgical management of neuroblastoma. In: Pochedly C, ed. *Neuroblastoma: tumor biology and therapy.* Boca Raton, FL: CRC Press, 1990:277–288.

118. Arma E, Byfield JE, Finkelstein JZ, Fonkalsrund EW. An experimental model for the therapy of mouse neuroblastoma. *J Pediatr Surg* 1973;8:757–762.

119. Ohnuma N, Kasuga T, Najiri I, Furuse. Radio-sensitivity of human neuroblastoma cell line (NB-1). *Gann* 1977;68:711–712.

120. Wheldon TE, O'Donaghue JA, Gregor A. Radiobiological rationale for hyperfractionation in the radiotherapy of neuroblastoma. *Int J Radiat Oncol Biol Phys* 1987;13:1430–1431.

121. Wheldon TE, O'Donaghue JA, Gregor A, Livingstone A, Wilson L. Radiobiological considerations in the treatment of neuroblastoma by total body irradiation. *Radiother Oncol* 1986;6:317–326.

122. Wheldon TE, Wilson L, Livingstone A, Russell J, O'Donaghue JA, Gregor A. Radiation studies on multicellular tumor spheroids derived from human neuroblastoma: absence of sparing effect of dose fractionation. *Eur J Cancer Clin Oncol* 1986;22: 563–566.

123. DeBernardi B, Rogers D, Carli M, et al. Localized neuroblastoma: surgical and pathologic staging. *Cancer* 1987;60:1066–1072.

124. O'Neill JA, Littman P, Blitzer P, Soper K, Chatten J,

Shimada H. The role of surgery in localized neuroblastoma. *J Pediatr Surg* 1985;20:708–712.

125. Matthay K, Stram D, Seeger RC, et al. A prospective children's cancer group study of stage II neuroblastoma treated with surgery alone. *Proc Am Soc Clin Oncol* 1993;12:414.

125a. Haase GM, Atkinson JB, Stram DO, Lukens JN, Matthay KK. Surgical management and outcome of locoregional neuroblastoma: comparison of the Children's Cancer Group and the international staging systems. *J Pediatr Surg* 1995;30(2):289–294.

*126. Kushner BH, Cheung NKV, LaQuaglia MP, et al. International neuroblastoma staging system stage 1 neuroblastoma: a prospective study and literature review. *J Clin Oncol* 1996;14:2174–2180.

127. Wittenborg MH. Roentgen therapy in neuroblastoma: a review of 73 cases. *Radiology* 1950;54:679–688.

128. Perez CA, Vietti T, Ackerman LV, Eagleton MD, Powers WE. Tumors of the sympathetic nervous system in children: an approval of treatment and results. *Radiology* 1967;88:750–760.

129. Thomas P, Lei J, Fineberg B, et al. An analysis of neuroblastoma at a single institution. *Cancer* 1984;53: 2079–2082.

130. Zucker JM, Margulis E. Radio-chemotherapy of post-operative minimal residual disease in neuroblastoma. *Rec Res Cancer Res* 1979;68:423–430.

131. McGuire WA, Simmons D, Grosfeld JL, Behner RL. Stage II neuroblastoma—does adjuvant irradiation contribute to cure? *Med Pediatr Oncol* 1985;13: 117–121.

131a. Ninane J, Pritchard J, Morris Jones PH, Mann JR, Malpas JS. Stage II neuroblastoma. Adverse prognostic significance of lymph node involvement. *Arch Dis Child* 1982;57(6):438–442.

132. Rosen EM, Cassady JR, Kretschmar C, Frantz CN, Levey R, Sallan SE. Influence of local-regional lymph node metastases on prognosis in neuroblastoma. *Med Pediatr Oncol* 1984;12:260–263.

133. Macklis RM, West DC, Shamberger RC, Kozakewish HP, Kriessman SG, Grier HE. Local control in stage III neuroblastoma patients over one year of age: the Joint Center/Children's Hospital/Dana Farber Cancer Institute experience. *Int J Radiat Oncol Biol Phys* 1993;27[Suppl 1]:132.

134. Green AA, Hayes FA, Hustu HO. Sequential cyclophosphamide and doxorubicin for induction of complete remission in children with disseminated neuroblastoma. *Cancer* 1981;48:2310–2317.

135. West D, Shamberger R, Macklis R, et al. Stage III neuroblastoma over 1 year of age at diagnosis: improved survival with intensive multimodality therapy including multiple alkylating agents. *J Clin Oncol* 1993;11:84–90.

136. Halperin EC. Radiotherapy in neuroblastoma. In: Pochedly C, Tebbi C, eds. *Neuroblastoma: tumor biology and therapy.* Chicago: CRC Press, 1989, 289–304.

137. Ingram SS, Halperin EC. Patterns of failure in neuroblastoma. *Radiology* 1993;189(supp):288.

138. Jacobson HM, Marcus RB Jr, Thar TL, Million RR, Graham-Pole JR, Talbert JL. Pediatric neuroblastoma: postoperative radiation therapy using less than 2000 rad. *Int J Radiat Oncol Biol Phys* 1983;9: 501–505.

139. Bowman L, Castleberry R, Altshuler G, et al. Therapy

based on DNA index (D1) for infants with unresectable and disseminated neuroblastoma (NB). Preliminary results of the Pediatric Oncology Group 'better risk' study. *Med Pediatr Oncol* 1990;18:364(abstr).

140. Strother D, Rao PV, Smith I, et al. Factors affecting outcome of therapy for regional neuroblastoma: a report of the pediatric oncology group. 1998 (submitted).

141. Strother D, Shuster JJ, McWilliams N, et al. Results of pediatric oncology group protocol 8104 for infants with stages D and DS neuroblastoma. *J Pediatr Hematol Oncol* 1995;17:254–259.

*142. Strother D, van Hoff J, Rao PV, et al. Event-free survival of children with biologically favourable neuroblastoma based on the degree of initial tumour resection: results from the pediatric oncology group. *Eur J Cancer* 1997;33:2121–2125.

143. Sagerman RH. Primary management of disseminated neuroblastoma by sequential segmental irradiation. *Radiology* 1968;90:352–353.

144. Helson L, Jereb B, Vogel R. Sequential hemi-body irradiation (HBI) in the treatment of advanced neuroblastoma: a pilot study. *Int J Radiat Oncol Biol Phys* 1981;7:531–534.

145. Kun LE, Casper JT, Kline RW, Piaskowski VD. Fractionated total body irradiation for metastatic neuroblastoma. *Int J Radiat Oncol Biol Phys* 1981;7: 1599–1602.

146. D'Angio GJ, Evans A. Cyclic low-dose total body irradiation for metastatic neuroblastoma. *Int J Radiat Oncol Biol Phys* 1983;9:1961–1965.

147. Finkelstein J, Klemperer M, Evans A, et al. Multiagent chemotherapy for children with metastatic neuroblastoma: a report of the Childrens' Cancer Study Group. *Med Pediatr Oncol* 1979;6:179.

148. Nitschke R, Cangir A, Crist W, Berry DH. Intensive chemotherapy for metastatic neuroblastoma: a Southwest Oncology Group Study. *Med Pediatr Oncol* 1980;8:281–288.

149. Pinkerton C, Pritchard J, Deraker J, et al. ENSG1 randomized study of high dose melphalan in neuroblastoma. In: Dicke K, Spitzer G, Jaganoth S, eds. *Autologous bone marrow transplantation.* Austin, TX: University of Texas Press, 1987:401.

150. Shafford EA, Rogers DW, Pritchard J. Advanced neuroblastoma: improved response rate using a multiagent regimen (OPEC) including sequential cisplatin and VM-26. *J Clin Oncol* 1984;2:742–747.

151. Lindsley K, LaQuaglia M, Kushner BH, Cheung KV, Bonilla MA. Hyperfractionated radiotherapy for consolidation of advanced stage neuroblastoma. *Int J Radiat Oncol Biol Phys* 1993;27(Suppl 1):132.

152. Ohnuma N, Takahashi H, Kaneko M, et al. Treatment combined with bone marrow transplantation for advanced neuroblastoma: an analysis of patients who were pretreated intensively with the protocol of the study group of Japan. *Med Pediatr Oncol* 1995;24: 181–187.

*153. Matthay KK. Neuroblastoma: a clinical challenge and biologic puzzle. *CA: Cancer J Clin* 1995;45:179–192.

154. Kushner B, O'Reilly R, Mandell L, Gulati S, LaQuaglia M, Cheung N. Myeloablative combination chemotherapy without total body irradiation for neuroblastoma. *J Clin Oncol* 1991;9:274–279.

*155. Shuster J, Cantor A, McWilliams N, et al. The prognostic significance of autologous bone marrow transplant in advanced neuroblastoma. *J Clin Oncol* 1991; 9:1045–1049.

*156. Sibley GS, Mundt AJ, Goldman S, et al. Patterns of failure following total body irradiation and bone marrow transplantation with or without a radiotherapy boost for advanced neuroblastoma. *Int J Rad Oncol Biol Phys* 1995;32:1127–1135.

*157. Graham Pole J, Casper J, Elfenbein G, et al. High-dose chemoradiotherapy supported by marrow infusions for advanced neuroblastoma: a Pediatric Oncology Group Study. *J Clin Oncol* 1991;9:152–158.

*158. Marcus KC, Tarbell NJ. The changing role of radiation therapy in the treatment of neuroblastoma. *Sem Rad Oncol* 1997;7:195–203.

*159. Seeger RC, Villablanca JG, Matthay KK, et al. Intensive chemoradiotherapy and autologous bone marrow transplantation for poor prognosis neuroblastoma. *Prog Clin Biol Res* 1991;336:527–534.

160. Seeger R, Matthay K, Villablanca J, et al. Intensive chemoradiotherapy and autologous bone marrow transplantation for high risk neuroblastoma. *Proc ASCO* 1991;10:310(abstr).

*161. Stram DO, Matthay KK, O'Leary M, et al. Consolidation chemoradiotherapy and autologous bone marrow transplantation versus continued chemotherapy for metastatic neuroblastoma: a report of two concurrent children's group studies. *J Clin Oncol* 1996;14: 2417–2426.

*162. Shuster JJ. The role of autologous bone marrow transplantation in advanced neuroblastoma. *J Clin Oncol* 1996;14:2413–2414.

163. Pinkerton CR. ENSG-1 randomized study of high-dose melphalan in neuroblastoma. *Bone Marrow Trans* 1991;7[Suppl 3]:112–113.

164. Suarez A, Hartmann O, Vassal G, et al. Treatment of stage IV-S neuroblastoma: a study of 34 cases treated between 1982 and 1987. *Med Pediatr Oncol* 1991;19: 473–477.

165. Bernardi B, Pianca C, Boni L, et al. Disseminated neuroblastoma (stage IV and IV-S) in the first year of life. *Cancer* 1992;70:1625–1633.

166. Stephenson SR, Cook BA, Mease AD, et al. The prognostic significance of age and pattern of metastasis in stage IV-S neuroblastoma. *Cancer* 1986;58: 372–375.

167. van Noesel MM, Hanlen K, Hakvoert-Cammel FGAJ, Egeler RM. Neuroblastoma 4S: a heterogeneous disease with variable risk factors and treatment strategies. *Cancer* 1997;80:834–843.

168. Blatt J, Deutsch M, Wollman M. Results of therapy in stage IV-S neuroblastoma with massive hepatomegaly. *Int J Radiat Oncol Biol Phys* 1987;13: 1467–1471.

169. Evans AE. Natural history of neuroblastoma. In: Evans AE, eds. *Advances in neuroblastoma research.* New York: Raven Press, 1980;3–12.

170. Halperin EC. Hepatic metastasis from neuroblastoma. *South Med J* 1987;80:1370–1373.

171. McWilliam NB. IV-S neuroblastoma: treatment controversy revisited. *Med Pediatr Oncol* 1986;14: 41–44.

*172. Bowman L, Hancock M, Santana F, et al. Impact of intensified therapy on clinical outcome in infants and children with neuroblastoma: the St Jude Children's Research Hospital Experience, 1962–1988. *J Clin Oncol* 1991;9:1599–1608.

173. Mugishima H, Iwata M, Okabe I, et al. Autologous bone marrow transplantation in children with advanced neuroblastoma. *Cancer* 1994;76:1295–1297.

*174. Kretschmar CS, Frantz CN, Rosen EM, Cassady JR, Levey R, Sallan SE. Improved prognosis for infants with stage IV neuroblastoma. *J Clin Oncol* 1984;2: 799–803.

175. Pepper W. A study of congenital sarcoma of the liver and suprarenal. *Am J Med Sci* 1901;1121:287–289.

176. Prassad KN, Sahu SK, Sinha PK. Cyclic nucleotides in the regulation of expression of differentiated functions in neuroblastoma cells. *J Natl Cancer Inst* 1976;57:619–631.

177. Cheung N, Heller G. Chemotherapy dose intensity correlates strongly with response, median survival, and median progression-free survival in metastatic neuroblastoma. *J Clin Oncol* 1991;9:1050–1058.

178. Anderson J, Coccia P. Is more better? Dose intensity in neuroblastoma. *J Clin Oncol* 1991;9:902–904.

179. Meresse V, Vassal G, Michon J, et al. Combined continuous infusion etoposide with high-dose cyclophosphamide for refractory neuroblastoma: a phase II study from the Societe Francaise d'Oncologie Paediatrique. *J Clin Oncol* 1993;11:630–637.

180. Hutchinson R, Sisson J, Miser J, et al. Long-term results of [^{131}I]Metaiodobenzylguanidine treatment of refractory advanced neuroblastoma. *J Nucl Biol Med* 1991;35:237–240.

181. Negrier S, Michon D, Floret E, et al. Interleukin-2 and lymphokine-activated killer cells in 15 children with advanced metastatic neuroblastoma. *J Clin Oncol* 1991;9:1363–1370.

*182. Mayfield JK, Riseborough EJ, Jaffe N, Nehme AME. Spinal deformity in children treated for neuroblastoma. *J Bone Joint Surg [Am]* 1981;63a:183–193.

183. Mitus A, Tefft M, Fellers FX. Long term follow-up of renal function of 108 children who underwent nephrectomy for malignant disease. *Pediatrics* 1969; 44:912–921.

*184. Peschel RE, Chen M, Seashore J. The treatment of massive hepatomegaly in stage IV-S neuroblastoma. *Int J Radiat Oncol Biol Phys* 1981;7:549–553.

185. Deacon JM, Wilson P, Steel GG. Radiosensitivity of neuroblastoma. In: Evans AE, D'Angio GJ, Seeger RC, eds. *Advances in neuroblastoma research.* New York: Alan R Liss, 1985:525–536.

186. Halperin EC. Response. *Int J Radiat Oncol Biol Phys* 1987;13:1430.

187. Jacobson GM, Sause WT, O'Brien RT. Dose response analysis of pediatric neuroblastoma to megavoltage radiation. *Am J Clin Oncol* 1984;7:693–697.

188. Fontanesi J, Bowman L, Hancock M, et al. Impact of irradiation on local control in advanced neuroblastoma. *Proc Annu Meet Am Assoc Cancer Res* 1992; 33:A1538(abstr).

189. Stella JR, Schweisquth O, Schlienger M. Neuroblastoma: a study of 144 cases treated in the Institut Gustave-Roussy over a period of 7 years. *AJR* 1970;108: 324–332.

190. Wyatt GM, Farber S. Neuroblastoma sympatheticum: roentgenological appearance and radiation treatment. *AJR* 1941;46:485–495.

191. D'Angio GJ, August C, Elkins W, et al. Metastatic

neuroblastoma managed by supralethal therapy and bone marrow reconstitution (BMRc). Results of a four-institution children's cancer study group pilot study. In: Evans AE, D'Angio GJ, Seeger RC, eds. *Advances in neuroblastoma research.* New York: Alan R Liss, 1985:557–563.

192. Probert JC, Parker BR, Kaplan HS. Growth retardation in children after megavoltage irradiation of the spine. *Cancer* 1973;32:634–639.

193. Philip T. Overview of current treatment of neuroblastoma. *Am J Pediatr Hematol Oncol* 1992;14:97–102.

194. Wright JH. Neurocytoma or neuroblastoma, a kind of tumor not generally recognized. *J Exp Med* 1910;12: 556–561.

195. Cushing H, Wolbach SB. The transformation of a malignant paravertebral sympathicoblastoma into a benign ganglioneuroma. *Am J Pathol* 1927;3:203–216.

196. Brodeur GM. Neuroblastoma—clinical applications of molecular parameters. *Brain Pathol* 1990;1:47–54.

197. Brodeur G. Neuroblastoma and other peripheral neuroectodermal tumors. In: Fernbach D, Vietti T, eds. *Clinical pediatric oncology,* 4th ed. St. Louis: Mosby-Year Book, 1991:437–464.

198. Nitschke R, Humphrey GB, Sexquer CL, Smith EI. Neuroblastoma: therapy for infants with good prognosis. *Med Pediatr Oncol* 1983;11:154–158.

199. Dini G, Lanino E, Garaventa A, et al. Myeloablative therapy and unpurged autologous bone marrow transplantation for poor-prognosis neuroblastoma: report of 34 cases. *J Clin Oncol* 1991;9:962–969.

200. Sawaguchi S, Kaneko M, Uchino J, et al. Treatment of advanced neuroblastoma with emphasis on intensive induction chemotherapy. *Cancer* 1990;66: 1879–1887.

201. Philip T, Zucker J, Bernard J, et al. Improved survival at 2 and 5 years in the LMCE1 unselected group of 72 children with stage IV neuroblastoma older than 1 year of age at diagnosis: is cure possible in a small subgroup? *J Clin Oncol* 1991;9:1037–1044.

202. Zucker J, Philip T, Bernard J, et al. Single or double consolidation treatment according to remission status after initial therapy in metastatic neuroblastoma. *Prog Clin Biol Res* 1991;366:543–551.

*203. Hartmann O, Benhamou E, Beaujean F, et al. Repeated high-dose chemotherapy followed by purged autologous bone marrow transplantation as consolidation therapy in metastatic neuroblastoma. *J Clin Oncol* 1987;5:1205–1211.

204. Matthay KK. Impact of myeloblative therapy with bone marrow transplantation in advanced neuroblastoma. *Bone Marrow Trans* 1996;18[Suppl 3]: S21–24.

205. Garaventa A, Rondelli R, Lanino E, et al. Myeloablative therapy and bone marrow rescue in advanced neuroblastoma. Report from the Italian bone marrow transplant registry. *Bone Marrow Trans* 1996;18: 125–130.

*206. McCowage GB, Vowels MR, Shaw PJ, Lockwood L, Mameghan H. Autologous bone marrow transplantation for advanced neuroblastoma using teniposide, doxorubicin, melphalan, cisplatin, and total-body irradiation. *J Clin Oncol* 1995;13:2789–2795.

7

Hodgkin's Disease

In 1832, Thomas Hodgkin (1) described seven patients with enlarged absorbent (lymphatic) glands not thought to result from inflammation. At the turn of the century, Sternberg and Reed each described the multinucleated giant cell characteristic of Hodgkin's disease (HD) (2). Shortly after the discovery of x-rays, Pusey (3), in 1902, demonstrated the radioresponsiveness of HD. In the 1930s, Gilbert (4) laid the foundation for its definitive treatment with radiotherapy, and additional definition of important principles was provided by Peters (5). During the war-years, the lympholytic effects of nitrogen mustard were recognized (6), and over the next two decades progress in safely combining multiple chemotherapeutic agents in treating HD led to DeVita's report on the use of nitrogen mustard, vincristine, procarbazine, and prednisone (MOPP) chemotherapy (7). Kaplan (2) systematically studied the role of radiotherapy for HD during these decades. Concurrently, advances were made in identifying different pathologic subtypes, determining staging criteria, improving diagnostic imaging capabilities, and developing effective chemotherapeutic regimens. When the clonality of the Reed-Sternberg (R-S) cell was finally established in the 1960s, controversy over the malignant versus inflammatory nature of HD abated (8).

Although the biology and natural history of HD in children is similar to that in adults, when irradiation techniques and doses suitable for controlling disease in adults were translated to the pediatric setting, substantial morbidities (primarily musculoskeletal growth inhibition) were produced (9,10). It is within this context that new strategies for the treatment of pediatric HD were developed by Donaldson and others (11–13). Historically, children were thought to have a worse prognosis than adults (2). It is now apparent that the converse is true (14–17).

BIOLOGY AND EPIDEMIOLOGY

Biology

HD persists in its elusiveness regarding clarification of such basic issues as the origin and evolution of the malignant cell, its relative rarity and distribution within pathologic material, the events that lead to disease development, and even whether the disease is a single entity or family of diseases (18). However, recent investigations provide insight. The R-S cell is most commonly a neoplastic clone that originates from B lymphocytes in lymphoid germinal centers. Clonality can be demonstrated at diagnosis and relapse through detection of unique nucleotide sequences, which essentially molecularly fingerprint the R-S cell clone; these sequences represent rearrangements of immunoglobulin variable-region (V) genes, which are B-cell derived (19,20). Complicating this scenario is the finding by Kanzler et al. (20), that flawed V genes, which would be lethal for normal B cells, are present in R-S cells and prevent them from expressing immunoglobulin. Such cells would be expected to die of apoptosis. Therefore, the genesis of classic Hodgkin's disease (cHD) must involve blockage of the apoptotic pathway for the R-S cell. This is where Epstein-Barr virus (EBV) and genes that monitor cell damage, such as p53, enter the picture, through rescue and repair of the R-S cell (20,21). EBV genome fragments can be found in R-S cells in 30% to 50% of HD specimens, most commonly in the mixed cellularity (MCHD) subtype, and rarely in the lymphocyte predominant type (LPHD) (22–24). The EBV genome is temporally stable because it can be found at diagnosis and relapse. Finally the R-S cell can also have characteristics of T lymphocytes and the interdigitating reticulum cell. Such evidence for a multilineage origin of the R-S cell may be explicable by postulating that the R-S cell is a hybridoma resulting from fusion of different cell lines, provoked by a virus or other agent. Cytogenetic data also show an unexpected frequency of B-cell translocation (14:18) and bcl-2 gene involvement in HD, but these may derive from bystander normal lymphocytes rather than the R-S cell (25,26). A pathogenetic model for HD is depicted in Fig.

1, which suggests that the R-S cells arises in a germinal-lymphoid center from a clone of antigen-stimulated B cells, and through genetic changes achieves immortality and malignant properties (18).

A curious characteristic of HD is the rarity (about 1%) of the malignant R-S cell in specimens, and the abundant reactive cellular infiltrate of lymphocytes, macrophages, granulocytes, and eosinophils. What accounts for the symptoms and signs of HD? This is due to the powerful cytokines that R-S cells secrete, which number at least 12 and include interleukin-1 and interleukin-6, and tumor necrosis factor (27,28). Interleukin-5 could be responsible for the eosinophilia in MCHD, and transforming growth factor-β for the fibrosis in the nodular sclerosis subtype. These cytokines also enable the cells to evade immunologic surveillance as well as promote their own replication (27).

The support for HD actually comprising a family of diseases includes the observation

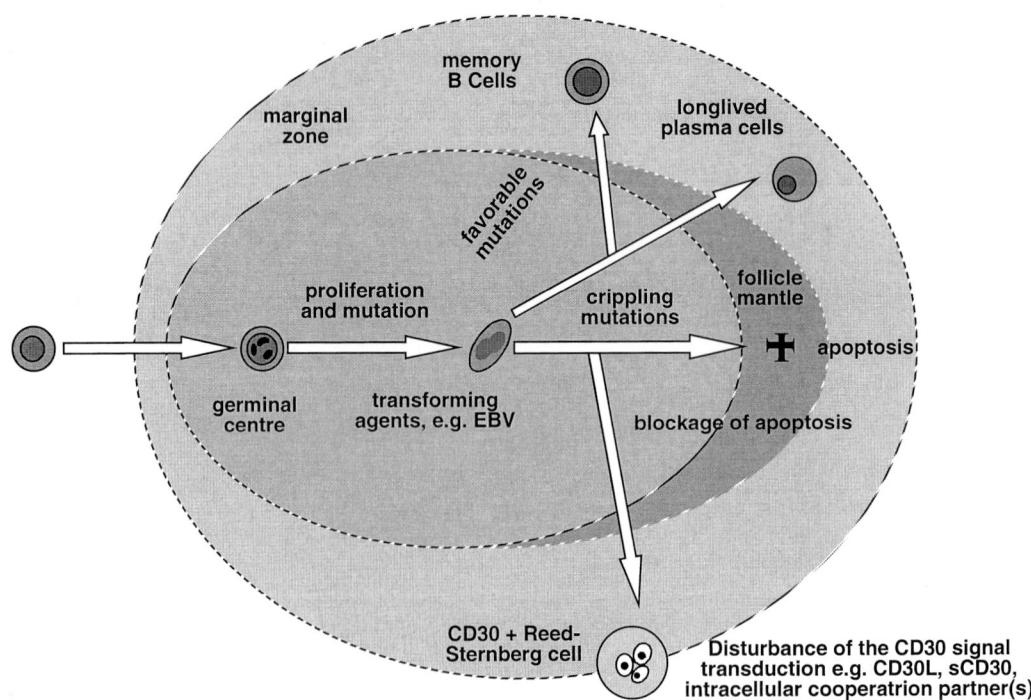

FIG. 1. Pathogenetic model for Hodgkin's disease. (From ref. 18, with permission.)

that R-S cells can rarely be derivatives of cytotoxic T cells, and that nodular lymphocyte predominant HD (nLPHD) is a distinctive and uncommon lymphoproliferative disorder. The lymphocytic and histiocytic (L&H) cells characteristic of nLPHD have folded and lobate nuclei, and lie in a background of small lymphocytes and histiocytes. The L&H cells are also B-cell derived, but harbor V gene alterations, which differ from those in R-S cells; whether the L&H cells are monoclonal is unclear (29,30). The clinical characteristics of nLPHD differ from the subtypes of classic HD by virtue of its indolence and excellent prognosis, as well as its epidemiology and (poor) response to chemotherapy. The revised European-American classification of lymphoid neoplasia (REAL) has proposed a schema that reflects the distinction of nLPHD from classic HD (31) (to be described in the Pathologic Classification section).

Epidemiology

HD comprises 6% of childhood cancers. A striking male:female predominance is found among children, with a ratio of 4:1 for 3- to 7-year-olds, 3:1 for 7- to 9-year-olds, and 1.3:1 (a ratio more similar to that of adults) for older children (14,32–34). The age-specific incidence curves for HD in the United States are bimodal, peaking in the 20s and then again after age 50 (35). The disease is uncommon before age 5, and, among children, is most common in adolescence.

Although evidence for HD being infectious or contagious was suggested by reports of case clusters (36), confirmatory data is lacking (37). However, the role of EBV in its pathogenesis is well established as discussed previously. In a recent report, EBV early RNA1 was expressed in R-S cells in 58% of childhood cases (38). Of particular interest is that expression was age dependent—75% of children under age 10 compared with 20% of older children. In addition, a past history of infectious mononucleosis increases the risk for HD, and anti-EBV titers are elevated prior to diagnosis of HD.

Evidence for a genetic predisposition exists and is relevant when counseling families. Siblings have a 2- to 5-fold increased incidence, and this is 9-fold increased in same sex siblings. Parent-child associations are reported (35,37,39). Mack et al. (40) reported a 99-fold increased risk in monozygotic twins of patients, but no increased risk in dizygotic twins. The status of the immune system in patients with HD deserves comment. A complex deficiency in cellular immunity exists, which includes a relative decrease in naive T cells, and an increased sensitivity of effector T cells to suppressor monocytes and T-suppressor cells (41,42). Of interest is that radiation results in a long-term dysregulation of T-cell subset homeostasis. Finally, it is unclear as to whether an increased frequency of HD is seen in patients with either congenital (e.g., ataxia-telangiectasia) or acquired immunodeficiency states, including AIDS (36,43). Against an association is that HD is rarely seen as a second malignancy. In HIV-positive patients, the disease is more commonly in an advanced stage with systemic symptoms, extranodal involvement, and a poor response to therapy (44).

CLINICAL PRESENTATION

HD appears to be unifocal in origin, with 90% of patients presenting in a pattern that suggests contiguous lymphatic spread (2,45). Most children are diagnosed on the basis of supradiaphragmatic lymph nodes, with painless cervical adenopathy in 80%. The nodes are generally firm and may be tender. Mediastinal involvement occurs in 76% of adolescents, but in only 33% of 1- to 10-year-olds. Mediastinal disease may produce symptoms such as dyspnea, cough, or superior vena cava (SVC) syndrome. Axillary adenopathy is less common (2). Associations exist between the mediastinum and neck, the neck and ipsilateral axilla, the mediastinum and hilum, and the spleen and abdominal lymph nodes (45). Isolated mediastinal or infradiaphragmatic HD is rare, occurring in less than 5% of patients. About one-third of the patients will have systemic "B" symptoms as defined in Table 1 (2,46).

TABLE 1. *Cotswold staging classification for Hodgkin's disease*

Stage	Description
I	Involvement of a single lymph node region or lymphoid structure, e.g., spleen, thymus, Waldeyer's ring, or single extralymphatic site (IE).
II	Involvement of two or more lymph node regions on the same side of the diaphragm, or localized contiguous involvement of only one extranodal organ/site and lymph node region on the same side of the diaphragm (IIE). The number of anatomic sites are indicated by a subscript (e.g., II$_3$).
III	Involvement of lymph node regions on both sides of the diaphragm (III), which may be accompanied by involvement of the spleen (III$_S$) or by localized contiguous involvement of only one extranodal organ site (IIIE) or both (IIISE).
III$_1$	With or without involvement of splenic hilar, celiac or portal nodes.
III$_2$	With involvement of paraaortic, iliac, or mesenteric nodes.
IV	Diffuse or disseminated involvement of one or more extranodal organs or tissues, with or without associated lymph node involvement.
Designations applicable to any disease stage	
A	No symptoms.
B	Fever (temperature >38°C), drenching night sweats, unexplained loss of >10% of body weight within the preceding 6 mo.
X	Bulky disease (a widening of the mediastinum by more than one-third or the presence of a nodal mass with a maximal dimension >10 cm).
E	Involvement of a single extranodal site that is contiguous or proximal to the known nodal site.
CS	Clinical stage.
PS	Pathologic stage (as determined by laparotomy).

Modified from ref. 165, with permission.

PATHOLOGIC CLASSIFICATION

The R-S cell is the essential malignant cell in HD (Fig. 2). It is large with abundant cytoplasm, two or three nuclei, and a prominent nucleolus. However, its frequency in pathologic specimens is greatly variable, due to the presence of numerous reactive cells including lymphocytes, eosinophils, and plasma cells. Moreover, the R-S cell, and in particular its mononuclear variant, is not pathognomonic for HD because cells simulating it can be found in other disorders that are reactive, infectious, or malignant (47). The diagnosis of HD must be established by lymph node biopsy. Aspiration cytology alone is not recommended because of the lack of stromal tissue, the small number of cells present in the specimen, and the difficulty of classifying HD into one of the four categories of the Rye classification. The Rye classification subcategorizes HD into the following types: nodular sclerosing (NS), mixed cellularity (MC), lymphocyte predominant (LP), and lymphocyte depleted (LD). With modern treatment the prognostic significance of these subtypes has diminished, although the presenting characteristics and natural history remain evident, particularly for the nodular subtype of LPHD. The importance of distinguishing nLPHD from the other types has led to the revised European-American classification (REAL) as described in Table 2 (31). The clinicopathologic characteristics are the same as in adults and, therefore, will only be briefly described.

• nodular lymphocyte predominant HD (48):

The distinctive cell is the lymphocyte and histiocytic (L&H) "popcorn" cell, which is CD20+ (B-lymphocyte marker), CD15-. Classic R-S cells (which are usually CD15+) are rare, as is the detection of EBV. Progressive transformation of the germinal centers of lymph nodes is often seen, and, in fact, can occur in the absence of nLPHD. It is, therefore, important to distinguish these entities.

nLPHD has a long natural history, both in its time to diagnosis and to relapse, reminiscent of indolent non-Hodgkin's lymphomas. It is relatively more common in

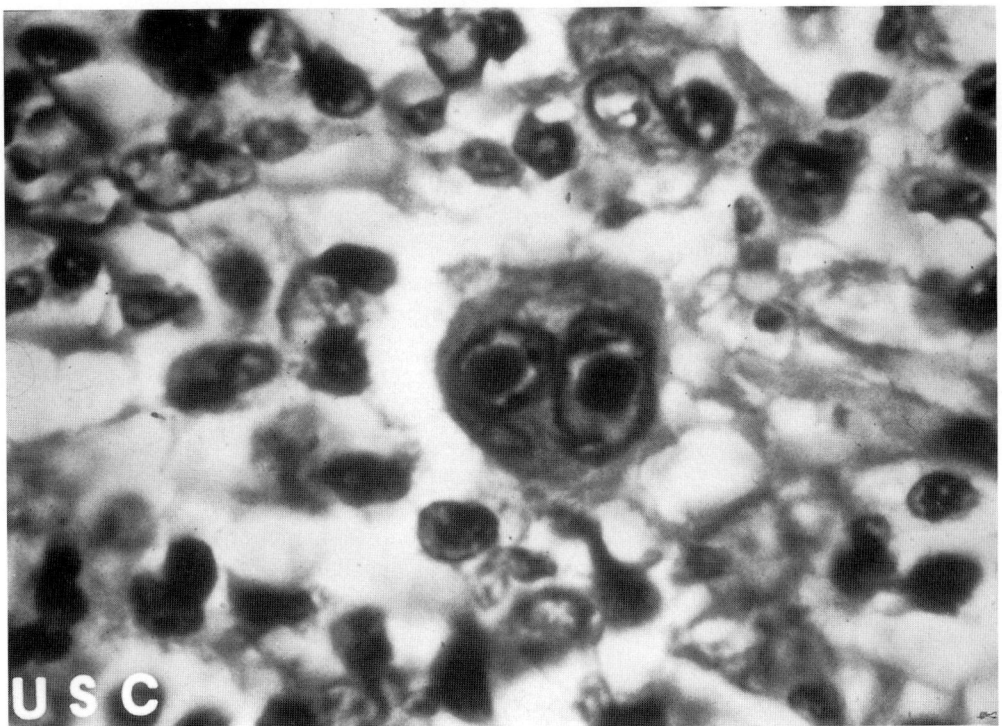

FIG. 2. Reed-Sternberg cell.

young children (33% of all patients are less than 15-years-old), has a high male:female ratio (4:1), and commonly involves a single lymph node region with sparing of the mediastinum (49).

• lymphocyte-rich (classic) HD:
    R-S cells (CD15+) are identifiable in a background predominantly of lymphocytes. Clinical behavior is similar to MCHD.

• mixed cellularity (classic) HD:
    R-S cells (CD15+) are frequent in a background of abundant normal reactive cells (lymphs, plasma cells, eosinophils, histiocytes). It can be confused with peripheral T-cell lymphoma. MCHD is less common in children, often accompanied by "B" symptoms, and commonly is stage III or IV.

TABLE 2. *Comparison of REAL and Rye classifications of Hodgkin's disease*

REAL classification	Rye classification
Lymphocyte predominance, nodular (with or without diffuse)	Lymphocyte predominance, nodular (most cases)
Classic disease	
Lymphocyte-rich classic disease	Lymphocyte predominance, diffuse (most cases)
	Lymphocyte predominance, nodular (some cases)
Nodular sclerosis	Nodular sclerosis
Mixed cellularity	Mixed cellularity (most cases)
Lymphocyte depletion	Lymphocyte depletion

Modified from ref. 165, with permission.

- nodular sclerosis (classic) HD:

  This subtype is distinctive due to the presence of collagenous bands that divide the lymph node into nodules, which often contain an R-S cell variant called the lacunar cell. It frequently occurs in children, involves supradiaphragmatic nodes, and spreads in an orderly manner.
- lymphocyte depleted (classic) HD:

  This subtype is rare and commonly confused with non-Hodgkin's lymphoma, particularly of the anaplastic large cell type. R-S and pleomorphic variants are common, relative to the number of background lymphocytes. It often is advanced at diagnosis, and has a poor prognosis.

Although the pathologic and immunohistochemical characteristics of HD are gener-ally sufficiently clear to establish a diagnosis, confusion with select subtypes of non-Hodgkin's lymphoma is at times problematic. In particular, classic HD and nLPHD can be confused with anaplastic large cell lymphoma and LPHD can be confused with T cell rich B-cell lymphoma (18,31) (Fig. 3).

The relative distribution of the subtypes in younger children differs from that in adolescents and adults, as shown in an analysis of 2,238 patients treated at Stanford University (14) (Table 3). LP is relatively more common (13%) in younger children (age less than 10 years), whereas LD is exceedingly rare. Although NS is the most common subtype in all age groups, it is more frequent in adolescents (77%) and adults (72%) than in younger children (44%). Conversely, MC is more common

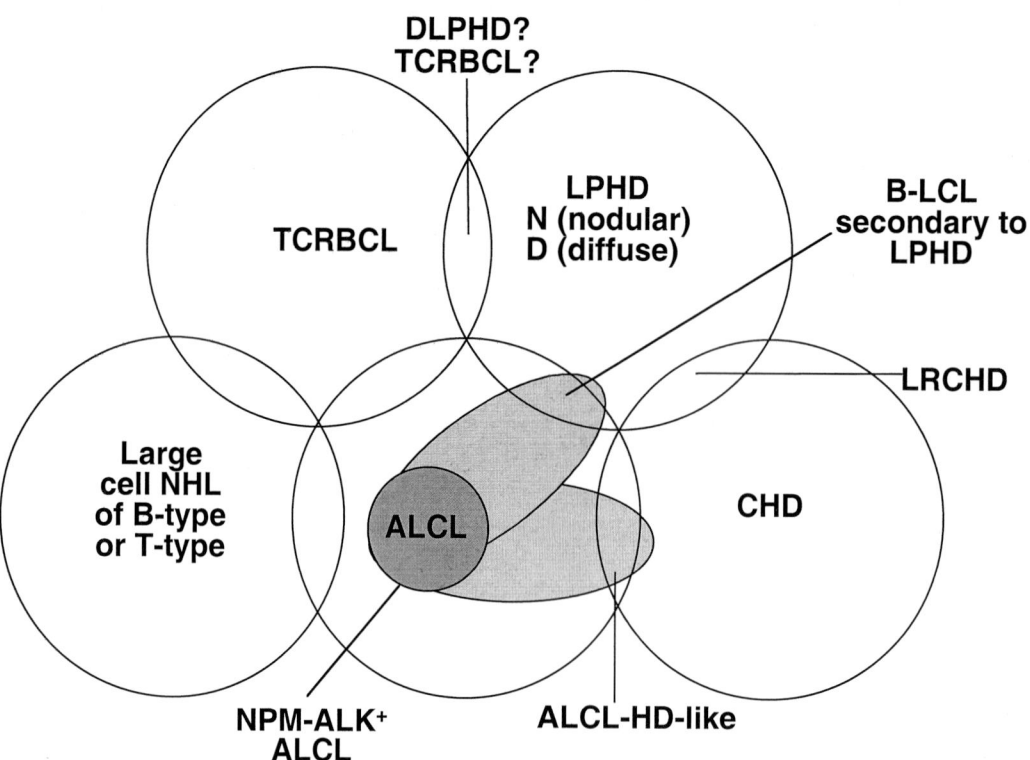

FIG. 3. Morphologic overlaps of Hodgkin's disease with anaplastic large cell lymphoma (ALCL) and other lymphomas. LPHD HD; B-LCL, B-cell large cell lymphoma; CHD, classic Hodgkin's disease; LRCHD, lymphocyte rich CHD; NHL, non-Hodgkin's lymphoma; TCRBCL, T-cell rich B-cell lymphoma. (From ref. 18, with permission.)

TABLE 3. *Distribution of pathologic subtypes according to patient age*

Age	≤10 years	10–16 years	≥17 years
Number of patients (%)	91 (4%)	235 (11%)	1912 (85%)
M:F ratio	4:1	1:1	3:2
Histology (%)			
Nodular sclerosis	44%	77%	72%
Mixed cellularity	33%	11%	17%
Lymphocyte predominance	13%	8%	5%
Lymphocyte depleted	0%	1%	1%
Unclassified/interfollicular	10%	3%	5%

Modified from ref. 14, with permission.

in younger children (33%) than in adolescents (11%) or adults (17%).

STAGING

Using anatomical groups of regional lymph nodes, the staging system was designed for all age groups, according to a modification of the system devised at the 1970 Ann Arbor Symposium. This was most recently revised at the Cotswolds Meeting, although not all suggestions from those recommendations are consistently used (46). In this system patients are assigned a clinical stage, and if staging laparotomy is performed, the patient is assigned a pathologic stage (2) (Table 1).

A relative weakness of the Ann Arbor system is its failure to consider disease bulk (either dimension or number of involved sites) or specific patterns of involvement. For this reason, subclassifications of the Ann Arbor staging system have been proposed, particularly for patients with large mediastinal adenopathy (LMA) or stage IIIA disease. LMA, most commonly defined as a mass exceeding one-third the transverse diameter of the chest (intrathoracic width measured at the dome of the diaphragm) on a standard posteroanterior (PA) chest radiograph, places a patient at a greater risk for disease recurrence after radiation alone. Patients with pathologic stage (PS) III disease limited to the spleen or splenic, celiac, or portal nodes are denoted anatomic substage III_1 and considered to have a more favorable prognosis than patients with involvement of paraaortic, iliac, or mesenteric nodes, denoted as III_2 (51). However, this system has not proven useful in some centers.

Data from Stanford University indicate that the presence of five or more nodules visible in the spleen on cut section is an adverse prognostic factor; patients are thus designated as either stage IIIAS + extensive or IIIAS + minimal (52).

The distribution of stages observed in children is somewhat different than that observed in adults. Among 2,238 consecutive patients with HD treated at Stanford, 4% were less than or equal to 10-years old and 11% were 11- to 16-years old. Stage I/II disease was present in about 60% of children. Stage I disease was slightly more common in younger children (18%) than in adolescents (8%), stage II disease occurred in 40% to 50% of all age groups, and stage IV disease was less common in younger children (3%) than in adolescents (15%). "B" symptoms occurred in 19% of younger children and in 30% of adolescents (14).

DIAGNOSTIC EVALUATION

After pathologic confirmation, the patient undergoes an extensive "clinical" staging. This begins with a detailed history for systemic symptoms and evidence for cardiorespiratory compromise or organ dysfunction. The patient's physical examination carefully records the location and size of all palpable lymph nodes. An evaluation of Waldeyer's ring, cardiorespiratory status, and organomegaly is vital. Laboratory studies include complete blood count (CBC) with platelets, erythrocyte sedimentation rate (ESR), and renal and liver function studies. Under investigation are serum makers such as CD8 and

CD30 antigen levels that, along with the ESR, may be associated with a worse prognosis or serve as indicators of disease activity (53–55). Patients with B symptoms or stage III to IV disease should have a bone marrow biopsy (56).

Imaging studies of the thorax should include a chest radiograph with a PA and lateral view. Computerized tomography (CT) scans help delineate the status of intrathoracic lymph node groups (including the hila and cardiophrenic angle), lung parenchyma, pericardium, pleura, and the chest wall, demonstrating abnormalities in about one-half of patients with unremarkable chest radiographs (17,57,58). Definition of disease involvement of some of these tissues will often dictate more aggressive therapy than would otherwise have been administered. Distinguishing normal (or hyperplastic) thymus from nodes in children can be problematic. Magnetic resonance imaging (MRI) can assist in treatment planning (coronal views) and offers the potential to better characterize the presence or absence of posttherapy disease activity (59). The usefulness of gallium scanning in childhood in evaluating supradiaphragmatic nodes has not been specifically established, although the procedure is useful in adults, particularly in assessing the response of mediastinal adenopathy to treatment (60–62).

Imaging of the abdomen and pelvis should include an abdominal/pelvic CT scan and optimally a bilateral lower-extremity lymphangiogram (LAG). LAG can guide the surgeon in subsequent laparotomy, assist the radiation therapist in abdominal radiation field design, and facilitate identification of recurrent disease on follow-up. Distinction of reactive lymph node hyperplasia from HD is problematic. Overall, of the 30% of patients who will have an abnormal LAG, approximately 19% have involvement with HD while 12% have reactive hyperplasia, which is more common in younger children than in adolescents (13,63). Older studies reported CT scanning to be less sensitive than LAG in detecting retroperitoneal HD, and suggested that the ac-

curacy of abdominal CT in children was less than that in adults because of the lack of fat, which provides contrast for the retroperitoneal lymph nodes (64). However, the quality of CT scanning has improved, increasing its sensitivity and specificity. Moreover, many centers are reluctant to perform LAG in young children because the procedure may require general anesthesia, and at some institutions expertise in LAG interpretation is lacking. Of interest, is a report from the Dana–Farber Cancer Institute on 247 children who presented with supradiaphragmatic HD and underwent laparotomy. LAG and CT had false-negative rates of 25% and 22%, respectively, and false-positive rates of 45% and 14%, respectively (65). In a Pediatric Oncology Group (POG) analysis of 216 children, intrinsic spleen lesions and abnormal portahepatic and celiac nodal areas were highly predictive CT findings, but infrequently observed (66). In an important sequence of studies (to be discussed under the Therapy section) from the German-Austrian Pediatric Hodgkin's Disease Study Group, the extent of staging has been progressively refined, including the frequency of laparotomy and splenectomy (67–70). Using ultrasound and CT, these investigators have determined splenic involvement as follows: (a) structural splenic abnormalities from imaging (95% predictive), (b) splenic nodules detected at laparotomy (greater than 95% predictive), and (c) enlargement of splenic hilar nodes (70% predictive). In the German and POG ongoing studies, the size of abdominal/pelvic lymph nodes on CT determine whether lymph node sampling should be performed. Nodes less than 1.5 cm and less than 2 cm, respectively, are considered to be negative, while nodes greater than 2 to 2.5 cm and greater than 3 cm, respectively, are considered positive; nodes falling in between these sizes are biopsied (68,71). A report from St. Jude Children's Research Hospital found MRI to be useful for abdominal imaging (72).

As demonstrated by this data, noninvasive (imaging) studies remain limited in determining splenic involvement in particular, and infradiaphragmatic involvement in general. Representative of other data (2,9,66,73–75), is the Dana–Farber Cancer Institute report (65) in which 25% of 202 clinical stage (CS) I or II children were upstaged, and 27% of 45 CS III or IV children were downstaged. Ninety-six percent of upstaged patients had splenic involvement, and 54% had positive nodes; the spleen was the only site involved in 42% of patients. Three groups had a less than 10% chance of restaging, including CS I to II patients with LPHD, CS I females, and CS III to IV females with non-LPHD histology. A review of the POG experience of the impact of laparotomy on stage change is provided in Table 4. When performed, staging laparotomy includes splenectomy, inspection and wedge biopsy of the liver, multiple lymph node biopsies, and, in the presence of pelvic disease, oophoropexy in females. Bilateral bone marrow biopsies should be performed while the patient is under general anesthesia. Complications following staging laparotomy include immediate postoperative morbidity (rare infection, bowel or ureteral obstruction), and a less than 4% risk of small bowel obstruction due to adhesion. Postoperative mortality is essentially unreported in the past 15 years (2,9,73,74). Historically, a high rate of postsplenectomy sepsis in children (especially less than 5-years old) was reported (9). Administration of pneumococcal vaccination before surgery and daily prophylactic antibiotics appears to have decreased this risk (12). Moreover, a review of 235 children followed after laparotomy and splenectomy for HD re-

vealed only five cases of bacterial sepsis with no fatalities (75). In the Dana–Farber series, 1% of patients were hospitalized for sepsis, and none died (65). The risk of infection appears to be related to the intensity of therapy rather than to splenectomy (9). Any relationship of splenectomy to second malignancies remains controversial (76).

The decision to use surgical staging should be carefully considered. Will the information obtained at laparotomy influence the treatment decision? Clearly this will depend on the philosophy of treatment or specific therapeutic protocol, which must take into account the limitations of clinical staging (66). Will radiotherapy be used and, if so, will it be directed only to sites of gross involvement, to sites of suspected involvement (based on imaging studies), or to sites of demonstrable (by surgical sampling) microscopic involvement? As will be discussed, ample data exist to support strategies that rely on chemotherapy alone to sites of (possible) occult disease (50,67,68,77–79). In general, it is inadvisable to devise new protocols that simultaneously minimize chemotherapy (choice of agents, number of cycles), radiation therapy (dose, volume), and also the thoroughness of staging (63). Therefore, the choice of therapy should dictate the extent of staging. For patients with early stage disease who will be treated with radiotherapy alone, freedom from relapse and overall survival are superior after surgical staging (10, 76,80). In addition, if the abdomen will be treated, then the amount of lung, heart, and

TABLE 4. *Incidence of stage change by laparotomy*

Clinical stage	No. of patients	Pathologic stage				Total stage changes	
		I/II	III₁[a]	III₂	IV	No.	%
I/II	181	13 13	36	9	3	48	27
III₁	9	2	3	4	—	6	67
III₂	9	—	2	7	—	2	22
IV	4	—	—	—	4	0	0

[a]Excludes 13 pathologic stage III₁ patients in whom clinical stage was not reported.
Modified from ref. 66, with permission.

kidney treated will be reduced. If a patient has CS III or IV or bulky mediastinal and pericardial disease and surgical staging will not alter the decision to use aggressive chemotherapy, then involved field radiotherapy based on clinical staging can be considered. If the chemotherapeutic regimen is reduced in intensity, then radiotherapy to all sites of known or suspected microscopic involvement must be considered (10,12,82). On balance, laparotomy with splenectomy has a small rate of morbidity, which argues against its routine use; however, if its results will influence the treatment strategy, it remains appropriate.

PROGNOSTIC FACTORS

As the treatment of HD has improved, characteristics that influence outcome have diminished in importance. However, several factors continue to influence the success and certainly the choice of therapy. These factors are interrelated in the sense that disease stage, bulk, and biologic aggressiveness are frequently codependent (83). Additionally complicating the determination of prognostic factors is that relevant variables are often dependent on staging evaluation and treatment. Most data is based on reports that primarily include adults.

- The *stage of disease* persists as the most important prognostic variable. Patients with advanced stage disease, especially stage IV, have an inferior outlook compared with patients with early stage disease (84).
- The *bulk of disease* is reflected by the disease stage but more specifically is determined by the volume of distinct areas of involvement, and the number of disease sites. Large mediastinal adenopathy (LMA), usually defined as a mass exceeding one-third the transverse diameter of the chest (intrathoracic width measured at the dome of the diaphragm) on a standard PA chest radiograph, places a patient at a greater risk for disease recurrence. For patients with PS I to

II disease with LMA treated with primary radiotherapy, disease-free survival is inferior to that in patients treated with combined modality therapy. However, overall survival remains high due to the effectiveness of salvage chemotherapy (2,17,85–89). Nevertheless, patients with LMA have a somewhat inferior survival rate (2,17,86). Patients (at least those staged only clinically) with *more sites* of involvement, generally defined as 4 or more, fare less well (17,86,89–91). Patients with *extensive splenic involvement* (5 or more nodules) have an inferior prognosis if treated with primary irradiation (52). Patients with stage IV disease who have *multiple organs* involved fare especially poorly.

- *Systemic ("B") symptoms,* which result from cytocrine secretion, reflect biologic aggressiveness and confer a worse prognosis. The constellation of symptoms appears to be relevant to this observation. That is, patients with night sweats only (at least among patients with PS I and II disease) appear to fare as well as PS I to IIA patients, while those with both fevers and weight loss have the worst prognosis (92).
- *Laboratory studies,* including the ESR, serum ferritin, hemoglobin level, serum albumen, and serum CD8 antigen levels have been reported to predict a worse outcome (53–55,83). This could reflect disease biology or bulk.
- *Histologic subtype* is relevant, at least among adults. Patients with pathologic stage I to II MCHD have an increased frequency of subdiaphragmatic relapse, and disease subtype independently influences survival in some reports (17,91). Patients with LDHD fare poorly. A recent report from the United Kingdom Children's Cancer Study Group assessing the relevance of histology in 331 children is revealing. Less than 1% had LDHD, obviating any meaningful assessment of its prognostic significance. For patients with other histologies treated with combined therapy, no difference in outcome was observed (93). As previously discussed, patients with nLPHD

have distinctive differences in disease-free and overall survival.

- *Age* is significant. Survival rates for children with HD approach 85% to 95%. In a report from Stanford, the 5- and 10-year survival for children with HD less than or equal to 10 years of age is 94% and 92%, respectively, compared with 93% and 86% for adolescents (aged 11- to 16-years old) and 84% and 73% for adults (14). Several features of the youngest patient group may influence their improved prognosis, including higher frequency of LP and MC subtypes and of stage I disease, a lower frequency of systemic symptoms, and the more common use of combined modality therapy. Multivariate analysis of this data showed that age, and stage, histology, and treatment modality (combined radiation and chemotherapy versus radiation alone) were all independent prognostic variables for survival (14). Although children less than 4 years of age with HD are uncommon, even these children would appear to have an excellent prognosis (16).

SELECTION OF THERAPY

HD is one of the pediatric malignancies that has an adult counterpart with a similar natural history and biology. Devising the optimal therapeutic approach for children with this disease is complicated by their increased risk for adverse effects. In particular, radiotherapy doses and fields used in adults can cause profound musculoskeletal retardation including intraclavicular narrowing, shortened sitting height, decreased mandibular growth, and decreased muscle development in the treated volume (9,10) (see Chapter 19). Therefore, while adults with early stage HD are often treated with full dose radiation as a single modality (17,86), this approach in prepubertal children, despite a similar success rate, produces unacceptable sequelae (10,88,94–96). Additionally complicating the treatment of children are gender-specific differences in chemotherapy-induced gonadal

injury. The desire to cure young children with minimal side effects has stimulated attempts to reduce staging procedures, the intensity and types of chemotherapy, and the radiation dose and volume. Because of the differences in the age-related developmental status of children, and the gender-related sensitivity to chemotherapy, there is no single method of treatment that is ideal for all pediatric patients.

Important studies using chemotherapy and low-dose radiation in children to effect cure with tolerable sequelae were done at Stanford University. Trials at Stanford have used chemotherapy in combination with lower doses of radiation therapy for young children with early-stage disease (2,11,12). Donaldson and Link (12) reported excellent results with local control with irradiation after using nitrogen mustard, vincristine, procarbazine, and prednisone (MOPP). Radiation doses were 15 Gy for patients with bone age 5 years or less, 20 Gy for those 6 to 10 years, and 25 Gy for those 11 to 14 years of age. Additional boosts were given to those who failed to achieve a complete remission or in those with bulky disease (greater than 6-cm nodes or LMA if mediastinal disease was present). The overall local control was 97% (12). Although growth deformity was decreased, full course MOPP is associated with a high risk of sterility and secondary leukemia (discussed in Chapters 19 and 20). Therefore, alternate regimens were subsequently used. In general, the use of radiation and chemotherapy broadens the spectrum of potential toxicities, while reducing the severity of individual (drug or radiation-related) toxicities. Current approaches, to be discussed subsequently, entail chemotherapy in conjunction with reduced radiation doses (12,97,98) (Tables 2 and 3). The extent of staging should be treatment dependent. The volume of radiation and the intensity/duration of chemotherapy is stage dependent. Results for patients with early and advanced stage HD are summarized in Tables 5 and 6 (data to be discussed in the following sections), and an outline of our therapeutic recommendations is presented in Table 7.

TABLE 5. *Treatment results in children with early-stage Hodgkin's disease[a]*

Group/Institution	No. Patients	Stage		RT (Therapy)	Chemo	Overall (% Survival)	Relapse	Follow-up interval (yr)	Ref.
Radiotherapy alone (full dose IF or EF)									
Children's Hospital of Philadelphia	31	PS	IA, IIA	EF		83	64	10	107
Joint Center/Harvard	50	PS	I, IIA	EF		97	82	11	10,34
St. Bartholomew's/ Great Ormond Street	28	CS[b]	I, II	IF		96	79	10	95
Stanford University	48	PS[c]	I, II	EF		86	82	10	95
Intergroup Hodgkin's Study	39	PS	I, II	IF		95	41	5	96
	58	PS	I, II	EF		96	67	5	96
University of Toronto	23	CS/PS	I	IF[d]		95	87	10	110
	42	PS	IIA, IIIA	EF		85	45	10	110
Full-dose RT + chemotherapy									
Hospital Saint-Louis	52	CS	I, II	IF	MOPP ×3–6	94	88	10	167
Intergroup Hodgkin's Study	97	PS	I, II	IF	MOPP ×6	90	95	5	96
St. Bartholomew's/ Great Ormond Street	39	CS[b]	I, II	IF	ChlVPP or MOPP or MVPP ×3–8	86	84	10	95
German (DAL) HD78	73	PS	I-IIA	EF	OPPA ×2	97	90	10	70
HD82	100	CS/PS	I, IIA	IF	OPPA ×2	100	96	12	69
HD85	53	CS/PS	I, IIA	IF	OPA ×2	98	85	5	69,70
Low-dose RT + chemotherapy									
Stanford University	27	PS	I, II		MOPP ×6	100	96	10	13
	44	CS/PS	I, II, III		MOPP ×3/ABVD ×3	100	100	10	106
University of Toronto	27	CS	II, III		MOPP ×6	93	89	10	110
Children's Hospital of Philadelphia	30	CS	I, II		COPP ×6 or ABVD ×6 or MOPP ×3/ ABVD ×3	90	68	10	107
German (DAL) HD87	104	CS/PS	I-IIA	IF[e]	OPA ×2	99	85	5	70
HD90	115f	CS	IA, IIA	IF[e]	OPPA ×2		96	5	67,68
	159m	CS	IA, IIA	IF[e]	OEPA ×2		93	5	67,68
Italian Multicenter Study	58	CS	IA, IIA	IF	ABVD ×3		95	7	79
French National Study	67	CS	IA, IIA	IF	MOPP ×2ABVD ×2		89	6	102
	65	CS	IA, IIA	IF[e]	ABVD ×4		[f]	6	102
	133	CS	I, II	IF[e]	VBVP ×4±OPPA ×2	96	92	3	102
St. Jude Children's Research Hospital	28	CS	I-IIB	IF	COP(P)×4–5 or ABVD×3–4	96	96	5	50
Chemotherapy alone									
Uganda	38	CS	I-II		MOPP ×6	100	100	5	119
Australia/New Zealand	38	CS	IA-IIIA		MOPP or ChlVPP ×6–8	94	92	4	117
Costa Rica	52	CS	IA-IIIA		CVPP ×6	100	90	5	168

[a]Modified from ref. 166, with permission.
[b]Some patients pathologically staged
[c]Some patients clinically staged
[d]Some patients received chemotherapy
[e]Boost to 35–40 Gy allowed
[f]The relapse-free survival was 89% for both therapy regimens combined

PS, pathologic stage; **CS**, clinical stage; Full-dose radiotherapy = minimum dose to any nodal field ≥30 Gy; Low-dose to any nodal field ≤25.5 Gy; **IF**, involved field; **EF**, extended field; **MOPP**, nitrogen mustard, vincristine, procarbazine, prednisone; **ChlVPP**, chlorambucil, vincristine, prednisone, procarbazine; **MVPP**, nitrogen mustard, vinblastine, procarbazine, prednisone; **OPPA**, vincristine, procarbazine, prednisone, doxorubicin; **OPA**, vincristine, prednisone, doxorubicin; **COPP**, cyclophosphamide, vincristine, procarbazine, prednisone; **ABVD**, adriamycin, bleomycin, vinblastine, and dacarbazine; **OEPA**, vincristine, etoposide, prednisone, doxorubicin; **VBVP**, vinblastine, bleomycin, vincristine, prednisone; **CVPP**, cyclophosphamide, vinblastine, procarbazine, prednisone

TABLE 6. *Treatment Results in Children with Advanced-Stage Hodgkin's Disease*[a]

Group/Institution	No. Patients	PS Stage	RT (Gy)	Chemo	Survival (%) Overall	Survival (%) Relapse-free	Follow-up interval (yr)	Ref.
Stanford University	28	III-IV	IF 15–25	MOPPx6	78	84	7.5	13
	13	IV	IF 15–25	MOPPx3/ABVDx3	85	69	10	106
German (DAL) HD82	53	IIB-IIIA	IF 30	2OPPA/2COP(P)		90	12	68
	50	IIIB-IV	IF 25–35	OPPAx2/COP(P)x4	72	85	12	68
German (DAL) HD90	57 f	IEA, IIB,	IF 25	OPPAx2/COPPx2		96	3	68
	66 m	IIEA		OEPAx2/COPPx2		90	3	
	86 f	IIEB,	IF 20	OPPAx2/COPPx4		91	3	
	92 m	IIIEA, IIIB, IV		OEPAx2/COPPx4		83	3	68
French (SFOP)	69	[b]IB, IIB, III-IV	IF+PA 20	MOPPx3/ABVDx3	95	93	2.5	105
Children's Hospital of Philadelphia	29	III-IV	EF 25–40	COPPx6, ABVDx6, or MOPPx3/ABVDx3	88	63	10	107
Children's Cancer Group (CCG 521)	111	III-IV	none	MOPPx6/ABVDx6 versus	[c]	77	3	101
			IF 21	ABVDx6	[c]	84	3	101
Pediatric Oncology Group	62	IIB-IV	TNI 21	MOPPx4/ABVDx4	91	77	3	108
	81	IIB, IIIA$_2$	none	MOPPx4/ABVDx4	96	79	5	71
	80[d]	IIIB, IV	IF 21	MOPPx4/ABVDx4	87	80		
University of Toronto	20	[b]III-IV	EF 20–30	MOPPx6	60	65	10	110
Joint Center/Harvard	96	III-IV	EF 25–40	MOPPx6	81	—	11	10,34
Australia/New Zealand	8	III-IV	none	MOPPx6-12	92	80	5	117
Italian Multicenter Study	38	IIIB, IV	EF 20–25	MOPPx5/ABVDx5		60	7	79
Int Soc Ped Onc (SIOP)	65	IV	IF 20	OPPAx2/COPPx4	93	78	8	68
St. Jude Children's Research Hospital	57	III-IV	IF 20	COP(P)x4-5/ABVDx3-4	93	93		50
Costa Rica	24	III-IV	none	CVPPx6/EBOx6	81	60	5	168

[a]Modified from ref. 166, with permission.
[b]Clinically staged
[c]Overall survival for both arms = 90%; of these 100% of stage III and 60% of stage IV were relapse-free
[d]g did not receive RT

PS = pathological stage; **CS** = clinical stage; **IF** = involved field; **EF** = extended field; **PA** = para-aortic + spleen (pedicle); **TNI** = total nodal irradiation; **MOPP** = nitrogen mustard, vincristine, procarbazine, prednisone; **ABVD** = adriamycin, bleomycin, vinblastine, and dacarbazine; **OPPA** = vincristine, procarbazine, prednisone, doxorubicin; **COPP** = cyclophosphamide, vincristine, procarbazine, prednisone; **OEPA** = vincristine, etoposide, prednisone, doxorubicin; **CVPP** = cyclophosphamide, vinblastine, procarbazine, prednisone; **EBO** = epirubicin, bleomycin, vincristine.

TABLE 7. *Guidelines for Treatment Selection in Pediatric Hodgkin's Disease[a]*

Stage	Clinical Presentation	Recommendations
IA, IIA	Post pubertal: Laparotomy negative, non-bulky mediastinal mass, no juxtapericardial disease	Standard dose RT (STNI generally)
	Prepubertal, pubertal, bulky mediastinal mass or juxtapericardial disease	Low-dose RT (IF)[b] + chemotherapy
IB, IIB	Post pubertal; laparotomy negative, non-bulky mediastinal mass, no juxtapericardial disease, and night-sweats ± fevers or weight loss	Standard dose RT (STNI generally) alternative: low-dose RT (IF) + chemotherapy
	Prepubertal, pubertal, bulky mediastinal mass or juxtapericardial disease, or fevers and weight loss	Low-dose RT (IF)[b] + chemotherapy
IIIA1, IIIA1S + (minimal)	Post pubertal: Non-bulky mediastinal mass, no juxtapericardial disease	Standard RT (STNI or TNI) or RT + CT Hepatic RT if spleen involved and RT only is used
	Prepubertal, or pubertal with bulky mediastinal mass or juxtapericardial disease	Low dose RT (IF) + chemotherapy
IIIA1S+ (extensive), IIIA2, IIIB, IVA, IVB		Chemotherapy + low dose RT (IF) (RT particularly recommended for bulky adenopathy)
Recurrent		Chemotherapy if none previously, otherwise consider BMT (RT ± CT in selected patients with nodal relapse >1 yr after CT alone)

[a]Modified from ref. 166, with permission.
[b]Some institutions always use a mantle field and/or standard dose for bulky mediastinal disease.
RT = radiation therapy; Standard dose RT = 35–36 Gy ± boost; Low-dose RT = ≤ 25 Gy; **STNI** = subtotal nodal irradiation; **IF** = involved field; **TNI** = total nodal irradiation; **BMT** = bone marrow transplant; S + (minimal) based on < 5 nodules; S + (extensive) based on ≥ 5 nodules; **CT** = Chemotherapy: 6 ABVD, 6–8 MOPP/ABVD, 6 OPPA/COP(P) or other experimental regimens. Less intensive therapy for early-stage disease is experimental as to the number of cycles and drug combinations.

Combined Chemotherapy and Radiotherapy

MOPP was the standard chemotherapy regimen used in the United States for many years after DeVita et al.'s 1972 report (7). The major toxicities include an associated risk of acute leukemia, azospermia in more than 90% of males treated at any age, and a risk of sterility in females, which increases with age (99). In 1987, Stanford investigators reported long-term follow-up of patients less than 14 years of age treated with 6 cycles of MOPP chemotherapy and low-dose involved field radiation; the actuarial sur-

vival rate was 89% with a local control rate of 97%. Long-term side effects included acute leukemias in 3 of 55 children and azoospermia in all 4 boys tested. Inhibition of soft tissue and bone growth was minimal with this approach (12). Subsequently, the effectiveness of adriamycin, bleomycin, vinblastine, and dacarbazine (ABVD) as front-line chemotherapy was established (100–102). Compared to MOPP, second malignancies and sterility were less common (103). The predominant adverse effects of ABVD are pulmonary toxicity related to bleomycin and cardiovascular toxicity secondary to adriamycin. These side effects may be exacerbated by the addition of mediastinal or mantle irradiation (104).

Reports on the use of combined ABVD and MOPP also document excellent disease control with diminished toxicity relative to MOPP alone (101,105–108). The intention is to decrease the number of cycles of MOPP and, therefore, potentially lower the risk of leukemogenesis and sterility, while also diminishing the side effects associated with 6 cycles of ABVD (105). In a report on 238 clinically staged patients from the French Society of Pediatric Oncology (SFOP), early stage (CS I to IIA) patients were treated with 4 cycles of ABVD, or 2 cycles each of MOPP and ABVD plus involved-field, low-dose (20 Gy) radiation therapy. For advanced disease (CS IB to IV), patients were treated with 3 cycles each of MOPP and ABVD plus extended-field low-dose radiotherapy. For patients with a poor response to chemotherapy, additional radiation therapy to achieve full dose was given. The 5-year disease-free survival rate is 86% and the actuarial survival for the entire group is 92% (102). The Children's Cancer Study Group compared alternating MOPP and ABVD (12 cycles) with ABVD (6 cycles) and low-dose irradiation (21 Gy) to regions of disease involvement for patients with advanced HD (stages III and IV). For stage III patients, the 3-year overall survival rate was 90%, while event-free survival (EFS) was 81% (77% for the MOPP/ABVD group, and 84% for the ABVD/radiation group). The 3-year EFS for 111 patients without LMA was 100%, for those with LMA it was 78%, and for stage IV patients it was 60% (101). Investigators at Stanford University treated 57 children younger than 16 years (1, stage I; 22, stage II; 21, stage III; 13, stage IV) with 6 cycles of alternating ABVD and MOPP, with involved field radiotherapy intercalated between cycles. The radiotherapy dose was 15 Gy, with a boost to 25 Gy to sites of bulky disease and to areas that failed to respond completely to 2 cycles of chemotherapy. Five and 10-year actuarial survival and freedom-from-relapse (FFR) rates are 96% and 93%. For the stage IV subgroup, the 5-year actuarial sur-

vival and FFR are 85% and 68%, respectively (106). A regimen that eliminates dacarbazine while administering ABV/MOPP each month has now been used in children with apparent success (78).

An important sequence of studies performed by the German-Austrian Pediatric Hodgkin's Disease Study Group progressively refined the extent of staging, and the intensity of chemotherapy and radiation (67–70). The nature and results of these studies (HD-82, 85, 87, 90) are summarized in Tables 5 and 6. Staging was reduced from systematic use of laparotomy (HD-78), to selective laparotomy and splenectomy (HD-82), to infrequent laparotomy without splenectomy (HD-90) (discussed fully in the Staging section). Stage-dependent chemotherapy and radiation dose/volume was also used. In the early studies, vincristine, procarbazine, prednisone, doxorubicin (OPPA) ± cyclophosphamide, vincristine, procarbazine, prednisone (COPP) were used. In HD-85 and HD-87 OPA (eliminating procarbazine) was used for boys in order to reduce testicular toxicity, but EFS declined. In HD-90, girls received OPPA ± COPP (depending on stage), while boys received OEPA ± COPP, adding etoposide to OPA.

Radiotherapy

As for adults, select adolescents with favorable early-stage HD are appropriately treated with full-dose radiotherapy, reserving chemotherapy for relapse (10,33,95,96,107, 109,110). Children appropriate for this approach are pubertal and fully grown, obviating concerns about muscle and bone development. Therefore, radiation therapy to mantle and paraaortic fields remains standard for surgically staged adolescents with supradiaphragmatic stage IA to IIA disease (111). Patients with LMA and/or extensive disease involving the pericardium or juxtapericardial nodes should usually not be treated with radiation alone because of the inferior prognosis as well as the unacceptable pulmonary and cardiac radiation doses. Exceptions include patients with LMA but no juxtapericardial disease or other adverse prognostic factors in whom sufficient lung and heart can be protected; meticulous technique with successive field reductions are necessary (2,17,85–88). Extended-field radiation to the mantle and paraaortic regions has been associated with an improved relapse-free survival when compared to more limited volumes in surgically staged patients (11,17,82). However, select patients (e.g., stage IA LPHD with cervical involvement) may be treated to more limited volumes. Radiotherapy alone for patients with clinical stage I and II disease and favorable prognostic factors (female sex, less than or equal to 3 sites, low ESR, LPHD or NSHD, no LMA) is now increasingly used, but specific long-term data for children are lacking (91,112,113). More recently, mantle field irradiation alone has been used for pathologically staged favorable patients, but this approach remains investigational in children (113).

Adolescents with stage IB and IIB disease may be considered for treatment with radiation alone. Hoppe et al. (90) reported a randomized prospective trial of children and adults who were treated for PS IB to IIB disease with total lymphoid irradiation (TLI) alone versus TLI plus MOP(P) or PAVe (procarbazine, mustard, vinblastine). The 10-year survivals were no different (approximately 80%). In an additional analysis of the Stanford and Harvard-Joint Center for Radiation Therapy PS IB to IIB patients, it continued to appear reasonable to treat many such patients with radiation alone. However, the presence of LMA or fever plus weight loss predicted a poor outcome, warranting combined modality therapy (92).

Can pelvic irradiation be safely omitted in children with laparotomy-proven supradiaphragmatic stage I and II disease (114)? Goodman et al. (115) reported 81 patients aged 6 to 59 years treated for supradiaphragmatic PS IA to IIA disease with mantle and paraaortic fields but no pelvic irradiation. There were no pelvic or inguinal recurrences. These results were confirmed by Kaplan (2). However, Mendenhall et al. (116) observed a 9% frequency of pelvic recurrence in pathologically staged I to II patients treated with mantle and paraaortic fields. In patients with IB or IIB disease, the addition of pelvic irradiation did not influence overall survival or FFR (92). In patients with supradiaphragmatic PS I to II disease, it is desirable to reduce bone marrow and gonadal irradiation and not treat the pelvis.

The treatment of fully grown children with TLI alone for stage IIIA disease is controversial. In combined adult-pediatric series the 5-year relapse-free survival rate ranges from 35% to 60%. Several investigators have tried to subclassify IIIA to identify (a) good prognosis groups suitable for treatment with TLI alone, and (b) bad prognosis groups more appropriate for combined modality therapy. These attempts include the University of Chicago system (better prognosis: IIIA1—upper abdominal nodes accompanying the celiac vessels; worse prognosis: IIIA2—lower abdominal nodes), the Yale system (better prognosis: CS I or II/PS III; worse prognosis: CS III/PS III), and the Stanford system (worse prognosis: greater than 5 splenic nodules) (51,52). LMA is also a poor prognostic sign (2,17,86). Differences in treatment techniques of individual institutions may make comparisons of these systems difficult. In grown children, however, TLI alone may be appropriate for minimal IIIA disease, although combined therapy is recommended at many centers and is always recommended for less favorable IIIA patients. The exact definition of minimal disease remains controversial.

Chemotherapy

The arguments that favor treatment with chemotherapy alone for all stages are that it eliminates the need for surgical staging, and that the dysmorphic and rare carcinogenic consequences of irradiation are avoided. The disadvantages of the use of chemotherapy alone are the risks of treatment-related fatality, infertility, and leukemogenesis (117), as well as an increased likelihood of disease recurrence in sites of bulk disease (84,118). The longest follow-up data are from the Uganda experience (119) with only a 67% 9-year survival. Subgroups included CS I to IIIA patients with a 75% survival, and CS IIIB to IV patients with a 60% and 47% survival at 5 and 10 years, respectively. Ekert et al. (117) reported a 90% 5-year survival for CS I to II children treated with MOPP or a similar program that substitutes chlorambucil for nitrogen mustard and vinblastine for vincristine (ChlVPP) (Table 5), but the disease-free and overall survival was 40% and 55%, respectively, for children with advanced disease. A report from The Netherlands describes 37 children treated with 6 cycles of MOPP for "small" lymph node disease (defined as less than or equal to 4 cm), with the addition of 25 Gy involved-field radiation therapy for children with "large" lymph node disease. The disease-free survival with a median follow-up of 62+ months is 90% for the former (21 children) and 85.5% for the latter (16 children) (120). In a recent report from the POG, children treated with 4 cycles each of MOPP and ABVD had an excellent outcome (71) (Table 6); the addition of radiation therapy did not improve disease-free or overall survival. However, statistical and quality assurance issues complicate interpretation of this data (121). Moreover, longer follow-up will be necessary to assess the toxicity from 8 cycles of chemotherapy. Could a beneficial effect of radiation therapy have been seen if the number of cycles of chemotherapy was decreased (122)? Other data in adults support the appropriateness of combined therapy rather than chemotherapy alone for patients with early and advanced stage disease (111,123,124).

Summary Recommendations for Primary Disease

Overall, for children who are prepubescent or have advanced-stage disease, chemotherapy plus low-dose radiation therapy appears to be the most appropriate treatment with excellent long-term survival (Table 7). Adolescents with favorable early-stage disease should be considered for radiation therapy alone. Future studies will define the optimal chemotherapeutic agents and number of cycles, chemotherapy/radiotherapy scheduling, and the necessary dose and volume of irradiation to maximize cure while decreasing the side effects of chemotherapy and radiation therapy.

Refractory/Relapsed Disease and Bone Marrow Transplantation

HD may still be cured even after initial treatment programs fail. Relapse occurs most often within 4 years, but late relapse is not rare. The choice of therapy for such patients is dependent on the initial treatment and the disease characteristics at the time of relapse.

A spectrum of treatment options exist, including (125):

- standard-dose chemotherapy, with either the same initial regimen, or an alternative regimen, which could be third-line (depending on previous regimens). If possible, radiation therapy can be added.
- radiation therapy alone
- high-dose chemotherapy (with or without radiation therapy), followed by stem-cell support. The source of the stem cells can be allogeneic or autologous bone marrow, or peripheral stem cells
- experimental therapy (e.g., radiolabeled antiferritin)
- palliative therapy

For patients who were initially treated with radiation therapy alone, salvage chemotherapy is effective, providing disease-free and overall survival in 55% to 80% (109,126, 127). If radiation therapy can be safely added to chemotherapy as salvage treatment, the outcome may be superior (125,127). Factors that independently predict a more favorable outcome include the following:

- site of relapse (nodal better than extranodal),
- the stage that could be assigned at relapse (early better than advanced)
- the histology (LP and NS better than MC).

For children who relapse after treatment that includes chemotherapy, conventional (standard-dose) salvage chemotherapy regimens are of limited success, providing disease-free and overall survival in only 10% to 50% (109,125,126). Fortunately, other strategies can be effective. The selection of the most appropriate salvage regimen is based on several considerations, including:

- did the patient ever achieve a complete remission, or was the disease refractory?
- if a CR was achieved, was it durable (longer than 1 year)?
- was the relapse in nodal or extranodal sites and, as a corollary, was the stage at relapse early or advanced?

The most favorable patients are those who have disease recurrence only at a prolonged interval after an initial CR, and in a limited nodal pattern. Some of these patients can, in fact, be cured by radiotherapy alone, often administered as TLI (128–131). TLI is difficult to administer, however, in patients who have had a significant marrow insult from aggressive chemotherapy. Regional irradiation (e.g., a mantle in a patient with mediastinal recurrence), with or without chemotherapy, is preferred in some centers (132). However, even these patients may have a superior outcome (EFS as high as 80%) if treated with high-dose chemotherapy and autologous stem cell rescue (133,134). On the opposite end of the spectrum, are those patients who have chemotherapy refractory disease, who are essentially never cured by conventional salvage chemotherapy.

Patients who relapse after regimens that include chemotherapy have been treated with high-dose chemotherapy and hematopoietic stem cell rescue (125,134–136). Three- to 5-year survival probabilities of 25% to 80%, depending on characteristics at relapse, have been reported (primarily in adults) following such treatment (100,133,135,137). Only one prospective study randomizing refractory or relapsed patients with HD to high-dose chemotherapy and stem cell rescue versus conventional dose chemotherapy has been performed. The British National Lymphoma Investigation Group randomized 40 patients to carmustine, etoposide, cytarabine, and melphalan (BEAM) with stem cell support versus lower dose (mini-) BEAM (138). Progression-free survival at 3 years was 53% versus 10%, respectively. Recently, investigators at Stanford compared patients with recurrent or relapsed HD who were treated with high-dose chemotherapy and autologous bone marrow transplant (AuBMT) (EFS 53%) to a matched group treated with conventional dose chemotherapy (EFS 27%) (139). Consistent with previous data, patients refractory or relapsing within 12 months of therapy benefited the most; conversely, an advantage was not observed for patients with a durable (more than 1 year) first remission. Data specific to children with recurrent HD is limited. However, an analysis of 81 pediatric HD patients who underwent AuBMT and were reported to the European Bone Marrow Transplant Group demonstrated a similar outcome to a case-matched group of adults similarly treated (Fig. 4) (140). Prognostic factors for a favorable outcome include the duration of initial response to chemotherapy, "B" symptoms at relapse, disseminated pulmonary or bone marrow disease at relapse, and more than minimal disease at the time of transplantation (133,141). A variety of preparative regimens provide similar outcome (136,141–143).

What are the possible roles for radiation therapy in the setting of high-dose chemotherapy and stem cell rescue for HD? The basis for including radiation therapy is essentially 2-fold: (a) these aggressive salvage programs still fail to cure a large proportion of patients, and (b) ample data exists which documents many patients with progressive/recurrent HD following chemotherapy do not exhibit a cross-resistance to radiation (125,128–131). Moreover, most patients relapse in sites of previous involvement, mostly nodal (133, 142,169). Radiation therapy can be administered, in combination with chemotherapy conditioning regimens, as total-body irradiation (TBI), involved field radiation therapy, and TLI. Typical preparative regimens that in-

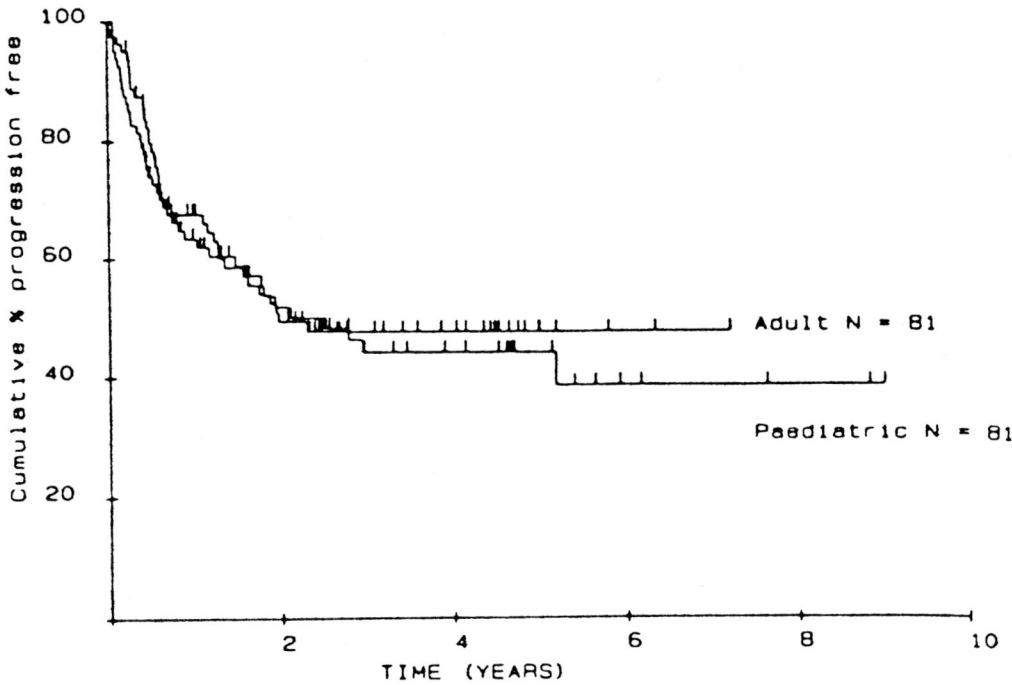

FIG. 4. Progression-free survival after allogeneic bone marrow transplant for Hodgkin's disease: comparison between pediatric and matched adult patients. $x = 0.2194$, $p = 0.6395$. (From ref. 140, with permission.)

clude TBI or TLI are cyclophosphamide with or without etoposide (125,141,144). The rationale for TBI (e.g., 12 to 14 Gy in 4 to 5 days at 1.5 to 2.5 Gy b.i.d.) or TLI (e.g., 18 Gy in 2 weeks at 0.9 Gy b.i.d.), is the associated tumor cell kill and immunosuppressive effects. However, TBI/TLI programs for patients who have previously been treated with mediastinal radiation therapy are associated with a significant increase in pulmonary complications (144,145). Pneumonitis and pulmonary alveolar hemorrhage are often fatal. Because there does not appear to be a difference in relapse-free survival between TBI/TLI preparative regimens and those which do not use magna field irradiation, one can make an argument to avoid TBI or TLI if prior mediastinal irradiation has been given or is contemplated as boost treatment.

In considering the role of involved field radiation therapy (IFRT) in the setting of high-dose chemotherapy and stem cell rescue,

three essential questions must be answered: (a) Does radiation therapy to sites of recurrent or refractory HD diminish relapse at these sites? (b) If so, then what is the impact on freedom from relapse, EFS, and overall survival? (c) Is the associated morbidity of IFRT acceptable? Data from several series support an affirmative answer to these questions (125,136,143,146–148). In a Stanford report, patients with stages I to III disease at relapse who received AuBMT and IFRT had a 3-year freedom from relapse of 100% and overall survival of 85%, compared with 67% and 60%, respectively, for patients not receiving IFRT (148). For patients not previously irradiated, IFRT was associated with an improved freedom from relapse of 85% and overall survival of 93%, in contrast to 57% and 55%, respectively, for those previously irradiated. Morbidity was similar to those not irradiated, although radiation therapy may have contributed to the peritransplant death of 2 patients. Central issues relating to the use of IFRT are the dose, target volume and timing with respect to the transplant. Radiation therapy doses are generally 20 to 36 Gy, in 1.5 to 2.0 Gy fractions. This variation relates to potential normal tissue toxicity as well as the consideration for higher radiation doses in patients with identifiable tumor that demonstrates radiation responsiveness (136,149). Radiation volume can vary and include treatment to all sites of initial disease, recurrent disease, persistent disease following salvage chemotherapy, persistent disease following the preparative regimen for transplant, or all nodal sites (125,134,136). TLI administered prior to transplant has been an effective program at Memorial Sloan-Kettering (144). IFRT can be administered prior to the high-dose chemotherapy program in order to place patients in a minimal disease state. Radiation therapy can also be administered after the high-dose chemotherapy program in order to decrease the potential for disease progression elsewhere during the time radiation therapy is being administered, and radiation therapy-related peritransplant morbidity such as esophagitis, pneumonitis, cardiomyopathy, and venoocclusive disease. Possible disadvantages of this approach include the loss of the pretransplant cytoreductive effect, and the theoretical carcinogenic effect of radiation therapy on the newly proliferating hematopoietic system (125,134,136).

RADIOTHERAPEUTIC MANAGEMENT

Success in the radiotherapeutic management of patients with HD requires excellent technique. The Patterns of Care studies (73,97,150) have helped define radiation therapy standards of practice. Results of treatment with radiation therapy alone were statistically better at institutions that treated a large number of HD patients. Factors associated with an increased risk of relapse included the use of small "involved" radiation fields as opposed to more extended fields, inadequate margins, cobalt-60 machines with a source-skin dis-

tance of less than 80 cm, and patients not undergoing treatment simulation. Although different institutions and radiation oncologists may use slightly different techniques, underlying principles and, in fact, most of the technical details are the same (2,151–153).

Volume considerations

The *mantle field* requires meticulous technique because of the distribution of lymph nodes and the critical adjacent normal tissues. This field can be simulated with the arms up over the head, or down with hands on the hips. The former pulls the axillary lymph nodes away from the lungs, allowing greater lung shielding. However, the axillary lymph nodes then move into the vicinity of the humeral heads, which should be blocked in growing children. Therefore, the position chosen involves weighing concerns regarding lymph nodes, lung, and humeral heads. Equally weighted anterior and posterior fields treated daily are used. Anteriorly weighted fields excessively irradiate the anterior heart with associated cardiac morbidity (154). Dose calculations should be based on the patient separation at the central axis. When a full mantle field is treated, nodes in the neck and axilla receive a higher dose because of the decreased patient thickness compared to the mid-thorax. Therefore, separate axillary, neck, and low mediastinal dosimetry should be performed. Extended source-to-skin distances decrease dose inhomogeneity in these different areas. Because of the increased dose to the neck and cervical spinal cord, a posterior cervical spine block extending from the top of the field down to below the level of the larynx may be added at a neck dose of 20 to 30 Gy. Blocking the thoracic cord is not recommended because it risks underdosing mediastinal nodes (153). Lung blocks should then be carefully drawn, allowing adequate (1 to 2 cm) margins around mediastinal disease. If chemotherapy has been given, then the width of the field is generally based on the postchemotherapy residual disease. As previously stated, humeral head blocks are appropriate unless bulky axillary adenopathy would thereby be shielded. Laryngeal and occipital blocks are also used unless disease is located in the vicinity of these structures; these blocks can be placed at the beginning of treatment or after some portion of it. Depending on the dose administered, field reductions may be possible. Because 10- to 15-Gy doses can cytoreduce HD, increasing the size of lung or cardiac blocks is often possible once or twice during the course of therapy. The entire heart or lungs are rarely treated above doses of 10 to 16 Gy, depending on the distribution of disease and chemotherapy used. More specifically, the indications for whole heart irradiation include pericardial involvement as suggested by a pericardial effusion or frank pericardial invasion with tumor; such patients will generally receive combined modality therapy and 10 to 15 Gy to the entire heart. Whole lung irradiation with partial transmission blocks is a consideration in the setting of overt pulmonary nodules, or hilar involvement. In the former setting, whole lung irradiation to 10 to 15 Gy is a consideration in patients who are treated with combined modality therapy. For patients with hilar involvement who are treated with radiation therapy alone, whole lung irradiation through partial transmission blocks is controversial (155). If a patient is treated to the whole lung and later requires chemotherapy due to disease recurrence, then the risk for pneumonitis escalates. In any case, most patients with hilar involvement will receive combined therapy; in this setting chemotherapy is presumed to be adequate for possible microscopic lymphatic involvement within the lung. Attempts should be made to position breast tissue under the lung/axillary blocking. A gap should be calculated when matching the paraaortic field (2,151).

When treating the *subdiaphragmatic region*, the spleen or pedicle must be included while minimizing the radiation dose to the kidneys. Usually the upper pole of the left kidney is within the irradiated volume. An intravenous pyelogram performed at the time of the simulation, a treatment planning CT, or

diagnostic information obtained from the CT or MRI (coronal slices from a thoracic MRI will reveal the relationship of the spleen to the kidney) are helpful in drawing the blocks. When treating the *pelvis*, special attention must be given to the ovaries and testes. The ovaries should be relocated, and marked with surgical clips, laterally along the iliac wings, or centrally behind the uterus. In this manner appropriate shielding may be used. The testes receive 5% to 10% of the administered pelvic dose, which is sufficient to cause transient or permanent azospermia, depending on the total pelvic dose. The greatest shielding can be afforded to the testes if the patient is placed in a frog-legged position with an individually constructed testes shield. If multileaf collimation is available, the multileaf can be placed over the testes, additionally decreasing the transmitted dose.

The appropriate treatment volume, as well as the radiation dose, essentially depends on whether the patient is being treated with radiation therapy alone or combined modality therapy. Additional considerations relate to the location of disease (e.g., pericardium, chest wall, etc.) In the presence of chemotherapy, involved fields or regions may be used. Definitions of such fields depend on the anatomy of the region in terms of lymph node distribution, patterns of disease extension into regional areas, and considerations for match line problems should disease recur. Field definitions are often protocol specific, but excessively small fields are usually inappropriate. For example, if only supraclavicular nodes are involved, at a minimum the ipsilateral cervical nodes should also be treated due to the anatomic continuity of these areas. Moreover, in a pre-pubertal child, consideration should be given to treating bilateral areas (e.g., both sides of the neck) to avoid growth asymmetry. However, this is less of a concern with low radiation doses. Other considerations relate to the risk of second malignant neoplasms. For example, a child with isolated mediastinal disease receiving combined modality therapy can be treated with shielding of the axilla and thus the breast tissue, and perhaps the thyroid gland. Clearly, careful planning and judgement are necessary.

Energy

Megavoltage energies are necessary. A 4- to 6-MV linear accelerator should be used for mantle fields, thereby ensuring adequate doses to the superficial nodes in the build-up region as well as to deep nodal areas such as the mediastinum. Higher energy machines (8 to 15 MV) are recommended for treating paraaortic nodes. If high-energy machines are used for treatment of the mantle field, some therapists introduce a beam spoiler or bolus on the neck and supraclavicular regions.

Dose considerations

Kaplan (2) constructed a radiation dose-response curve for HD, but limitations of its current applicability include its use of kilovoltage data. Reports demonstrate that lower radiation doses provide excellent local control with variables including tumor size and fractionation schedule (73,97,98,150,152,156). In the absence of chemotherapy, subclinical disease is reliably (95%) controlled with 25 to 30 Gy, small bulk disease (variously defined but less than 5 cm in most reports) requires 30 to 35 Gy, and large bulk disease an additional 5 to 10 Gy. The doses per fraction should be 1.5 to 1.8 Gy daily, five times a week. Patients treated with large volumes may only tolerate 1.5 Gy fractions. In the setting of combined therapy, certainly the intensity of the chemotherapy is important to consider in the choice of the radiation dose and volume. However, doses of 15 to 30 Gy are typical with shrinking fields and boosts individualized (Tables 6 and 7). In a recently reported randomized trial by the German Hodgkin Lymphoma Group (157), patients with stage I to IIIA disease with intermediate prognosis received 20, 30, or 40 Gy to nonbulky or uninvolved sites following 4 months of chemotherapy. Bulk (greater than 7.5 cm) disease always received 40 Gy. With this constraint, no difference was observed for the various doses.

Sequence of therapy

The most effective sequence of therapy in the setting of combined chemotherapy and irradiation is not unequivocally established. However, chemotherapy is usually the first modality. This allows assessment of drug response, maximization of the amount of drug treatment as well as shrinkage of disease and more limited fields of irradiation. Occasionally, focal irradiation prior to chemotherapy will be necessary because of airway obstruction.

RESULTS

In assessing the results of therapy for HD, specific reports must be evaluated for the following:

- definitions of survival (e.g., event-free, relapse-free, freedom-from-progression, overall, etc.)
- characteristics of the patient population regarding evaluation and prognostic factors
- treatment regimens and techniques, including chemotherapy dose intensity, etc.
- mortality of therapy

The actuarial 10-year survival for children with early-stage disease is 85% to 95%, and for children with advanced stage disease it is 70% to 90% (Tables 5 and 6). The data for early stage patients (Table 5) indicate a similar overall survival for patients treated with full dose radiotherapy, combined full dose radiotherapy and chemotherapy, and low-dose radiotherapy and chemotherapy. This was illustrated in a report by Donaldson et al. (95) comparing results in early-stage disease from Stanford (pathologic staging, extended-field radiation therapy alone or combined chemotherapy and involved-field radiation therapy) with those from St. Bartholomew's/Great Ormond Street (clinical staging, involved/regional-field full-dose radiation therapy). Overall survival from each institution was 91% at 10 years, although the disease-free survival for stage I patients at St. Bartholomew's/Great Ormond Street was somewhat lower than that at Stanford. However, the toxicities vary greatly among the treatment strategies, which underlie the recommendations present in Table 7. Size of mediastinal disease is an important prognostic factor. The overall relapse-free survival is 53% for LMA patients treated with radiotherapy alone, in contrast to 86% for small or no mediastinal disease. Overall survival is not significantly different (88% and 93%, respectively)—because of the use of salvage chemotherapy. This high rate of relapse, however, does make the use of initial chemotherapy with consolidative radiation therapy a more rational ap-

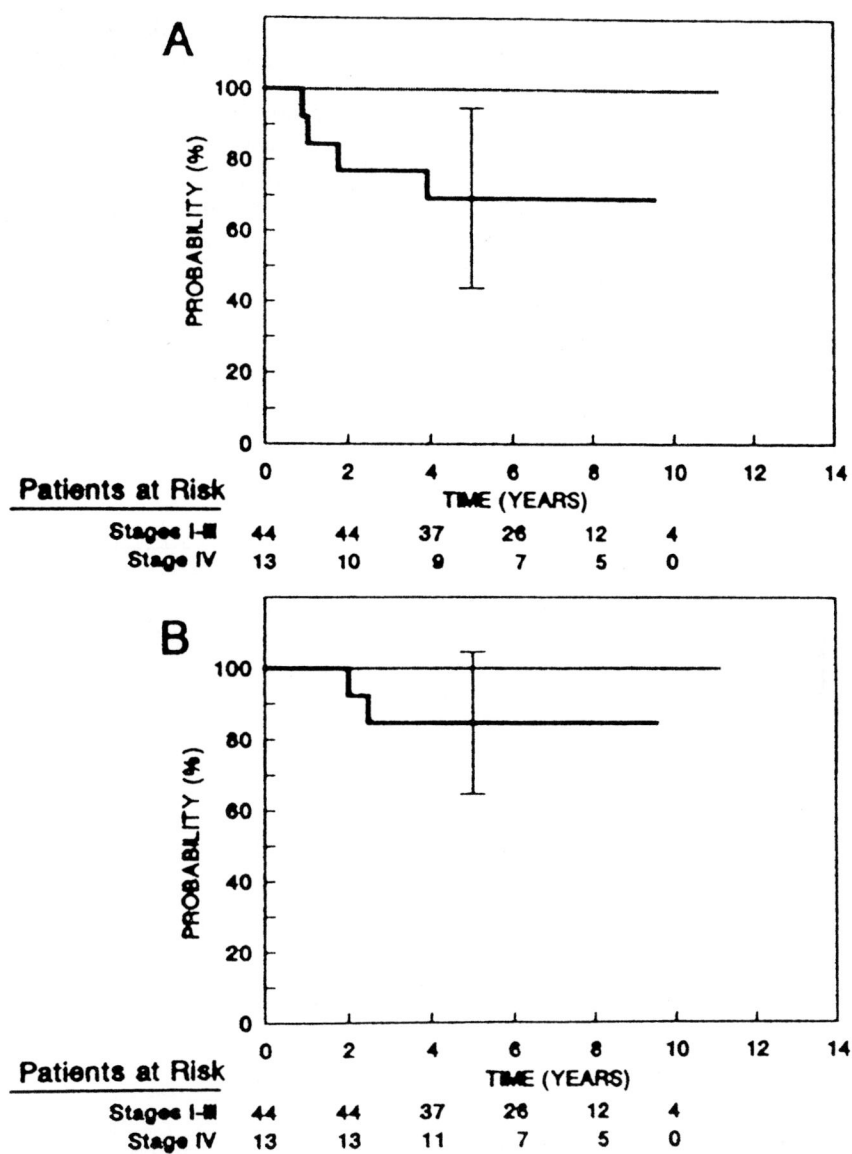

FIG. 5. Comparison of treatment outcome by stage. **A:** Event-free survival and **(B)** survival for patients with stages I to III disease (upper line) vs. stage IV (lower line). Bars denote 95% confidence interval at 5 years for stage IV patients. The number of patients at risk at each time point is listed below each graph. (From ref. 106, with permission.)

proach in patients with LMA. Although re-
lapse-free and overall survival remain excel-
lent for patients with advanced disease when
all are analyzed together, patients with stage
IV disease continue to fare poorly (Table 6).
This is highlighted by the results from the
Stanford group for 57 children (less than 16-
years old) treated with 6 chemotherapy cycles
(3 ABVD/3 MOPP) and 15 to 25 Gy IFRT.
The contrasting results for patients with stage
I to III versus stage IV disease are depicted in
Fig. 5.

It is critical to appreciate the extent to
which death from causes other than recurrence of HD compromises overall survival.
Although HD is the main cause of death during the first 10 to 15 years following therapy,
other causes (e.g., second malignancy, cardiovascular disease) of death are predominant at
even longer follow-up times. This is particularly dramatic for early stage patients, as
shown by data from Hancock and Hoppe
(146) on 1,440 patients with stage I/II HD

(Fig. 6). The estimated risk of death relative to
that expected in a general population (relative
risk) from causes other than HD ranges from
2.09 to 5.3 (146). In a recent report of 694
children treated at Stanford for HD, monitored for 1 to 31.6 years (mean 13.1 years),
147 (21%) have died. Causes of death were as
follows: HD 54%, second cancers 20%, accidents or other causes 26% (158).

COMPLICATIONS

Acute side effects seen during mantle irradiation include temporary loss or change in
taste, low posterior scalp epilation, xerostomia, skin erythema (particularly on the neck
and shoulders), and occasionally nausea and
vomiting requiring antiemetics. Long-term
complications are discussed in Chapter 19.
Mantle irradiation can cause pulmonary, cardiac and thyroid damage, and impair muscle
and bone development. These effects are less
common with the use of modern treatment

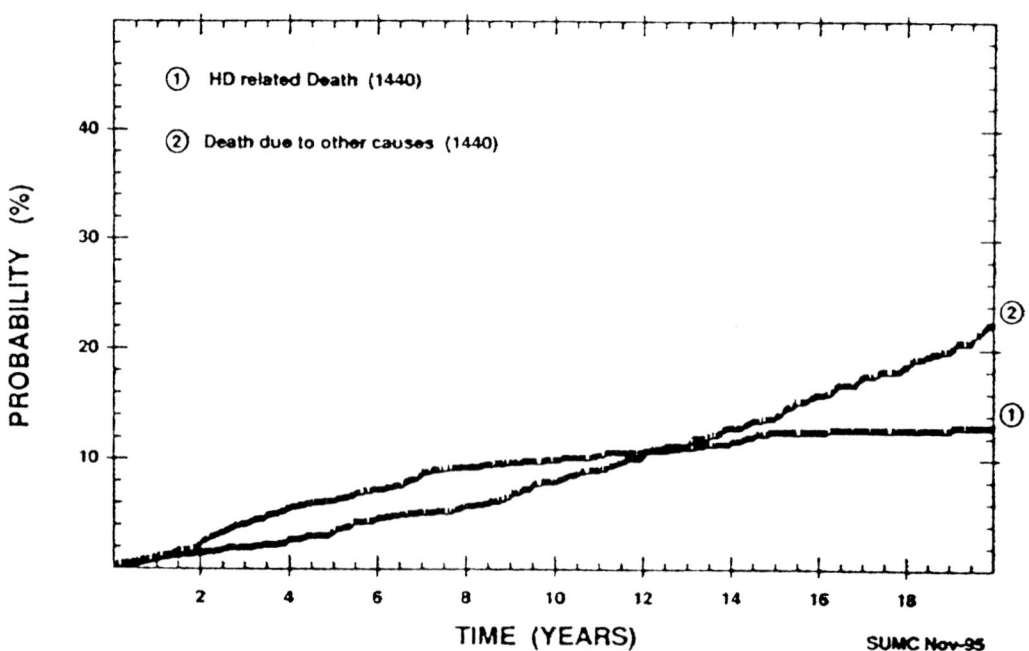

FIG. 6. Actuarial probability of death due to Hodgkin's disease (curve 1) or death due to other causes (curve 2) among 1,440 patients presenting with stage I or II Hodgkin's disease. (From ref. 146, with permission.)

programs (Fig. 4) (9,10,159–162) (see Chapter 19).

Acute effects of paraaortic irradiation are uncommon, but nausea and vomiting can occur. Late effects of paraaortic irradiation are also infrequent. Small bowel obstruction after both surgical staging and irradiation requiring surgical intervention is rare and is related to the total dose given: 1% for doses less than 35 Gy and 3% for doses greater than 35 Gy (73). Gonadal injury including infertility and impaired secretion of sex hormones are potential but generally preventable complications of pelvic irradiation.

The 15-year actuarial risk of second tumors is approximately 15% (see Chapter 20, "Secondary Tumors") (34,146,158,163). The risk of solid tumors does, however, increase with time. The risk of leukemia is associated primarily with the use of alkylating agents. Several reports on treated pediatric Hodgkin's patients (34,146,158,163) described an increased observed/expected risk ratio of second tumors for women compared with men, primarily due to breast cancer.

FUTURE INVESTIGATIONS

Devising new strategies for the treatment of children with HD is problematic due to the overall success of current treatment regimens. However, grouping patients into different risk categories allows investigators to construct protocols intended to diminish therapy-induced toxicity for "favorable" patients, improve treatment effectiveness for "unfavorable" patients, and aim for both goals in patients who are intermediate in their prognosis. Unfortunately, the ability to conduct clinical trials in which the differences in survival among treatment arms are likely to be small is compromised by the large patient numbers necessary to detect such differences. If a reduction in treatment toxicity is the intended goal of a new regimen, then many years of follow-up are necessary to prove effectiveness. Some generalizations regarding ongoing efforts in clinical trials for pediatric HD are as follows:

1. Patients with early stage disease (I, IIA without bulk disease and perhaps patients with IIB disease with sweating as the only systemic symptom) have an excellent prognosis and, therefore, "negative" questions can be asked. Can the intensity and duration of chemotherapy be decreased, selecting agents which are associated with less severe side effects? Concomitantly, can the volume and perhaps dose of radiotherapy be reduced? Can the amount of chemotherapy be based on the response to the initial cycles? Will chemo- and radioprotectants prove useful?

2. Patients with disease of an intermediate stage or with characteristics indicating that their prognosis is of an intermediate nature (II with bulky disease, IIB with fevers and/or weight loss, IIIA) are appropriate for study questions which intend to increase efficacy without increasing toxicity. Generally, this entails modification of existing chemoradiotherapy programs.

3. Patients with advanced stage disease (IIIB, IV) require more effective treatment regimens. This might be attainable by increasing dose intensity or the rate of drug delivery, and by combining agents into regimens that are new. The use of hemopoietic growth factors may assist in drug delivery. Definition of the role of radiotherapy in such trials will continue to be an important objective.

Of interest are the current early and advanced-stage studies in the Pediatric Oncology Group. For patients with IA, IIA, and IIIA disease who do not have large mediastinal disease, 2 to 4 cycles of 4-drug therapy are given dependent on the response to radiation therapy. For other patients (advanced disease), 3 to 5 cycles of dose-intense 6-drug therapy are given, also dependent on response to radiation therapy. Granulocyte-macrophage colony-stimulating factor is used, and patients are randomized to a cardioprotectant.

Finally, immunotherapeutic approaches are under development and investigation, such as the use of antiferritin antibody jointed with yttrium-90 (164), and EBV-specific T lymphocytes (81).

REFERENCES

References particularly recommended for further reading are indicated by an asterisk.

1. Hodgkin T. On some morbid appearances of the absorbent gland and spleen. *Medico-Chir Trans* 1832; 17:68–114.
*2. Kaplan HS. *Hodgkin's disease.* Cambridge: Harvard University Press, 1980:689.
3. Pusey W. Cases of sarcomas and of Hodgkin's disease treated by exposures to x rays: a preliminary report. *JAMA* 1902;38:166–170.
4. Gilbert R. Radiotherapy in Hodgkin's disease (malignant granulomatosis): anatomic and clinical foundations, governing principles, results. *AJR* 1939;41: 198–241.
5. Peters MV. A study of survival in Hodgkin's disease treated radiologically. *AJR* 1950;63:299–311.
6. Goodman L, Wintrobe M, Dameshek W, et al. Nitrogen mustard therapy: use of methyl-bis-(choroethyl)amine hydrochloride for Hodgkin's disease, lymphosarcoma, leukemia and certain allied and miscellaneous disorders. *JAMA* 1946;132:126–131.
7. DeVita VT Jr, Canellos GP, Moxley JH. A decade of combination chemotherapy of advanced Hodgkin's disease. *Cancer* 1972;30:1495–1504.
8. Seif G, Spriggs A. Chromosome changes in Hodgkin's disease. *J Natl Cancer Inst* 1967;39: 557–570.
*9. Donaldson SS, Kaplan HS. Complications of treatment of Hodgkin's disease in children. *Cancer Treat Rep* 1982;66:977–989.
*10. Mauch PM, Weinstein H, Botnick L, et al. An evaluation of long-term survival and treatment complications in children with Hodgkin's disease. *Cancer* 1988;51:925–932.
*11. Donaldson SS, Glatstein E, Rosenberg SA, et al. Pediatric Hodgkin's disease. II. Results of therapy. *Cancer* 1976;37:2436–2447.
12. Donaldson SS, Link MP. Combined modality treatment with low-dose radiation and MOPP chemotherapy for children with Hodgkin's disease. *J Clin Oncol* 1987;5:742–749.
13. Donaldson SS, Link MP. Hodgkin's disease: treatment of the young child. *Pediatr Clin North Am* 1991; 38:457–473.
*14. Cleary S, Link M, Donaldson S. Hodgkin's disease in the very young. *Int J Radiat Oncol Biol Phys* 1994; 28:77–84.
15. Kennedy BJ, Loeb V, Peterson V, et al. Survival in Hodgkin's disease by stage and age. *Med Pediatr Oncol* 1992;20:100–104.
16. Kung FH. Hodgkin's disease in children 4 years of age or younger. *Cancer* 1991;67:1428–1430.
17. Mauch P, Tarbell NJ, Weinstein H, et al. Stage IA-IIA

supradiaphragmatic Hodgkin's disease: prognostic factors in surgically staged patients. *J Clin Oncol* 1988;6:1576–1583.
*18. Stein H, Hummel M, Durkop H, et al. Biology of Hodgkin's disease. In: Canellos G, Lister T, Sklar J. eds. *The lymphomas.* Philadelphia: WB Saunders Co., 1998:287–304.
19. Jox A, Zander T, Diehl V, et al. Clonal relapse in Hodgkin's disease [Letter]. *N Eng J Med* 1997;337: 499.
20. Kanzler H, Kuppers R, Hansmann M, et al. Hodgkin and Reed-Sternberg cells in Hodgkin's disease represent the outgrowth of a dominant tumor clone derived from (crippled) germinal center B cells. *J Exp Med* 1996;184:1495–1505.
21. Gupta R, Patel K, Bodmer W, et al. Mutation of p53 in primary biopsy material and cell lines from Hodgkin's disease. *Proc Natl Acad Sci USA* 1993;90: 2817–2821.
22. Ambinder R, Browning P, Lorenzana I, et al. Epstein-Barr virus and childhood Hodgkin's disease in Honduras and the United States. *Blood* 1993;81:462–467.
23. Klein G. Epstein-Barr virus-carrying cells in Hodgkin's disease. *J Am Soc Hematol* 1992;80: 299–301.
24. Weiss L, Movahed L, Warnke R, et al. Detection of Epstein-Barr viral genomes in Reed-Sternberg cells of Hodgkin's disease. *N Engl J Med* 1989;302:502–506.
25. Gupta RK, Whelan JS, Lister TA, et al. Direct sequence analysis of the (14, 18) chromosomal translocation in Hodgkin's disease. *Blood* 1992;79: 2084–2088.
26. Poppema S, Kaleta J, Hepperle B. Chromosomal abnormalities in patients with Hodgkin's disease: evidence for frequent involvement of the 14q chromosomal region but infrequent bcl-2 gene rearrangement in Reed-Sternberg cells. *J Natl Cancer Inst* 1992;84: 1789–1792.
27. Gruss HJ, Pinto A, Duyster J, et al. Hodgkin's disease: a tumor with disturbed immunological pathways. *Immunol Today* 1997;18:156–163.
28. Schwartz R. Hodgkin's disease—time for a change. *N Engl J Med* 1997;337:495–496.
29. Marafioti T, Hummel M, Anagnostopoulos I, et al. Origin of nodular lymphocyte-predominant Hodgkin's disease from a clonal expansion of highly mutated germinal-center B cells. *N Engl J Med* 1997;337: 453–458.
30. Ohno T, Stribley J, Wu G, et al. Clonality in nodular lymphocyte-predominant Hodgkin's disease. *N Engl J Med* 1997;337:459–465.
*31. Harris N, Jaffe E, Stein H. A revised European-American classification of lymphoid neoplasms: a proposal from the International Lymphoma Study Group. *Blood* 1994;84:1361–1392.
32. Miller RW. Mortality in childhood Hodgkin's disease: an etiologic clue. *JAMA* 1966;198:1216–1217.
33. Spitz MR, Sider JG, Johnson CC, et al. TI Ethnic patterns of Hodgkin's disease incidence among children and adolescents in the United States, 1973–82. *J Natl Cancer Inst* 1986;76:235–239.
34. Tarbell N, Gelber R, Weinstein H, et al. Sex differences in risk of second malignant tumours after Hodgkin's disease in childhood. *Lancet* 1993;341: 1428–1432.

35. MacMahon B. Epidemiological evidence on the nature of Hodgkin's disease. *Cancer* 1957;10: 1045–1054.

36. Vianna N, Polan A. Epidemiologic evidence for transmission of Hodgkin's disease. *N Engl J Med* 1973;289:499–502.

37. Grufferman S, Delzell E. Epidemiology of Hodgkin's disease. *Epidemiol Rev* 1984;6:76–106.

38. Razzouk B, Gan Y, Mendonca C, et al. Epstein-Barr virus in pediatric Hodgkin disease: age and histiotype are more predictive than geographic region. *Med Pediatr Oncol* 1998;28:248–254.

39. Robertson S, Lowman J, Gutterman S. Familial Hodgkin's disease: a clinical and laboratory investigation. *Cancer* 1987;59:1314–1319.

40. Mack T, Cozen W, Shibata D, et al. Concordance for Hodgkin's disease in identical twins suggesting genetic susceptibility to the young-adult form of the disease. *N Engl J Med* 1995;332:413–418.

41. Slivnick D, Nawrocki J, Fisher R. Immunology and cellular biology of Hodgkin's disease. *Hematol Oncol Clin North Am* 1989;3:205–220.

42. Watanabe N, DeRosa S, Cmelak A, et al. Long-term depletion of naive T cells in patients treated for Hodgkin's disease. *Blood* 1997;90:3662–3672.

43. Filipovich AH, Mathur A, Kamat D, et al. Primary immunodeficiencies: genetic risk factors for lymphoma. *Cancer Res* 1992;52:5465s–5476s.

44. Rubio R. Hodgkin's disease associated with human immunodeficiency virus infection: a clinical study of 46 cases. *Cancer* 1994;73:2400–2407.

*45. Mauch P, Kalish L, Kadin M, et al. Patterns of presentation of Hodgkin's disease. *Cancer* 1993;71: 2062–2071.

*46. Lister TA, Crowther D, Sutcliffe SB, et al. Report of a committee convened to discuss the evaluation and staging of patients with Hodgkin's disease: Cotswolds meeting. *J Clin Oncol* 1989;7:1630–1636.

47. Jackson H, Parker F. Hodgkin's disease II-pathology. *N Engl J Med* 1994;231:35(abst).

*48. Ferry J, Harris N. The pathology of Hodgkin's disease: what's new? *Sem Radiat Oncol* 1996;6:121–130.

49. Karayalcin G, Behm F, Gieser P, et al. Lymphocyte predominant Hodgkin's disease: clinico-pathologic features and results of treatment—the Pediatric Oncology Group Experience. *Med Pediatr Oncol* 1997; 29:519–525.

*50. Hudson M, Greenwald C, Thompson E. Efficacy and toxicity of multiagent chemotherapy and low-dose involved-field radiotherapy in children and adolescents with Hodgkin's disease. *J Clin Oncol* 1993;11: 100–108.

51. Farah R, Weichselbaum R. Substaging of stage III Hodgkin's disease. *Hematol Oncol Clin North Am* 1989;3:277–286.

52. Hoppe RT, Cox RS, Rosenberg SA, et al. Prognostic factors in pathologic stage III Hodgkin's disease. *Cancer Treat Rep* 1982;66:743–750.

53. Friedman S, Henry-Amos M, Casset JM, et al. Evaluation of erythrocyte sedimentation rate as predictor of early relapse in post-therapy, early-stage Hodgkin's disease. *J Clin Oncol* 1988;6:598–602.

54. Gause A, Pohl C, Tschiersch A, et al. Clinical significance of soluble CD30 antigen in the sera of patients with untreated Hodgkin's disease. *Blood* 1988;77: 1983–1988.

55. Pui CH, Ip S, Thompson E, et al. Increased serum CD8 antigen level in childhood Hodgkin's disease relates to advanced stage and poor treatment outcome. *Blood* 1989;73:209–213.

56. Mahoney D, Schreuders L, Gresik M, et al. Role of staging bone marrow examination in children with Hodgkin's disease. *Med Pediatr Oncol* 1998;7: 175–177.

57. Castellino RA, Blank N, Hope Cho C. Hodgkin's disease: contributions of Chest CT in the initial staging evaluation. *Radiol* 1986;160:603–605.

58. Rostock RA, Giangreco A, Wharam MD, et al. CT scan modification in the treatment of mediastinal Hodgkin's disease. *Cancer* 1982;49:2267–2275.

59. Nyman R, Rehn S, Gimelius B, et al. Residual mediastinal masses in Hodgkin's disease: prediction of size with MR imaging. *Radiology* 1989;170:435–440.

60. Hagenmeister F, Feses S, Lamki L, et al. Role of gallium scan in the disease. *Cancer* 1990;65: 1090–1096.

61. Lally KP, Arnstein M, Siegel S, et al. A comparison of staging methods for Hodgkin's disease in children. *Arch Surg* 1986;121:1125–1127.

62. Salloum E, Brandt D, Caride V. Gallium scans in the management of patients with Hodgkin's disease: a study of 101 patients. *J Clin Oncol* 1997;15: 518–527.

63. Donaldson SS. Making choices in the staging of children with Hodgkin's disease. *Med Pediatr Oncol* 1991;19:211–213.

64. Castellino RA, Marglin SI. Imaging of abdominal and pelvic lymph nodes: lymphography or computed tomography? *Invest Radiol* 1982;17:433–443.

*65. Breuer C, Tarbel N, Mauch P, et al. The importance of staging laparotomy in pediatric Hodgkin's disease. *J Pediat Surg* 1994;29:1085–1089.

*66. Mendenhall N, Cantor A, Williams J, et al. With modern technique is staging laparotomy necessary in pediatric Hodgkin's disease? A pediatric oncology group study. *J Clin Oncol* 1993;11:2218–2225.

67. Schellong G. The balance between cure and late effects in childhood Hodgkin's lymphoma: the experience of the German-Austrian Study-Group since 1978. *Ann Oncol* 1996;7:567–572.

*68. Schellong G. Treatment of children and adolescents with Hodgkin's disease: the experience of the German-Austrian Paediatric Study Group. *Baillieres Clin Haematol* 1996;9:619–634.

69. Schellong G, Bramswig J, Hornig-Franz I. Treatment of children with Hodgkin's disease: results of the German Pediatric Oncology Group. *Ann Oncol* 1992; 3:73–76.

*70. Schellong G, Bramswig J, Hornig-Franz I, et al. Hodgkin's disease in children: combined modality treatment for stages IA, IB and IIA. Results of 356 patients of the German-Austrian Paediatric Study Group. *Ann Oncol* 1994;5:113–115.

71. Weiner M, Leventhal B, Brecher M, et al. Randomized study of intensive MOPP-ABVD with or without low-dose total nodal radiation therapy in the treatment of stages IIB, IIIA2, IIIB, and IV Hodgkin's disease in pediatric patients: a Pediatric Oncology Group study. *J Clin Oncol* 1997;15:2769–2779.

72. Hanna S, Fletcher B, Boulden T, et al. MR imaging of infradiaphragmatic lymphadenopathy in children and adolescents with Hodgkin's Disease: comparison with lymphography and CT. *J Magn Reson Imaging* 1993;3:461–470.

73. Coia LR, Hanks GE. Complications from large field intermediate dose infradiaphragmatic radiation: an analysis of the patterns of care outcome studies for Hodgkin's disease and seminoma. *Int J Radiat Oncol Biol Phys* 1988;15:29–35.

74. Green DM, Ghoorah J, Douglass HO Jr, et al. Staging laparotomy with splenectomy in children and adolescents with Hodgkin's disease. *Cancer Treat Rev* 1983;10:23–28.

75. Hays DM, Ternberg JL, Chen TT, et al. Postsplenectomy sepsis and other complications following staging laparotomy for Hodgkin's disease in childhood. *J Pediatr Surg* 1986;21:628–632.

*76. Mendenhall N. Diagnostic procedures and guidelines for the evaluation and follow-up of Hodgkin's disease. *Sem Radiat Oncol* 1996;6:131–146.

77. Behrendt H, Brinkhuis M, Van Leeuwen E. Treatment of childhood Hodgkin's disease with ABVD without radiotherapy. *Med Pediatr Oncol* 1996;26:244–248.

78. Khan S, Gilchrist G, Arndt C, et al. Vancouver hybrid: preliminary experience in the treatment of Hodgkin's disease in childhood and adolescence. *Mayo Clin Proc* 1994;69:949–954.

79. Vecchi V, Pileri S, Burnelli R, et al. Treatment of pediatric Hodgkin's disease tailored to stage, mediastinal mass, and age. *Cancer* 1993;72:2049–2057.

80. Garden AS, Woo SY, Fuller LM, et al. Results of a changing treatment philosophy for children with stage I Hodgkin's disease: a 35-year experience. *Med Pediatr Oncol* 1991;19:214–220.

81. Rooney C, Smith C, Ng C, et al. Use of viral-specific cytotoxic lymphocytes to control Epstein-Barr virus-related lymphoproliferation. *Lancet* 1995;345:9–13.

82. Fuller LM, Sullivan MP, Butler JJ. Results of regional radiotherapy in localized Hodgkin's disease in children. *Cancer* 1973;32:640–645.

*83. Specht L. Prognostic factors in Hodgkin's disease. *Sem Radiat Oncol* 1996;6:146–161.

84. Bader S, Weinstein H, Mauch P, et al. Pediatric stage IV Hodgkin's disease: long-term survival. *Cancer* 1993;72:249–255.

85. Behar RA, Hoppe RT. Radiation therapy in the management of bulky mediastinal Hodgkin's disease. *Cancer* 1990;66:75–79.

86. Hoppe RT. Stage I-II Hodgkin's disease: current therapeutic options and recommendations. *Blood* 1983; 62:32–36.

*87. Hoppe RT. The management of stage II Hodgkin's disease with a large mediastinal mass: a prospective program emphasizing irradiation. *Int J Radiat Oncol Biol Phys* 1985;11:349–355.

88. Maity A, Goldwein JW, Lange B, et al. Mediastinal masses in children with Hodgkin's disease. An analysis of the Children's Hospital of Philadelphia and the Hospital of the University of Pennsylvania experience. *Cancer* 1992;69:2755–2760.

89. Sprecht L, Nordentoft A, Cold S. Tumor burden as the most important prognostic factor in early stage Hodgkin's disease. Relations to other prognostic factors and implications for choice of treatment. *Cancer* 1988;61:1719–1727.

90. Hoppe RT, Coleman CN, Cox RS, et al. The management of stage I-II Hodgkin's disease with irradiation alone or combined modality therapy: the Stanford experience. *Blood* 1982;59:455–465.

91. Tubiana M, Henry-Amar M, Hayat M. Toward comprehensive management tailored to prognostic factors of patients with clinical stages I and II in Hodgkin's disease. The EORTC Lymphoma Group controlled clinical trials: 1964–1987. *Blood* 1989;73:47–56.

*92. Crnkovich MJ, Leopold K, Hoppe RT, et al. Stage I and IIB Hodgkin's disease: the combined experiences at Stanford University and the Joint Center for Radiation Therapy. *J Clin Oncol* 1987;5:1041–1049.

93. Shankar A, Ashley S, Radford M, et al. Does histology influence outcome in childhood Hodgkin's disease? Results from the United Kingdom Children's Cancer Study Group. *J Clin Oncol* 1997;15:2622–2630.

94. Barrett A, Crennan E, Barnes J, et al. Treatment of clinical stage I Hodgkin's disease by local radiation therapy alone. A United Kingdom Children's Cancer Study Group study. *Cancer* 1990;66:670–674.

*95. Donaldson S, Whitaker S, Plowman N, et al. Stage I-II pediatric Hodgkin's disease: long-term follow-up demonstrates equivalent survival rates following different management schemes. *J Clin Oncol* 1990;8: 1128–1137.

96. Gehan EA, Sullivan MP, Fuller LM, et al. The intergroup Hodgkin's disease in children. A study of stage I and II. *Cancer* 1990;65:1429–1437.

97. Hanks GE, Kinzie JJ, White RL, et al. Patterns of care outcome studies: results of the national practice in Hodgkin's disease. *Cancer* 1983;51:560–573.

98. Schewe KL, Reavis J, Kun LE, et al. Total dose, fraction size and tumor volume in the local control of Hodgkin's disease. *Int J Radiat Oncol Biol Phys* 1988;15:25–28.

99. Horning SJ, Hoppe RT, Kaplan HS, et al. Female reproductive potential after treatment for Hodgkin's disease. *N Engl J Med* 1981;304:1377–1382.

100. Fryer CJ, Hutchinson RJ, Krailo M, et al. Efficacy and toxicity of 12 courses of ABVD chemotherapy followed by low-dose regional radiation in advanced Hodgkin's disease in children: a report from the Children's Cancer Study Group. *J Clin Oncol* 1990;8: 1971–1980.

101. Hutchinson R, Krailo M, Fryer C. Prognostic factor analysis in advanced Hodgkin's disease (stages III and IV). Results of the CCG 521 trial. *Med Pediatr Oncol* 1993;21:61(abst).

102. Oberlin O, Leverger G, Pacquement M, et al. Low-dose radiation therapy and reduced chemotherapy in childhood Hodgkin's disease: the experience of the French Society of Pediatric Oncology. *J Clin Oncol* 1992;10:1062–1068.

103. Santoro A, Bonadonna G, Valagussa P, et al. Long-term results of combined chemotherapy-radiotherapy approach in Hodgkin's disease: superiority of ABVD plus radiotherapy versus MOPP plus radiotherapy. *J Clin Oncol* 1987;5:27–37.

104. Lamonte C, Yeh S, Straus D. Long-term follow-up of cardiac function in patients with Hodgkin's disease treated with mediastinal irradiation and combination chemotherapy including doxorubicin. *Cancer Treat Rep* 1986;70:439–444.

105. Dionet C, Oberlin O, Habriand JL, et al. Initial chemotherapy and low dose radiation in limited fields in

childhood Hodgkin's disease: results of a joint cooperative study by the French Society of Radiation Oncology (SFOP) and Hospital Saint-Louis. Paris. *Int J Radiat Oncol Biol Phys* 1988;15:341–346.

*106. Hunger S, Link M, Donaldson S. ABVD/MOPP and low-dose involved-field radiotherapy in pediatric Hodgkin's disease: the Stanford experience. *J Clin Oncol* 1994;12:2160–2166.

107. Maity A, Goldwein JW, Lange B, et al. Comparison of high-dose and low-dose radiation with and without chemotherapy for children with Hodgkin's disease: an analysis of the experience at the Children's Hospital of Philadelphia and the Hospital of the University of Pennsylvania. *J Clin Oncol* 1992;10:929–936.

108. Weiner MA, Leventhal BG, Marcus R, et al. Intensive chemotherapy and low-dose radiotherapy for the treatment of advanced-stage Hodgkin's disease in pediatric patients: a Pediatric Oncology Group study. *J Clin Oncol* 1991;9:1591–1598.

109. Bit GP, Cimino G, Cartoni C, et al. Extended field radiotherapy is superior to MOPP chemotherapy for the treatment of pathologic stage I-IIA Hodgkin's disease: eight-year update of an Italian prospective randomized study. *J Clin Oncol* 1992;10:378–382.

110. Jenkin D, Doyle J, Berry M, et al. Hodgkin's disease in children: treatment with MOPP and low-dose extended field irradiation without laparotomy late results and toxicity. *Med Pediatr Oncol* 1990;18:265–272.

*111. Mauch PM. Controversies in the management of early stage Hodgkin's disease. *Blood* 1994;83:318–329.

112. Gospodarowicz MK, Sutcliffe SB, Clark RM, et al. Analysis of supradiaphragmatic clinical stage I and II Hodgkin's disease treated with radiation alone. *Int J Radiat Oncol Biol Phys* 1992;22:859–865.

*113. Jones E, Mauch P. Limited radiation therapy for selected patients with pathological stages IA and IIA Hodgkin's disease. *Sem Radiat Oncol* 1996;6:162–171.

114. Hartsell WF, Farah R, Murthy A, et al. Is pelvic irradiation necessary in stage IIIA Hodgkin's disease? *Int J Radiat Oncol Biol Phys* 199;19:715–719.

115. Goodman RL, Piro AJ, Hellman S. Can pelvic irradiation be omitted in patients with pathologic stages IA and IIA Hodgkin's disease? *Cancer* 1976;37:2834–2839.

116. Mendenhall NP, Taylor B, Marcus R, et al. The impact of pelvic recurrence and elective pelvic irradiation on survival and treatment morbidity in early-stage Hodgkin's disease. *Int J Radiat Oncol Biol Phys* 1991;21:1157–1165.

117. Ekert H, Waters KD, Smith PJ, et al. Treatment with MOPP or CHIVPP chemotherapy only for all stages of childhood Hodgkin's disease. *J Clin Oncol* 1988;6:1845–1850.

118. Yahalom J, Ryu J, Straus D, et al. Impact of adjuvant radiation on the patterns and rate of relapse in advanced-stage Hodgkin's disease treated with alternating chemotherapy combinations. *J Clin Oncol* 1991;9:2193–2201.

119. Olweny CLM, Katongole-Mdidde E, Kiire C, et al. Childhood Hodgkin's disease in Uganda—a ten-year experience. *Cancer* 1978;42:787–792.

120. Behrendt H, van Bunning en BNFM, van Leewen W. Treatment of Hodgkin's disease in children with or without radiotherapy. *Cancer* 1987;59:1870–1873.

121. Donaldson S, Lamborn K. Radiation in pediatric Hodgkin's disease [Letter]. *J Clin Oncol* 1998;16:391–392.

122. Constine L. Should MOPP-ABVD alone be standard for childhood Hodgkin's? [Letter]. *J Clin Oncol* 1998;16:1235

123. Fabian C, Mansfield C, Dahlberg S, et al. Low-dose involved field radiation after chemotherapy in advanced Hodgkin's disease: a Southwest Oncology Group Randomized study. *Ann Intern Med* 1994;120:903–912.

*124. Mendenhall N, Bennett J, Lynch J. Is combined modality therapy necessary for advanced Hodgkin's disease? *Int J Rad Oncol Biol Phys* 1997;38:583–592.

*125. Yahalom J. Management of relapsed and refractory Hodgkin's disease. *Sem Radiat Oncol* 1996;6:210–224.

126. Healey E, Tarbell N, Kalish L, et al. Prognostic factors for patients Hodgkin's disease in first relapse. *Cancer* 1993;71:2613–2620.

127. Roach M, Brophy N, Cox R, et al. Prognostic factors for patients relapsing after radiotherapy for early-stage Hodgkin's disease. *J Clin Oncol* 1990;8:623–629.

128. Pezner RD, Lipsett JA, Vora NJ, et al. Radical radiotherapy as salvage treatment for nodal relapse of Hodgkin's disease initially treated by chemotherapy. *Int J Radiat Oncol Biol Phys* 1993;27:298(abst).

129. Roach M, Kapp DS, Rosenberg SA, et al. Radiotherapy with curative intent: an opinion in selected patients relapsing after chemotherapy for advanced Hodgkin's disease. *J Clin Oncol* 1987;5:550–555.

130. Uematsu M, Tarbell N, Silver B, et al. Wide-field radiation with or without chemotherapy for patients with Hodgkin's disease in relapse after initial combination chemotherapy. *Cancer* 1993;72:207–212.

131. Wirth A, Corry J, Laidlaw C, et al. Salvage radiotherapy for Hodgkin's disease following chemotherapy failure. *Int J Radiat Oncol Biol Phys* 1997;39:599–607.

132. van den Berg H, Stuve W, Behrendt H. Treatment of Hodgkin's disease in children with alternating mechlorethamine, vincristine, procarbazine, and prednisone (MOPP) and adriamycin, bleomycin, vinblastine, and dacarbazine (ABVD) courses without radiotherapy. *Med Pediatr Oncol* 1997;29:23–27.

133. Reece D, Connors J, Spinelli J. Intensive therapy with cyclophosphamide. carmustine. etoposide ± usplatin and autologous bone marrow transplantation for Hodgkin's disease in first relapse after combinations chemotherapy. *Blood* 1994;83:1193–1199.

134. Yahalom J. Do not miss a second (and possibly last) chance to cure Hodgkin's disease. *Int J Radiat Oncol Biol Phys* 1997;39:595–597.

135. Bierman P, Vase J, Armitage J. Antologous transplantation for Hodgkin's disease: coming of age? *Blood* 1994;83:1161–1164.

*136. Constine L, Rapoport A. Hodgkin's disease, bone marrow transplantation, and involved field radiation therapy: coming full circle from 1902 to 1996. *Int J Radiat Oncol Biol Phys* 1996;36:253–255.

137. Desch E, Lasala MR, Smith TJ, et al. The optimal timing of autologous bone marrow transplantation in Hodgkin's disease patients after a chemotherapy relapse. *J Clin Oncol* 1992;10:200–209.

138. Linch D, Winfield D, Goldstone A, et al. Dose intensification with autologous bone-marrow transplantation in relapsed and resistant Hodgkin's disease: results of a BNLI randomized trial. *Lancet* 1993;341:1051–1054.

*139. Yuen A, Rosenberg S, Hoppe R, et al. Comparison between conventional salvage therapy and high-dose therapy with autografting for recurrent or refractory Hodgkin's disease. *Blood* 1997;89:814–822.

*140. Williams C, Goldstone A, Pearce R, et al. Autologous bone marrow transplantation for pediatric Hodgkin's disease: a case-matched comparison with adult patients by the European Bone Marrow Transplant Group Lymphoma Registry. *J Clin Oncol* 1993;11: 2243–2249.

*141. Horning S, Chao N, Negrin R, et al. High-dose therapy and autologous hematopoietic progenitor cell transplantation for recurrent or refractory Hodgkin's disease: analysis of the Stanford University Results and Prognostic indices. *Blood* 1997;89:801–813.

142. Anderson J, Litzow M, Applebaum F, et al. Allogeneic, syngeneic, and autologous marrow transplantation for Hodgkin's disease: the 21-year experience. *J Clin Oncol* 1993;11:2342–2350.

143. Rapoport A, Rowe J, Korides P, et al. One hundred autotransplants for relapsed or refractory Hodgkin's disease and lymphoma: value of pretransplant disease states for predicting outcome. *J Clin Oncol* 1993;11: 2351–2361.

144. Yahalom J, Gulati S, Shank B, et al. Total lymphoid irradiation, high-dose chemotherapy and autologous bone marrow transplantation for chemotherapy resistant Hodgkin's disease. *Int J Radiat Oncol Biol Phys* 1989;17:915–922.

145. Jules-Elysee K, Stover DE, Yahalom J, et al. Pulmonary complication in lymphoma patients treated with high-dose therapy and autologous bone marrow transplantation. *Am Rev Respir Dis* 1992;1246:485–591.

*146. Hancock S, Hoppe R. Long-term complications of treatment and causes of mortality after Hodgkin's disease. *Sem Radiat Oncol* 1996;6:225–242.

147. Mundt AJ, Sibley G, Williams S, et al. Patterns of failure following high-dose chemotherapy and autologous bone marrow transplantation with involved field radiotherapy for relapsed/refractory Hodgkin's disease. *Int J Radiat Oncol Biol Phys* 1995;33:261–270.

*148. Poen J, Hoppe R, Horning S. High-dose therapy and autologous bone marrow transplantation for relapsed/refractory Hodgkin's disease: the impact of involved field radiotherapy on patterns of failure and survival. *Int J Radiat Oncol Biol Phys* 1996; 36:3–12.

149. Brasacchio R, Constine L, Rapoport A, et al. Dose escalation of consolidation radiation therapy (involved field) following autologous bone marrow transplant for recurrent Hodgkin's disease and lymphoma. *Int J Radiat Oncol Biol Phys* 1996;36:171(abst).

150. Kinzie JJ, Hanks GE, MacLean CJ, et al. Patterns of care study: Hodgkin's disease relapse rates and adequacy of portals. *Cancer* 1983;52:2223–2226.

*151. Hoppe RT. Treatment planning in the radiation therapy of Hodgkin's disease. *Front Radiat Ther Oncol* 1987;21:270–287.

*152. Nautiyal J, Weichselbaum R, Vijayakumar S. Radiation therapy techniques in the treatment of Hodgkin's disease. *Sem Radiat Oncol* 1996;6:172–184.

153. Prosnitz L, Brizel D, Light K. Radiation techniques for the treatment of Hodgkin's disease with combined modality therapy or radiation alone. *Int J Radiat Oncol Biol Phys* 1997;39:885–895.

154. Gottdiener JS, Katin MJ, Borer JS, et al. Late effects of therapeutic mediastinal irradiation. Assessment by echocardiography and radionuclide angiography. *N Engl J Med* 1983;308:569–572.

155. Tarbell N, Thompson L, Mauch P. Thoracic irradiation in Hodgkin's disease: disease control and long-term complications. *Int J Radiat Oncol Biol Phys* 1990;18:275–281.

156. Sears J, Greven K, Ferree C, et al. Definitive irradiation in the treatment of Hodgkin's disease. *Cancer* 1997;79:145–151.

157. Loeffler M, Diehl V, Pfreundschuh M, et al. Dose-response relationship of complementary radiotherapy following four cycles of combination chemotherapy in intermediate-stage Hodgkin's disease. *J Clin Oncol* 1997;15:2275–2287.

*158. Wolden S, Lamborn K, Cleary S, et al. Second cancers following pediatric Hodgkin's disease. *J Clin Oncol* 1998;16:536–544.

159. Constine LS, Donaldson SS, McDougall IR, et al. Thyroid dysfunction after radiotherapy in children with Hodgkin's disease. *Cancer* 1984;53:878–883.

160. Hancock S, Donaldson S, Hoppe R. Cardiac disease following treatment of Hodgkin's disease in children and adolescents. *J Clin Oncol* 1993;11:1208–1215.

161. Tarbell NJ, Mauch P, Hellman S. Pulmonary complications of Hodgkin's disease treatment: radiation pneumonitis, fibrosis, and the effect of cytotoxic drugs. In: Lacher M, Redman J. eds. *Hodgkin's disease: the consequences of survival*. Philadelphia: Lea & Febiger, 1990:296–305.

162. Willman K, Cox R, Donaldson S. Radiation induced height impairment in pediatric Hodgkin's disease. *Int J Radiat Oncol Biol Phys* 1994;28:85–92.

163. Bhatia S, Robison L, Oberlin O, et al. Breast cancer and other second neoplasms after childhood Hodgkin's disease. *N Engl J Med* 1966;334:745–751.

164. Bierman P, Vose J, Leichner P, et al. Yttrium 90-labeled antiferritin followed by high-dose chemotherapy and autologous bone marrow transplantation in poor-prognosis Hodgkin's disease. *J Clin Oncol* 1993;11:698–703.

165. DeVita VT Jr, Mauch PM, Harris NL. Hodgkin's disease. In: DeVita VT Jr, Hellman S, Rosenberg SA, eds. *Cancer principles and practice of oncology*. Philadelphia: Lippincott-Raven, 1997:2242–2283.

166. Constine LS, Quazi R, Rubin P. Malignant lymphomes. In: Rubin P, McDonald S, Quazi R, eds. *Clinical oncology: a multidisciplinary approach for physicians and students*. Philadelphia: WB Saunders, 1993:217–250.

167. Bayle-Weisgerber C, Lemercier N, Teillet T, Asselain B, Gout M, Schweisguth O. Hodgkin's disease in children. Results of therapy in a mixed group of 178 clinical and pathologically staged patients over 13 years. *Cancer* 1984;54(2):215–22.

168. Lobo-Sanahuja F, Garcia I, Barrantes JC, Barrantes M, Gonzalez M, Jimenez R. Pediatric Hodgkin's disease in Costa Rica: twelve years' experience of primary treatment by chemotherapy alone, without staging laparotomy. *Med Pediatr Oncol* 1994;22(6):398–403.

8

Non-Hodgkin's Lymphoma

Malignant lymphoma was described by Hodgkin in 1832 (1), and was distinguished from leukemia by Virchow in 1845 (2). Progress in the management of children with non-Hodgkin's lymphoma (NHL) mirrors the recognition of the systemic nature of the disease and underlying biology. Response to therapy and overall prognosis depend on the underlying cell type, primary site, and the extent of disease (3,4). Historically, local therapy resulted in an overall survival of 10% to 30% (5). New multiagent protocols result in overall survivals of 70% to 90% (6–8).

Childhood NHL is distinguished from adult NHL by differing frequencies of immuno-histopathologic types and by the relatively greater frequency of extranodal presentations (9,10). The three major histologic categories of NHL in children are lymphoblastic, small noncleaved cell or Burkitt's, and large-cell lymphoma. There is a greater tendency of childhood NHL to disseminate noncontiguously, evolve into leukemia, and involve the central nervous system (CNS) at relapse (10).

EPIDEMIOLOGY AND ETIOLOGY

Malignant lymphomas are the third most common malignancy in children under 15 years of age. They are rare under the age of 3 years, peaking in incidence from age 7 to 11 years. There is approximately a 3:1 male:female ratio (5,7,11). Lymphomas account for approximately 10% of all childhood cancers; 60% are NHL and 40% are Hodgkin's disease (11). However, their occurrence varies in different geographic regions. For example, in equatorial Africa, 50% of childhood cancers are NHL, primarily Burkitt's lymphoma. In this setting, an association with the Epstein-Barr virus (EBV) is observed, along with specific chromosomal breakpoints (resulting in a characteristic 8:14 chromosomal translocation) (12,13). EBV has long been associated with endemic Burkitt's lymphoma, and more recently with hairy leukoplakia, nasopharyngeal carcinoma, and leiomyosarcomas in children with HIV. The role of EBV in the pathogenesis of Burkitt's lymphoma and other malignancies is unknown. NHL occurs in association with genetically determined immunodeficiency syndromes (such as X-linked lymphoproliferative syndrome, ataxia telangiectasia, Wiscott-Aldrich syndrome, common variable immune deficiency disease), presumably due to host defects in immunoregulation or gene rearrangement (14–16). Immunosuppressive therapy and acquired immunological disorders including acquired immunodeficiency secondary to HIV infection also increase the risk for NHL (17). These are predominantly large B cell or Burkitt in subtype.

CLINICAL PRESENTATION

Patients generally present with one of a number of syndromes, which are associated with certain histopathologies (Table 1). Symptoms leading to diagnosis are usually of short duration. Approximately 25% of children with NHL present with mediastinal disease (usually lymphoblastic histology with T-cell markers), with malaise and cough progressing to dyspnea. The majority of these

TABLE 1. *Important features of childhood NHLs and their correlates with histologic subtype*

Histology	Cases (%)	Phenotype	Cytogenic markers	Common clinical presentations
Lymphoblastic	28.1	T-cell, early pre-B cell, TdT[+]	14q11, 7q34	Mediastinal mass, pleural effusion, lymphadenopathy superior vena cava syndrome, respiratory distress
Small noncleaved	38.8	B-cell sIg[+]	8q24	Abdominal primary, tumor lysis syndrome, jaw tumors (African)
Large cell	26.3	B-cell, T-cell	t(2;5)(p23;q35)	Extranodal sites common (i.e., lung, face, brain, skin, bone)

From ref. 63, with permission.

patients are adolescents, and their presentation may pose a medical emergency (18). Primary gastrointestinal involvement occurs in about 30% (usually undifferentiated or small noncleaved histology), commonly presenting as an abdominal mass with ascites, an acute abdomen, intussusception, or a malnutrition syndrome with colitis symptoms (7,12). In 20% to 30% of children, the head and neck, including Waldeyer's ring or cervical lymph nodes, is the site of origin. The remainder of patients have miscellaneous primary sites, including bone, breast, skin, epidural space, or noncervical lymph nodes (7). Involvement of the bone marrow at diagnosis is common, occurring in 20% to 30% of patients with undifferentiated or lymphoblastic histology. Overt CNS involvement at diagnosis is most frequent in children with head and neck sites, advanced disease, or endemic (African) Burkitt's lymphoma (19). African Burkitt's lymphoma usually presents in the jaw, in contrast to the abdominal presentation typical of nonendemic Burkitt's lymphoma (20).

EVALUATION

Surgical biopsy establishes the diagnosis. Although histology continues to be the primary determinant of therapy, morphologic analysis is supplemented by immunophenotypic, enzymatic, and cytogenetic studies. The workup includes complete blood count with platelets, routine chemistries with electrolytes, uric acid, chest radiograph, bone scan, bone marrow aspirates and biopsy (which may obviate the need for lymph node biopsy) (21), and a lumbar puncture with cytocentrifugation. Abdominal, thoracic, and head and neck computerized tomographic (CT) scans should be obtained depending on the presenting site (22). Laparotomy is not indicated for staging and is only performed for abdominal presentations requiring surgical intervention.

STAGING AND CLASSIFICATION

Originally, the Ann Arbor staging for Hodgkin's disease was used for NHL (see Chapter 7, Table 1) (23). The usefulness of this system in pediatric NHL is limited and an alternative staging system proposed by Murphy has become widely accepted (Table 2) (24). This system recognizes typical patterns of disease presentation and has greater prognostic utility than the Ann Arbor system. In Burkitt's lymphoma the Ziegler staging system is used (Table 3). It classifies patients according to tumor burden, which correlates with prognosis (20).

Pediatric NHL histology generally falls into one of three categories. There are several classification systems utilized to name these histologic categories. These include the Rappaport system, the Lukes-Collins classifications, the Kiel system, and the Working Formulation (3,25–28). The Revised European-American Classification of Lymphoid neoplasms (REAL) is gaining increased accep-

TABLE 2. *Murphy/St. Jude Children's Research Hospital staging system for childhood NHLs[a]*

Stage I	A single tumor (extranodal) or single anatomical area (nodal), with the exclusion of mediastinum or abdomen
Stage II	A single tumor (extranodal) with regional node involvement
	Two or more nodal areas on the same side of the diaphragm
	Two single (extranodal) tumors with or without regional node involvement on the same side of the diaphragm
	A primary gastrointestinal tract tumor, usually in the ileocecal area, with or without involvement of associated mesenteric nodes only[b]
Stage III	Two single tumors (extranodal) on opposite sides of the diphragm
	Two or more nodal areas above and below the diaphragm
	All the primary intrathoracic tumors (mediastinal, pleural, thymic)
	All extensive primary intraabdominal disease[b]
	All paraspinal or epidural tumors, regardless of other tumor sites
Stage IV	Any of the above stages with initial CNS or bone marrow involvement[c]

[a]See refs. 7, 10, 24, 59, 67, 68.

[b]A distinction is made between apparently localized gastrointestinal tract lymphoma and more extensive intraabdominal disease. Stage II disease typically is limited to a segment of the gut plus or minus the associated mesenteric nodes only, and the primary tumor can be completely removed grossly by segmental excision. Stage III disease typically exhibits spread to paraaortic and retroperitoneal areas by implants and plaques in mesentery or peritoneum, or by direct infiltration of structures adjacent to the primary tumor. Ascites may be present, and complete resection of all gross tumor is not possible.

[c]If marrow involvement is present initially, the number of abnormal cells must be 25% or less in an otherwise normal marrow aspirate with normal peripheral blood picture.

tance as the preferred classification system (29).

Almost all pediatric NHL is diffuse and high-grade (7,9). The most common subtypes are *precursor T-lymphoblastic lymphoma* and *precursor B-lymphoblastic lymphoma,* also called diffuse lymphoblastic lymphoma (30% of cases, precursor T-cell is the more common type), *Burkitt's lymphoma* and *high-grade B-cell, Burkitt-like* lymphoma also called diffuse small noncleaved cell lymphoma (including undifferentiated Burkitt's and non-Burkitt's types deriving from relatively mature B cells; 35% to 40% of cases), and *diffuse large B-cell lymphoma,* also called large-cell (diffuse histiocytic or immunoblastic) lymphoma (usu-

ally B-cell or non-B, non–T-cell; sometimes T-cell; 25% to 30% of cases), and *anaplastic large cell* [CD30 + lymphoma (T-cell and null-cell types)] (Fig. 1).

Precursor B-lymphoblastic lymphoma consists of cells with round or convoluted nuclei, fine chromatin, inconspicuous nuclei, and scant, faintly basophilic cytoplasm. Tumor cell are characteristically TdT+, CD19+, CD79a+ (29). Lymphoblastic lymphomas share many clinical and biologic features with acute lymphoblastic leukemia (ALL) (30,31). When the bone marrow is involved with lymphoblasts, the distinction between lymphoma and leukemia is difficult and generally determined by the percentage of blast cells in the bone marrow, with 25% the most commonly used cutoff (30). The biologic correlate to this distinction is unclear but appears to involve the degree of differentiation of the neoplastic cell. Malignancies with an immature phenotype most frequently present as leukemia, whereas those with a more mature phenotype characteristically present with less marrow involvement but accumulations of cells in other areas.

Burkitt's lymphoma tumor cells are monomorphic, medium-sized cells with round nu-

TABLE 3. *Clinical staging of Burkitt's lymphoma[a]*

Stage	Extent of tumor
A	Single extraabdominal site
B	Multiple extraabdominal sites
C	Intraabdominal tumor
D	Intraabdominal tumor with extraabdominal sites
AR	Stage C but with >90% of tumor surgically resected

[a]See refs. 13, 20.

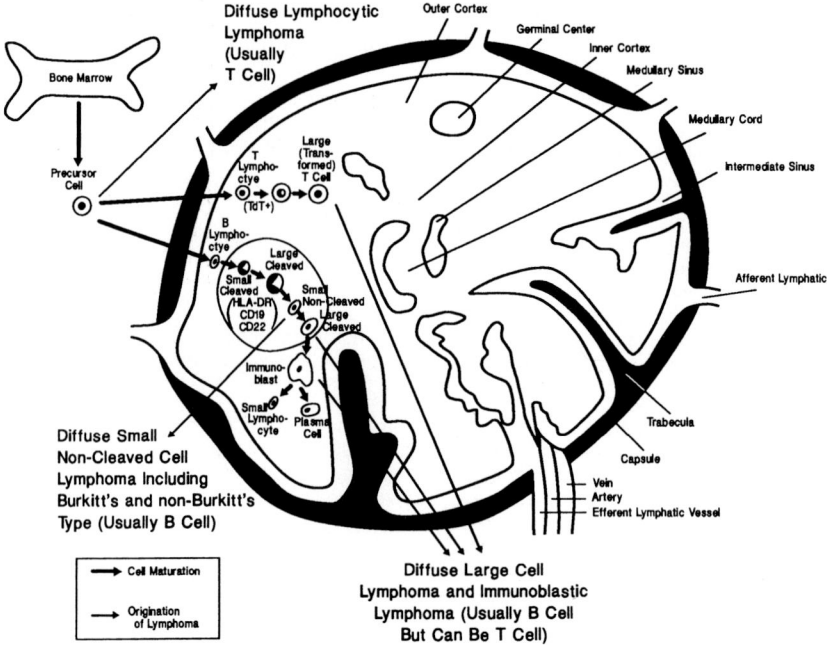

FIG. 1. Classification of the pediatric non-Hodgkin's lymphomas according to the functional anatomy of the lymph node and the process of lymphocyte transformation. Lymphoblastic lymphoma is thought to arise from the paracortical areas of the lymph node from small noncleaved T cells. The Burkitt's and non-Burkitt's types of small noncleaved cell lymphoma are generally of B-cell origin. Most of the non-Hodgkin's lymphomas formerly referred to as histiocytic have been shown to be derived from transformed lymphocytes. Diffuse large-cell lymphoma and immunoblastic lymphoma are usually of B-cell or non-B, non-T-cell origin. (Diagram based on concepts presented in refs. 66 and 68.)

clei, multiple nucleoil, and basophilic cytoplasm. A "starry-sky" pattern is the result of benign macrophages that have ingested apoptotic tumor cells. Cells are typically sIgM+, CD19+, CL20+, CD22+, CD79a+, CD10+. *High-grade B-cell lymphoma, Burkitt-like* has features intermediate between large-cell and Burkitt's lymphoma (29).

Diffuse large B-cell lymphoma consists of large cells with vesicular nuclei, basophilic cytoplasm, and a moderate to high proliferation fraction (29).

PROGNOSTIC FACTORS

The most prominent prognostic determinant in childhood NHL is the tumor burden at presentation (7,32). The clinical stage is also predictive, but in turn is based on the tumor burden and disease extent. In general, patients with stage I and II disease have localized lymphomas and a better prognosis than those with extensive or disseminated disease or with tumors located in unfavorable sites (mediastinum, thymus, CNS). Bone marrow involvement has been associated with a poor prognosis but, with intensive therapy, it may no longer be prognostically significant (33–35). Serum concentrations of lactic dehydrogenase and the interleukin-2 receptor have a strong correlation with prognosis; it is likely that they reflect tumor bulk, although other explanations may exist (7,36).

CNS involvement will develop in 30% to 35% of children with NHL, particularly lymphoblastic subtypes. Therefore, prophylactic CNS treatment is required (7,37–39). This is especially true in patients at high risk of CNS disease, such as those with advanced-stage lymphoblastic lymphoma. Overt CNS involvement may present with headache, increased intracranial pressure, and focal neurologic deficits.

SELECTION OF THERAPY

Chemotherapy

Because of the high likelihood of disseminated disease, all children, regardless of stage or histology, receive systemic chemotherapy. Childhood NHL responds to a wide range of agents, but different combinations and schedules are optimal for particular histologies, stages, and primary sites. Active drugs include adriamycin, methotrexate, vincristine, prednisone, mercaptopurine, cyclophosphamide, and cytosine arabinoside. Table 4 lists some of the commonly reported systemic regimens, their acronyms, and treatment outcome.

For stages I and II nonlymphoblastic disease, COMP (cyclophosphamide, vincristine, methotrexate, and prednisone) and ACOP [and modifications of these regimens with either deletion of some agents and the addition of others (i.e., cytarabine)] produce excellent results (6,33,40–43). Relapse-free survivals approximate 90%. Current studies are evaluating the possibility of decreased therapy without maintenance for this favorable group (44). For stages I and II lymphoblastic disease, the use of ALL therapy is quite effective, with approximately 80% disease-free survival (33,45).

In patients with stages III or IV disseminated lymphoblastic NHL, less than 40% were cured with "standard risk" ALL treatment (33). The APO (doxurubicin, prednisone, and vincristine) and LSA2-L2 regimens were two of the early successful protocols for children with high-risk ALL and advanced stage lymphoblastic lymphoma (33,43,46). Both protocols included preventive CNS therapy. These protocols resulted in approximately 65% survival. The use of more intensive ALL chemotherapy regimens appears to additionally improve the outcome for these children (8,47).

Approximately 30% of pediatric large-cell lymphomas are classified as anaplastic large cell (ALCL) in the REAL classification. The remainder are diffuse large B-cell, and the rare peripheral T-cell lymphoma. Children with localized large-cell lymphoma have a very favorable prognosis. The COMP and CHOP (cyclophosphamide, doxorubicin, vincristine, prednisone) regimens that are effective in early-stage lymphoblastic and Burkitt's lymphoma also result in 85% survival for these children. The results of CHOP with or without involved irradiation were similar.

Large-cell lymphoma constitutes approximately 30% of childhood NHL. For advanced-stage large-cell histology APO, CHOP and modified ACOP regimens are also effective (32,48–50). Because of the similar outcomes after APO and ACOP+ therapy and concerns of second malignancy and gonadal failure after cyclophosphamide. Pediatric Oncology Group (POG) study 8615 compared APO [adriamycin, prednisone, vincristine, 6-mercaptopurine, asparaginase, and intrathecal (IT) and intravenous (IV) methotrexate] to ACOP+ (APO with cyclophosphamide but without asparaginase) in large-cell NHL. The 2-year disease-free survival is 79% for APO and 70% for ACOP+ (51).

Conclusions about the safety of omitting cyclophosphamide await confirmatory studies as well as a detailed analysis of various subsets of patients. Most protocols for children with advanced-stage large-cell lymphoma do not include involved field radiotherapy, but no controlled trials have addressed this issue (52). The risk of an isolated CNS relapse is rare, but nevertheless pediatric protocols include IT chemotherapy for these patients.

Recent studies suggest that undifferentiated Burkitt's and non-Burkitt's lymphoma have a similar response to therapy and a similar relapse-free and overall survival (12,32,53,54). Most current protocols treat undifferentiated Burkitt's and non-Burkitt's lymphoma in the same manner. Rapid sequencing of high doses

TABLE 4. *Survival of childhood NHL patients with modern therapy*

Protocol	Chemotherapy	Radiation to tumor bulk	CNS prophylaxis	Stage	Number of patients	CR (%)	Survival (%)	Median follow-up	Reference
Lymphoblastic NHL NHL-75 SJCRH	VCR, PDNCTX, ADR, 6MP, MTX	Randomized in stage III and IV	CR RT, IT MTX	III, IV	20	88	40 (DFS)	7 years	68
LSA₂-L₂	CTX, VCR, PDN, DNR, MTX, araC, TG, ASP, BCNU,HU	Yes	IT MTX	III	9	88	88 (DFS)	70+ months	46
LSA₂-L₂ (modified POG-7615)	As above (with modification)	Yes	IT MTX	III	24	96	57 (FFS)	3 years	39
LSA₂-L₂ (modified CCG-551)	As above (with modification)	Yes	IT MTX	III, IV	31	—	76 (FFS)	2 years	69
BFM-75/81	PDN, VCR, DNR, ASP, araC, MTX, 6MP	No	CR RT, IT MTX	III, IV	42	—	78 (FFS)	4+ years	70
X-H	VM-26, araC, PDN, VCR, ASP, MTX, 6MP	No	CR RT, IT MTX	III, IV	22	96	73 (DFS)	4 years	47
APO	VCR, ADR, PDN, ASP, 6MP, MTX	Yes	CR RT, IT MTX	III, IV	21	95	58 (DFS)	3 years	43
77-04	CTX, ADR, VCR, PDN, HD MTX	No	IT MTX, HD MTX	III	10	100	70 (DFS)	4 years	71
A-COP+[a]	ADR, VCR, PDN, CTX, MTX, HC	Yes	CR RT, IT MTX	III	33	—	54 (DFS)	3 years	49
SNCC NHL Total B	CTX, ADR, VCR, araC, HD MTX	No	IT MTX, IT araC, HD MTX	III IV[b]	17 12	93 20	81 20 (DFS)	2 years 2 years	67
LMBO 281	HD CTX, HD MTX, araC, VCR, PDN, ASP ADR	No	IT MTX	III IV	72 42	84	73 48	2 years 2 years	34
HD MTX/HD CTX	HD CTS, HD MTX, VCR, PDN	No	IT MTX, It araC, IT HC	I–IV	22	9	75[a]	30+ months	73
BFM 81/86	CTX, PDN, VM-26, araC, HD MTX, ADR	No	CR RT, IT MTX	III IV	75 15	—	73 57	21 months 21 months	70
7704	CTX, ADR, VCR, PDN, HD MTX	No	IT MTX, HD MTX	III[c] IV	38 9	—	60 28	4 years 4 years	71
COMP	CTX, VCR, HD MTX, PDN	Yes	IT MTX	III, IV	24	—	26 (FFS)	2 years	69

From ref. 72, with permission.

VCR, vincristine; PDN, prednisone; CTX, cyclophosphamide; ADR, doxorubicin; 6MP, 6-mercaptopurine; MTX, methotrexate; IDMTX, intermediate-dose methotrexate ($\geq$300 mg/m^2); HDMTX, high-dose methotrexate (2.7 g/m^2); IT MTX, intrathecal methotrexate; DNR, daunomycin; araC, cytarabine; TG, thioguanine; ASP, asparaginase; HU, hydroxyurea; CR complete response; DFS, disease-free survival; FFS, failure-free survival; CR RT, cranial irradiation.

[a]Actual survival.
[b]Includes patients with B-cell ALL.
[c]Includes patients with large-cell lymphoma.

of active drugs (usually including cyclophosphamide, methotrexate, and cytosine arabinoside) are frequently used for this rapidly growing tumor. The survival rates for stages A and B are excellent. Survivals for stages C and D are poor (12,32). A recent intense regimen of shortened duration for advanced-stage undifferentiated lymphoma, which includes cyclophosphamide, vincristine, methotrexate, and cytosine arabinoside has provided excellent results (42). Decreasing the length of therapy in childhood NHL of all histologies from 2 to 3 years to 6 to 18 months or even less appears to provide similar outcomes (32–34,39,40,55).

In the course of treatment for Burkitt's lymphoma a tumor lysis syndrome may develop. This can result in elevated serum uric acid, uric acid nephropathy, and renal failure requiring the temporary use of dialysis. Careful management of hydration with monitoring of uric acid and electrolyte balance is required. The risk of renal failure is closely related to oliguria immediately before and after the initiation of chemotherapy (56).

Radiotherapy

The role of radiotherapy in the management of all childhood NHL has decreased as chemotherapeutic regimens have become more effective (6,7,48). As treatment programs were developed, it was clear that the combination of chemotherapy plus irradiation resulted in significant improvements in survival (33). Trials assessing the need for radiotherapy followed. Reports from POG demonstrate successful local and systemic control with chemotherapy alone for children with Murphy/SJCRH stages I and II disease regardless of histology (6). There also does not appear to be any benefit to the addition of radiation therapy either to the primary site or for CNS prophylaxis for Burkitt's NHL (20,30,37,38). The addition of localized radiation therapy to chemotherapy has also shown no benefit for patients with advanced-stage disease (7).

The role of radiation therapy for primary NHL of bone in children has also diminished. These cases were specifically excluded from the POG randomized trials of early-stage pediatric NHL, which showed no benefit to local irradiation (6). In these studies, all cases of bone NHL received local radiation therapy. There are data that demonstrate good results for pediatric NHL of bone when radiotherapy is omitted. These data will need confirmation, at least for large-cell nonlymphoblastic histologies (57).

The current *indications for radiation therapy outside the CNS* in pediatric NHL are: (a) emergency treatment for mediastinal disease or spinal cord compression (a hyperfractionated regimen should be considered), (b) treatment for patients who fail to obtain a complete remission after induction chemotherapy, (c) palliation of pain or mass effect, and (d) for consolidation to regions of local disease prior to or following bone marrow transplantation in patients with recurrent disease.

Emergency radiation therapy for superior vena cava syndrome, acute airway compromise, or spinal cord compression can provide rapid relief of symptoms. The response is particularly dramatic with lymphoblastic lymphoma. Symptoms usually are relieved within 48 hours of treatment. Usually 1.5 to 2 Gy per fraction for a total dose of 6 to 7.5 Gy is adequate to relieve symptoms. Hyperfractionated regimens (1.2 to 1.5 Gy per fraction twice each day for a total dose of 6 to 10 Gy) can also be used. There will be rare occasions when emergency radiotherapy will be appropriate in the absence of a histologic diagnosis. Because of the rapid response to radiation, the histologic diagnosis may be lost and selection of the appropriate definitive therapy will depend either on biopsy of other disease or on a presumed diagnosis (58).

The *CNS* requires prophylactic treatment in the majority of children with NHL, thereby reducing the otherwise high risk of CNS relapse (38,59). The results of a randomized trial of CNS prophylaxis in stage II to IV pediatric NHL confirm this view. A 1977 report from Uganda and Kenya described 22 children with Burkitt's NHL. All received systemic chemotherapy and 11 were randomized to have prophylactic craniospinal irradiation. No benefit in CNS disease control or overall freedom from relapse was attributable to radiotherapy (19). It is now generally agreed that in most situations prophylactic CNS treatment will consist of systemic and IT chemotherapy. Mandell et al. (37) reported only one isolated CNS relapse in 58 evaluable children treated with an LSA2-L2-based protocol, which used IT methotrexate without cranial irradiation regardless of histology or stage. In a Children's Cancer Study Group report of children treated with COMP or a modified LSA2-L2 protocol using IT methotrexate without cranial irradiation, the incidence of isolated CNS relapse was only 6% in patients without CNS disease at diagnosis (33). Therefore, cranial irradiation is not warranted for the majority of patients. Indications for 18 to 24 Gy of cranial irradiation are currently limited to (a) patients with overt CNS lymphoma at diagnosis or relapse, and (b) patients with leukemic transformation at diagnosis (38, 60). These indications are based on a high rate of CNS relapse with chemotherapy alone and the proven efficacy of IT methotrexate plus cranial radiation in these settings (35). Finally, patients with cranial nerve palsies at diagnosis or subsequently should receive radiation to the skull base or whole cranium. This may improve survival and functional recovery (61).

Some patients will be irradiated to regions of *local residual disease* after failing to achieve a complete remission on chemotherapy, or for *relapse* with local disease only. Both of these situations are rare. Care should be taken to use modest dose per fraction schedules and to avoid exceeding normal tissue tolerance doses because patients may be eligible for bone marrow transplantation requiring total-body irradiation (TBI) as a component of the preparative regimen.

Children with refractory or relapsed NHL can experience prolonged disease-free survival following treatment with high-dose chemotherapy or high-dose chemoradiotherapy followed by autologous or allogeneic bone marrow transplant (62–64) (Table 5). When TBI is a component of the preparatory regimen, fractionated courses to total doses of 12 to 14 Gy are common (see Chapter 2). Disease recurrence rather than the morbidity of transplant is the predominant cause of failure in this setting. The strategy of irradiating the local site(s) of initial disease recurrence prior to or following transplant, whether or not TBI is used, has proved to be effective in adults and should be considered (22,62,64,65). Doses to these sites (usually at least 20 Gy) are constrained by normal tissue tolerances.

TABLE 5. *Autologous bone marrow transplantation for NHl*

Center	Number of patients	Preparative regimen	Status of BMT	Projected disease-free survival (%)
Dana—Farber (22)	100	Cy/TBI	All in CR or sensitive relapse	50
Center Leon, Bernard, and others (65)	100	Various	50% advanced relapse	19
Seattle (64)	101	Cy/TBI, araC/TBI, others	73% advanced relapse	11
Johns Hopkins (74)	20	Cy/TBI	15% advanced relapse, others in second CR or sensitive relapse	50
Middlesex (75)	50	Various chemotherapy	Most advanced relapse	14
Tours/St. Antoine (76)	46	Various	29% advanced relapse	60

From ref. 71, with permission.
BMT, bone marrow transplant; Cy, cyclophosphamide; TBI, total-body irradiation

TABLE 6. *Influence of potentially significant prognostic factors on event-free survival in childhood NHL estimated by Cox regression model*

Factor	Univariate analysis			Multivariate analysis		
	X^2	df	P value	X^2	df	p value
Era of treatment	42.9	2	<0.0001	53.8	2	<0.0001
Stage	40.4	3	<0.0001	10.6	3	0.014
Log LDH	26.3	1	<0.0001	11.1	1	0.0008
Primary site	26.2	4	<0.0001	7.8	4	0.10
Histology	3.2	3	0.4	4.3	3	0.2
Sex	0.2	1	0.6	0.2	1	0.6
Age	0.6	2	0.7	1.5	1	0.5
Race	0.1	1	0.7	0.1	1	0.7

From ref. 7, with permission.

RESULTS OF THERAPY

Prior to 1975, when therapy was directed to the identifiable gross tumor, few children survived. The small number of patients who did survive had favorable presentations, including (a) limited resectable abdominal disease, or (b) involvement of a single nodal region or extranodal site. With current intensive multiagent regimens, survival is generally excellent except for patients with disseminated disease and adverse prognostic factors such as large tumor bulk, CNS involvement, and high serum lactate dehydrogenase (LDH) (Table 6).

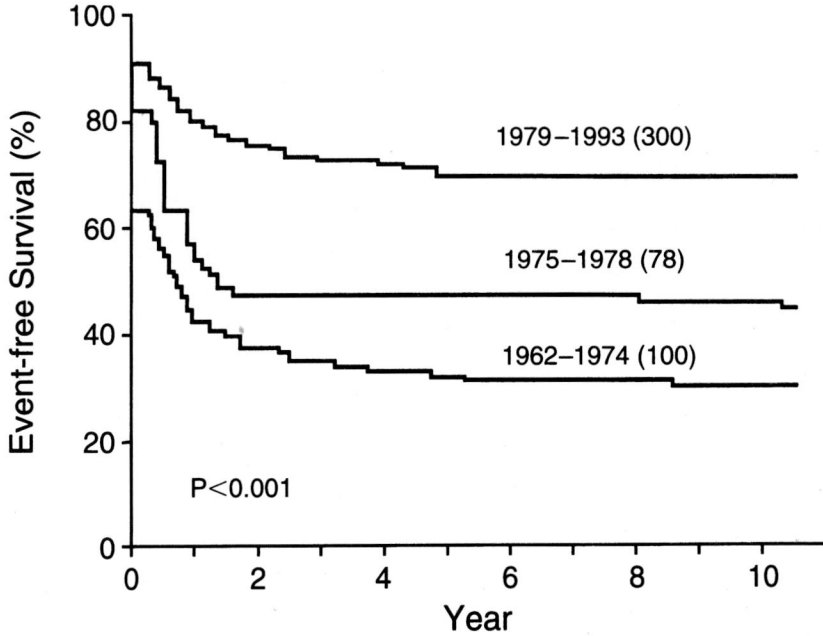

FIG. 2. Event-free survival of patients with non-Hodgkin's lymphoma treated from 1962 to 1993 at St. Jude Children's Research Hospital. The numbers in parentheses are the total number of patients. Because some patients were not in complete remission at year 0, the curves do not begin at 100%. From 1962 to 1974 a variety of chemotherapy programs were utilized along with some use of local irradiation. From 1975 to 1978, a single combined modality protocol was used. From 1979 to 1993 treatment was based on the stage and histologic type of lymphoma. (Reproduced from ref. 77, with permission.)

Most relapses occur within 12 months of diagnosis, and are uncommon beyond 2 years (40).

Children with stage I to II disease have 2-year disease-free survival rates of 70% to 90% (6,7,33,40–42). Children with nonlymphoblastic histologies may have a somewhat better outlook than those with lymphoblastic disease (45). Children with stage III disease have a 60% to 80% 2-year disease-free survival. Those with stage IV disease fare less well: results for children with lymphoblastic lymphoma (T-cell) range from 60% to 80%, and those for children with nonlymphoblastic (especially small noncleaved) histologies range from 35% to 55% (7,12,32,39,42,46,48, 49,53,54) (Fig. 2). Deaths from second malignancies can occur at prolonged time intervals and modify survival curves (66).

Patients undergoing transplantation early in their disease course—that is, after first relapse or second complete remission—have 2-year DFS approaching 50%, whereas those with refractory disease fare less well (5% to 20%) (62–64) (Table 5).

REFERENCES

References particularly recommended for further reading are indicated with an asterisk.

1. Hodgkin T. On some morbid appearances of the absorbent gland and spleen. *Medico-Chir Trans* 1832;17: 68–114.
2. Virchow R. Weisses Blu, Neue notizen aus dem Gebiete der Natur and Heikkunde (Frorip's neue notizen). 1845;36:151–156.
3. Gasparini M, Lombardi F, Gianni C, Lattuada A, Rilke F, Fossati-Bellani F. Childhood non-Hodgkin's lymphoma: prognostic relevance of clinical stages and histologic subgroups. *Am J Pediatr Hematol Oncol* 1983; 5(2):161–171.
4. Schutt S, Seeger K, Schmidt E. Immunoglobulin and T-cell receptor gene rearrangements in childhood acute lymphoblastic leukemia and non-Hodgkin's lymphoma. *Haematol Blood Transfus* 1990;33:56–61.
5. Lemerle M, Gerard-Marchant R, Sancho H, Schweisguth O. Natural history of non-Hodgkin's malignant lymphomata in chldren: a retrospective study of 190 cases. *Br J Cancer* 1975;31:324–331.
*6. Link M, Donaldson S, Berard C, Shuster JJ, Murphy S. Results of treatment of childhood localized non-Hodgkin's lymphoma with combination chemotherapy with or without radiotherapy. *N Engl J Med* 1990;322: 1169–1174.
*7. Murphy SB, Fairclough DL, Hutchison RE, Berard CW. Non-Hodgkin's lymphomas of childhood: an analysis of the histology, staging and response to treatment of 338 cases at a single institution. *J Clin Oncol* 1989;7:186–193.
8. Reiter A, Schrappe M, Parwasesch R, et al. Non-Hodgkin's lymphomas of childhood and adolescence: results of a treatment stratified for biologic subtypes and stage: a report of the Berlin-Frankfort-Munster Group. *J Clin Oncol* 1995;13:359–372.
9. Frizzera G, Murphy SB. Follicular (nodular) lymphoma in childhood: a rare clinical-pathological entity. Report of eight cases from four cancer centers. *Cancer* 1979;44:2218–2235.
*10. Murphy SB. Classification, staging, and end results of treatment of childhood nonHodgkin's lymphomas: dissimilarities from lymphomas in adults. *Semin Oncol* 1980;1:332–339.
11. Young JL Jr, Miller RW. Incidence of malignant tumors in U.S. children. *J Pediatr* 1975;86:254–158.
*12. Magrath IT. Biology and treatment of small noncleaved cell lymphoma. *Oncology* 1989;3:41–55.
13. Ziegler JL, Magrath IA, Olweny CLM. Cure of Burkitt's lymphoma. Ten-year follow-up of 157 Ugandan patients. *Lancet* 1979;2:936–938.
14. Filipovich AH, Mathur A, Kamat D, Shapiro RS. Primary immunodeficiencies: genetic risk factors for lymphoma. *Cancer Res* 1992;52[Suppl]:5465s–5476s.
15. Grundy GW, Creagan ET, Fraumeni JF. Non-Hodgkin's lymphoma in childhood: epidemiologic features. *J Natl Cancer Inst* 1973;51:767–776.
16. Taylor A, Metcalfe J, Thick J, Mak Y. Leukemia and lymphoma in ataxia telangiectasia. *Blood* 1996;87: 423–438.
17. Reynolds P, Saunders LD, Lavefsky ME, Lemp GF. The spectrum of acquired immuno-deficiency syndrome (AIDS) associated malignancies in San Francisco, 1980–1987. *Am J Epidemiol* 1993;137:19–30.
18. Weinstein HJ, Vance ZB, Jaffe N, Buell D, Cassady JR, Nathan DG. Improved prognosis for patients with mediastinal lymphoblastic lymphoma. *Blood* 1979;53: 687–694.
19. Olweny CLM, Atine I, Kaddu-Mukasa A, et al. Cerebrospinal irradiation of Burkitt's lymphoma. Failure in preventing central nervous system relapse. *Acta Radiol Ther* 1977;16:225–231.
20. Ziegler JL, DeVita VT Jr, Graw RG, et al. Combined modality treatment of American Burkitt's lymphoma. *Cancer* 1976;38:2225–2231.
21. Haddy TB, Parker RL, Magrath IT. Bone marrow involvement in young patients with non-Hodgkin's lymphoma: the importance of multiple bone marrow samples for accurate staging. *Med Pediatr Oncol* 1989;17: 418–423.
22. Freedman AS, Takvorian T, Anderson K, et al. Autologous bone marrow transplantation in B-cell non-Hodgkin's lymphoma: very low treatment mortality in 100 patients in sensitive relapse. *J Clin Oncol* 1990;8: 784–791.
23. Carbone PP, Kaplan HS, Musshoff K, Smithers DW, Tubiana M. Report of the Committee on Hodgkin's Disease staging classification. *Cancer Res* 1971;31: 1860–1861.
24. Murphy SB. Management of childhood non-Hodgkin's lymphoma. *Cancer Treat Rep* 1977;61(6):1161–1173.
25. Griffith RC, Kelly DR, Nathwani BN, et al. A morphologic study of childhood lymphoma of the lym-

phoblastic type. The Pediatric Oncology Group experience. *Cancer* 1987;59:1126–1131.

26. Lukes R, Collins RD. Immunologic characterization of human malignant lymphomas. *Cancer* 1972;34: 1488–1503.

27. Nathwani BN, Kim H, Rappaport H, Solomon J, Fox M. Non-Hodgkin's lymphoma. A clinicopathologic study comparing two classifications. *Cancer* 1978;41: 303–325.

28. Wilson JF, Jenkin RD, Anderson JR, et al. Studies on the pathology of non-Hodgkin's lymphoma of childhood. I. The role of routine histopathology as a prognostic factor. A report from the Children's Cancer Study Group. *Cancer* 1984;53(8):1695–1704.

*29. Harris N, Jaffe E, Stein H, et al. A revised European-American classification of lymphoid neoplasms: a proposal from the International Lymphoma Study Group. *Blood* 1994;84:1361–1392.

30. Duque-Hammershaimb L, Wollner N, Miller DR. LSA2-L2 protocol treatment of stage IV non-Hodgkin's lymphoma in children with partial and extensive bone marrow involvement. *Cancer* 1983;52(1): 39–43.

31. Bernard A, Boumsell L, Reinherz E, et al. Cell surface characterization of malignant T cells from lymphoblastic lymphoma using monoclonal antibodies: evidence for a phenotypic difference between malignant T cells from patients with acute lymphoblastic leukemia and lymphoblastic lymphoma. *Blood* 1981;57:1105–1110.

32. Magrath IT, Janus C, Edwards BK, et al. An effective therapy for both undifferentiated (including Burkitt's) lymphomas and lymphoblastic lymphomas in children and young adults. *Blood* 1984;63:1102–1111.

33. Anderson JR, Jenkin RD, Wilson JF, et al. Long-term follow-up of patients treated with COMP or LSA²L² therapy for childhood NHL: a report of CCG-551 from the CCG. *J Clin Oncol* 1993;11:1024–1032.

34. Patte C, Philip T, Rodary C, et al. Improved survival rate in children with stage III and IV B cell non-Hodgkin's lymphoma and leukemia using multiagent chemotherapy: results of a study of 114 children from the French Pediatric Oncology Society. *J Clin Oncol* 1986;4:1219–1226.

35. Pullen DJ, Sullivan MP, Falletta JM, et al. Modified LSA2-L2 treatment in 53 children with E-rosette-positive T-cell leukemia: results and prognostic factors (a Pediatric Oncology Group study). *Blood* 1982;60: 1159–1168.

36. Pui CH, Ip SH, Kung P, et al. High serum interleukin-2 receptor levels are related to advanced disease and a poor outcome in childhood non-Hodgkin's lymphoma. *Blood* 1987;70(3):624–628.

*37. Mandell LR, Wollner N, Fuks Z. Is cranial radiation necessary for CNS prophylaxis in pediatric NHL? *Int J Radiat Oncol Biol Phys* 1987;13(3):359–363.

*38. Murphy SB, Bleyer WA. Cranial irradiation is not necessary for central nervous system prophylaxis in pediatric non-Hodgkin's lymphoma. *Int J Radiat Oncol Biol Phys* 1987;13:467–468.

39. Sullivan MP, Boyett J, Pullen J, et al. Pediatric oncology group experience with modified LSA2- L2 therapy in 107 children with non-Hodgkin's lymphoma (Burkitt's lymphoma excluded). *Cancer* 1985;55(2): 323–336.

*40. Meadows AT, Sposto R, Jenkin RDT, et al. Similar efficacy of 6 and 18 months of therapy with four drugs (COMP) for localized non-Hodgkin's lymphoma of children: a report from the Children's Cancer Study Group. *J Clin Oncol* 1989;7:92–99.

*41. Nachman J. Therapy for childhood non-Hodgkin's lymphomas, nonlymphoblastic type. *Am J Pediatr Hemat Oncol* 1990;12:359–366.

42. Schwenn MR, Blattner SR, Lynch E, Weinstein HJ. HiC-COM: a 2-month intensive chemotherapy regimen for children with stage III and IV Burkitt's lymphoma and B-cell acute lymphoblastic leukemia. *J Clin Oncol* 1991;9:133–138.

43. Weinstein HJ, Cassady JR, Levey R. Long-term results of the APO protocol (vincristine, doxorubicin [adriamycin], and prednisone) for treatment of mediastinal lymphoblastic lymphoma. *J Clin Oncol* 1983;1(9): 537–541.

44. Murphy S, Bowman W, Abromowitch M, et al. Results of treatment of advanced stage Burkitt's lymphoma and B-cell (SIg+) acute lymphoblastic leukemia with high-dose fractionated cyclophosphamide and coordinated high-dose methotrexate and cytarabine. *J Clin Oncol* 1986;4:1732–1739.

45. Jenkin RD, Anderson JR, Chilcote RR, et al. The treatment of localized non-Hodgkin's lymphoma in children: a report from the Children's Cancer Study Group. *J Clin Oncol* 1984;2(2):88–97.

46. Wollner N, Burchenal JH, Lieberman PH, Exelby GP, D'Angio G, Murphy ML. Non-Hodgkin's lymphoma in children: a comparative study of two modalities of therapy. *Cancer* 1976;37:123–134.

47. Dahl G, Rivera G, Pui CH, et al. A novel treatment of childhood lymphoblastic non-Hodgkin's lymphoma: early and intermittent use of teniposide plus cytarabine. *Blood* 1985;66:1110–1114.

48. Camitta BM, Lauer SJ, Casper JT, et al. Effectiveness of a six-drug regimen (APO) without local irradiation for treatment of mediastinal lymphoblastic lymphoma in children. *Cancer* 1985;56(4):738–741.

*49. Hvizdala EV, Berard C, Callihan T, et al. Nonlymphoblastic lymphoma in children—histology and stage-related response to therapy: a Pediatric Oncology Group study. *J Clin Oncol* 1991;9:1189–1195.

*50. Hvizdala EV, Berard C, Callihan T, et al. Lymphoblastic lymphoma in children—a randomized trial comparing LSA2-L2 with the A-COP+ therapeutic regimen: a Pediatric Oncology Group study. *J Clin Oncol* 1988; 6(1):26–33.

51. Pick T, Weinstein HJ, Schwenn M, et al. Treatment of advanced stage large cell non-Hodgkin's lymphoma in childhood: a Pediatric Oncology Group study (8615). *Blood* 1993;82:333a.

52. Sandlund JT, Santana V, Abromowitch M, et al. Large cell non-Hodgkin's lymphoma of childhood: clinical characteristics and outcome. *Leukemia* 1994;8:30–34.

*53. Hutchinson RE, Murphy SD, Fairclough EL, et al. Diffuse small noncleaved cell lymphoma in children, Burkitt's versus non-Burkitt's types. *Cancer* 1989;64: 23–28.

54. Kelly DR, Nathwani BN, Griffith RC, et al. A morphologic study of childhood lymphoma of the undifferentiated type. The Pediatric Oncology Group experience. *Cancer* 1987;59:1132–1137.

55. Link M, Shuster JJ, Berard C, Murphy S. Nine weeks

of chemotherapy without radiotherapy is sufficient treatment for most children with localized non-Hodgkin's lymphoma (NHL). *Proc Ann Meet Soc Clin Oncol* 1993;12:AT309.

56. Stapleton F, Strother D, Roy S, Wyatt R, McKay C, Murphy S. Acute renal failure at onset of therapy for advanced stage Burkitt lymphoma and B cell acute lymphoblastic lymphoma. *Pediatrics* 1988;82:863–868.

57. Haddy TB, Keenan AM, Jaffe ES, Magrath IT. Bone involvement in young patients with non-Hodgkin's lymphoma: efficacy of chemotherapy without local radiotherapy. *Blood* 1988;72:1141–1147.

58. Loeffler JS, Leopold KA, Recht A, Weinstein HJ, Tarbell NJ. Emergency prebiopsy radiation for mediastinal masses: impact on subsequent pathologic diagnosis and outcome. *J Clin Oncol* 1986;4:716–721.

59. Murphy SB. Current concepts in cancer: childhood non-Hodgkin's lymphoma. *N Engl J Med* 1978; 299(26):1446–1448.

*60. Loeffler JS, Ervin TJ, Mauch P, et al. Primary lymphoma of the central nervous system: patterns of failure and factors that influence survival. *J Clin Oncol* 1985;3:490–494.

61. Ingram LC, Fairclough DL, Furman WL, et al. Cranial nerve palsy in childhood acute lymphoblastic leukemia and non-Hodgkin's lymphoma. *Cancer* 1991;67:2262–2268.

62. Armitage JO. Bone marrow transplantation in the treatment of patients with lymphoma. *Blood* 1989;73: 1749–1758.

*63. Kurtzberg J, Graham M. Non-Hodgkin's lymphoma: biologic classification and implications for therapy. *Pediatr Clin North Am* 1991;38:443–456.

64. Petersen FB, Applebaum FR, Hill R, et al. Autologous marrow transplantation for malignant lymphoma: a report of 101 cases from Seattle. *J Clin Oncol* 1990;8: 638–647.

65. Philip T, Armitage J, Spitzer G, et al. High-dose therapy and autologous bone marrow transplantation after failure of conventional chemotherapy in adults with intermediate grade or high-grade non-Hodgkin's lymphoma. *N Engl J Med* 1987;316:1493–1498.

66. Ingram L, Mott MG, Mann JR, Faafat F, Darbyshire PJ, Morris Jones PH. Second malignancies in children treated for non-Hodgkin's lymphoma and T-cell leukemia with the UKCCSG regimens. *Br J Cancer* 1987;55(4):463–466.

67. Murphy SB, Bowman WP, Abromowitch M, et al. Results of treatment of advanced stage Burkitt's lymphoma and B-cell (SIg+) acute lymphoblastic leukemia with high-dose fractionated cyclophosphamide and coordinated high-dose methotrexate and cytarabine. *J Clin Oncol* 1986;4:1732–1739.

68. Murphy SB, Hustu HO, Rivera G, Berard CW. End results of treating children with localized non-Hodgkin's lymphomas with a combined modality approach of lessened intensity. *J Clin Oncol* 1983;1(5):326–330.

69. Anderson JR, Wilson JF, Jenkin DT, et al. Childhood non-Hodgkin's lymphoma: the results of a randomized therapeutic trial comparing a 4-drug regimen (COMP) with a 10-drug regimen (LSA2-L2) *N Engl J Med* 1983;308:559–565.

70. Muller-Weihrich S. Childhood B-cell lymphomas and leukemias. Improvement of prognosis by a therapy developed for B-cell neoplasms by the BMF study group. *Onkologie* 1984;7:205–208.

71. Magrath IT, ed. *The non-Hodgkin's lymphomas.* Baltimore: Williams & Wilkins, 1990.

72. Sandlund J, Hutchison R, Crist W. Non-Hodgkin's lymphoma. In: Fernback D, Vietti T, eds. *Clinical pediatric oncology,* 4th ed. St. Louis: Mosby-Year Book, 1991:337–353.

73. Sullivan M, Ramirez I. Curability of Burkitt's lymphoma with high-dose cyclophosphamide—high dose methotrexate therapy and intrathecal chemoprophylaxis. *J Clin Oncol* 1985;3:627–636.

74. Braine HG, Santos GW, Kaizer H, et al. Treatment of poor prognosis non-Hodgkin's lymphoma using cyclophosphamide and total body irradiation regimens with autologous bone marrow rescue. *Bone Marrow Trans* 1987;2:7–14.

75. Gribben JG, Golston AH, Linch DC, et al. Effectiveness of high-dose combination chemotherapy and autologous bone marrow transplantation for patients with non-Hodgkin's lymphoma who are still responsive to conventional dose therapy. *J Clin Oncol* 1989;7: 1621–1629.

76. Colombat P, Gorin N-C, Lemonnier M-P, et al. The role of autologous bone marrow transplantation in 46 adult patients with non-Hodgkin's lymphoma. *J Clin Oncol* 1990;8:630–637.

77. Sandlund J, Downey JR, Crist WM. Non-Hodgkin's lymphoma in childhood. *N Engl J Med* 1996;334: 1328–1348.

9

Ewing's Sarcoma

James Ewing (1866–1943) first described the bone tumor that bears his name in 1921 (1). Ewing characterized the tumor as either an endothelioma or endothelial myeloma of bone. He observed that the malignancy was most common in teenagers, occurred in the metaphyseal/diaphyseal region of long bones or in the flat bones, was associated with pain and often fever, had a histologic appearance of highly vascular sheets of small round cells, and was quite sensitive to radiation (2) (Fig. 1).

Ewing was, in his time, a leading authority on cancer. He became Professor and Chairman of Pathology at Cornell Medical School in New York City at 33 years of age and went on to serve as Director of the Memorial Hospital—playing a crucial role in the growth of what is now known as the Memorial Sloan-Kettering Cancer Center. His definitive textbook, *Neoplastic Diseases,* was first published in 1919 and went through four editions. Ewing's accomplishments, including over 160 publications, are even more remarkable in light of the fact that his life was marked by considerable personal difficulty: the death of his wife from toxemia of pregnancy after only a brief marriage, and his own battles with osteomyelitis and trigeminal neuralgia (for which he was operated on by Harvey Cushing in 1926) (2).

Ewing's sarcoma is the second most common childhood primary bone tumor. The tumor is slightly less frequent than osteosarcoma and represents 3% of pediatric cancer. Approximately 200 cases occur annually in the United States. Although presenting in the pubertal age range in 40% of patients, the age at diagnosis is more variable than osteosarcoma: 30% of cases occur in children less than 10-years old, and 5% occur in young adults over age 20 years. Boys are affected more often than girls, in a ratio of 1.5 to 2:1. Age at diagnosis parallels the earlier onset of puberty in girls, with a median time of onset 3 to 4 years younger than in boys. Ewing's sarcoma is rare in children of Asian or African descent (3).

PATHOLOGY

Ewing's sarcoma consists of monomorphic sheets of small, round malignant cells with hyperchromatic nuclei and relatively little cytoplasm. There is a relative dearth of associated stroma. Cells are usually periodic acid-Schiff (PAS) positive, indicating the presence of glycogen granules. Glycogen within the tumor cells and the demonstration of the MIC2 gene product on the tumor cell membrane help identify Ewing's sarcoma (4,5). The tumor cells are also uniformly vimentin-positive and frequently cytokeratin-positive, indicating origin from epithelial and neuronal elements (6).

There has been much debate over the cell of origin of Ewing's sarcoma. Ewing contended that the tumor was of endothelial origin. The most recent data suggests derivation from primitive neuroepithelial tissue (2). Primitive neural features have been described in peripheral primitive neuroectodermal tumors of soft tissue (PNET) and Ewing's sarcoma (7). It is sometimes difficult to distin-

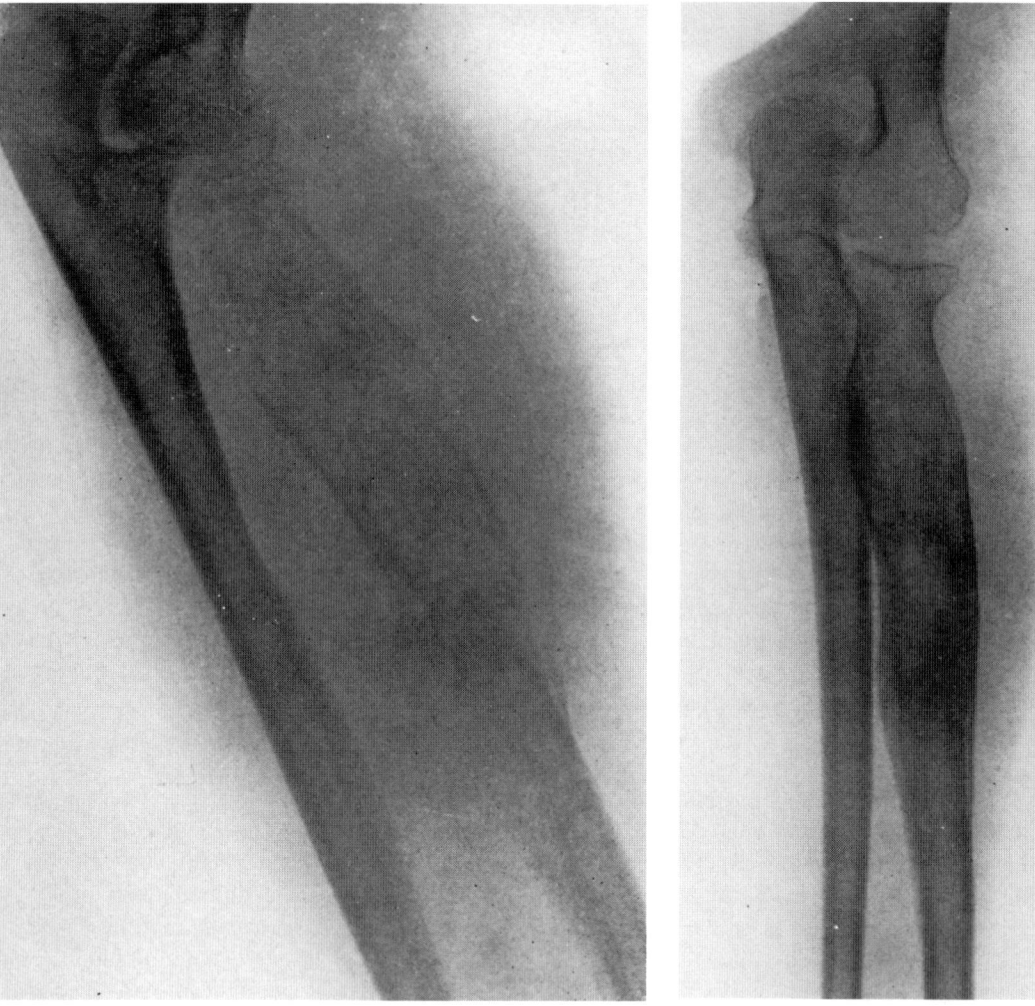

FIG. 1. A: In the fourth edition of his textbook, *Neoplastic Diseases* (1940), James Ewing of the Memorial Hospital, New York, described a "diffuse endothelioma of radius. Diffuse absorption without destruction of shaft. Spontaneous fracture. Wide invasion of muscle. Duration 1 year." Ewing wrote that " the first indication is for treatment by radiation in full doses, and over considerable periods. This recommendation is based on the reported cure of certain cases . . . by radiation alone, and on the clinical disappearance of the disease by variable periods in many more cases. The response to radiation also confirms the diagnosis. The danger of metastases occurring while this treatment is in progress is probably negligible, since the tumor tissue generally undergoes rapid liquefaction and necrosis." **B:** Ewing illustrated the excellent response of the tumor to radiotherapy.

guish Ewing's sarcoma and PNET from other small round cell tumors. The two entities are both primitive with few specific ultrastructural, enzymatic, or cell surface characteristics. The diagnosis is often made by excluding other possibilities. On a cellular level, however, most Ewing's sarcoma and PNET have several things in common. Both tumors have high levels of choline acetyltransferase, an enzyme important in the biosynthesis of cholonergic neurotransmitters. Some but not all, of Ewing's sarcoma express neurofilament proteins. In addition, some Ewing's tumors have neuroantigens on the cell membrane (4,5,8). PNETs are typically neuron-specific enolase (+) S100 positive and vimentin positive in contrast to classic Ewing's, which is neuron-specific enolase (−), S100 variable, and vimentin (+) (4–6,8–13) (see also Chapter 11).

Ewing's sarcoma and PNET have been linked to the specific chromosomal abnormalities involving a reciprocal translocation between chromosome 11 and 22: (t) (11;22) (q24;q12). This genetic rearrangement is detectable in 86% to 90% of tumors. Approximately 5% to 10% of Ewing's sarcomas do not contain (t) (11;22) but instead have a translocation between chromosome 21 and 22 (t) (21;22) (q21;q12). It is of importance, however, that this alternate rearrangement has similar molecular consequences as (t) (11;22) (14).

The 11;22 translocation juxtaposes the EWS gene with the FLI gene, a member of the ETS transcription factor family. The 21;22 translocation juxtaposes the EWS gene to another ETS family member, ERG. There are structural similarities between these two translocations suggesting that they bind to similar DNA target sites. EWS/FLI can produce malignant transformation of some, but not all, cell lines. The EWS/FLI gene appears to act as an transcription factor. Its mechanism of action appears to be a modulation of transcription of target genes. The Ewing's sarcoma/PNET translocation seems to fall within a developing class of tumor-associated chromosomal tranlocations that form chimeric transcription factors (14). We may conclude that the probable mechanism of carcinogenesis in Ewing's sarcoma is a translocation that produces an aberrant transcription factor. If Ewing's sarcoma shares this transcription mechanism with PNET, then the cell of origin in Ewing's might be related to a primitive neuroectodermal cell. Therefore, Ewing's sarcoma cytogenetics may help us to understand oncogenic mechanisms.

Two recent publications have shown that the t(11;22) breakpoint location, and, therefore, the exact amino acid composition of the resultant EWS-FLI fusion oncoproteins, might have prognostic relevance (9,13,15).

Therefore, the importance of the availability of specimens for genetic analysis cannot be overemphasized (15).

CLINICAL PRESENTATION

Pain is the most common presenting symptom, noted in approximately 90% of cases. Local swelling or mass effect related to the bone tumor is apparent in a majority of children. A distinct soft-tissue mass can be appreciated clinically in one-third of cases. Significant limitation of movement has been described in 25% of presentations. Neurologic symptoms or signs occur in 15% of children, either as spinal cord compression or peripheral nerve compression. The latter is most often apparent with lesions of the pelvis or about the knee. Fever is present in 10% of cases and has been related to tumor size and metastatic disease at diagnosis.

The diagnostic evaluation of the patient with Ewing's sarcoma is shown in Table 1. Laboratory findings include high leukocyte count and/or elevated erythrocyte sedimentation rate (ESR). The former has been related to increased risk of tumor recurrence (15,16). Pretreatment serum lactate dehydrogenase (LDH) is of prognostic significance, and the degree of LDH elevation has been related to tumor volume (16).

The diagnostic features of Ewing's sarcoma are radiographically defined as a per-

TABLE 1. *Clinical evaluation of the patient with Ewing's sarcoma*

Pathology
Biopsy with routine histology
Electron microscopy
Immunohistochemistry
Cytogenetics
Radiography
CT and MRI of the local tumor extent
Chest CT
Bone scan
Bone marrow aspirate and biopsy
Laboratory
Routine chemistries, including LDH

CT, computerized tomography; MRI, magnetic resonance imaging; LDH, lactate dehydrogenase.

meative, destructive lesion of bone. In long bones, the tumor most often presents along the metaphyseal region or within the diaphysis (i.e., at the mid-shaft level). The periosteum is often displaced by the underlying tumor, resulting in the clinical sign of Cottman's triangle representing a bone-expansile lesion. Although bone expansion occurs commonly, new bone formation beyond the periosteal margin is relatively rare. An associated soft-tissue mass is typical, occurring in over 50% of long-bone neoplasms (17,18). Both computerized tomography (CT) and magnetic resonance imaging (MRI) appear necessary for most sites and are complementary. Using both studies has added substantially to the determination of disease extent, identifying extraosseous involvement and the degree of marrow infiltration linearly (Fig. 2). CT has been valuable in outlining the bone and soft tissue extent of central Ewing's sarcoma (Fig. 3), and more accurate definition of tumor extent by CT scans is credited with improvement in control of pelvic Ewing's sarcoma (19). MRI has additionally added to this definition of tumor (20) (Fig. 4). Radionuclide bone scan may also be of value although it may exaggerate the linear tumor extent. MRI may show edema. Whether there is direct microscopic extension of tumor associated with the edema is unknown at present.

Approximately 53% of Ewing's sarcoma has a primary site in an extremity and 47% have central primaries. Ewing's sarcoma presents in the proximal extremities in 20% to 30% and distal extremities in 30% to 40% of cases (21–23). Metastases are present at diagnosis in 21% to 23%.

Primary lesions of the rib are associated with direct pleural extension and significant extraosseous soft-tissue mass in a majority of cases (24,25). The original description by Askin et al., in 1979 (26), of thoracopulmonary malignant tumors characterized small round cell tumors in this location as a separate clinicopathologic entity—called, by many, Askin's tumor. He described a female predominance and a short median survival (8 months). These tumors tend to have a large

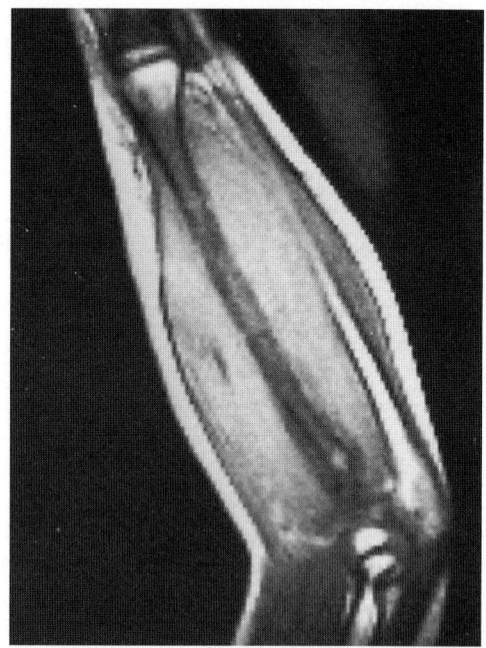

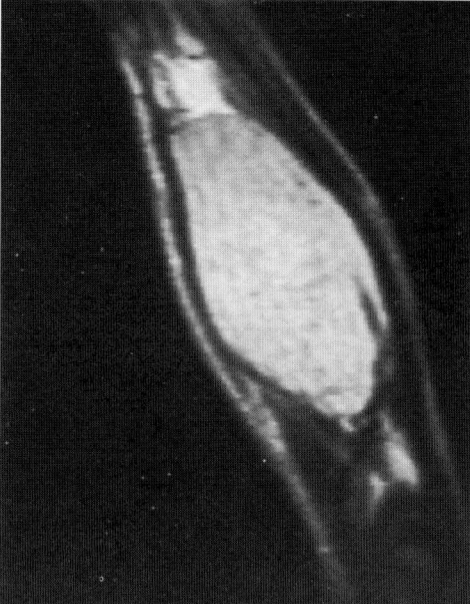

FIG. 2. Ewing's sarcoma of the left radius **(A)** with extensive infiltration of the surrounding soft tissue **(B)**.

soft-tissue component that can displace most of one lung with or without much rib involvement. This patient group has special management issues, which are discussed under irradiation technique (27).

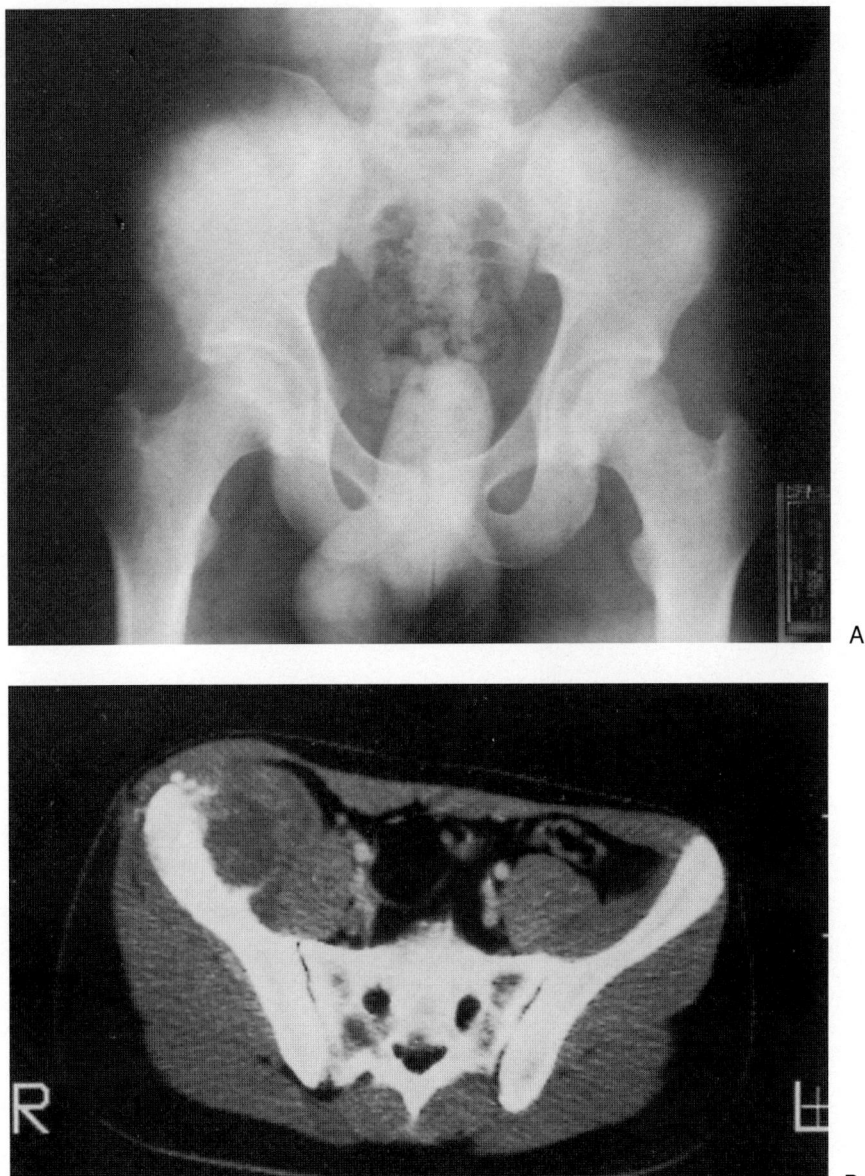

FIG. 3. Pelvic Ewing's sarcoma, involving the right ileum. Plain films **(A)** show only mottled destruction of the lateral aspect of the right ilium. **B:** CT study shows the extensive associated soft-tissue mass.

The frequency of overt metastasis is estimated at 25% to 30% for pelvic primaries and less than 8% to 10% for tumors of the extremities or ribs. The sites of metastatic disease at diagnosis parallel the distribution noted with treatment failure, most often involving the lungs (40%) or bones (40%), with less frequent disease involving the bone marrow, lymph nodes, soft tissue, visceral sites, or, rarely, the central nervous system (28).

No formal staging system has been recognized for Ewing's sarcoma. The disease factors most recognized as prognostically signif-

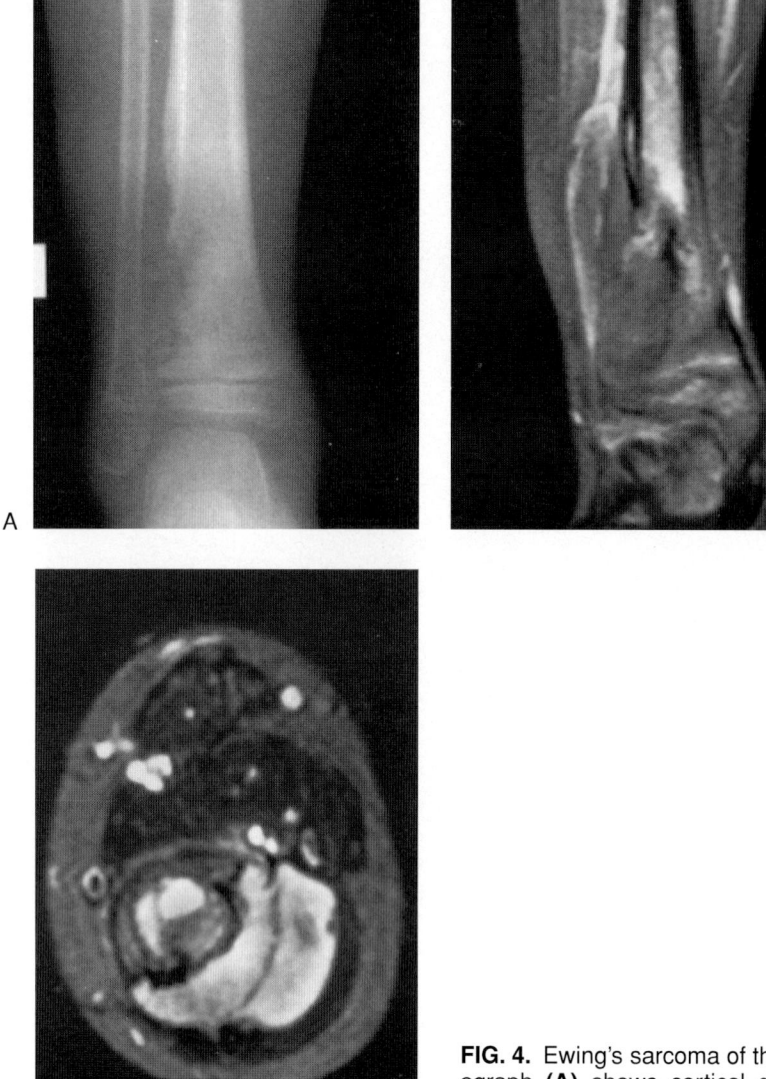

A

B

C

FIG. 4. Ewing's sarcoma of the tibia seen on a plain radiograph **(A)** shows cortical disruption, "onion skinning," and a suggestion of soft tissue involvement. Coronal and axial MRI show extensive soft-tissue infiltration (**B** and **C**).

icant include the bone of origin or primary site, tumor size, presence or degree of soft-tissue extension, and identification of hematogenous metastasis at diagnosis (Table 2). Smaller tumors (less than 100-mL volume) and distal extremity tumors tend to be favorable (23,29). At present, the most important prognostic factor at diagnosis appears to be the presence of metastasis. Reports suggest that the response to initial chemotherapy may be of significance as well (30). The prognostic importance of the EWS-FLI fusion in Ewing's sarcoma will need additional study (9, 13).

TABLE 2. *Prognostic factors in Ewing's sarcoma: disease-related parameters*

Disease factors	Favorable prognosis	Unfavorable prognosis	References
Site	Distal extremity (tibia, fibula, radius, ulna, hands, feet)	Central lesions (especially pelvic bones) relatively less favorable: proximal extremity (humerus, femur), ribs	6,10,17,30,57, 67,84
Size	<5–8 cm in greatest diameter or <100–500 mL estimated volume	Tumors of greater dimension	17,54,62,85
Soft tissue extension	Absence of radiographically identifiable soft tissue extension	Presence of soft tissue extension by radiograph or significant extension by CT	17,22

SELECTION OF TREATMENT

Local Control

The relative roles of surgery and radiation therapy for local treatment of Ewing's sarcoma have long been debated. In 1953, Wang and Schulz (31) reported 5-year survival in 6 of 36 children treated with wide-field irradiation, as compared to 1 of 14 treated by primary surgical resection. Using 50 Gy to the entire bone, Phillips and Sheline (32) documented survival in 5 of 21 cases in 1969. Following these reports, Ewing's was generally treated with radiation therapy except for small tumors in expendable bones. Reviews have indicated an overall rate of local tumor control of 75% to almost 95% following primary radiation therapy (3,21,33–37).

Historically, radiotherapy has been the local treatment of choice. Developments have led to a reconsideration of the role of surgery. These important developments include the recognition that the local failure rate for Ewing's sarcoma, following radiotherapy, ranges from 9% to 25%. This is shown by a survey of the literature in Table 3. In addition, the development of innovative surgical techniques allowing preservation of limb and structural bone function have contributed to utilizing surgery as an alternative to radiation. The routine use of cytoreductive chemotherapy, as will be discussed later in this chapter, often produces a significant decrease in the soft-tissue component rendering tumors more readily resectable.

One must interpret the data, however, concerning local control with radiotherapy alone with caution. Difficulties in assessing response to radiation therapy are evident in the slow rate of resolution of CT, MRI, and radionuclide bone scan findings following irradiation. The significance of residual soft-tissue abnormalities and persistent areas of increased uptake on technitium scans are un-

TABLE 3. *The roles of surgery and radiation therapy in the local management of Ewing's sarcoma*

Series (reference)	Number of patients	Relapse-free survival	Local failure	Percentage of patients treated with surgical resection
IESS-1 (16)	333	47%	15%	6%
IESS-2 (60,55)	214 (nonpelvic)	65%	9%	43% (complete resection 27%)
IESS-2 (60,55)	59 (pelvic)	55%	12%	33% (complete resection 19%)
National Cancer Institute (86)	94	44%	17%	
Memorial Sloan-Kettering Cancer Center (5)	67	79%	21% radiotherapy, 0% surgery	50%
Massachusetts General Hospital (46)	45	50%	21%	25%

Modified from ref. 55

certain (21,22,30,38). In patients who have hematologic metastasis, the implication of residual recurrent tumor at the primary site confirmed by biopsy or autopsy is uncertain because of the possibility of reseeding from the primary tumor (19,39).

Several other fundamental factors make it difficult to interpret the data comparing surgery and radiotherapy for local treatment. The local recurrence rate following radiotherapy is strongly correlated with the primary tumor site. Local failure of extremity lesions is on the order of 5% to 10% versus a local failure rate for pelvic lesions of 15% to 70%. Local recurrence following radiotherapy of pelvic lesions is expected to improve with improved tumor imaging and the widespread use of computerized radiotherapy treatment planning. Therefore, old data may be of more limited use in contemporary management. One must also note that tumor size affects local control. Local control for tumors less than 8 cms in diameter is on the order of 80% compared to 90% for those larger than 8 cms in diameter. Because it is more likely that larger tumors will be treated with radiotherapy, instead of surgery, this considerably modifies the results of modalities.

Some patients are treated with combination of surgery and radiotherapy. Several factors make it difficult to interpret this data. These include the important effect of quality of radiotherapy on local control. In many "surgical" series, one is not really comparing surgery to radiotherapy but, rather radiotherapy to radiotherapy plus surgery. This is analogous to many other cell tumors that are treated with radiotherapy plus resection.

Many surgical series include patients who are "lower risk." These include individuals who have undergone ray resection of the hands and feet, removal of the wing of the ileum, lower sacrectomy (lower than the S3 bone), ribs, clavicle, or body of the scapula. One must also consider the relative functional deficits that will be experienced during high dose irradiation versus surgery alone versus surgery plus irradiation. In this context, when selecting local treatment for childhood Ew-

ing's sarcoma, one must consider the rehabilitation capacity, and the psychological adjustment of the patient with these local treatments (24,40,41).

Fundamentally, when attempting to compare surgery to radiotherapy in the management of Ewing's sarcoma, the problem one faces is that of case selection. Studies are not strictly comparable and one may, therefore, think of surgery and radiotherapy not as competitive but as complementary. One additional matter must be considered, however, in comparing radiotherapy to surgery: the risk of second malignant neoplasms. As we will describe later in this chapter, radiotherapy and alkylating agents combine to create an increased risk of second malignant neoplasms after the treatment of Ewing's sarcoma. Studies indicate that the relative risk of sarcomas in the treatment field is related to the radiotherapy dose as well as the extent of exposure to alkylating agents.

One must also consider the relative functional deficits that will be experienced during high dose irradiation versus surgery alone versus surgery plus irradiation. In this context, when selecting local treatment for childhood Ewing's sarcoma, one must consider the rehabilitation capacity and the psychological adjustment of the patient with these local treatments (4,36,42).

Surgery

The role of surgical resection in combined modality treatment was addressed by Rosen when reporting the experience at Memorial Sloan-Kettering Cancer Center (22,43). With overall disease-free survival approaching 80% at 3.5 years, Rosen described local treatment failure in 34 (21%) patients following radiation therapy and aggressive multiagent chemotherapy, compared to 0 of 33 patients who underwent surgical resection in addition to chemotherapy. In an influential review of the Mayo Clinic experience with Ewing's sarcoma, Wilkins et al. (23) related a significant impact of surgical resection on overall survival: 74% at 5 years compared to 27% in patients treated without surgery. Other reports have also described improvement in local control with the addition of surgery (21,24, 36,40,44–46). However, the studies to date reflect *selected* surgical intervention. For example, in a review by Wilkins et al. (47) of 27 children with microscopically complete resection in a total series of 65 cases, the analysis included 11 cases treated with radiotherapy and no adjuvant chemotherapy. These 11 were included in the analysis of the "nonoperated group" and were compared to the patients receiving surgery plus chemotherapy, clearly biasing the results to favor the surgical group (47). In a more balanced comparison, Brown et al. (21) described improvement in local control with surgery in extremity lesions. There were local recurrences in 0 of 5 resected cases compared to 3 of 15 treated with primary radiation therapy. Brown et al.'s analysis pointed out the selected use of surgery in 35 of 67 patients, clearly selecting cases with distal and smaller lesions for surgery.

Treatment results following surgical resection when combined with chemotherapy have been excellent, recognizing the selection factors inherent with the surgical subsets. In cases with complete or "good partial" response to preoperative chemotherapy, Hayes et al. (48) described disease-free survival in 11 of 11 cases with negative operative margins and no added irradiation. Most other series addressing the impact of surgery have incorporated postoperative radiation therapy, often at reduced dose levels (24,40, 42,46,47,49,50). The addition of surgery for "dispensable bones" (e.g., fibula, rib, smaller lesions of the hands or feet) is often considered a significant addition to therapy with little attendant functional deficit, although excellent results have also been reported with irradiation (39). Options for surgical management have also been considered primarily in the very young population in whom radiation late effects would be more significant (50–53).

Appropriate comparison of surgical results for Ewing's sarcoma requires attention to the adequacy of radiation therapy in the "control arm" (22,38). The German Cooperative Group Study (CESS) reported a significant difference in local control and survival favoring the cases operated on in the CESS-81 trial (19,36,50). On review, the high rate of local failure in the radiation therapy group was attributed to a substantial number of cases with inadequate irradiation volume. In fact, a report by Sauer et al. (50), on the same cohort, showed equivalent results of surgery or radiation therapy in small lesions. In addition, the CESS initiated a quality assurance program in 1984. The results of the subsequent study (CESS-86) demonstrate a marked improvement in local control with irradiation compared to the previous trial. From 1986 to 1991, 177 patients with localized Ewing's sarcoma were treated with chemotherapy plus radical surgery or surgery plus radiation (45 Gy) or irradiation alone (60 Gy total) with a central treatment planning review for quality assurance. Results are now comparable to the surgery group (3-year relapse-free survival 67% after irradiation, 65% after surgery, and 62% after resection plus irradiation) (33,37,38,44, 54,55). If the functional results are similar, the potential for second malignancies in patients treated with irradiation for Ewing's sarcoma would favor surgery as the treatment of choice for small extremity lesions, dispensable bones, or very young children. High-risk lesions may benefit from combined surgery and radiotherapy (33,56).

Chemotherapy

Early studies established the role of chemotherapy in primary management of Ewing's sarcoma (16,45,57). Multiagent regimens incorporating cyclophosphamide (C) and vincristine (V) with dactinomycin (A) and/or adriamycin (Ad) resulted in overall survival rates of 50% to 75% for patients without metastasis at diagnosis (16,21,35, 49,58). The value of multiagent therapy is also apparent in the studies described from the National Cancer Institute (35). In Intergroup Ewing's Sarcoma Group Study 1 (IESS-1) patients were randomized to three forms of adjuvant therapy: one arm with vincristine, actinomycin-D, cyclophosphamide, and adriamycin, (VACA); the second arm with vincristine, actinomycin-D, cyclophosphamide; and the third arm were these three drugs plus prophylactic bilateral lung irradiation (16,59). The 5-year relapse-free survival for VACA was 60% compared to 20% for VAC and 44% for VAC plus lung irradiation. VACA was superior to VAC or VAC plus lung irradiation when comparing survival. The 5-year results for VACA were 65% compared to 28% for VAC and 53% for VAC plus lung irradiation.

The results of IESS-1 must be interpreted with some caution. Patients were not randomized at each individual institution between the three arms of the study. Rather, there were two-part randomizations at individual institutions, i.e., either VACA versus VAC, VAC versus VAC plus lung irradiation, or VACA versus VAC plus lung irradiation. When the data is analyzed for statistical significance within randomization groups by relapse-free survival, VACA was superior to VAC plus lung irradiation, (62% versus 47%, $p = 0.06$). VACA was superior to VAC (55% versus 21%, $p = 0.01$) and VAC plus lung irradiation was superior to VAC (41% versus 21%, $p = 0.16$).

In IESS-2, patients with nonmetastatic and nonpelvic primary tumors were randomized to high dose, intermittent VACA and moderate dose continuous VACA (34,60). The 5-year relapse-free survival for high-dose intermittent VACA was 73% versus 66% for the moderate dose, continuous four drug combination ($p = 0.03$). For primary, nonmetastatic pelvic sites patients were treated with high-dose intermittent VACA and the 5-year relapse-free survival was 55%. When patients were grouped by local control and modality, the 5-year relapse-free survival rate for patients treated with amputation was 66%, 63% for those treated with complete surgical resection, 64% for those with incomplete resection, and 63% for those treated with radiotherapy after biopsy only.

When one compares IESS-1 to IESS-2, the 5-year relapse-free survival and survival rates are considerably improved in IESS-2. Local failure rate was 12% in IESS-2, significantly better than the 28% local failure rate seen in IESS-1.

The German Cooperative Ewing's Sarcoma study, CESS-81, was conducted from 1981 to 1985 (36,54,61,62). Patients received VACA × 2 cycles followed by local therapy and two additional cycles of the four drug chemotherapy program. The result of this study as analyzed by local therapy, which was not randomized, showed a 5-year relapse-free survival of 54% for those patients treated with surgery only, 68% for those treated with surgery and postoperative irradiation, and 43% for those treated with radiotherapy alone. The local failure rate, as stated earlier in this chapter, was quite strikingly different: 6% for surgery alone, 17% for surgery and postoperative irradiation, and 50% for radiotherapy alone. The high local failure rate secondary in the radiotherapy alone arm was clearly, however, secondary to major radiotherapy volume deviations. The local failure rate declined following institution of central radiotherapy treatment planning reviewed midway through the trial.

The response of the primary tumor to chemotherapy as an important prognostic factor has been demonstrated in patients undergoing surgery following initial chemotherapy. Picci et al. (53) studied 118 patients between 1983 and 1993, and graded the surgical specimens from grade I to III, with grade I having gross visible tumor, grade II microscopic tumor, and grade II being specimens with total necrosis. The 5-year disease-free survival ranged from 34% for grade I patients to 95% in the grade III group (53).

The proportion of patients failing with distant metastasis is another measure of chemotherapeutic responsiveness. In Marcus and co-workers' analysis of the impact of tumor size on survival, the dominant pattern of failure for large tumors remained distant metastasis despite aggressive chemotherapy (20). Jurgens et al. (36) described distant metastasis in 29% of the CESS-I cases; isolated distant metastasis occurred in 10%. The updated results of IESS-II demonstrated a 63% survival at 5 years with 25% of patients developing distant metastases only (60).

The Cooperative German Ewing's Sarcoma Study CESS-86, included 177 patients from 1986 to 1991 (19,36,54,61,62). Patients whose primary tumors were judged to be smaller than 100 cms^3 received induction VACA. Those with larger tumors received VAIA, ifosfamide substituted for the cyclophosphamide. Local therapy, at the discretion of the treating physician, was given at week 10. This was then followed, for the smaller tumors, with four courses of VACA and for the larger tumors with four courses of VAIA.

When a curative resection was possible, and conducted, then no additional radiation was given if there were no significant risk factors for local recurrence such as positive margins. If, however, the operative bed was at risk for local persistence of tumor, patients were randomized to once versus twice per day postoperative irradiation as described below for primary irradiation. For those patients for whom a curative resection was possible, but there was only small residual disease following induction chemotherapy, then surgery was not performed and patients were randomized to once versus twice a day radiation. When a tumor resection was not undertaken and there was substantial tumor, patients were randomized to either 45 Gy of conventional irradiation, once per day, to a larger field with a 15 Gy cone down boost to a total of 60 Gy versus 44.8 Gy of twice per day radiation to a larger field followed by a 16 Gy boost with twice daily irradiation.

In CESS-86, 22% of the patients were treated locally with surgery, 53% with surgery plus radiotherapy, and 25% with radiotherapy. The results of this trial are shown in Table 4. While those patients treated with surgery alone had a low rate of local failure, they had a higher rate of distant metastases. Local treatment did not influence survival. In addition, there appeared to be no difference between once versus twice per day irradiation.

The completed Children's Cancer Study Group (CCG) 7881/Pediatric Oncology Group Study 8850 is of considerable importance in assessing the modern use of chemotherapy in the management of Ewing's sarcoma (63). This trial is an evaluation of VACA with and without ifosfamide and etoposide in the treatment of newly diagnosed Ewing's sarcoma or primitive neuroectodermal tumors. This Phase III trial was open from 1983 to 1994. The trial appears to show, both in terms of increased survival and overall survival, the superiority of six drug chemotherapy to four drug chemotherapy for localized disease (Table 5). However, no benefit was attributable to six drug chemotherapy for metastatic disease.

TABLE 4. *Cooperative Ewing's Sarcoma study 86 (CESS86)*

Patient group	Survival	Local failure	Distant metastases
Entire patient population	69%		
The 22% of the patients treated locally with surgery[a]		0%	26%
The 53% of the patients treated locally with surgery + radiotherapy[a]		5%	29%
The 25% of the patients treated locally with radiotherapy		14%	16%
Of the patients treated locally with radiotherapy only, a comparison of once per day irradiation vs. twice per day[a]	63% qid 65% bid	18% qid 14% bid	
Of the patients treated locally with surgery + radiotherapy, a comparison of once per day irradiation vs. twice per day	69% qid 71% bid		

[a]Local therapy was not randomized. The results, therefore, are a result of case selection.
From ref. 33, 54, with permission.
The design of this study is described in the text.

TABLE 5. *Children's Cancer Group study 7881/Pediatric Oncology study 8850*

Patient characteristics of 398 patients enrolled

Characteristic	Distribution
Primary site	Pelvic 24%
	Femur 18%
	Rib 14%
	Tibia 10%
	Humerus 7%
	Other 27%
Local therapy	Surgery 44%
	Radiotherapy 44%
	Both 12%
3 Year event-free survival for patients with local disease	4 drugs 50% vs. 6 drugs 69%, $p = 0.0005$
3 Year overall survival for patients with local disease	4 drugs 56% vs. 6 drugs 80%, $p = 0.0007$
Event-free survival for patients with metastatic disease	22%, no difference between the two arms

From ref. 63, with permission.
Biopsy patients were randomized to receive either vincristine, adriamycin, cyclophosphamide, and actinomycin-D or these four drugs plus ifosphamide and etoposide. The therapy lasted a total of ~51 weeks. Local therapy was administered at weeks 9–15.

In the management of metastatic disease at presentation, little progress appears to have been made during serial studies. For example, in IESS-1 patients with metastatic disease were treated with VACA for a 5-year survival of 30%. In IESS-2 drugs were VACA plus 5-FU (5-fluorouracil) and the 5-year survival was 28%. In the aforementioned CCG-POG trial recently completed, the 2-year survival was 22%.

Radiotherapeutic Management

The role of radiation therapy in primary management of Ewing's sarcoma is evolving. As previously discussed, there is controversy concerning irradiation versus surgery with pre- or postoperative irradiation (20,38,46,55,64).

Volume

Local control of tumor with irradiation improved following the general acceptance of a target volume encompassing the entire medullary cavity to moderately high dose levels (28,65). Suit (66) summarized the experience of the 1950s and 1960s in recommending irradiation to the entire involved bone with a higher dose "boost" to the primary tumor site. He noted few instances of marginal or distant intramedullary recurrence with such treatment.

Assessment of the primary target volume requires attention to intraosseous and adjacent soft-tissue tumor extent. The traditional volume included a 3- to 5-cm margin beyond the known soft-tissue extension and inclusion of the entire medullary cavity. In analyzing the radiation therapy results of IESS-I, Tefft et al. (59) reported an overall increase in local recurrence with fields that had not included the opposite epiphysis. Although failure increased from 7% local recurrence to 20% with marginal or inadequate treatment fields, the differences were not statistically significant and, apparently, were obviated in the subset treated with adriamycin in addition to standard three-drug therapy (32,59,67). Subsequent studies have reported irradiation results based largely on treatment techniques that have not included the opposite epiphysis, noting no marginal recurrences despite high variable rates of local tumor control (20,44, 68).

The importance of adequate treatment volume cannot be overemphasized. The results of the CESS-I study indicated an excessive rate of local recurrence attributed to poor quality control for radiation therapy. Protocol modification to include central planning for radiation therapy diminished the frequency of local failure (50,68).

Brown et al. (21) analyzed the sites of local recurrence, describing consistent failure within the primary tumor volume for patients with lesions of the extremities and pelvis. Marginal failures occurred infrequently, limited to patients with rib primaries. In a study reducing treatment volume and dose, Hayes et al. (48) found a high rate of local recurrence (25% isolated, 35% overall). Treatment failures, however, were localized within the primary target volume in 13 of 14 instances using a limited, postchemotherapy tumor extent to define the soft-tissue component of the irradiation fields.

Data addressed the efficacy of diminished treatment volumes (29,69). Local or "tailored" fields encompassing the primary tumor with a 3- to 5-cm margin rather than the whole bone have been studied (Fig. 5). Marcus and Million (29) reported excellent local control using tailored fields, noting the ability to spare a component of the long bones in tumors smaller than 8 cm in diameter while frequently requiring full-bone irradiation to achieve a 4-cm margin about larger tumors. Despite the higher overall rates of local failure in the St. Jude Children's Research Hospital (SJCRH) study, Hayes et al. (48) also noted local control in 12 of 14 patients with lesions smaller than 9 cm in diameter using smaller target volumes.

A seminal study in the determination of the proper field size for the irradiation of localized Ewing's sarcoma was Pediatric Oncology Group (POG) Study 8346. Between 1983 and 1988, 184 children were entered on the study. Of this group, 179 were truly eligible for the study and 79% had localized disease while 21% had metastases. Induction treatment was cyclophosphamide/adriamycin followed by local treatment with either surgery or radiation therapy. This was followed by actinomycin-D/vincristine. Patients treated to the local site with radiotherapy were randomized to whole bone irradiation to 39.6 Gy + a 16.2 Gy boost or involved field irradiation to 55.8 Gy. For the 104 patients with localized disease who were irradiated, the 5-year event-free survival was 42% with no difference in event-free survival between those randomized to large versus small fields. There was only a 45% local control for those not treated to the protocol specified volume (70).

In postoperative irradiation, the appropriate target volume has not been adequately defined. Based on the data supporting local volume for primary radiation therapy, one would recommend treatment to the preoperative tumor bed with adequate margins, later reducing the treatment fields to documented sites of tumor residual in incompletely resected lesions. In all cases with residual tumor in the operative specimen, encompassing the surgical incision appears to be important.

Dose

Early reports established the efficacy of radiation doses about 50 to 60 Gy at 180 to 200 cGy per fraction, describing improvement in local control compared to total dose of less than 45 Gy (6,71). Dose recommendations have included 40 to 45 Gy to the entire medullary cavity with "boost" to the primary site to cumulative levels of 55 to 60 Gy (37,38,66).

The IESS-I results indicated no dose response between 40 and 68 Gy (43,72). Using 50 Gy per 25 fractions, the National Cancer Institute reported clinically apparent local recurrence in 20% of cases (39). Whether the lower frequency of local recurrence in the IESS and selected single institution series using 60 Gy reflects a dose-response relationship is uncertain based on available data (38,43,72).

Alterations in total dose and the time-dose relationship have been reported by the University of Florida utilizing hyperfractionated irradiation (29,73,74). Patients were treated with 120 cGy b.i.d. to 36 Gy for initial target volumes encompassing the primary tumor in 4-cm margins. Subsequent reduced fields were utilized to cumulative levels of 50.4 Gy (with total resolution of the soft-tissue component by preirradiation chemotherapy) and 55.2 Gy (with no response to chemotherapy). For patients with a lesion smaller than 8 cm in diameter, local recurrence was documented in only 1 of 11 children (75). In the review of the University of Florida series patients treated between 1969 and 1987, those with tumors smaller than or equal to 8 cms treated with b.i.d. irradiation had a local control rate of 88% versus 92% for once per day radiation. However, for those with tumors larger than 8 cm, local control rate for b.i.d. radiation was 88% versus 58% for once per day irradiation. Evaluation

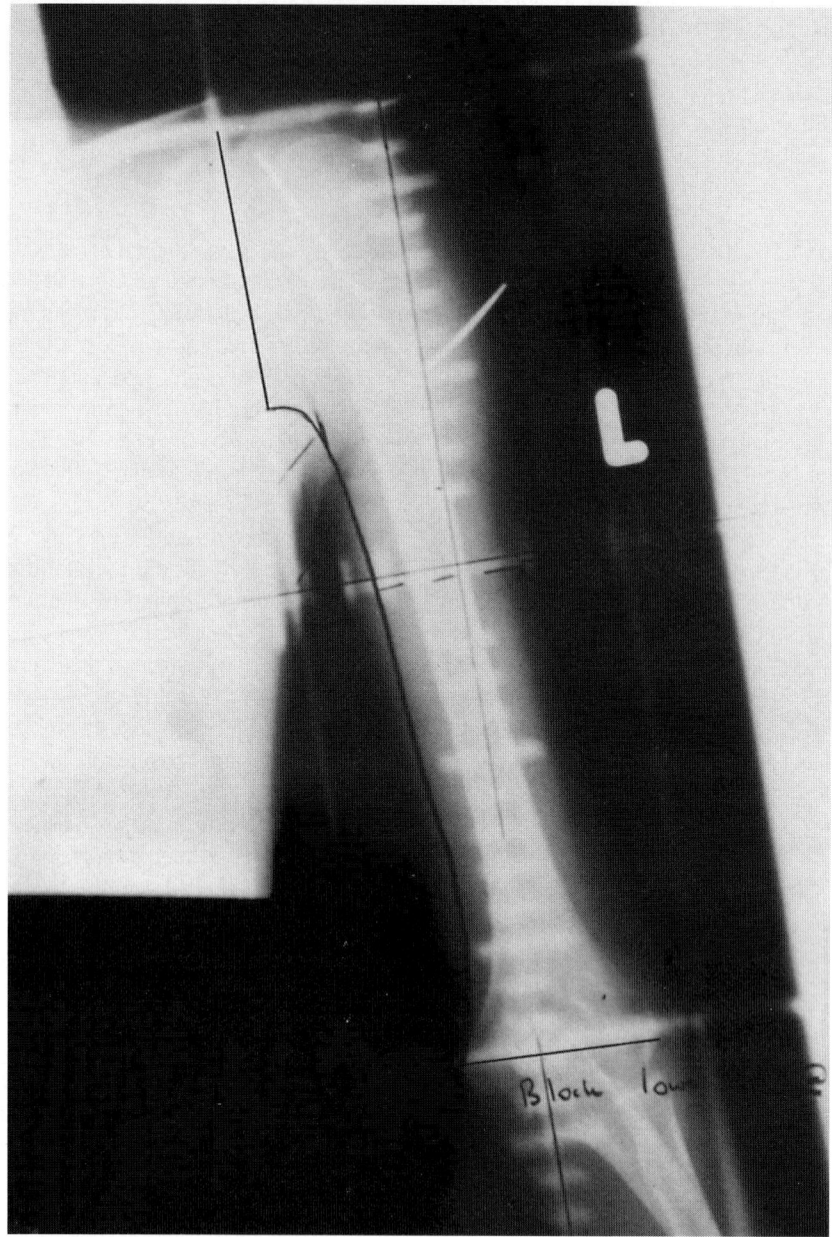

A

FIG. 5. Changes in treatment volume for Ewing's sarcoma. **A:** Field encompassing the entire length of the medullary cavity for a tumor involving the proximal left humerus.

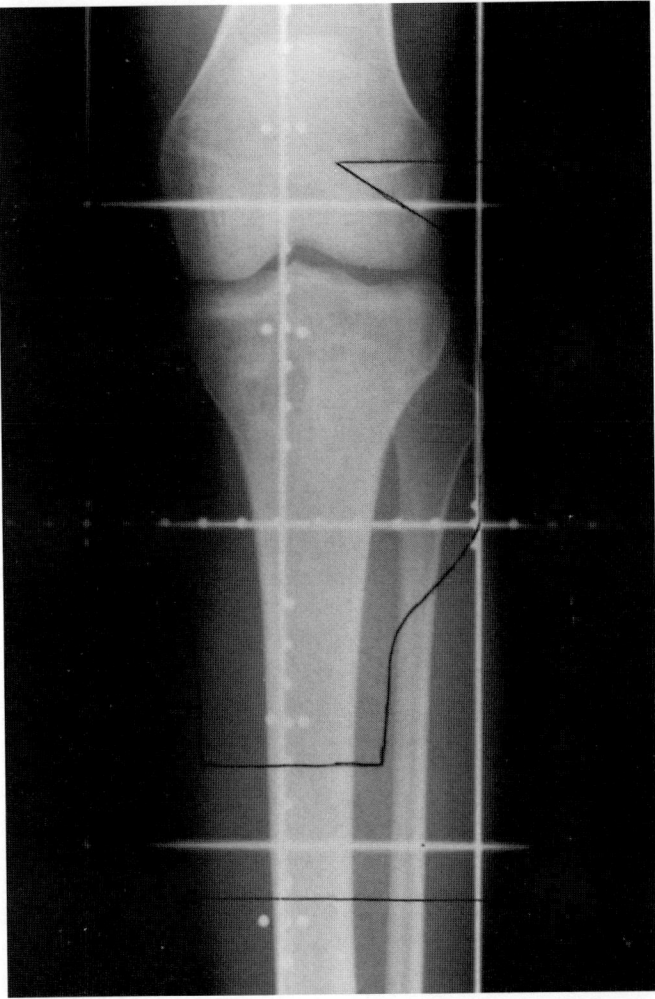

B

FIG. 5. *Continued.* **B:** "Tailored field" encompassing only the proximal aspect of the leg for a relatively limited tumor of the left tibia; there is a 5-cm distal margin beyond known bone involvement as demonstrated by all imaging procedures. In recent years, national protocols have called for a 3-cm margin.

of this data, must be tempered by the previously cited randomized trial of CESS, which did not show a benefit to multiple fraction per day irradiation (36,54). With larger lesions, more aggressive systemic therapy and TBI (400 cGy daily × 2) have resulted in improved local and overall disease control (20).

An interesting evaluation of the possibility of using reduced doses for selected primary presentations is shown in the review from the St. Jude's Children's Research Hospital detailed in Table 6. The data suggests that local control may be obtained with lower dose irradiation for tumors smaller than 8 cm in individuals who are excellent responders to induction chemotherapy. The number of patients, however, is small and must be interpreted with caution. However, local control is quite poor for tumors larger than or equal to 8 cm treated with low-dose irradiation.

TABLE 6. *The St. Jude Children's Hospital Ewing's sarcoma series 1978–1988, 60 patients*

Cyclophosphamide + BCNU/adriamycin; local therapy + vincristine actinomycin-D;
cyclophosphamide/adriamycin + vincristine/actinomycin-D

Patient group	Five-year event-free survival	Local control
Total group of 60 patients	59%	68%
14 patients treated locally with surgery alone and 3 treated with surgery with microscopic residual tumor + postoperative irradiation	75%	100%
Patients treated with local irradiation, either low dose (see below) or high dose (50–60 Gy) to those with proven residual disease after partial or no response to induction chemotherapy or, after 1985, to all tumors >8 cm in greatest dimension	54%	58%
tumor <8 cm ($n = 11$)	73%	94%
tumor ≥8 cm ($n = 31$)	44%	44%
31 patients treated with low dose local irradiation (30–36 Gy) for complete responders to induction chemotherapy, partial or nonresponders with negative biopsies following induction chemotherapy, and cases with no soft tissue extension at diagnosis)		
tumor <8 cm ($n = 10$)	54%	90%
tumor ≥8 cm ($n = 31$)	58%	52%

From ref. 69, with permission.

Technique

Definition of the primary target volume requires care in interpreting multiple imaging studies to accurately outline both the osseous and soft-tissue extent. The minimal target volume should encompass the primary lesion with 3-cm margins around the bone and soft tissue.

Sophisticated radiation therapy techniques will achieve maximal local tumor control while minimizing treatment-related complications. For extremity lesions, a sparing of strip of linear soft tissue is fundamental. Avoidance of circumferential irradiation limits the likelihood of significant late fibrosis and limitation of function (38,76). To achieve adequate coverage, treatment plans incorporating obliqued opposed fields or angled pairs with compensating wedges may be necessary. Conventional opposed anterior/posterior or lateral field configurations may be ideal if adequate soft tissue can be spared. The use of immobilizing casts or molds are important for daily reproducibility and accuracy during treatment (see Chapter 22).

Large-extremity lesions often require irradiation of the adjacent joint. With the same attention to normal tissue sparing, the major late problem associated with joint irradiation appears to be greater growth alterations if both epiphyses of the joint are included, particularly at the knee (37,76).

Lesions of the distal extremities, including the ankle, feet, and hands, present individualized problems regarding treatment planning. The use of tissue compensation, immobilizing devices, and detailed attention to dosimetry are critical to achieving excellent tumor control and functional integrity (22,71). The use of a water bath to achieve dose homogeneity has been suggested. Alternatively, a single photon beam incident on the contralateral surface of the hand or foot may be combined with an ipsilateral electron field.

For pelvic lesions, techniques to avoid full-dose irradiation of the bladder are often possible with oblique or multifield configurations. Caution to include the soft-tissue extent, often more impressive on CT or MRI studies, will ensure maximal tumor control. For vertebral Ewing's sarcoma, uniform irradiation of the adjacent vertebrae will minimize late effects (see Chapter 20). The use of weighted opposed anterior/posterior fields or a wedged pair technique will generally ensure adequate coverage of the vertebrae, of necessity including the spinal canal.

There is a limited experience with brachytherapy for Ewing's sarcoma. Potter et al. have described six patients treated with chemotherapy, external beam irradiation, and intraoperative high-dose rate brachytherapy for close surgical resection margins. All six children are alive and well (77).

Rib lesions (Askin's tumor) are generally sizable tumors with frequent extension to the pleural surfaces. This site warrants special consideration because it is frequently associated with a large soft-tissue component (62). It is important that the surgeon does not attempt to remove the tumor initially prior to chemotherapy. After biopsy, chemotherapy should be given for large lesions because it induces shrinkage of the tumor (27). In thoracic rib and soft-tissue primaries, the post-chemotherapy volume appears adequate to define the irradiation volume. If resection is done first, margins may be positive and may require a much larger volume of irradiation. The radiation volume is frequently limited by organ toxicity such as the heart in left-sided lesions. Resection following chemotherapy may be adequate if operative margins are clearly negative following "near-complete" response to chemotherapy. More often, local irradiation is important to increase the likelihood of local tumor control (21,25,27,48). Inclusion of the pleural cavity in patients with cytologically positive effusions has been recommended because the pattern of failure as described by Askin et al. (26) included the pleura in a significant number of cases. There is also a risk of pleural relapse in patients with Askin's tumor and no initial pleural effusion. Some clinicians attempt to treat the pleural surface, but spare the lung, by using external beam electrons. An alternative technique is intrapleural radioisotope application. A small amount of dye is placed in the pleural cavity with saline and the patient is rotated. Free flow is confirmed by fluoroscopy. As an alternative a tracer amount of radioactivity may be used to confirm free flow in the pleural space with a gamma camera. After free flow is confirmed a therapeutic dose of P^{32} is instilled to irradiate the pleural surface. The patient is turned periodically to distribute the isotope (27).

Radiation Therapy for Metastatic Disease

The efficacy of low-dose irradiation in controlling pulmonary micrometastases is documented in the IESS-I study. The frequency of pulmonary relapse was diminished and survival improved with "prophylactic" pulmonary irradiation in comparison to triple-drug chemotherapy alone (16,43,52,72,78). (See discussion earlier in this chapter.)

For patients with metastatic Ewing's sarcoma to the lung, local irradiation to the lungs and primary site are of value in overall disease control (28,61). An interesting review addressed the role of lung irradiation for Ewing's sarcoma with pulmonary metastases at diagnoses (61). In patients accessioned to CESS studies from 1981 to 1992, there were 42 patients who presented with pulmonary metastases. One died of progressive disease prior to irradiation. The other patients either had a complete radiographic remission after chemotherapy ($n = 25$) or chemotherapy plus resection of the lung metastases ($n = 4$). Twenty-two patients received bilateral lung irradiation with doses of 12 to 21 Gy. Six had no additional treatment after chemotherapy and/or surgery and one had a bone marrow transplantation. Of the 10 patients in complete remission, 9 had received lung irradiation and 1 had undergone complete resection of lung metastases. Overall, 1 of 6 patients was in complete remission without lung irradiation versus 4 of 10 who received 12 to 16 Gy versus 5 out of 6 who received 18 to 21 Gy. This data suggests a value to lung irradiation for a patient with pulmonary metastases at diagnosis of Ewing's sarcoma and appears consistent with the suggestion from IESS-1 of the ability of pulmonary irradiation to sterilize micrometastatic disease in the well oxygenated lungs.

The treatment strategy for patients presenting with bone metastases is under investigation. Treatment of the primary site utilizing a "tailored field" is recommended.

Total-Body Irradiation/Bone Marrow Transplantation

Total-body irradiation (TBI) has been utilized in advanced Ewing's sarcoma since the late 1960s (39). Improvement in survival using TBI led the Princess Margaret Hospital group to studies incorporating sequential hemibody irradiation in addition to a relatively attenuated three-drug chemotherapy regimen (79). The use of low-dose, fractionated TBI (15 cGy twice weekly to cumulative levels of 150 cGy) at the NCI has been followed by studies utilizing "intensification TBI" (400 cGy daily × 2), both at NCI and the University of Florida (20,35). These initial reports have yielded different results with a positive impact in the University of Florida series (10) and minimal or no impact in the NCI series. The NCI series has been updated and the long-term results continue to demonstrate no benefit to this approach (80).

Burdach et al. has reported using TBI (12 Gy, 1.5 b.i.d.) and simultaneous high-dose melphalan, followed by etoposide and stem-cell rescue. Their results (17 patients) are encouraging, with 7 of 17 patients disease-free, 45% ± 12% at 6 years, compared with 2% ± 2% for the historic control group (81). Two recent reports using a non-TBI regimen appear to yield similar results (18,78). Therefore, improvement in overall survival for patients with advanced local and/or metastatic disease has been reported, although the specific contribution of TBI in such regimens is difficult to assess.

CURE RATES AND SIDE EFFECTS OF TREATMENT

Current experience with Ewing's sarcoma indicates 5-year disease-free survival in 50% to 75% of patients with localized disease at diagnosis (16,24,46,60). A limited number of single institution reports indicate higher dis-

ease-free survival (20,36,49). Survival clearly parallels initial disease extent (34). Disease-free survival in excess of 75% to 85% has been documented for limited volume Ewing's sarcoma involving the distal extremities. Survival rates of only 25% to 35% are achieved with large central lesions (21,34,36,46).

Overall functional results following treatment of Ewing's sarcoma have correlated closely with the degree of attention to detailed local management. Selection of primary surgery for lesions permitting function-preserving resection with negative or microscopically positive margins may decrease late effects of high-dose irradiation, particularly in prepubertal youngsters (24,45,46).

With appropriate radiation therapy, patients treated for Ewing's sarcoma of the extremities had excellent functional results in over 60% of cases. The NCI late-effects review noted minor alterations in leg length or minimal symptoms of soft-tissue change in another 20% of cases (76). Significant treatment-related morbidity occurred in 20% of the NCI cases and was related primarily to larger primary lesions or posttreatment fracture of the femur. Significantly increased morbidities have been reported in series combining systemic chemotherapy with doses greater than 60 Gy (21,76,46). In a limited number of patients treated with 70 Gy to the primary site, severe functional deterioration was reported in 26% of patients (49).

The risk of posttreatment fracture has also been related to total dose. Fracture appears to correlate more directly with the extent of cortical disruption at the time of biopsy, in addition to tumor size and younger age at presentation (16,19,45,51).

Limited changes have been reported following primary irradiation of tumors of the upper extremities. Some degree of hip dysfunction and potential growth disturbances is documented in long-term follow-up of patients with pelvic Ewing's sarcoma. Combined cyclophosphamide-irradiation cystopathy has also been noted in such cases (21,37). One of the primary concerns regarding irradiation is the impact on bone growth. Morphologic changes of the irradiated epiphysis have been reviewed in the NCI series (76). Quantitatively, reduction and subsequent growth relates to the site(s) of epiphyseal irradiation and the age at treatment. Overall functional results are less favorable in the very young child (37,76). (See Chapter 19.)

The high incidence of secondary tumors in Ewing's sarcoma was originally suggested in the combined reporting of the Late Effect Study Group (LESG), assessing the frequency of secondary bone sarcomas in 9,170 children surviving more than 2 years after treatment for cancer. The rate of carcinogenesis in the Ewing's sarcoma population was second only to that in retinoblastoma in this study. There was a sharp dose-response after doses to the bone of more than 60 Gy. With the current standard in Ewing's of 45 to 55 Gy, this risk of second tumors appears to be less than the original reports. In contrast to the 22% actuarial risk of second tumors reported by LESG (82), more recent data demonstrate a cumulative incidence of any second malignancy of 9.2%, and for secondary sarcoma 6.5% (41). Here again, a dose-response relationship was demonstrated with no secondary sarcomas seen with a dose of less than 48 Gy.

TABLE 7. *Second malignancies after treatment for Ewing's sarcoma in patients treated in the German Cooperative Ewing's sarcoma studies CESS 81 and CESS 86*

Type of local treatment in a total population of 674 patients followed for a median of 7 years	Cumulative risk of any second malignancy after 15 years
All patients	4.6%
Local treatment with surgery alone	0.9%
Local treatment with surgery and postoperative irradiation to 36–46 Gy	6.1%
Local treatment with definitive irradiation to 46–60 Gy	6.7%

From ref. 83, with permission.

In an overall review of second malignancies after treatment for Ewing's sarcoma in the CESS-81 and CESS-86 studies, the addition of radiotherapy to surgery or treatment with radiotherapy alone was associated with an increased cumulative risk of second malignancies (83) (Table 7).

REFERENCES

References particularly recommended for further reading are indicated by an asterisk.

1. Ewing J. Diffuse endothelioma of bone. *Proc NY Pathol Soc* 1921;21:17–24.
2. Roberts KB. Ewing's sarcoma. *N C Med J* 1991;52:319.
3. Miller RW. Contrasting epidemiology of childhood osteosarcoma, Ewing's tumor, and rhabdomyosarcoma. *Natl Cancer Inst Monogr* 1981;56:9–14.
4. Ambros IM, Ambros PF, Strehl S, et al. MIC2 is a specific marker for Ewing's sarcoma and peripheral primitive neuroectodermal tumors. Evidence for a common histogenesis of Ewing's sarcoma and peripheral primitive neuroectodermal tumors from MIC2 expression and specific chromosome aberration. *Cancer* 1991;67:1886.
5. Delattre O, Zucman J, Melot T. The Ewing family of tumors—a subgroup of small-round-cell tumors defined by specific chimeric transcripts. *N Engl J Med* 1994;331:294–299.
6. Moll R, Lee I, Gould V, Berndt R, Roessner A, Franke WW. Immunocytochemical analysis of Ewing's tumors. *Am J Pathol* 1987;127:288–304.
7. Whang-Peng J, Triche TJ, Knutsen T. Chromosome translocation in peripheral neuroepithelioma. *N Engl J Med* 1984;311:584–585.
8. Kretschmar C. Ewing's sarcoma and the "peanut" tumors. *N Engl J Med* 1994;331:325–327.
9. de Alava E, Kawai A, Healey JH, et al. *EWS-FLI1* fusion transcript is an independent determinant of prognosis in Ewing's sarcoma. *J Clin Oncol* 1998;16:1248–1255.
10. Hartman KR, Triche TJ, Miser JS. Prognostic value of histopathology in Ewing's sarcoma-long term follow up of distal extremity primary tumors. *Cancer* 1991;67:1:163–171.
11. Schmidt D, Hermann C, Jurgens H, Hanns D. Malignant peripheral neuroectodermal tumor and its necessary distinction from Ewing's sarcoma: a report from the Kiel pediatric tumor registry. *Cancer* 1991;68:10:2251–2259.
12. Shimada H, Newton WA Jr, Soule EH, et al. Pathologic features of extraosseous Ewing's sarcoma: a report from the intergroup rhabdomyosarcoma study. *Hum Pathol* 1988;19:442–453.
13. Zoubek A, Dockhorn-Dworniczak B, Delattre O, et al. Does expression of different EWS chimeric transcripts define clinically distinct risk groups of Ewing tumor patients? *J Clin Oncol* 1996;14:1245–1251.

14. Denny CT. Gene rearrangements in Ewing's sarcoma. *Cancer Invest* 1996;14:83–88.

15. Fletcher JA. Ewing's sarcoma oncogene structure: a novel prognostic marker? *J Clin Oncol* 1998;16: 1241–1243.

*16. Nesbit ME, Gehan EA, Burget O, et al. Multimodal therapy for the management of primary nonmetastatic Ewing's sarcoma of bone; a long-term follow-up of the first intergroup study. *J Clin Oncol* 1990;8: 1664–1674.

17. Braun BS, Frieden R, Lessnick SL, May WA, Denny CT. Identification of target genes for the Ewing's sarcoma EWS/FLI fusion protein by representational difference analysis. *Mol Cell Biol* 1995;15:4623–4630.

18. Ladenstein R, Lasset C, Pinkerton R, et al. Impact of megatherapy in children with high-risk Ewing's tumours in complete remission: a report from the EBMT Solid Tumour Registry. *Bone Marrow Trans* 1995;15: 697–705.

19. Jenkin RDT. Ewing's sarcoma: radiation treatment at the primary site. *Int J Rad Oncol Biol Phys* 1995;32: 1253–1254.

20. Marcus RB Jr, Graham-Pole JR, Springfield DS, et al. High-risk Ewing's sarcoma: end-intensification using autologous bone marrow transplantation. *Int J Radiat Oncol Biol Phys* 1988;15:53–59.

21. Brown AP, Fixsen JA, Plowman PN. Local control of Ewing's sarcoma: analysis of 67 patients. *Br J Radiol* 1987;60:261–268.

22. Kinsella TJ, Loeffler JS, Fraass BA, Tepper J. Extremity preservation by combined modality therapy in sarcomas of the hand and foot: analysis of local control, disease free survival and functional result. *Int J Radiat Oncol Biol Phys* 1983;9:1115–1119.

23. Mendenhall CM, Marcus RB Jr, Enneking WF, Springfield DS, Thar TL, Million RR. The prognostic significance of soft tissue extension in Ewing's sarcoma. *Cancer* 51:913–917.

24. Anne P, Efird JT, Spiro IJ, Gebhardt M, Suit HD. Ewing's sarcoma: comparison of local treatment with radiation or radiation plus surgery. *Int J Radiat Oncol Biol Phys* 1993;27[Suppl 1]:295–296.

25. Thomas PRM, Foulkes MA, Gilula LA, et al. Primary Ewing's sarcoma of the ribs: a report from the intergroup Ewing's sarcoma study. *Cancer* 1983;51: 1021–1027.

*26. Askin FB, Rosa J, Sibley RK, Dehner LP, McAlister WH. Malignant small cell tumor of the thorocopulmonary region in childhood. A distinctive clinicopathologic entity of uncertain histogenesis. *Cancer* 1979;43:2438–2451.

27. Shamberger RC, Grier HE, Weinstein HJ, Perez-Atayde AR, Tarbell NJ. Chest wall tumors in infant and childhood. *Cancer* 1989;63:774–785.

28. Vietti TJ, Gehan EA, Nesbit ME Jr, et al. Multimodal therapy in metastatic Ewing's sarcoma: an intergroup study. *Natl Cancer Inst Monogr* 1981;56:279–284.

29. Marcus RB Jr. Current controversies in pediatriac radiation oncology. *Orthop Clin North Am* 1996;27(3): 551–557.

30. Murphy WA. Imaging bone tumors in the 1990's. *Cancer* 1991;67:1169–1176.

31. Wang CC, Schultz MD. Ewing's sarcoma. *N Engl J Med* 1953;248:571–576.

32. Phillips TL, Sheline GE. Radiation therapy of malignant bone tumors. *Radiology* 1969;92:1537–1545.

33. Dunst J, Jürgens H, Sauer R, et al. Radiation therapy in Ewing's sarcoma: an update of the CESS 86 trial. *Int J Radiat Oncol* 1995;32:919–930.

*34. Evans RG, Nesbit ME, Gehan EA, et al. Multimodal therapy for the management of localized Ewing's sarcoma of pelvic and sacral bones: a report from the Second Intergroup Study. *J Clin Oncol* 1991;8: 1173–1180.

35. Horowitz ME, Kinsella TJ, Wexler LH, et al. Total body irradiation and autologous bone marrow transplant in the treatment of high-risk Ewing's sarcoma and rhabdomyosarcoma. *J Clin Oncol* 1993;11: 1911–1918.

36. Jürgens H, Exner U, Gadner H, et al. Multidisciplinary treatment of primary Ewing's sarcoma of bone. A 6-year experience of a European Cooperative Trial. *Cancer* 1988;61:23–32.

37. Thomas PRM, Perez CA, Neff JR, Nesbit ME, Evans RG. The management of Ewing's sarcoma: role of radiotherapy in local tumor control. *Cancer Treat Rep* 1984;68:703–710.

38. Kinsella TJ, Lichter AS, Miser J, Gerber L, Glatstein E. Local treatment of Ewing's sarcoma: radiation therapy versus surgery. *Cancer Treat Rep* 1984;68: 695–710.

39. Jenkin RDT, Rider WD, Sonley MJ. Ewing's sarcoma adjuvant total body irradiation, cyclophosphamide and vincristine. *Int J Radiat Oncol Biol Phys* 1976;1: 407–413.

40. Bacci G, Picci P, Gitelis S, Borghi A, Companacci M. The treatment of localized Ewing's sarcoma: the experience at the Istituto Ortopedico Rizzoli in 163 cases treated with and without adjuvant chemotherapy. *Cancer* 1982;49:1561–1570.

*41. Kuttesch JF Jr, Wexler LH, Marcus RB, et al. Second malignancies after Ewing's sarcoma: radiation dose-dependency of secondary sarcomas. *J Clin Oncol* 1996;14:2818–2825.

42. Aurias A, Rimbaut C, Buffe D, Dubousset J, Mazabraud A. Chromosomal translocations in Ewing's sarcoma. *N Engl J Med* 1983;309:496–497.

43. Perez CA, Tefft M, Nesbit ME Jr, et al. Radiation therapy in the multimodal management of Ewing's sarcoma of bone: report of the intergroup Ewing's sarcoma study. *Natl Cancer Inst Monogr* 1981;56: 263–271.

44. Barbieri E, Emiliani E, Zini G, et al. Combined therapy of localized Ewing's sarcoma of bone; analysis of results in 100 patients. *Int J Radiat Oncol Biol Phys* 1990;19:1165–1170.

*45. Neff JR. Nonmetastatic Ewing's sarcoma of bone: the role of surgical therapy. *Clin Orthop* 1986;204–111.

46. Sailer SL, Harmon DC, Mankin HJ, Truman JT, Suit HD. Ewing's sarcoma: surgical resection as a prognostic factor. *Int J Radiat Oncol Biol Phys* 1988;15: 43–52.

47. Wilkins RM, Pritchard DJ, Burgert EO Jr, Unni KK. Ewing's sarcoma of bone: experience with 140 patients. *Cancer* 1986;58:2551–2555.

48. Hayes FA, Thompson E, Meyer WH, et al. Therapy of localized Ewing's sarcoma of bone. *J Clin Oncol* 1989; 7:208–213.

49. Rosen G, Caparros B, Nirenberg A, et al. Ewing's sarcoma: ten-year experience with adjuvant chemotherapy. *Cancer* 1981;47:2204–2213.

50. Sauer R, Jürgens H, Burgers JMV, Dunst J, Hawlicek R, Michaelis J. Prognostic factors in the treatment of Ewing's sarcoma. *Radiother Oncol* 1987;10: 101–110.

51. Hayes FA, Thompson EI, Parvey L, et al. Metastatic Ewing's sarcoma: remission induction and survival. *J Clin Oncol* 1987;5:1199–1204.

52. Newton WA, Meadows AT, Shimada H, Brunin GR, Vawter GF. Bone sarcomas as second malignant neoplasms following childhood cancer. *Cancer* 1991;67: 193–201.

53. Picci P, et al. Chemotherapy-induced tumor necrosis as a prognostic factor in localized Ewing's sarcoma of the extremities. *J Clin Oncol* 1997;15:1553–1559.

*54. Dunst J, Sauer R, Burgers JM, et al. Radiation therapy as local treatment in Ewing's sarcoma—results of the Cooperative Ewing's Sarcoma Studies CESS-81 and CESS-86. *Cancer* 1992;67:2818–2825.

*55. Horowitz ME, Neff JR, Kun LE. Ewing's sarcoma. Radiotherapy versus surgery for local control. *Pediatr Clin North Am* 1991;38:365–380.

56. Scully SP, Temple HT, O'Keefe RJ, et al. Role of surgical resection in pelvic Ewing's sarcoma. *J Clin Oncol* 1995;13:2336–2341.

57. Hayes FA, Thompson EI, Hustu HO, Kumar M, Coburn T, Webbert B. The response of Ewing's sarcoma to sequential cyclophosphamide and adriamycin induction therapy. *J Clin Oncol* 1983;1:45–51.

58. Fellinger EJ, Garinchesa P, Triche TJ, Huvos AG, Rettig WJ. Immunohistochemical analysis of Ewing's sarcoma cell surface of antigen P30/32 MIC2. *Am J Pathol* 1991;138:L317–L325.

59. Tefft M, Razek A, Perez C, et al. Local control and survival related to radiation dose and volume and to chemotherapy in nonmetastatic Ewing's sarcoma of pelvic bones. *Int J Radiat Oncol Biol Phys* 1978;4: 367–372.

60. Burgert EO, Nesbitt ME, Garnsey LA, et al. Multimodal therapy for the management of nonpelvic, localized Ewing's sarcoma of bone; Intergroup Study IESS-II. *J Clin Oncol* 1990;8:1514–1524.

61. Dunst J, Paulussen M, Jürgens H. Lung irradiation for Ewing's sarcoma with pulmonary metastasis at diagnosis: results of the CESS-studies. *Strahlenther Onkol* 1993;169:621–623.

62. Jürgens H, Bier V, Harms D, et al. Malignant peripheral neuroectodermal tumors, a retrospective analysis of 42 patients. *Cancer* 1988;61:349–357.

63. Grier H, Krailo M, Link, et al. Improved outcome in non-metastatic Ewing's sarcoma (EWS) and PNET of bone with the addition of ifosfamide and etoposide to vincristine. Adriamycin, cyclophosphamide and actinomycin. *ASCO Abstracts* 1994;13:421.

64. Marcove RC, Rosen G. Radical en bloc excision of Ewing's sarcoma. *Clin Orthop* 1980;153:86–91.

65. Pomeroy TC, Johnson RE. Integrated therapy of Ewing's sarcoma. *Front Radiat Ther Oncol* 1975;10: 152–166.

66. Suit HD. Role of therapeutic radiology in cancer of bone. *Cancer* 1975;35:930–935.

67. Reinus WR, Gilula LA, Donaldson S, Shuster J, Glicksman A, Viletti TJ. Prognostic features of Ewing Sarcoma in plain radiograph and computed tomography scan after initial treatment. A Pediatric Oncology Group Study (8346). *Cancer* 1993;72(8):2503–2510.

68. Prindull G, Jürgens H, Jentsch F, Sauer R, Lasson U. Radiotherapy for non-metastatic Ewing's sarcoma. *J Cancer Res Clin Oncol* 1985;110:127–130.

69. Arai Y, Kun LE, Brooks MT, et al. Ewing's sarcoma: local control and patterns of failure following limited-volume radiation therapy. *Int J Radiat Oncol Biol Phys* 1991;21:1501–1508.

70. Donaldson S, et al. A multi-disciplinary study investigating radiotherapy in Ewing's sarcoma—a final report of POG. *Int J Rad Oncol Biol Phys* 1997;39 [Suppl]:141.

71. Shirley SK, Askin FB, Gilula LA, et al. Ewing's sarcoma in bones of the hands and feet: a clinicopathologic study and review of the literature. *J Clin Oncol* 1985;3:686–697.

72. Perez CA, Tefft M, Nesbit M, et al. The role of radiation therapy in the management of non-metastatic Ewing's sarcoma of bone. Report of the intergroup Ewing's sarcoma study. *Int J Radiat Oncol Biol Phys* 1981;56:263–271.

73. Bolek TW, et al. Local control and functional results after twice-daily radiotherapy for Ewing's sarcoma of the extremities. *Int J Rad Oncol Biol Phys* 1996;35: 678–692.

74. Marcus RB Jr, et al. Local control and function after twice-a-day-radiotherapy for Ewing's sarcoma of bone. *Int J Rad Oncol Biol Phys* 1991;21: 1509–1515.

75. Kushner BH, Meyers PA, Gerald WL, et al. Very-high-dose short-term chemotherapy for poor-risk peripheral primitive neuroectodermal tumors, including Ewing's sarcoma, in children and young adults. *J Clin Oncol* 1995;13:2796–2804.

76. Jentzsch K, Binder H, Cramer H, et al. Leg function after radiotherapy for Ewing's sarcoma. *Cancer* 1981; 47:1267–1278.

77. Potter R, et al. Brachytherapy in the combined modality treatment of pediatric malignancies. Principles and preliminary experience with treatment of soft tissue sarcoma. (recurrence) and Ewing's sarcoma. *Klin Padiatr* 1995;207:164–173.

78. Ozkaynak MF, Matthay K, Cairo M, et al. Double-alkylator non-total-body irradiation regimen with autologous hematopoietic stem-cell transplantation in pediatric solid tumors. *J Clin Oncol* 1998;16: 937–944.

79. Berry MP, Jenkin RDT, Harwood AR, et al. Ewing's sarcoma: a trial of adjuvant chemotherapy and sequential half-body irradiation. *Int J Radiat Oncol Biol Phys* 1986;12:19–24.

80. McKeon C, Thiele CJ, Ross RA, et al. Indistinguishable pattern of protooncogene expression in two distinct but closely related tumors, Ewing's sarcoma and neuroepithelioma. *Cancer Res* 1988;48: 4307–4311.

81. Burdach S, Jürgens H, Peters C, et al. Myeloablative radiochemotherapy and hematopoeitic stem-cell rescue in poor-prognosis Ewing's sarcoma. *J Clin Oncol* 1993;11:1482–1488.

82. Tucker MA, D'Angio GJ, Boice JD Jr, et al. Bone sar-

comas linked to radiotherapy and chemotherapy in children. *N Engl J Med* 1987;317:588–593.

83. Ahrens S, Dunst J, Rübe C, et al. Second malignancy after treatment for Ewing's sarcoma. *Int J Rad Oncol Biol Phys* 1997;39[Suppl 2]:142.

84. Meyer WH, Kun L, Marina N, et al. Ifosfamide plus etoposide in newly diagnosed Ewing's sarcoma of bone. *J Clin Oncol* 1992;10:1737–1742.

85. Lanza LA, Miser JS, Pass HI, Roth JA. The role of resection in the treatment of pulmonary metastases from Ewing's sarcoma. *J Thorac Cardiovas Surg* 1987;94: 181–187.

86. Tepper J, Glaubiger D, Lichter A, Wackenhut J, Glatstein E. Local control of Ewing's sarcoma of bone with radiotherapy and combination chemotherapy. *Cancer* 1980;46:1969–1973.

10

Osteosarcoma

Osteosarcoma is the most common primary malignant bone tumor in children. The tumor derives from bone-forming mesenchyme (1–9). The majority of cases occur in the second decade of life, and there is a male predominance. The incidence rate is one to three new cases per million per year (10) (Fig. 1).

Inactivation of the retinoblastoma (Rb) gene may be important for osteosarcoma formation. Rb is a tumor suppressor gene that is discussed in more detail in Chapter 5. A frequent karotype change in osteosarcoma is deletion of the short arm of chromosome 17, where the p53 gene is localized; p53 is a nuclear phosphoprotein with properties of a tumor suppressor gene (11). Second malignant neoplasms can occur in osteosarcoma patients treated with surgery alone or surgery and chemotherapy—perhaps related to these genetic abnormalities (12–14). Osteosarcoma may develop in long-term survivors of heritable retinoblastoma. These secondary osteosarcomas may arise in or out of the irradiated field and in children treated without radiotherapy (also see Chapters 5 and 20).

SIGNS, SYMPTOMS, EVALUATION, AND STAGING

Osteosarcoma usually occurs in the metaphyses of the long bones, especially around the knee joint. The bones most commonly involved are the femur (approximately 40% of cases), tibia (15%), and humerus (15%) (1,3,4,10,15) (Fig. 2). The usual clinical presentation is swelling and/or pain. A few patients present with a pathologic fracture.

The tumor has a typical appearance on conventional radiographs. There are poorly defined margins, interrupted periosteal new bone, and soft-tissue invasion. Where the bony cortex is penetrated at the edge of a tumor, there may be a periosteal elevation and vertical spicule formation (Codman's triangle) (3,4,15). Computerized tomography (CT) and magnetic resonance imaging (MRI) help delineate the intramedullary extent of tumor as it tracks along the marrow cavity as well as the soft-tissue extent of tumor (4,16). The bone scan has nearly 100% sensitivity for the presence of malignant bone tumor, although the specificity is less. One may observe, on the bone scan, osteoblastic activity within the shaft of the long bone proximal to the primary tumor. This may represent reactive change and not be indicative of the presence of malignancy (4). The most common sites of distant metastases are the lungs and bones (6,15,17,18). Chest CT is used for the detection of metastatic pulmonary nodules (3,16).

If we are to improve the treatment of osteosarcoma, it will be important to adapt therapy to the individual patient's prognostic factors (19). The conventional means of doing this, of course, is via a staging system. The presence or absence of metastases and the use of histologic subtyping do help predict prognosis. A system for subclassification by histopathologic evaluation and site of tumor origin is shown in Table 1. A variety of factors have been investigated as potential

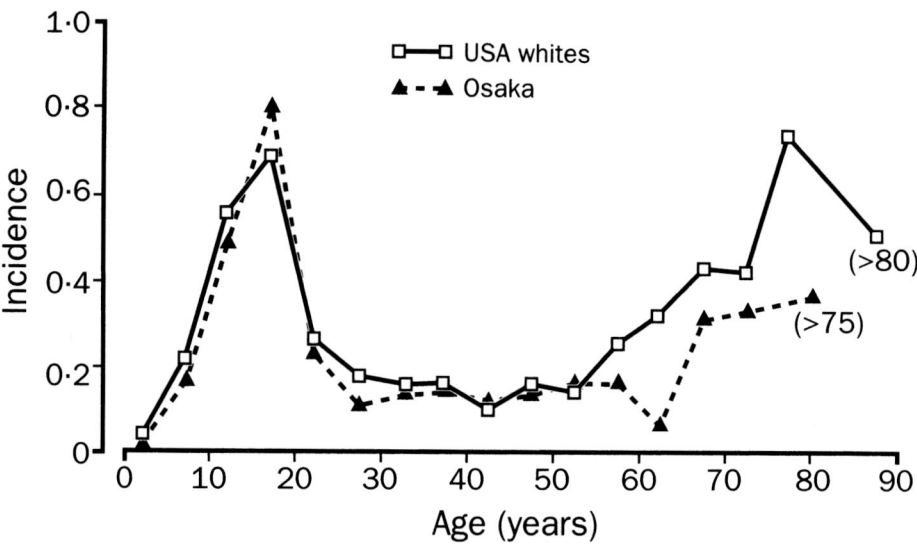

FIG. 1. Osteosarcoma incidence per 100,000 population per year by age. The peak for older individuals is associated with Paget's disease. (Reproduced from Ishikawa Y, et al., *Lancet* 1996;347: 1559, with permission.)

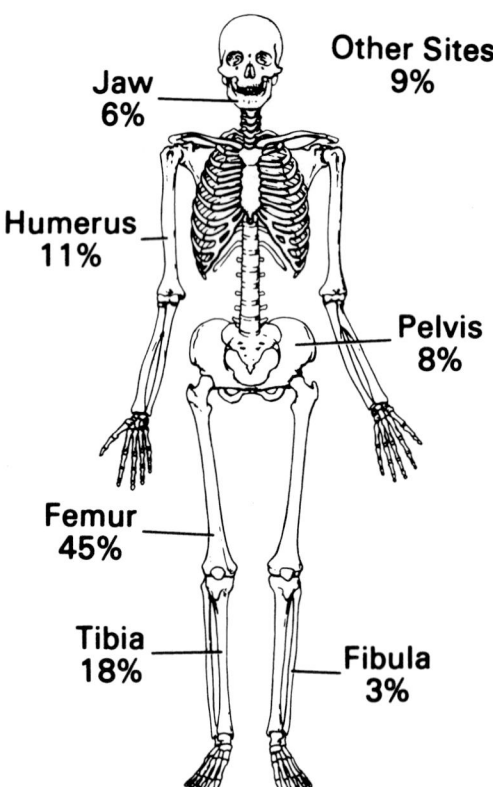

FIG. 2. Osteosarcoma: sites of occurrence. (From ref. 3, with permission.)

prognostic factors. As will be discussed later in this chapter, histologic response to neoadjuvant chemotherapy is useful in predicting outcome. Information of this type, however, is available only after administration of chemotherapy and surgery. Clinical features providing predictive value in determining outcome include: the duration of presenting symptoms (shorter is worse), tumor size (larger is worse), location of the primary tumor (head, spine, rib, and pelvic sites are worse), and weight loss more than 10 lbs. Tumor size seems strongly predictive of outcome and may be calculated as either absolute tumor length (+10 cm), relative tumor length given as the proportion of tumor length to the overall length of the involved bone (+one-third of the involved bone), or absolute tumor volume (+70 or 150 cm^3) (19,20).

There is no widely used staging system for osteosarcoma. Some clinicians simply separate patients into those with localized disease and those with metastatic disease. The system developed by Enneking and adopted by the Musculoskeletal Tumor Society is used

TABLE 1. *A system for subclassification of osteosarcoma by histology and origin*

The death rates per 100 patient-years, correlated with histologic group and calculated by Taylor et al. (96), are shown in **bold** type,

Centrally located tumor
Primary tumors
  Conventional: About 75% of patients fall within this category. This group may be additionally subdivided
    based on the predominant matrix pattern into the following three subgroups:
      Osteoblast, **14.4**
      Chondroblastic, **9.6**
      Fibroblastic (spindle cell stroma with a herring-bone pattern similar to that seen in fibrosarcoma), **10.7**
  Telangiectatic (characterized by a purely lytic radiographic appearance and a macroscopic and microscopic
    resemblance to aneurysmal bone cyst), **14.5**
  Small cell
  Malignant fibrous histiocytoma subtype
  Low-grade intraosseus (a rare low-grade fibroosseous lesion often confused with fibrous dysplasia)
  Multicentric
  Gnathic
Secondary tumors
  Associated with Paget's disease, **64.2**
  Radiation-induced
  Associated with other benign preexisting condition (i.e., fibrous dysplasia)
Juxtacortical tumor, **1.0**
  Parosteal (often arises from the posterior distal femur in older patients. Generally it is a low-grade spindle
    cell tumor with well-formed, parallel trabecular bone. Some patients may dedifferentiate into a higher grade
    lesion)
  Periosteal (typically involves femur or tibia)
  High-grade surface

As shown in the **bold** type, the death rates for the three subtypes of conventional osteosarcoma are similar. There is some controversy in the literature concerning the prognostic importance of the telangiectatic variant. Most authorities now feel that with aggressive therapy, there is no prognostic difference attached to this diagnosis variant. It is generally agreed that the prognosis for juxtacortical patients is better and that the prognosis for tumor associated with Paget's disease, an entity seen in adults, is decidedly worse.
  From refs. 1,4,7,9,22,96, with permission.

by some orthopedic oncologists. There are, however, relatively few "low grade" osteosarcomas so that the vast majority of patients are, in this system, stage II or III (Table 2).

TABLE 2. *The Enneking staging system for osteosarcoma*

Stage I—Low grade
  IA. Confined to bone of origin
  IB. Extension beyond bone of origin
Stage II—High grade
  IIA. Confined to bone of origin
  IIB. Extension beyond bone of origin
Stage III—Metastatic disease
  IIIA. Confined to bone of origin
  IIIB. Extension beyond bone of origin

Modified from ref. 27.

SELECTION OF THERAPY

Surgery

Local disease

Selection of the biopsy site should be made in order to have access to the infiltrating edge of the tumor. It is, in general, recommended that either no or minimal cortical bone be removed in order to reduce the risk of pathologic fracture (6,21–25).

The classic definitive operative procedure is either an amputation above the region of the affected bone or a disarticulation at the joint above the lesion. Traditional teaching is that if one resects the bone beyond the site defined by all radiographs as the most proximal extent of disease, and if the margins are pathologically negative, the chance of stump recurrence is negligible (6,23,24). In recent years surgical treatment for local osteosarcoma has changed. New limb-salvage procedures have been performed with gratifying results (26).

Limb-sparing operations may be selected if there is no evidence of neurologic or vascular compromise by the local tumor, if the surgeon believes that they can obtain an adequate margin around the primary osteosarcoma, and if there is a plan for reconstruction that will provide better function than amputation. Relative contraindications to limb sparing include the presence of a pathologic fracture, a poor response to neoadjuvant chemotherapy, or skeletal immaturity that will lead to significant limb growth discrepancies (27).

What is an adequate surgical margin for local management of osteosarcoma? A "radical margin" implies removal of the entire bone of origin with accompanying soft tissue involvement—such as what is achieved by a hip disarticulation for a distal femoral tumor. A "wide margin" is defined as excision of the tumor with a cuff of surrounding normal tissue and a "marginal margin" describes excision of the tumor and its surrounding reactive pseudocapsule. Local control is improved both by the adequacy of the surgical margin as well as the response to neoadjuvant chemotherapy. Therefore, a good chemotherapeutic response may allow the surgeon to have a tighter margin on the primary tumor and exclude more normal tissue from the resection. However, in order to know, prior to surgery, whether a marginal excision is reasonable, one must have an idea of what tumor response was achieved by chemotherapy. Unfortunately, there is no single imaging study that can reliably provide this information—although plain x-ray films, CT, bone scan, and MRI can be used to obtain a reasonable prediction (27).

The reconstruction technique elected after limb-sparing procedures depends on the location of the osteosarcoma, whether or not there is joint involvement, the extent of bone and soft-tissue resection, the patient's age, the functional demands of the patient and the family, and the prospects for rehabilitation.

When the excision is intraarticular (within or involving a joint), reconstruction options include custom segmental total joint replacement, whole segment osteoarticular allograft (i.e., from a cadaveric donor), allograft-prosthetic composite reconstruction, arthrodesis (surgical fixation of a joint; artificial ankylosis) with autologous or allogeneic bone, or arthrodesis with a porous prosthesis allowing host bone ingrowth and bone graft. If a joint is not involved, one can reconstruct with autologous or allogeneic bone, a prosthesis, or a segmental prosthetic spacer. Rotation plasty is also an option in certain situations (2, 27–29).

It is generally accepted that limb-sparing surgery has a slightly greater risk of local tumor recurrence than does amputation. Amputation has a slightly greater risk of local recurrence than does disarticulation. A multi-institutional review by the Musculoskeletal Tumor Society compared local control rates of three different operations for osteosarcoma of the distal femur. This was not, however, a randomized study. Local recurrence was greater among patients receiving nonablative procedures (Table 3), while survival and metastatic rates were no different between the three surgical groups (30).

It is gratifying that, in modern pediatric oncology practice, the child with osteosarcoma may be offered limb sparing options for local treatment beyond the traditional amputation or hip disarticulation. The previous discussion has cited indications and relative contraindications to limb sparing surgery, the risk of local recurrence after various forms of surgery, op-

TABLE 3. *Comparison of surgical treatments for osteosarcoma of the distal femur: a Musculoskeletal Tumor Society study (30)*

	Limb sparing operation	Above the knee amputation	Hip disarticulation
Number of patients	73	115	39
Local recurrence rate	11%	8%	0%

tions for reconstruction after tumor resection, and the need for adequate surgical margins. While it is reasonably clear that limb function, following limb-sparing surgery, is better for patients than that achieved after amputation, the clinician is well advised that limb sparing surgery is not for everyone faced with osteosarcoma. Case selection by a skilled orthopedic oncologist, invocation of sound oncologic principles, and adequate rehabilitative services postoperatively are all necessary to achieve the best possible result in terms of function and of cancer control.

Metastatic Disease

Surgery also plays a role in the treatment of osteosarcoma metastatic to the lung. At presentation, some patients will have a primary tumor along with limited pulmonary involvement. Aggressive multiagent chemotherapy, surgical management of the primary tumor, and thoracotomy for resection of pulmonary metastases appears to have significantly increased survival in what had been close to a hopeless situation (31).

The most common sites of metastases in the relapse of initially localized osteosarcoma are lung and bone (Fig. 3). When tumor relapses in the lung, surgical resection of pulmonary nodules may result in a prolonged disease-free interval and occasional cures (6, 12,18,23,24,32). In some patients, repeated thoracotomies appear to have prolonged survival in the face of multiple episodes of pulmonary metastases (33). Thoracic CT, by diagnosing pulmonary recurrences earlier and with limited tumor bulk, may either open the possibility for a beneficial effect of surgery or simply create a lead-time bias (31).

Several variables need to be considered when using mastastectomy for pulmonary metastases. These include the aggressiveness of the proposed operation, whether they are unilateral versus bilateral, the interval between the development of the metastases and the treatment of the primary, the extent of vascular invasion, the presence or absence of hilar lymph node involvement, and whether ad-

ditional "salvage" chemotherapy is available following surgery (27,34,35). The role of the bony metastastectomy is not well defined—undoubtedly because the occurrence of bony metastases in the setting of potentially salvageable osteosarcoma is far less frequent than that of pulmonary metastases (27).

Radiation Therapy

Prebiopsy

Low-dose irradiation prior to the initial biopsy (approximately 10 Gy) was administered by Sweetnam (23) to 29 patients in the hope of reducing the viability of cells that might be disseminated into the bloodstream by the biopsy. The 20% overall survival rate, no different than that of historical controls, discouraged additional investigation. Only 2 of 19 patients survived when treated with amputation without prior biopsy.

Primary and Preoperative Treatment

The "Cade" Technique

In the era prior to adjuvant therapy, physicians were distressed by the practice of treating the primary lesion with amputation or disarticulation—only to have the young patient die within 6 months of pulmonary metastases. Because the survival rate with surgical ablation alone was only 20%, many limbs were sacrificed in vain. Surgeons and radiotherapists reasoned that if high-dose local irradiation could obtain at least temporary control of the primary tumor, a time interval would be obtained that would allow the selection of those cases suitable for a radical surgery. Those patients who develop pulmonary metastasis in a 4- to-6-month waiting period following irradiation would be spared an unnecessary amputation. Those patients who did not develop pulmonary metastasis after the waiting period would undergo extirpation of the primary tumor. This philosophy was promulgated by the English physician Sir Stanford Cade and is referred to as the "Cade technique." The 5-year survival rates of 15% to

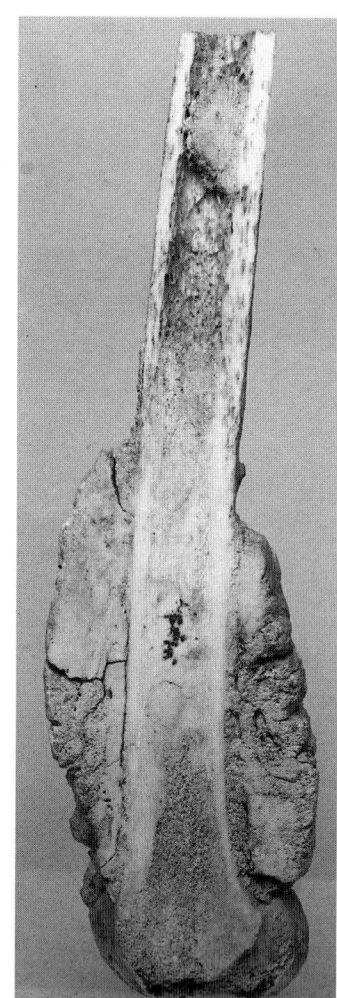

A

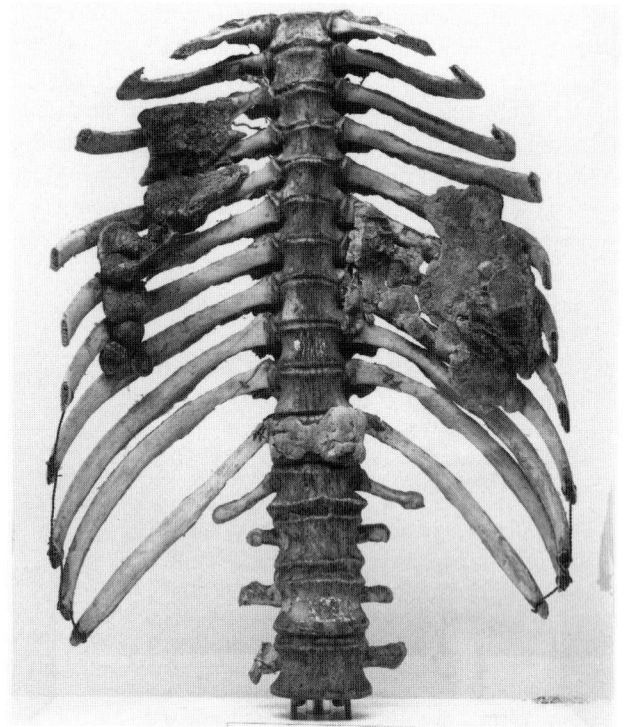

B

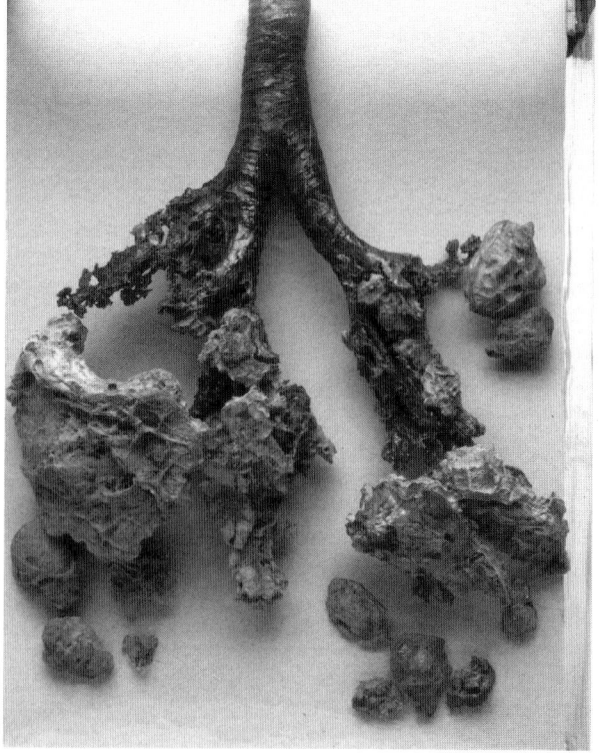

C

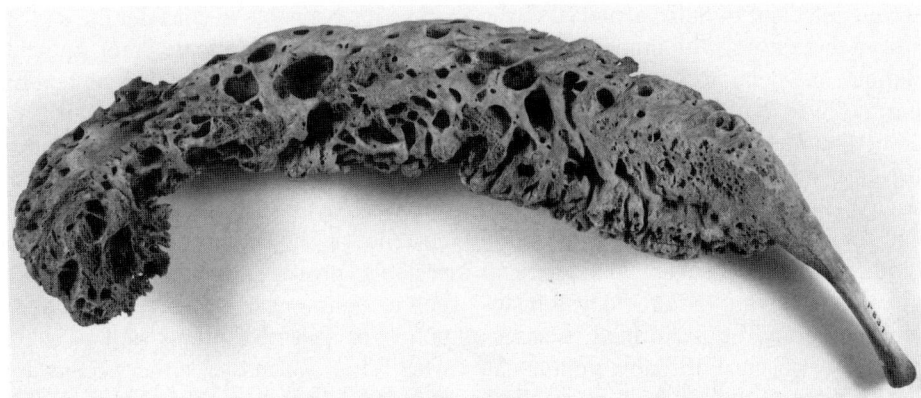

D

FIG. 3: John Hunter (1728–1793) was an extraordinary surgeon, anatomist, teacher, and collector. He investigated, by dissection and experiment, human and comparative anatomy. His magnificent collection of scientific specimens was purchased by Parliament and placed in the custody of the Company of Surgeons—renamed the Royal College of Surgeons in 1800. These illustrations of osteosarcoma, taken from The Hunterian Museum, Lincoln's Inn Fields, London, were selected by one of the authors (ECH) and appear by kind permission of the President and Council of The Royal College of Surgeons of England. In November 1786, Hunter encountered a patient at St. George's Hospital with "a hard swelling of the lower part of the thigh, as it were beginning from the knee . . . the part began evidently to enlarge . . . and was attended with more pain as it enlarged . . . and the pain was now exhausting him much. . . ." An amputation was done. Hunter described an "osteoid sarcoma" of the distal femur **(A)** and also noted the now classically described intramedullary spread of the tumor: "A short distance below the site of amputation there is a second hemispherical tumour in the medullary canal . . . above the main growth, the disease having extended within the canal, in this case, for an unusual distance beyond the limits of the external swelling."

Four weeks after the amputation the patient "began to complain of a difficulty in breathing, but not attended with the least pain . . . he began to lose his flesh and sink gradually, his breathing being more and more difficult . . . he died; living only seven weeks after the operation." On autopsy "bony tumors were found in the cellular membrane of the lungs, upon the pericardium, and some very large ones of the pleura, adhering to the ribs, and upon the anterior surface of the vertebrae of the back" **(B and C)**.

Hunter noted that "when the leg was amputated he had not the least symptom of any disease in the chest" but deduced that the lung metastases "had taken place a considerable time before the symptoms took place."

As for the osteoid appearance of the tumor, Hunter wrote that "one can figure to themselves a reason why the tumour which formed on the outer surface of the thigh-bone might become bony, because it might acquire that disposition from the bone it surrounded; but, from these tumours formed in the chest becoming bone, shows it was the nature of the tumours themselves."

The remaining figure **(D)** is "the osseous part of an osteosarcomatous tumour" from "the rib of a Horse" from Hunter's collection.

(Descriptions of this material are found in *Descriptive catalogue of the pathological series in the Hunterian Museum of the Royal College of Surgeons of England. Parts I and II*. Edinburgh and London: E. & S. Livingstone, 1972; Part I:133–138; Part II:75–77. Biographical material concerning Hunter is from Allen, Elizabeth. *Hunterian Museum* (pamphlet), Royal College of Surgeons, 1974.)

20% were equivalent to those achieved in the preadjuvant therapy era with immediate surgical ablation. The delay in surgery appears to have cost no lives that might have been saved (10,32,36–44). There generally was a reduction in pain and swelling at the tumor site after the first 20 Gy. This response tended to continue for several weeks after completion of radiotherapy. In patients who underwent limb ablation following radiotherapy, a histologic analysis could be performed to assess the presence or absence of viable tumor. The majority of patients had a good or excellent local response (Table 4). There were some long-term survivors following aggressive treatment with radiation therapy alone (6,43).

Modern Series

In modern radiotherapy practice, it is rare to be asked to use radiotherapy as the primary local treatment for osteosarcoma except for lesions in unaccessible sites. The data acquired with the Cade technique, however,

make it reasonable to consider the use of radiation in certain situations. Preoperative radiotherapy has been given, in the context of a research protocol, to reduce tumor viability prior to surgery, increase the probability of performing limb-sparing surgery instead of amputation, and/or reduce the risk of local recurrence (32,44). In patients with nonresectable primary tumors such as difficult pelvic bone sites, vertebral column, frontal bones, or base of skull, as well as in patients who refuse definitive surgery, consideration should be given to precision high-dose irradiation. Modern techniques use three-dimensional computerized treatment planning. Neutron or proton beams offer an improved possibility of local control in certain circumstances (45). There is also precedent for high-dose preoperative irradiation and rapid surgery, preoperative radiotherapy with local hyperthermic perfusion (46), intraoperative electron beam therapy (47), and radiotherapy with intraarterial infusion of a radiosensitizer (48).

TABLE 4. *The "Cade" technique: management of osteosarcoma with primary irradiation or primary irradiation and selected delayed amputation (excluding parosteal tumors)*

Authors (listed in the order of increasing dose)	Dose (Gy)	Clinical or pathological local response	Survival
Jenkin et al. (41,42)	50–60	Complete 11% Partial 63% None 26%	2-yr: 16%
van den Brenk et al. (97)	60–70, then 40–50 every 6 mo	Severe limb deformity in long-term survivors	5-yr: 12% (includes cases of chondrosarcoma and fibrosarcoma)
Lee (32,43)	70–80	1/3 totally destroyed 1/3 doubtful viability 1/3 capable, in part, of growth and perhaps dissemination	5-yr: 22%
Poppe et al. (10)	70–80	70% considerable radiation effect 19% moderate effects 11% slight or no effect	5-yr: 18%
Gaitan-Yanguas (40)	10–100	44% no residual tumor 56% residual tumor	
Allen and Stevens (37)	79–100	Pain relief 6/7 Reclassification 6/10 Tumor sterilization 6/7	60% NED at 30–114 months
Caceres and Zaharia (38)	80–120	16% remaining viable tumor 56% severe radiation damage 28% total tumor destruction	5-yr: 18% (no difference from historical surgical controls 22%)
Phillips and Sheline (44)	50–120	35% no tumor in destruction 65% tumor in specimen	

Data on photon irradiation as primary treatment for osteosarcoma, in lieu of surgery and in conjunction with aggressive chemotherapy, is available from Albrecht et al. from Berlin (36). They have described seven patients with osteosarcoma who were treated from 1977 to 1992 according to contemporary COSS protocols (Table 5). Six patients refused the appropriate amputation or rotation plasty. One had a primary tumor described as inoperable. Each patient received 50 to 70 Gy of conventionally fractionated photon irradiation. The patient with the inoperable tumor died within one year of initiation of treatment. The remaining six patients are alive without evidence of recurrent disease from 2 to 18 years following treatment (mean follow-up 11 years). Three of the six survivors ultimately suffered a pathologic fracture from 8 to 12 months following 50 to 70 Gy and one of these subsequently had an amputation. This small clinical series may be used to argue that photon radiotherapy in conjunction with chemotherapy may be used in the management of osteosarcoma if appropriate surgery is impossible or refused (36). Whether such patients are best treated with photons or neutrons or protons (vide infra) is a matter for debate.

Hirano et al. (29) from Nagasaki University sandwiched 30 Gy (2 to 3 Gy per fraction) between preoperative chemotherapy in 15 osteosarcoma patients. Histology of the resected specimens showed a considerable tumoricidal effect in nine patients and a fair effect in three.

Maxilla and Mandible

Some surgeons feel that a wide surgical excision of osteosarcoma of the maxilla or mandible is difficult because the functional consequences are considerable. Local recurrence and death following intralesional resection or resection with a positive margin is the rule (49,50). Chambers and Mahoney (51) reported 33 patients treated with preoperative brachytherapy. Implantation was accomplished by drilling holes in the mandible and placing radium needles. The dose was 100 to 160 cGy. Wide surgical excision of the involved hemimandible and adjacent soft tissue was performed 2 to 4 weeks after irradiation. Ten of 11 children were long-term survivors with follow-up from 4 to 15 years. Suit (21,22) has reported an additional three cases (two of the mandible and one of the maxilla) locally controlled with a similar technique. Heroic brachytherapy should rarely be necessary in modern practice. With radical surgical resection of the tumor, followed by reconstruction, local control of facial bone osteosarcoma is to be expected (52).

Lung

Whole-lung irradiation (WLI) has been used for the treatment of overt and subclinical pulmonary metastases in osteosarcoma. When used for overt pulmonary metastases, one would expect little effect. Individual lung lesions may respond to high-dose "rifle shot" fields (24,42). Weichselbaum et al. (53) have reported an aggressive program for the treatment of metastatic osteosarcoma with chemotherapy, WLI, and boost irradiation to individual metastases. Three of 10 patients were alive without evidence of disease. Equivalent or better results have been achieved with chemotherapy, thoracotomy, and no WLI (31).

Of considerably more interest is the use of WLI as adjuvant treatment to prevent the development of overt pulmonary metastases from subclinical disease. It was reasoned that relatively low doses of irradiation (15 to 20 Gy) could eliminate well-oxygenated groups of tumor cells if the number of tumor cells did not exceed 104 to 105 (17).

Table 6 summarizes clinical studies of WLI. The EORTC radiotherapy/chemotherapy group, comprised mainly of French, Belgian, and Dutch centers, conducted the two most important initial trials of WLI. The first study, Study 02, collected 6 patients. The use of local therapy plus 17.5 Gy of WLI achieved a superior, although not statistically significant, improvement in 5-year survival versus local therapy alone. The subsequent trial, "Control trial on adjuvant therapy on the

TABLE 5. *Significant recent cooperative group trials addressing the management of localized osteosarcoma*

Study name/ number of eligible patients	Primary objective	Treatment arms	Results	Comment (ref.)
Pediatric Oncology Group (POG)				
(POG) 8651 $n = 101$	To determine whether chemotherapy administered prior to and after definitive surgery is superior to surgery followed by adjuvant chemotherapy.	Arm A: HDM + A/P; then surgery; then HDM+BCD+ADR+A/P Arm B: Surgery; then HDM +A/P+BCD	The projected 5-yr event-free survival is 61% for patients assigned to neoadjuvant chemotherapy and 67% for patients treated with the more traditional approach.	At present, there is no evidence to suggest an advantage in terms of event-free survival for either treatment arm. (99)
POG 9351/CCG 7921 Currently open study	To compare the results of the two chemotherapy programs (± ifosfamide and ± a derivative of BCG) and to determine whether histologic response assessed after prolonged therapy predicts disease-free survival.	Arm A: AP + HDTMX; then surgery; then AP + HDMTX ± MTP-PE Arm B: AI + HDMTX; then surgery; then AP+MDMTX+I + MTP-PE	Study activated 1993; no results yet	(99, 100, 101)
European Osteosarcoma Intergroup (A combination of the European Organization for Research and Treatment of Cancer and the Medical Research Council)				
EOI 80831 $n = 307$ registered, 207 evaluable, 163 completed allotted chemotherapy	This study began as a randomized phase II toxicity and response trial of two short intensive chemotherapy programs. It accrued patients rapidly and was expanded into a phase III trial of survival and disease-free survival.	Surgery, randomization of chemotherapy of AP vs. AP + MTX	6-yr survival: AP 65% vs. AP + MTX 50% ($p = 0.10$); 6-year disease-free survival: AP 58% vs. AP + MTX 40% ($p = 0.02$)	The dose intensity of AP was greater in the two drug arm than the three drug arm. This may have produced the superior outcome. Disease-free survival was better for patients planned for conservation surgery than amputation. (102)
EOI 80861 $n = 407$ 391 eligible	To compare short, intensive chemotherapy vs. a complex, longer duration program based on the Rosen T10 program	Arm A: AP for 3 cycles, then surgery, then 3 more cycles. Arm B: ADR + V + HDMTX, then surgery, then BCD + ADR + V + HDMTX + AP	The median follow-up is 5.6 years. Survival in both groups is almost identical. 5-yr progression-free survival is 44%.	AP appears equally effective to the more complicated program at a lower cost. (99,103)

276

The Children's Cancer Group

CCG-741 n = 166	To compare HDMTX vs. moderate dose MTX in the context of a multiagent chemotherapy program.	Surgery, ADR then randomize to Arm A: HDMTX + AV or Arm B: Moderate dose MTX + AV	38% disease-free survival at 48 mos. No difference between the two arms (p>0.5)	Decrease disease-free survival was associated with the presence of spontaneous tumor necrosis at presentation. (104)
CCG-782 n = 232	To use histologic response of the primary tumor to neoadjuvant chemotherapy to determine postoperative chemotherapy.	Biopsy then HDMTX + AV + BCD; then surgery. All patients without local progression received BCD + AV + HDMTX. Then, if <95% necrosis receive BCD + HDMTX + AV	4-yr disease-free survival was 58%. Overall survival was 70%. Patients with local disease progression in the induction phase had 48% 3-yr event-free survival.	A poor prognosis is associated with an elevated alkaline phosphatase at diagnosis and/or a primary tumor in the proximal humerus or proximal femur. (104)

The Cooperative Osteosarcoma Study (COSS) Group of the German Society of Pediatric Oncology (GPO)

COSS-77 n = 68	Improved survival from adjuvant chemotherapy	Surgery then HDMTX + AV	46% 14-yr metastasis-free survival	(71, 105)
COSS-80 n = 101	Improved survival with neoadjuvant chemotherapy	Arm A: ADR + HDMTX + P, then surgery, then ADR + HDMTX + P ± B; ADR + HDMTX + BCD ± B-IFN	68% 10-yr metastasis-free survival	There was no difference in outcome between the two chemotherapy arms. There was no difference associated with the use of B-IFN. (71, 105)
COSS-86 n = 153	Chemotherapy was stratified by risk group. High risk was large tumor and/or chondroid matrix and/or poor bone scan response at week 5.	**Low Risk:** ADR + HDMTX + P, then surgery, then ADR + HDMTRX + P. **High Risk:** Arm A: ADR + HDMTX + intraarterial IP, then surgery, then ADR + HDMTX + IP. Arm B: Same as arm A except IP is intravenous	77% 5-year metastasis-free survival	Response rate is >76% better than previous COSS studies (105)

Abbreviations: ADR = Adriamycin, BCD = Bleomycin, Cyclophosphamide, Actinomycin D, AP = Adriamycin + Cisplatinum, P = Cisplatinum, IP = Ifosfamide + Cisplatinum, HDMTX = High dose methotrexate B- IFN = Beta-Interferon, AV = Adriamycin + Vincristine, MTX = Methotrexate, V = Vincristine, MTP-PE = Liposome encapsulated muramyl tripeptide-phosphatidylethanolamine.

TABLE 6. *Prophylactic lung irradiation in the treatment of osteogenic sarcoma*

Authors	Technique	Number of patients	Survival	Comment
Breur et al. (17)	Local therapy of surgery, Cade technique, or radiotherapy; then randomized: 17.5 Gy WLI	44	5-yr: 55%	$p = 0.18$; metastasis-free survival 43% versus 28% ($p = 0.059$)
	Control	42	40%	
Burgers et al. (64)	Local therapy of surgery, Cade technique, or radiotherapy; then randomized:		5-yr:	No difference between the treatment arms
	Chemotherapy	65	30%	
	20 Gy WLI	73	25%	
Ellis et al. (55) Springfield et al. (20)	Local surgical therapy; 16 Gy WLI with partial heat block, adriamycin	53 or 57	~60% metastasis-free survival	Follow-up duration not clear
Jenkin et al. (41–42)	Cade technique; 15 Gy WLI ± actinomycin			All six developed lung metastases in 2–6 mos.
Lougheed et al. (98)	15 Gy irradiation to one lung only; actinomycin	8		Four patients developed metastases in the untreated lung, one in the treated lung
Newton (97)	Radiation and delayed amputation for primary tumor; 19.5 Gy adjuvant WLI	14	43%	Minimum 52 mos. follow-up; survival better than that of historical controls
Rab et al. (81)	Local therapy of surgery, Cade technique, or radiotherapy; then randomized: 15 Gy WLI + actinomycin	26	42%	WLI did not influence survival
	Control	27	38%	WLI did not influence survival
Zaharia et al. (82)	Local therapy was surgery, nonrandomized: 20 Gy WLI	7	241-d median	$p \leq 0.33$
	20 Gy WLI + adriamycin	29	843-d survival	

treatment of osteosarcomas; Protocol 20781" permitted patients to have therapy with either definitive surgery, delayed technique, or radiotherapy. Among the 205 patients, 19% underwent radiotherapy as treatment for the primary tumor, 52% had amputation, and 29% had disarticulation. In the first arm of the study, adjuvant chemotherapy consisting of adriamycin, vincristine, and methotrexate were given every 2 weeks for the first 12 weeks. This was then followed by a consolidation phase in which these drugs were alternated with cyclophosphamide every 4 weeks for 6 months. The total adjuvant chemotherapy period was 41 weeks. The second treatment arm was identical to that of Study 02 with no chemotherapy but, instead, WLI to a total dose of 20 Gy after air correction. In the third treatment arm, the chemotherapy of arm 1 was utilized followed after 12 weeks by WLI. The 5-year overall survival, for this study, was 43% with no significant difference between the three treatment arms. The disease-free survival at 5 years was 24% (54). In an unpublished analysis, cited by Burgers, it is asserted that "the localization of pulmonary metastases was mainly behind the dome of the diagram behind the heart and mediastinum in those patients who were irradiated. These areas had received a smaller dose, as the irradiation passes partly through non-aerated tissue." No other assertions similar to this, appear in the literature (54).

Between 1979 and 1984, approximately 57 patients with osteogenic sarcoma were enrolled in a University of Florida protocol in which patients had definitive surgical treatment of the primary tumors. Within 7 days of the surgery, all patients received WLI to a total dose of 16 Gy in 10 fractions with parallel opposed anterior and posterior fields with 8 MV photons. An anterior heart block was utilized. Following WLI patients received five courses of adriamycin. Detailed results of the efficacy of this program have not been published. In reports published 4 and 8 years after the study was closed to patient accrual, the crude survival is approximately 67%, and the crude metastases-free survival is about 56% (55,56).

There have been cases reported of breast cancer developing in long-term survivors following elective WLI for osteosarcoma (57, 58). There may also be an increased risk of breast cancer in women who have had osteosarcoma but who never had WLI (58a). In light of the association of osteosarcoma with abnormalities of tumor suppressor genes (see previous text), concern is warranted about radiation-induced malignancy.

Chemotherapy

For many years it was accepted that the long-term survival of osteosarcoma treated with radical surgical ablation alone was approximately 20%. A 1978 M.D. Anderson Cancer Center trial utilized cyclophosphamide, vincristine, melphalan, and adriamycin and achieved a 2-year survival rate of 50% (59). Subsequent pediatric trials from M.D. Anderson utilized preoperative intraarterial cisplatin, surgery, and postoperative programs of adriamycin, methotrexate, cisplatin, and cyclophosphamide in various combinations. Limb-salvage patients had a 58%, 110-month disease-free survival. Amputation patients had a 54% disease-free survival (difference not significant). Optimum

survival (80%) was found in patients with greater than 90% tumor necrosis, induced by the preoperative chemotherapy, at the time of amputation. Survival was also correlated with smaller primary tumor volumes (60). In a separate report from the M.D. Anderson group, covering the years 1979 to 1982, reporting 37 patients 16 years of age or older with extremity lesions, preoperative adriamycin and intraarterial cisplatin was followed postoperatively by the same drugs. Those patients who suffered cisplatin toxicity received DTIC (dacarbazine) as a substitute. Sixty additional patients, treated from 1983 to 1988, received intensified preoperative intraarterial cisplatin. Postoperatively, complete responders received adriamycin plus cisplatin (or DTIC) while partial or poor responders were changed to an alternating program of methotrexate, adriamycin/DTIC, and bleomycin/cyclophosphamide/actinomycin. Patients treated from 1979 to 1982, had a 54%, 5-year disease-free survival. Those treated from 1983 to 1988 had a 69%, 3-year disease-free survival (61).

Pratt et al. (62) from St. Jude Children's Research Hospital, reported 76 patients who received adriamycin, cyclophosphamide, and methotrexate at two different dose levels, following amputation, in studies open from 1973 to 1981. The actuarial 10-year survival was 46% and 56% for two chemotherapy protocols compared to 18% to 25% for historical controls who received no or ineffective chemotherapy following amputation ($p < 0.001$).

Sequential chemotherapy trials were conducted at New York's Memorial Sloan-Kettering Cancer Center from 1976 to 1986. Patients received preoperative high-dose methotrexate with leucovorin rescue (some patients were randomized to additionally receive vincristine) and postoperative cyclophosphamide, bleomycin, adriamycin, and actinomycin-D. In recent years, patients who had a poor response to methotrexate received adriamycin and cisplatin. The 10-year survival of 279 patients was 73%. As in the M.D. Anderson and other series, histologic response of the primary tumor to neoadjuvant chemotherapy was an important predictor of survival (13,61,63–71).

The apparent successes of adjuvant chemotherapy trials were challenged by the assertion of a research team at the Mayo Clinic. This group suggested that there might be a change in the natural history of osteosarcoma. While the Mayo Clinic noted a 20% survival rate from ablative surgery in patients treated from 1963 to 1965, a comparable group treated from 1972 to 1974, without chemotherapy, had a 50% overall survival rate (72). A randomized prospective trial reported by the Mayo Clinic Group showed that high-dose methotrexate as adjuvant therapy, in comparison to a group of patients treated with no chemotherapy, offered no benefit: survival in both groups was 52% (61,73–75).

Two randomized prospective trials attempted to resolve the argument over the value of adjuvant chemotherapy. The University of California at Los Angeles (UCLA) trial randomized 59 patients with nonmetastatic osteosarcoma. All patients received preoperative adriamycin. Thirty-two patients were randomized to adjuvant postoperative high-dose methotrexate, adriamycin, bleomycin, cyclophosphamide, and actinomycin-D. Twenty-seven patients received no adjuvant chemotherapy. Of the patients who received adjuvant chemotherapy, 55% remained disease free at a median of 2 years following excision of the primary tumor. Of the patients who received no adjuvant chemotherapy, only 20% remained free of disease ($p < 0.01$). Of 18 control patients treated prior to the trial, the overall disease-free survival was not significantly different from the 27 randomized control patients treated without chemotherapy from 1981 to 1984. Overall survival for randomized patients did not differ significantly between the two arms (76). If the larger group of patients who chose their therapy was combined with the randomized group, there was a significant overall survival benefit favoring chemotherapy at 6 years (73).

Link et al. (68) reported a randomized chemotherapy trial in 36 patients. At 2 years, the actuarial relapse-free survival was 17% in the control group and 66% in the group receiving adjuvant cyclophosphamide, bleomycin, actinomycin, methotrexate with leucovorin rescue, doxorubicin, and cisplatin ($p < 0.001$). A similar benefit to chemotherapy was observed among 77 patients who declined to undergo randomization but elected observation or chemotherapy.

Several large cooperative group studies have been reported addressing the role of chemotherapy in the clinical management of osteosarcoma. In Table 5, we summarize studies by the Pediatric Oncology Group, European Osteosarcoma Intergroup, Children's Cancer Group, and the Cooperative Osteosarcoma study of the German Society of Pediatric Oncology. The data indicates that surgery plus modern chemotherapy should achieve approximately a 60% to 70% 5-year event-free survival. It is not clear that neoadjuvant chemotherapy is superior to postoperative chemotherapy.

RADIOTHERAPEUTIC TECHNIQUE

Dose

Osteosarcoma has developed the reputation of being radioresistant. This reputation, however, is unjustified. Because radiotherapy was formerly used for the treatment of bulky tumors, it is no surprise that there were frequently local failures. The Do values of human and rodent osteosarcoma cell lines are reported to be similar to those of most other mammalian tumors, perhaps with a higher Dq (44,77).

In a dose-response study of patients treated with Cade technique, Gaitan-Yanguas (40) produced uniform tumor sterilization with doses of 80 to 100 Gy and always found persistent tumor at less than or equal to 50 Gy. Phillips and Sheline (44) found viable tumor in 1 of 10 patients receiving less than 100 Gy and in 2 of 7 patients receiving at least 100 Gy.

Lombardi et al. (78) administered 36 Gy/6 Gy per fraction/3 fractions per week/2 weeks to 21 osteosarcoma sites irradiated for palliation in 14 patients. There was a clinical response (disappearance of pain, decrease in tumor size, improvement in function) and/or radiological response at 18 of the 21 sites. Of eight primary sites irradiated because of synchronous metastases, all showed a clinical or radiographic response. In five patients, radiotherapy was given where preoperative chemotherapy had not rendered the patient suitable for limb-sparing surgery. Surgery following radiotherapy revealed 95% to 100% tumor necrosis in all cases. Limb-sparing surgery was performed in 3 of 5 cases, but, because of infectious complications related to soft-tissue damage, all limbs were eventually amputated.

Caceres et al. (65) from Peru gave 60 Gy in 6 weeks to 15 patients in conjunction with chemotherapy. Postradiotherapy biopsy showed no evidence of active tumor in 12 of 15 (80%) patients. The whole specimen was studied, because of amputation or autopsy, in five patients. No viable tumor was found. Complications were common, including pathological fracture, soft-tissue fibrosis or necrosis, local infection, and moist desquamation. The degree of tumor necrosis seen by Caceres et al. is in contrast with an earlier report from the same group of less impressive tumor destruction following 80 to 120 Gy at 10 to 12 Gy per fraction (Table 4) (38). If radiotherapy is to be used alone as definitive treatment for a small (less than 5 cm) osteosarcoma in an unresectable location such as the base of skull or vertebral body, or in a patient who refuses surgery, the dose should be carried as high as normal tissue tolerance allows—that is, 60 to 75 Gy at conventional fractionation in progressive shrinking field technique (79,80).

When radiotherapy is used for prophylactic treatment of the lungs, the dose is 15 to 19.5 Gy at 1.5 Gy per fraction. These doses have generally been reported without lung correction factors being applied (17,33,81,82).

Volume

The treatment volume is determined by plain x-ray films, bone scan, CT, and MRI. It is customary to define the tumor volume based on the largest volume of these studies (the "worst-case volume"). A margin is then allowed.

Prophylactic WLI is directed to the entire substance of the lung. Particular attention must be paid to coverage of the apices of the lung and to the areas of the lung that curve over the surfaces of the diaphragms.

Technique

An immobilization device is generally required. The field should be contoured specifically to the anatomic problem for the individual patient. In most cases, multiple fields will be used. In order to maintain a functional limb after irradiation, a strip of skin should be spared and one should avoid high-dose irradiation to the full width of the joint.

Some investigators have attempted to improve the local control rates of osteosarcoma by altering tumor and normal tissue oxygenation. The tourniquet technique attempts to produce anoxia in both tumor and normal limb tissues to remove any advantage the tumor may have by virtue of hypoxic areas. Using this technique, patients have received fractionated irradiation up to total doses of 75 to 160 Gy. In those patients who were long-term survivors, the functional result was poor (69). One group reported local response rates of approximately 70% and reasonable limb function with tourniquet anoxia and high-dose per fraction treatment (i.e., 25 Gy × 3). Radiation treatment under hyperbaric oxygen conditions has also been investigated (83). A group of investigators from Stanford University have reported a series of patients with unresectable osteosarcomas, or who refused amputation, treated with 42 to 48 Gy at 6 Gy per fraction, one fraction every 5 days, and pulsed 5'-bromodeoxyuridine (BUdR) infusion as a radiosensitizer

(45). Local control was achieved in 7 of 9 patients, 4 of whom were long-term survivors. Significant soft-tissue injury occurred in five patients (48).

Neutron Therapy

Neutrons are a form of high linear energy transfer radiation. They offer several advantages over conventional photon or electron radiotherapy. These include: (a) neutrons are better able to kill hypoxic cells than photons. The oxygen enhancement ratio (OER) for neutrons is on the order of 1.6, compared to 2.5 to 3.0 for photons. (b) Repair of radiation-induced sublethal and potentially lethal damage is less readily accomplished following neutron compared to conventional irradiation. (c) Neutrons are toxic throughout the phases of the cell cycle (M, G1, S, G2) compared to photons, which are more toxic in late G2/M (84,85).

Kubota et al. (77) compared the biological effects of 13 MeV neutrons to ^{137}Cs gamma rays in MG-63 human osteosarcoma cells in plateau phase growth and in multicellular spheroids. The relative biological effectiveness varied slightly with the measurement technique but was in the range of 1.9 to 2.29 (77). If one accepts the assertion that osteosarcomas are rapidly growing tumors with areas of necrosis and, potentially, hypoxic ar-

eas and that they are relatively radioresistant to photon irradiation, then one might conclude that they would be more effectively irradiated by neutrons.

There is a small clinical experience with the use of neutrons for local control of osteosarcomas. Many of the patients treated had inoperable tumors or refused amputations (86). The results of neutron treatment are shown in Table 7. The 77 patients cited have an overall local control rate of 44 of 77 (58%). At first glance, this appears to be better than the historically quoted local control rate with photon irradiation of approximately 20% (discussed previously in this chapter). There are, however, clearly risks from combining the results of eight series to draw a conclusion. The local control rates of the individual series ranges from 0% to 100%, and they contain patients with tumors at a variety of locations. Dense fibrotic reactions can occur following neutron treatment leading to severe complications and leading, in some patients, ultimately to amputation (87,88). For an osteosarcoma patient who absolutely refuses definitive surgery or is medically or technically inoperable, it is reasonable to consider the use of neutrons. Part of the informed consent for such treatment, however, must include a discussion of the potential for serious late ill effects of such treatment.

TABLE 7. *Literature Review of the Local Control Rates for Osteosarcomas After Neutron Therapy*

Year of Report	First Author	Reporting Institution	Number of Patients	Local Control
1979	Ornitz (106)	MANTA	1	1/1
1980	Salinas (107)	Texas A&M Variable Energy Cyclotrol (TAMVEC)	1	0/1
1981	Batterman (108)	Amsterdam	3	0/3
1982	Tsunemoto (109)	National Institute of Radiological Sciences, Chiba	41	33/41
1984	Cohen (87)	Fermilab, Batavia	9	2/9
1986	Duncan (88)	Western General Hospital, Edinburgh	5	1/5[a]
1989	Laramore (85)	University of Washington, Seattle	13	3/13[b]
1994	Carrie (76)	Centre Hospitalier d'Orleans, Orleans	4	4/4[c]

[a]A persistent mass and calcification were considered a local failure. For this reason, local control rates may be underestimated.

[b]This is two-year actuarial data.

[c]These patients received combined local therapy with photons and neutrons.

This table is based on material found in the cited references and on the work of Chauvel, Laramore, et al., and Wambersie (27, 85, 86)

Charged Particle Therapy

Osteosarcoma of the skull base and axial skeleton pose a particularly difficult problem for the pediatric radiation oncologist. These tumors are more difficult to extirpate at surgery. An initial gross and microscopic tumor resection is inhibited by the proximity of brainstem, spinal cord, cranial nerves, nerve roots, and/or vessels. These normal tissue structures, however, also prevent the radiation oncologist from using their modality as an alternative to surgery because tumoricidal doses for osteosarcoma exceed the tolerance of critical neural tissue (89). While three-dimensional treatment planning with multiple noncoplanar photon beams may be used in an attempt to achieve an acceptable dose distribution, the penetrance and divergence of photons presents significant limitations.

Protons and other charged particle beams (such as neon, helium, or carbon ions) have a finite dose range with steep dose fall-off beyond the Bragg peak. This property engenders a treatment beam that has little exit dose beyond the deposition of energy in the target volume—making these beams distinctly different from photons. The advantage of protons resides solely in this physical difference because proton beams have no significant biologic advantage over megavoltage photons (89). Other charged particle beams have both the advantage of rapid Bragg peak dose fall-off as well as an increase in relative biological effectiveness (77). Charged particles can be used to shape a dose distribution around an osteosarcoma of the skull base or vertebral body with the possibility of maintaining the dose to the adjacent brain or spinal cord within acceptable limits.

The Radiation Oncology Department at the Massachusetts General Hospital in collaboration with the Harvard Cyclotron Laboratory, treated 15 osteosarcoma patients with combined proton/photon irradiation (anatomic sites were base of skull, 7; cervical spine, 3; lumbar spine, 2; sacrum, 3). Doses of 61.1 to 80 Cobalt Gray Equivalent were administered and 14 of the 15 patients also received che-

motherapy. At 5 years, the actuarial local control rate was 59% and the overall survival rate was 44% (89). In a series that includes skull base tumors of various histologies, Castro et al. reported that 20% of disease-free survivors following charged particle therapy had Grade III, IV, or V complications such as cranial nerve or vascular injuries (90).

Intraoperative Therapy

A combined specialty team at the Universidad de Navarra, Spain, has treated 22 osteosarcoma patients with preoperative chemotherapy, surgical excision, a 15- to 20-Gy intraoperative radiation therapy (IORT) electron beam boost to the tumor bed area, and postoperative chemotherapy (47). Five patients also received pre- and postoperative external beam radiotherapy. There was only one local recurrence among the 22 patients with a median follow-up of 18 months. Local recurrence following definitive surgery for osteosarcoma is infrequent, and it is not clear that the IORT was helpful.

An additional 32 patients with osteosarcoma were treated with intraoperative radiation by Yamamuro and Kotoura (91). Prior to 1984, treatment consisted apparently solely of exposing the primary tumor site and administering 50 to 60 Gy of IORT with 12 to 26 MeV electron beams. Subsequent to 1984, patients received cisplatinum and adriamycin in combination with IORT. The clinical results from this relatively small series spread out over many years (1978 to 1990) must be interpreted with caution. Ten patients underwent limb amputation or prosthetic replacement 2 to 10 months after IORT. Eight patients had complete necrosis of the tumor cells throughout the specimen except for a "few scattered, markedly altered, presumably non-viable tumor cells in small clusters." Two patients showed local-regional tumor recurrence in nonirradiated areas and one failed in the radiation field (a juxtacorticol osteosarcoma). Joint function was reported as being satisfactory; five patients had some evidence of moderate to severe skin necrosis, but "among the patients who underwent neither limb amputation nor prosthetic replacement and survived longer than one year after IORT, about 58% sustained pathologic fracture through the lesions. All attempts of osteo synthesis failed to fuse the fracture site" (91).

These two series must be interpreted cautiously. It is possible that IORT, in combination with surgery and chemotherapy, may reduce the already low local recurrence rate for most cases of osteosarcoma. This is a testable hypothesis. As for the use of IORT as the definitive local control measure, as described by Yamuro and Kotura (91), this must be considered investigational therapy with, apparently, a high risk of subsequent fracture.

Radioisotope Therapy

Bone seeking therapeutic radio pharmaceuticals are an early stage of investigation in the treatment of osteoblastic osteosarcoma. The uptake of radio pharmaceuticals in adult skeletal metastatic lesions such as breast and prostate cancer is due to an osteoblastic response in the normal bones surrounding the metastases. Osteosarcoma, however, often has the property of producing bone matrix within the target. A radio isotope that hones into bone and gives off radioactivity for a sufficiently long period of time may produce the therapeutic benefit. There is a preliminary report of a single palliative case treated with 153SmEDTPM (92) and an evaluation of the use of strontium 89 (93).

Palliation

It is reasonable to consider radiotherapy as treatment for the palliation of painful bony sites and in the treatment of spinal cord compression (41,42,78). The literature documenting the palliative efficacy of radiotherapy in osteosarcoma is, unfortunately, relatively sparse. The 1964 report by Lee and Mackenzie of the Westminster Hospital, London, describes the results with the administration of 7,000 to 8,000 R with a 2 MeV Vandegraft electrostatic generator. The authors note that, "clinical response of the tumour was very variable. Sometimes there was apparent worsening: there might be sudden increase in the size of the tumor, with more pain. Such changes might be the result of hemorrhage, or fracture, or disintegration of bone. More often there was a gradual reduction of pain and swelling, starting after some 2,000 R (sometimes much later) and continuing for several weeks after completion of treatment" (43). In 1975, deMoor from Johannesburg described the use of radiation for palliation and noted that "pain relief or reduction in swelling was experienced generally, and often within the first two to three weeks of treatment" (94).

The series of Beck et al. from the University of California at San Francisco (95), indicates that there were 44 patients with adequate information "to assess whether the treatment represented even a short term subjective gain for the patient. In 19 (43%) there was definite palliation. Twenty-five (57%) had either no change or worsening of symptoms. Those who survived experienced relief only after surgery." These authors used conventionally fractionated radiation with total doses ranging from 5,000 to 8,000 cGy (95). In contrast, Lombardi et al. (78) administered 6 Gy, 3 times per week for a total of 36 Gy in 6 fractions over 2 weeks. In 14 patients with 21 evaluable sites, there was a clinical response in 18 (86%).

REFERENCES

References particularly recommended for further reading are indicated with an asterisk.

1. Carter JR, Abdul-Karim FW. Pathology of childhood osteosarcoma. *Perspect Pediatr Pathol* 1987;9:133–170.
2. Chung EB, Enzinger FM. Extraskeletal osteosarcoma. *Cancer* 1987;60:1132–1142.
3. Kumar R, David R, Madwell JE, Lindell MM Jr. Radiographic spectrum of osteogenic sarcoma. *AJR* 1978;148:767–772.
4. Miller JH, Ettinger LJ. Osteosasrcoma. In: Miller JH,

ed. *Imaging in pediatric oncology*. Baltimore: Williams & Wilkins, 1985:378–388.

5. Spjut HJ, Ayala AG. Skeletal tumors in childhood and adolescence. In: Finegold M, ed. *Pathology of neoplasia in children and adolescents*. Philadelphia: WB Saunders, 1986:265–281.

6. Sweetnam R. Osteosarcoma. *Br Med J* 1979;2: 536–537.

7. Ueda Y, Roessner A, Grundmann E. Pathological diagnosis of osteosarcoma: the validity of the subclassification and some new diagnostic approaches using immunohistochemistry In: Humphrey GB, Koops HS, Molenaar WM, Postma A, eds. *Osteosarcoma in adolescents and young adults: new developments and controversies*. Boston: Kluwer Academic Publishers, 1993:109–124.

8. Unni KK, Dahlin DC. Osteosarcoma: pathology and classification. *Semin Roentgenol* 1989;25:143–152.

9. Ushigome S, Nakamori K, Nikaido T, Takagi M. Histologic subclassification of osteosarcoma: differential diagnostic problems and immnohistochemical aspects. In: Humphrey GB, Koops HS, Molenaar WM, Postma A, eds. *Osteosarcoma in adolescent and young adults: new developments and controversies*. Boston: Kluwer Academic Publishers, 1993:125–137.

10. Poppe E, Liverrud K, Efskind J. Osteosarcoma. *Acta Chir Scand* 1968;134:549–556.

11. Diller L, Kassel J, Nelson CE, et al. p53 Functions as a Cell Cycle Control Protein in Osteosarcoma. *Mol Cell Biol* 1990;10:5772–5781.

12. Beattie EJ, Harvey JC, Marcove R, Martini N. Results of multiple pulmonary resections for metastatic osteogenic sarcoma after two decades. *J Surg Oncol* 1991;46:154–155.

13. Glasser DB, Lne JM, Nuvos AG, Marcove RC, Rosen G. Survival, prognosis, and therapeutic response in osteogenic sarcoma. *Cancer* 1991;69:698–708.

14. Tillotson C, Rosenberg A, Gebhardt M, Rosenthal DI. Post-radiation multicentric osteosarcoma. *Cancer* 1988;62:65–71.

15. Jaffe N, Link MP, Cohen D, et al. High-dose methotrexate in osteogenic sarcoma. *Natl Cancer Inst Monogr* 1981;56:201–206.

16. Aisen AD, Martell W, Braunstein EM, McMillin KI, Phillips WA, Cling TF. MRI and CT evaluation of primary bone and soft issue tumors. *AJR* 1986;146: 749–756.

17. Breur K, Cohen P, Schwiesguth O, Hart AMM. Irradiation of the lungs as an adjuvant therapy in the treatment of osteosarcoma of the limbs. An EORTC randomized study. *Eur J Cancer* 1978;14:461–471.

18. Marion J, Burgers V, Breur K, van Doddendurgh A, et al. Role of metastatectomy without chemotherapy in the management of osteosarcoma in children. *Cancer* 1980;45:1664–1668.

19. Beiling P, Rehan N, Winkler P, et al. Tumor size and prognosis in aggressively treated osteosarcoma. *J Clin Oncol* 1996;14:848–858.

20. Springfield DS, Schmidt R, Graham-Pole J, Marcus RB Jr, Spanier SS, Enneking WF. Surgical treatment for osteosarcoma. *J Bone Joint Surg* 1988;70-A: 1124–1130.

21. Suit HD. Radiotherapy in osteosarcoma. *Clin Orthop* 1975;111:271–275.

22. Suit HD. Radiation therapy for osteosarcoma, chor-

doma and chondrosarcoma. In: Kumar S, ed. *Advances in medical oncology, research, and education Vol 10: Clinical cancer principle sites 1*. New York: Pergamon Press, 1979:181–185.

23. Sweetnam R. Tumors of bone and their management. *Ann R Coll Surg Engl* 1974;54:63–66.

24. Sweetnam R. The surgical management of primary osteosarcoma. *Clin Orthop* 1975;111:57–64.

25. White VA, Fanning CV, Ayala AG, Raymond AK, Carrasco CH, Murray JA. Osteosarcoma and the role of fine-needle aspiration: a study of 51 cases. *Cancer* 1988;62:1238–1246.

26. Wong ACW, Akahoshi Y, Takeuchi S. Limb-salvage procedures for osteosarcoma: an alternative to amputation. *Int Orthop* 1986;109:245–251.

*27. Damaron JA, Pritchard DJ. Current combined treatment of high-grade osteosarcomas. *Oncology* 1995; 9:327–350.

28. Button S. Rotation plasty for childhood osteosarcoma. *Nurs Times* 1987;83:49–51.

29. Hirano T, Iwasaki K, Kimashiro T, Suzuki R. Low dose irradiation for limb salvage in malignant bone tumors. *Int Orthop* 1991;115:381–385.

30. Simon MA, Asxhliman MA, Thomas N, et al. Limb-salvage treatment versus amputation for osteosarcoma of the distal end of the femur. *J Bone Joint Surg* 1986;68-A:1331–1337.

31. Marina NM, Pratt CB, Rao BN, Shema SJ, Meyer WH. Improved prognosis of children with osteosarcoma metastatic to the lung at the time of diagnosis. *Cancer* 1992;70:2722–2727.

32. Lee ES. Treatment of bone sarcoma. *Proc R Soc Med* 1971;64:1179–1181.

33. Marcove RC, Martini N, Rosen G. The treatment of pulmonary metastasis in osteogenic sarcoma. *Clin Orthop* 1975;111:65–70.

34. Meyer WH, Schell MJ, Kumar APM, et al. Thoracotomy for pulmonary metastatic osteosarcoma: an analysis of prognostic indicators of survival. *Cancer* 1987;59:374–379.

35. Suttow WW, Herson J, Perez C. Survival after metastasis in osteosarcoma. *Cancer Inst Monogr* 1981;56: 227–231.

36. Albrecht MR, Henze G, Habermalz HJ, Ruhl U. Osteosarcoma—a radioresistant tumor? Long term evaluation after multidrug chemotherapy and definitive irradiation of the primary instead of radical surgery. Unpublished scientific meeting presentation, Philadelphia: Radiation Therapy for Children with Cancer. July 24, 1994.

37. Allen CF, Stevens KR. Preoperative irradiation for osteogenic sarcoma. *Cancer* 1973;31:1364–1366.

38. Caceres E, Zaharia M. Massive preoperative radiation therapy in the treatment of osteogenic sarcoma. *Cancer* 1972;30:634–638.

39. Farrell C, Raventos A. Experience in treating osteosarcoma at the Hospital of the University of Pennsylvania. *Radiology* 1964;83:1080–1083.

40. Gaitan-Yanguas M. A study of the response to osteogenic sarcoma and adjacent normal tissues to radiation. *Int J Radiat Oncol Biol Phys* 1981;7:593–595.

41. Jenkin RDT. Radiation treatment of Ewing's sarcoma and osteogenic sarcoma. *Can J Surg* 1977;20: 530–536.

42. Jenkin RDT, Allt WEC, Fitzpatrick PJ. Osteosar-

coma: an assessment of management with particular reference to primary irradiation and selective delayed amputation. *Cancer* 1972;30:393–400.

43. Lee ES, MacKenzie DH. Osteosarcoma: a study of the value of preoperative megavoltage radiotherapy. *Br J Surg* 1963;51:252–274.

44. Phillips TL, Sheline GE. Radiation therapy of malignant bone tumors. *Radiology* 1969;92:1537–1545.

45. Goffinet DR, Kaplan HS, Donaldson SS, Bagshaw MA, Wilbur JR. Combined radiosensitizer infusion and irradiation of osteogenic sarcomas. *Radiology* 1975;117:211–214.

46. Cavaliere R. Hyperthermic treatment of osteogenic sarcoma. *Chemother Oncol* 1978;2:190–196.

47. Calvo FA, deUrbina DO, Sierrasesumaga L, et al. Intraoperative radiotherapy in the multidisciplinary treatment of bone sarcomas in children and adolescents. *Med Pediatr Oncol* 1991;19:478–485.

48. Martinez A, Goffinet DR, Donaldson SS, Bagshaw MA, Kaplan HS. Intra-arterial infusion of radiosensitizer (RUdr) combined with hypofractionated irradiation and chemotherapy for primary treatment of osteogenic sarcoma. *Int J Radiat Oncol Biol Phys* 1985; 11:123–128.

49. Bieling F, Dallera P, Bacchini P, Marchetti C, Campobassi A. The Instituto Rizzoli-Beretta experience with osteosarcoma of the jaw. *Cancer* 1991;68: 1555–1563.

50. Panizzoni GA, Gasparini G, Clauser L, Barasti P, Pozza F, Curioni C. Osteosarcoma of the facial bones. *Ann Oncol* 1992;3:S47–S50.

51. Chambers RG, Mahoney WD. Osteogenic sarcoma of the mandible: current management. *Am Surg* 1970; 36:463–471.

52. Saunders WM, Chen GTY, Austin-Seymour M, et al. Precision high dose radiotherapy. II. Helium ion treatment of tumors adjacent to critical central nervous system structures. *Int J Radiat Oncol Biol Phys* 1985;11:1339–1347.

53. Weichselbaum RR, Cassady JR, Jaffe N, Filler RM. Preliminary results of aggressive multimodality therapy for metastatic osteosarcoma. *Cancer* 1977;40: 78–83.

54. Burgers JMV. Experience of the EORTC radiotherapy/chemotherapy group in osteosarcoma trials. In: Humphrey GB, Koops HS, Molenaar WM, Postma A, eds. *Osteosarcoma in adolescent and young adults: new developments and controversies.* Boston: Kluwer Academic Publishers, 1993:173–175.

55. Ellis ER, Marcus RB Jr, Cicale MJ, et al. Pulmonary function tests after whole-lung irradiation and doxorubicin in patients with osteogenic sarcoma. *J Clin Oncol* 1992;10:459–463.

56. Springfield DS, Schakel ME Jr, Spanier SS. Spontaneous necrosis in osteosarcoma. *Clin Orthop* 1991;263:233–237.

57. Ivins JC, Taylor WF, Wold LE. Elective whole-lung irradiation in osteosarcoma treatment: appearance of bilateral breast cancer in two long-term survivors. *Skeletal Radiol* 1987;16:133–135.

58. Thompson DK, Li FP, Cassady JR. Breast cancer in a man 30 years after radiation for metastatic osteogenic sarcoma. *Cancer* 1979;44:2362–2365.

58a. Russo CL, McIntyre J, Goorin AM, Link MP, Gebhardt MC, Friend SH. Secondary breast cancer in patients presenting with osteosarcoma: possible involvement of germline p53 mutations. *Med Pediatr Oncol* 1994;23:354–8.

59. Suttow WW, Gehan EA, Dymen TPJ, et al. Multidrug adjuvant chemotherapy for osteosarcoma: interim report of the southwest oncology group studies. *Cancer Treat Rep* 1978;62:265–270.

60. Hudson M, Jaffe MR, Jaffe N, et al. Pediatric osteosarocoma: therapeutic strategies, results, and prognostic factors derived from a 10-year experience. *J Clin Oncol* 1990;12:1988–1997.

61. Benjamin RS, Chawla SP, Carrasco CH, et al. Preoperative chemotherapy for osteosarcoma with intravenous adriamycin and intra-arterial therapy in the treatment of osteosarcoma. *Radiology* 1976;120: 163–165.

62. Pratt CB, Champion JE, Fleming ID, et al. Adjuvant chemotherapy for osteosarcoma of the extremity. *Cancer* 1976;38:939–942.

63. Bacci G, Springfield D, Capanna R, et al. Neoadjuvant chemotherapy for osteosarcoma of the extremity. *Clin Orthop* 1987;224:268–276.

64. Burgers JM, van Glabbeke M, Bussan A, et al. Osteosarcoma of the limbs. Report of the EORTC-SIOP 03 trial 20781 investigating the value of adjuvant treatment with chemotherapy and/or prophylactic lung irradiation. *Cancer* 1988;61:1024–1031.

65. Caceres E, Zaharia M, Valdivia S, et al. Local control of osteogenic sarcoma by radiation and chemotherapy. *Int J Radiat Oncol Biol Phys* 1984;10:35–39.

66. Silberman A, Elber FR, Giuliano AE, et al. Adjuvant chemotherapy of osteosarcoma. *J Clin Oncol* 1987;5: 982–984.

67. Goorin AM, Perrz-Atayade A, Gebhardt M, et al. Weekly high-dose methotrexate and doxorubicin for osteosarcoma: the Dana Farber Cancer Institute/The Children's Hospital—Study III. *J Clin Oncol* 1987; 15:381–385.

*68. Link MP, Goorin M, Miser AW, et al. The effect of adjuvant chemotherapy on relapse-free survival in patients with osteosarcoma of the extremity. *N Engl J Med* 1986;314:1600–1606.

69. Saeter G. Alvegard TA, Elomaa I, Stenwig AE, Holmstrom T, Solheim OP. Treatment of osteosarcoma of the extremities with the T-10 protocol, with emphasis on the effects of preoperative chemotherapy with a single-agent high-dose methotrexate: a Scandinavian Sarcoma Group Study. *J Clin Oncol* 1991;9:1766–1775.

70. Thorpe WP, Reilly JJ, Rosenberg SA. Prognostic significance of alkaline phosphative measurements in patients with osteogenic sarcoma receiving chemotherapy. *Cancer* 1979;43:2178–2181.

71. Winkler K, Beran G, Delling G, et al. Neoadjuvant chemotherapy of osteosarcoma: results of a randomized cooperative trial (Coss-82) with salvage chemotherapy based on histological tumor response. *J Clin Oncol* 1988;6:329–337.

72. Taylor WF, Ivins JC, Pritchard DJ, Dahlin DC, Gilchrist GS, Edmonson JH. Trends and variability in survival among patients with osteosarcoma: 7 year update. *Mayo Clin Proc* 1985;60:91–104.

73. Bentzen SM, Paulsen HS, Kaae S, et al. Prognostic factors in osteosarcomas: a regression analysis. *Cancer* 1988;62:194–202.

74. Edmonson JH, Green SJ, Ivins JC, et al. A controlled pilot study of high-dose methotrexate as post surgical adjuvant treatment for primary osteosarcoma. *J Clin Oncol* 1987;5:21–26.

75. Holland JF. Adjuvant chemotherapy of osteosaocma: no runs, no hits, two men left on base. *J Clin Oncol* 1987;5:4–5.

76. Carrie C, Bretau N, Negrier S, et al. The role of fast neutron therapy in unresectable pelvic osteosarcoma: preliminary report. *Med Pediatr Oncol* 1994;22: 355–357.

77. Kubota N, Suzuke M, Furusawa Y, et al. A comparison of biological effects of modulate carbon-ions and fast neutrons in human osteosarcoma cells. *Int J Radiat Oncol Biol Phys* 1995;33:135–141.

78. Lombardi F, Gandola L, Fossati-Bellani F, Gianni MC, Rottoli L, Gasparine M. Hypofractionated accelerated radiotherapy in osteogenic sarcoma. *Int J Radiat Oncol Biol Phys* 1991;24:761–765.

79. Suit HD. Role of therapeutic radiology in cancer of bone. *Cancer* 1975;35:930–935.

80. Urtasun RC, McConnachie PR. Disappearance of osteogenic sarcoma after irradiation: immunologic observations. *J Assoc Can Radiol* 1976;27:80–83.

81. Rab GT, Ivins JC, Childs DS Jr, Cupps RE, Pritchard DJ. Elective whole lung irradiation in the treatment of osteogenic sarcoma. *Cancer* 1976;38: 939–942.

82. Zaharia M, Caceres E, Valdivia S, Moran M, Tejada F. Postoperative whole lung irradiation with or without adriamycin in osteogenic sarcoma. *Int J Radiat Oncol Biol Phys* 1986;12:907–910.

83. van den Brenk HAS, Kerr RC, Madigan JP, Cass NM, Ritcher W. Results from tourniquet anoxia and hyperbaric oxygen techniques combined with megavoltage treatment of sarcomas of bone and soft tissues. *AJR* 1966;96:760–776.

84. Chauvel P. Osteosarcomas and adult soft tissue sarcomas: is here a place for high LET radiation therapy? *Ann Oncol* 1992;3:S107–S110.

85. Laramore GE, Griffith JT, Boespflug M, et al. Fast neutron radiotherapy for sarcomas of soft tissue, bone, and cartilage. *Am J Clin Oncol* 1989;12: 320–326.

86. Wambersie A. Fast neutron therapy at the end of 1988—a survey of the clinical data. *Stahlenther Onkol* 1990;166:52–60.

87. Cohen L, Hendrickson F, Mansell J, et al. Response of sarcomas of bone and soft tissue to neutron beam therapy. *Int J Radiat Oncol Biol Phys* 1984;10: 821–824.

88. Duncan W, Arnott SJ, Jack WJL. The Edinburgh experience of treating sarcomas of soft tissues and bone with neutron irradiation. *Clin Radiol* 1986;37: 317–320.

89. Hug EB, Fitzek MM, Liebsch NJ, Menzenrider JE. Locally challenging osteo- and chondrogenic tumors of the axial skeleton: results of combined proton and photon radiation therapy using three-dimensional treatment planning. *Int J Radiat Oncol Biol Phys* 1995;31:467–476.

90. Castro JR, Linstadt DE, Bahary J-P, et al. Experience in charged particle irradiation of tumors of the skull base: 1977–1992. *Int J Radiat Oncol Biol Phys* 1994; 29:647–655.

91. Yamamuro T, Kotoura Y. Intraoperative radiation therapy for osteosarcoma. In: Humphrey GB, Koops HS, Molenaar WM, Postma A, eds. *Osteosarcoma in adolescents and young adults: new developments and controversies.* Boston: Kluwer Academic Publishers, 1993:177–183.

92. Bruland OS, Skretting A, Solhein OP, Aas M. Targeted radiotherapy of osteosarcoma using [153]Sm-EDTMP: a new promising approach. *Acta Oncol* 1996;35:381–384.

93. Blake GM, Zivanovic MA, McEwan AJ, Condon BR, Ackery M. Strontium-89 therapy: strontium kinetics and dosimetry in two patients treated for metastasizing osteosarcoma. *Br J Radiol* 1987;60: 253–259.

94. deMoor NG. Osteosarcoma: a review of 72 cases treated by megavoltage radiation therapy with or without surgery. *S African J Surg* 1975;13:137–146.

95. Beck JC, Wara WM, Bovil EG Jr, Phillips TL. The role of radiation therapy in the treatment of osteosarcoma. *Radiology* 1976;120:163–165.

96. Taylor WF, Ivins JC, Unni KK, Beabout JW, Golenzer HJ, Black LE. Prognostic variables in osteosarcoma: a multi-institutional study. *J Natl Cancer Inst* 1989;81:21–30.

97. Newton KA. Prophylactic irradiation of the lung in bone sarcoma. In: Price CHG, Ross FGM, eds. *Bone—certain aspects of neoplasia.* London: Butterworths, 1972:307–311.

98. Lougheed MN, Palmer JD, Henderson I, McIntyre JM. Radiation and regional chemotherapy in osteogenic sarcoma. *Excerpta Med Int Cong Ser* 1965; 105:1124–1128.

99. Anonymous. Osteosarcoma chemo regimens debated. *Oncol News Internat* 1995;4:1–26.

100. Link MP. Commentary of the use of presurgical chemotherapy. In: Humphrey GB, Koops HS, Molenaar WM, Postma A, eds. *Osteosarcoma in adolescents and young adults: new developments and controversies.* Boston: Kluwer Academic Publishers, 1993:383–385.

*101. Link MP. The multi-institutional osteosarcoma study: an update. In: Humphrey GB, Koops HS, Molenaar WM, Postma A, eds. *Osteosarcoma in adolescents and young adults: new developments and controversies.* Boston: Kluwer Academic Publishers, 1993: 261–267.

102. Craft AW, Burgers JMW. The European osteosarcoma intergroup (E.O.I.) studies in 1980–1991. In: Humphrey GB, Koops HS, Molenaar WM, Postma A, eds. *Osteosarcoma in adolescents and young adults: new developments and controversies.* Boston: Kluwer Academic Publishers, 1993:279–286.

103. Souhami RL, Craft AW, Vander EI, et al. Randomized trial of two regimens of chemotherapy in operable osteosarcoma: a study of the European osteosarcoma intergroup. *Lancet* 1997;350:911–917.

*104. Miser JS, Krailo M. The children's cancer group (CCG) studies. In: Humphrey GB, Koops HS, Molenaar WM, Postma A, eds. *Osteosarcoma in adolescents and young adults: new developments and controversies.* Boston: Kluwer Academic Publishers, 1993:287–291.

*105. Winkler K, Bielack SS, Belling G, Jurgens H, Kotz R, Salzer-Kuntschik M. Treatment of osteosarcoma: experience of the cooperative osteosarcoma study group

(COSS). In: Humphrey GB, Koops HS, Molenaar WM, Postma A, eds. *Osteosarcoma in adolescents and young adults: new developments and controversies.* Boston: Kluwer Academic Publishers, 1993:269–277.

106. Ornitz R, Herskovic A, Schell M, Fender F, Rogers CC. Treatment experience: locally advanced sarcomas with 15 MeV fast neutrons. *Cancer* 1980;45: 2712–2716.

107. Salinas R, Hussey DH, Fletcher GH, et al. Experi-

ence with fast neutron therapy for locally advanced sarcomas. *Int J Radiat Oncol Biol Phys* 1980;6: 267–272.

108. Batterman JJ, Bruer K. Fast neutron therapy for locally advanced sarcomas. *Int J Radiat Oncol Biol Phys* 1981;7:1051–1053.

109. Tsunemoto H, Arai T, Morita S, et al. Japanese experience with clinical trials of fast neutrons. *Int J Radiat Oncol Biol Phys* 1982;8:2169–2172.

11

Rhabdomyosarcoma

Rhabdomyosarcoma (RMS) is a highly malignant neoplasm that arises from embryonal mesenchyme with the potential for differentiating into striated muscle (1). Although the cells will show differentiation along rhabdomyoblastic lines, RMS is not limited to cells with recognizable muscle cross-striations (2,3). Although RMS was initially described in 1854 by Weber (4), progress in our understanding and treatment of this complex neoplasm accelerated with Stout's landmark descriptive series in 1946 (5), and the delineation by Horn and Enterline in 1958 of the four classic forms of RMS (6). It can arise almost anywhere in the body, is locally invasive, and rapidly disseminates early in its course. Early in this century, the only cures were accomplished with radical surgery, and these cures were only possible in the few fortunate children without metastases. Significant disfigurement and loss of function were common sequelae. High-dose radiation therapy increased the potential for local control but caused a different set of morbidities (7–9). As chemotherapy has become increasingly effective in eliminating micrometastatic disease and assisting in local control, the need for aggressive surgery and large-volume irradiation has diminished (10). Overall survival rates have concomitantly increased from 15% to 25% to as high as 70% (1,10–19).

RMS is a rare tumor with clinical and biologic heterogeneity. Consequently, multiinstitutional trials were necessary to develop and refine treatment approaches. A paramount role in this progress has been played by investigators comprising the Intergroup Rhabdomyo-

sarcoma Studies (IRS), which is now in its fifth generation of protocols. The difficulty of this undertaking is clear in view of the myriad of sites, stages, and histologies of RMS, which are associated with different natural histories and prognoses (20). Beyond this, advances in imaging, changes in endpoints, and the need for mature data all increased the difficulty in conducting and comparing randomized, controlled clinical studies of patients with RMS. With this view, IRS was established through the collaboration of three multidisciplinary cancer treatment study groups (Cancer and Leukemia Group B, Children's Cancer Study Group, and the Pediatric Branch of the Southwest Oncology Group, which later became the Pediatric Oncology Group). Intergroup Rhabdomyosarcoma Study I (IRS-I) was open for patient entry from 1972 to 1978 (17). With an overall 5-year survival rate of 55% in IRS-I, IRS-II was designed to improve survival for the patient subgroups with poor outcomes, and to refine treatment for the remaining patients (16). IRS-II ran from 1978 to 1984, and IRS-III from 1984 to 1991. IRS-IV opened in 1991 and is still in progress. Although the previous generations of IRS studies were based on a surgically oriented clinical grouping system dependent on the tumor that remained after initial surgery, IRS-IV is based on a more biologically oriented staging system, discussed later in this chapter. The entire series of studies, each based on the results of its predecessor, have provided a database of approximately 3,000 patients. Other multiinstitutional group studies have also provided important data (21). Of particular note are the International Society

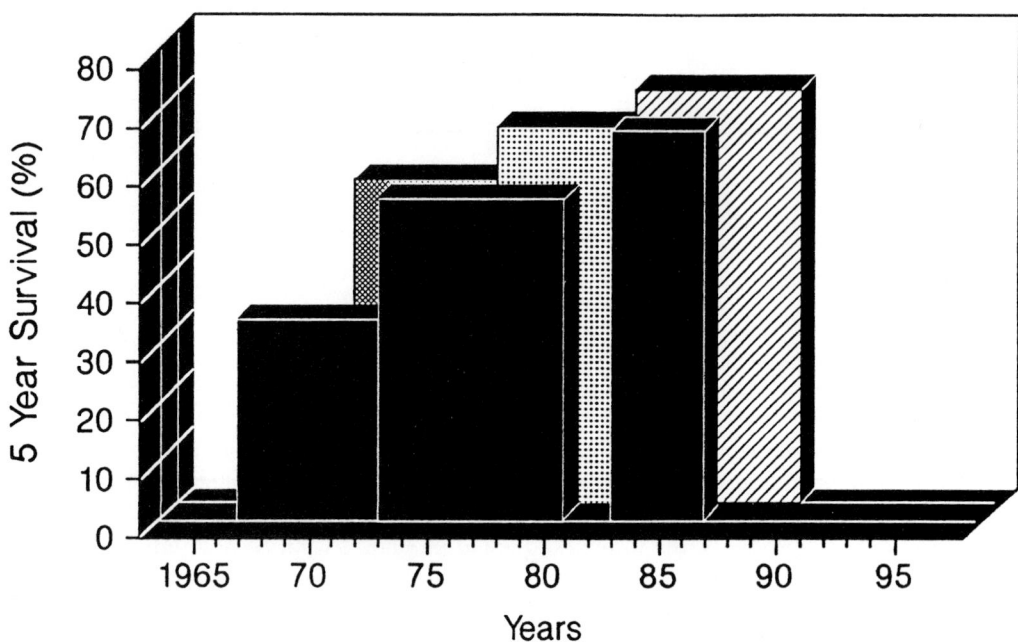

FIG. 1. Improvement in 5-year survival of children with RMS treated between 1967 and 1991 in IRS trials (light dots, IRS-I; heavy dots, IRS-II; diagonal slashes, IRS-III) and compared with data from the Epidemiology and End Results Section of the National Cancer Institute (solid bars). (From ref. 30, with permission.)

of Pediatric Oncology (SIOP) and the Children's Solid Tumor Group (CSTG); the latter was initially set up by the St. Bartholomew's and the Royal Marsden Hospitals in the United Kingdom (14,22). Finally, many single-institution studies have also been quite informative regarding RMS (7,10,23,24). The progress in treating RMS is exemplified by the improvement in overall 5-year survival in the IRS studies: 56% in IRS-I, 63% in IRS-II, and 71% in IRS-III (11,12,16,17) (Fig. 1).

EPIDEMIOLOGY AND BIOLOGY

Epidemiology

Soft-tissue sarcomas account for 4% to 8% of all malignant disease in children less than 15 years of age (1). RMS comprises one-half of these sarcoma cases. The annual incidence of RMS is 4.4 per million in white children and 1.3 per million in black children. There is a slight male predominance (1.4:1). Seventy percent of cases occur before the age of 10 years, with a peak incidence at 2 to 5 years of age (Fig. 2). Congenital anomalies have been identified in a large proportion of children with RMS—most commonly involving the gastrointestinal, genitourinary, cardiovascular, and central nervous systems (25).

Environmental factors in the development of RMS are undefined, but some suggestive influences are under study. For example, a national case-control report of 332 children with RMS enrolled into IRS-III, demonstrated an association of RMS with maternal and paternal marijuana and cocaine use (26). Of particular note is that the pattern of cancers in relatives of children with RMS is consistent with the Li-Fraumeni syndrome in which germline mutations of P53 exist, supporting a genetic etiology (27). An increased frequency of RMS is also present in children with neurofibromatosis type 1 and the Beckwith-Wiedemann syndrome (28).

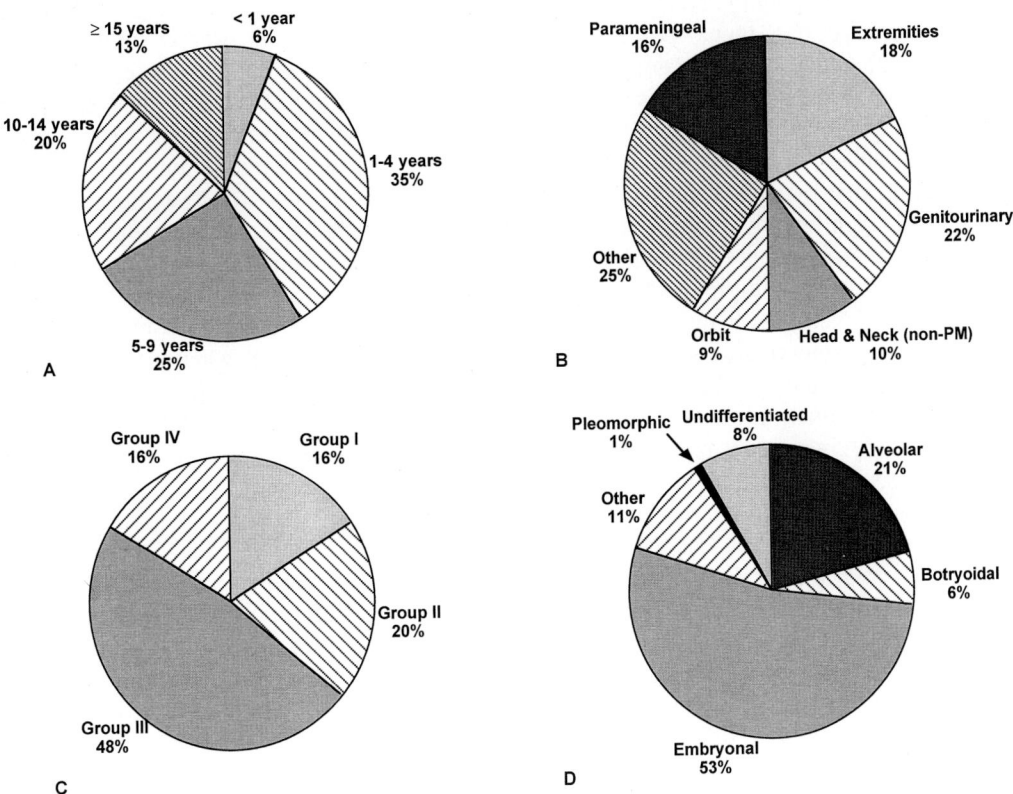

FIG. 2. Clinical features of RMS from IRS-I,-II,-III pooled data. **A:** Age at presentation. **B:** Site of primary tumor. **C:** Clinical group. **D:** Histology. (Modified from ref. 100, with permission.)

Biology

Although the etiology and genetics of RMS remain unclear, observations provide direction for additionally understanding this tumor. The relevance of this to the clinician should be clear.

If we can determine the tumor characteristics that predict radiochemotherapy responsiveness or, conversely, tumor resistance to therapy and a propensity to disseminate, then we will be able to select those patients in whom more or less toxic therapy should be used. Moreover, we may also devise novel biologic maneuvers to treat such tumors that avoid some of the normal tissue damage. Areas in which progress has come include the genetic control of myogenesis, tumor suppressor genes, the influence of the percentage of

cells in S phase of the cell cycle, and the role of proto-oncogenes and their protein products (29,30).

Cytogenetics

The t(2:13)(p35:q14) or t(1:13)(p36:q14) translocation exists in approximately 70% of children with alveolar RMS, which results in the fusion of a transcriptional regulator (PAX3 or PAX7, respectively) to a transcription factor (FKHR on chromosome 13) (31,32). This may induce cell proliferation via transcriptional deregulation, and its presence may aid in the diagnosis of alveolar RMS, which has a worse prognosis than the embryonal subtype (33). Loss of heterozygosity at the 11p15.5 locus characterizes embryonal RMS. Chromosomal ploidy also appears relevant to prognosis of

RMS (34). A report from the Netherlands suggests that diploid DNA index may be correlated with unfavorable tumor location and advanced TNM (tumor-node-metastasis) stage (35). Conversely, an analysis of 20 patients with unresectable, nonmetastatic group III RMS showed that patients with hyperdiploid tumors had significantly improved overall (greater than 90%) event-free survival as compared with those with diploid tumors ($p <$ 0.0001) (36). Patients with tumors that converted from aneuploid to diploid at the time of relapse were more likely to die of disease than those who maintained a persistent favorable DNA index (35). In a recent report identification of the PAX3-FKHR fusion transcript using reverse transcriptase Polymerase Chain Reaction (PCR) can denote residual submicroscopic disease in alveolar RMS (37).

Cell Cycle Control

Myogenesis involves differentiation of the mesenchymal fibroblast into skeletal muscle under the control of a series of gene products including the Myo D protein family (Myogenin, MYF5, and MYF6). These gene products also serve to halt cell cycling. Expression of the Myo D proteins, which can be determined by an anti-Myo D antibody, has become the "gold standard" to demonstrate that malignant cells have characteristics of skeletal muscle differentiation and, therefore, represent RMS (Fig. 3). It is possible that there is some tumor suppressor factor present in the normal fibroblast that, when combined with the RMS cell and the Myo D gene product, can drive the cell toward differentiation as well as halt cell proliferation.

Proto-oncogenes

The *myc* gene can contribute to uncontrolled cell proliferation via several pathways including insertion mutations, translocations, retro-viral transductions, and amplification. Two reports involving 20 patients showed 50% of those with alveolar RMS had n-*myc*

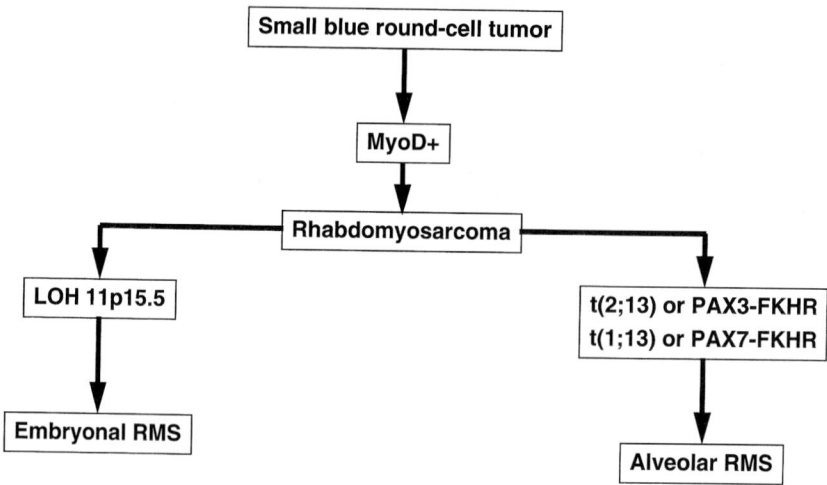

FIG. 3. Molecular diagnosis of RMS. Expression of MyoD is specific for cells of myogenic origin, including RMS, and rules out other major categories of small blue round-cell tumors. Loss of heterozygosity (LOH) at the 11p15.5 locus characterizes embryonal RMS, whereas two specific translocations, t(2;13) and t(1;13), characterize the alveolar subtype. These translocations respectively fuse the PAX3 or PAX7 genes to the FKHR gene on chromosome 13. Reverse transcriptase polymerase chain reaction can readily detect these fusion transcripts. (Modified from ref. 99, with permission.)

amplification, in contrast to its uniform absence in patients with embryonal RMS (38,39). Impressively, among the patients with alveolar RMS, n-*myc* amplification predicted a fatal outcome.

Tumor Suppressor Genes

P53 mutations can be demonstrated in a significant proportion of childhood RMS (40). In the presence of damaged DNA normal P53 produces G1 arrest and prevents the cell with damaged DNA from undergoing any proliferation. P53, in conjunction with *myc*, drives such damaged cells toward apoptosis. This might explain why some forms of RMS which escape cure by radiochemotherapy become progressively more virulent—they generate resistant clones of tumor cells.

CLINICAL PRESENTATION AND EVALUATION

Primary Sites and Clinical Presentations

RMS occurs in any anatomic location of the body where there is skeletal muscle, as well as in locations where skeletal muscle is not normally found (Fig. 2) (16). The most common locations are genitourinary and head and neck. Genitourinary sites include the bladder, prostate, vagina, uterus, urethra, and paratesticular region. Head and neck lesions are divided into parameningeal sites (nasopharynx, nasal cavity, paranasal sinuses, middle ear and mastoid region, infratemporal fossa, pterygopalatine and parapharyngeal areas) and other head and neck sites (parotid region, cheek, masseter muscle, oral cavity, oropharynx, larynx, hypopharynx, scalp, face, and pinna) (41). An equally large group is the extremity, followed by the orbit (analyzed separately from other head and neck sites due to its excellent prognosis) as the next most frequent site. The rank order of primary sites varies slightly between the cooperative groups—the result of differing referral patterns (14).

RMS commonly presents as an asymptomatic mass with poorly defined margins, but specific presentations relate to the primary disease site. A mass in the *genitourinary system* may cause urinary tract or rectal obstruction. On occasion, the mass may protrude from the cervix, vagina, or urethra. When the protruding tumor has the gross appearance of a cluster of grapes, it is called *sarcoma botryoid* ("grape-like"). Prostate and bladder RMS may also have a botryoid appearance and protrude into the lumen of the bladder. Hematuria, urinary frequency, or retention may occur. Paratesticular RMS can appear as a hydrocele, incarcerated hernia, testicular torsion, or mass. In the *extremities,* RMS will often be palpable and cause pain or limitation of motion. *Parameningeal* RMS may present with airway obstruction or a palpable mass. As the tumor grows, it may cause erosion of the base of skull and cranial nerve palsies. Penetration into the brain can occur and mimic an intracranial mass, with headache, vomiting, and diplopia. RMS of the cheek or larynx will cause obstruction of the aerodigestive track or a discernible mass; other symptoms or signs referable to the *head and neck* region include hoarseness, polyps, decreased hearing, persistent otitis, sinusitis, or parotitis. Patients with *orbital* RMS usually present with proptosis, discoloration, or limitation of extraocular motion. RMS of the *trunk* can present as a mass simulating a hernia or hematoma, or causing a classic superior vena cava syndrome. In the *retroperitoneum,* RMS can cause gastrointestinal discomfort or other mass-related symptoms.

Diagnostic Evaluation

The history and physical exam should focus on the extent of local disease and the possible presence of metastases. RMS may extend locally and infiltrate along fascial planes and into surrounding tissues. Tumor margins are often indistinct. The local tumor will, depending on the site, generally be imaged by some combination of computerized tomography (CT), magnetic resonance imaging (MRI), and plain radiography. Genitourinary RMS is often investigated initially by ultrasound and barium enema, voiding cystourethrogram, cystoscopy, or pelvic examination under anesthesia will occasionally be indicated. The draining lymphatics, in genitourinary primary sites, are evaluated with CT and lymphangiography (42,43). The most common sites of metastases are lung, bone, bone marrow, and lymph nodes (43). Chest CT is the optimal evaluation for lung metastases. A nuclear medicine bone scan is performed to detect bony metastases but is not reliable to determine base of skull involvement in parameningeal tumors, which is evaluated with CT or MRI. Other sites of distant metastasis are evaluated with liver chemistries, nuclear medicine scans, and bone marrow biopsy and aspirate. Cerebrospinal fluid (CSF) cytology is performed to evaluate central nervous system (CNS) involvement by parameningeal tumors (44). MRI or myelography is, or course, used to evaluate spinal cord-related symptoms.

CLASSIFICATION AND STAGING

Histologic Classification

Most RMS subtypes are soft, fleshy tumors with variation in the extent of invasion and necrosis. Cross-striations and periodic acid-Schiff positivity (from cytoplasmic glycogen) may be seen by light microscopy. Intracytoplasmic filaments and Z-band material may be identified by electron microscopy. More recently, the use of immunohistochemical techniques, including antidesmin and antimuscle-specific actin (anti-MSA), has been shown to enhance diagnostic capabilities (3), and the detection of the muscle regulatory gene MyoD1 may be even more sensitive than desmin (Fig. 3).

Four histologic subtypes of RMS are classically described: embryonal, alveolar, pleomorphic, and mixed (Fig. 2). However, the lack of agreement in classification among pathologists and the need to develop a single prognostically significant system prompted formation of an international panel to devise a new system, the International Classification of Rhabdomyosarcoma (ICR) (45,46).

Table 1 denotes this system and associated outcome.

Superior Prognosis

Botryoid

This "grape-like" polypoid variant of embryonal RMS occurs in mucosa-lined organs including the bladder, vagina, nasopharynx, middle ear, and biliary tree. The stroma is loose with a myxoid character, and a condensed tumor cell or cambial layer must be identifiable. The tumor cells may be small or large, with varying degrees of myogenesis. These tumors are generally localized and noninvasive (2,45,46).

Spindle cell

This variant is exclusively composed of spindle-shaped cells and has a low cellularity. It can be collagen rich or poor, with the former having a storiform pattern. Its most common site is paratesticular.

Intermediate prognosis

Embryonal

This form is composed of blastemal mesenchymal cells that tend to differentiate into

TABLE 1. *International classification of rhabdomyosarcoma*

	Frequency (%)	Actuarial 5-yr survival (%)
I. Superior prognosis		
a. Botryoid rhabdomyosarcoma	6	95
b. Spindle cell rhabdomyosarcoma	3	88
II. Intermediate prognosis		
a. Embryonal rhabdomyosarcoma	79	66
III. Poor prognosis		
a. Alveolar rhabdomyosarcoma	32	54
b. Undifferentiated sarcoma	1	40
Other	9	

Data taken from ref. 46, with permission.

cross-striated muscle cells. Although it resembles normally developing skeletal muscle in the 7- to 10-week fetus, great variation in the degree of differentiation can exist. Cellularity is moderate and the stroma is loose and myxoid in most cases. The cells are generally fusiform or stellate, often admixed with primitive round cell forms. Cross-striations are present in about one-third of cases (2). Periodic acid-Schiff staining, actin/desmin positive reactivity, and Z-band material is usually present. Loss of heterozygosity at 11p15.5 may be identifiable (see the Biology section). The pathologic differential diagnosis often includes lymphoma, Ewing's sarcoma, and neuroblastoma.

Poor Prognosis

Alveolar

The alveolar form of RMS resembles developing skeletal muscle in the 10- to 20-week-old fetus. The cells are round with scanty eosinophilic cytoplasm which is occasionally vacuolated. Cross-striations are quite rare. The name *alveolar* is derived from the pattern produced by the tendency of cells to line connective tissue septa reminiscent of alveoli. Variable arrangement of trabeculae may cause the tumor cells to be arranged in strands, clefts, sheets, and clusters (2). The characteristic translocations are discussed in the Biology section. A "solid" variant has been identified, which grows as solid masses of closely aggregated cells with scarce or no discernible alveolar arrangement.

Undifferentiated

These tumors are generally diffuse, with no specific features other than primitive non-committed mesenchymal cells. It is defined by its negativity of the common antigenic markers and, therefore, is a diagnosis of exclusion. Patients with this variant had a better prognosis is IRS-III than in IRS-I/II (47).

The previously designated "pleomorphic" variant is rare and many of these cases would currently be classified as malignant fibrous histiocytoma.

The IRS review of pathologic material disclosed a number of tumors classified as *Extraosseous Ewing's sarcoma.* This is a tumor that has the same morphologic and cytologic features as Ewing's sarcoma but arises next to, and not in, bone. The tumor is composed uniformly of small undifferentiated cells with immature nuclei and abundant cytoplasmic glycogen. By virtue of the presence of glycogen, it is not possible to distinguish this category histologically from osseous Ewing's sarcoma. Broad bands of dense collagen may be seen as disorganized septa within the tumor (2,48). These patients are currently managed as Ewing's sarcoma (see Chapter 9).

Staging and Grouping

RMS has been staged according to multiple systems developed in different institutions or multiinstitutional groups, both in this country and elsewhere (14) (also see Table 2, Chapter 12). The initial system used by the IRS was a clinicopathologic "grouping" based on the extent of disease at the time of treatment, which essentially corresponded to the completeness of surgery (Table 2, Fig. 2). Because therapeutic decisions made prior to study entry affected the assigned group, this system did not accurately reflect the biology of RMS

TABLE 2. *The IRS grouping system*

Group I: Localized disease, completely resected
  a. Confined to muscle or organ of origin.
  b. Infiltration outside the muscle or organ of origin.
Group II: Total gross resection with:
  a. Microscopic residual disease.
  b. Regional lymphatic spread, resected.
  c. Both.
Group III: Incomplete resection with gross residual disease
  a. After biopsy only.
  b. After major resection (>50%).
Group IV: Distant metastatic disease present at onset

TABLE 3. *TNM pretreatment staging classification for IRS-IV*

Stage	Sites	T	T size	N	M
1	Orbit Head and neck (excluding parameningeal) GU-Nonbladder/Nonprostate	T1 or T2	a or b	any N	M0
2	Bladder/prostate Extremity Head and neck parameningeal Other (including trunk, retroperitoneum, etc)	T1 or T2	a	N0 or NX	M0
3	Same as Stage 2	T1 or T2	a b	N1 any N	M0
4	All	T1 or T2	a or b	any N	M1

T, tumor: 1, confined to anatomic site of origin; 2, extension; a, ≤ 5 cm in diameter; b, >5 cm in diameter; N, regional nodes; NX, clinical status unknown; N0, not clinically involved; N1, clinically involved; M, metastasis; M0, none; M1, present.

(18,49,50). Moreover, the emphasis on surgical reduction of tumor bulk implicit in this system led surgeons to perform unnecessarily morbid surgery at inappropriate times. In addition, the surgical approach was not uniformly applied, which obfuscated interpretation of results (49). With the advent of IRS-III, a pretreatment staging system was developed based on the TNM-UICC system used by SIOP, which reflected the disease characteristics at diagnosis (Table 3). However, the older grouping system was used to assign treatment until IRS-IV was organized. This currently used TNM staging system emphasizes tumor size and invasiveness (a/b, T1/T2, respectively), nodal status and identifiable metastasis. Because the site of disease influences prognosis and treatment, the staging system incorporates this parameter. Essentially stage 1 tumors are in favorable sites. Stage 2 tumors are in unfavorable sites but are small (less than 5 cm) with negative lymph nodes. Stage 3 tumors are in unfavorable sites and of large size or with positive lymph nodes. Stage 4 tumors are of any site with hematogenous metastasis. This staging system determines the chemotherapeutic regimen to be used, while the older IRS clinical grouping system is used to determine the radiotherapeutic guidelines.

A report from the International Rhabdomyosarcoma Workshop based on data from the IRS, the SIOP, and the German and Italian multiinstitutional group studies supports the validity of the new classification system (18). Significant by univariate analysis were tumor invasiveness (T), size (a/b), lymph node status (N), and site, and by multivariate analysis, tumor invasiveness and primary site. Recently, the IRS compared the predictive value of the pretreatment staging system on patients from IRS-II (retrospective) and IRS-III (prospective) (50) (Table 4). Of note was that the survival of patients with small lesions at unfavorable anatomic sites without clinically involved lymph notes (stage 2) was similar to that of patients with tumors at favorable anatomic sites (stage 1). In addition, stage 1 patients with N1 disease had a poorer 5-year survival (65%) than the stage 1 patients who were N0 (92%) ($p < 0.001$), but similar to the stage 3 N1 patients (69%). Therefore, the new

TABLE 4. *Percent survival at 5-years by clinical group and pretreatment stage*

	IRS-I	IRS-II	IRS-III
Clinical group			
I	83	81	93
II	71	80	81
III	52	65	73
IV	21	27	30
All	55	63	71
Pretreatment stage			
I		91	89
II		73	86
III		52	69
IV		23	30

Data taken from refs. 11,12,16,17,50, with permission.

system was not completely predictive of the IRS-III patient outcome, which the authors concluded could be due to differences in the management strategy used for IRS-III or the statistical variability in the model-fitting process used to develop the system. Consequently, this system will need to be continually reevaluated.

PROGNOSTIC VARIABLES

Clinical Group

Implicit in the discussion of the grouping and staging systems is the importance of accurately identifying prognostic variables. Most of these variables are interrelated. A wealth of data supports the relevance of the

clinical group of the patient, which in essence is the postsurgical disease extent at the time chemotherapy is initiated. Data from the three analyzed IRS studies support this (11,12,16,17) (Table 4, Fig. 4). Although the clinical group reflects either the absence (group I) or presence of microscopic disease (group II), gross disease (group III), or metastatic disease (group IV), the clinical group also reflects the disease site (in terms of resectability) and the biological invasiveness of the tumor (also in terms of resectability).

Primary Site and Lymphatic Spread

The *primary site* is a strong determinant of outcome, as verified by data from IRS-II and

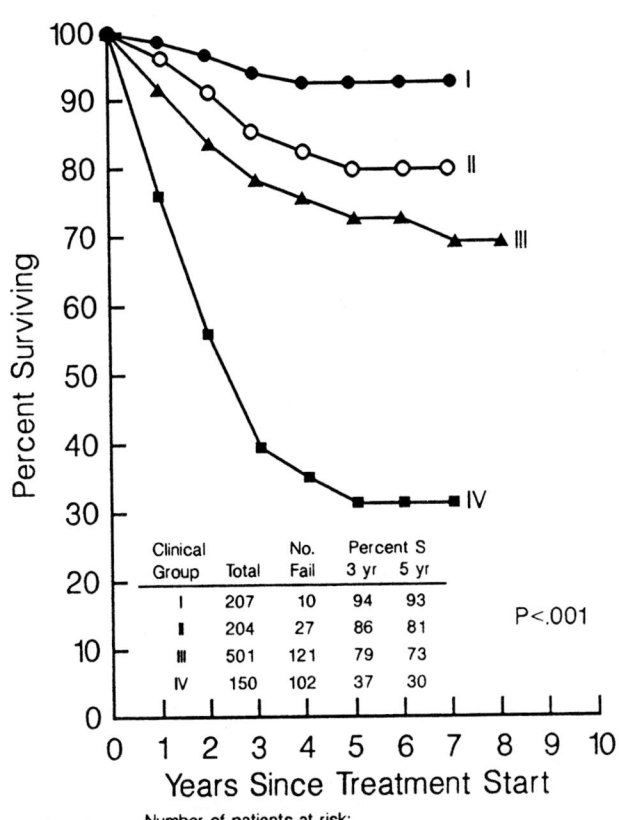

Clinical Group	Total	No. Fail	Percent S 3 yr	Percent S 5 yr
I	207	10	94	93
II	204	27	86	81
III	501	121	79	73
IV	150	102	37	30

P<.001

Number of patients at risk:

Clin. Grp. I	189	151	97	68	42	15	7	-	-	-
Clin. Grp. II	189	154	105	73	41	21	6	-	-	-
Clin. Grp. III	444	381	324	265	179	92	22	1	-	-
Clin. Grp. IV	110	79	55	45	23	13	4	-	-	-

FIG. 4. Survival by clinical group for all patients treated in IRS-III. (From ref. 12, with permission.)

IRS-III (11,12,16,17) (Fig. 5). This relates, at least in part, to the association of site with other tumor and treatment variables. The primary site generally dictates resectability, which in turn determines the IRS grouping (16). Resectability relates to tumor invasiveness and the morbidity that would attend resection. Most orbital lesions are in group III (73.5% in IRS-I, IRS-II, and IRS-III) (51); this is also true for parameningeal (which are never in group I) and genitourinary-bladder/prostate lesions. Conversely, most genitourinary-nonbladder/nonprostate tumors are in group I, and most extremity tumors are in group I or II, or are metastatic (group IV) at diagnosis. Other factors are also relevant to the association of primary site with prognosis.

For example, the tumor location determines the presenting signs and symptoms, which are often related to the rapidity of diagnosis. *Tumor size* (less than or equal to 5 cm versus more than 5 cm), by multivariate analysis, is associated with survival time ($p < 0.001$) (46). Size is also related to tumor site due to presenting symptoms and signs. Primary site influences the propensity for *lymphatic spread* (43) (Table 5). Whereas genitourinary, abdominal/pelvic, and extremity tumors commonly involve regional lymph nodes, tumors in the head and neck, trunk, and female genital organs rarely do so. However, the frequency of lymph node involvement is almost certainly underestimated by IRS data because the assessment of nodal status has not been

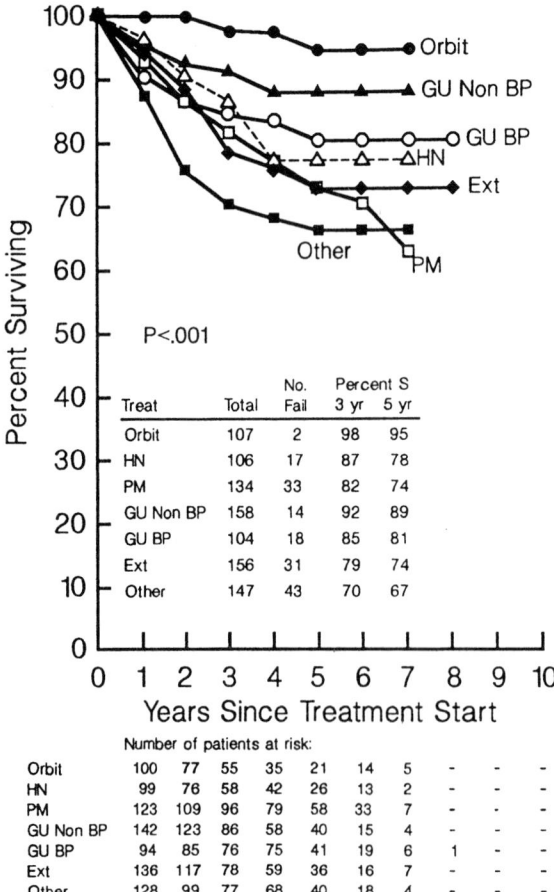

Treat	Total	No. Fail	Percent S 3 yr	5 yr
Orbit	107	2	98	95
HN	106	17	87	78
PM	134	33	82	74
GU Non BP	158	14	92	89
GU BP	104	18	85	81
Ext	156	31	79	74
Other	147	43	70	67

Number of patients at risk:

Orbit	100	77	55	35	21	14	5	-	-	-
HN	99	76	58	42	26	13	2	-	-	-
PM	123	109	96	79	58	33	7	-	-	-
GU Non BP	142	123	86	58	40	15	4	-	-	-
GU BP	94	85	76	75	41	19	6	1	-	-
Ext	136	117	78	59	36	16	7	-	-	-
Other	128	99	77	68	40	18	4	-	-	-

FIG. 5. Survival by primary site for all patients treated in IRS-III. GU Non BP, genitourinary tract non-bladder/prostate; GU BP, genitourinary tract bladder/prostate; HN, head and neck, nonparameningeal; Ext, extremities; PM, parameningeal sites. (From ref. 12, with permission.)

TABLE 5. *Lymph node metastasis by primary site for 592 patients with visibly resected disease[a] from IRS-I and IRS-II[b]*

Site	Number of patients	Number and percentage with nodal metastases
Extremity		
Upper	74	12 (16%)
Lower	107	10 (9%)
Total	181	22 (12%)
Genitourinary organs		
Paratesticular	107	28 (26%) $p = 0.001$[c]
Bladder	29	6 (21%)
Prostate	12	5 (42%) $p = 0.03$
Female genital organs	17	1 (6%)
Other	1	—
Total	166	40 (24%)
Head and neck		
Orbit	39	0 (0%)
Other	96	8 (8%) $p = 0.06$
Total	135	8 (6%)
Other		
Anus-perineum	15	2 (13%)
Pelvis-retroperitoneum	22	5 (23%)
Trunk	65	2 (3%) $p = 0.01$
Abdomen-thorax	8	2 (25%)
Total	110	11 (10%)
Totals	592	81 (14%)

[a]Microscopic or no residual disease.
[b]From ref. 43, with permission.
[c]*p*-values relate to comparison of frequency of nodal metastases for this site compared with the 14% for all 592 patients.

systematic. Data from Stanford and Memorial-Sloan Kettering support the prognostic significance of *lymph node involvement* (24,52). Pedrick et al. (24) showed that 88% of patients presenting with involved nodes had primary tumors that were invasive and extended beyond the site or organ of origin. IRS-IV intends to more consistently document lymph node status.

Histology

The prognosis of RMS has traditionally been associated with *histology*, a finding supported by IRS data (2,11,16,17) and international including SIOP data (18). The estimated percentages of patients surviving for 5 years in IRS-II are, in decreasing order by histology, botryoid RMS 89%, embryonal RMS 68%, alveolar RMS 52%, and all others 55% (16). Histology-associated prognosis was pivotal in construction of the new ICR system

(46) (see "pathology" and Table 1). However, analysis of IRS-III data did not show that, *within the different clinical groups*, histology exerted a prognostic influence (12). This may be due to the more intense chemotherapy administered to patients with alveolar tumors. The distribution of tumor histology also varies by primary site. The more aggressive alveolar type represents about 21% of all RMS cases. It contributes, however, approximately one-half of extremity and perineal tumors. Conversely, over 80% of orbital tumors are the better prognosis embryonal type. Over 90% of genitourinary tumors are embryonal type or sarcoma botryoides (2,16).

Biology

Prognostically relevant *biologic* characteristics of RMS are discussed under "Biology." Briefly, tumor-cell ploidy is related to histologic subtype and treatment outcome. Patients with diploid tumors appear to have a worse prognosis than patients with hyperdiploid tumors (35,36,53). Within the alveolar and embryonal tumor subtypes, tumor-cell ploidy remained an important determinant of survival, even after adjusting for disease stage and anatomic site. Cytogenetic findings of note include specific translocations such as t(2;13), and n-*myc* amplification in alveolar RMS, which portend an extremely poor prognosis (33,38,39).

Other

A variety of other factors have prognostic significance, some of which are general and others specific to certain tumor subgroups. IRS data show that lymphocyte count, patient sex, and age are prognostically relevant (11). Although younger *age* is associated with an improved outcome (52), the specific subgroup of children younger than 1 year with alveolar histology have a significantly poorer survival than do older children, a finding not seen for infants with the embryonal subtype (54,55). Some site specific variables influence outcome. In the head and neck, risk factors that predict tumor access to the cranial subarachnoid space (skull base erosion, cranial nerve palsy, intracranial extension) decrease the likelihood of disease-free survival (51% versus 81% if no risk factors) (44,56, 57). In extremity sites, the presence of lymph node involvement is strongly associated with a high incidence of relapse in metastatic sites and inferior survival (58).

GENERAL PRINCIPLES OF THERAPY

The therapeutic struggle for clinicians managing children with RMS, to cure while minimizing functional and cosmetic deficits, is heightened by the difficulty in eradicating local as well as systemic disease. The spectrum of sites and histologies complicates determination of treatment strategies due to differences in the propensity for local and systemic control as well as treatment sequelae. It is clear that multidisciplinary therapy is

necessary. Aggressive surgery and radiation therapy alone have been curative in less than 25% of children, with the exception of patients with orbital or genitourinary primary sites (59). Conversely, chemotherapy alone is associated with high local failure rates, a lesson learned by attempts to manage orbital or genitourinary tumors by chemotherapy alone (60,61). The judicious use of chemotherapy to eradicate micrometastatic disease and reduce the extent of local disease, and radiation therapy to increase the potential for local control, has led to a decrease in aggressive surgery except in selected situations (10). Progress in treating children with RMS is illustrated by increasing survival rates accomplished by the secession IRS trials from 1967 to 1991 (Fig. 1). The current challenge is to develop approaches to additionally enhance the complementary actions of all three treatment modalities in terms of intensity and sequence.

Surgery

Prior to the advent of radiation and chemotherapy, complete resection of RMS was the clear goal of surgical treatment. This may have involved pelvic exenteration, radical prostatectomy, cystectomy, amputations, and orbital exenterations. Even so, less than 10% of children were amenable to complete resection and curable due to the absence of metastatic disease. Beyond this, most of these children had severe compromise of their quality of life functionally, cosmetically, and psychologically. Select sites that were more frequently curable by aggressive surgery included the orbit and bladder. Using pooled data from IRS-I, IRS-II, and IRS-III, if those patients with overt metastatic disease (group IV) are excluded, then 16% of children have RMS that is minimally invasive and in an accessible site such that complete resection is possible (group I); 20% can undergo a subtotal resection leaving microscopic disease (Fig. 2). In general, achievement of local control and organ preservation with nonradical surgery, radiotherapy, and chemotherapy is the appropriate goal. Although this is often compatible with a complete surgical resection, qualifications and frank exceptions now exist. As discussed, exenterative surgery remains appropriate in certain situations, particularly for salvage therapy.

Reoperation for microscopic residual disease following an initial excision, or when the first operation was performed without knowledge of the type of neoplasm involved, may be indicated prior to additional management. This is called "pretreatment reexcision" or PRE in the IRS guidelines; this is site-dependent. Reoperation following chemotherapy as a "second-look" procedure has proven to be an attractive option (62). Many of these patients will have had a "pathologic" complete response and have a survival similar to patients who had an initial complete resection.

The role of lymph node dissection as a component of surgical therapy continues to evolve. Should clinically involved lymph nodes be resected? Should elective dissections of clinically uninvolved regions be performed? Current guidelines are site specific due to the variability in the frequency of lymph node involvement and outcome data relating to its significance. Genitourinary and extremity RMS have a 10% to 40% incidence of lymph node metastases (43) (Table 5). The prognosis for extremity tumors is influenced by an elective lymph node dissection and is, therefore, indicated. In select patients with paratesticular tumors, routine lymph node sampling but not dissection is advised. This topic will be additionally considered in later sections, because considerations are site specific.

Overall, the extent and timing of surgical excision will depend on the site of tumor and overall treatment strategy, balancing cure with functional outcome.

Chemotherapy

Prior to the 1960s, chemotherapy in RMS was largely reserved for the treatment of metastatic disease. Several investigators reported responses to vincristine and actino-mycin used alone or in combination (VA) and with cyclophosphamide (VAC) (1). Various groups then began to report that the adjuvant administration of chemotherapy for totally or subtotally resected localized disease contributed to an increase in survival probability from 10%–40% to 60%–80% (63). In 1974, Heyn et al. (10) randomized 32 children with completely resected RMS to adjuvant therapy with VA versus no adjuvant therapy. There were 8 deaths among the 15 children in the control group and 2 deaths in the 17 treated children. All children with microscopic residual disease received chemotherapy, and survival rates were excellent.

With the widespread adoption of chemotherapy as part of the therapy of RMS, several trials were undertaken to establish the optimum drug combinations. IRS-I tested whether VAC was superior to VA in group II disease and whether "pulse" VAC plus adriamycin was superior to "pulse" VAC alone in groups II and III disease (Table 6). The study found no benefit to cyclophosphamide in group II diseases, nor did it find a benefit to the addition of adriamycin in groups III and IV (17).

IRS-II built on the results of IRS-I (16) (Table 7). Patients in group I received VAC or VA. Disease-free survival was similar. IRS-II showed no benefit to pulse VAC versus cyclic sequential VA for group II. In groups III and IV, pulse VAC was better than a VAC + adriamycin combination, but not statistically significantly better.

IRS-III began in 1984 and ended in 1991; it separated patients by histology into either a favorable (embryonal) or unfavorable (alveolar, anaplastic, and monomorphous cell types) category. The assignment of therapy according to specific subgroups, results, and lessons learned are outlined in Table 8 (12). Several drug pairs (adriamycin + DTIC, actinomycin-D + VP-16, actinomycin-D + DTIC) appear to have been associated with gain in survival (12).

IRS-IV began in August 1991 and uses the new staging system to assign drug therapy, as previously discussed.

TABLE 6. *Design and results of IRS-I, 1972–1978 (686 patients)*

Clinical group	Chemotherapy regimen	Conventional RT	5-Year survival	Entire group survival
I	VAC × 2 yrs	No	93%	83%
	VAC × 2 yrs	Yes	81%	
II	Cyclic-sequential VA × 1 yr	Yes	73%	71%
	VAC × 2 yrs	Yes	70%	
III	Pulse VAC × 2 yrs	Yes	53%	52%
	Pulse VAC + Adr × 2 yrs	Yes	51%	
IV	Pulse VAC × 2 yrs	Yes	14%	21%
	Pulse VAC + Adr × 2 yrs	Yes	26%	
Overall			55%	

A, dactinomycin; Adr, doxorubicin; C, cyclophosphamide; RT, radiation therapy; V, vincristine.
Modified from ref. 15, with permission.

Overall, in addition to VAC, several drugs are active in RMS. These include DTIC, cisplatin, melphalan, methotrexate, VP-16, and ifosfamide. Doxorubicin continues to be used in European studies. The challenge remains to identify those drug combinations with the most favorable therapeutic ratio when used in combination with the other modalities, and to determine the optimal sequences, doses, and routes of administration.

Radiation Therapy

If one asks the question, "*What prevents cure of RMS?*," a component of the answer is *local/regional disease resistance*. The goal of radiation therapy (RT) is to provide local/regional control, with or without surgery but, currently, always in conjunction with chemotherapy. The optimal multimodal strategy would coordinate RT with these other therapies so as not to impair surgical healing or drug administration. Major considerations would, therefore, include the primary site of the tumor, the extent of surgery, the interaction of RT with chemotherapeutic agents, and any emergent contingencies. An analysis of IRS-II data for group III patients, discussed subsequently, underscores the difficulty that still exists in obtaining local/regional control (19).

TABLE 7. *Design and results of IRS-II, 1978–1984 (1003 patients)*

Clinical group	Chemotherapy	Conventional R	5-Year survival	Entire group survival
I[a]	VA × 1 yr	No	85%	
				81%[b]
	VAC × 2 yrs	No	84%	
II[a]	Cyclic-sequential VA × 1 yr	Yes	88%	
				80%[b]
	Repetitive pulse VAC × 1 yr	Yes	79%	
III	Repetitive pulse VAC × 2 yrs	Yes	66%	
				65%
	Repetitive pulse VAdrC-VAC × 2 yrs	Yes	65%	
IV	Repetitive pulse VAC × 2 yrs	Yes	26%	
				27%
	Repetitive pulse VAdrC-VAC × 2 yrs	Yes	27%	
Overall			62%	63%

A, dactinomycin; Adr, doxorubicin; C, cyclophosphamide; RT, radiation therapy; V, vincristine.
[a]Alveolar/extremity patients excluded in groups I and II; treated with repetitive pulse vincristine/actinomycin-D/cyclophosphamide × 1 to 2 years ± conventional radiotherapy.
[b]Includes extremity alveolar treated differently.
Modified from refs. 15 and 16, with permission.

TABLE 8. *Therapy and outcomes according to specific patient subgroups in IRS-III, 1984–1991 (1032 patients)*

Risk subgroup	Treatment	5-Year progression-free survival, %	5-Year survival, %	Progress (IRS III vs. II)
Group I (favorable histology)	VA × 1 yr	83	93	C not necessary
Group II (favorable histology)	VA × 1 yr + RT	56	54	Need for Adr not proven
	VAdrA × 1 yr + RT	77	89	due to small patient numbers, different histologies compared with IRS-I
Group I and II (unfavorable histology)	VAdrC-VAC + CDDP × 1 yr + RT	71	80	Better than IRS-II due to intense chemo
Group II (paratesticular)	VA × 1 yr + RT	81	81	C not necessary
Group II and III (orbit and head)	VA × 1 yr + RT	78	91	C not necessary
Group III (except special pelvic, orbit, and head sites)	VAC × 2 yrs + RT	70	70	Differences not statistically significant but better than IRS-II due to intense induction chemo, 2nd-look surgery.
	VAdrC-VAC + CDDP × 2 yrs[a] + RT	62	63	
	VAdrC-VAC + CDDP + VP16 × 2 yrs[a] + RT	56	64	
Group III (special pelvic sites)	VAdrAC-VAC + CDDP + VP16 × 2 yrs ± RT ± surgery	74	83	Better than IRS-II due to intense chemo, early RT, 2nd-look surgery. The bladder salvage rate more than doubled (60% vs 25%)
Group IV	VAC × 2 yrs + RT	27	27	No significant differences and no better than IRS-II
	VAdrAC-VAC + CDDP × 2 yrs + RT	27	31	
	VAdrAC-VAC + CDDP + VP16 × 2 yrs + RT	30	29	

A, dactinomycin; Adr, doxorubicin; C, cyclophosphamide; CDDP, cisplatin; reg, regimen; RT, radiation therapy; V, vincristine; VP16, etoposide; DTIC, imidazole carboxamide.

[a]Second-look surgery recommended at week 20, if partial response, patients received Adr + DTIC or A + VP16 or A + DTIC.

Modified from ref. 101, with permission.

The responsiveness of RMS to radiotherapy was established in the 1940s and 1950s (8). Relatively high doses of 50 to 65 Gy were thought to be necessary to achieve local control of the primary tumor regardless of the nature of the surgical procedure. In the setting of postoperative microscopic residual disease, these doses were demonstrated to achieve local control in 90% of cases (9,59,63–66). Because RMS was known to extensively infiltrate tissues, large radiation volumes were initially used as was appropriate for other soft-tissue sarcomas. As the efficacy of chemotherapy for micrometastatic disease became established, and the risk of normal tissue damage due to combined modality therapy was recognized, investigators considered whether equivalent local control rates could be obtained with lower radiation doses and less generous volumes (9). Beyond this, the need for any RT following wide local tumor resection with negative margins was questioned. The IRS studies attempted to systematically examine the issues of radiation dose and volume within the limits imposed by the many chemotherapy questions that were also asked.

IRS-I patients in group I were randomized to receive postoperative RT versus no RT, whereas all other patients were irradiated (Table 6). The dose was adjusted to the patient's age and ranged from 40 to 60 Gy. Daily fractions were 1.5 to 2 Gy, and RT was administered immediately following surgery and protocol randomization for group I patients, and after 6 weeks of chemotherapy for groups III and IV. At 5 years, approximately 80% of the patients in both group I study arms were continuously disease-free. Overall survival was 93% (control) versus 81% (irradiated group, $p = 0.67$) (9,17), which prompted the deletion of RT in group I favorable histology cases for IRS-II. Overall, in IRS-I (9), the dose required for local control appeared to be related to patient age and tumor size. A 32% local recurrence rate was seen after doses less than 40 Gy versus a 12% rate after doses greater than 40 Gy ($p = 0.41$) in the subgroup of children 6 years of age and older. A dose relationship for local control also existed in children who had tumors with a diameter of 6 cm or greater (9). These data were corroborated by the CSTG (22). IRS-I found no dose-response relationship when patients were stratified solely by clinical group (9). The treatment volume was also analyzed for its impact on local failure. Patients who received RT to less than the entire muscle bundle were compared to those whose RT encompassed the entire bundle. In patients younger than 6 years, local control rates were 84% versus 92%, respectively, and in older children rates were 91% versus 85%; these differences were nonsignificant. RT to clinically uninvolved lymph nodes was not encouraged, whereas it was recommended for involved nodal regions. Local control was better in genitourinary sites than in the extremity.

In IRS-II the RT guidelines were modified based on IRS-I results (Table 7). The minimum tumor doses were 40 Gy and 45 Gy for younger (less than 6 years of age) and older children, respectively, but tumors 5 cm or larger received 50 to 55 Gy. The treatment volume was reduced to 5 cm beyond evident tumor. Analyses of local and regional failure have been performed for IRS-II, with local failure defined as initial failure to achieve complete response as well as local relapse following an initial response (16,19). Regional failure is defined as tumor recurrence in lymph nodes adjacent to the primary site or in the same anatomic compartment. For group I patients, those with an unfavorable alveolar histology had a significantly higher frequency of locoregional recurrence than those with favorable histology (65). Although the frequency of local failure was only 10% in group II, it was at 20% for group III (excluding "special pelvic" sites) and 41% for group IV. When local relapse was analyzed as a percentage of all relapses, it accounted for 46% of relapses in group I (despite "complete" surgical removal of tumor) and 36%, 53%, and 20% of relapses in groups II, III, and IV, respectively (16,19). Moreover, the local relapse rate was greater (and survival rates inferior) for patients with unfavorable versus favorable histologic features (41% versus 13%) and for lesions greater than 5 cm versus smaller than 5 cm (34% versus 23%) (64). Locoregional relapse rates were also higher in all groups, and greater than distant relapse rates in all but group IV patients (16). In the recent analysis by Wharam et al. (19), for group III patients, prognostic factors for local failure were identified. Patients with primary tumors in the chest, pelvis, extremity or trunk, or with tumors greater than 10 cm (diameter) had a local failure rate of 35% versus 15% for all other patients. Patients at high risk, 23%, for regional (nodal) failure had node involvement at diagnosis and a primary site other than orbit, parameningeal, or trunk; other patients had a 9% rate. The relevance of radiation dose to local control was suggested by an analysis by Wharam et al. (41) for patients with nonparameningeal head and neck tumors. An increased relapse rate occurred at doses less than 40 Gy, although these data must be interpreted with caution insofar as this was not a randomized dose study. Local control for all patients receiving more than 40 Gy was 93%.

In IRS-III, which accrued 1,062 patients between 1984 and 1991, therapy was assigned or randomized not only by clinical group, but also by histology (with unfavorable types, comprising those with alveolar, anaplastic, and monomorphous cells/patterns) and primary site (Table 8). Postoperative RT was administered to all patients except (a) those in group I with FH tumors, and (b) those in group III with special pelvic sites in complete pathologic remission after primary chemotherapy. The RT dose for group I and II patients was 41.4 Gy. For patients with gross residual disease, the dose was dependent on patient age and tumor size: 41.4 Gy was given for children less than 6-years old with tumors less than 5 cm, 50.4 Gy was given for children 6-years old or older with tumors greater than or equal to 5 cm, and an intermediate dose of 45 Gy was given for children who were either older or had larger tumors, but not both. The overall survival at 5 years is 71%, which is superior to that in IRS-II (63%) and IRS-I (55%) (Table 4) (12). For group III patients, the respective rates are 73% versus 65% versus 52%. Although local control rates of 90% were achieved for patients in groups I and II, local recurrence in patients with group III disease remained unacceptably high, as in IRS-II.

IRS-IV began in August 1991, using the new pretreatment TNM-staging system for the determination of chemotherapy and using the clinical grouping system for assigning radiotherapy. Because of the unsatisfactory local control rates for patients with gross residual disease (group III) in IRS-II and IRS-III, and because of the normal tissue toxicities associated with radiation doses higher than those used in the previous studies, hyperfractionated radiotherapy is being prospectively tested (1.1 Gy b.i.d. to 59.4 Gy versus 1.8 Gy q.i.d. to 50.4 Gy) (13); preliminary data supports its safety. Data from Memorial-Sloan

Kettering (67) and St Jude et al. (68) support the efficacy of this approach.

Although patients will optimally be treated in appropriate institutional or multiinstitutional studies, occasional patients will not be entered into such trials. Until such studies are complete, most cases of bulky local RMS should be treated to at least 50 Gy, and postoperative microscopic disease should be treated to at least 40 Gy (23). A report from St. Jude Children's Research Hospital found that local control was maintained in 10 of 10 evaluable patients who received a mean/median dose of 40 Gy for microscopic residual (IRS group II) disease, which had been cytoreduced from gross disease (group III) using chemotherapy with or without delayed surgery (68). The local control rate for orbital RMS is 93%, and 45 to 50 Gy seems quite satisfactory (66). In cervix, vaginal, and head and neck sites, brachytherapy will allow the administration of a high local dose of irradiation—often with an acceptable risk of morbidity (22,69). It is imperative that when radiotherapy is used in this infiltrative tumor, the prechemotherapy tumor volume is covered with an adequate margin to avoid marginal misses. Margins are based on the confidence with which this volume can be identified and on the location of critical normal tissues that should be excluded. In the setting of surgical reduction of gross disease and multiagent chemotherapy, a 2-cm margin as determined by the prechemotherapy CT or MRI scan is generally appropriate. Every effort is made to shield epiphyses as long as this is consistent with adequate tumor coverage. Brachytherapy may be appropriate in select situations (70).

SPECIFIC SITES

Bladder

Bladder RMS usually arises as a pedunculated mass in the submucosa (see Table 9 for treatment recommendations). Although the tumor may remain intravesical for some period of time, it ultimately develops a broad

TABLE 9. *Therapy recommendations for IRS-IV, 1991–present[a]*

Site	TNM Stage	Clinical Group	Radiation Therapy[b]	Chemotherapy[c]	Operative/RT considerations
Orbit and eyelid	1	I	None	VA	Nonexcisional biopsy appropriate. RT to tumor + margin, not whole orbit.
		II	CRT	VA	
		III	CRT vs HFRT	VAC vs VAI vs VIE	
Other head and neck lymph (nonparameningeal)	1	I	None	VAC vs VAI vs VIE	Cosmetic and functional outcome determine extent of surgery, both at diagnosis or "2nd look". Biopsy suspicious nodes; if (+), consider excision.
		II	CRT	VAC vs VAI vs VIE	
		III	CRT vs HFRT	VAC vs VAI vs VIE	
Paratesticular	1	I	None	VA	Orchidectomy, resect entire spermatic cord via inguinal incision. Sample abdominal/pelvic nodes except if Group I. (+) inguinal nodes denote distant spread (Stage 4). If scrotal skin involved or violated, area is resected and irradiated.
		II	CRT	VAC vs VAI vs VIE	
		III	CRT vs HFRT	VAC vs VAI vs VIE	
Vulva and vagina	1	I	None	VAC vs VAI vs VIE	"Radical" excision inappropriate. Gross excision often possible at "2nd look" at week 9. Biopsy suspicious nodes but dissection inappropriate. Brachytherapy may be used.
		II	CRT	VAC vs VAI vs VIE	
		III	CRT	VAC vs VAI vs VIE	
Uterus/Cervix	1	I	None	VAC vs VAI vs VIE	Hysterectomy only if necessary. Preserve ovaries and vagina if possible.
		II	CRT	VAC vs VAI vs VIE	
		III	CRT vs HFRT	VAC vs VAI vs VIE	
Cranial parameningeal	2/3	I	None for Stage 2 CRT for Stage 3	VAC vs VAI vs VIE	Cosmetic and functional outcome determine extent of surgery, both at diagnosis or "2nd look". Biopsy suspicious nodes; if (+), consider excision. RT at day 0 for limited intracranial extension, base of skull erosion, or cranial neuropathy. Otherwise RT at wk 9. Use 2 cm margin on intracranial disease.
		II	CRT	VAC vs VAI vs VIE	
		III	CRT vs HFRT	VAC vs VAI vs VIE	

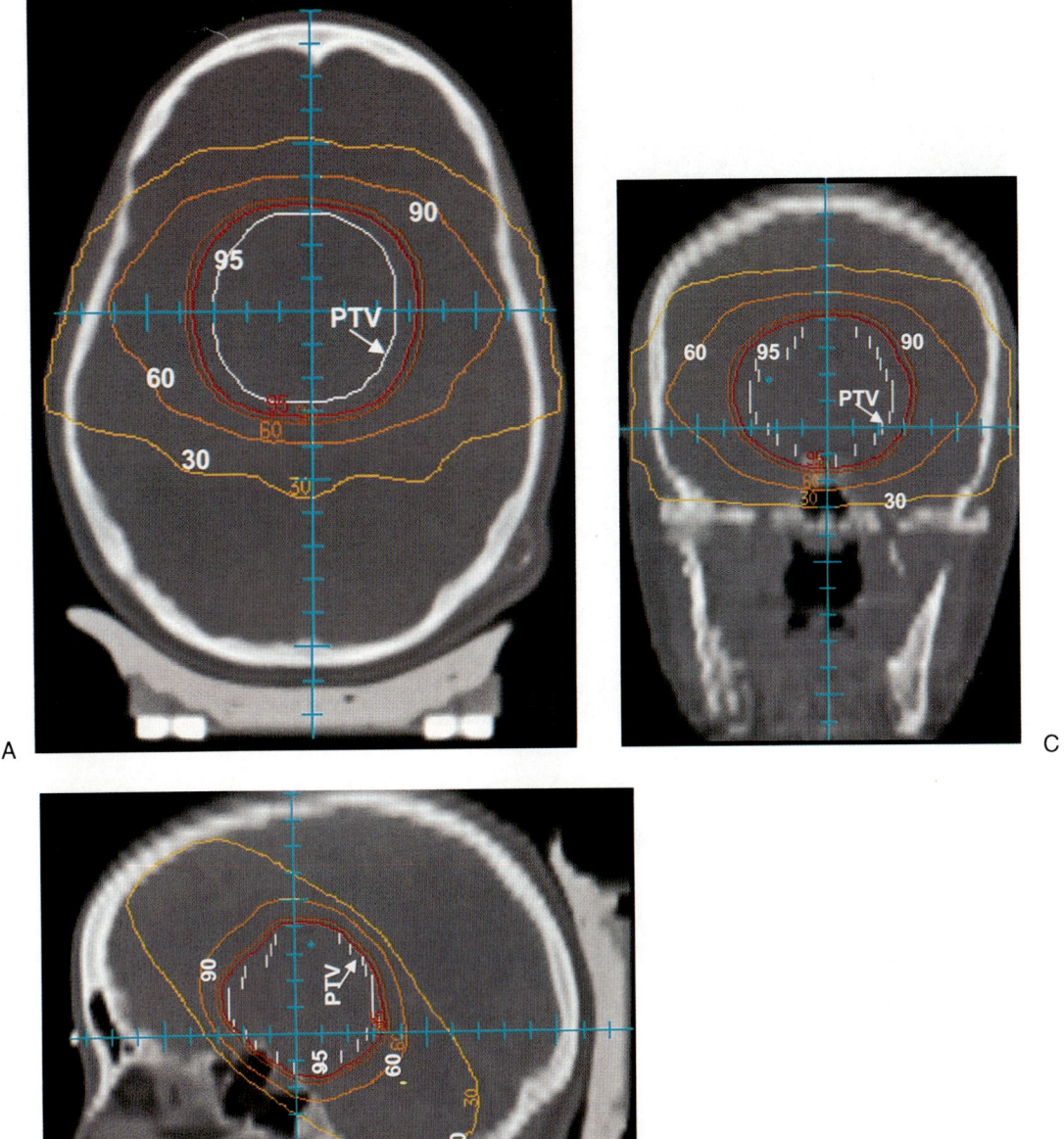

COLORPLATE 1. (A, B, C) Three-dimensional conformal planning for central diencephalic astrocytoma, an approach that achieves conformation of dose (here 54 Gy) to the lesion through six noncoplanar fields.

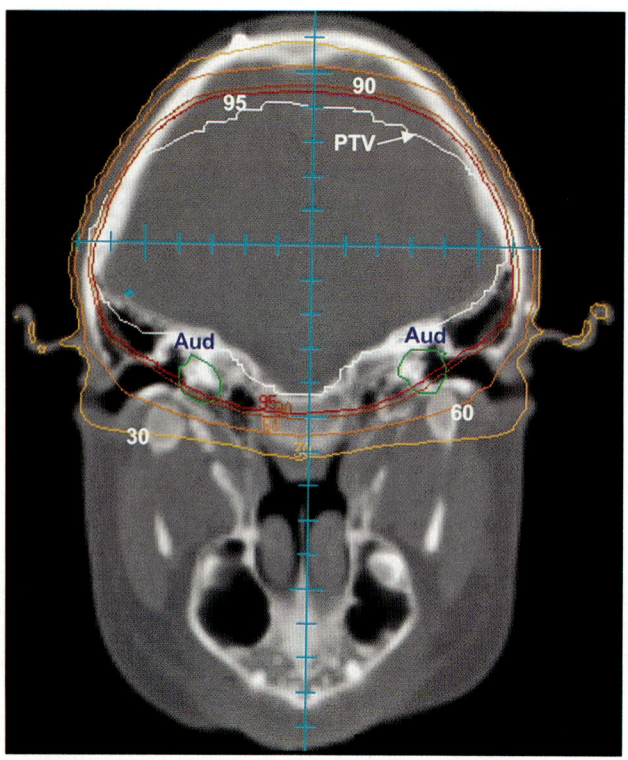

A

COLORPLATE 2. (A, B) Three-dimensional conformal approach to encompass the posterior fossa, utilizing four noncoplanar fields; note the dose distribution in the region of the hearing apparatus is relatively diminished for this component of therapy.

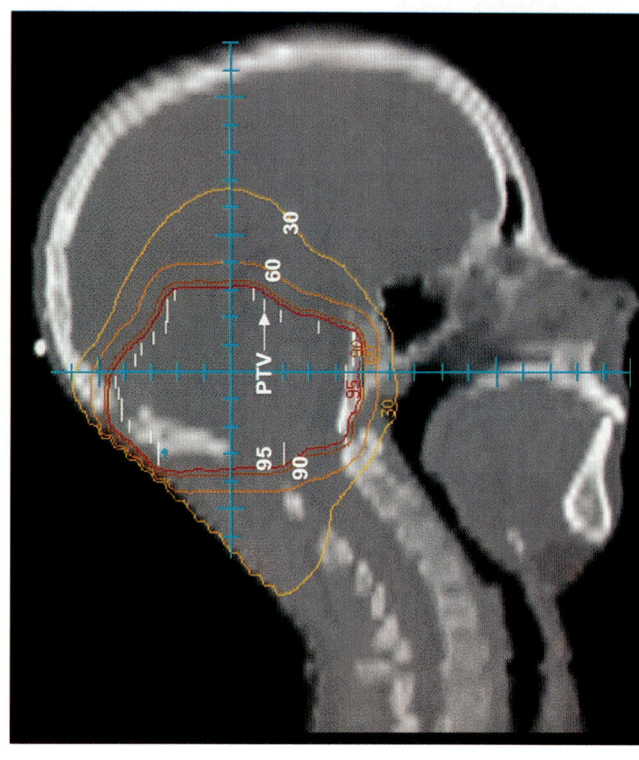

B

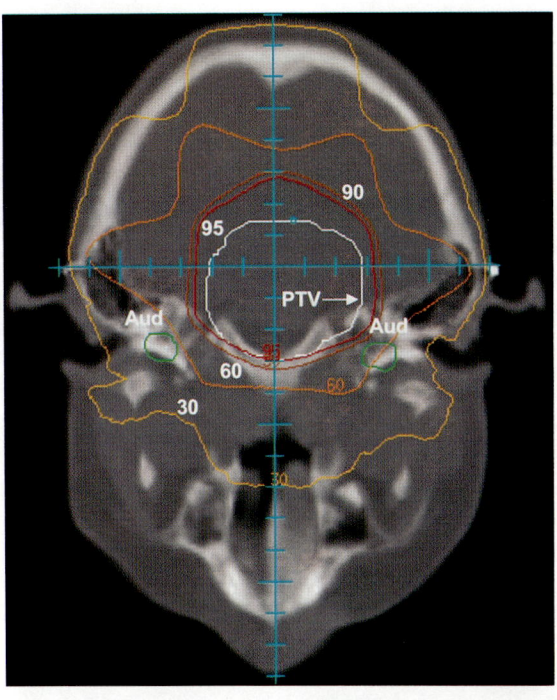

A

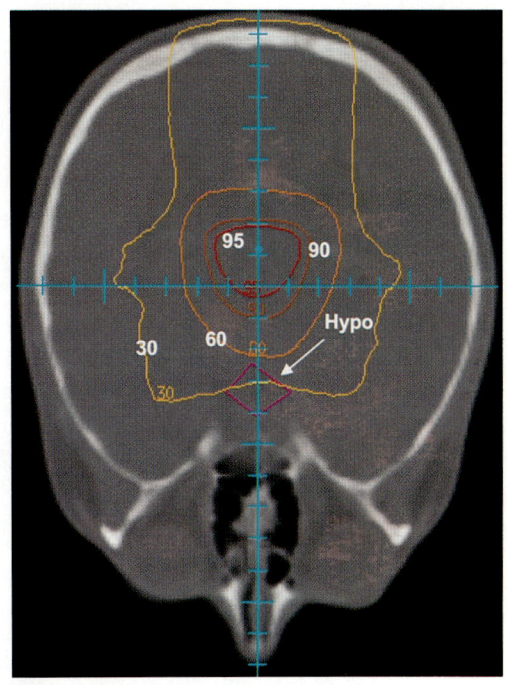

B

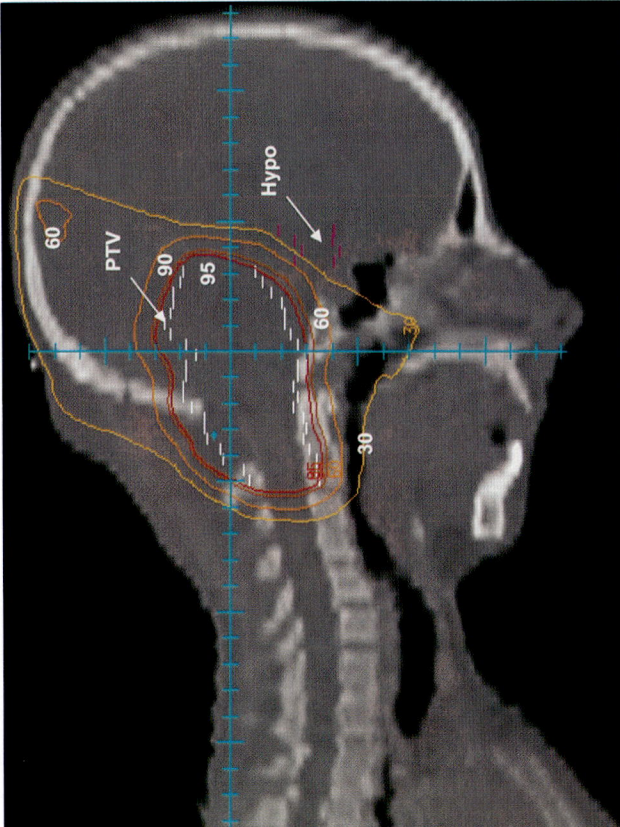

C

COLORPLATE 3. (A, B, C) Three-dimensional conformal approach for treating ependymoma following near total resection, targeting the tumor bed with a 1.5 cm margin (defining the somewhat broader PTV). The 3-field noncoplanar approach achieves relative dose conformation and relatively spares the hearing apparatus (Aud), as well as the pituitary-hypothalamic region (Hypo).

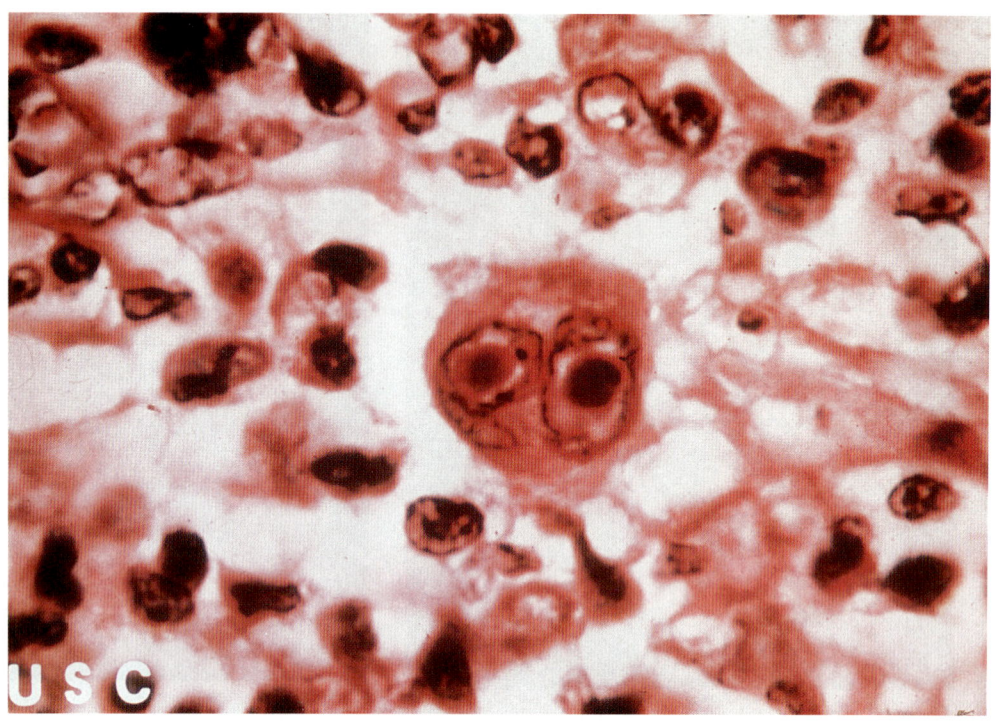

COLORPLATE 4. Reed-Sternberg cell.

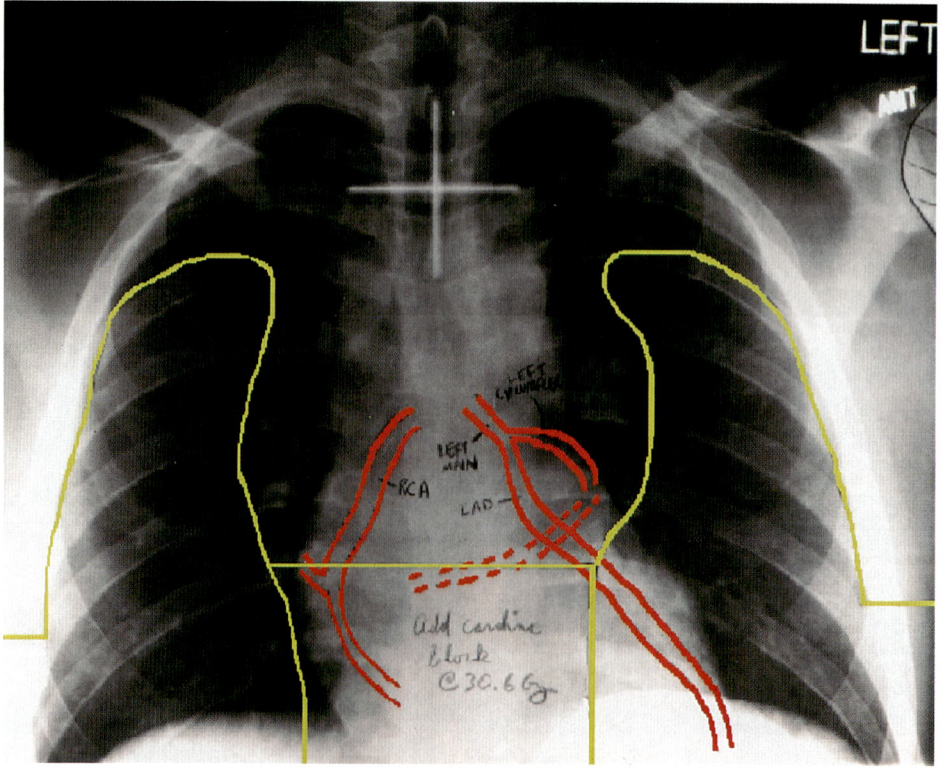

COLORPLATE 5. Location of the coronary vessels (red lines) on a standard mantle field is illustrated. The blocks are outlined in yellow.

Site		Group	RT	Chemotherapy	Surgery/Comments
Extremity	2/3	I	None for Stage 2, CRT for Stage 3	VAC vs VAI vs VIE	Wide or radical limb-sparing resection to remove gross and microscopic tumor. Sample regional nodes. If (+), sample more proximal group. Involvement of supraclavicular or iliac/paraaortic nodes denotes distant spread (Stage 4). 2cm margins advised but avoid circumferential RT.
		II	CRT	VAC vs VAI vs VIE	
		III	CRT vs HFRT	VAC vs VAI vs VIE	
Genitourinary (bladder and prostate)	2/3	I	None for Stage 2, CRT for Stage 3	VAC vs VAi vs VIE	Goal is preservation of bladder and urethral function. Total resection with partial cystectomy if possible, either at diagnosis or "2nd look" after chemo/RT. Extirpative surgery may be necessary if residual disease post chemo/RT. Node sampling (iliac and paraaortic) only if laparotomy.
		II	CRT	VAC vs VAI vs VIE	
		III	CRT vs HFRT	VAC vs VAI vs VIE	
Chest wall, trunk, retroperitoneum, and other	2/3	I	None for Stage 2, CRT for Stage 3	VAC vs VAI vs VIE	Wide excision if feasible, either at diagnosis, as reexcision pre-chemo, or "2nd look". RT for abdominal tumors usually entails multiple cone downs.
		II	CRT	VAC vs VAI vs VIE	
		III	CRT vs HFRT	VAC vs VAI vs VIE	
Any site	4	I	CRT	Adr/I vs V/Mel vs I/E	For gross residual disease, RT begins at week 18.5 (except for select parameningeal tumors.) Whole lung RT for nodules with boost if possible. Pulmonary nodules can be resected post chemo/RT if acceptable lung function is preserved.
		II	CRT	Adr/I vs V/Mel vs I/E	
		III	CRT	Adr/I vs V/Mel vs I/E	

[a]Modified from ref. 100, with permission.
[b]CRT for any Group I or Group II patient is 41.4 Gy; CRT for any Group III patient is 50.4 Gy; HFRT for any Group III patient is 59.4 Gy.
[c]All chemotherapy regiments followed by VAC.
A, actinomycin D; C, cyclophosphamide; E, etoposide; I, ifosfamide; V, vincristine; Adr, doxorubicin; Mel, melphalan; CRT, conventional fractionation; HFRT, hyperfractionation.

base and invades the bladder wall. In most boys, the tumor arises in the bladder neck and then invades the prostate, making difficult the distinction between primary bladder and prostate RMS on clinical findings alone. RMS in these two sites account for about one-half of pelvic RMS and usually occurs in younger children. Urinary abnormalities—including dysuria, polyuria, and, in particular, retention—are early signs. Ultrasound can greatly assist in defining the tumor, and cystoscopy frequently allows histologic diagnosis (1). Over 90% of tumors are embryonal, including the botryoid subtype, which accounts for one-third. Regional lymph node involvement is documented in about 20% (16). The hypogastric or external iliac nodes are most commonly involved, although spread to lumboaortic nodes may occur, even in isolation. Only 15% have demonstrable metastases at diagnosis. It was clearly demonstrated in the prechemotherapy era that 10% to 40% of patients could be cured by exenteration alone (71). Treatment programs were subsequently designed to improve the cure rate and to increase bladder preservation (42).

The SIOP attempted to achieve local control of bladder (and prostate) RMS with a program emphasizing chemotherapy alone; however, complete responses were not achieved. Small single-institution studies have generally used surgery, chemotherapy, and RT.

IRS-I provided data that suggested that limited surgery (partial cystectomy or "tumorectomy") followed by RT and chemotherapy might allow preservation of the bladder with excellent cure rates (72). Although one-third of patients underwent pelvic exenteration, most patients who underwent bladder preserving surgery ultimately retained their bladder. IRS-II adopted a strategy using more vigorous primary chemotherapy with the intention of using minimal surgery to remove residual tumor (followed by additional chemotherapy) and avoiding the morbidity of pelvic irradiation. RT was added in the setting of residual (postsurgical) disease or if an exenterative procedure would be required. Almost all patients eventually required either RT, surgery,

or both to achieve a complete remission. Although the 3-year survival for these patients was similar (70%) to that in IRS-I (78%), the 3-year disease-free survival rate was significantly inferior (52% versus 70%). Although the bladder preservation rate was initially higher in IRS-II (97%) than in IRS-I (58%), the percentage of patients who retained their bladder and were alive at 3 years was only 22%, compared with 23% in IRS-I (72,73). The delay of irradiation to week 16 was a negative prognostic factor, impairing the likelihood of local control (9,22).

IRS-III investigators approached the problem of bladder tumors with a view of what appeared to limit successful bladder preservation in IRS-I and IRS-II; therefore, RT was routinely administered to all patients at week 6, after induction chemotherapy, except those in whom complete removal of all tumor was possible without total cystectomy. Surgery was then performed to document a complete response or to excise residual tumor while attempting to maintain bladder function. The results of IRS-III have been gratifying: the bladder retention rate at 4 years was 60% and survival was 90% for patients presenting with local/regional disease. An analysis of the 28 group III patients by Heyn et al. (74) showed that 15 (54%) ultimately retained their bladder. Induction chemoradiotherapy induced a complete loss of tumor cells in 46%; in cystectomy specimens tumor cellularity was reduced and tumor cell maturation occurred. Of interest is that cellular maturation was greater in tumor specimens of patients who retained their bladder (74).

Table 10 demonstrates how the treatment philosophies of IRS-I, IRS-II, and IRS-III converted into an influence on clinical grouping. The number of patients in groups I and II fell significantly during successive studies. This was the result of an increasing emphasis on primary chemotherapeutic approaches in an attempt to preserve the bladder and a move away from aggressive up-front surgery.

In determining the optimum therapeutic approach for bladder tumors, the site of the lesion is relevant; tumors in the dome are more

TABLE 10. *Distribution of patients with localized bladder and prostate tumors by clinical group in IRS-I, IRS-II, and IRS-III*

Study/ group	I	II	III	Total
IRS-I	13(20%)	21(32%)	32(48%)	66
IRS-II	1(1%)	3(3%)	91(96%)	95
IRS-III	9(9%)	7(7%)	88(85%)	104
Total	23(9%)	31(12%)	211(80%)	265

The numbers in parentheses are % of the individual row totals.

From refs. 12,36,53,60,71,75,102, with permission.

commonly resectable at diagnosis than trigone or bladder neck tumors. IRS-IV also recommends bladder preserving surgery at "second look" after induction chemoradiotherapy, if possible (60). However, if viable RMS persists after induction therapy, then extirpative surgery may be necessary. The RT technique for pelvic tumors is somewhat controversial. Many radiotherapists utilize a four-field box or arcs similar to those used in adults. In children, however, high-energy megavoltage photon fields with anteroposterior-posteroanterior technique often give good dosimetry. The use of simple anterior and posterior fields allows shielding of the femoral epiphyseal plates and proximal femurs. Multiportal technique may not improve upon the dose distribution obtained with the simpler technique (22). Careful, long-term follow-up of patients is necessary in order to diagnose and manage treatment-related normal tissue damage (75).

Prostate

While bladder RMS could, on occasion, be cured with radical surgery alone, prostatic RMS is far less amenable to this approach. Not only do primary prostate tumors tend to be more locally invasive, they also tend to disseminate earlier (22). Symptoms are similar to those of bladder tumors through compression of the base of the bladder and infiltration of the bladder neck and urethra.

In IRS-I, 14 patients had nondisseminated prostatic primary tumors and were treated with exenteration. Only one patient died, and this death was therapy-related. Eleven patients were treated with a primary chemotherapy program without radical surgery. Two patients died of RMS and two of the survivors later required urinary diversion or exenteration, leaving 7 of the 11 with normal bladder function (71).

The treatment strategy in IRS-II was the same as that for patients with bladder RMS, but the 3-year survival was inferior (59%) to that of patients with prostate RMS in IRS-I (82%) and also inferior to that of patients with primary bladder RMS in either study (70% to 81%) (73). In addition, approximately one-half of all patients had lost their bladder by 3 years. It is, however, also noteworthy that patients with pelvic primary tumors who had the botryoid subtype had a higher survival rate than those with the solid embryonal subtype. This is relevant because botryoid tumors were almost exclusively found in patients with vaginal and bladder primaries, and nonbotryoid tumors were found in patients with prostate primaries. Beyond this, the prostatic lesions tended to be larger than their counterparts in the vagina and bladder (73). This experience suggests that children with prostatic RMS have a worse outlook than those with other pelvic primary RMS, and that definitive local control measures should not be delayed for primary chemotherapy (Table 11).

TABLE 11. *Three-year treatment results for patients with bladder and prostate tumors in IRS-I, IRS-II, and IRS-III*

Study/ outcome	Overall survival	Disease-free survival	Alive with functioning bladder
IRS-I	75%	68%	23%
IRS-II	71%	56%	22%
IRS-III	81%	73%	60%[a]

[a]In IRS-III the data is presented as "bladder salvage rate"; presumably at 5 years, for bladder, prostate, vagina, and other central pelvic sites. A "bladder salvage rate" for those cured of 64% has been reported for prostate patients.

From refs. 12,60,71,72,73,75,102,103,104,105,106, with permission.

Paratesticular

Intrascrotal paratesticular RMS usually arises in the distal area of the spermatic cord and may invade the testis or surrounding tissues, although primary RMS of the epididymis or tunics can also occur (1). It frequently spreads through the lymphatics to the paraaortic nodes, following the course of the spermatic cord into the renal hilar retroperitoneal space. It often presents as a unilateral painless scrotal swelling, and may grow to a considerable size before the patient is diagnosed. An orchiectomy is performed through an inguinal incision with a high ligation of the spermatic cord at the level of the inguinal ring.

Lymphangiography and CT are used to detect gross nodal involvement, but may fail to demonstrate microscopic infiltration in some patients. Consequently, it has been the practice in the United States to perform a unilateral (transabdominal) nerve-sparing retroperitoneal lymph node dissection. Twenty-six percent of patients in IRS-I and IRS-II had retroperitoneal lymph node involvement at diagnosis, and 16% had positive ipsilateral inguinal nodes; contralateral nodal involvement is rare (22,76). A similar percentage of patients in IRS-III had nodal disease (77). Patients with group II disease on the basis of positive nodes receive RT to the nodal areas in the IRS studies, in contrast to patients with negative lymph node dissections.

It is not absolutely certain that a lymph node dissection or nodal irradiation in the absence of involvement by imaging studies is necessary. In the United Kingdom CSTG, 14 paratesticular RMS cases treated with VAC did not have a lymph node dissection, and undissected nodes did not appear to be a high-risk site of regional relapse (22). SIOP investigators have successfully used multiagent chemotherapy alone to sterilize micrometastases. However, preliminary data from IRS-IV suggest that CT imaging indicates lymph node involvement in less than 10% of patients, and these patients have an inferior progression-free survival than surgically staged patients (42). Current IRS-IV recommendations are that systematic sampling of ipsilateral high and low infrarenal and bilateral iliac nodes be performed, except in group I patients. Positive inguinal lymph nodes are considered to represent distant spread.

If a transcrotal biopsy is performed instead of using the inguinal approach, then the patient is considered to have group II disease and the hemiscrotum is irradiated. Resection of the violated scrotal tissue is necessary, and even hemiscrotectomy should be considered. The contralateral testicle can be transposed laterally into the thigh prior to irradiation and later reimplanted into the scrotum.

The 5-year survival of patients treated for paratesticular RMS exceeds 80% (12,22,76).

Vagina and Vulva

RMS of the vagina most commonly occurs in very young children (90% less than 5 years of age). It commonly presents as a mass or discharge, and is almost exclusively the embryonal (usually botryoid) subtype. The mean age of girls with vulvar tumors is 8 years (78). Vulval inflammation and genital bleeding are the most common presenting signs. Vulvar RMS is most commonly found as a firm nodule embedded in the labial folds or in a periclitoric location and is often of the alveolar subtype (1). Vaginal tumors most commonly arise from the anterior wall, are frequently multicentric, and can invade the vesicovaginal septum or bladder wall. Regional nodal involvement is uncommon (1). The classic surgical technique for treatment of vaginal tumors was an anterior exenteration with urinary diversion. Occasionally, this was accompanied by resection of the adjacent colon. Unfortunately, less than 20% of patients could be cured with surgery alone (79), and only 25% with chemotherapy alone. Survival rates did improve to 60% to 80% when chemotherapy was added to extirpative surgery, with or without RT. Attempts to minimize the surgical procedure, in the absence of adjuvant RT, led to an unacceptably high rate of local recurrence. Vulvar tumors are frequently localized and curable with wide excision, usually hemivulvectomy, followed by chemotherapy with or without RT (80).

In order to better integrate all three treatment modalities, IRS-II adopted a strategy that included second-look surgery at either week 8 or 16, depending on the response to chemotherapy. The use of RT depended on the completeness of the surgical procedure. Limited surgery (partial vaginectomy) was preferred when the procedure was expected to result in the removal of all visible tumor (73). Using this treatment approach, 18 of 21 (86%) patients were surviving at 3 years (73). Current guidelines are similar; limited surgery is preferred, and can be performed as a second look at week 9. Suspicious nodes are biopsied but dissections are inappropriate. Complete surgical excision for these patients is more likely than in those with bladder or prostate tumors, and RT is not given if excision is complete. When radiation is required, teletherapy is most common, although intracavitary or interstitial brachytherapy may be possible (22,81). This approach has been successful at the Institut Gustave-Roussy (69). Either technique should strive to minimize the RT dose to the ovaries (which at times should be transposed outside the primary radiation volume), hips, and pelvic organs. Over 90% of children are expected to survive.

Uterus and Cervix

Uterine/cervix RMS is much less common than vaginal RMS, and it tends to occur in adolescent girls near the time of puberty. Patients may present with pedunculated polyps with vaginal extrusion of tumor tissue, or with a pelvic mass due to diffuse intramural involvement; bleeding is common (81,82). When uterine tumors occur in younger children, distinction from a vaginal tumor may be difficult. Sometimes this is possible only after regression of the tumor following chemotherapy.

In IRS-I and IRS-II, 13 patients had uterine (5 patients) or cervical (8 patients) primaries. In patients who presented with localized poly-poid tumors, polypectomy and adjuvant chemotherapy were highly curative. When hysterectomy/vaginectomy successfully removed all gross tumor, cure was also likely. Conversely, patients with group III or IV RMS died (78,81). Brand et al. (82) reviewed 21 cases of sarcoma botryoides of the uterine cervix. Most received chemotherapy and eight received pelvic irradiation. Eighty percent of these patients survived.

Currently, treatment of uterine/cervix RMS is intended to preserve pelvic organs when possible. Patients with initially resectable disease are placed in group I or II by surgery, followed by chemotherapy, and then RT only if microscopic residual disease is proven to persist. For those with group III disease, primary chemotherapy is given followed by a second-look laparotomy. If there is gross residual that cannot be completely resected or if microscopic disease is found after resection, the patient then receives RT and continues on chemotherapy. If the second-look exploration shows no demonstrable tumor or tumor that is completely resected, then no radiotherapy is given and the patient continues on chemotherapy alone. Survival rates should approximate those of the vagina and vulva (42,83).

Extremity

Extremity lesions have a relatively poor prognosis (Fig. 1). Approximately one-half of these lesions are unfavorable histology alveolar RMS (Table 3). In IRS-I and IRS-II, regional lymph node involvement occurred in 15% and 9% of patients with upper- and lower-extremity lesions, respectively (43,84).

The prognosis for patients with extremity RMS is compromised by the high frequency (50%) of the alveolar subtype, of lymphatic metastasis at diagnosis, and of metastasis to any site at diagnosis (27% versus 18% in all RMS patients) (85). Although there is no evidence that amputation is more often curative than wide local excision, this procedure retains a role in patients where limited excision and high-dose irradiation would produce unacceptable functional results, in patients with distal (alveolar) extremity lesions where gross removal is otherwise impossible, and in patients with massive local recurrences following conservative therapy (1). The preferred operative procedure for primary management is wide excision with negative margins and adjacent lymph node group sampling. In IRS-IV, the axilla or inguinal regions are explored even in the absence of clinically evident nodal involvement. Chemotherapy is always given. RT is omitted only for patients with completely resected small (less than 5 cm) tumors with negative nodes. The tumor is treated with a 2 cm margin, and regional lymph nodes only when involved. One should spare a strip of soft tissue along the extremity to avoid late radiation-induced extremity edema.

Parameningeal

Parameningeal (PM) RMSs include those arising in the skull base and, therefore, can extend intracranially and produce neoplastic meningitis, which occurs in about 35% (44,86). In IRS-III, PM RMS comprised 41% of head and neck tumors, and 15% of all tumors. Most patients were under age 10 years (72%) (12). Middle ear tumors extend through the tegmen tympani to middle cranial fossa meninges, or through the posterior mastoid to the posterior cranial fossa. Tumors of the nasal cavity, paranasal sinus, and nasopharynx extend to meninges through the basal foramina or sinus roofs. Nasopharyngeal RMS invades the base of skull in 35% of patients, involving the cavernous sinus and causing cranial nerve palsies (1,56,86). Although lymph node involvement was previously thought to be common, in IRS-III, less than 20% were classified as node-positive (1,44). The ratio of embryonal to alveolar histology is 4:1. Meningeal penetration and leptomeningeal tumor cell seeding must be assessed in PM patients. Complete surgical extirpation of the primary with a satisfactory cosmetic and functional result is almost never possible; in IRS-III 76% of patients were group III. The role of surgery, therefore, is confined to establishing a diagnosis with a

biopsy and/or a subtotal excision. Cervical lymph node dissection (radical neck) is rarely appropriate because of the morbidity and relatively low frequency of subclinical nodal involvement; conversely, suspicious nodes should be examined. Prior to the use of chemotherapy, less than 20% of patients survived despite intense irradiation (63,86).

For patients with PM RMS, the volume and timing of RT are critical. The volume of irradiation appropriate for parameningeal lesions has required reevaluation in light of the experience in IRS and advances in imaging. Meningeal extension is associated with a high risk of CNS relapse and a 90% chance of death. In IRS-I, meningeal extension following radiotherapy appeared to be associated with inadequately small fields and doses less than 50 Gy (57,86). These findings prompted a call for the use of local treatment plus cranial or craniospinal irradiation (CSI). Follow-up analysis of the IRS-I patients suggested that part of the risk of CNS relapse was engendered by fields that were too tight but that widespread use of full cranial irradiation was unlikely to increase disease control and would increase morbidity, a conclusion supported by non-IRS data (87). In IRS-III, if there was no evidence of intracranial extension, CSF cytology was negative, and bone erosion or cranial nerve palsies were absent, then the primary lesion was irradiated with a 5-cm margin—including treatment of the adjacent meninges. Patients not meeting these criteria received IT chemotherapy. If the CT or MRI demonstrated in continuity intracranial extension of the primary tumor, but the CSF cytology was negative, prophylactic whole-brain irradiation was given along with treatment to the primary tumor. Finally, for positive CSF cytology, CSI was given. Results are as follows: (a) 69% 5-year progression-free survival, (b) 15% local failure for group III patients, and (c) a 4.7% contiguous CNS relapse (44). Based on IRS-II data, three risk factors for tumor access to the cranial subarachnoid space were determined: skull base erosion, cranial nerve palsy, and intracranial extension. Patients with any risk factor had a 51% 3-year progression-free survival, versus 81% for other patients. In IRS-IV the radiation margin is reduced to 2 cm, and only patients with diffuse intracranial meningeal extension or multiple sites of brain parenchymal disease are treated to the entire cranial cavity. When there is clear evidence of meningeal (including base of skull erosion or nerve palsies) or intracranial extension, RT is given at the beginning of the treatment course. Otherwise, chemotherapy is given first with RT given at week 9. RT is omitted only for patients with completely resected small (less than 5 cm) tumors with negative nodes. The extent of surgery is determined by the potential cosmetic and functional outcome, and second-look procedures may be effectively performed (88). Of interest is a recent analysis comparing outcome for PM RMS treated on IRS and three European cooperative groups. For low-risk patients, 5-year survival was superior in IRS, possibly due to early routine RT, the IRS quality assurance program, and inclusion of patients with smaller tumors without involved lymph nodes (89).

Other Head and Neck Sites

Parotid region, oral cavity, oropharynx, and larynx RMSs generally have an embryonal histology. Cheek and scalp lesions have a high frequency of alveolar histology (41). Superficial lesions may be marginally or, at times, widely resected with satisfactory cosmesis and function—a situation that less often appertains for deeper tumors. Optimal cosmesis with excellent disease control may best be obtained with a marginal resection and subsequent RT. For the deeper tumors (oral cavity, buccal mucosa, larynx, parapharyngeal, or parotid region), RT is generally necessary. Because of the relatively favorable outlook for patients with nonparameningeal head and neck tumors, such patients are classified as stage I in IRS-IV and, therefore, receive less intense chemotherapy than do the PM head and neck tumors. However, if a nonparameningeal head and neck tumor extends to and invades a parameningeal region, then it should be treated as a PM RMS.

Although the early experience with head and neck RMS suggested that lymph node involvement was uncommon (8% in IRS-I and IRS-II), this may have resulted from less than thorough assessments. In support of this is that lymph nodes were in fact positive in 20% of patients in whom lymph node status was reported (41). Donaldson et al. (63) reported a similar incidence. Involved lymph node groups may be resected as well as irradiated.

Orbit

Because of the accessibility of the orbit to examination, and the sensitivity of ocular function to mass effect, orbital RMS is often diagnosed relatively early. Eyelid swelling and globe displacement are common presenting signs. Orbital exenteration was the standard treatment to the mid-1960s, but rarely achieved local control or survival. In the late 1960s, Cassady and co-workers (7,59) observed that RT afforded local control in 5 of 5 patients following a biopsy. RT has now assumed a major role in the treatment of orbital RMS. Approximately two-thirds of cases are group III. Treatment is with biopsy, chemotherapy, and RT. The volume need not include the entire orbit if the tumor is small. In the IRS study, local control has been 94% with RT and is increased to 98% with surgical salvage (66). Of note is that orbital RMS can also invade meninges via erosion of the superior orbital fissure. A recent analysis of IRS data suggested a relationship of histology to outcome. For the 84% with embryonal histologies, the 5-year survival was 94%. However, for the 10% of children with alveolar RMS, this rate was 74%, and all five infants with alveolar disease died (51). Because of the favorable outcome of patients with orbital RMS, investigators have attempted to use chemotherapy alone (61). Local control and survival are compromised by this strategy.

The late adverse effects of orbital irradiation are considerable, because the minimum irradiated volume appropriately includes all bony limits of the orbit—larger if there is extension into adjacent soft tissue or bone (see

Table 5 in Chapter 19) (90). It is important to treat the child with the eye open to avoid the bolus effect of the lids.

Trunk

Truncal sites include the chest wall, paraspinal area, and the abdominal wall, in decreasing order of frequency. Scapular and buttock lesions are considered to be extensions of the extremity, and retroperitoneal and perineal tumors are considered separately. An early IRS report focused on 30 children with soft-tissue sarcoma of the trunk (91). Ten of the 14 children with chest wall primaries had group I to III disease, and five were long-term survivors. None of the four children with metastases at diagnosis survived.

Paraspinal tumors were rare (3.3%) in IRS-I and IRS-II. They tended to be greater than 5 cm in diameter, often invaded the spinal extradural space, and were commonly of an undifferentiated or extraosseous Ewing's subtype. Survival at 5 years was approximately 50% in both studies (92). Local and distant relapses were frequent, and patients with embryonal subtypes fared no better than others.

Current guidelines include as wide a surgical resection as is feasible, either at diagnosis, or after chemoradiotherapy as a second look. For patients with an initial excision that was less aggressive than feasible, or of an uncertain nature, a primary reexcision should be considered. RT is given to all patients except those with completely excised small tumors and uninvolved lymph nodes. RT fields encompass the original disease extent, and chemotherapy is always used (91,92).

Retroperitoneal

Retroperitoneal tumors are frequently large at diagnosis, probably due to the considerable room for expansion prior to causing symptoms (93). These tumors are technically difficult to resect, and lymph node involvement is common (23% in IRS-I, IRS-II for retroperitoneal pelvic tumors). Therefore, most patients have group III or IV disease. Not only is resection problematic, but the aggressiveness of RT is compromised by the tolerance of normal tissue, in terms both of volume and dose. In the IRS, 39% of patients with retroperitoneal RMS had difficulties in delivery of the specified RT. All these factors combine to render the prognosis for retroperitoneal RMS worse than for most others sites; 5-year survival was approximately 40% in IRS-II (16,93) (Fig. 1). Guidelines are essentially the same as those noted previously for truncal tumors. Because of normal tissue tolerance, RT usually involves multiple reductions in field size.

Perineal

Perineal tumors, in IRS-I and IRS-II, were most commonly alveolar (56%) or embryonal (30%), and patients were equally likely to have negative or microscopic versus gross residual disease after surgery (94). The 3-year survival was 59%, which was somewhat inferior to that of patients with disease in other sites (16,94). The approach to these patients also entails as complete a resection as "functionally" acceptable followed by chemotherapy and RT as appropriate.

Hepatobiliary Tree

The common bile duct, the common, right, or left hepatic duct, and the ampulla of Vater may also be sites for RMS. An early IRS report on ten cases noted that all had embryonal histology with varying degrees of botryoid features. The most common presentation included intermittent obstructive jaundice with or without abdominal distention, fever, pain, and loss of appetite. Resection of the mass with only microscopic or minimal gross residual disease was possible in six cases. Chemotherapy and RT consistent with the IRS protocols was given postoperatively; four patients, all of whom had relatively successful surgical resections, are disease-free survivors (95). Local recurrence with extension to the liver was the most common pattern of failure.

Metastatic Disease

Fewer than 10% of patients with bone marrow metastases at diagnosis achieve long-term survival. Patients with metastatic disease not involving the bone marrow are more likely to survive (25% to 30%) (12,16,17).

Chemotherapy is the dominant treatment modality for patients with metastatic disease. Because extirpative surgery is usually not appropriate, RT assumes the major role in obtaining local control of both primary and metastatic lesions, which are imagable and localizable. Respecting normal tissue tolerances, the volume used includes that which existed prior to chemotherapy, and the dose is up to 40 to 50 Gy (although this must often be modified). Low-dose whole-lung irradiation is used as part of the treatment of pulmonary metastasis. If there are a few isolated lung metastases, not encompassing an excessive volume of lung, they may be boosted by a "rifle shot" field. In addition, lung nodules can be resected after chemoradiotherapy if acceptable lung function is preserved. Unfortunately, high-dose cytotoxic therapy with bone marrow rescue has not yet proven to be effective for patients with metastatic or recurrent disease (96).

Painful or obstructing metastatic lesions may be treated with palliative RT.

AREAS FOR FUTURE INVESTIGATION

As is generally true for children with cancer, the goal of future investigations is to optimize outcome, in terms of tumor eradication and normal tissue damage.

Therapeutic Maneuvers

The ability to safely administer more intensive RT using hyperfractionated and/or accelerated courses is under study (13,67). Conversely, identifying settings in which lower RT doses are effective will decrease late effects. Optimally sequencing RT and chemotherapy to improve efficacy, safety, and protocol compliance continues to be explored. Administering short, intensive chemotherapy regimens, with growth factor support, is another area of study. High-dose cytotoxic therapy with bone marrow rescue may yet prove to be effective. RT must strive to improve the local control rates for bulky RMS without engendering high morbidity from damage to normal tissue. Among the areas meriting additional investigation are multiple fraction per day treatment, hyperthermia, brachytherapy, intraoperative teletherapy, chemical radiosensitizers, and radioprotectors.

Diagnostic and Biologic Investigations

As suggested in the earlier sections of this chapter, advances in molecular genetics, immunohistochemistry, and diagnostic imaging may permit a deeper understanding of the nature of RMS and identification of new prognostic factors that will allow improved tailoring of existing therapies and the discovery of new treatment approaches. For example, insulin-like growth factor (IGF)-2 is a proto-oncogene protein product that has been evaluated in RMS. Five out of six RMS tumors, as well as one cell line, were shown to have abnormalities of IGF-2, and both embryonal and alveolar RMS overproduce IGF-2 (97). Work by Helman and others at the National Cancer Institute suggests an intriguing pathway toward treating RMS by taking advantage of this (98). IGF-2 acts through autocrine stimulation of the IGF-1 receptor, which regulates cdc2 mRNA, a critically important gene in the control of cell cycling. Blocking the receptor with the monoclonal antibody alpha IR-3 decreases tumor growth and final mass. The IGF receptor can also be competitively inhibited by the drug suramin and by the T-cell immunosuppressant rapamycin. Flow cytology analysis of the extent of cell proliferation has been suggested to be of value in the therapy of adult female breast cancer. Analogous efforts have been undertaken in RMS. In one study, patients were grouped into those whose percentage of cells in S phase were greater than or equal to 15% as opposed to those who had less than 15% of cells in S phase. The prognosis of those with low S phase fractions was significantly better than those with a high fraction ($p = 0.03$) (35).

REFERENCES

References particularly recommended for further reading are indicated by an asterisk.

*1. Maurer H, Ruymann F, Pochedly C. *Rhabdomyosarcoma and related tumors in children and adolescents*, Boca Raton, FL: CRC Press, 1991.
2. Newton WA Jr, Soule EH, Hamoudi AB, et al. Histopathology of childhood sarcomas, Intergroup Rhabdomyosarcoma Studies I and II: clinicopathologic correlation. *J Clin Oncol* 1988;6:67–75.
3. Parham E, Webber B, Holt H, et al. Immunohistochemical study of childhood rhabdomyosarcomas and related neoplasms. Results of an Intergroup Rhabdomyosarcoma Study Project. *Cancer* 1991;67: 3072–3080.
4. Weber CO. Anatomische untersuchung einer hypertrophische zunge nebst bemerkungen ueber die neubildung quergestreifter muskelfasern, virchow. *Arch Pathol Anat* 1954;7:115–121.
5. Stout A. Rhabdomyosarcoma of the skeletal muscle. *Ann Surg* 1946;123:447–472.
6. Horn R Jr, Enterline H. Rhabdomyosarcoma: a clinicopathologic study and classification of 39 cases. *Cancer* 1958;11:181–199.
7. Cassady B, Sagerman RH, Tretter P, et al. Radiation therapy for rhabdomyosarcoma. *Radiol* 1968;91: 116–120.
8. Stobbe GC, Dargeaon HW. Embryonal rhabdomyosarcoma of the head and neck in children and adolescents. *Cancer* 1950;3:826–836.
9. Tefft M, Lindberg R, Gehan E. Radiation therapy combined with systemic chemotherapy of rhabdomyosarcoma in children: local control in patients enrolled into the Intergroup Rhabdomyosarcoma Study. *Natl Cancer Inst Monogr* 1981;56:75–81.
*10. Heyn RM, Holland R, Newton WA Jr, et al. The role of combined chemotherapy in the treatment of rhabdomyosarcoma. *Cancer* 1974;34:2128–2142.
*11. Crist W, Garnsey L, Beltangady M, et al. Prognosis in children with rhabdomyosarcoma: a report of the Intergroup Rhabdomyosarcoma Studies I and II. *J Clin Oncol* 1990;8:443–452.
*12. Crist W, Gehan E, Ragab A, et al. The Third Intergroup Rhabdomyosarcoma Study. *J Clin Oncol* 1995; 13:610–630.
13. Donaldson S, Asmar L, Breneman J, et al. Hyperfractionated radiation in children with rhabdomyosarcoma—results of the Intergroup Rhabdomyosarcoma pilot study. *Int J Radiat Oncol Biol Phys* 1995;32: 903–911.
14. Kingston JE, McElwain TJ, Malpas JS. Childhood rhabdomyosarcoma: experience of the Children's Solid Tumor Group. *Br J Cancer* 1983;48:195–207.
*15. Mandell L. Ongoing progress in the treatment of childhood rhabdomyosarcoma. *Oncology* 1993;7(1): 71–83.
*16. Maurer H, Gehan E, Beltangady M, et al. The Intergroup Rhabdomyosarcoma Study-II. *Cancer* 1993; 71:1904–1923.
*17. Maurer HM, Beltangady M, Gehan EA, et al. The Intergroup Rhabdomyosarcoma Study-I: a final report. *Cancer* 1988;61:209–220.
18. Rodary C, Gehan E, Flamant F, et al. Prognostic factors in 951 non-metastatic rhabdomyosarcoma in children: a report from the international rhabdomyosarcoma workshop. *Med Pediatr Oncol* 1991;19: 89–95.
*19. Wharam M, Hanfelt J, Tefft M, et al. Radiation Therapy for rhabdomyosarcoma: local failure risk for clinical group III patients on Intergroup Rhabdomyosarcoma Study II. *Int J Radiat Oncol Biol Phys* 1997;38: 797–804.
20. Womer R. The Intergroup Rhabdomyosarcoma Studies come of age. *Cancer* 1993;71:1719–1721.
21. Koscielniak E, Jurgens H, Winkler K, et al. Treatment of soft tissue sarcoma in childhood and adolescence. A report of the German Cooperative Soft Tissue Sarcoma Study. *Cancer* 1992;70:2557–2567.
22. Plowman PN. Radiotherapy of pediatric genitourinary tumors. In: Broecker BH, Klein FA, eds. *Pediatric tumors of the genitourinary tract*. New York: Alan R Liss, 1988;263–281.
*23. Mandell L, Ghavimi R, Peretz T, et al. Radiocurability of microscopic disease in childhood rhabdomyosarcoma with radiation doses less than 4000 cGy. *J Clin Oncol* 1990;8:1536–1542.
*24. Pedrick R, Donaldson S, Cox R. Rhabdomyosarcoma: the Stanford experience using a TNM staging system. *J Clin Oncol* 1986;4:370–378.
25. Ruymann FB, Maddux HR, Ragab A, et al. Congenital anomalies associated with rhabdomyosarcoma: an autopsy study of 115 cases. A report from the Intergroup Rhabdomyosarcoma Study Committee (representing the Children's Cancer Study Group, the Pediatric Oncology Group, the United Kingdom Children's Cancer Study Gruop, and the Pediatric Intergroup Statistical Center). *Med Pediatr Oncol* 1988;16:33–39.
26. Grufferman S, Schwartz A, Ruymann F, et al. Parents' use of cocaine and marijuana and increased risk of rhabdomyosarcoma in their children. *Cancer Causes Control* 1993;4:217–221.
27. Birch J, Hartley A, Blair V, et al. Cancer in the families of children with soft tissue sarcoma. *Cancer* 1990;66:2239–2248.
28. McKeen E. Rhabdomyosarcoma complicating multiple neurofibromatosis. *J Pediatr* 1987;93:992–993.
*29. Constine S, Marcus RB, Halperin EC. The future of therapy for childhood rhabdomyosarcoma: clues from molecular biology. *Int J Radiat Oncol Biol Phys* 1995;32:1245–1249.
*30. Pappo A, Shapiro D, Crist W, et al. Biology and therapy of pediatric rhabdomyosarcoma. *J Clin Oncol* 1995;12:2123–2139.
31. Barr F, Chatten J, D'Cruz C, et al. Molecular assays for chromosomal translocations in the diagnosis of pediatric soft tissue sarcomas. *JAMA* 1995;273: 553–557.
*32. McManus A, Gusterson B, Pinkerton C, et al. The

molecular pathology of small round-cell tumours: relevance to diagnosis, prognosis and classification. *J Pathol* 1996;178:116–121.

33. Whang-Peng J, Knutsen T, Theil K, et al. Cytogenetic studies in subgroups of rhabdomyosarcoma. *Genes Chromosomes Cancer* 1997;5:299–310.

34. De Zen L, Sommaggio A, d'Amore E, et al. Clinical relevance of DNA ploidy and proliferative activity in childhood rhabdomyosarcoma: a retrospective analysis of patients enrolled onto the Italian Cooperative Rhabdomyosarcoma Study RMS88. *J Clin Oncol* 1997;15:1198–1205.

35. Wignaendts LCD, van der Linden JC, van Diest PJ, et al. Prognostic importance of DNA flow cytometric variables in rhabdomyosarcoma. *J Clin Pathol* 1993; 46:948–952.

36. Pappo A, Crist W, Kuttesch J, et al. Tumor-cell DNA content predicts outcome in children and adolescents with clinical group III embryonal rhabdomyosarcoma. *J Clin Oncol* 1993;11:1901–1905.

37. Kelly K, Womer R, Barr F. Minimal disease detection in patients with alveolar rhabdomyosarcoma using a reverse transcriptase-polymerase chain reaction method. *Cancer* 1996;78:1320–1327.

38. Dias P, Kuma P, Marsden H, et al. N-myc gene is amplified in alveolar rhabdomyosarcomas (RMS) but not in embryonal RMS. *Int J Cancer* 1990;45: 593–596.

39. Driman D, Thorner P, Greenberg M, et al. MYCN gene amplification in rhabdomyosarcoma. *Cancer* 1994;73:2231–2237.

40. Felix CA, Kappel CC, Mitsudomi T, et al. Frequency and diversity of p53 mutations in childhood rhabdomyosarcoma. *Cancer Res* 1992;52:2243–2247.

41. Wharam M, Beltangady MS, Heyn RM, et al. Pediatric orofacial and laryngopharyngeal rhabdomyosarcoma: an Intergroup Rhabdomyosarcoma Study report. *Arch Otolaryngol Head Neck Surg* 1987;113: 1225–1227.

*42. Breneman J. Genitourinary rhabdomyosarcoma. *Sem Radiat Oncol* 1997;7:217–224.

*43. Lawrence W Jr, Hays D, Heyn R, et al. Lymphatic metastases with childhood rhabdomyosarcoma: a report from the Intergroup Rhabdomyosarcoma Study. *Cancer* 1987;60:910–915.

*44. Wharam M. Rhabdomyosarcoma of paramenigeal sites. *Sem Radiat Oncol* 1997;7:212–216.

45. Asmar L, Gehan E, Newton W, et al. Agreement among and within groups of pathologists in the classification of rhabdomyosarcoma and related childhood sarcomas. *Cancer* 1994;74:2579–2588.

*46. Newton W, Gehan E, Webber B, et al. Classification of rhabdomyosarcomas and related sarcomas. *Cancer* 1995;76:1073–1085.

47. Pawel B, Hamoudi A, Asmar L, et al. Undifferentiated sarcomas of children: pathology and clinical behavior—an Intergroup Rhabdomyosarcoma Study. *Med Pediatr Oncol* 1997;29:170–180.

48. Shimada H, Newton WA Jr, Soule EH, et al. Pathologic features of extra-osseous Ewing's sarcoma: a report from the Intergroup Rhabdomyosarcoma Study. *Hum Pathol* 1988;19:442–453.

*49. Donaldson S, Belli J. A rational clinical staging system for childhood rhabdomyosarcoma. *J Clin Oncol* 1984;2:135–139.

50. Lawrence W, Anderson J, Gehan E, et al. Pretreatment TNM staging of childhood rhabdomyosarcoma. *Cancer* 1997;80:1165–1170.

51. Kodet R, Newton W, Hamoudi A, et al. Orbital rhabdomyosarcomas and related tumors in childhood: relationship of morphology to prognosis—an Intergroup Rhabdomyosarcoma Study. *Med Pediatr Oncol* 1997;29:51–60.

52. LaQuaglia M, Heller G, Ghavimi F, et al. The effect of age at diagnosis on outcome in rhabdomyosarcoma. *Cancer* 1994;73:109–117.

53. Shapiro E, Parham D, Douglass E, et al. Relationship of tumor-cell ploidy to histologic subtype and treatment outcome in children and adolescents with unresectable rhabdomyosarcoma. *J Clin Oncol* 1991;9: 159–166.

54. Ragab AH, Heyn R, Tefft M, et al. Infants younger than 1 year of age with rhabdomyosarcoma. *Cancer* 1986;58:2606–2610.

55. Salloum E, Flamant F, Rey A, et al. Rhabdomyosarcoma in infants under one year of age: experience of the Institut Gustave-Roussy. *Med Pediatr Oncol* 1989;17:424–428.

56. Mandell L, Massey V, Ghavimi F. The influence of extensive bone erosion on local control in non-orbital rhabdomyosarcoma of the head and neck. *Int J Radiat Oncol Biol Phys* 1989;17:649–653.

*57. Raney R Jr, Tefft M, Newton W, et al. Improved prognosis with intensive treatment of children with cranial sarcoma arising in non-orbital parameningeal sites. A report from the Intergroup Rhabdomyosarcoma Study. *Cancer* 1987;59:147–155.

58. Mandell L, Ghavimi F, LaQuaglia M, et al. Prognostic significance of regional lymph node involvement in childhood extremity rhabdomyosarcoma. *Med Pediatr Oncol* 1990;18:466–471.

59. Sagerman RH, Cassady JR, Tretter P. Radiation therapy for rhabdomyosarcoma of the orbit. *Trans Am Acad Ophthalmol Otolaryngol* 1968;72: 849–854.

60. Hays D, Raney B, Wharam M, et al. Children with vesical rhabdomyosarcoma treated by partial cystectomy with neoadjuvant or adjuvant chemotherapy, with or without radiotherapy. *J Pediatr Hematol Oncol* 1995;17:46–52.

61. Rousseau P, Flamant F, Quintana E, et al. Primary chemotherapy in rhabdomyosarcoma and other malignant mesenchymal tumors of the orbit. Results of the International Society of Pediatric Oncology MMT 84 Study. *J Clin Oncol* 1994;12:516–521.

*62. Wiener E, Lawrence W, Hays D, et al. Survival is improved in clinical group III children with complete response established by second look operations in the Intergroup Rhabdomyosarcoma Study III [Abstract]. *Med Pediatr Oncol* 1991;19:399.

63. Donaldson SS, Castro JR, Wilbur JR, et al. Rhabdomyosarcoma of the head and neck in children: combination treatment by surgery, irradiation and chemotherapy. *Cancer* 1973;31:26–35.

64. Tefft M, Wharam M, Gehan E. Local and regional control of rhabdomyosarcoma by radiation in IRS-II. *Int J Radiat Oncol Biol Phys* 1988;15[Suppl 1]:159 (abst).

65. Tefft M, Wharam M, Ruymann F, et al. Radiotherapy (RT) for rhabdomyosarcoma (RMS) in children: a re-

port from the Intergroup Rhabdomyosarcoma Study #2 (IRS-2). *Proc ASCO* 1985;4:234(abst).

*66. Wharam M, Beltangady M, Hays D, et al. Localized orbital rhabdomyosarcoma: an interim report of the Intergroup Rhabdomyosarcoma Study Committee. *Ophthalmol* 1987;94:251–254.

67. Merchant T. Delayed-accelerated hyperfractionated radiation therapy for advanced-stage or high-risk rhabdomyosarcoma. *Med Pediatr Oncol* 1997;29: 45–50.

68. Regine WF, Fontanesi J, Kumar P, et al. A phase II trial evaluating selective use of altered radiation dose and fractionation in patients with unresectable rhabdomyosarcoma. *Int J Radiat Oncol Biol Phys* 1995; 31:799–805.

69. Flamant F, Gebaulet C, Nihoul-Fekete D, et al. Long-term sequelae of conservative treatment by surgery, brachytherapy, and chemotherapy for vulvar and vaginal rhabdomyosarcoma in children. *J Clin Oncol* 1990;8:1847–1853.

70. Nag S, Martinez-Monge R, Ruymann F, et al. Innovation in the management of soft tissue sarcomas in infants and young children: high-dose-rate brachytherapy. *J Clin Oncol* 1997;15:3075–3084.

71. Hays DM, Raney B Jr, Lawrence W Jr, et al. Bladder and prostatic tumors in the Intergroup Rhabdomyosarcoma Study (IRS-I): results of therapy. *Cancer* 1982;50:1472–1482.

*72. Hays D, Lawrence W Jr, Crist W, et al. Partial cystectomy in the management of rhabdomyosarcoma of the bladder: a report from the Intergroup Rhabdomyosarcoma Study. *J Pediat Surg* 1990;25:719–723.

*73. Raney R Jr, Gehan E, Hays D, et al. Primary chemotherapy with or without radiation therapy and/or surgery for children with localized sarcoma of the bladder, prostate, vagina, uterus, and cervix. *Cancer* 1990;66:2072–2081.

74. Heyn R, Newton W, Raney R, et al. Preservation of the bladder in patients with rhabdomyosarcoma. *J Clin Oncol* 1997;15:69–75.

75. Raney RB Jr, Heyn R, Hays D, et al. Sequelae of treatment in 109 patients followed for 5 to 15 years after diagnosis of sarcoma of the bladder and prostate. A report from the Intergroup Rhabdomyosarcoma Study Committee. *Cancer* 1993;71: 2387–2394.

*76. Raney RB Jr, Tefft M, Lawrence WJ, et al. Paratesticular sarcoma in childhood and adolescence: a report from the Intergroup Rhabdomyosarcoma Studies I and II, 1973–1983. *Cancer* 1987;60:2337–2343.

77. Wiener E, Lawrence W, Hays D, et al. Retroperitoneal node biopsy in paratesticular rhabdomyosarcoma. *J Pediat Surg* 1994;29:171–177.

78. Hays D, Shimada H, Raney B Jr, et al. Clinical staging and treatment results in rhabdomyosarcoma of the female genital tract among children and adolescents. *Cancer* 1988;61:1893–1903.

79. Friedman M, Peretz BA, Nissenbaum M, et al. Modern treatment of vaginal embryonal rhabdomyosarcoma. *Obstet Gynecol Surv* 1986;41:614–618.

80. Andrassy R, Hays D, Raney R, et al. Conservative Surgical management of vaginal and vulvar pediatric rhabdomyosarcoma: a report from the Intergroup Rhabdomyosarcoma Study III. *J Pediat Surg* 1995; 30:1034–1037.

81. Hays DM, Shimada H, Raney RB Jr, et al. Sarcomas of the vagina and uterus: the Intergroup Rhabdomyosarcoma Study. *J Pediat Surg* 1985;20:718–724.

82. Brand E, Berek J, Nieberg RK, et al. Rhabdomyosarcoma of the uterine cervix. *Cancer* 1987;60: 1552–1560.

83. Corpon C, Andrassy R, Hays D, et al. Conservative management of uterine pediatric rhabdomyosarcoma: a report from the Intergroup Rhabdomyosarcoma Study III and IV pilot. *J Pediat Surg* 1995;30: 942–944.

*84. Heyn R, Beltangady M, Hays D, et al. Results of intensive therapy in children with localized alveolar extremity rhabdomyosarcoma: a report from the Intergroup Rhabdomyosarcoma Study. *J Clin Oncol* 1989; 7:200–207.

85. Lawrence W, Hays E, Heyn R, et al. Surgical lessons from the Intergroup Rhabdomyosarcoma Study (IRS) pertaining to extremity tumors. *World J Surg* 1988; 12:676–684.

86. Tefft M, Fernandez C, Donaldson M, et al. Incidence of meningeal involvement by rhabdomyosarcoma of the head and neck in children: a report of the Intergroup Rhabdomyosarcoma Study (IRS). *Cancer* 1978;42:253–258.

87. Gasparini M, Lombardi M, Gianni M, et al. Questionable role of CNS radioprophylaxis in the therapeutic management of childhood rhabdomyosarcoma with meningeal extension. *J Clin Oncol* 1990;8: 1854–1857.

88. Blatt J, Synderman C, Wollman M, et al. Delayed resection in the management of non-orbital rhabdomyosarcoma of the head and neck in childhood. *Med Pediatr Oncol* 1997;29:294–298.

89. Benk V, Rodary C, Donaldson S, et al. Parameningeal rhabdomyosarcoma: results of an international workshop. *Int J Radiat Oncol Biol Phys* 1996;36:533–540.

90. Heyn R, Ragab A, Raney RB Jr, et al. Late effects of therapy in orbital rhabdomyosarcoma in children: a report from the Intergroup Rhabdomyosarcoma Study. *Cancer* 1986;57:1738–1743.

91. Raney RB Jr, Ragab AH, Ruymann FB, et al. Soft-tissue sarcoma of the trunk in childhood: results of the Intergroup Rhabdomyosarcoma Study. *Cancer* 1982; 49:2612–2616.

92. Ortega J, Wharam M, Gehan E, et al. Clinical features and results of therapy for children with paraspinal soft tissue sarcoma: a report of the Intergroup Rhabdomyosarcoma Study. *J Clin Oncol* 1991; 9:796–801.

93. Crist WM, Raney RB, Tefft M, et al. Soft tissue sarcomas arising in the retroperitoneal space in children: a report from the Intergroup Rhabdomyosarcoma Study (IRS) Committee. *Cancer* 1985;56: 2125–2132.

94. Raney R Jr, Crist W, Hays E, et al. Soft tissue sarcoma of the perineal region in childhood. A report from the Intergroup Rhabdomyosarcoma Studies I and II, 1972 through 1984. *Cancer* 1990;65: 2787–2792.

95. Ruymann FB, Raney RB Jr, Crist WM, et al. Rhabdomyosarcoma of the biliary tree in childhood: a report from the Intergroup Rhabdomyosarcoma Study. *Cancer* 1985;56:575–581.

96. Kinsella R, Miser J, Triche R, et al. Treatment of

high-risk sarcomas in children and young adults: analysis of local control using intensive combined modality therapy. *Natl Cancer Inst Monogr* 1988;6: 291–296.

97. Zhan S, Shapiro DN, Helman LJ. Activation of an imprinted allele of the insulin-like growth factor II gene implicated in rhabdomyosarcoma. *J Clin Oncol* 1994; 94:445–448.

98. Kalebic T, Tsokos M, Helman L. In vivo treatment with antibody against IGF-1 receptor suppresses growth of human rhabdomyosarcoma and down regulates p34. *Cancer Res* 1994;54:5531–5534.

99. Scrable H, Witte D, Shimada H, et al. Molecular differential pathology of rhabdomyosarcoma. *Genes Chromosomes Cancer* 1989;1:23–25.

100. Wexler LH, Helman LJ. Rhabdomyosarcoma and the undifferentiated sarcomas. In: Pizzo PA, Poplack DG. eds. *Principles and practice of pediatric oncology.* Philadelphia: Lippincott-Raven, 1997:799–829.

101. Pappo A. Rhabdomyosarcoma and other soft tissue sarcomas of childhood. *Curr Opin Oncol* 1995;7: 361–366.

102. Geary ES, Gong MC, Shortliffe LMD. Biology and treatment of pediatric genitourinary tumors. *Curr Opin Oncol* 1995;6:292–300.

103. Fryer CJH. Pelvic rhabdomyosarcoma: paying the price of bladder preservation. *Lancet* 1995;345: 141–142.

104. Heij HA, Vos A, de Kraker J, Voute PA. Urogenital rhabdomyosarcoma in children: is a conservative surgical approach justified? *J Urol* 1993;150:165–168.

105. Lobe TE, Wiener E, Andrassy RJ, et al. The argument for conservative delayed surgery in the management of prostatic rhabdomyosarcoma. *J Pediatr Surg* 1996; 31:1084–1087.

106. Yeung CK, Ward HC, Ransley PG, Duffy PG, Pritchard J. Bladder and kidney function after cure of pelvic rhabdomyosarcoma in childhood. *Br J Cancer* 1994;70:1000–1003.

12

Soft-Tissue Sarcomas Other Than Rhabdomyosarcoma; Desmoid Tumor

Soft-tissue sarcomas are defined as all those malignant tumors of nonepithelial, extra-skeletal tissues including the peripheral and autonomic nervous system but excluding the hematopoietic system, glia, and supporting tissues of specific organs and viscera. Soft-tissue sarcomas constitute approximately 6.5% to 7% of childhood cancer. Within this 6.5% to 7%, approximately one-half to two-thirds of cases are rhabdomyosarcoma (1–3). Non-rhabdomyosarcoma soft-tissue sarcoma (NRSTS), therefore, constitutes 2% to 4% of childhood cancer cases (4).

For most children with NRSTS, the etiology of the tumor will be unknown. Some cases may be traced to prior radiation exposure (see Chapter 20), chemical exposure, iatrogenic or disease-caused immunosuppression, and neurofibromatosis, with the latter group having a 7% to 10% lifetime risk of developing malignant neurofibrosarcoma. The association of sarcomas with neurofibromatosis indicates that some sarcomas are associated with chromosomal deletions and translocations and the presence of abnormalities of tumor suppressor genes (5). Homozygous gene deletions occur in both the long and short arms of chromosome 17 in neurofibrosarcomas type 1. Candidate tumor suppressor genes include 17 q11 (the neurofibromatosis tumor suppressor gene) and p53 (17p13) (1,5). Rhabdomyosarcoma and NRSTS also occur as part of the familial Li-Fraumeni syndrome.

PATHOLOGY

The frequency of the different histologic subgroups of the NRSTS of childhood varies between reporting institutions (Table 1). These differences may be attributable to variations in referral patterns and to the relatively small numbers in each series. In addition, NRSTS are often difficult for pathologists to classify, and there is considerable intraobserver variation (6). In an M.D. Anderson Hospital series of sarcomas of the head and neck in children and adolescents, histologic diagnoses were changed in 22% of patients (7). Several other studies have assessed discrepancy rates between the original diagnosis of soft-tissue tumors and the diagnosis made by expert reviewers when patients are referred to specialty centers for entry on the therapeutic trials. About 5% to 10% of cases having the original diagnosis of sarcoma are revised to nonsarcoma and 16% to 32% of those patients with a sarcoma have a revision of the histologic subtype of the sarcoma. Where grade was analyzed, there was disagreement in up to 40% of the cases (8). Malignant fibrous histiocytoma (MFH), for example, was first described as a separate entity in the 1960s. General recognition of this tumor's existence, distinct from other classifications followed. The reported incidence of MFH in adults, therefore, sharply increased while that of fibrosarcoma fell (9). MFH is unusual in childhood.

TABLE 1. *The most frequent types of childhood nonrhabdomyosarcoma soft-tissue sarcoma in recent clinical series*[a]

Histology	St. Jude Children's Research Hospital (64)	Harvard–Joint Center for Radiation Therapy[b] (23)	Children's Hospital of Philadelphia (3)	Baylor/Texas Children's Hospital (4)	Children's Hospital and Medical Center, Seattle (1)	M.D. Anderson Hospital–head and neck sarcomas (7)	SEER data (34)	Italian cooperative study of childhood soft-tissue sarcoma (19)	Pediatric Oncology Group (114)
Primitive neuroectodermal tumor + extraosseous Ewing's sarcoma + Askin's tumor				**32%**	**40%**			**36%**	
Neurogenic sarcoma/neurofibrosarcoma	20%	**30%**	**38%**	9%		**17%**		**15%**	10%
Synovial sarcoma	**30%**	**16%**	**10%**	**6%**	10%	4%	10%	**14%**	**42%**
Alveolar soft part sarcoma	**10%**		2%	2%				2%	
Sarcoma not otherwise specified	8%	**14%**	2%	**30%**		**26%**	**15%**	8%	
Malignant fibrous histiocytoma	8%	11%	15%			4%		4%	**12%**
Hemangiopericytoma	8%				2%			1%	
Liposarcoma	7%			2%				5%	5%
Dermatofibrosarcoma protuberans	2%				c	4%			
Fibrosarcoma	7%	9%	**18%**	4%	**20%**	**17%**	**48%**	**14%**	**13%**
Mixed mesenchymoma			2%	**6%**					
Angiosarcoma and Hemangiosarcoma			2%			4%		3%	
Epitheliod sarcoma			8%					2%	
Extrarenal rhabdoid sarcoma								3%	
Clear cell sarcoma								1%	
Leiomyosarcoma								1%	4%
Other	20%			4%					**12%**

[a] In each series, the three most common histologic types are indicated **by bold type.**

[b] This series does not include children with metastatic disease.

[c] This series combines dermatofibrosarcoma protuberans with fibrosarcoma.

Many of the childhood NRSTS have characteristic cell types. *Neurogenic sarcoma* is also known as neurofibrosarcoma, malignant peripheral nerve sheath tumor, malignant schwannoma, or malignant neurilemmoma. It is a malignant neoplasm that arises in a peripheral nerve sheath. In children, from one-fifth to two-thirds of cases of neurogenic sarcoma are associated with neurofibromatosis (10–12). The morphology is characterized by fascicles of spindle cells with either a herringbone or storiform pattern. One may observe evidence of schwannian differentiation (13). There can be areas of significant nuclear hyperchromatism and abundant mitotic figures (14). These tumors are usually positive for S-100, vimentin and neuron specific enolase. Biphasic *synovial sarcoma,* the more common type, also has spindle-shaped cells. These are mixed with oval and keratin-positive epithelial cells. Pseudoglandular spaces or slits and clefts mimic synovium (15–17). The rare monophasic type has recently become an accepted entity (18). About two-thirds of cases involve the lower extremity and one-third the upper. Synovial sarcomas differ from other NRSTS in that they have a significant risk of lymph node metastases (1). The biphasic type has a better prognosis. Synovial sarcomas may have a t(x;18) translocation (19). *Liposarcomas* originate from primitive mesenchymal cells rather than from mature adipose tissue (20). Some have a myxoid appearance, whereas others resemble benign lipomas (21). The pleomorphic type may resemble fibroblastic, myoblastic, and/or synovial sarcomas (22). *Leiomyosarcoma* originates from smooth muscle. The well-differentiated lesions usually have a centrally located blunt-ended nucleus ("cigar-shaped") (20,21). *Fibrosarcoma* is an infiltrative, fibrous neoplasm composed of interlocking bundles of spindle cells (23,24). The tumor usually stains positive for vimentin (19).

There are two clinically different forms of fibrosarcoma in children. One is a lesion appearing in the first 5 years of life with a low rate of distant spread. This type of fibrosarcoma, called the *congenital type,* is treated by excision (1,6,23). In children under 5 years of age this tumor may be referred to as *infantile fibrosarcoma.* The other occurs in children over 10 years of age and has a more ominous prognosis (24). This classic or adult-type fibrosarcoma is treated according to the principles outlined for other NRSTS. *Low-grade fibromyxoid sarcoma* is an indolent tumor that rarely occurs in children. It consists of spindle and stellate cells with uniform nuclei arranged in a whorled pattern with alternating areas of fibrous and myxoid stroma (25). *Malignant fibrous histiocytomas* are pleomorphic sarcomas often characterized by a whorled growth pattern (20). They are thought to arise from histiocytic cells acting as facultative fibroblasts. *Hemangiopericytomas* arise from pericytes, the modified smooth muscle cell with contractile function located on the internal surface of venous capillaries and postcapillary venules (26). The *malignant mesenchymoma* has two or more cell types—any of which, taken by itself, might be considered a malignant neoplasm (27,28).

There are several childhood NRSTS that have a characteristic microscopic picture but where the cell of origin is uncertain. The *epithelioid sarcoma* is a tumor of the subcutaneous tissue, tendons, and fascia—usually of the upper extremity, including the hand (29). There is a nodular arrangement of plump, polygonal to round, epithelioid cells interspersed with spindle-shaped cells (2,30). Central degeneration or necrosis is often present. The tumor tends to spread within fascial planes or aponeuroses and may grow along the neurovascular bundle and encroach on large vessels or nerves. Regional lymph node metastasis may occur in association with high-grade tumors and tumors larger than 5 cm (31). The tumor generally stains positive for keratin (19). *Alveolar soft part sarcomas* have a characteristic crystalline material seen with periodic acid-Schiff (PAS) stain (32,33). The tumor is positive for vimentin on immunohistochemistry (19). The tumor cells typically have an organoid or nestlike arrangement. Vascular invasion is always seen. Of 11

children with alveolar soft part sarcoma seen at St. Jude Children's Research Hospital in a 32-year period, 6 had localized disease and 5 had unresectable or metastatic disease. Recent cytogenetic studies indicate that 17q25 abnormalities are common (34). *Extraskeletal Ewing's sarcoma* and peripheral *primitive neuroectodermal tumor (PNET)* are characterized by cohesive, uniform, small hyperchromatic cells in a fibrous background. Dense clumping of chromatin, mitotic figures, and rosette formation are typical of PNET. On immunohistochemistry analysis extraosseous Ewing's sarcoma are generally positive for vimentin and HBA-17. PNET is generally positive for neuron specific enolase and other neural-related markers such as S-100 protein, neurofilament, or HNK-1. Both PNET and extraosseous Ewing's sarcoma are associated with a particular chromosome translocation t(11;22) (q24; q12). The progenitor cell for these two "small round blue cell" NRSTS is not established. They may arise for neural crest, primordial germ cells, or perhaps, mesenchymal stem cells (1,19,35). When PNET or extraosseous Ewing's sarcoma arises within the thoracic cavity it is referred to as Askin's tumor.

A fair proportion of NRSTS show no cellular differentiation. These are called *undifferentiated sarcomas* or *sarcomas not otherwise specified* (NOS).

PRESENTATION, WORKUP, AND STAGING

Most NRSTS present as a painless swelling. NRSTS may also present with signs and symptoms of vascular compression, neurologic impairment from nerve compression, or bowel dysfunction when tumors arise from the retroperitoneum.

The radiographic workup begins with the *plain radiograph.* One looks for evidence of soft-tissue mass, calcification, and destruction of adjacent bone. *Radionuclide bone scanning* is used to assess metastatic bone involvement, activity in bone adjacent to the tumor, and active vascular activity in the tumor

itself. *Arteriography* is advocated for its delineation of the tumor's blood supply—a matter of concern to the surgeon or to the direct infusional chemotherapist. *Xeroradiography* has a few proponents who believe that its outline of soft-tissue extent of disease in the neck or extremities is superior. *Computerized tomography (CT)* and/or *magnetic resonance imaging (MRI)* are the essential studies for clear definition of tumor extent, patterns of infiltration, evaluation of adjacent bone, and planning surgical and radiotherapeutic approaches. MRI often shows a larger area of involvement than does CT (Fig. 1). The evaluation for distant metastasis focuses on the most common site, the lungs, with *chest radiograph and thoracic CT scanning* (5,11,12, 36–39). Metabolic scanning techniques, such as *thallium scans* and *positron emission tomography (PET)*, are under active investigation. Fluorine-1-fluorodeoxyglucose (FDG) PET measures glucose utilization rate in sarcomas and may be used to assess lesion grade and to monitor neoadjuvant therapeutic response (40) (Fig. 2).

NRSTS in childhood may be staged by one of two systems. Some investigators use the rhabdomyosarcoma grouping system, although their number is shrinking (see Table 3 in Chapter 11). This system is convenient and relies on surgical resectability as an important prognostic factor. There is no doubt that tumor size and resectability are important in predicting outcome in NRSTS of children. The histologic tumor grade, however, is also quite important and is not directly considered in the rhabdomyosarcoma grouping system (6,41–43). Sarcoma grade assessment incorporates pleomorphism, spontaneous necrosis, and number of typical and atypical mitoses per 10 high-power fields (5). In the 1940s, Broders and colleagues at the Mayo Clinic developed a grading system for sarcomas based on the degree of nuclear atypia. In 1969, the American Joint Commission (AJC) on Cancer Staging described a staging system for soft-tissue sarcoma that utilizes grade, tumor size, nodal involvement, and presence of metastases as the determinants of

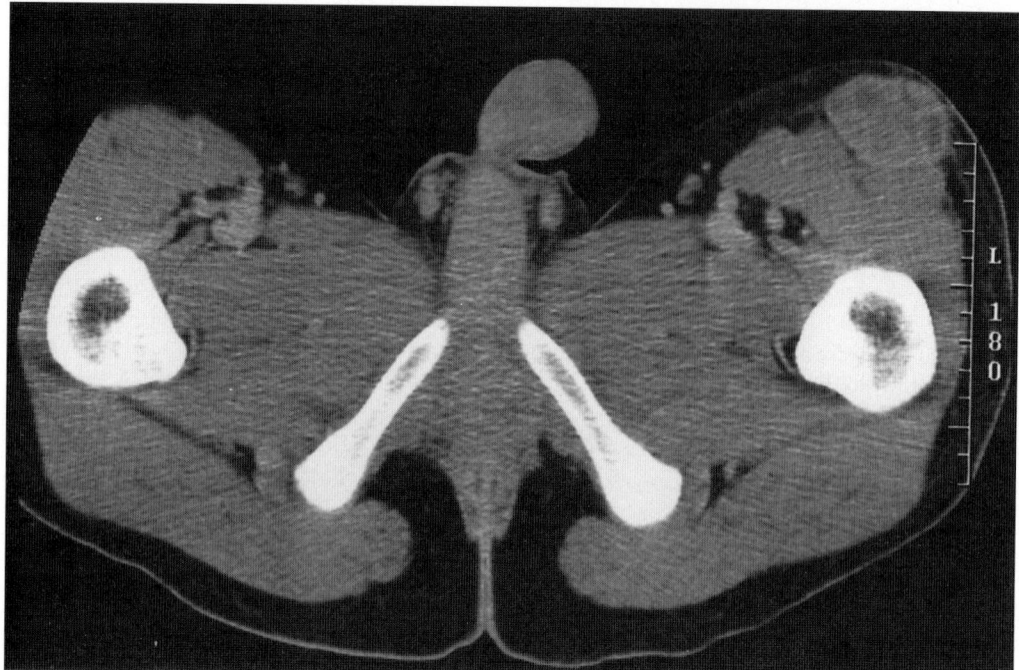

FIG. 1. This 17-year-old white male presented to medical attention with a 7-month history of a mass, noted on self-examination, of the left thigh. The mass eventually grew to 4 cm in size. The MRI demonstrated a mass without involvement of bone. PET scan showed increased metabolic activity. On pathology, the tumor was "hypercellular highly vascularized neoplastic proliferation of generally small round to oval nuclei with evenly distributed chromatin and small nucleoli. Immunohistochemical stains are positive for vimentin, negative for leukocyte antigen; most consistent with extra skeletal Ewing's sarcoma/primitive neuroectodermal tumor." The patient was treated with tumor excision, involved field irradiation, and systemic chemotherapy.

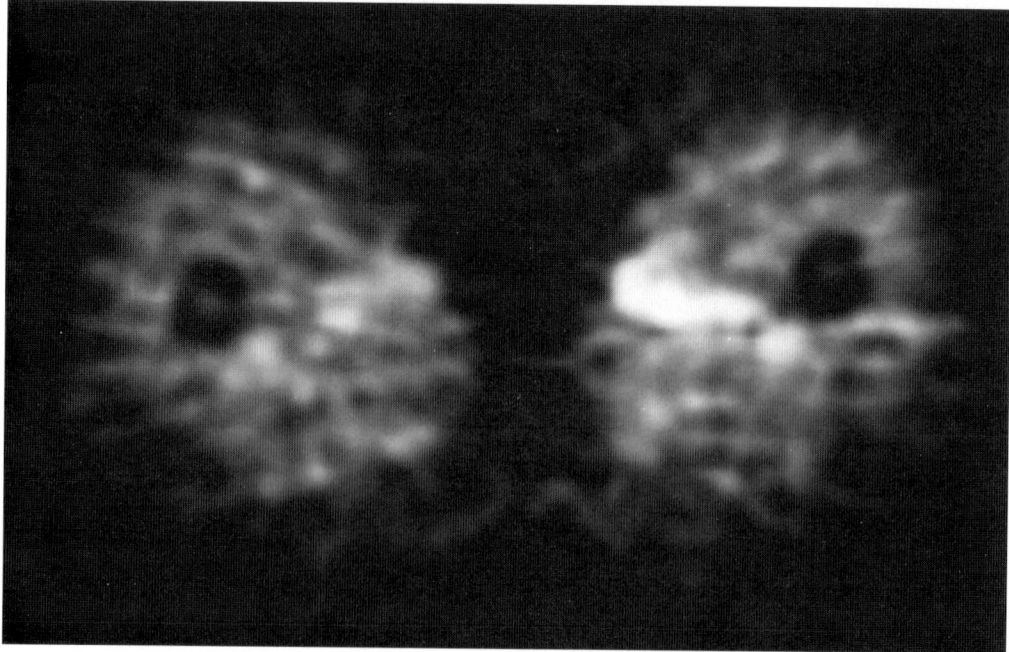

FIG. 2. A PET scan showing increased metabolic activity in a limb PNET.

TABLE 2. *The American Joint Committee staging system for sarcoma of soft tissue[a]*

T—Primary tumor
  Tx   Primary tumor cannot be assessed
  T0   No evidence of primary tumor
  T1   Tumor <5 cm in greatest dimension
    T1a Superficial tumor[a]
    T1b Deep tumor[a]
  T2   Tumor >5 cm in greatest dimension
    T2a Superficial tumor[a]
    T2b Deep tumor[a]
N—Regional lymph nodes
  Nx   Regional lymph nodes cannot be assessed
  N0   No regional lymph node metastasis
  N1   Regional lymph nodes metastasis
M—Distant metastasis
  Mx   Distant metastasis cannot be assessed
  M0   No distant metastasis
  M1   Distant metastasis
G—Histopathological grading
  Gx   Grade cannot be assessed
  G1   Well differentiated
  G2   Poorly differentiated
  G4   Undifferentiated
Stage
  Stage IA G1–2 T1a–1b NOMO
  Stage IB G1–2 T2a NOMO
  Stage IIA G1–2 T2b MO
  Stage IIB G3–4 T1a–1b NOMO
  Stage IIC G3–4 T2a NOMO
  Stage III G3–4 T2B NOMO
  Stage IV any G only T, N1, and/or MI

[a]Superficial = above superficial fascia without invasion of the fascia; Deep = located either beneath the superficial fascia or superficial to the fascia with invasion of or through the fascia. Retroperitoneal, mediastinal, and pelvic sarcomas are classified as deep.
From Sobin LH, Wittekind Ch. *TNM: classification of malignant tumours, fifth edition.* New York: Wiley-Liss, 1997, with permission.

stage (5) (Table 2). In the AJC system, grade is determined by evaluation of the degree of cellularity, cellular anaplasia or pleomorphism, mitotic activity, expansive or infiltrative growth, and necrosis (32).

Histologic grading is an important way to predict outcome of NRSTS. There are various strategies for grading. One system, developed by the Pediatric Oncology Group (POG), labels Grade 1 as tumor that has little propensity for malignancy. Grade 2 are those with less than 5 mitoses per 10 high powered fields or less than 15% geographic necrosis, and grade 3 tumors are those known to be clinically aggressive by virtue of histologic diag-

nosis and with greater than 4 mitoses per 10 high powered fields at more than 15% geographic necrosis (44). A review of this POG grading system found a 73% mortality in Grade 3 lesions as compared to 15% mortality in Grade 1 and 2 tumors (45).

Frequency of distant metastases increases and the survival probability decreases with increasing size of the primary tumor (42). About 15% of patients have metastatic disease at presentation (1).

SELECTION OF THERAPY

Surgery

Every biopsy should be planned in order to be consistent with the subsequent treatment plan. The two techniques for the biopsy are either needle or open incisional. Needle biopsy techniques include fine-needle aspiration (of variable accuracy and dependent on the experience of the cytopathologist) or core needle biopsy (1). The incision for an open incisional biopsy should be small (the minimum that is technically feasible), and homeostasis should be secure. Incisions on the extremity should be in the long axis (39). Muscle compartments should not be crossed—one does not wish to contaminate adjacent areas with tumor. The biopsy should be placed so that the entire surgical tract will be removed at the time of the definitive operation.

Complete surgical excision is the mainstay of therapy. NRSTS may infiltrate widely. Sarcomas tend to expand and infiltrate adjoining tissue spaces, producing a pseudocapsule comprised of compressed normal tissue intermingled with microscopic extensions of the tumor (5). A system for assessing the adequacy of surgical margins in sarcoma surgery was described by Enneking et al. An *intralesional* surgical margins is through tumor, with gross or microscopic contamination. A *margin* resection is through the reactive or inflammatory zone. A *wide* excision is through normal tissue outside of the inflammatory zone. A *radical* excision is outside of the anatomic compartment containing the tumor

(46). A wide excision or amputation is often required to obtain the microscopic-free margin needed for control. Clinical experience, primarily in adults, has shown that the local failure rate for simple excision of malignant soft-tissue sarcomas is 60% to 90% (11,12,36). This failure rate falls to 18% to 30% when simple excision is replaced by radical resection, radical compartmental resection, or amputation above the proximal joint (5,6,39,47–50). For low-grade lesions, wide excision with negative margins may be curative as the sole treatment (5,48).

There are some patients for whom limb-sparing treatments may be considered (49–53). Limb-sparing surgery removes a soft-tissue sarcoma while preserving the extremity with a satisfactory functional and cosmetic result. In order to achieve results comparable to radical procedures, most limb-sparing procedures involve the planned use of pre- or postoperative external beam irradiation, brachytherapy, and/or intraarterial or systemic chemotherapy. Some patients clearly are not appropriate for limb-sparing. These patients include: (a) young children who may deal with an amputation better than with the limb-length discrepancy which may occur with limb-sparing procedures; (b) extremity lesions where it is not possible to acquire adequate surgical margins and where radiotherapy may produce major long-term complications; (c) lesions that involve major vessels or nerves where resection will severely compromise function; and (d) where a fracture has occurred from tumor and the limb is already useless as well as painful (47,53).

Surgery also plays a role in the management of NRSTS in the treatment of pulmonary metastases. With proper patient selection, long-term survival is possible for individuals undergoing removal of pulmonary metastases. Preoperative evaluation with chest radiograph and thoracic CT scanning is performed to determine the number and location of the metastases. Tumor may be resected via a median sternotomy or lateral thoracotomy—generally with double-lumen endotracheal anesthesia. Two studies in the litera-

ture, both of which included adult and pediatric patients, evaluated the important prognostic factors predicting survival after pulmonary metastasectomy. Improved survival appears to be associated with complete resection of all metastases, the presence of relatively few lesions (i.e., 1 to 3), and a long disease-free interval before the development of metastases. Patients rendered free of disease in the series of Jablons et al. (54) had a median survival of 26.8 months. A similar group in the series of Casson et al. (55) had a median survival of 28 months. It is only fair to note that there are no randomized series in the literature comparing surgery to observation or chemotherapy without resection. Therefore, it cannot be proven that the apparent prolongation of survival of operated on patients is attributable to the surgical therapy as opposed to relatively good tumor biology (54).

Radiotherapy

We have previously noted that the local control rate for NRSTS increases as the extent of surgical resection increases. This is undoubtedly because more radical surgery extirpates microscopic extension of tumor. It is well known that radiation can also sterilize microscopic extensions of tumor (56). We may infer that radiation can be used to accomplish that which is achieved by increasing the extent of surgery (39). The judicious combination of limited surgery plus radiotherapy should be able to achieve local control rates equivalent to those of radical surgery with, in many cases, a superior functional result. Most of the available data support this line of reasoning (5,39,52,56–58).

POG protocol 8653 was designed to study the role of adjuvant chemotherapy in children with resectable NRSTS (59). Local therapy was standardized to include surgery only for patients with wide or radical margins and surgery plus postoperative irradiation for marginal excisions. Protocol guidelines were imperfectly followed. The results, shown in Table 3, indicate improved local control for marginal excisions in high-grade tumors (22).

TABLE 3. *POG Protocol 8653. Local control by surgical margins and radiotherapy.*

Surgical margins	IRS group	Low grade		High grade	
		Surgery alone n (%)	Surgery + radiotherapy n (%)	Surgery alone n (%)	Surgery + radiotherapy n (%)
Marginal	II	2/2 (100%)	10/11 (91%)	1/4 (25%)	10/11 (91%)
Wide	I	18/18 (100%)	3/3 (100%)	14/16 (88%)	2/2 (100%)
Radical	I	1/1 (100%)	no data	6/6 (100%)	no data

Modified from 22, with permission.

There will be situations where radical surgery is either not recommended for children or recommended and declined because of unacceptable functional, cosmetic, emotional, or psychological consequences. Radiotherapy may play a crucial role in these patients by allowing more conservative surgery with equivalent rates of local control.

In retrospective reviews of adult patients with NRSTS, treatment with conservative surgery and postoperative irradiation for microscopic extension of tumor yields local failure rates of 10% to 20%—comparable to radical surgery (39,49,50). In an analysis of 132 patients, largely adults, treated with preoperative radiation and conservative resection at the Massachusetts General Hospital the local control results were 97% for patients with negative surgical margins and 82% for those with positive margins (59a). In a series confined to children, the local control rate for patients who had no or microscopic residual disease following surgery and who were treated with postoperative irradiation was 79% (23). Tumor grade and size are the most important predictors of local failure in these series. The randomized prospective National Cancer Institute (NCI) trial, including adults and children, compared limb-sparing surgery and postoperative irradiation versus amputation. The 5-year disease-free survival for the limb-spared group was 69% compared to 72% for the amputated group ($p = 0.7$). The local failure rate was higher in the limb-conservation group, and several patients had to undergo salvage surgery (50,60). Psychological tests indicate that the amputees fared as well as those having limb-sparing surgery (61). A retrospective review of a large number of NCI patients who underwent limb-sparing surgery with radiotherapy for extremity NRSTS indicates that the most common long-term complications are contracture, limb edema, decreased range of motion, and decreased muscle strength. Certain radiotherapy technical factors were associated with a higher risk of complications: inclusion of more than 50% of a joint in the portal, doses over the equivalent of 63 Gy at 1.8 Gy/fraction, and large portals that encompassed more than 75% of the extremity diameter (62).

Several retrospective reviews, confined to children, have suggested a role for postoperative irradiation of NRSTS. Radiotherapy has been used, in accordance with the standards of the Intergroup Rhabdomyosarcoma Study, in group II (grossly complete tumor resection with microscopic residual disease or involved but completely resected regional nodes) and group III (incomplete resection with gross residual disease) NRSTS patients (2,11,12, 23,36,43,60,63).

Acceptable indications for radiotherapy in childhood NRSTS are: (a) localized, incompletely resected tumor with gross residual disease; and (b) palliation of metastasis. Palliation of pain or compressive syndromes requires on the order of 35 to 50 Gy (47); (c) as part of a planned limb-sparing procedure, and (d) following an attempt at gross total tumor removal when there is microscopic residual tumor or positive regional lymph nodes.

Chemotherapy

The use of adjuvant chemotherapy in childhood NRSTS has been defended on the basis of (a) the significant risk of metastatic disease and local recurrence in high-grade lesions, (b) retrospective comparisons, and (c) the success of chemotherapy in rhabdomyosarcoma. The most active single agents are adriamycin and ifosfamide. Other active agents are DTIC (dacarbazine), actinomycin D, vincristine, etoposide, and cyclophosphamide (3,5,6,11, 36,43,48,60,63–65).

The best clinical results for extraosseous Ewing's sarcoma and PNET are related to aggressive treatment with chemotherapy, radiotherapy, and surgery. In the past, these tumors were typically treated under the programs of the Intergroup Rhabdomyosarcoma Studies (see Chapter 11). Following biopsy a five-drug program, as described in Chapter 9, for Ewing's sarcoma of bone or one of the chemotherapy arms of Intergroup Rhabdomyosarcoma Study is administered. Local control is obtained with subsequent radiotherapy and/or surgery.

At least three factors prompt the use of adjuvant chemotherapy in childhood NRSTS. These factors include: (a) the significant risk of metastatic disease and local recurrence and high-grade lesions. This occurrence of metastatic disease naturally leads to the need for agents, which can interfere with the growth and development of metastatic deposits. (b) The considerable success of chemotherapy in rhabdomyoscaroma has stirred interest in the use of chemotherapy in NRSTS. (c) Some retrospective reviews suggest a role for adjuvant chemotherapy in NRSTS.

Cooperative Group Studies of Chemotherapy and NRSTS Exclusive of PNET, Extraosseous Ewing's Sarcoma, and Askin's Tumor

POG protocols 8653 and 8654 were open to patients younger than 21 years of age at diagnosis with any biopsy proven soft-tissue sarcoma other than rhabdomyosarcoma, extraosseous Ewing's sarcoma, or undifferentiated round cell sarcoma. Children who were treated with surgical resection with complete extirpation of tumor, surgical excision of the tumor with postoperative irradiation, or

biopsy, preoperative irradiation and secondary surgery obtaining complete resection, were randomized to adjuvant vincristine, adriamycin, cyclophosphamide versus observation. This randomization, constituting Protocol 8653, would be analogous, were one to use the rhabdomyosarcoma grouping system for NRSTS, to groups 1, 2, and 3 rendered resectable by radiation (59).

Protocol 8654 was for patients who were judged to have inoperable tumors or for those with metastatic disease. These patients were randomized to receive either vincristine, adriamycin, and cyclophosphamide or those three agents plus DTIC. Involved field radiation was used to the primary tumor site.

Study 8653 was open from June 1986 to May 1992. Study 8654 was open from June 1986 through April 1994. However, there was approximately a 1-year period where all patients in Study 8654 were treated with vincristine, actinomycin, cyclophosphamide due to a shortage of DTIC.

There were 31 patients randomized on Protocol 8653; 16 received chemotherapy, 15 were observed. The 2-year event-free survival was 75% for the chemotherapy arm and 87% for the observation arm ($p = 0.07$). There were 54 patients who were not randomized. The 3-year event-free survival for those treated with chemotherapy (20 patients) was 74% whereas for the observation arm (34 patients) it was 88%. There was, therefore, no discernible benefits to the use of chemotherapy. For study 8654, the 3-year event-free survival for those patients receiving vincristine, actinomycin D, cyclophosphamide, was 25% whereas it was 21% for the three drugs plus DTIC ($p = 0.625$) (66).

The German soft-tissue sarcoma study, CWS-81, was initiated in 1981 under the auspices of the German Society of Pediatric Oncology. This study was open to children with rhabdomyosarcoma, undifferentiated sarcoma, extraosseous Ewing's sarcoma, synovial sarcoma, lyomyosarcoma, pleural/neural extodermal tumors, fibro-sarcoma, hemangiosarcoma, neurofibrosarcoma, and liposarcoma. For the purposes of this chapter, we will confine our discussion to the available results concerning

NRSTS exclusive of extraosseous Ewing's sarcoma and PNET. Patients with localized disease, completely resected, received vincristine, actinomycin D, cyclophosphamide, and adriamycin. Patients with grossly resected tumor with microscopic residual disease with no evidence of regional node involvement received the same chemotherapy but also had involved field irradiation. These patients were then continued with vincristine, actinomycin D, and cyclophosphamide. Patients with grossly resected tumor with microscopic residual disease and regional nodal involvement or those with incomplete resection or biopsy with gross residual disease received four drug chemotherapy initially. Those who were good responders continued on this chemotherapy and received involved field irradiation ultimately having the adriamycin dropped. Those who were poor initial responders received involved field irradiation but had ifosphamide substituted for the cyclophosphamide. Patients who had stage IV disease received vincristine, actinomycin D, ifosphamide, and adriamycin. In 1984, ifosphamide was also added for patients with stage III disease who failed to respond to preoperative chemotherapy. Detailed information is available concerning the 30 children and adolescents with synovial sarcomas treated on this study (67). A survival rate of 70% was observed with a median observation time of 34 months. Those patients with synovial sarcoma of the extremities had a disease-free survival rate of 88%. Six of 8 patients who had their tumors resected with no residual disease are disease free survivors, 7 out of 9 patients who had disease resected with microscopic residual are disease-free survivors, 6 of 8 patients who have had their tumor resected with gross residual disease are disease-free survivors, and 3 of 5 patients with metastatic disease at presentation (stage IV) were disease-free survivors. Obviously, the German study was not a head-to-head trial of chemotherapy versus observation and it is not clear what the survival would have been if patients were treated with local therapy alone.

The International Society of Pediatric Oncology (SIOP) has conducted two protocols for NRSTS. The treatment program consisted of a primary complete tumor excision if feasible without mutilation. For those patients who were not resectable initially, neoadjuvant chemotherapy was administered. Initial chemotherapy was ifosphamide, vincristine, and actinomycin D. Second line chemotherapy on study MMT84 was cyclophosphamide, doxorubicin, and in study MMT89 it was epirubicin, doxyrubicin, carboplatinum, and VM26. Patients were then taken to surgery if possible. Radiosurgery was used for macroscopic residual tumor after surgery. For those patients who had initial primary excision, adjuvant chemotherapy was given with ifosphamide, vincristine, and actinomycin D. In nonmetastatic patients an initial complete excision was obtained in 24% of patients, complete response was obtained in 30% of patients by initial partial excision followed by chemotherapy, a complete response was obtained in 30% of patients by an initial biopsy, neoadjuvant chemotherapy, and second surgery, in 8% of patients a complete tumor response was obtained by surgery, chemotherapy, and radiotherapy, and in 8% of patients by surgery, chemotherapy, second surgery, and radiotherapy. Therefore, 16% of patients received radiotherapy. The overall survival rate in study MMT84 was 73% at 5 years for nonmetastatic patients, and in MMT89 it was 84%. Survival was only 15% for metastatic patients. The 5-year survival rate was 60% for fibr-sarcoma, leiomyosarcoma, and synovial sarcoma and other classified sarcomas and 50% for PNET and extraosseous Ewing's sarcoma (68,74).

In summary, the small study that randomized patients within NRSTS to chemotherapy versus observation showed no benefits of chemotherapy. The studies that have randomized patients to various chemotherapy arms have, to date, not shown a substantive difference from those results with local therapy alone.

Large Scale Studies of Adjuvant Chemotherapy in Adults with NRSTS

There are at least 14 randomized prospective trials of mostly adult patients evaluating adjuvant chemotherapy for NRSTS. These studies include the evaluation of adriamycin as a single agent versus observation as well as trials of adriamycin, cyclophosphamide, DTIC, vincristine versus observation; adriamycin, vincristine, cyclophosphamide, dactinomycin, DTIC versus observation; adriamycin, cyclophosphamide, methotrexate versus observation; adriamycin, cyclophosphamide, vincristine, DTIC versus observation; adriamycin and ifosphamide versus observation. The majority of these studies are quite equivocal as to the benefit of adjuvant chemotherapy. We will, briefly, summarize some of the larger ones.

The National Cancer Institute Trial was conducted for patients with stages IIA through IIIB extremity soft-tissue sarcoma. Patients either underwent amputation or limb-sparing surgery followed by radiotherapy. They were then randomized to observation versus adriamycin and cyclophosphamide. After achieving a maximum cumulative dose of adriamycin chemotherapy was switched to methotrexate with leucovorin rescue. At a median follow up of 7.1 years the 5-year relapse-free survival is better for patients who receive chemotherapy ($p = 0.04$); the difference in overall survival is, however, not particularly significant (5,48,60,69).

The Scandinavian Sarcoma Group randomized 240 patients with high-grade sarcomas to receive either adriamycin or no systemic treatment. No significant difference was seen between the adriamycin and the control group with respect to local recurrence, relapse-free survival, or overall survival either for the 181 evaluable patients or the 240 randomized patients (69,70).

The European Organization for the Research and Treatment of Cancer, soft-tissue and bone sarcoma group conducted a phase III trial following local therapy of histologically proven soft-tissue sarcoma in adults with either surgery or radiotherapy. Randomization was to treatment with cyclophosphamide, vincristine, adriamycin, and DTIC versus observation. Between 1997 and 1998,

468 patients entered the study, 151 patients were considered ineligible. The mean follow-up duration is 80 months. Relapse-free survival with chemotherapy was 56% versus 43% for controls ($p = 0.006$), local recurrence was reduced in the chemotherapy arm (17% vs. 31%, $p = 0.0041$), but overall survival did not differ significantly between the two arms (66% for chemotherapy vs. 55% for observation, $p = 0.64$). In patients with extremity tumors no significant improvement was seen with chemotherapy in terms of local recurrence, metastases, or survival. In contrast, local recurrence was less with chemotherapy for head and neck and trunk sarcomas (71).

The remaining approximately 11 randomized trials for adult NRSTS in general, do not show clear benefits to the use of adjuvant chemotherapy. Between 1991 and 1997, we are aware of 4 meta-analyses that have attempted to derive some information from combining the results of the extent randomized trials. A 1997 meta-analysis has been published that evaluates randomized prospective trials of adjuvant chemotherapy for soft-tissue sarcomas in adults. Of the 1,568 patients included in 14 analyzed trials, less than 1% of the patients were younger than 15-years old. The randomized trials accrued patients from 1973 to 1990 and included patients treated, on the chemotherapy arm of the various studies, with adriamycin (Adria) only or that drug with either vincristine, actinomycin, cyclophosphamide (Adria + VAC); Adria + VAC + DTIC; Adria + cyclophosphamide and methotrexate; Adria + cyclophosphamide, vincristine, and DTIC; or Adria + ifosfamide. About two-thirds of the analyzed patients had high-grade tumors, and one-half received radiotherapy. The meta-analysis indicated that adjuvant chemotherapy statistically significantly improved the local recurrence-free survival from 75% to 81% at 10 years, the distant recurrence-free survival from 60% to 70%, and the overall recurrence-free survival from 45% to 55%. The overall survival increased from 50% to 54%, which was not statistically significant (72–76).

Patients with metastatic disease are infrequently cured. A recent study of adults with NRSTS from institutions participating in the Scandinavian Sarcoma Group described a highly select group of 38 patients with metastatic NRSTS or locally advanced disease and who had achieved a complete response with chemotherapy alone or chemotherapy followed by surgery. The drug programs used were either VIG (vincristine, ifosfamide, mesna, G-CSF), VIG + doxorubicin, or ifosfamide, vincristine, doxorubicin, DTIC, and mesna. The 2-year disease-free survival, even in this select group, was only 34%. In general, the complete response rate to chemotherapy in advanced NRSTS is less than 10% and the combined complete and partial response rate is less than 50% (77).

The drugs utilized for the adjuvant treatment of NRSTS, particularly adriamycin, have significant toxicities. With the data currently available, chemotherapy is probably not the appropriate adjuvant therapy for low-grade NRSTS that had appropriate local therapy. For high-grade lesions, trials are ongoing to evaluate new drug combinations such as adriamycin/ifosfamide. It has been argued that improved staging and better local control techniques have been the major contributing factors to improved survival in NRSTS—as opposed to any benefits of chemotherapy. Adjuvant therapy for NRSTS is best given in the context of a clinical trial. Chemotherapy is often given as a component of the treatment of metastatic disease.

RADIOTHERAPEUTIC MANAGEMENT

Radiotherapy for childhood NRSTS may be administered after biopsy but prior to definitive surgery (preoperatively), postoperatively, or intraoperatively. The arguments for preoperative irradiation include the following: (a) preoperative treatment will produce partial regression of the tumor, and the resection may be less extensive than if the surgery had been done initially; (b) preoperative treat-

ment may decrease the risk of autotransplantation of the tumor in the surgical bed and may also decrease the risk of intravascular seeding; and (c) in preoperative treatment the clinically and radiographically demonstrable areas of risk are treated. Other tissues are shielded (21,78). In addition, because postoperative treatment must cover all surgically manipulated areas, the irradiated volume is often larger.

Some of the results in combined adult and pediatric series of NRSTS are quite promising. Suit and co-workers (39,49) achieved an 88% 5-year actuarial local control rate and a 66% survival with limited surgery and radiotherapy in 258 patients with extremity and head and neck primaries. These results have been echoed in other studies (41,79). Eilber et al. (52) administered preoperative external beam irradiation and intra-arterial adriamycin (30 mg per day × 3 days) followed by limb-sparing surgery for extremity sarcomas. The local control rate was 96% for patients who received 35 Gy, 90% to 95% for those who received 28 Gy, and 82% for individuals who received 17.5 Gy. Preoperative radiotherapy plus hyperthermia for NRSTS is being investigated. Local control rates are quite good when thermoradiotherapy is followed by conservative surgery (80). It is not uncommon to find no remaining viable tumor at the time of resection. External microwave hyperthermia is generally only appropriate in older and more cooperative children.

The disadvantages of preoperative therapy include: (a) a delay in the start of definitive surgery, (b) loss of ability to examine the whole tumor specimen for stage and grade, and (c) loss of the ability to surgically assess the extent of the disease. Therefore, many radiotherapists and surgeons favor postoperative treatment. Postoperative radiotherapy must be delayed until adequate wound healing has occurred (39,49). A retrospective review of pre- versus postoperative external beam irradiation from the University of Minnesota for adults with NRSTS found no significant difference in overall or relapse-free survival or local control. Wound complications, however, were more common in preoperative radiotherapy patients (31% vs. 8%, p = 0.0014) (21). Several other centers have done retrospective comparisons of pre- versus postoperative irradiation in series of largely adult patients. Some of the literature favors preoperative treatment (39,81), others do not (82). Most agree that wound complications are higher with preoperative treatment (81,83). When the therapeutic plan includes external beam radiotherapy and surgery for the local treatment of NRSTS, it is generally preferable to completely excise small lesions and treat with postoperative irradiation. Large lesions are, in most cases, better treated with biopsy, preoperative irradiation, and then excision.

Intraoperative brachytherapy may play an important role in limb-sparing surgery. Brachytherapy is often, but not always, given in combination with pre- or postoperative external beam treatment. The potential advantages of brachytherapy include: (a) improved radiobiologic effectiveness due to the administration of high dose of irradiation over a few days rather than several weeks; (b) an intense dose is given deep within the tumor bed; (c) relative sparing of surrounding normal tissue and overlying skin due to the rapid falloff of the dose; and (d) patient convenience due to short treatment time, therefore, avoiding the problems of travel and housing for protracted external beam therapy (57,84,85). Conventional afterloading brachytherapy is suitable for children capable of doing self-care. It is often too difficult, from a nursing standpoint, in younger children. New techniques of remote high-dose rate afterloading, utilizing machines especially designed for this purpose, eliminate the problem of personnel exposure during brachytherapy. Sources are in-place only for a short time each day. In most cases the high-dose rate sources are introduced for a brief period of time daily for several days. Therefore, high-dose rate brachytherapy can be used in young children. Intraoperative external beam electron treatment has been de-scribed for the treatment of NRSTS in adults (86). It can also be used in children.

Volume

Extremity NRSTS tend to grow in a longitudinal fashion by following muscle groups. Generous proximal and distal margins beyond the tumor volume (5 to 10 cm) are appropriate. Because the lesions usually do not cross muscle compartments, the circumferential margins may be more modest (50). A limb CT or MRI scan, followed by a computerized treatment plan, is extremely helpful. The treatment of sarcomas is often a venue for the demonstration of the benefits of three-dimensional treatment-planning techniques, tissue compensators, wedges, customized blocking, and rigid immobilization for reproducible treatments. One should avoid high-dose irradiation of the entire width of a limb in order to avoid severe lymphedema (radiation-induced elephantiasis) (47). Blocking should be used to avoid the ankylosis attendant to the high-dose irradiation of the full width of a joint (56). Growth plates should be shielded when possible (although it is usually better to fully treat a growth plate and shorten a limb rather than asymmetrically irradiate a growth plate and angulate a limb). In nonextremity lesions the tumor volume must be covered with as generous a margin as is feasible.

Epitheliod sarcoma and synovial sarcoma may metastasize to lymph nodes in 10% to 20% of cases (2,36,73,87–89). Elective lymph node irradiation is given by some physicians for these lesions—particularly high-grade tumors. Its efficacy is unknown.

Dose

Modern radiobiologic evidence gives little credence to the assertion that NRSTS are inherently radioresistant. The available retrospective reviews suggest that a minimum of 40 Gy is necessary for the postoperative control of microscopic NRSTS in children (11,12). At these doses, however, there is a substantial chance of local failure. More aggressive treatment is generally warranted. Most investigators would favor a dose of 50 to 60 Gy using a shrinking field technique (23,39,47). Some clinicians favor the use of twice-a-day irradiation, i.e., 1.1–1.2 Gy b.i.d. to 66–72 Gy (47). Similar doses are used for preoperative treatment. There were no local failures in either POG Protocol 8653 or in the University of Florida series for excised tumors treated with greater than or equal to 55 Gy (22). When intraoperative boosts with brachytherapy or electrons are given as part of a combined approach, the dose is usually 10 to 20 Gy. Gross residual sarcoma requires 65 to 72 Gy by external beam and implant (23,49,50). Some adult patients with unresectable lesions have been treated with external beam and intravenous radiosensitizers or external beam plus hyperthermia (4,90).

Brachytherapy

In the treatment of NRSTS, brachytherapy may be used as a boost following or prior to external beam radiotherapy or as the sole form of irradiation. The afterloading catheters are placed at the time of surgical excision. After tumor excision, the operative bed is inspected by the radiation oncologist and surgeon and the implant is planned. Parallel plastic catheters are placed, approximately 1 cm apart, throughout the entire tumor bed— usually with a 1- to 2-cm margin. For extremity lesions, some radiation oncologists place the catheters parallel to the axis of the limb (i.e., parallel to the incision), whereas others place catheters perpendicular to the axis of the incision and limb. Postoperative radiographs are taken with dummy sources to calculate the dose distribution and rate. Initial wound healing is allowed to begin, and the catheters are not loaded with iridium-192 (the most commonly used isotope in this situation) until the sixth postoperative day. Earlier loading is associated with a significant risk of wound complications—up to a 44% incidence (15,91). When the situation warrants it, catheters may be placed adjacent to bone

and/or neurovascular bundles. In general, little irradiation is given via the implant to the superficial incision.

When brachytherapy is the sole form of irradiation to be given, surgical drain sites are usually not implanted. If 45 to 50 Gy of external irradiation is given as part of a course of treatment, the brachytherapy boost is generally 10 to 20 Gy at about 50 cGy per hour. If brachytherapy is the sole form of irradiation used in combination with surgery, then 40 to 50 Gy in 4 to 5 days is given. A randomized trial at Memorial Sloan-Kettering Cancer Center for patients 16 years of age or older with NRSTS demonstrated improved local control with surgery + brachytherapy versus surgery alone. The difference was due to the effect on high-grade lesions (92,93). Patients with high-grade NRSTS with a negative margin had, in two studies, an 89% and 94% local control rate when treated with brachytherapy versus 59% and 77% in those with a positive margin. In patients with high-grade tumors and positive margins treated with brachytherapy and external beam irradiation the local control rate was 90% (15,92,93). Slightly less satisfactory results with brachytherapy + external beam were obtained by Burmeister et al. from Australia in patients with large high-grade sarcomas with close or positive margins (91). When brachytherapy is used as the only form of radiotherapy, some of the local failures are due to marginal misses (5,57,85,92,94). In the Institut Gustave-Roussy series 14 of 16 local failures were marginal or distant from the high-dose brachytherapy region (22).

While the role of brachytherapy in adult NRSTS has been evaluated in several retrospective reviews, some randomized prospective trials are particularly of note. Between 1982 and 1987, 126 patients, mostly adults, with soft-tissue sarcoma were entered into a prospective randomized trial at Memorial Sloan-Kettering Cancer Center. Patients underwent a grossly complete resection with a limb-sparing operation for NRSTS of the extremity or superficial trunk. Intraoperatively, after the resection was complete, patients were randomized to receive either adjuvant brachytherapy or no adjuvant therapy. Those patients who received the implant had a dose of 42 to 45 Gy administered with iridium-192 over a 4- to 6-day period. The median follow-up of this trial is 76 months. The 5-year actuarial local control rate for high grade tumors was 89% for brachytherapy treated patients versus 66% for controls ($p = 0.0025$). There was no local control benefit in the low-grade tumor group. The improved local control with brachytherapy in high-grade tumors did not translate into an overall decrease in distant metastasis. Even in the high-grade tumor the freedom from distant metastases was approximately 70% at 5 years in both the brachytherapy and the control arm (92,95). This trial is of interest not only because it demonstrated a benefit to adjuvant brachytherapy, but also because it showed a benefit to a form of therapy that, in contrast to adjuvant external beam irradiation, generally does not irradiate the full surgical scar, does not irradiate the drain site, is shorter in duration (10 to 14 days hospitalization vs. 6 to 7 weeks outpatient treatment), and is slightly less costly.

The team from Memorial Sloan-Kettering elected to explore the use of brachytherapy in low-grade tumors in more detail insofar as their initial randomized trial did not include a large number of patients with low-grade NRSTS. From 1982 to 1992, they randomized 45 patients with low-grade tumors to brachytherapy versus observation. There was no benefit to brachytherapy in terms of local recurrence (about 76% local control in each arm, $p = 0.60$) or in overall survival ($p = 0.38$) (93). These two randomized trials argue, in the view of the investigators, in favor of adjuvant brachytherapy for resected high-grade tumors, for surgery alone as the treatment for resected low-grade tumors smaller than 5 cm, and for consideration of external beam for resected low-grade tumors 5 cm or larger because of the remaining high risk of local recurrence in these tumors, i.e., 20% to 25%. In the early years of the Memorial Sloan-Kettering trials, there was a substantially higher rate of wound complications in the brachytherapy treated patients compared to controls (44% vs. 14%, $p = 0.0006$). The increased rate of complications has been alleviated by a policy of not loading patients with radioactivity until the fifth postoperative day (95).

What are we to conclude, on the basis of these adult NRSTS studies, concerning the role of brachytherapy in pediatric patients? Based on common histology, patterns of spread, and risk of recurrence, brachytherapy should be considered as an option in the treatment of children. It has the ability to deliver a highly localized dose with considerable sparing of normal tissue. In children, however, brachytherapy poses considerable problems of in-patient management: Can the child provide for their own feeding, bodily care, and immediate needs while radioactive? If not, will there be an unacceptable exposure to nursing personnel or to the parent(s) during the implant? Several solutions have been proposed. One is to utilize a remote afterloading brachytherapy machine. If a high-dose rate remote afterloader is used, the duration of the radiation exposure is short and personnel exposure is minimized. The drawback, however, is that the dose rate is so high that some of the normal tissue sparing benefits of brachytherapy may be lost. To address this latter concern, some physicians "fractionate" the brachytherapy, i.e., use multiple exposures. As an alternative, one can use a remote afterloader with conventional activity sources. In this way, the duration of the implant is no different than with conventional afterloading. The sources, however, may be withdrawn whenever nursing personnel or a parent enters the room for a planned feeding, wound care, bathing the child, etc. A third way of dealing with the particular problems of brachytherapy in a child is to utilize [125]Iodine instead of [192]Iridium. The treatment energy for [125]Iodine is 28 keV versus 380 keV for [192]Iridium. The lower energy of [125]Iodine reduces exposure to clinical staff and family, allows more efficacious shielding with lead drapes, and reduces exposure to normal tissue at a distance from the implant. Unfortunately, [125]Iodine is more expensive and, currently, the seeds have to be individually constructed into an afterloading catheter (95).

Hyperthermia

Hyperthermia has been demonstrated to be an effective radiosensitizer in a variety of clinical situations. Cells that are hypoxic, in S phase, or low pH are particularly sensitive to heating—the converse of conventional radiation. It is not surprising that hyperthermia plus radiation has been evaluated for the preoperative treatment of NRSTS and the primary treatment of inoperable tumors. Uno et al. from Tokyo treated eight patients with NRSTS with external beam irradiation, doxorubicin infusion, and radiofrequency hyperthermia. Five of the 8 patients had a gross recurrent tumor after prior surgical excisions, there were two complete responses and three partial responses. Five of the 8 had no local tumor progression until death or last follow-up (96).

A trial of preoperative radiotherapy plus hyperthermia for NRSTS in adults at Duke University Medical Center was opened in 1984. Forty-four patients with deep non-metastatic high-grade NRSTS received 50 Gy of radiotherapy plus microwave hyperthermia. Negative surgical margins were obtained in 40 patients. The local control rate was 98%, the 3-year overall survival 72%, and 3-year disease-free survival 58%. Patients with tumor median pO_2 less than 10 mm Hg had an 18-month actuarial disease-free survival of 35% v. 70% for patients with a median tumor pO_2 of more than 10mm Hg (p = 0.01) (97–99).

Radiotherapy plus hyperthermia plus surgery seems capable of achieving high local control rates. It has not, to date, shown an ability to reduce distant metastases. The modality is largely untested in children.

Neutrons

Radiobiologists and clinical radiotherapists have been intrigued by the therapeutic uses of neutrons. High linear energy transfer neutrons, by virtue of a low oxygen enhancement ratio and lack of cell cycle cytotoxicity preference, are quite toxic and have been used for the treatment of bulky tumors of various histologies and sites. There is data available from the United States, Europe, and Japan concerning the use of neutrons for the treatment of bulky sarcomas of adults and children. Although definitions of local tumor control vary among reports, the local control rate for neutron treatment of inoperable or residual soft tissue sarcomas is about 50% (100). In a retrospective comparison, Larramore et al. (18) found the local control rate of bulky sarcomas superior with neutrons compared with photons/electrons (53% vs. 38%). Between November 1980 and June 1981, 14 patients, presumably adults, were entered on a prospective trial of postoperative photons versus fast neutrons (15.6 Gy) for NRSTS. Two of the 9 (63 Gy) patients treated with photons relapsed locally as did 2 of the 5 patients treated with neutrons. The trial was halted due to unacceptable late tissue damage in the neutron-treated patients (20).

RESULTS

When NRSTS in children is localized and amenable to definitive surgical excision or limited excision plus radiotherapy, the survival probability is 60% to 90%. The 5-year disease-specific survival for children with NRSTS of the head and neck in the M.D. Anderson Hospital series was 75% (7). For stage I to III NRSTS patients treated on SIOP Trial MMT 84 the 5-year survival rate was 73%; it was 80% for Trial MMT 89 (34). A multivariate analysis of predictive factors for local tumor recurrence in the Royal Marsden series of NRSTS (adults + children) showed significant worsening of the risk for local recurrence with retroperitoneal versus lower limb tumors, high- versus low-grade, and inadequate surgical margins. Metastases were predicted by tumor size larger than 5 cm, high-grade, local recurrence, or the presence of involved lymph nodes (47). In POG Study 8653/8654 the 5-year overall survival for IRS Group I to II NRSTS was 82%, event-free survival 71%, for IRS Group III to IV disease the overall survival was 26%, event-free survival 19% (66). Unresectable or metastatic disease carries a dismal prognosis. Unresectable NRSTS are rarely cured by radiotherapy plus chemotherapy and the local control rate is also poor (22). The 5-year survival rate for children with stage IV NRSTS treated on SIP Trials MMT 84 and MMT 89 was 15% (34).

DESMOID TUMORS

There are a variety of childhood mesenchymal tumors of fibroblastic and/or myofibroblastic derivation that are generally regarded as benign in the sense that these tumors have no potential for metastases. The group includes infantile myofibromatosis, digital fibromatosis, fibromatosis colli, and desmoid tumors (10,101). In addition to the term *desmoid tumor,* these lesions are referred to as

extraabdominal desmoid, well-differentiated nonmetastasizing fibrosarcoma, aggressive fibromatosis, and *Grade I fibrosarcoma (desmoid)* (10,32,102). The usual presenting complaint is a deep-seated, firm mass arising in muscles or soft tissues (32,101,103–105) (Fig. 3). These lesions tend to extend along fascial planes. Histologically, spindle cells with an abundant collagenous background form interlacing bundles and infiltrate surrounding tissue. Mitoses are rare (10,32,106, 107). A small fraction of desmoid tumors are associated with Gardner's syndrome.

Desmoid tumors almost never metastasize. The goal of treatment is to obtain local control. The probability of local control with surgery alone is highly debatable. A review of the literature will disclose wide range of local control rates (10,32,101,102,108,109). The consensus view, however, is that local failures occur in about 20% to 50% of individuals treated primarily with wide surgical resection

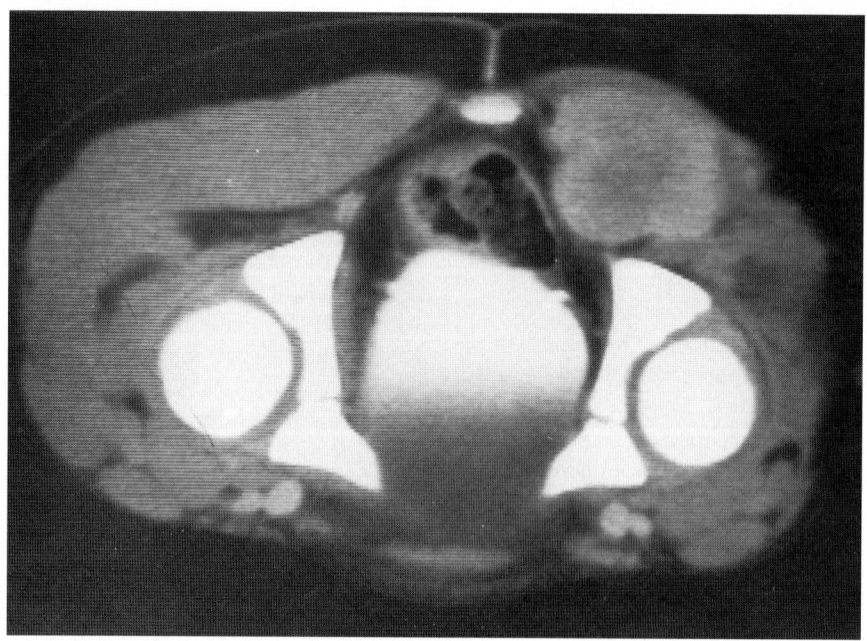

FIG. 3. A right-buttock desmoid tumor in a child. The lesion was excised and recurred. Postoperative irradiation (49.6 Gy) was given following a re-excision of gross disease. Angled photon fields were used to minimize rectal dose. Local control has been maintained. There is partial atrophy of the right-buttock musculature, and the bones of the right hemipelvis are smaller than those of the left hemipelvis. Follow-up of 10 years.

TABLE 4. *Local control rates in combined pediatric and adult series of radiotherapy with or without surgery for the management of desmoid tumors*

Institution	Year of the most recent update of the series	Number of patients	Dose (Gy)	Disease status	Local control
Harvard–Joint Center (17)	1981	9	30–68.6	8 gross disease	87%
				1 postoperative	100%
University of California–San Francisco (115)	1983	19	40.8–61.2	13 gross disease	69%
				6 microscopic	67%
Netherlands Cancer Institute (104)	1986	21	60	11 status post subtotal resection	91%
				8 status post gross total resection	87%
				2 gross disease	100%
Westminister Hospital (58)	1988	38	27–64	29 postoperative	76%
				9 gross disease	67%
Institut Curie (116)	1988	16	45–65	3 postoperative for microscopic disease	100%
				4 postoperative for macroscopic disease	75%
				9 radical radiotherapy for extensive disease	67%
M.D. Anderson Hospital (106)	1990	45	50–76.2	14 gross disease	71%
				31 postoperative	77%
Memorial Sloan–Kettering (111)	1991	38	^{192}Ir brachytherapy (20–60.55 Gy) and, often, supplemental external beam radiotherapy	38 postoperative	66%
Duke (102)	1993	16	49.6–56.2	15 gross disease	93%
				1 postoperative	
Groningen University Hospital (117)	1995	17	50–60	14 resection with postoperative treatment	92%
				2 gross disease	100%
				1 reexcision with brachytherapy	100%
Memorial Sloan–Kettering (112) Only pediatric patients	1995	11	30–50	2 of 11 were treated preoperatively	64%
Mayo Clinic (118)	1996	13	~50.4–64.8	Operation and radiation therapy	100%
				2 wide resection	75%
				4 marginal resection	75%
				4 intralesional resection	33%
				3 radiation therapy only	
University of Florida (110,119)	1996	53	35–70	29 microscopic residual disease	79%
				24 gross disease	88%
Massachusetts General Hospital (101,105,109)	1997	56	22–70.9	15 radiation therapy alone	92%
				41 radiation therapy + surgery	79% primary tumors, 67% recurrent tumors

Table from a concept originally in ref. 102; updated and modified, with permission.

and negative margins and 75% of patients with partial resections. Several factors contribute to this wide range of local control frequencies. Because desmoids can occur in a variety of locations, the degree of resectability is variable. Lesions in accessible sites, which are not adjacent to vital structures, are more amenable to gross total excision than those adjacent to major nerves or vessels. About two-thirds of desmoids are amenable to gross total excision. Even if the surgical margins are minimally positive, many patients will not have a recurrence. Miralbell et al. (105) reported 26 individuals, mostly children, with uncertain or histologically minimally positive margins in areas that were amenable to close follow-up. Seventeen of these 26 patients have not recurred with mean follow-up of 6 years (74%). Where feasible, gross total resection of the tumor is the treatment of choice.

Several types of patients are at high risk for local recurrence/progression: those with unresectable lesions, those who have undergone resection with gross tumor left behind, those who have undergone resection with large areas of clearly positive histologic tumor margins, and those who have already suffered one or more local recurrences following primary surgical therapy. It is clear that radiotherapy can be used to good effect in these cases.

Several retrospective series, combining pediatric and adult patients, have demonstrated that fractionated external beam irradiation or external beam plus brachytherapy can locally control approximately 75% of desmoid tumors (Table 4). Complete or partial resolution may require 2 to 3 years following completion of a course of treatment (102,106). For some patients "local control" will mean cessation of growth rather than tumor regression.

Desmoids can widely infiltrate. When external beam is utilized, treatment portals should be generous. McCullough et al. (110) and Zelefsky et al. (111) found that postradiotherapy relapses often occurred at the margin or beyond the irradiated volume. MRI studies of desmoids frequently show an infiltrative margin. At surgery, microscopic tumor has been found to extend beyond the volume defined by MRI (102). All available evidence from the physical examination, surgical report, CT, and MRI should be integrated to determine the tumor volume. Generous margins should then be used around this volume. Daily fractionations of 1.8 to 2 Gy are used. There may be an increased local recurrence when doses less than 45 to 50 Gy are used. In 1984, Kiel and Suit (101) suggested that doses greater than 60 Gy may be associated with a greater incidence of local control and have treated some patients with 70 Gy—often using photons and protons. Neutron boosts have also been used (106). Evidence indicates that a total dose of 50 to 55 Gy is appropriate and that higher doses may increase the risk of complications without commensurate gain in local tumor control (102,105,106,109). Brachytherapy has been reported as a treatment for desmoids, either alone or with external beam therapy, by one institution (111). Because of concerns about the assessment of tumor margins and their coverage, we believe that the role of brachytherapy is quite limited in children with desmoids.

In young children with desmoids, radiation's effects on growing bone, the risk for subsequent soft-tissue fibrosis, and the potential for secondary malignancy may prompt consideration of alternative therapies. Some efficacy has been reported in children treated with vincristine, actinomycin D, and cyclophosphamide (79,112). Obviously, cytotoxic chemotherapy has the potential for serious short- and long-term ill effects. Antiestrogen therapy, nonsteroidal anti-inflammatory agents, and immunotherapy have also been attempted with occasional benefit (101,102,113).

REFERENCES

References particularly recommended for further reading are indicated by an asterisk.

1. Conrad EU, Bradford L, Chansky HA. Pediatric soft-tissue sarcomas. *Orthop Clin North Am* 1996;17:655–664.
2. Greenberg J. Epithelioid sarcoma. *Med Pediatr Oncol* 1982;10:497–500.
3. Raney B Jr. Soft-tissue sarcoma in adolescents. In:

Tebbi CK, ed. *Major topics in adolescent oncology.* Mount Kisco, NY: Futura Publishing, 1987:221–240.

4. Hayani A, Mahoney DH Jr, Hawkins HK, Steuber CP, Hurwitz R, Fernbach DJ. Soft-tissue sarcomas other than rhabdomyosarcoma in children. *Med Pediatr Oncol* 1992;20:114–118.

5. Antman KH, Eilber FR, Shiu MH. Soft tissue sarcomas: current trends in diagnosis and management. *Curr Prob Cancer* 1989;13:340–369.

6. Horowitz ME, Pratt CB, Webber BL, et al. Therapy for childhood soft tissue sarcomas other than rhabdomyosarcoma: a review of 62 cases treated at a single institution. *J Clin Oncol* 1986;4:559–564.

7. Lyos AT, Goepfert H, Luna MA, Jaffe N, Malpica A. Soft tissue sarcoma of the head and neck in children and adolescents. *Cancer* 1996;77:193–200.

8. Harris M, Hartley AL. Value of peer review of pathology to soft tissue sarcomas. In: Verweij J, Pinedo HM, Suit HD, eds. *Soft tissue sarcomas: present achievements and future prospects.* Boston: Kluwer Academic Publishers, 1997:1–8.

9. Scott SM, Reiman HM, Pritchard DJ, Ilstrup DM. Soft tissue fibrosarcoma: a clinicopathologic study of 132 cases. *Cancer* 1989;64:925–931.

10. Coffin CM, Dehner LP. Soft tissue neoplasms in children: a clinicopathologic overview. In: Finegold M, ed. *Pathology of neoplasia in children and adolescents.* Philadelphia: WB Saunders, 1986:223–255.

11. Raney B, Schnaufer L, Ziegler M, Chatten J, Littman P, Jarrett P. Treatment of children with neurogenic sarcoma: experience at the Children's Hospital of Philadelphia, 1958–1984. *Cancer* 1987;59:1–5.

12. Raney RB Jr, Littman P, Jarrett P, Waldman MTG, Chatten J. Results of multimodal therapy for children with neurogenic sarcoma. *Med Pediatr Oncol* 1979;7:229–236.

13. Ducatman BS, Scheithauer BW, Piepgras DG, Reiman HM, Ilstrup DM. Malignant peripheral nerve sheath tumors: a clinicopathologic study of 120 cases. *Cancer* 1986;57:2006–2021.

14. Coffin CM, Dehner LP. Peripheral neurogenic tumors of the soft tissues in children and adolescents: a clinicopathologic study of 108 examples in 103 patients. *Pediatr Pathol* 1989;11:559–588.

15. Alekhteyar KM, Leung DH, Brennan MF, Harrison LB. The effect of combined external beam radiotherapy and brachytherapy on local control and wound complications in patients with high-grade soft tissue sarcomas of the extremity with positive microscopic margin. *Int J Radiat Oncol Biol Phys* 1996;36:321–324.

16. Frey E, Niggli F, Stauffer U, Pluss HJ. Primary resection of soft-tissue sarcomas: yes and no. *Eur J Pediatr Surg* 1997;7:227–229.

17. Greenberg HM, Goebel R, Weichselbaum RR, Greenberger JS, Chaffey JT, Cassady JR. Radiation therapy in the treatment of aggressive fibromatoses. *Int J Radiat Oncol Biol Phys* 1981;7:305–310.

18. Larramore GE, Griffith JT, Boespflug M, et al. Fast neutron radiotherapy for sarcomas of soft tissue, bone, and cartilage. *Am J Clin Oncol* 1989;12:320–326.

19. Carli M, Guglielmi M, Sotti G, Cecchetto G, Ninfo V. Soft tissue sarcoma. In: Pinkerton CR, Plowman PN, eds. *Paediatric oncology: clinical practice and controversies,* second edition. London: Chapman & Hall Medical, 1997:380–416.

20. Glaholm J, Harmer C. Soft-tissue sarcoma: neutrons versus photons for postoperative irradiation. *Br J Radiol* 1988;61:829–834.

21. Cheng EY, Dusenbery KE, Winters MR, Thompson RC. Soft tissue sarcomas: preoperative versus posoperative radiotherapy. *J Surg Oncol* 1996;61:90–99.

*22. Marcus RJ. Current controversies in pediatric radiation oncology. *Orthop Clin North Am* 1996; 27: 551–557.

23. Brizel DM, Weinstein H, Hunt M, Tarbell NJ. Failure patterns and survival in pediatric soft tissue sarcoma. *Int J Radiat Oncol Biol Phys* 1988;15:37–41.

24. Neifeld JP, Berg JW, Godwin D, Salzberg AM. A retrospective epidemiologic study of pediatric fibrosarcomas. *J Pediatr Surg* 1978;13:735–739.

25. Canpolat C, Evans HL, Corpron C, et al. Fibromyxoid sarcoma in a four-year old child: case report and review of the literature. *Med Pediatr Oncol* 1996;27:561–564.

26. Staples JJ, Robinson RA, Wen B-C, Hussey DH. Hemangiopericytoma—the role of radiotherapy. *Int J Radiat Oncol Biol Phys* 1990;19:445–451.

27. Nash A, Stout AP. Malignant mesenchymomas in children. *Cancer* 1961;14:524–533.

28. Newman PL, Fletcher CDM. Malignant mesenchymoma: clinicopathologic analysis of a series with evidence of low-grade behaviour. *Am J Surg Pathol* 1991;15:607–614.

29. Gross E, Rao BN, Pappo AS, et al. Soft tissue sarcoma of the hand in children: clinical outcome and management. *J Pediatr Surg* 1997;32(5):698–702.

30. Womer RB, Sinniah D. Soft tissue sarcomas. In: D'Angio GT, Sinniah D, Meadows AT, Evans AE, Pritchard J, eds. *Practical pediatric oncology.* New York: Wiley-Liss, 1992:318–325.

31. Gross E, Rao BN, Papo A, et al. Epithelioid sarcoma in children. *J Pediatr Surg* 1996;31(12):1663–1665.

32. Enzinger FM, Weiss SW. *Soft tissue sarcomas.* St. Louis: CV Mosby, 1983.

33. Kim TH, Bell BA, Mauer HM, Ragab AH. Sarcomas of soft tissues and their benign counterparts. In: Fernbach DJ, Vietti TJ, eds. *Clinical pediatric oncology,* 4th ed. St. Louis: Mosby-Year Book, 1991:517–544.

34. Pappo AS. Rhabdomyosarcoma and other soft tissue sarcomas in children. *Curr Opin Oncol* 1996;8: 311–316.

35. Dehner LP. Primitive neuroectodermal tumor and Ewing's sarcoma. *Am J Surg Path* 1993;17:1–13.

36. Raney RB Jr. Synovial sarcoma. *Med Pediatr Oncol* 1981;91:41–45.

37. Raney RB Jr. Chemotherapy for children with aggressive fibromatosis and Langerhans' cell historytosis. *Clin Orthop* 1987;59:1–5.

38. Salloum E, Flamant F, Caillaud JM, et al. Diagnostic and therapeutic problems of soft tissue tumors other than rhabdomyosarcoma in infants under 1 year of age: a clincopathological study of 34 cases treated at the Institut Gustave-Roussy. *Med Pediatr Oncol* 1991;18:37–43.

*39. Suit HD, Mankin HJ, Wood WC, Proppes KH. Preoperative, intraoperative, and postoperative radiation in the treatment of primary soft tissue sarcoma. *Cancer* 1985;55:2659–2667.

40. Jones DN, McCowage GB, Sostman HD, et al. Monitoring of neoadjuvant therapy response of soft-tissue and musculoskeletal sarcoma using fluorine-18-FDG PET. *J Nucl Med* 1996;37:1438–1444.

41. LeVay J, O'Sullivan B, Cotton C, et al. Outcome and prognostic factors in soft tissue sarcoma. *Int J Radiat Oncol Biol Phys* 1992;24[Suppl 1]:182–183.

42. Miser JS, Triche TJ, Pritchard DJ, Kinsella T. Ewing's sarcoma and the nonrhabdomyosarcoma soft tissue sarcomas of childhood. In: Pizzo PA, Poplack DG, eds. *Principles and practice of pediatric oncology.* Philadelphia: JB Lippincott, 1989:659–688.

43. Wenger J, Davidson R. Fibrosarcoma of the leg. *Med Pediatr Oncol* 1984;12:209–211.

44. Parham DM, Webber BL, Jenkins JJ, Cantor AB, Maurer HM. Nonrhabdomyosarcomatous soft tissue sarcomas of childhood: formulation of a simplified system for grading. *Mod Pathol* 1995;8:705–710.

45. Rao BN. Nonrhabdomyosarcoma in children: prognostic factors influencing survival. *Semin Surg Oncol* 1993;9:524–531.

46. Enneking WF, Spanier SS, Goodman MA. A system for the surgical staging of musculoskeletal sarcomas. *Clin Ortho* 1980;153:106–120.

47. Harmer C. Management of soft tissue sarcomas. In: Selby P, Bailey C, eds. *Cancer and the adolescent.* London: BMJ Publishing Group, 1996:69–89.

*48. Mazanet R, Antman KH. Adjuvant therapy for sarcomas. *Semin Oncol* 1991;18:603–612.

*49. Suit HD. The George Edelstyn Memorial lecture: radiation in the management of malignant soft tissue tumours. *Clin Oncol* 1989;1:5–10.

*50. Tepper JE, Suit HD. The role of radiation therapy in the treatment of sarcoma of soft tissue. *Cancer Invest* 1985;3:587–592.

51. Delaney TF, Stinson SF, Greenberg J, et al. Effects on limb function of combined modality limb-sparing therapy for extremity soft tissue sarcoma. *Proc ASCO* 1991;10:350.

52. Eilber FR, Guiliana AE, Huth J, Mirra J, Morton DL. High grade soft-tissue sarcomas of the extremity: UCLA experience with limb-sparing. *Prog Clin Biol Res* 1985;201:59–74.

53. National Institutes of Health Consensus Development Conference Statement. Limb-sparing treatment of adult soft-tissue sarcomas and osteosarcomas. *National Health Cons Dev Conf State,* NIH, Bethesda, MD. 1985;3:1–8.

54. Jablons D, Steinberg SM, Roth J, Pittaluga S, Rosenberg SA, Pass HI. Metastasectomy for soft tissue sarcoma: further evidence for efficacy and prognostic indicators. *J Thorac Cardiovasc Surg* 1989;97:695–705.

55. Casson AG, Putman JB, Natarajan G, et al. Efficacy of pulmonary metastasectomy for recurrent soft tissue sarcoma. *J Surg Oncol* 1991;47:1–4.

56. Kalnicki S. Radiation therapy in the treatment of bone and soft tissue sarcomas. *Orthop Clin North Am* 1989;20:505–512.

57. Schray MF, Gunderson LL, Sim FH, Pritchard DJ, Shives TC, Yeakel PD. Soft tissue sarcoma: integration of brachytherapy, resection, and external irradiation. *Cancer* 1990;66:451–456.

58. Stockdale AD, Casson AM, Coe MA, et al. Radiotherapy and conservative surgery in the management of musculo-aponeurotic fibromatosis. *Int J Radiat Oncol Biol Phys* 1988;15:851–857.

59. POG (Pediatric Oncology Group) Protocol 8653/8654: A study of childhood soft tissue sarcoma (STS) other than rhabdomyosarcoma and its variations. Chicago, IL: Pediatric Oncology Group, 1986.

59a. Spiro IJ, Gebhardt MC, Jennings LC, Mankin HJ, Marmon DC, Suit HD. Prognostic factors for local control of sarcomas of the soft tissues managed by radiation and surgery. *Semin Oncol* 1997;24(5):540–6.

60. Rosenberg SA, Glatstein E, Chang AE. The role of adjuvant chemotherapy in the treatment of soft tissue sarcomas: review of the National Cancer Institute studies. In: van Oosteram AT, van Unnik JAM, eds. *Management of soft tissue and bone sarcomas.* New York: Raven Press, 1986:201–214.

61. Chang AE, Sugarbaker PH, Rosenberg SA. Quality of life after different treatment modalities for soft tissue sarcoma: review of National Cancer Institute studies. In: van Oosteram AT, van Unnik JAM, eds. *Management of soft tissue and bone sarcomas.* New York: Raven Press, 1986:225–232.

62. Stinson SF, Dellancy TF, Greenberg J, et al. Acute and long-term effects on limb function of combined modality limb sparing therapy for extremity soft tissue sarcoma. *Int J Radiat Oncol Biol Phys* 1991;21:1493–1499.

63. Raney RB Jr, Allen A, O'Neill J, Handler SD, Uri A, Littman P. Malignant fibrous histiocytoma of soft tissue in childhood. *Cancer* 1991;262:58–63.

64. Horowitz M, Pratt C, Webber B, et al. Childhood malignant soft tissue sarcomas (STS) other than rhabdomyosarcoma: results of therapy. *Proc ASCO* 1984;3:84.

65. Meyer WH, Pratt CB, Thompson EI, et al. Ifosfamide/etoposide (Ifos/VP-16) in patients with previously untreated Ewing's sarcoma (ES) or primitive neuro-ectodermal tumors (PNET). *Proc ASCO* 1991;10:307.

66. Koscielniak E, Jugens H, Winkler K, et al. Treatment of soft tissue sarcoma in childhood and adolescence. *Cancer* 1992;70:2557–2567.

67. Treuner J, Jurgens H, Winkler K, et al. The treatment of 30 children and adolescents of synovial sarcoma in accordance with the protocol of the German multicenter study for soft tissue sarcoma. *Proc ASCO* 1987;6:215.

68. Sommelet-Olive D. Non-rhabdo malignant mesenchymal tumors in children. *Med Pediatr Oncol* 1995;25:273.

69. Verweij J, Pinendo HM. Adjuvant chemotherapy of soft tissue sarcomas. In: Verweig J, Pinedo HM, Suit HD, eds. *Soft tissue sarcomas: present achievements and future prospects.* Boston: Kluwer Academic Publishers, 1997:173–188.

70. Alvegard TA, Sigurdsson H, Mourdisen H, et al. Adjuvant chemotherapy with doxorubicin and high grade soft tissue sarcoma: a randomized trial of the Scandinavian Sarcoma Group. *J Clin Oncol* 1989;7:1504–1513.

*71. Bramwell V, Rouesse J, Steward W, et al. Adjuvant CYVADIC Chemotherapy for adult soft tissue sarcoma-reduced local recurrence but no improvement in survival: a study of the European Organization for Research and Treatment of Cancer Soft Tissue and Bone Sarcoma Group. *J Clin Oncol* 1994;12: 1137–1149.

72. Newton WA Jr, Soule EH, Hamoudi AB, et al. A prospective study of nonrhabdomyosarcoma soft tissue sarcomas in the pediatric age group. *J Pediatr Surg* 1992;27:241–245.

73. Womer RB. Problems and controversies in the management of childhood sarcomas. *Br Med Bull* 1996;4: 826–843.

74. Sommelet-Olive D, Oberlin O, Flamant F, Stevens M. Non-rhabdo malignant mesenchymal tumors in children, results of SIOP MMT 84 and 89 Protocols. *Proc ASCO* 1995;14:446.

*75. Sarcoma Meta-Analysis Collaboration. Adjuvant chemotherapy for localised resectable soft-tissue sarcoma of adults: meta-analysis of individual data. *Lancet* 1997;350:1647–1654.

76. Tierney JF, Mosseri V, Stuart LA, Souhami RL, Parmer MKB. Adjuvant chemotherapy for soft tissue sarcoma: review and meta-analysis of the published results of randomized clinical trials. *Br J Cancer* 1995;72:469–475.

77. Wiklund T, Saeter G, Strander H, Alvegard T, Blomqvist C. The outcome of advanced soft tissue sarcoma patients with complete tumour regression after either chemotherapy alone or chemotherapy plus surgery. The Scandinavian Sarcoma Group Experience. *Eur J Cancer* 1997;33:357–361.

78. Tanabe K, Sherman N, Pollock R, Romsdahl M. Local control of extremity sarcomas treated with preoperative radiotherapy and limb sparing surgery. *Proc ASCO* 1991;10:351.

79. Keus RB, Rutgers EJ Th, Ho GH, Gortzok E, Albus-Lutter C, Hart AA. Limb sparing therapy of extremity soft tissue sarcomas: treatment outcome and long-term functional results. *Eur J Cancer* 1994;30A: 1459–1463.

80. Hiraoka M, Nishimura Y, Nagata Y, et al. Hyperthermia combined with radiotherapy in the treatment of soft tissue tumors. *Int J Radiat Oncol Biol Phys* 1992;24[Suppl 1]:297–298.

*81. Suit HD, Spiro I. Role of radiation in the management of adult patients with sarcoma of soft tissue. *Semin Surg Oncol* 1994;10:347–356.

82. Sawyer TE, Peterson IA, Pritchard DJ, et al. Prognostic factors in extemity soft tissue sarcomas treated with limb salvage therapy. Joint Meeting of European Musculo-skeletal Oncology Society and American Musculo-Skeletal Tumor Society. Florence, Italy, May 8, 1995.

83. Barkley H Jr, Martin RG, Romsdahl MM, et al. Treatment of soft tissue sarcomas by preoperative irradiation and conservative surgical resection. *Int J Radiat Oncol Biol Phys* 1988;14:693–699.

84. Gerbaulet A, Panis X, Flamant F, Chassagne D. Iridium afterloading curitherapy in the treatment of pediatric malignancies: the Institut Gustave-Roussy experience. *Cancer* 1958;56:1274–1279.

85. Shiu MH, Hilaris BS, Harrison LB, Brennan MF. Brachytherapy and function-saving resection of soft tissue sarcoma arising in the limb. *Int J Radiat Oncol Biol Phys* 1991;21:1485–1492.

86. Willett CG, Suit HD, Tepper JE, et al. Intraoperative electron beam radiation therapy for retroperitoneal soft tissue sarcoma. *Cancer* 1991;68:278–283.

87. MacKenzie DH. Synovial sarcoma: a review of 58 cases. *Cancer* 1966;19:169–180.

88. Pratt J, Woodruff JM, Marcove RC. Epithelioid sarcoma: an analysis of 22 cases indicating the prognostic significance of vascular invasion and regional lymph node metastasis. *Cancer* 1978;41: 1472–1487.

89. Santavirta S. Synovial sarcoma: a clinicopathological study of 31 cases. *Arch Orthop Trauma Surg* 1992; 111:155–159.

90. Kinsella TJ, Glatstein E. Clinical experience with intravenous radiosensitizers in unresectable sarcomas. *Cancer* 1987;59:908–915.

91. Burmeister BH, Dickinson I, Bryant G, Doody J. Intra-operative implant brachytherapy in the management of soft-tissue sarcomas. *Aust N Z J Surg* 1997; 67:5–8.

92. Harrison LB, Franzese F, Gaynor J, et al. Long term results of a prospective randomized trial of adjuvant brachytherapy in the management of completely resected soft tissue sarcoma of the extremity and superficial trunk. *Int J Rad Oncol Biol Phys* 1993;27: 259–265.

93. Pisters PWT, Harrison LB, Woodruff JM, Gaynor JJ, Brennan MF. A prospective randomized trial of adjuvant brachytherapy in the management of low-grade soft tissue sarcomas of the extremity and superficial trunk. *J Clin Oncol* 1994;6:1150–1155.

94. Habrand JL, Gerbaulet A, Pejovic MH, et al. Twenty years experience of interstitial iridium brachytherapy in the management of soft tissue sarcomas. *Int J Radiat Oncol Biol Phys* 1991;20:405–411.

95. Devlin PM, Harrison LB. Brachytherapy for soft tissue sarcomas. In: Verweig J, Pinedo HM, Suit HD, eds. *Soft tissue sarcomas: present achievements and future prospects.* Boston: Kluwer Academic Publishers, 1997:107–128.

96. Uno T, Itami J, Kato H. Combined chemo-radiation and hyperthermia for locally advanced soft tissue sarcoma: response and toxicity. *Anticancer Res* 1995;15: 2655–2658.

97. Brizel DM, Scully SP, Harrelson JM, et al. Radiation therapy and hyperthermia improve the oxygenation of human soft tissue sarcomas. *Cancer Res* 1996;56: 5347–5350.

98. Leopold KA, Harrelson J, Prosnitz L, Samulski TV, Dewhirst MW, Oleson JR. Preoperative hyperthermia and radiation for soft tissue sarcomas: advantage of two vs. one hyperthermia treatments per week. *Int J Rad Oncol Biol Phys* 1989;16:107–115.

99. Scully SP, Oleson JR, Leopold KA, Samulski TV, Dodge R, Harrelson JM. Clinical outcome after neoadjuvant thermoradiotherapy in high grade soft tissue sarcomas. *J Surg Oncol* 1994;57:143–151.

100. Rhomberg W, Hassenstein EOM, Gefeller D. Radiotherapy vs. radiotherapy and razoxane in the treatment of soft tissue sarcomas: final results of a randomized study. *Int J Radiat Oncol Biol Phys* 1996; 36:1077–1084.

101. Kiel KD, Suit HD. Radiation therapy in the treatment of aggressive fibromatoses (desmoid tumors). *Cancer* 1984;54:2041–2055.

*102. Acker JC, Bossen EH, Halperin EC. The management of desmoid tumors. *Int J Radiat Oncol Biol Phys* 1993;26:851–858.

103. Benninghoff D, Robbins R. The nature and treatment of desmoid tumors. *AJR* 1964;91:132–137.

104. Keus R, Bartelink H. The role of radiotherapy in the treatment of desmoid tumors. *Radiother Oncol* 1986; 7:1–5.

*105. Miralbell R, Suit HB, Mankin H, Zuckerberg LR, Stracher M, Rosenberg AE. Fibromatoses: from post-surgical surveillance to combined surgery and radiation therapy. *Int J Radiat Oncol Biol Phys* 1990;18: 535–540.

106. Sherman NE, Romsdahl M, Evans H, Zagars G, Oswald MJ. Desmoid tumors: a 20 year radiotherapy experience. *Int J Radiat Oncol Biol Phys* 1990;19:37–40.

107. Spicer RD. Neonatal soft tissue tumours. *Br J Cancer* 1992;18[Suppl]:580–583.

108. Reitamo JJ. The desmoid tumor. *Arch Surg* 1983;118: 1318–1322.

109. Suit HD, Spiro IJ, Speer M. Benign and low grade tumors of the soft tissues: role for radiation therapy. In: Verweig J, Pinedo HM, Suit HD, eds. *Soft tissue sarcomas: present achievements and future prospects.* Boston: Kluwer Academic Publishers 1997:95–106.

110. McCullough WM, Parson JT, van der Griend R, Enneking WF, Heare T. Radiation therapy for aggressive fibromatosis. *J Bone Joint Surg* 1991; 73A(5):717–725.

111. Zelefsky MJ, Harrison LB, Shiu MH, Armstrong JG, Hajdu SI, Brennan MF. Combined surgical resection and iridium 192 implantation for locally advanced and recurrent desmoid tumors. *Cancer* 1991;67: 380–384.

*112. Faulkner LB, Hajdu SI, Kher U, et al. Pediatric desmoid tumor: Retrospective analysis of 63 cases. *J Clin Oncol* 1995;13:2813–2818.

113. Lackner H, Urban C, Kerbi R, Schwinger W, Beham A. Noncytotoxic drug therapy in children with unresectable desmoid tumors. *Cancer* 1997;80:334–340.

114. Dillon P, Maurer J, Jenkins J, et al. A prospective study of nonrhabdomyosarcoma soft tissue sarcomas in the pediatric age group. *J Pediatr Surg* 1992;27:241–245.

115. Leibel SA, Wara WM, Hill DR, et al. Desmoid tumors: local control and patterns of relapse following radiation therapy. *Int J Radiat Oncol Biol Phys* 1983; 9(8):1167–1171.

116. Bataini JP, Belloir C, Mazabraud A, et al. Desmoid tumors in adults: the role of radiotherapy in their management. *Am J Surg* 1988;155:754–760.

117. Plukker JT, Oort IV, Vermey A, et al. Aggressive fibromatosis (non-familial desmoid tumour): therapeutic problems and the role of adjuvant radiotherapy. *Br J Surg* 1995;82:510–514.

118. Pritchard DJ, Nascimento AG, Petersen IA. Local control of extra-abdominal desmoid tumors. *J Bone Joint Surg* 1996;78-A;848–854.

119. Kamath SS, Parsons JT, Marcus RB, Zlotecki RA, Scarborough MT. Radiotherapy for local control of aggressive fibromatosis. *Int J Radiat Oncol Biol Phys* 1996;36:325–328.

Wilms' Tumor

HISTORY

The first description of a Wilms' tumor was from Thomas F. Rance in his 1814 report *Case of fungus haematodes of the kidnies* (1). In 1828, Dr. Ebenezer Gairdner, Fellow of the Royal College of Physicians, Edinburgh, published the second case. The patient was a 3-year-old girl named "Agnes B" who died of a left renal tumor that weighed 5 pounds 3 ounces (2). In 1879, the renowed physician William Osler described two cases of "myosarcoma of the kidney"—one of which had tumor extension into the right heart and pulmonary artery (3). Max Wilms (1867–1918), who was trained in pathology, internal medicine, and surgery thoroughly reviewed the pertinent literature and added seven new patients in his 1899 monograph *Die Misch-geschwuelste*. In addition to renal tumors, Wilms described the histologically "mixed tumors" of the ovary, testicle, head and neck, bladder, and other organs (4). It was because of Wilms' exceptional monograph that his name became connected with this childhood tumor (5) (Fig. 1).

EPIDEMIOLOGY

Wilms' tumor (nephroblastoma) is an embryonic kidney tumor. It is the most common abdominal tumor in children and represents 6% of childhood cancer. The incidence rate in white children younger than 15 years of age is 8.1 new cases per million population (6). There were approximately 470 new cases in the United States in 1996 (7,8). Wilms' tumor is bilateral at presentation in 4% to 8% of cases (9–11).

The median age at diagnosis is 41.5 months for males with unilateral tumors and 46.9 months for females with unilateral tumors. For bilateral tumors the median age at presentation is 29.5 months for males and 32.6 months for females (7). Over 75% of patients present before 5 years of age (12). The male to female ratio is 0.92 for unilateral tumors and 0.6 for bilateral tumors (7). The incidence rate is approximately three times higher for blacks in the United States and Africa than for East Asians. Rates for the white populations in Europe and North America are intermediate between those of blacks and East Asians (6). Children tend to present with more advanced stage disease in less developed nations (13–15).

MOLECULAR BIOLOGY

In Chapter 5 of this text, we discussed the Knudson "two-hit" hypothesis of the origins of retinoblastoma. This hypothesis explained the earlier age of onset and bilateral presentation of familial retinoblastoma compared to sporadic cases. Subsequent research confirmed the veracity of the two-hit hypothesis for retinoblastoma and showed that it could be explained by the inactivation of both alleles of a tumor-suppressor gene on the long arm of chromosome 13 (abbreviated 13q). After vetting his hypothesis for retinoblastoma, Knudson proposed a similar model for Wilms' tumor in 1972 (16,17).

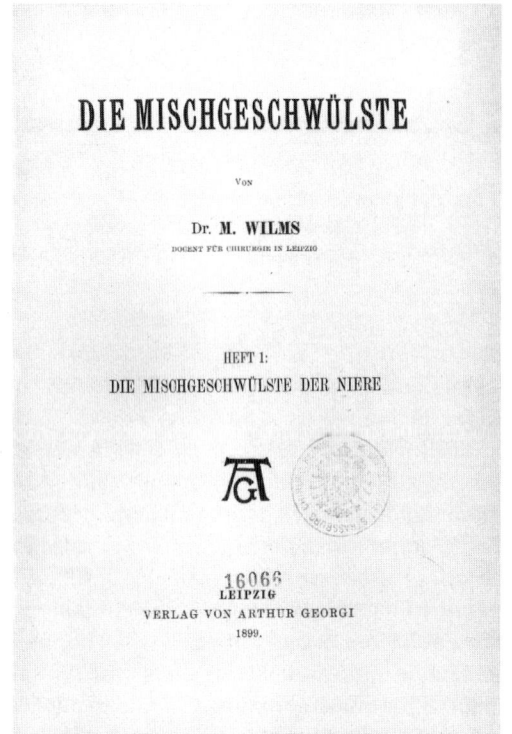

A

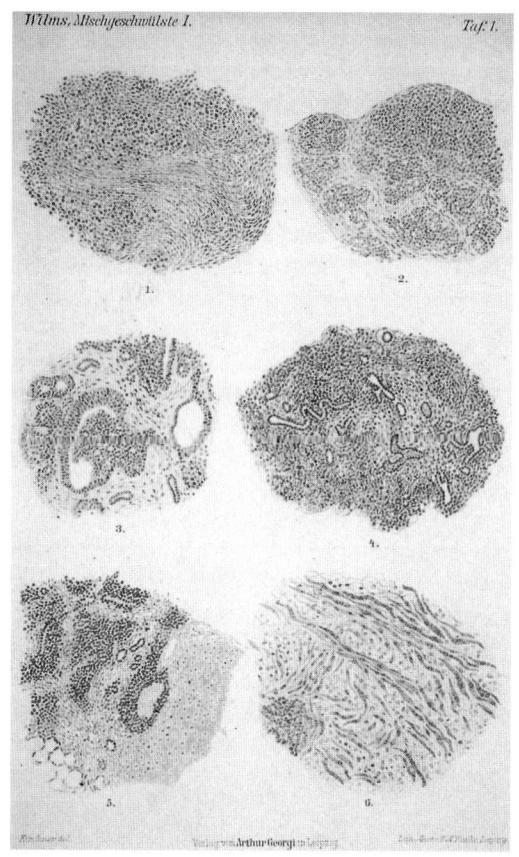

C

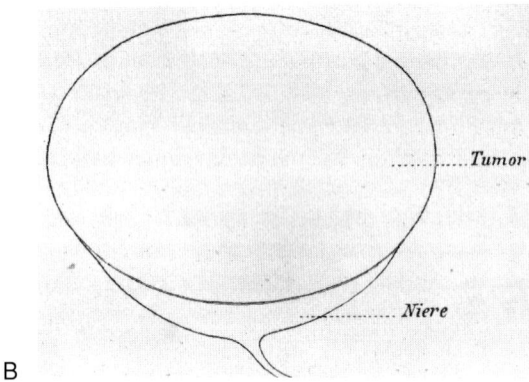

B

FIG. 1. A and B: In his monograph, *Die Mis-chgeschwulste Der Niere* (The mixed tumor of the kidney), published in Leipzig in 1899, Max Wilms described, as his first illustrative case, "niven tumor von einem 3 jahrien Madchen" (renal tumor of a 3-year-old little girl). **C:** Wilms described the blastemal, epithelial (tubules), and stromal elements seen on microscopic examination of "mixed" renal tumor.

Just as retinoblastoma, Wilms' tumor may be unilateral or bilateral. The 4% to 8% occurrence of bilateral disease, appearing at an earlier age than unilateral disease and associated with a greater frequency of other hereditary anomalies, supports the concept of a specific predisposing constitutional chromosomal deletion. It should be noted that fewer familial and bilateral cases of Wilms' tumor than retinoblastoma were available for analysis due to the lower incidence of familial Wilms' tumor and the poor disease survival at that time (18,19).

Wilms' tumor is associated with congenital anomalies in 10% to 13% of cases (13,14,20, 21). Aniridia is present in 1% of children with Wilms' tumor; hemihypertrophy is noted in 2% to 3% (21–23). Other genitourinary malformations are identified in 5% of cases, primarily cryptorchidism, hypospadias, double collecting system, or fused kidney (14,23,24).

It seemed reasonable to look for candidate Wilms' tumor genes in association with these congenital anomalies.

The next major clue to the molecular genetics of Wilms' tumor was found from the **WAGR** syndrome—**W**ilms' tumor with **A**niridia, **G**enitourinary malformations, and mental **R**etardation. Karyotypic analysis of WAGR children showed a deletion on the short arm of chromosome 11, band 13 (abbreviated 11p13). This deletion encompasses the aniridia gene *PAX6* and the Wilms' tumor suppressor gene *WT1*. *WT1* is a developmentally regulated transcription factor of the zinc finger family. Analysis of sporadic Wilms' tumors, however, shows evidence of *WT1* mutation in only 5% to 10% of cases. Therfore, although *WT1* appears to be a tumor suppressor gene, it accounts for a minority of Wilms' tumors (18,19).

Wilms' tumor also occurs with increased frequency in the Beckwith-Wiedemann syndrome (25). This familial condition variably includes macrosomia or hemihypertrophy, macroglossia, omphalocele, abdominal organomegaly, and ear pits or creases. The genetic locus of this syndrome is also on the short arm of chromosome 11 (11p15). The putative second Wilms' tumor suppressor gene, located at this site, is called *WT2* (18,19).

In addition to the tumor suppressor genes associated with Wilms' tumor, there is evidence for genetic loci that may be related to more malignant or aggressive Wilms' tumors. In a study of 232 children with Wilms' tumor registered on the National Wilms' Tumor Studies 3 and 4, loss of chromosomal material (called loss of heterozygosity or LOH) on the long arm of chromosome 16 (16q) was associated with a statistically significantly poorer 2-year relapse-free and overall survival. (If there is no LOH for 16q, 2-year relapse-free survival is 90%, vs. 78% if present.) The difference remained when the analysis was adjusted for stage or histologic subgroup. Loss of chromosomal material from the short arm of chromosome 1 (1p) was also associated with poorer relapse-free and overall survival—although of borderline statistical

significance (chromosomal material from 1p is absent, 2-year relapse-free survival is 88%, vs. 64% if present) (7,26). The prognostic importance of loss of material on 1p and 16q are prospectively evaluated in national Wilm's Tumor Study 5 (vide infra). They are appropriately called *Wilms' tumor progression genes*.

Identification of the genes associated with Wilms' tumor will, it is hoped, add to our knowledge of tumor suppressor genes, allow for more precise genetic counseling, and help predict outcome of treatment for this tumor and identify those children in need of more aggressive therapy (19,26).

PATHOLOGY

The two popular childhood kidney tumor pathology classification systems are those of the National Wilms' Tumor Study (NWTS) and the International Study of Pediatric Oncology (Societe Internationale d'Oncologie Pediatrique, SIOP) (Table 1).

Mesoblastic Nephroma

Mesoblastic nephroma is the most common renal tumor encountered in the first month of

TABLE 1. *Classification of pediatric renal tumors*

SIOP	NWTS
I. Low risk	
Cystic partially differentiated Wilms'	Mesoblastic nephroma
Mesoblastic nephroma	
Wilms' tumor with fibroadenomatous structures	
Highly differentiated epithelial Wilms' tumor	
II. Intermediate risk	
Nonanaplastic Wilms' tumor with its varients (excluding low risk types)	Favorable histology Wilms' tumor
III. High Risk	
Anaplastic Wilms' tumor	Anaplastic Focal Diffuse
Clear cell sarcoma	Clear cell sarcoma
Rhabdoid tumor	Rhabdoid tumor

Modified from (ref. 32, with permission.)

life. Its median age at presentation is 3 months. It is distinguished from Wilms' tumor by its usually benign behavior, a preponderance of mesenchymal derivatives, and a lack of the malignant epithelial components seen in Wilms'. The tumor consists of spindle-shaped cells in interlacing bundles adjacent to renal parenchyma where there are foci of cystic or dysplastic tubules. The treatment of choice is nephrectomy. Local recurrence is unusual. Nonetheless, adequate margins of resection should be obtained—although recurrence even following operative rupture or positive margins at resection are still rare. Distant metastases are also rare. The actuarial 2-year survival is excellent: 98% (27–29).

Nodular Renal Blastema and Nephrogenic Rests

A spectrum of "pre-Wilms' tumor" entities have been described. Nodular renal blastema are small but visible subcapsular nodules composed of benign embryonic rests. Nephrogenic rests may be limited to the periphery of the renal cortex (perilobar) or randomly distributed throughout the renal lobe (intralobar). Multifocal or diffuse nephrogenic rests are called nephroblastomatosis.

Wilms' Tumor

Wilms' tumor is a triphasic embryonal neoplasm, which includes blastemal, epithelial (tubules), and stromal elements. Each element may exhibit a variety of patterns of aggregation or lines of differentiation (25,30, 31). The proportion of the three components varies from tumor to tumor. If one of the components comprises more than two-thirds of the tumor sample, the pattern is designated according to the predominant component. The mixed type is most common (41% of Wilms' tumor) followed closely by the clinically more aggressive blastemal predominant (39%), the more indolent epithelial predominant (18%), and the stromal predominant (1%), which behaves like the mixed type (32).

Wilms' tumor's gross pathologic features are its general occurence as a single unilateral tumor—although multicentric growth and bilateral disease can occur. The tumor is typically solid, lobulated, and not calcified. Soft and cystic areas may, however, be encountered.

Histopathologic studies in the NWTS identified factors that correlate with prognosis. In the first NWTS, 88% of cases were categorized as *favorable histology* (FH), defined as having typical histologic features of Wilms' tumor without anaplastic or sarcomatous components (33,34). The frequency of this pattern was upheld in the third NWTS, with 89% of cases being FH on central pathology review (35).

Three entities have traditionally been grouped under the general term *unfavorable histology* in the NWTS: anaplastic Wilms' tumor, clear cell sarcoma, and rhabdoid tumor (31). The later two are no longer considered to be variants of Wilms' tumor but are distinct entities (25,30).

Anaplasia is defined as (a) significant enlargement of nuclei within the stromal, epithelial, or blastemal cell lines to at least three times the diameter of adjacent nuclei of the same cell type; (b) hyperchromatism of these enlarged nuclei; and (c) multiple mitotic figures (25,30,32,36). DNA indices greater than 1.5 are associated with anaplastic histology (37). Anaplasia was noted in 4% of all NWTS-3 entries and in 5% of the SIOP study (32,35,36). Anaplastic tumors are extremely rare in infants, uncommon before two years of age, and make up about 10% of Wilms' tumor diagnosed after 5 years of age (32). Anaplasia appears to be associated with increased resistance to chemotherapy rather than increased aggressiveness of Wilms' tumor. The 4-year survival in NWTS-3 for anaplastic histology patients was 82%, but was less in earlier studies (14,34–36,38).

Anaplastic Wilms' tumor may be focal or diffuse. When this distinction was originally drawn, the term *diffuse anaplasia* was applied to tumors with anaplastic nuclear changes in more than 10% of ×400 microscopic fields.

Focal anaplasia was applied to the remainder of anaplastic tumors. Using this distinction focal anaplasia was associated with a more favorable outcome than diffuse anaplasia in the first NWTS but this difference did not obtain statistical significance and was not confirmed in the second and third NWTS (39).

The original distinction between focal and diffuse anaplasia did not consider distribution of tumor throughout the kidney, which might affect the likelihood of complete resection. In a recently revised definition, focal anaplasia refers to anaplasia that is sharply localized within the primary tumor, without significant nuclear or mitotic atypia in the remainder of the lesion. Diffuse anaplasia is either nonlocalized anaplasia, localized anaplasia with severe nuclear unrest elsewhere in the tumor, anaplasia outside the tumor capsule or in metastases, or where a random biopsy taken from the tumor reveals anaplasia.

Using the new criteria, and on review of patients entered on NWTS-3 and NWTS-4, patients with focal anaplasia had a statistically significantly superior 4-year survival to those with diffuse anaplasia (97% vs. 50%). This difference did not exist for stage I tumors (100% survival for focal or diffuse), but did exist for stages II (90% vs. 55%), III (100% vs. 45%), and IV (100% vs. 4%) (32,39).

Rhabdoid Tumor of the Kidney

Rhabdoid tumor is a highly malignant tumor characterized by uniform cellular infiltrates initially interpreted as rhabdomyoblastic or sarcomatous elements. The tumor is unrelated to rhabdomyosarcoma or Wilms' tumor and may be of neural crest origin (25,31,40). Rhabdoid cells are characterized by eosinophilic cytoplasm that contains hyaline globular inclusions. On electron microscopy, these inclusions are found to be intermediate filaments—most contain vimentin and cytokeratin. The nuclei are large, round, and vesicular—frequently containing a centrally placed eosinophilic nucleolus (32).

Most rhabdoid tumors of the kidney are diagnosed in the first 2 years of life. Rhabdoid

tumors have also been reported as primary extrarenal lesions; there is a known association between rhabdoid tumor of the kidney and primary central nervous system neoplasms (25). Children with rhabdoid tumors have responded poorly to the therapies of the NWTS. The 4-year relapse-free survival for patients treated with vincristine, actinomycin D, and adriamycin on NWTS-3 was 23.1% and the 4-year overall survival rate was 25% (14,35,41).

Clear Cell Sarcoma of the Kidney

Clear cell sarcoma of the kidney (CCSK) is a primitive mesenchymal neoplasm that comprises 4% of childhood renal tumors. The cell of origin is unknown. The lesion is distinguished by cells with poorly stained cytoplasm. The cell boundaries are indistinct, and cytoplasmic vaculation may be prominent. The classic histologic pattern has a characteristic feature of an arborizing network of thinwalled capillary blood vessels that separates groups of cells (32). In NWTS-3, 23% of CCSK children developed bone metastases compared to 0.3% of all other children entered in the study (20).

Response of CCSK to therapy had been poor until adriamycin and local irradiation were added to the treatment program. The 4-year relapse-free survival rate for patients with stage I to IV CCSK treated with vincristine, adriamycin, and actinomycin D on NWTS-3 was 71%.

CLINICAL PRESENTATION AND WORKUP

As we have already noted, there are several clinical syndromes that are risk factors for the development of Wilms' tumor. These include aniridia, the Beckwith-Wiedemann syndrome (exomphalos-macroglossia-gigantism), and hemihypertropia. If somatic changes of these kinds are known to exist, then routine screening in an attempt to make the early diagnosis of Wilms' tumor is appropriate (8,42). A physical examination and periodic ultrasound are indicated. It is interesting to note that in Germany, 10% of Wilms' tumor patients are diagnosised at infant and childhood screening examinations—conducted for known predisposing syndromes as well as at routine "well baby" examinations (42).

The majority of children who are diagnosed with Wilms' tumor is in response to a medical complaint causing a visit to the doctor; the clinical presentation is generally an abdominal mass (83%), fever (23%), or hematuria (21%). Abdominal pain (37%) may be the result of local distention, spontaneous intralesional hemorrhage, or peritoneal rupture. In one major series, abdominal pain correlated with poorer 5-year survival (43). Less common presenting signs and symptoms include hypertension, varicocele, hernia, enlarged testicle, congestive heart failure, hypoglycemia, Cushing's syndrome, hydrocephalus, pleural effusion, and an acute abdomen (44).

The presence and character of the abdominal pain, the previous medical history, and the family history are important aspects of the medical interview. Physical examination is of value in assessing abdominal status and identifying associated congenital anomalies.

The optimum diagnostic imaging workup for Wilms' tumor is a matter of some controversy. Evaluation of disease extent classically included intravenous pyelogram (IVP) and chest radiograph. Current imaging protocols largely replace the IVP with abdominal ultrasound. Ultrasound will usually allow determination of the origin of a childhood abdominal mass, identify a contralateral kidney, and demonstrate the presence or absence of tumor extension into the renal vein or inferior vena cava (7).

When an abdominal mass is identified or suspected, abdominal computerized tomography (CT) is utilized to (a) assess the volume of tumor involvement in one or both kidneys, renal function, retroperitoneal lymph nodes, and invasion of the collecting system or renal vein; (b) evaluate the margin between tumor, kidney, and surrounding structures; (c) assess hepatic metastasis (although many children thought to have invasion of the liver from a right-sided Wilms' tumor are found, at surgery, to have hepatic compression rather than invasion); and (d) to demonstrate lesions in the opposite kidney, which may represent either bilateral Wilms' tumor or nephrogenic rests (7) (Fig. 2). The evaluation of the contralateral kidney has become a matter of discussion in the surgical literature. Some authorities believe that preoperative CT and MRI can be used to rule-in or rule-out bilateral Wilms' tumor. Others, however, feel that imaging is useful but not definitive and that a surgical exploration of the contralateral kidney remains essential during the time of surgical approach to the primary tumor (42).

Plain chest radiograhps should be obtained to determine if pulmonary metastases are present. Some centers recommend thoracic CT to detect pulmonary metastasis that might be missed on chest radiograph. CT-positive, chest radiograph-negative lung metastases do occur—albeit infrequently (7). There had been considerable uncertainty regarding appropriate therapy for pulmonary disease documented only by CT in the presence of normal plain chest films (45). Data from NWTS-3 shows no significant difference in 4-year event-free survival between 18 favorable histology patients with CT-positive, chest radiograph-negative lungs treated with whole-lung irradiation (WLI; 88% event-free survival) and 9 favorable histology patients treated without WLI (88% event-free survival) (46). These results, while interesting, are obviously from a small number of patients. NWTS-4 recommendations were to treat with WLI in CT-positive, chest radiograph-negative FH patients only if disease is unresponsive to chemotherapy. Biopsy proof of intrathoracic disease was recommended for strong consideration (12). NWTS-5 recommendations are that pulmonary nodules not detected on chest radiographs but visible on chest CT do *not* mandate treatment with WLI. While the decision to adminster WLI is at the discretion of the investigator, excisional biopsy of suspected pulmonary metastatic lesions is strongly recommended to confirm the diagnosis.

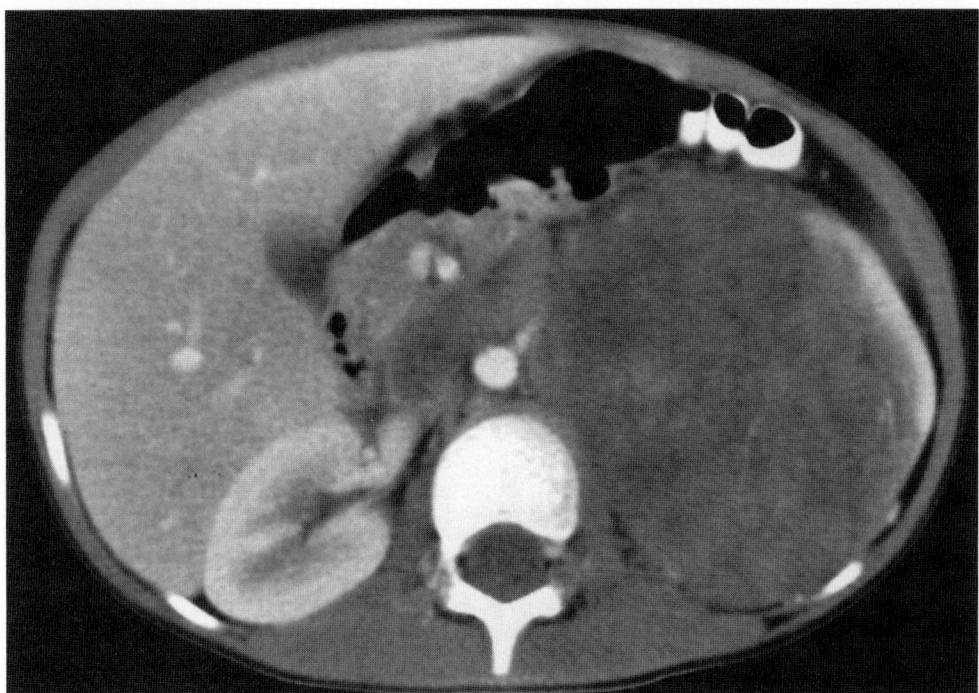

FIG. 2. A 5-year-old female presented to medical attention with intermittent sharp abdominal pain, nausea, vomiting, weight loss, and hematuria. Abdominal CT scan showed a 7 × 9 × 12.5 cm mass at the left renal region, beginning immediately subdiaphragmatically and extending to just below the aortic bifurcation. There was a calcified rim superiorly and a heterogeneous parenchymal enhancement. Left renal vein invasion and inferior vena cava thrombosis were observed. On exploratory laparotomy tumor was palpated within the inferior vena cava. The tumor was resected with some tumor spillage from a weak point on Gerota's fascia. Tumor thrombus was removed from the inferior vena cava. Pathology showed a favorable histology Wilms' tumor, 13.5 cm in greatest diamater, invading through the renal capsule to the inked surgical margin. Rupture of the renal capsule was identified. Tumor was present at the renal vein margin of the tumor thrombosis with focal invasion of the vein wall. No lymph nodes were involved. For pathological stage III Wilms' tumor, favorable histology, the child was treated with chemotherapy and flank irradiation. She is without evidence of persistent or recurrent tumor 3 years following diagnosis.

Radionuclide bone scan is indicated in CCSK and renal rhabdoid tumor. Bone scan and skeletal survey are complementary in CCSK. If only one technique is used, metastases may be missed (47). Cranial CT is of value with rhabdoid tumors and, perhaps, in Wilms' tumor with overt pulmonary involvement at diagnosis.

STAGING

A staging system for Wilms' tumor was first published by Cassady et al. in 1973, building on prognostic factors identified in a review from Garcia et al. (48–50). The Cassady system remains useful for the identification of young children with early stage disease who may be appropriate for therapy with surgery alone. For tumor confined to the kidney and completely excised in children younger than 2 years of age at diagnosis and with tumors that weigh less than 550 g the prognosis is excellent. Such patients may be treated appropriately with surgery alone and are referred to as stage I (48,49). The absence of an inflammatory pseudocapsule, renal sinus invasion, capsular invasion, and intrarenal vessel invasion in such patients are additional factors that mitigate against the risk of relapse when treated with nephrectomy alone (7).

The NWTS proposed initial staging criteria to prospectively address tumor-related factors. The first two NWTS studies were based upon a system of surgically identified groups (10) (Table 2).

Beginning with the third NWTS trial in 1979, a new staging system was adopted (Table 3). Specific disease-related parameters noted to be prognostically significant in analyses of NWTS-1 and NWTS-2 led to modifications of the system of "groups" to "stages." A closed or open biopsy permitted categorization as stage II (rather than group III), assuming subsequent total tumor removal. Local spill of tumor during surgery was downstaged from group III to stage II, reflecting data indicating that such cases had excellent tumor control even with limited irradiation and chemotherapy in NWTS-1 and NWTS-2 (24,51).

The more recent NWTS staging system upstages all previous group II cases with lymph node metastasis to stage III, even when all visible disease has been completely resected. The adverse impact of lymph node involvement, both on abdominal recurrence and on

TABLE 2. *Grouping system used in National Wilms' Tumor Study 1 and 2*

Group I. Tumor limited to kidney and completely excised (intact surface of the renal capsule; tumor not ruptured before or during removal; no residual tumor apparent beyond excision margins).

Group II. Tumor extent beyond the kidney but is completely excised (penetration into the perirenal soft tissues or para-aortic lymph node involvement; renal vessels outside the kidney infiltrated or contained tumor thrombus; no residual tumor apparent beyond the margins of excision).

Group III. Residual nonhematogenous tumor confined to abdomen (tumor has undergone biopsy or rupture before or during surgery; implants on peritoneal surfaces; lymph nodes involved beyond the periaortic region; tumor incompletely removed due to local infiltration into vital structures).

Group IV. Hematogenous metastasis (deposits beyond group III; e.g., lung, liver, bone, brain).

Group V. Bilateral renal involvement either initially or subsequently.

TABLE 3. *Staging system used in National Wilms' Tumor Study 3 and 4*

I. Tumor limited to kidney and completely excised. The surface of the renal capsule is intact. Tumor was not ruptured before or during removal. There is no residual tumor apparent beyond the margins of resection.

II. Tumor extends beyond the kidney but is completely removed. There is regional extension of the tumor—that is, penetration through the outer surface of the renal capsule into perirenal soft tissues.
 Vessels outside the kidney substance are infiltrated or contain tumor thrombus. The tumor may have been biopsied, or there has been local spillage of tumor confined to the flank. There is no residual tumor apparent at or beyond the margins of excision.

III. Residual nonhematogenous tumor confined to abdomen. Any one or more of the following occur:
 a. Lymph nodes on biopsy are found to be involved in the hilus, the periaortic chains, or beyond.
 b. There has been diffuse peritoneal contamination by tumor such as by spillage of tumor beyond the flank before or during surgery, or by tumor growth that has penetrated through the peritoneal surface.
 c. Implants are found on the peritoneal surfaces.
 d. The tumor extends beyond the surgical margins either microscopically or grossly.
 e. The tumor is not completely resectable because of local infiltration into vital structures.

IV. Hematogenous metastases. Deposits beyond stage III (e.g., lung, liver, bone, and brain).

V. Bilateral renal involvement at diagnosis: an attempt should be made to stage each side according to the above criteria on the basis of extent of disease before biopsy.
 Staging, which is on the basis of gross and microscopic tumor distribution, is the same for tumors with favorable and with unfavorable histologic features. The patient should be characterized, however, by a statement of both criteria—for example, stage II (favorable histologic features) or stage III (unfavorable histologic features).
 Tumors of unfavorable type are those with focal or diffuse anaplasia, or those of sarcomatous histology.

ultimate relapse-free survival, has been documented (13,24,38,43,52).

In the SIOP Wilms' tumor Trial 1, investigators compared preoperative radiotherapy to primary surgery. The staging system used in this trial is shown in Table 4. SIOP subsequently began using NWTS grouping/staging—with the proviso that the NWTS systems were not

TABLE 4. *Staging system used in SIOP trial 1*

Stage I: The tumor is limited to the kidney and is completely excised.
Stage II. The tumor extends outside the kidney, but is completely excised.
Stage III: Incomplete excision of the tumor, but without hematogenous metastatic spread.
Stage IV: Hematogenous metastases are present.
Stage V: Bilateral renal tumors.

specifically designed for the preoperative therapy frequently used by SIOP (see subsequent text) (53,54). For this reason, outcomes between the NWTS and SIOP should not be compared stage-for-stage (37,55,56). In addition, SIOP uses a "stage II, node negative" and "stage II, node positive" distinction and, therefore, includes some NWTS stage III patients in the stage II infradiaphragmatic SIOP stage.

NWTS, SIOP, AND THE MANAGEMENT OF WILMS' TUMOR

A considerable body of information has been compiled concerning the clinical management of Wilms' tumor by the NWTS, SIOP, and the United Kingdom Children's Cancer Study Group (USCCSG). The most widely quoted studies are those of NWTS and SIOP. A review of the major studies of these two groups follows.

The NWTS and SIOP Strategies

The SIOP studies began with the presumption that treatment with radiation therapy and/or chemotherapy prior to surgery would render a Wilms' tumor less vulnerable to intraoperative rupture and surgery-related tumor seeding. By downstaging the tumor, it was also hoped to reduce treatment related morbidity due to a reduced total amount of treatment (55,56). In accordance with this philosophy, the initial strategy of SIOP was to evaluate the roles of radiotherapy and chemotherapy prior to definitive surgery based on clinical diagnosis. Subsequently, treatment was assigned according to the extent of disease found at surgery. The advantages attributed to the SIOP

were the aforementioned arguments that preoperative treatment may diminish the risk of operative tumor rupture, seeding, and/or nonresectability. One disadvantage is the risk of misdiagnosis and mistreatment (i.e., treating a tumor other than Wilms' tumor or treating benign disease). In addition, the SIOP approach runs the risk of obscuring important prognostic clues in individual patients (57). Lymph node involvement and histologic subtype may be affected by preoperative therapy. Because prognosis and subsequent therapy are influenced by histology and lymph node involvement, the SIOP approach may theoretically render therapy less precise by interfering with histology obtained at the time of definitive surgery. Supporting this contention was a review of data from two SIOP studies indicating that necrotic changes were more frequently seen in patients pretreated with radiotherapy than in those pretreated with chemotherapy. However, an analysis of posttreatment histology in these two SIOP studies as well as in 83 patients who underwent prenephrectomy chemotherapy in NSTS-3 showed no evidence that prenephrectomy therapy altered the detection of anaplastic histology (53,54,56). It appears that the SIOP presurgical therapy approach does not substantively influence histology.

The NWTS strategy is to forego preoperative therapy in order to obtain the maximum amount of information concerning prognostic factors and tailor therapy accordingly. Therefore, the local extent of the primary tumor, degree of anaplasia, presence of unusual histology, and presence or absence of lymph node involvement are assessed in the absence of the confounding influence of preoperative chemotherapy or radiotherapy, in order to select therapy. The benefit of the NWTS approach is the obvious generation of a large body of information concerning prognostic clues, the avoidance of misdiagnosis, and the customization of therapy. The disadvantages include the necessity of a hospital providing the full clinical services necessary for major pediatric surgery and pathology. In addition, there is the risk that the patient who might benefit from preoperative therapy would be denied it by the demand for surgery (57). Finally, the complexity of the NWTS prognostic and treatment algorithm may discourage the participation of some physicians and inhibit patient accrual to clinical trials.

We will review the major clinical trials and their outcomes in turn.

SIOP Wilms' Tumor Studies

SIOP Study 1 (1971–1974) has been reported to have registered 397 patients from 42 participating centers: 194 were eligible and randomized, and 203 were excluded from the randomization but were followed. The nonrandomized patients included 44 errors in diagnosis (10%, most commonly neuroblastoma and cysts), 62 children less than 1 year of age, and 54 with metastases. In patients older than 1 year and less than 15 years of age at diagnosis, the randomized trial was designed to ascertain the following: (a) Is preplus postoperative primary tumor site irradiation superior to postoperative irradiation only? (b) Is a single postoperative course of actinomycin D equal to multiple courses? To answer the first question, 73 children were randomized to receive 20 Gy before surgery versus immediate surgery for 64 children. Utilizing SIOP staging (Table 4), stage I patients randomized to preoperative irradiation received no additional irradiation while stage II and III patients were given an additional 15 Gy. Children who were randomized to the postoperative irradiation arm received 20 Gy for stage I and were given 30 Gy for stages II and III, with provision for additional boosts for bulky stage III. Three of 72 evaluable patients who received preoperative radiotherapy had tumor rupture during surgery (4%), whereas 20 of 60 patients who received no preoperative irradiation suffered from tumor rupture (33%, $p = 0.001$). The 5-year recurrence-free survival was 51% for those without tumor rupture and 27% for those with rupture ($p = 0.01$), with no difference in eight-year overall survival (66% vs. 61%) between the two groups (8). In the randomization between

one and seven courses and actinomycin D (15 μmg/kg/d × 5 days), there was no survival difference (55,56,58,59).

SIOP Trial 2 (1974–1976) was a nonrandomized study of 86 patients receiving 20 Gy of irradiation with 5 days of actinomycin D prior to surgery compared to a concurrent group of 52 children treated with primary surgery. Tumor rupture occurred in 5% of the preoperatively treated patients and in 20% of the other group ($p = 0.0025$) (53,54,56). The main reason for not giving preoperative therapy was small tumor size. Survival was only 61% in those patients with larger tumors who received preoperative and postoperative irradiation. SIOP Trials 1 and 2 demonstrated that presurgical treatment with radiotherapy reduced the number of tumor ruptures. This, in turn, reduced the need for whole-abdominal irradiation and its attendant ill effects in young children (56,59).

SIOP Trial 5 (1977–1980) was designed to ascertain if preoperative actinomycin D (two 3-day courses 15 μmg/kg) and vincristine (four weekly injections, 1.5 mg/m^2) was equally effective preoperative therapy when compared to the previously used program of 20 Gy plus actinomycin D. Following surgery the preoperatively irradiated patients were given an additional 15 Gy for NWTS group II or III disease, whereas those treated preoperatively only with chemotherapy received 30 Gy for group II or III disease. All patients received postoperative maintenance VCR and AMD. An analysis of the 172 randomized patients showed no significant difference in the reduction in tumor size, incidence of tumor rupture, stage distribution, mean weight of the tumor specimen, or 3-year recurrence-free survival (89% for preoperative chemotherapy alone vs. 83% for chemotherapy plus radiotherapy). Major histologic changes such as massive necrosis were significantly less frequent after preoperative chemotherapy than preoperative chemoradiotherapy (54,56, 58,59) (Table 5).

SIOP Trial 6 (1980–1987) adopted the prenephrectomy chemotherapy used in SIOP Trial 5. All patients received actinomycin D and vincristine. If, at the time of surgery, the

TABLE 5. *Effect of preoperative treatment—SIOP trial 5[a]*

Effect	Chemotherapy	Chemotherapy + radiotherapy	p value
Major clinical reduction in tumor size (%)	84%	88%	NS
Mean weight of the specimen (g)	519	473	NS
Tumor rupture (%)	9%	6%	NS
Stage (% of cases)			
I	43%	52%	NS
II	36%	32%	NS
III	21%	16%	NS
Major change in pathologic pattern (% of cases)	17%	53%	p<0.001
3-year recurrence-free survival			
Stage I	43%	52%	
Stage II	36%	32%	
Stage III	21%	16%	
Overall 3-year survival	89%	83%	NS

From refs. 81 and deKraker and Jereb, with permission.

patient had stage I disease they were randomized to receive either postoperative vincristine and actinomycin D for 17 weeks or 38 weeks. All lymph node negative stage II patients received 38 weeks of vincristine and actinomycin D and were randomized to receive or not receive 20 Gy of involved field irradiation. Stage II node positive patients and stage III patients were randomized to receive either vincristine, actinomycin D with intensified vincristine or the two drugs with doxorubicin. The stage distribution for the 396 SIOP Trial 6 patients was stage I (56%), stage II node negative (27%), stage II node positive + stage III (17%). Tumor rupture was found in 6% of cases.

In the radiotherapy randomization for stage II node negative patients in SIOP Trial 6 there were eight relapses among 50 nonirradiated patients. Of these 8, 7 had subdiaphragmatic regrowths of tumor and in 6 the tumor bed was the site of first relapse. This was in contrast to only 1 local recurrence of the 58 patients given postoperative irradiation. Twelve of the 58 children, however, developed lung metastases. Three of the 50 nonirradiated patients died and 5 of the 58 irradiated patients died—all of disseminated Wilms' tumor. The overall survival of the two groups at 4 years was not different: 90% of the nonirradiated patients and 85% of the irradiated patients (56,58,59).

SIOP Trial 9 (1987–1993) had, as its primary question, the appropriate duration of prenephrectomy chemotherapy. One-half of the patients with disease confined to the abdomen received 4 weeks of actinomycin D and vincristine and one-half received 8 weeks. After nephrectomy, those patients with multicystic, tubular, and nephroblastoma with fibroadenomatous-like structures received no additional therapy. Those patients with unfavorable histology received actinomycin D, epidoxorubicin, vincristine, ifosfamide and, generally, irradiation. Those patients with favorable histology received, postoperatively: stage I, actinomycin D and vincristine; stage II node negative, actinomycin D, vincristine, and epidoxorubicin; stage II node positive and stage III, actinomycin D, vincristine, and epidoxorubicin; along with local irradiation (15 Gy to the tumor bed with an optional boost to residual disease up to 30 Gy). Infants younger than 6-months old underwent up-front nephrectomy. Children with a preoperative diagnosis of stage IV disease received actinomycin D, vincristine, and epidoxorubicin. This was followed by nephrectomy and possible metastatectomy. Those rendered free of disease continued on actinomycyin D, vincristine, and epidoxorubicin. Those with persistent metastatic disease received ifosfamide, vincristine, and actinomycin D and irradiation. Available results show that the duration of prenephrectomy chemotherapy has not influenced the stage distribution at the time of surgery. There is also no difference in toxicity between the 4-week and 8-week chemotherapy arms (56,58,59).

SIOP Trial 93-01 opened in 1993. Patients are classified into three histologic groups as shown in Table 1. Because the available results show no difference between 4-week and 8-week preoperative chemotherapy, 4 weeks has been adopted as the standard. As nephrectomy, patients with stage I low-grade histology receive no additional therapy.

Patients with stage I intermediate or high-grade tumors are randomized to a 4-week postoperative program of vincristine plus actinomycin-D versus a 6-week program. All stage II and III patients with intermediate grade tumors receive therapy as per SIOP Trial 9. Stage II and III high-grade tumors are treated with ifosfamide, etoposide, and carboplatin.

A summary of SIOP's data shows that 4-weeks of prenephrectomy chemotherapy, without irradiation, results in 56% of patients having stage I disease at surgery. These patients go on, in most cases, to receive postoperative che-

motherapy and have a survival rate of more than 90%. Stage II node positive and stage III patients have approximately a 61% relapse-free survival and a 75% overall survival (37). A diminishing number of patients have received radiotherapy in the sequential SIOP Trials. The estimated percent of patients who received irradiation is: SIOP 1, 90%; SIOP 2, 90%; SIOP 5, 72%, SIOP 6, 34%, SIOP 9, 24% (58). If one excludes metastatic patients, then only about 16% of SIOP patients receive irradiation (56).

The National Wilms' Tumor Studies (NWTS)

NWTS-1 (1969–1974) asked several important treatment questions: (a) Is postoperative radiotherapy necessary in group I disease? (b) Is single-agent chemotherapy with either vincristine or actinomycin D equivalent to combining these drugs for group II and III disease? (c) Is preoperative vincristine of value in group IV disease? The study is shown schematically in Fig. 3, and the results are summarized in

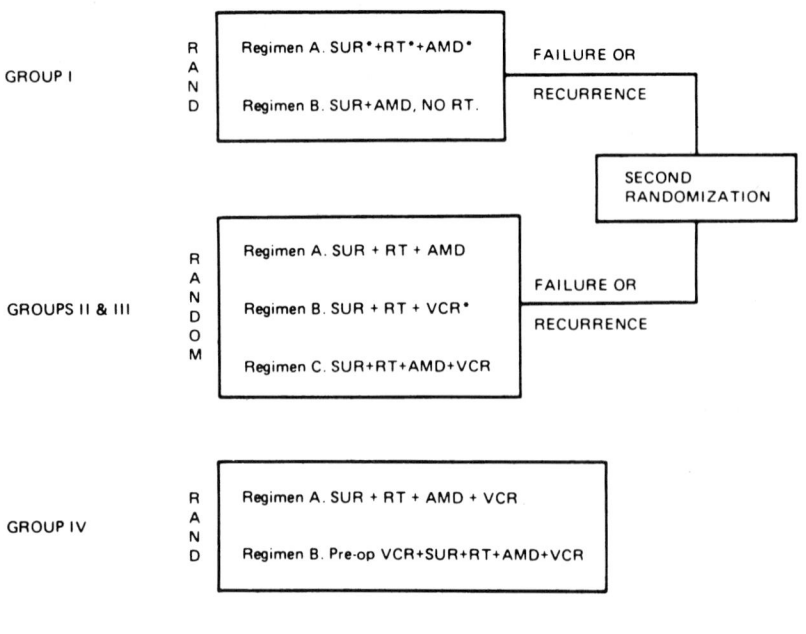

*SUR = Surgery   RT = Radiotherapy   AMD = Actinomycin D   VCR = Vincristine   PRE-OP = Preoperative

FIG. 3. The design of NWTS-1. (From ref. 12, with permission.)

Table 6 (12,39,50). Radiotherapy doses were age-adjusted (Birth to 18 months of age, 18 to 24 Gy; 18 to 30 months of age, 24 to 30 Gy; 31 to 40 months of age, 30 to 35 Gy; 41 months of age or older, 35 to 40 Gy). Radiotherapy appeared to be unnecessary in group I babies, combined drug therapy was superior in group II and III, and preoperative VCR was not helpful in group IV (10,34,59).

NWTS-1 also generated additional important information. The study demonstrated the significance of the unfavorable histology versus favorable histology distinction, with the 2-year unfavorable histology relapse-free survival being 29% versus 89% for favorable histology (33,34). Large tumor size, lymph node involvement, and age over 2 years were confirmed as poor prognostic factors. No radiation dose response was discerned within the 10- to 40-Gy administered range; delays of up to 10 days in initiation of postoperative irradiation appeared acceptable, and whole-abdominal irradiation was not found to be necessary for tumor spills confined to the flank or for prior tumor biopsy (10,51). In these patients, limited radiotherapy fields sufficed.

NWTS-1 had shown an advantage for patients over 2 years of age with group I tumors

TABLE 6. *NWTS-1 results*

Group and therapy	n	Four-year relapse-free survival (%)	Four-year survival (%)
I <2-yrs old			
A (radiotherapy)	38	89	94
B (no radiotherapy)	41	88	90
I ≥2-yrs old			
A (radiotherapy)	42	76	98
B (no radiotherapy)	42	57	81
II and III			
A (AMD)	63	56[a]	71[a]
B (VCR)	44	57[a]	71[a]
C (AMD + VCR)	63	79	84
IV			
A (immediate surgery)	13		83[a,b]
B (pre-op VCR)	13		29[a,b]

[a]$p \leq 0.02$
[b]Two-year survival.
From refs. 14,34,44,61, with permission.

treated with irradiation. It was noted, however, that patients with group II tumors receiving actinomycin D plus vincristine seemed to do as well as those with group I disease. It was postulated that postoperative vincristine plus actinomycin D could substitute for postoperative radiotherapy plus actinomycin D. Investigators also were interested in the potential value of adriamycin in the initial treatment of Wilms' tumor—the drug having been effective in recurrent disease (59).

NWTS-2 (1974–1979) explored three major questions: (a) can vincristine and actinomycin D substitute for radiotherapy in older children with group I disease? (b) Is adjuvant vincristine + actinomycin D for protracted periods helpful in group I? (c) Is the addition of adriamycin to actinomycin D and vincristine of value in groups II to IV? The study is shown schematically in Fig. 4 (60). Flank irradiation was given in group II to IV disease according to the same age-dependent scale as NWTS-1. Whole-abdominal irradiation was reserved for diffuse peritoneal seeding. Lung metastases were initially treated with 14 Gy of WLI, but when a 10% incidence of pneumonitis occurred the dose was scaled back to 12 Gy. Study results are summarized in Table 7. About 85% of the patients were favorable histology and 15% unfavorable (59). Two-year survival rates were 54% for unfavorable histology, 90% for favorable histology, 54% for lymph node positive, and 82% for lymph node negative. Excellent survival rates appeared to be achievable without irradiation in group I, and adriamycin added considerable benefit in groups II to III favorable histology and some benefit in groups II to III unfavorable histology and group IV. The 2-year relapse-free survival for all NWTS-2 patients was 88% for group I, 78% for group II, 70% for group III, and 49% for group IV (14, 60–62).

NWTS-3 (1979–1985) incorporated two major changes in treatment planning: Patients were stratified by *stages* rather than by *groups* (Tables 3 and 4), and the distinction between favorable and unfavorable histology was incorporated into the treatment algorithm (Fig. 5).

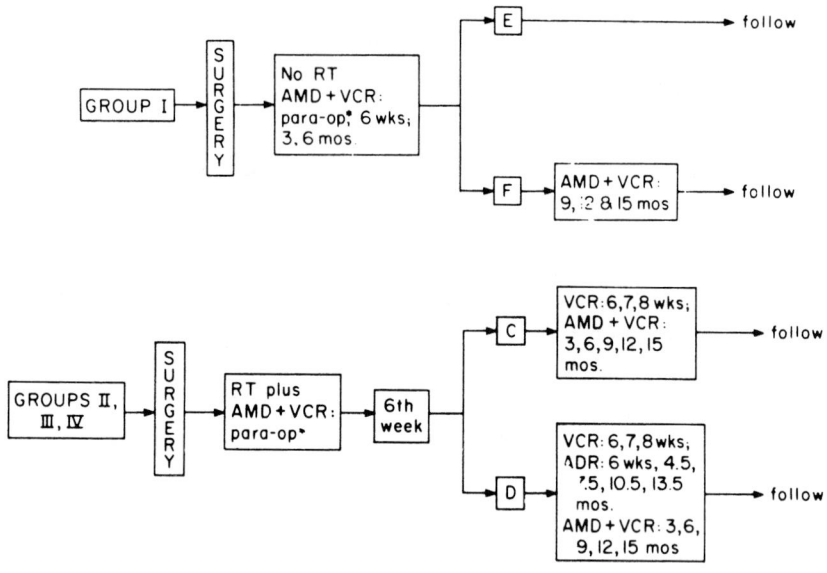

* para-op = day 1: AMD - 15 mcg/Kg/d x 5
days 7, 14, 21, 28, 35: VCR - 1.5 mg/m²

subsequent courses = AMD: doses as above; VCR: days 1 & 5, doses as above
ADR: 60 mg/m²

FIG. 4. The design of NWTS-2. (From ref. 34, with permission.)

TABLE 7. *NWTS-2 results*

Group and therapy	n	Three-year relapse-free survival (%)	Three-year survival (%)
I			
E (6 m ADR, VCR)	88	89	97
F (15 m ADR, VCR)	91	84	92
II and III FH			
C (VCR, AMD)	121	70[a]	82
D (VCR, AMD, ADR)	111	88	92
II and III UH			
C (VCR, AMD)	16	35	38
D (VCR, AMD, ADR)	19	42	78
IV			
C (VCR, AMD)	22	43[a]	44
D (VCR, AMD, ADR)	27	60[a]	60
Lymph node status			
Negative/not examined	383	82[b]	
Positive	84	54	

[a] $p \leq 0.05$

[b] Two-year survival.

(From refs. 14, 34, 61, 62, with permission).

Although data from NWTS-1 and NWTS-2 had been analyzed by histology, histology had not been used to stratify treatment (7,63).

NWTS-3 considered five major questions: (a) can the duration of chemotherapy be shortened for stage I favorable histology? (b) Can radiotherapy be eliminated for stage II favorable histology? (c) What is the minimum effective radiotherapy dose for stage III favorable histology? (d) Is cardiotoxic adriamycin clearly beneficial and, therefore, necessary in stages II and III favorable histology? (e) Will the addition of cyclophosphamide improve survival in stages I to III unfavorable histology and in stage IV favorable histology and unfavorable histology?

NWTS-3 results are summarized in Table 8. Short-course therapy appeared equivalent to long-course therapy in stage I favorable histology. Patients in this group can be treated successfully with a 10-week program of vin-

NATIONAL WILMS' TUMOR STUDY-3

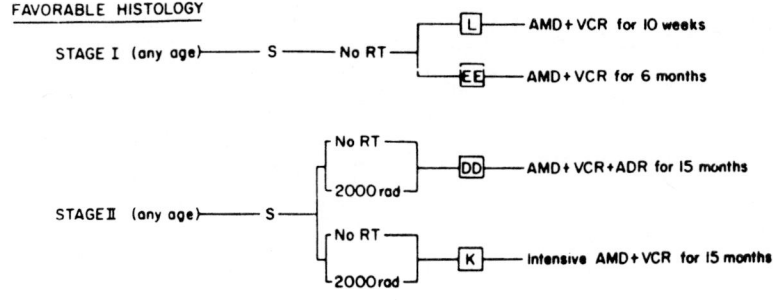

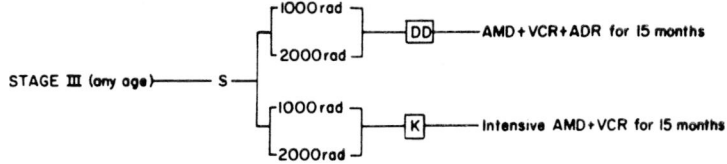

UNFAVORABLE HISTOLOGY, AND ALL STAGE IV

* All FH Stage IV receive 2000 rad flank RT and RT to other sites as in NWTS-2

All UH, all stages receive age-adjusted flank RT and to other sites as in NWTS-2

FIG. 5. The design of NWTS-3. (From ref. 60, with permission.)

cristine and actinomycin D without irradiation and achieve a 4-year relapse-free survival of 89% and overall survival of 96%. Elimination of radiotherapy was acceptable in stage II favorable histology. The 4-year relapse-free and overall survival for the patients not receiving irradiation were 87% and 91%, respectively. Ten Gy was equivalent to 20 Gy in stage III favorable histology. There was no statistically significant difference in frequency of intraabdominal relapse between 10 and 20 Gy although the trend favored the use of adriamycin or irradiation (intraabdominal relapse for vincristine, actinomycin D and 10 Gy, 7/61 or 11%; vincristine, actinomycin D and 20 Gy, 3/68 or 4%; vincristine, actinomycin D, adriamycin, and 10 Gy, 3/70 or 4%. The addition of adriamycin was not clearly beneficial in stage II but seemed to be of benefit in stage III favorable histology. Cyclophosphamide did not benefit stage IV favorable histology. The 4-year survival rate for stage IV favorable histology treated with vincristine, actinomycin D, adriamycin, abdominal and lung irradiation was 81%. The use of cyclophosphamide seemed to help pa-

TABLE 8. *NWTS-3 results*

Stage and therapy	n	Four-year relapse-free survival (%)	Four-year survival (%)
Stage I FH			
L (10 weeks ADR, VCR)	306	89	96
EE (6 m ADR, VCR)	301	92	97
Stage II FH			
DD (No radiotherapy; AMD, VCR, ADR)	70	88	94
DD2 (20 Gy; AMD, VCR, ADR)	71	87	90
K (No radiotherapy; AMD, VCR)	67	87	91
K2 (20 Gy; AMD, VCR)	70	90	95
Stage III FH			
DD1 (10 Gy; AMD, VCR, ADR)	68	82	91
DD2 (20 Gy; AMD, VCR, ADR)	66	86	87
K1 (10 Gy; AMD, VCR)	71	71	85
K2 (20 Gy; AMD, VCR)	70	77	85
Stage IV FH[a]			
DD (AMD, VCR, ADR)	64	72	78
J (AMD, VCR, ADR, CPM)	56	78	87
Stages I–III UH[a]			
DD (AMD, VCR, ADR)	69	67	68
J (AMD, VCR, ADR, CPM)	61	62	68
Stage IV UH[a]			
DD (AMD, VCR, ADR)	12	58	58
J (AMD, VCR, ADR, CPM)	17	53	52
Anaplastic[a]			
DD (AMD, VCR, ADR)	31	1:80	
II–IV: 37	1:78		
II–IV: 38[b]			
J (AMD, VCR, ADR, CPM)	17	1:100	
II–IV: 83	1:100		
II–IV: 82[b]			
CCSK[a]			
DD (AMD, VCR, ADR)	25	71	75
J (AMD, VCR, ADR, CPM)	25	60	76
Rhabdoid[a]			
DD (AMD, VCR, ADR)	13	23	25
J (AMD, VCR, ADR, CPM)	18	27	26

[a]Radiotherapy also given—not a randomized radiotherapy question.
[b]$p \leq 0.05$.
From refs. 35 and 83, with permission.

tients with focal anaplasia. CCSK patients did relatively well, whereas those with rhabdoid tumors continued to do poorly (12,14,24,35,63).

NWTS-4 (1986–1994) addressed issues of minimization of therapy (and, hopefully, therapy-related toxicity) as well as customization of therapy by stage and histology. The trial was the first study of a pediatric population to evaluate the economic impact of two different treatment approaches, one of which required fewer clinic visits. By the end of NWTS-3 it had been shown that 62% of Wilms' tumor patients (stages I to II, favorable histology) needed neither irradiation nor adriamycin. The study was designed to compare the relapse-free and overall survival rates of stage I and II favorable histology and stage I anaplastic patients treated with conventional actinomycin D + vincristine versus pulsed, intensive actinomycin D + vincristine. Stages III and IV favorable histology and stage I to IV clear cell sarcoma were treated with conventional actinomycin D + vincristine + adriamycin versus pulsed, intensive actinomycin D + vincristine + adriamycin; all patients received radiotherapy (for favorable histology 10.8 Gy to the abdomen; 12 Gy whole-lung irradiation where appropriate; for stage II to IV anaplastic tumors a sliding scale of radiation dose, as per NWTS-1, was used). Stages II to IV anaplastic Wilms' tumor were treated with appropriate irradiation followed by actinomycin D + vincristine + adriamycin versus these three drugs plus cyclophosphamide. Stages II to IV favorable histology and stages I to IV clear cell sarcoma were treated with 26 weeks versus 54 weeks of chemotherapy (Fig. 6).

The results of NWTS-4 were reported in abstract form just as this edition of *Pediatric Radiation Oncology* was in final preparation (7,64,65). The results are expected to be published in the peer-reviewed literature shortly. For children with stages I to II favorable histology or stage I focal anaplastic tumors the 2-

year relapse-free survivals were 91.6% for those treated with conventional actinomycin D and vincristine versus 91.3% for those treated with the pulse-intensive program ($p = 0.95$). The 2-year overall survivals were 98.6% for conventional chemotherapy and 97.8% for the pulse intensive program ($p = 0.27$). For children with stages III to IV favorable histology or stages I to IV CCSK the 2-year relapse-free survival percentages were 89.4% for those treated with conventional chemotherapy and 87.4% for pulse-intensive chemotherapy ($p = 0.94$). Overall survival was 95.9% for conventional chemotherapy and 95.6% for pulse-intensive ($p = 0.99$).

For stages II to IV favorable histology and stages I to IV clear cell sarcoma, there was a second randomization to 22 to 26 weeks of chemotherapy versus 65 to 66 weeks. The 2-

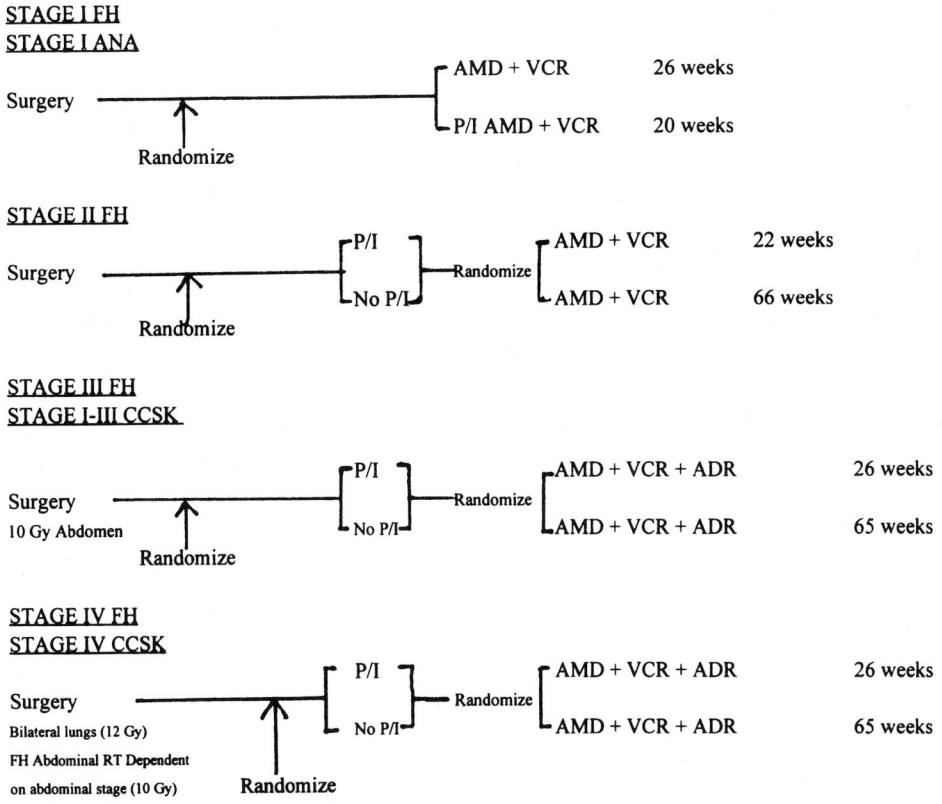

FIG. 6. NWTS-4 simplified schema. Stage IV anaplastic tumors continued the randomization as per NWTS-3. (From ref. 59, with permission.)

year relapse-free survival for children who were randomized to receive conventional actinomycin D and vincristine initially and then got a shorter course of chemotherapy was 87.7% versus 92.2% for initial conventional chemotherapy and a longer course of subsequent treatment ($p = 0.29$). The 2-year relapse-free survival for children who were initially randomized to receive pulse-intensive actinomycin D and vincristine and then got a 22 to 26 week course of chemotherapy was 87.2% versus 88.9% for those who got the 65 to 66 week course of chemotherapy ($p = 0.74$).

The evidence from NWTS-4 is that pulse-intensive initial chemotherapy is as effective as a longer program. Shorter course subsequent chemotherapy appears as effective as a longer program. Overall survival rates are excellent and relatively few patients are irradiated (64).

NWTS-5 (1995 to present) treats stage I favorable and anaplastic histology and stage II favorable histology with 18 weeks of actinomycin D and vincristine. Stage I favorable histology in children younger than 24 months of age and with tumor weight less than 550 g is treated with surgery alone. Stage III to IV favorable histology and Stages II to IV focal anaplasia (see definition in the histology section of this chapter, *vide supra*) are treated with 24 weeks of actinomycin D, vincristine, and adriamycin and local and whole-lung irradiation as appropriate (see Table 9). Stages II to IV diffuse anaplastic and Stage I to IV clear cell sarcoma of the kidney are treated with cyclophosphamide, vincristine, adriamycin, and etoposide along with local and whole-lung irradiation as appropriate. Stages I to IV rhabdoid tumor of the kidney is treated with carboplatinum, etoposide, cyclophosphamide, and radiotherapy (NWTS-5, Thomas). NWTS-5 has, as major objectives, an assessment of the importance of loss of heterozygosity for chromosome 1p and 16q markers for prognosis. (This issue is discussed earlier in this chapter.)

TABLE 9. *A simplified scheme of radiation therapy used in NWTS-5*

Stage	Favorable histology	Anaplastic tumors	Clear cell sarcoma of the kidney and rhabdoid tumor
I–II	No irradiation	No irradiation for stage I. For stage II, follow the guidelines for favorable histology, stage III.	Follow the guidelines for favorable histology, stage III.
III	If the tumor involved the renal hilar nodes, gross or microscopic residual disease confined to the flank, or the paraaortic nodes, irradiate the flank, crossing the midline to include the bilateral paraaortic nodes. If there was peritoneal seeding, gross residual abdominal disease, preoperative intraperitoneal tumor rupture, or diffuse abdominal tumor spill, irradiate the whole abdomen. Administer 10.8 Gy in 6 fractions. Boost tumor >3 cm in maximum diameter an additional 10.8 Gy.	Follow the guidelines for favorable histology, stage III.	Follow the guidelines for favorable histology, stage III.
IV	Treat the abdomen per the guidelines for the intraabdominal stage, i.e., irradiate the abdomen for local Stage III but not I–II. Whole lung irradiation to 12 Gy. Boost persistent lung metastases to 19.5 Gy or resect them. In certain circumstances, liver metastases are irradiated.	As for stage IV favorable histology	As for stage IV favorable histology except that stage I and II abdominal disease is also locally irradiated.

From ref. 80 after a concept in (ref. 59), with permission.

SELECTION OF THERAPY

Surgery

If one follows the NWTS philosophy, 90% to 95% of intraabdominal tumors are resectable at diagnosis and surgery is the initial definitive treatment. Operative approaches have included a vertical incision or a thoracoabdominal exposure. The current preferred approach is a wide transverse abdominal incision (14,57,66). The incision is extended to the thorax when needed for adequate exposure. This is infrequently necessary and the thoracoabdominal incision has been associated with higher complication rates (8). Total resection is generally achievable with the transverse transperitoneal incision. Data regarding the value of adjuvant irradiation and chemotherapy for those with small deposits of residual tumor demonstrate that "heroic" attempts at tumor removal are not indicated (67). A recent analysis of NWTS-1, 2, and 3 shows no significant reduction in survival rates with direct extension or contiguous involvement of the liver in comparison to other stage III presentations. Survival is diminished with hematogenous intraparenchymal liver metastasis (68).

In NWTS-3, surgeons encountered renal vein involvement in 10% of patients. Extension into the inferior vena cava and atrium occurs in up to an additional 5%. En bloc removal of the kidney and renal vein tumor thrombus is possible in most children, and separate removal is possible in others. In some cases the thrombus is "milked" from the inferior vena cava to the renal vein prior to removal. With meticulous surgery, renal vein involvement does not adversely affect prognosis (8,69).

Surgical staging is important in determining treatment and prognosis. Palpation and visual assessment of the opposite kidney and liver are routine (although, as noted earlier in this chapter, some surgeons believe that preoperative imaging studies, particularly MRI, can exclude contralateral kidney involvement with tumor). The prognostic importance of lymph node involvement has been established and discussed previously (Table 7). Only 56% of patients in whom the surgeon thought that the nodes were involved by tumor in fact had pathologic confirmation of nodal tumor. If the surgeon thought the nodes were negative, 11% proved to be positive. Because the presence of nodal involvement upstages from II to III, it is important to sample the nodes and obtain pathologic confirmation (70).

As previously discussed, the incidence of operative rupture or spill of generally sizable, often "soft" tumors ranges from 15% to 30% (38,61,62,71). Most cases of operative spill are "focal" (limited to the operative site) rather than "diffuse" (contamination of the peritoneal cavity) (51). The risk of abdominal relapse and mortality has been significantly greater following surgical spill (33,38,54). In cases with marginally operable tumors or with large areas of central necrosis, preoperative radiotherapy or chemotherapy may be preferable to attempted resection with spill (72). As noted earlier in this chapter, the SIOP philosophy, using preoperative chemotherapy, has significantly impacted the risk of operative spill and tumor rupture.

Inoperability is primarily due to massive tumor with direct involvement of the liver and/or retroperitoneal structures. Some surgeons will recommend preoperative chemotherapy to improve the chance of resectability. Those who subscribe to the viewpoints of the SIOP studies will, of course, come to the patient's bedside predisposed to using preoperative chemotherapy without a biopsy. For those who feel uncomfortable with a diagnosis made by physical findings and diagnostic imaging, percutaneous biopsy is indicated and tumor resection is planned following response to preoperative chemotherapy (68). A needle biopsy may require general anesthesia or heavy sedation with local anesthesia. Ultrasound or contrast-enhanced CT scans may be used to localize the biopsy site. A proper biopsy must provide an adequate, representative specimen (38,61). Subtumor capsular bleeding is a possible biopsy-related complication. For this reason, some clinicians prefer a posterior approach for the biopsy so that bleeding will be more locally confined and less likely to spill into the abdominal cavity.

In the 1930s, nephrectomy alone achieved cure in 15% to 30% of children (48,73). Recent experience with the management of highly selected small intrarenal primary WT suggests that one can identify a group of patients at extremely low risk of systemic micrometastasis potentially treatable with surgery alone (67,74). In a pilot study at Children's Hospital in Boston, eight patients less than 2-years old with unilateral, nonmetastatic, small (less than 550 g total tumor and kidney specimen weight) favorable histology tumors (stage I) (48,49) underwent nephrectomy with no additional therapy. With mean follow-up of 5 years, all eight children are alive. Seven are continuously disease-free; one developed a metachronous bilateral tumor and was successfully treated (67). Other investigators have found that the risk of tumor recurrence in stage I favorable histology is negligible if the following factors are absent: inflammatory pseudocapsule, renal sinus invasion, capsular invasion, and intrarenal vessel invasion (75). A review of children treated on NWTS-1, 2, and 3 supports the hypthesis that changes in the NWTS regimens have not improved upon the excellent prognosis of children <2 years of age at diagnosis with tumors less than 550 g (63). In NWTS-5 this group of children is treated with surgery only.

Radiation Therapy

In 1950 Gross and Neuhauser of Boston Children's Hospital reported that 10 of 31 (32%) patients treated for Wilms' tumor from 1931 to 1939 appeared to be cured of their tumors compared to 18 of 38 (47%) cured when treated between 1940 and 1947. The authors suspected that the difference was explicable on the basis of the radiotherapy administered to 36 of the 38 patients in the later period. It was customary to irradiate children in the immediate postoperative period i.e. shortly after leaving the operating room. Doses of 200 roentgen per day were given to a total dose of 4,000 to 5,000 roentgen (76).

At present approximately 70% to 75% of children with Wilms' tumor will be treated without radiation therapy. The number rises to 80% to 85% if metastatic disease is excluded. The NWTS and SIOP trials that have lead to this restricted use of radiation therapy are described earlier in this chapter. When irradiation is employed, it is successful in limiting the frequency of abdominal relapse to 0% to 4% of children with favorable histology (62).

There are additional single-institution data concerning the role of radiotherapy for nonmetastatic WT. For example, studies at St. Jude Children's Research Hospital (SJCRH) eliminated radiation therapy for stage II disease after 1979 and began using reduced-dose irradiation for stage III (12 Gy; whole-abdomen irradiation until 1985, local-field irradiation since 1985 for FH without diffuse peritoneal contamination) (77). Abdominal disease control was obtained in 97% of patients. Utilizing a neoadjuvant chemotherapy protocol at the Hospital for Sick Children, Toronto, 15 of 54 patients with localized disease at presentation required radiation therapy (27%), 9 for stage III or anaplastic disease, and 6 for recurrence (56).

Chemotherapy

In 1966, Sidney Farber (73) reported improved results in the treatment of recurrent and metastatic Wilms' tumor. His series included 16 patients with recurrent disease and 15 with metastatic disease at diagnosis. Patients were treated primarily with actinomycin D and, to a limited degree, vincristine. The 2-year survival was 58%.

The addition of effective chemotherapy has substantially improved the overall results in Wilms' tumor within the past two decades. The NWTS and SIOP studies that have substantivally established the indications for chemotherapy are discussed earlier in this chapter.

RADIOTHERAPEUTIC MANAGEMENT

The current guideline for external beam radiation therapy on NWTS Trial 5 are summarized in Table 9 (12,57,59,77–79). Indications for radiation therapy in the current SIOP trial are summarized earlier in this chapter.

The timing of postoperative irradiation is important. Delayed initiation of treatment beyond 10 days following surgery has been related to increased risk of abdominal recurrence in several, but not all, studies (35,51,61, 62). Most relapses related to delayed start of therapy have been in patients with unfavorable histology (62). NWTS-5 recommends that postoperative irradiation begin no later than the ninth postoperative day.

Volume

Local-regional irradiation treatment fields include the "tumor bed," importantly differentiated from the "renal bed," to include the entire preoperative tumor extent within the abdomen. The tumor bed is defined as the outline of the kidney and any associated tumor. The tumor volume is established by careful review of the surgical findings, IVP, CT, ultrasound, and/or MRI. The superior margin of the field is placed at the upper pole of the kidney with an additional 1-cm margin in a child with a lower-pole neoplasm, while the inferior portal margin encompasses the lower margin of the tumor with a 1-cm margin. The field should extend to the dome of the diaphragm only in those patients in whom the tumor is known to have extended that far superiorly (80). A variable proportion of the liver will be necessarily included to adequately encompass the initial tumor extent for right-sided lesions. Medially, the target volume should encompass the entire width of the vertebral bodies with adequate contralateral extension to include the entire paraaortic lymph node chain but exclude the remaining kidney. The choice of the medial margin reflects the importance of lymph node radiation therapy. In addition, homogeneous irradiation of the vertebral bodies will avoid one mechanism of late scoliosis by equally affecting growth on each side of the vertebral body. Laterally, the treatment field tangentially includes the abdominal wall. Parallel opposed anterior and posterior fields are used.

For patients with preoperative intraperitoneal tumor rupture, intraoperative rupture with diffuse dissemination of tumor, diffuse peritoneal implants, or massive abdominal disease, irradiation must address the entire abdominal cavity. The target volume includes all of the peritoneal surfaces, defined superiorly by the diaphragms and inferiorly through the lower pelvic region generally at the bottom of the obturator foramen (80). The acetabulum and femoral heads are blocked. Attempts to limit irradiation by blocking the contralateral pelvic region of the peritoneal cavity have been associated with abdominal recurrence when abdominal irradiation was appropriate (81).

Whole-lung irradiation requires care to encompass both apices as well as the posterior inferior extent of the lungs. The average field extends above the clavicles and down to L1. The shoulders are excluded from the field by blocks. Care should be taken not to irradiate the uninvolved kidney in the whole-lung field (82).

There will be some clinical situations, which call for whole-lung irradiation plus flank irradiation—for example, anaplastic Wilms' tumor (stage II) in the abdomen, with lung metastases (overall stage IV). Some patients can be treated with one large field, reducing off the lungs at approximately 12 Gy to continue the flank irradiation. Usually the lungs and flank are irradiated separately. Field matching with appropriate gaps and feathering are important in avoiding excessive liver irradiation in right-sided disease as well as to avoid irradiation of the remaining kidney in the lower border of the whole-lung irradiation field.

Dose for Abdominal Disease

Earlier data regarding radiation control of abdominal disease recommended local irradiation to 24 to 30 Gy (48,72,81). The first two NWTS trials incorporated an age-dependent scale of doses ranging from 18 to 40 Gy

(10,57). Review of these trials showed an overall rate of initial abdominal failure of 2% to 4% with favorable histology in groups II and III (63). Details of radiation therapy showed no apparent dose response, with equal frequency of abdominal recurrence at dose levels of 18 to 20 Gy, 20 to 24 Gy, and 24 to 40 Gy (10,63).

NWTS-3 randomly assigned stage III cases to receive 10 or 20 Gy postoperatively, including an option for supplemental doses up to 10 Gy for regions of gross residual disease (35,83). This "boost" was utilized in only 2% of the stage III favorable histology patients (35). As shown in Table 8, the NWTS notes no difference in survival or relapse-free survival between the 10- and 20-Gy arms. The current NWTS-5 trial incorporates a "boost" at the investigator's option from 10.8 Gy to a cumulative dose of 21.6 Gy for patients with residual disease larger than 3 cm in diameter (80). SJCRH used 12 Gy postoperatively for patients with stage III disease. Two-year disease-free survival for patients with stage III FH and for those with stage IV favorable histology was 88% and 71%, respectively. Abdominal failure occurred in 3 of 52 patients (77).

The frequency of abdominal recurrence following protocol-directed therapy has been impressively reduced by the use of radiotherapy with adriamycin, actinomycin D, vincristine, and cyclophosphamide for patients with anaplastic Wilms' tumor (Table 8). A dose response for anaplastic Wilms' tumor has not clearly been identified. The frequency of infield recurrence at low doses has led some investigators to recommend an age-modulated dose scheme: less than 12 m, 12 to 18 Gy; 13 to 18 m, 18 to 24 Gy; 19 to 30 m, 24 to 30 Gy; 31 to 40 m, 30 to 35 Gy; greater than or equal to 41 m, 35 to 40 Gy. This is not because of an age-related dose response, but because of a fear of toxicity in the young.

In recent SIOP trials local-regional radiation therapy is given to patients who, after preoperative chemotherapy and nephrectomy, are found to have stage II node positive tumors, stage III, or unfavorable histology. These categories comprise approximately 25% of patients. The dose to the tumor bed is 15 Gy with an optional boost to localized areas of tumor as needed (56,58).

Brachytherapy and Intraoperative Radiation

Three cases of bilateral Wilms' tumor have been reported in which afterloading brachytherapy was utilized to treat renal disease in the remaining kidney following nephrectomy on one side and spare, to the extent possible, surrounding normal tissue. Brachytherapy may be of use in highly selected cases (84,85). Intraoperative radiation, including *ex vivo* bench surgery irradiation, has also been used in selected cases (52).

Bilateral Wilms' Tumor

Stage V or bilateral WT is found in 4% to 8% of patients (4,33,19). The 2-, 5-, and 10-year survival is 83%, 73%, and 70%, respectively (9,11,86,87). The majority of bilateral cases present with simultaneous or synchronous involvement in both kidneys. As with bilateral retinoblastoma, the extent of disease in each kidney is often quite disparate, frequently including a sizable unilateral tumor and scattered nodules involving the contralateral kidney. Unfavorable histology is found in 10%, and discordant histology (i.e., unfavorable histology on one side and favorable histology on the other) is found in 4% (9). The presence of unfavorable histology, older age at diagnosis, and the most advanced stage of the individual tumors are the most important prognostic factors (11,86–89).

There are a variety of therapeutic approaches to stage V disease. The goal of therapy is cure with preservation of renal function. Radical nephrectomy should almost never be performed as part of the initial surgical procedure. Rather, the initial operation defines the extent of tumor in each kidney, obtains bilateral biopsies to histologically confirm the diagnosis, and biopsies suspicious lymph nodes. Subsequently, the child should be treated with chemotherapy. If

NWTS-5 guidelines are followed, the chemotherapy is tailored to the worst histology (favorable or unfavorable) and the stage of the primary tumors (i.e., more aggressive chemotherapy if one of the tumors is intrabdominal stage III, less agressive if both tumors are stage I). After this inital chemotherapy, the child is returned to the operating room for second look surgery. If tumor can be removed with preservation of renal function, it should. If surgery successfully removes the tumors and there is no gross or pathological evidence of persistent or residual disease, chemotherapy is contined appropriate to the surgical stage. If there is gross or microscopic residual intraabdominal tumor following second look surgery, the patient is switched to alternative chemotherapy. If abnormalities persist in the kidneys on repeat imaging, a third operation may be attempted to finally excise the tumors. The reader will appreciate the general strategy: alternating between chemotherapy and surgery to achieve sufficient cytoreduction of tumor to achieve successful cancer surgery with preservation of functioning kidney(s) (9,67,80,88,89).

The indications for radiation therapy in stage V Wilms' tumor are: (a) when definitive surgery has been accomplished and one or both of the primary tumors are found to be stage III favorable histology or stages II to III anaplastic tumors or stages I to III clear cell sarcoma of the kidney or rhabdoid tumor. (b) When preoperative chemotherapy and one or two surgeries have not achieved successful extirpation of cancer, preoperative low-dose irradiation, 12 to 16 Gy, may produce sufficient tumor shrinkage to achieve tumor removal (80,90).

Metachronous or asynchronous bilateral disease has a decidedly less favorable outcome than does synchronous disease. Malcolm et al. (91) reported 0 of 4 survivors with metachronous disease compared to 10 of 16 with simultaneous presentations; speculatively, the less favorable results with metachronous involvement may be interpreted as representing a pattern of relapse rather than independent tumor development. Jones et al.

(66; also see ref. 92) confirmed a less favorable outcome with metachronous bilateral tumors: 39% 2-year survival in contrast to 87% with simultaneous presentations.

Metastatic Disease

The ability to control overt pulmonary metastasis represented the major advance consequent to the addition of actinomycin D to irradiation in the management of Wilms' tumor (44,48,72,73). In stage IV with pulmonary metastasis at diagnosis, conventional NWTS management begins with nephrectomy, postoperative chemotherapy, abdominal irradiation if appropriate, and whole lung irradiation. The indications for infradiaphragmatic irradiation are dictated by the degree of abdominal disease. Abdominal irradiation is given for stage IV patients with in-the-abdomen stage III favorable histology, stages II to III anaplastic histology, and stages I to III CCSK and rhabdoid tumor. For patients with pulmonary metastasis by chest radiograph at diagnosis, the addition of lung radiation therapy is standard (7,13,63,67,79,93). Although earlier reports documented excellent control dose levels of 16 to 18 Gy, the impressive results in recent series utilizing doses limited to 12 Gy at 1.5 Gy per fraction approach the control rates for abdominal disease with attenuated dose levels (35,38,77,79). A "boost" to local sites of residual pulmonary nodules to cumulative levels of 30 Gy is appropriate if permitted by the lung volumes. Stage IV favorable histology with lung metastases has an 80% 4-year survival rate on NWTS-3 whereas survival for those with stage IV unfavorable histology is about 55% (12,14,94).

In the current SIOP protocol Stage IV disease is treated with preoperative chemotherapy. Nephrectomy is then performed. Radiation therapy is adminstered per SIOP guidelines for intraabdominal disease (discussed eariler in this chapter). While lung irradiaton is reserved for those who do not have a complete pulmonary tumor response and are not rendered free of disease by metastectomy (56,58).

Is whole-lung irradiation necessary in stage IV (pulmonary) Wilms' tumor? In a United Kingdom Children's Cancer Group Study, stage IV favorable histology patients were spared whole-lung irradiation if they had complete resolution of pulmonary metastases after chemotherapy. Thirty-five of 39 patients were treated without whole-lung irradiation. The 6-year disease-free survival was 50%, overall survival 65% (94). These results appear to be somewhat worse than the NWTS and may be used to argue in favor of whole-lung irradiation. In a SIOP study, 36 stage IV FH patients received chemotherapy with abdominal irradiation given for stage III and/or node-positive stage II (37). Chemotherapy produced a complete disappearance of lung disease in 27 of 36 patients. Six additional patients were cleared of lung metastases with surgery. Only seven children ultimately received whole-lung irradiation: 7 for recurrent tumor, 1 immediately after nephrectomy for inoperable multiple metastases, and 2 following complete tumor clearance by chemotherapy. Five-year actuarial disease-free survival is 83% (7,37,56,58,63).

Radiation therapy had been considered fundamental for control of stage IV Wilms' tumor. From the date described above, one may assert that this view might have to be modified for children whose lung metastases completely respond to chemotherapy with supplemental surgery in selected cases, as well as for patients with minimal disease—for example, CT-positive, chest radiograph-negative disease (46). One hopes that future studies will help identify those patients with stage IV disease who, on the basis of biologic markers, require whole-lung irradiation and those who may be spared it with equivalent high survival probabilities (7).

It is important to take account of prior abdominal irradiation in patients who require thoracic irradiation. One must respect liver tolerance when adjoining fields that encompass the hepatic region. One must also respect the upper pole of the remaining kidney in delineating thoracic irradiation fields in a child with previous abdominal irradiation.

Liver metastases may be treated by hepatic irradiation in addition to chemotherapy. Whole-liver irradiation is sometimes given for diffuse disease with supplementary boosts to gross disease (12,57,61). When possible, however, more limited radiotherapy fields are used if the disease is more localized in the liver.

RECURRENT WILMS' TUMOR

A considerable body of evidence has been developed concerning the important prognostic factors for outcome following relapse of Wilms' tumor. The major prognostic factors will be considered in turn.

Site of Recurrence

Patients who relapse in the abdomen may, in general, be separated into two groups: (a) those having recurrences in previously irradiated fields. These individuals have resistant disease. In NWTS-3 the 3-year post relapse survival for such patients was 15%. (b) Intra-abdominal recurrences after surgery and chemotherapy only. These patients are amenable to retreatment and the 3-year postrelapse survival is 77% (81,95–97).

The lung is a common site of recurrence of Wilms' tumor. Relapse confined to the lung has a 44% 3-year postrelapse survival. Relapse in the liver portends a worse prognosis: 14% at 4-years postrelapse (38,91,96). There are some survivors of a solitary metastases to brain or liver (98,99).

Initial Stage of Disease

The prognosis following relapse is related to the inital stage. In both the NWTS trials and the United Kingdom Children's Cancer Study Group Wilms' tumor trials, group I patients had a better ultimate survival following relapse than did groups II or III. In NWTS-2 and 3 the 3-year postrelapse survival was 57% for initial stage I, 36% for initial stage II and III, and 17% for initial stage IV (7,96,100).

Histology

The survival following relapse of patients with favorable histology is two- to four-fold greater than that of patients with unfavorable histology (18,96). The United Kingdom Children's Cancer Study Group has reported only 17 survivors out of 71 patients (24%) who relapsed during or after treatment. Fifteen of 51 (29%) patients with relapsed favorable histology survived compared to 2 of 20 (10%) with unfavorable histology (99,101).

Time of Relapse

Relapse following initial therapy is demonstrated within 1 year of diagnosis in 75% of cases with ultimate failure. Less than 3% of proven relapses have been documented beyond 2 years after diagnosis (61,62). The longer the time between diagnosis and the development of recurrent disease, the better the ultimate outcome (7). The 3-year postrelapse survival for NWTS-2 and 3 patients who relapsed 0 to 5 months following diagnosis was 18%, 6 to 11 months following diagnosis was 30%, and longer than or equal to 12 months following diagnosis was 41% (96,100).

Nature of Prior Therapy

Patients who relapse following initial therapy that included adriamycin of abdominal irradiation fare worse than those who did not receive such therapy (7,96). Presumably this is the result both of the use of adriamycin and radiotherapy being surrogate markers for initially more advanced disease as well as the possibility that tumor that recurs after such therapy represents more resistant disease.

The rate of success in achieving secondary disease-free survival varies inversely with the intensity of the initial treatment regimen. Data reporting "salvage" in the NWTS studies demonstrate lower rates of secondary control that parallel the selective use of more aggressive treatment in high-risk patients. Serial reduction in the actual rate of demonstrated pulmonary metastases has paralleled reduction in later control of metastatic disease. Secondary disease-free survival has been reported in 51% of relapsed cases from NWTS-1, 40% from NWTS-2, and 34% from NWTS-3 (38,102).

When tumor relapses in the lung a surgical biopsy or excision is performed to confirm the diagnosis. Surgical excision of metastases, however, does not reduce the risk of second relapse (7). Chemotherapy and whole-lung irradiation are generally given.

When favorable histology relapses in the abdomen in a child with inital stage I or II disease who did not receive prior irradiation, the treatment generally includes preoperative chemotherapy, tumor excision, and involved field irradiation (Thoms, Green, Miser). A local relapse of initial stage III disease calls for preoperative chemotherapy, tumor excison, and re-irradiation (96).

TOXICITIES

The late effects of treatment of childhood cancer and the causes and frequency of treatment-induced second malignant neoplasms are considered, in detail, in Chapters 19 and 20. In this section we will briefly review those late ill effects, including induced neoplasms, particularly associated with the treatment of Wilms' tumor.

Complications Attributable to Surgery

Small bowel obstruction occurred in 7% of children who underwent primary nephrectomy in NWTS-3. Factors contibuting to obstruction include tumor rupture, intravascular extension of tumor, the necessity of resecting other organs at the time of nephrectomy, and the presence of postoperative residual tumor. Other complications attributable to surgery include extensive intraoperative hemorrhage (6%), vascular injuries (1%), injuries to uninvolved organs (1%), and death (0.5%) (8, 103). The operative mortality rate in the United Kingdom Children's Cancer Wilms' Tumor Study was 1% (104).

Hematologic Toxicity

Review of the data from NWTS-3 indicates a rate of clinically significant acute hematologic toxicities. Fatal toxicities occur in a small proportion of patients. Depending on the drugs given, severe hematologic toxicity occurs in 6% to 64% of patients over a 6-week course of treatment. Toxicity and infections account for 15% of the deaths of NWTS children, producing a 1% treatment-related mortality rate (12).

Hepatic Effects

Hepatotoxicity from Wilms' tumor therapy may be ascertained by an increase in transaminases and/or hyperbilirubinemia. Veno-occlusive disease consists of the clinical triad of hepatomegaly, ascites, and icterus. In unirradiated NWTS-4 patients the frequency of hepatic toxicity related to actinomycin D (SGOT, SGPT elevations) rose from 2.8% in patients receiving 15 μmg/kg of standard divided-dose therapy to 3.7% in those receiving pulse-intensive 45 μmg/kg and 14.3% in those receiving 60 μmg/kg pulse-intensive therapy. These data prompted replacement of the 60 μmg/kg treatment with the 45-μmg/kg dose (98). A review of patients accrued via the German Pediatric Oncology Hematology Group to SIOP Trial 9 studies 58 patients who received chemotherapy and abdominal irradiation. Eleven of these 58 patients developed signs of hepatotoxicity, four of them with venoocclusive disease. There was a predominance of children with right-sided tumors in the group with hepatic injury (9/33, 27% vs. 2/24, 8%). This is probably a reflection of the larger volume of liver irradiated in right sided tumors. Plowman from St. Bartholomew's Hospital/The Hospital for Sick Children, London, has described the use of a partial transmission block to reduce the radiation dose administered to the liver in right-sided Wilms' tumor and, therefore, reduce the risk of late toxicity (105).

Orthopedic Effects

In long-term follow-up studies of Wilms' tumor survivors, scoliosis and musculoskeletal abnormalities have been found more frequently in irradiated patients than in those not treated with radiotherapy. Rate et al. identified 31 children with Wilms' tumor who received abdominal irradiation between 1970 and 1984 and were followed past skeletal maturity. Ten of the children were irradiated with ortholovoltage and 21 with megavoltage. Of the children irradiated with megavoltage, the most frequent orthopedic abnormalities were lower rib hypoplasia (57%) and mild scoliosis (10° to 20°) (48%). In the orthovoltage patients lower rib hypoplasis occurred in 50%, mild scoliosis in 40%, severe scoliosis (greater than 20°) in 40%, and limb length inequality in 20% (106,107). Scoliosis as a late ill effect of abdominal irradiation for Wilms' tumor was confirmed by a report from the University of Helsinki where 21 of 24 patients (88%) had some degree of scoliosis. Most patients had been irradiated with Cobalt 60 (108). Abdominal irradiation can also produce significant reduction in sitting height and a more modest decrease in standing height. These effects are more pronounced the younger the patient is at the time of radiotherapy (109).

Renal Effects

After unilateral nephrectomy in childhood, the remaining kidney generally adjusts its function and size—this is called compensatory hypertrophy of the kidney. One year after nephrectomy for Wilms' tumor the glomerular filtration rate and effective renal plasma flow are approximately 90% of normal values for age-matched children with two normal kidneys. Children treated with surgery plus chemotherapy also have close to normal values. The addition of radiation to chemotherapy results in a diminished renal function—approximately 73% of normal glomerular filtration rate (110).

Treatment-induced neoplasms

Initial reports concerning the risk of second malignant neoplasms following treatment of Wilms' tumor indicated that the cumulative incidence 10 years following diagnosis was 1% (83,111,112). A recent update of long-term survivors indicates a significant increased of second malignancies as assessed by an observed: expected relative risk ratio (8.4). Patients who received both adriamycin and higher dose irradiation (35 Gy) had the highest relative risk (36.3) (113).

REFERENCES

References particularly recommended for further reading are indicated by an asterisk.

1. Rance TM. Case of fungus haematodes in kidnies. *Med Phys* 1814;32:19.
2. Gairdner E. Case of fungus haematodes in the kidneys. *Edinburgh Med Surg J* 1828;29:312–315.
3. Osler W. Two cases of striated myosarcoma of the kidney. *J Anat Physiol* 1879;14:229.
4. King SC. Wilms' tumor. *N C Med J* 1991;52:74.
5. Zantinga AR, Coppes MJ. Historical aspects of the identification of the entity Wilms tumor, and its management. *Hematol Oncol Clinc North Am* 1995;9:1145–1155.
6. Green DM, Breslow N, Li YI, et al. The role of surgical excision in the management of relapsed Wilms' tumor patients with pulmonary metastases. *J Pediatr Surg* 1991;26:728–733.
*7. Green DM. Wilms' tumor. *Eur J Cancer* 1997;33:409–418.
8. Haase GM. Current surgical management of Wilms' tumor. *Curr Opin Pediatr* 1996;8:268–275.
9. Blute ML, Kelalis PP, Offord KP, Breslow N, Beckwith JB, D'Angio GJ. Bilateral Wilms' tumor. *J Urol* 1987;138(2):968–973.
*10. D'Angio GJ, Breslow N, Beckwith JB, et al. Treatment of Wilms' tumor: results of the Third National Wilms' Tumor Study. *Cancer* 1989;64:349–360.
11. Montgomery BT, Kelalis PP, Blute MD, et al. Extended follow-up of bilateral Wilms' tumor: results of the National Wilms' Tumor Study. *J Urol* 1991;146:514–518.
12. D'Angio GJ. Informational bulletin #19. National Wilms' Tumor Study, 1991. Seattle, WA: NWTS Data and Statistical Center.
13. Breslow NE, Churchill G, Nesmith B, et al. Clinico-pathologic features and prognosis for Wilms' tumor patients with metastases at diagnosis. *Cancer* 1986;58:2501–2511.
*14. Green DM, Finkelstein JZ, Breslow NE, Beckwith JB. Remaining problems in the treatment of patients with Wilms' tumor. *Pediatr Clin North Am* 1991;38:475–488.
15. Hadley GP, Jacobs C. The clinical presentation of Wilms' tumour in black children. *S Afr Med J* 1990;77:565–567.
16. Knudson AG. Hereditary cancer, oncogenes, and antioncogenes. *Cancer Res* 1985;45:1437–1443.
17. Knudson AG, Strong LC. Mutation and cancer: a model for Wilms' tumor of the kidney. *J Natl Cancer Inst* 1972;48:313–324.
18. Grundy P, Coppes M. An overview of the clinical and molecular genetics of Wilms' tumor. *Med Pediatr Oncol* 1996;27:394–397.
19. Grundy P, Coppes MJ, Haber D. Molecular genetics of Wilms tumor. *Hematol Oncol Clin North Am* 1995;9:1201–1215.
20. Douglass EC, Look AT, Webber B, et al. Hyperdiploidy and chromosomal rearrangements define the anaplastic variant of Wilms' tumor. *J Clin Oncol* 1986;4:975–981.
21. Riccardi VM, Hittner HM, Francke U, et al. The aniridia- Wilms' tumor association: the critical role of chromosome band 11p13. *J Cancer Genet Cytogenet* 1980;2:131–137.
22. Palmer N, Evans AE. The association of aniridia and Wilms' tumor: methods of surveillance and diagnosis. *Med Pediatr Oncol* 1983;11:73–75.
23. Pendergrass TW. Congenital anomalies in children with Wilms' tumor: a new survey. *Cancer* 1976;37:403–409.
24. Breslow NE. Epidemiological features of Wilms' tumor: results of the National Wilms' Tumor Study. *J Natl Cancer Inst* 1982;68:429–436.
*25. Beckwith JB. Wilms' tumor and other renal tumors of childhood. *Hum Pathol* 1983;14:481–492.
26. Coppes MJ, Ritchey ML, D'Angio GJ. Preface. *Hematol Oncol Clin North Am* 1995;9:xiii–xvii.
27. Howell CG, Othersen HB, Kiviat NE, Norkool P, Beckwith JB, D'Angio GJ. Therapy and outcome in 51 children with mesoblastic neophroma: a report of the National Wilms' Tumor Study. *J Pediatr Surg* 1982;17:826–831.
28. Puri P, Kalidasan V. Mesoblastic nephroma and Wilms' tumour. In: Puri P, ed. *Neonatal tumours*. London: Springer, 1996:43–48.
*29. Walterhouse D. Mesoblastic nephroma. *Med Pediatr Oncol* 1990;18:64–67.
30. Beckwith JB. Wilms' tumor and other renal tumors in childhood. In: Finegold M, ed. *Pathology of neoplasia in children and adolescents.* Philadelphia: WB Saunders, 1986:313–332.
31. Beckwith JB, Palmer NF. Histopathology and prognosis of Wilms' tumor: results from the First National Wilms' Tumor Study. *Cancer* 1978;41:1937–1948.
*32. Schmidt D, Beckwith JB. Histopathology of childhood renal tumor. *Hematol Oncol Clin North Am* 1995;9:1179–1200.
33. Breslow NE, Palmer NF, Hill LR, Buring J, D'Angio JD. Wilms' tumor: prognostic factors for patients without metastases at diagnosis: results of the National Wilms' Tumor Study. *Cancer* 1978;41:1577–1589.
34. D'Angio GJ, Tefft M, Breslow N, Meyer JA. Radiation therapy of Wilms' tumor: results according to dose, field, post-operative timing and histology. *Int J Radiat Oncol Biol Phys* 1978;4:769–780.
35. D'Angio GJ, Evans AE, Breslow N, et al. The treatment of Wilms' tumor: results of the National Wilms' Tumor Study. *Cancer* 1976;38:633–646.
36. Bonadio JF, Storer B, Norkool P, Farewell VT, Beckwith JB, D'Angio GJ. Anaplastic Wilms' tumor: clinical and pathologic studies. *J Clin Oncol* 1985;3:513–520.
37. de Kraker J, Lemerle J, Voute PA, Zucker JM, Tournade MF, Carli M, for the International Society of Pediatric Oncology Nephroblastoma Trial and Study

Committee. Wilms' tumor with pulmonary metastases at diagnosis: the significance of primary chemotherapy. *J Clin Oncol* 1990;8:1187–1190.

38. Breslow N, Churchill G, Beckwith JB, et al. Prognosis for Wilms' tumor patients with nonmetastatic disease at diagnosis—results of the Second National Wilms' Tumor Study. *J Clin Oncol* 1985;3:521–531.

*39. Faria P, Beckwith JB, Mishra K, et al. Focal versus diffuse anaplasia in Wilms tumor–new definitions with prognostic significane: a report from the national Wilms tumor study group. *Am J Surg Pathol* 1996;20:909–920.

40. Haas JE, Bonadio JF, Beckwith JB. Clear cell sarcoma of the kidney with emphasis of ultrastructural studies. *Cancer* 1984;54:2978–2987.

*41. Green DM, Thomas PRM, Shochat S. The treatment of Wilms' tumor: results of the National Wilms' tumor studies. *Hematol Oncol Clin North Am* 1995;9:1267–1274.

42. Gutjahr P. Progress and controversies in modern treatment of Wilms' tumor. *World J Urol* 1995;13:209–212.

43. Leape L, Breslow N, Bishop H. Surgical resection of Wilms' tumor: results of the National Wilms' Tumor Study. *Ann Surg* 1978;181:351–356.

44. Green DM, Jaffe N. Wilms' tumor—model of a curable pediatric malignant solid tumor. *Cancer Treat Rev* 1978;5:143–172.

45. Wilimas JA, Douglass EC, Magill L, Fitch S, Hustu HO. Significance of pulmonary computed tomography at diagnosis in Wilms' tumor. *J Clin Oncol* 1988;6:1144–1146.

46. Flentje M, Weirich A, Potter R, Ludwig R. Hepatotoxicity in irradiated nephroblastoma patients during postoperative treatment according to SIOP9/GPOH. *Radiol Oncol* 1994;31:222–228.

47. Feusner JH, Beckwith JB, D'Angio GJ. Clear cell sarcoma of the kidney: accuracy of imaging methods for detecting bone metastases. Report from the National Wilms' Tumor Study. *Med Pediatr Oncol* 1990;18:225–227.

48. Cassady JR, Tefft M, Filler RM, Jaffe N, Paed D, Hellman S. Considerations in the radiation therapy of Wilms' tumor. *Cancer* 1973;32:598–608.

49. Cassady JR, Jaffe N, Paed D, Filler RM. The increasing importance of radiation therapy in the improved prognosis of children with Wilms' tumor. *Cancer* 1977;39:825–829.

50. Garcia M, Douglass C, Schlosser JV. Classification and prognosis in Wilms' tumor. *Radiology* 1963;80:574–580.

51. Tefft M, D'Angio GJ, Grant W. Post-operative radiation therapy for residual Wilms' tumor: review of Group III patients in the National Wilms' Tumor Study. *Cancer* 1976;37:2768–2772.

52. Jereb B, Tournade MF, Lemerle J, et al. Lymph node invasion and prognosis in neophroblastoma. *Cancer* 1980;45:1632–1636.

53. Lemerle J, Voute PA, Tournade MF, et al. Preoperative versus postoperative radiotherapy, single versus multiple courses of actinomycin D, in the treatment of Wilms' tumor. *Cancer* 1976;38:647–654.

54. Lemerle J, Voute PA, Tournade MF, et al. Effectiveness of preoperative chemotherapy in Wilms' tumor: results of an International Society of Pediatric Oncol-

ogy (SIOP) clinical trial. *J Clin Oncol* 1983;1:604–610.

55. De Kraker J. Commentary on Wilms' tumor. *Eur J Cancer* 1997;419–420.

*56. De Kraker J, Weitzman S, Voute PA. Preoperative strategies in the managment of Wilms' tumor. *Hematol Oncol Clin North Am* 1995;9:1275–1285.

57. D'Angio GJ. Editorial: SIOP and the management of Wilms' tumor. *J Clin Oncol* 1983;1:595–596.

*58. Jereb B, Burgers JMV, Tournade M-F, et al. Radiotherapy in the SIOP (international society of pediatric oncology) nephroblastoma studies: a review. *Med Pediatr Oncol* 1994;22:221–227.

*59. Thomas PRM. Wilms' tumor: changing role of radiation therapy. *Semin Radiat Oncol* 1997;7:204–211.

60. D'Angio GJ, Evans A, Breslow N, et al. The treatment of Wilms' tumor: results of the Second National Wilm's Tumor Study. *Cancer* 1981;47:2302–2311.

*61. Tefft M, D'Angio GJ, Beckwith B, Farewell V, Meyer JA. Patterns of intra-abdominal relapse (IAR) in patients with Wilms' tumor who received radiation: analysis by histopathology, a report of National Wilms' Tumor Studies 1 and 2 (NWTS-1 & 2). *Int J Radiat Oncol Biol Phys* 1980;6:663–667.

*62. Thomas PR, Tefft M, Farewell VT, Norkool P, Storer B, D'Angio GJ. Abdominal relapses in irradiated second national Wilms' tumor study patients. *J Clin Oncol* 1984;2:1098–1011.

*63. Green DM, Coppes MJ. Future directions in clinical research in Wilms' tumor. *Hematol Oncol Clin North Am* 1995;9:1329–1339.

64. Green DM. Disease committee chair update: Wilms' tumor. *POG Perspectives* 1997;Fall:10–11.

65. Green D, Breslow N, Beckwith J, et al. A comparison between single dose and divided dose administration of dactinomycin and doxorubicin: a report from the national Wilms' tumor study group. *Med Pediatr Oncol* 1998;16:237–245.

66. Jones B, Hrabovsky E, Kiviat N, Breslow N. Metachronous bilateral Wilms' tumor: National Wilms' Tumor Study. *Am J Clin Oncol* 1982;5:545–550.

67. Larsen E, Perez-Atayde A, Green DM, Retik A, Clavell LA, Sallan SE. Surgery only for the treatment of patients with stage I (Cassady) Wilms' tumor. *Cancer* 1990;66:264–266.

68. Thomas PR, Sochat SJ, Norkool P, Breslow NE, D'Angio GJ. Prognostic implications of extension, invasion or metastases to the liver at diagnosis of Wilms' tumor. *Proc Am Soc Clin Oncol* 1988;7:255.

69. Ritchey ML, Othersen HB Jr, de Lorimier AA, Kramer SA, Benson C, Kelalis PO. Renal vein involvement with nephroblastoma: a report of the National Wilms' Tumor Study—3. *Eur Urol* 1990;17:139–144.

70. Othersen HB Jr, DeLarimer A, Hrabovsky E, Kelalis P, Breslow N, D'Angio GJ. Surgical evaluation of lymph node metastases in Wilms' tumor. *J Pediatr Surg* 1990;25:330–331.

71. Gonzalez-Chirinas P, Aguilar M, Rivera M. Preoperative vincristine (VCR) in children with Wilms' tumor. *Proc ASCO* 1991;10:314.

*72. Burgers JMV, Tournade MF, Bey P, et al. Abdominal recurrences in Wilms' tumours: a report from the

SIOP Wilms' tumour trials and studies. *Radiother Oncol* 1986;5:175–182.

73. Farber S. Chemotherapy in the treatment of leukemia and Wilms' tumor. *JAMA* 1966;138:826–836.

74. Hughes E, Klavell L, Cassady JR, Sallen S. Wilms' tumor treated by surgery without chemotherapy. *Proc Am Soc Clin Oncol* 1985;4:241.

75. Weeks DA, Beckwith JB, Luckey DW. Relapse-associated variables in stage I favorable histology Wilms' tumor: a report of the National Wilms' Tumor Study. *Cancer* 1987;60:1202–1204.

76. Gross RE, Neuhauser EBD. Treatment of mixed tumors of the kidney in childhood. *Pediatrics* 1950;6: 843–852.

77. Tobin RL, Fantanesi J, Kun LE, et al. Wilms' tumor: reduced-dose radiotherapy in advanced-stage Wilms' tumor with favorable histology. *Int J Radiat Oncol Biol Phys* 1990;19:867–871.

*78. Thomas PR, Tefft M, D'Angio GJ, Norkool P. Validation of radiation dose reductions used in the Third National Wilms' Tumor Study (NWTS-3). *Proc Am Soc Clin Oncol* 1988;29:227.

79. Wilimas JA, Douglass EC, Lewis S, et al. Reduced therapy for Wilms' tumor: analysis of treatment results from a single institution. *J Clin Oncol* 1988;6: 1630–1635.

80. Pediatric Oncology Group. POG 9440/CCG 4941. National Wilms' Tumor Study-5: Therapeutic Trial and Biology Study, Chicago, IL, August 16, 1995.

81. Jeal P, Jenkins RDT. Abdominal irradiation in the treatment of Wilms' tumor. *Int J Radiat Oncol Biol Phys* 1980;6:655–661.

82. Donaldson SS, Moskowitz PS, Canty EL, Fajardo LF. Combination radiation-adriamycin therapy: renoprival growth, functional and structural effects in the immature mouse. *Int J Radiat Oncol Biol Phys* 1980;6:851–859.

83. D'Angio GJ. Results of the Third National Wilms' Tumor Study (NWTS-3): a preliminary report. *AACR* 1984;723(abst).

84. Duckett CP, Zderic S, Goldwein J, Duckett JW. Brachytherapy for residual intra-renal Wilms' tumor. *Med Pediatr Oncol* 1997;28:316–320.

85. Thoms WW Jr, Goldwein JW, D'Angio G. A technique for the use of afterloading [137]brachytherapy in renal-sparing irradiation of bilateral Wilms' tumor. *Int J Rad Oncol Biol Phys* 997;39:1121–1124.

86. Longaker MT, Harrison MR, Adzick NS, et al. Nephron-sparing approach to bilateral Wilms' tumor: *in situ* or *ex vivo* surgery and radiation therapy. *J Pediatr Surg* 1990;25:411–414.

87. Malcolm AW, Jaffe N, Folkman MJ, Cassady JR. Bilateral Wilms' tumor. *Int J Radiat Oncol Biol Phys* 1980;6:167–174.

88. Laberge J-M, Nguyen LT, Homsy YL, Doody DP. Bilateral Wilms' tumors: changing concepts in management. *J Pediatr Surg* 1987;22:730–735.

*89. Ritchey ML, Coppes MJ. The management of synchronous bilateral Wilms tumor. *Hematol Oncol Clin North Am* 1995;9:1303–1315.

90. Ritchey ML, Kelalis PP, Haase GM, Shochat SJ, Green DM, D'Angio G. Preoperative therapy for intracaval and atrial extension of Wilms' tumor. *Cancer* 1993;71:4104–4110.

91. Jereb B, Issac R, Tournade MF, et al. Survival of pa-

tients with metastases from Wilms' tumor (SIOP 1, SIOP 2, SIOP 5). *Eur Paediatr Haematol Oncol* 1985;2:71–76.

92. Bishop HC, Tefft M, Evans AE, D'Angio GJ. Survival in bilateral Wilms' tumor—review of 30 national Wilms' tumor study cases. *J Pediatr Surg* 1977;12:631–638.

93. Sutow WW, Breslow NE, Palmer NF, D'Angio GJ, Takashima J. Prognosis in children with Wilms' tumor metastases prior to or following primary treatment: results from the First National Wilms' Tumor Study (NWTS-1). *Am J Clin Oncol* 1982;5: 339–347.

94. Green D, Fernbach D, Narkool P, Kollia G, D'Angio G. The treatment of Wilms' tumor patients with pulmonary metastases detected only with computerized tomography. A report from the National Wilms' Tumor Study. *Proc ASCO* 1991;10:309.

95. Green DM, Finkelstein JZ, Tefft ME, Norkool P. Diffuse interstitial pneumonitis after pulmonary irradiation for metastatic Wilms' tumor: a report from the National Wilms' Tumor Study. *Cancer* 1989;63: 450–453.

*96. Miser JS, Tournade MF. The management of relapsed Wilms tumor. *Hematol Oncol Clin North Am* 1995;9: 1287–1302.

97. Thoms WW Jr, Vega R, Abramowsky C, Ricketts R, Wyly B. Multimodal management of recurrent Wilms' tumor: the role of radiation therapy. *Med Pediatr Oncol* 1996;27:179–184.

98. Green DM, Narkool P, Breslow NE, Finkelstein JZ, D'Angio GJ. Severe hepatic toxicity after treatment with vincristine and dactinomycin using single-dose or divided-dose schedules: a report from the National Wilms' Tumor Study. *J Clin Oncol* 1990;8: 1525–1530.

99. Groot-Loonen JJ, Pinkerton CR, Morris-Jones PH, Pritchard J. How curable is relapsed Wilms' tumor? *Arch Dis Child* 1990;65:968–970.

100. Grundy P, Breslow NE, Green DM, et al. Prognostic factors for children with recurrent Wilms' tumor: results from the second and third Wilms' tumor study. *J Clin Oncol* 1989;7:638–647.

101. Pinkerson CR, Groot-Loonen JJ, Morris-Jones PH, Pritchard J. Response rates in relapsed Wilms' tumor: a need for new effective agents. *Cancer* 1991;67: 567–571.

102. Larsen E, Griffin GC, Grundy P, Green DM. Phase II upfront therapy for recurrent Wilms' tumor. Concept sheet, Pediatric Oncology Group, St. Louis, 1991.

103. Ritchey ML, Kelalis PP, Etzioni R, Breslow N, Shochat S, Haase GM. Small bowel obstruction after nephrectomy for Wilms' tumor: a report of the national Wilms' tumor study 3. *Ann Surg* 1993;218: 654–659.

*104. Pritchard J, Imeson J, Cotterill S, et al. Results of the United Kingdom children's cancer study group first Wilms' tumor study. *J Clin Oncol* 1995;13: 124–133.

105. Plowman PN. Hepatotoxicity in irradiated nephroblastoma patients. *Radiother Oncol* 1994;31:191.

106. Rate WR, Butler MS, Roibertson WW Jr, D'Angio GJ. Late orthopedic effects in children with Wilms' tumor treated with abdominal irradiation. *Med Pediatr Oncol* 1991;19:265–268.

107. Westerinki HP, Alberts AS. Letter to the editor. *Med Pediatr Oncol* 1992;21:382.

108. Makipernaa A, Heikkila JT, Merikanto J, Marttinen E, Siimes MA. Spinal deformity induced by radiotherapy for solid tumours of childhood: a long-term follow up study. *Eur J Pediatr* 1993;152:197–200.

109. Wallace WHB, Shalet SM, Morris-Jones PH, Swindell R, Gahameneni HR. Effect of abdominal irradiation on growth in boys treated for a Wilms' tumor. *Med Pediatr Oncol* 1990;18:441–446.

110. De Graaf SSN, van Gent H, Reitsma-Bierens WCC, van Luyk WHJ, Dolsma WV, Postma A. Renal function after unilateral nephrectomy for Wilms' tumour: the influence of radiation therapy. *Eur J Cancer* 1996;32A:465–469.

111. Breslow NE, Norkool PA, Olshan A, Evans A, D'Angio GJ. Second malignant neoplasms in survivors of Wilms' tumor: a report from the National Wilms' Tumor Study. *J Natl Cancer Inst* 1988;80: 592–595.

112. Kovalic JJ, Thomas PRM, Beckwith JB, Feusner JH, Narkool P. Hepatocellular carcinoma as second malignant neoplasms in successfully treated Wilms' tumor patients: a National Wilms' Tumor Study Report. *Cancer* 1991;67:342–344.

113. Breslow NE, Takashima JR, Whitton JA, et al. Second malignant neoplasms following treatment for Wilms' tumor: a report from the national Wilms' tumor study group. *J Clin Oncol* 1995;13: 1851–1859.

14

Tumors of the Liver and Biliary Tree

Childhood primary malignant liver tumors (PMLTs) constitute between 0.5% and 2% of pediatric cancer in Europe and the United States. They are more frequent in Japan, Southeast Asia, and sub-Sahara Africa (1–3). A cure is dependent upon the ability to achieve a surgical extirpation of the tumor. Chemotherapy plays a supportive role to surgery in curative treatment. There are several types of benign liver tumors in children. These benign tumors are either treated with surgery or observed (4,5). On rare occasion there will be a role for radiotherapy or invasive radiologic procedures. Rhabdomyosarcoma of the biliary tree may occur in children (6). Primary biliary adenocarcinoma, primary hepatic sarcoma, and primary hepatic malignancy with rhabdoid features in childhood are extremely rare (7,8). External beam, intraoperative, or intraluminal radiotherapy and chemotherapy are usually used with surgery in these cases.

CLINICAL PRESENTATION, STAGING, AND WORKUP

Children with PMLTs will present with an abdominal mass or generalized abdominal enlargement. The child may have pain localized to the right upper quadrant, fever, anorexia, weight loss, jaundice, or vomiting. The first presentation may, on occasion, be an acute abdominal crisis due to tumor rupture and hemoperitoneum. Paraneoplastic syndromes have been associated with PMLTs (9).

Hepatoblastoma (HBL) is the most common PMLT occurring in the first 20 years of

life and accounts for about 43% to 51% of malignant liver tumors in the pediatric age group (9–11). The median age at diagnosis is 1 year. As with all PMLTs, there is a male predominance (3,9,12–14). HBL has been reported to be associated with a host of other conditions, including Beckwith-Wiedemann syndrome, Wilms' tumor, adrenal cortical tumors, fetal alcohol syndrome, familial adenomatous polyposis, precocious puberty in males due to human chorionic gonadotropin (HCG) secretion, and thrombocytosis (2,7, 11–13,15–20).

HBL may be histologically subclassified into six patterns (Table 1). Conventional HBLs contain fetal hepatoblasts, embryonal hepatoblasts, or a mixture of the two cell types (Fig. 1). Fetal-type hepatoblasts recapitulate the cytoarchitecture of the normal human fetal liver. Cells of the early fetal liver and the cells of fetal HBL are of similar size and configuration. Both proliferate as cuboidal cells with trabeculae one to two cells thick. Both display strong positivity for alphafetoprotein (AFP). Both tissues also display sinusoidal hematopoesis and a lack of intrahepatic bile ducts (21). Fetal cells are slightly smaller than normal hepatocytes and have a low nuclear-to-cytoplasm ratio. In contrast, embryonal hepatoblasts have a higher nuclear-to-cytoplasm ratio than do fetal cells, and they also have a compact basophilic cytoplasm. This gives a light-microscopic impression of a higher cell density (3,14,22–24). Small-cell undifferentiated or anaplastic HBL contains sheets and nests of medium-sized cells, with little or no evidence of hepatoblas-

TABLE 1. *Histologic classification of hepatoblastoma*

Epithelial type (56%)	Mixed epithelial and mesenchymal type (44%)
Fetal pattern (31%)	Without teratoid features (34%)
Embryonal and fetal pattern (19%)	With treated features (10%)
Macrotrobecular pattern (3%)	
Small-cell undifferentiated pattern (3%)	

Modified from ref. 21, with permission.

tic differentiation. There is scant cytoplasm and a high mitotic rate. Mixed epithelial and mesenchymal HBL is composed of typical areas of fetal epithelial and embryonal type cells mixed with primitive mesenchyme and various mesenchymally derived tissue (21). In long-term survivors of HBL the most common histology is the conventional type with a predominately fetal cell pattern (13). While conventional epithelial tumors constitute 60%

of all HBLs, they represent 85% of those children who have undergone complete tumor resection and who are long-term survivors (3,22). Almost no children with anaplastic HBL survive the disease. A Pediatric Oncology Group (POG)-Children's Cancer Study Group (CCSG) trial convincingly showed the distinction between fetal HBL and other histologic subtypes to be of prognostic importance in stage I disease (3-year progression-free survival of 79% versus 56%, $p = 0.11$) (25). Not all investigators, however, have confirmed the prognostic importance of histologic subtyping in all stages (14).

Hepatocellular carcinoma (HCC), the second most common PMLT in children, accounts for about one-fourth to one-third of pediatric hepatic malignancies (1,9). HCC is unusual in children less than 5 years of age (Fig. 2). The median age of presentation for pediatric HCC is 12 years (9,22). Approximately 25% of cases in children are associated with cirrhosis (13). Etiologies of this cir-

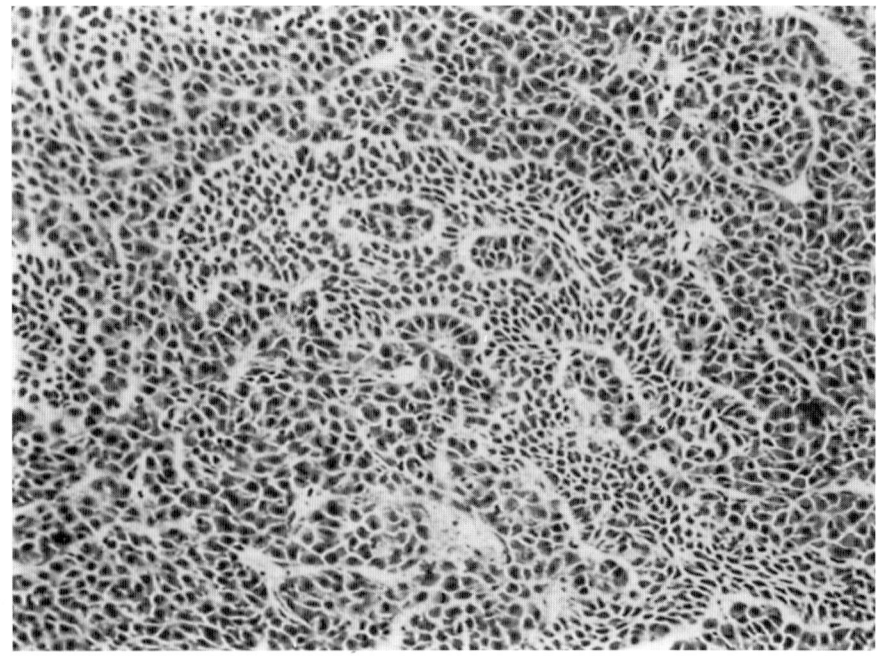

FIG. 1. Hepatoblastoma. In this example of a mixed cellular pattern the elongated tumor cells are between nodules of darker-staining larger cells resembling fetal hepatocytes (hematoxylin and eosin; ×365). (From ref. 57, with permission.)

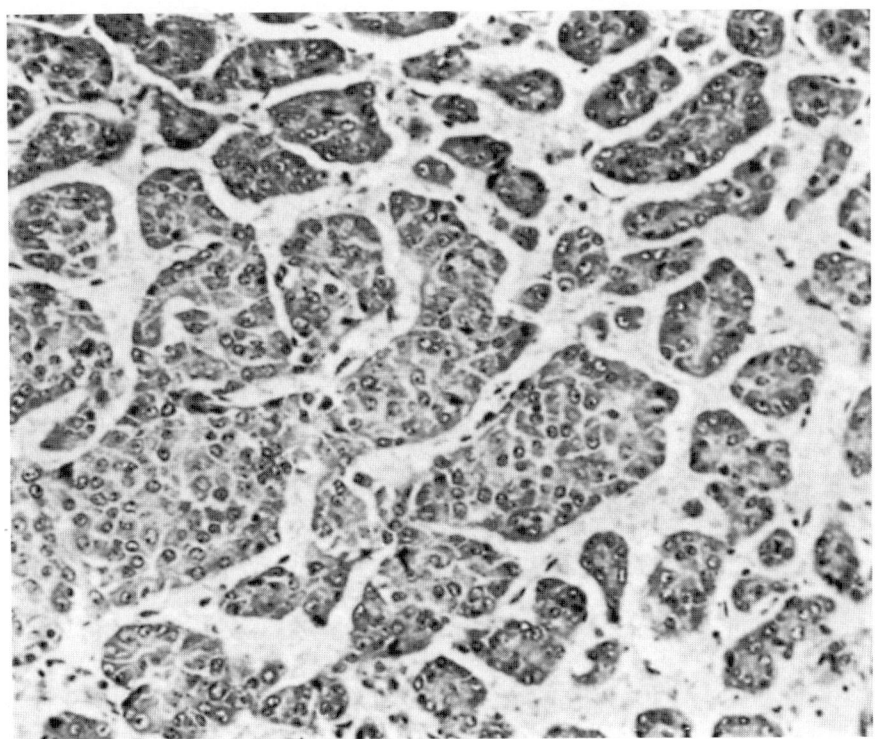

FIG. 2. Hepatocellular carcinoma: large cells with abundant cytoplasm in a trabecular configuration (hematoxylin and eosin; ×100). (From ref. 57, with permission.)

rhosis include biliary atresia, Fanconi's anemia, glucose-6-phosphatase deficiency, and hereditary tyrosinemia. HCC has also been reported in association with hemihypertrophy, anomalies of the abdominal venous drainage system, and the use of oral contraceptives. The tumor occurs in areas with a high prevalence of hepatitis B viral infection (10,26,27). Molecular hybridization studies have shown that viral DNA is integrated into the DNA of cellular lines derived from human HCC and into morphologically nonmalignant adjacent liver cells (9). There is a fibrolamellar (FL) histologic variant of HCC, which occurs in the noncirrhotic livers of older children. This variant is characterized by large polygonal neoplastic hepatocytes and lamellar bundles of collagen. The mean age at presentation of FL HCC is 20 years (9). This tumor is associated with an increased frequency of resectability and a good probability of cure (2,14,15,28,29).

Together, HBLs and HCCs constitute 75% to 90% of PMLTs of childhood. Malignant mesenchymoma, undifferentiated embryonal sarcoma, primary hepatic malignant tumor with rhabdoid features, leiomyosarcoma, angiosarcoma, hepatic sinusoid tumor simulating neuroblastoma, carcinoid, and primary hepatic and hepatosplenic non-Hodgkin's lymphoma have also been reported (7,8,12, 30–34).

Benign tumors account for approximately one-third of all liver tumors of childhood. The benign tumors may be classified by their cell of origin as either mesenchymal (hemangioma, hemangioendothelioma, and hematoma) or epithelial (cysts, focal nodular hyperplasia, and adenoma) (4,5,35–37).

Bile duct adenocarcinoma (cholangiocarcinoma) is extremely unusual before the age of 30. It has, however, been reported in a few adolescents (38). This tumor has been associated with congenital cystic dilatation of the bile ducts, ulcerative colitis, biliary atresia, Carali disease, cystic fibrosis, and sclerosing cholangitis (39). Rhabdomyosarcoma may arise in the walls of the extrahepatic biliary tree. The botryoid projections of the tumor may cause partial or complete biliary obstruction (6,27,40). Rhabdomyosarcoma is discussed in Chapter 11 and will not be additionally considered in this chapter.

If a hepatic or biliary tumor produces biliary obstruction, there may be elevations of serum hepatic enzymes or bilirubin (30,41). During the imaging evaluation, an excretory urogram may be performed. This will help to determine that the mass is not of renal origin and that it lies within the peritoneal cavity. An ultrasound examination helps to establish the presence of a hepatic mass and differentiates cystic from solid lesions. Ultrasound permits evaluation of the adrenals and the kidneys, helps to exclude these organs as possible primary sites of tumor metastatic to the liver, and allows evaluation of the inferior vena cava for tumor thrombus. Color Doppler ultrasound may be performed to demonstrate the relationship of the tumor to hepatic vessels (42). The technetium-90m sulfur colloid scan is of value in localizing the tumor to the liver and defining its boundaries. It is a sensitive test, but not specific (12). Computerized tomography (CT) or magnetic resonance imaging (MRI) provides superior delineation of the mass and shows evidence of multifocality. The operating surgeon may request an angiogram to obtain information concerning the origin and distribution of the right and left hepatic arteries to allow an informed decision concerning resectability (2,9,18). Routine chest radiographs and thoracic CT scans are mandatory because approximately 10% of patients with HBL or HCC have lung metastasis at the time of diagnosis (20,43).

A valuable test in the evaluation of PMLT is the serum AFP. The clinician should note that AFP, synthesized by the fetal liver, may be detected in pregnant women. AFP levels are high in the normal newborn infant but drop rapidly by 1 month of age. AFP should be barely detectable by 2 years of age (20).

Approximately two-thirds of children with HBL and HCC have an elevated AFP (41). The clinician should be cautioned, however, that AFP is not always elevated in HBL or HCC and that this protein may be slightly elevated in benign hamartomas. Absence of AFP elevation may be a poor prognostic sign in HBL; it is associated with the small cell (anaplastic) histologic type and responds poorly to therapy (44). For those patients with elevated AFP, it may be of value in monitoring the course of therapy (42). Complete resection of HBL or HCC should result in a normal AFP by 2 months postoperatively (17). No change in an elevated AFP following surgery indicates either residual tumor or regenerating normal liver. The diagnosis of growing tumor will depend on confirmatory imaging studies (2,18). An elevation in the AFP during the follow-up period generally heralds a local tumor recurrence or metastasis (41).

Staging systems for PMLT are based on resectability and, to a lesser extent, histology (45,46). The CCSG, Intergroup, and POG staging systems are shown in Tables 2 and 3. The clinician must be wary of the pitfalls in the extant staging systems. At least two important drawbacks of the systems shown in Tables 2 and 3 are: (a) the systems are applied at initial diagnosis. If up-front chemotherapy

TABLE 2. *CCSG staging system for primary malignant liver tumors[a]*

Stage	Description
I	Complete excision
A	Favorable histology (fetal HBL)
B	Unfavorable histology (embryonal HBL, HCC)
II	Microscopic residual disease
A	In liver
B	Extrahepatic
III	Gross residual disease ± node involvement ± spilled tumor
A	Tumor completely removed; tumor spilled, residual gross disease in nodes, or both
B	Gross tumor not completely removed ± positive nodes ± spill
IV	Metastatic disease
A	Primary tumor completely excised
B	Primary tumor not completely excised

[a]Adapted from refs. 2 and 42, with permission.

TABLE 3. *POG staging system for primary malignant liver tumors[a]*

I	Complete resection achieved
II	Microscopic residual tumor remaining
III	Gross residual tumor remaining
IV	Metastatic disease present at diagnosis

[a]From ref. 39, with permission.

is given and if it produces a substantive tumor response prior to delayed surgery, then the initial stage may no longer be pertinent. (b) A surgeon's determination of "resectability" is somewhat subjective and differs between practitioners (42). There is no generally accepted staging system for bile duct adenocarcinoma.

SELECTION OF THERAPY

Surgery

Localized HBL or HCC is curable with complete surgical excision of the tumor. It is also possible to achieve a cure with a near-complete excision in conjunction with adjuvant therapy that is able to sterilize residual tumor. Tumor resectability is determined by tumor size, the existence of bilobar involvement necessitating more than three liver segments for hepatic resection, vascular invasion, or distant metastases (47).

Some surgeons believe that therapy begins with an attempt at resection rather than biopsy. Between one-half and two-thirds of HBL patients have resectable tumors at presentation (48). These are typically fetal HBL (25). Only 30% of the cases of HCC are amenable to complete resection at presentation because of multilobar involvement or massive tumor size. In the FL variant of HCC, 50% to 75% of cases may be resectable (1,14). Relatively few PMLTs, however, are readily resectable at diagnosis (48).

Many cases will be managed with preoperative chemotherapy. Therefore, the surgeon must first deal with the question of whether to (a) perform a biopsy before chemotherapy is administered in order to histologically confirm the presence of PMLT, or (b) accept the diagnosis based on a characteristic clinical presentation, supportive diagnostic imaging, and an elevated AFP (2,18). Most clinicians prefer to have a histologic diagnosis. The classic way to obtain tissue is via an open-wedge biopsy. Some controversy exists over the use of CT or ultrasound-directed needle biopsy as an alternative to the wedge biopsy. There are those who voice concern over the possibility that a needle biopsy will cause a significant hemorrhage by disruption of a highly friable PMLT. Other authorities believe that the risk is minimal (2,12).

Preoperative chemotherapy reduces the tumor burden in the majority of HBL cases and in a significant number of HCC patients (1,18). Many children with initially unresectable HBL may be rendered resectable by preoperative chemotherapy. Many surgeons are also of the opinion that PMLTs, following chemotherapy, are less friable and more often relatively encapsulated. For those patients who have tumors that are unresectable at presentation, chemotherapy is clearly indicated in an attempt to render the tumor resectable. Radiotherapy may succeed in rendering an unresectable tumor resectable if this goal is not achieved by chemotherapy (vide infra) (1).

When the patient comes to surgery, an extensive incision allowing a large area of exposure is often performed (49). A simple tumorectomy with adequate margins is rarely possible. Rather, hepatic lobectomy or extended lobectomy is required. Perioperative mortality had been reported to be as high as 18% to 33% (13,43,50,51), but is now on the order of 5% to 10% in specialized centers (52). Surgical complications include severe bleeding, bile leakage, pleural effusion, rupture of the inferior vena cava, cardiac arrest, convulsions, and subhepatic abscess (53). Improved surgical techniques such as vascular reconstruction, ultrasonic aspiration, and dissection under vascular exclusion as well as improvements in anesthesia, blood product replacement, and postoperative intensive care have produced the significant reduction in operative and perioperative mortality (1).

In stage IV disease surgical resection of pulmonary metastases can be considered if they persist after preoperative chemotherapy and if the primary tumor has been rendered resectable by drug treatment (52). In patients with stage I disease at initial diagnosis who recur with isolated pulmonary disease, surgical resection may result in extended survival. Feusner et al. reported 6 patients with pulmonary relapses of stage I HBL. Three had concurrent relapses in brain, bone, or abdomen and died of metastatic disease. Three of the 6, having recurrence only in the lung, were long-term survivors (less than 5 years) following metastasectomy and chemotherapy (54).

Because it is difficult to resect some PMLTs, there has been interest in the use of total hepatectomy and liver transplantation (12,39,41). Tagge et al. (55) reported 18 children who underwent laparotomy for a possible hepatectomy and liver transplantation for HBL or HCC. Thirteen were transplanted. Five of the 6 transplanted HBL patients are survivors (83%) and 3 of the 7 HCC patients are survivors (44%) (55). Superina and Bilik from the Hospital for Sick Children, Toronto, selected patients suitable for transplant based on absence of lymph node disease and tumor confined to the liver without breech of the capsule. Of three transplanted HBL patients, two are alive at 2 and 2.5 years. Of five HCC patients, three are alive at 1, 3, and 5 years of follow-up; for two patients the follow-up is short (56). In those children who undergo liver transplantation primarily for end-stage nonneoplastic liver disease, but who have an incidental PMLT identified, survival is quite good.

The diagnosis of biliary adenocarcinoma is usually made at exploratory laparotomy. A gross total resection with reestablishment of biliary flow should be attempted. Resection is often not possible. Liver transplantation has not been curative because the tumor tends to disseminate in response to immunosuppression (39). Undifferentiated embryonal sarcoma of the liver in childhood is rare; less than 100 cases have been reported. The usual

dismal prognosis is favorably influenced if a radical tumor resection is achieved (7). Hepatic malignant rhabdoid tumor is almost invariably fatal (8).

Radiation Therapy

Radiation therapy has been used preoperatively and postoperatively in the curative treatment of HBL and HCC. Its preoperative use has been intended to reduce the tumor burden and increase the probability of resection. Contemporary practice favors using chemotherapy alone for preoperative therapy (see subsequent text) (13,17,30,45). In those children who have unresectable tumors after initial chemotherapy, radiotherapy is warranted (1,15,57). POG Study 8697, described in the chemotherapy section of this chapter, included five patients treated with radiotherapy because they remained unresectable after chemotherapy. Three became resectable (39, 58).

Some evidence exists that postoperative radiotherapy is valuable in children who have residual disease following an attempt at resection. A combined CCSG-POG protocol studied 177 children with HBL or HCC. Patients with microscopic residual disease (stage II) received postoperative chemotherapy and 45 Gy to the tumor bed. Those unable to undergo complete excision following preoperative chemotherapy received 30 Gy whole liver irradiation. The 3-year progression-free survival was 60% for stage II and 22% for stage III (25). The Institut Gustave-Roussy administered preoperative chemotherapy, performed surgical resection, and then gave radiotherapy and additional chemotherapy if there was micro- or macroscopic persistent tumor at surgery. A dose of 25 to 45 Gy was given, targeted to the area of postoperative disease only. Seven of nine children are disease-free with 22 to 98 months of follow-up. One died with a local failure, and one died with a local-plus-distant failure (1). Habrand et al. described eight cases treated after incomplete resection (4 with gross and 4 with microscopic disease) with combined radiation and chemotherapy.

Six are free of disease with 4 to 83 months of follow-up (1,17). The evidence in favor of the use of irradiation for residual disease is not unequivocal, and we cannot prove that chemotherapy by itself would have failed to control persistent microscopic disease. No dogmatic policy may be adopted based on current evidence (13,15,17).

Is whole lung irradiation (WLI) appropriate in metastatic HBL? There is sparse data on the subject. Patients with metastatic disease to the lung only can be cured with surgical resection of the metastatic deposits plus chemotherapy. There is, however, a risk of subsequent pulmonary relapse (54). This may be used as an argument in favor of WLI to treat presumed small deposits of well oxygenated metastatic disease. Reasoning, for example, from Wilms' tumor, Ewing's, or osteosarcoma data, a total dose of 12 to 13 Gy would be sound.

Radiotherapy may be used for palliative treatment of unresectable PMLT. In primary hepatic non-Hodgkin's lymphoma, consolidative irradiation to the primary site, in conjunction with vigorous chemotherapy, may be warranted (31).

Hemangiomas of the liver are often asymptomatic and require no treatment. They may, however, produce congestive heart failure from arteriovenous shunting, rupture and bleed, cause pain, produce an abdominal mass, coagulopathy, or respiratory distress. The preferred treatments include steroids, arterial embolization, lobectomy, interferon alfa-2, cyclophosphamide, and hepative artery ligation. External radiotherapy has been successful in situations where other treatments were not appropriate (5,10,35,36, 59,60).

Chemotherapy

Chemotherapy has been used preoperatively in an attempt to improve the probability of resection of HCC and HBL. It has also been used postoperatively, either as adjuvant therapy when there is no apparent residual disease or for treatment of obvious residual disease. In the presence of metastatic disease, chemotherapy has been utilized in attempts to prolong survival (13,17,19,60,61).

CCG Trial 831, opened to patient accrual in 1972, gave no adjuvant chemotherapy to stage I disease. Patients with residual tumor in one hepatic lobe received actinomycin-D, vincristine, and cyclophosphamide plus involved field irradiation. Patients with disseminated tumors received only chemotherapy. No patients responded to drug alone. Of 40 patients entered on the study, the only 7 long-term survivors were children either with stage I disease or those with minor residual tumor who had been irradiated (63).

CCG Trial 881 added doxorubicin and 5-fluorouracil to the three drugs used in Trial 831. Twelve (44%) of 27 patients with measurable disease achieved a response with a median duration of 18 months. Adjuvant chemotherapy was given to 24 patients who did not have measurable disease following surgery. Of these, 83% were disease-free survivors with median follow-up of 30 months (63).

CCG Trial 823F used doxorubicin and cisplatin for four courses following histologic diagnosis but prior to definitive surgery for disease confined to the liver. Thirty-three children with HBL and 14 with HCC were entered on the study. Of the 26 patients with HBL who completed the prescribed four courses of chemotherapy, 25 achieved a response and were eligible for second-look surgery, 22 were taken to the operating room, and 16 had complete resections. There was no viable tumor in 9 of these patients. Of these 16 children, 15 are alive without evidence of disease. Of the 25 children who completed the chemotherapy and were eligible for surgery, 19 (78%) are alive and disease free. The estimated 2-year survival for the initial 33 HBL patients is 67%. Of the 14 patients with HCC, 12 died of progressive disease, and 2 remain free of disease. Only 14% of the HCC patients had complete removal of the tumor at second look laparotomy (63).

The Pediatric Intergroup Hepatoma Study (CCG881/POG 8945) enrolled 173 patients with HBL. Ninety-one patients were randomized to receive cisplatin, vincristine, and 5-fluorouracil and 82 were randomized to receive cisplatin and doxorubicin. The later program was more toxic—patients had a higher probability of neutropenia, thrombocytopenia, need for parenteral nutrition, and toxic deaths. As shown in Table 4, the chemotherapy programs were equally effective in terms of overall and event-free survival ($p = 0.219$). The results for stage I to III HBL were reasonably good. Patients with more advanced disease did quite poorly (64,65). For patients with HCC there was also no difference between the two programs for either event-free survival ($p = 0.88$) or overall survival ($p = 0.68$). All 7 stage I patients were event-free survivors (64). Clearly better therapy is required for advanced stage HCC.

Stringer et al. have reported 40 children with HBL, treated with the intent to cure, from the Hospital for Sick Children, London. Two received surgery only, 26 received preoperative chemotherapy (most commonly cisplatin/doxorubicin); postoperative chemotherapy (usually cisplatin/doxorubicin also) was given to 12 patients, 11 of whom were suspected of having residual disease. Of the 40 patients, 26 are disease-free survivors following surgery and chemotherapy, 1 is alive and well following a partial response to chemotherapy and a liver transplant, 1 died perioperatively, 11 died with tumor, and 1 is alive with disease at the time of reporting (66).

The German Cooperative Pediatric Liver Tumor Study HB-89 treated 60 HBL and 10 HCC patients. Seventeen patients were treated with total resections alone. Four children with subtotal resections and 39 others received ifosfamide, cisplatin, and adriamycin. In cases of insufficient tumor response, high dose cisplatin and adriamycin were added. An initial complete resection was achieved in 4 of the 10 cases of HCC. With a maximum follow-up of 4 years, 82% of the HBL patients are in complete remission as are 30% of the HCC patients (53).

POG study 8697 enrolled 60 evaluable patients with HBL. Children with POG stage I favorable histology were followed. Children with stage I unfavorable histology or stage II received cisplatin/vincristine/5-fluorouracil. Patients with stage III or IV disease were evaluated for resection after five cycles of chemotherapy. Those who remained unresectable received 33 to 39 Gy of local irradiation plus additional chemotherapy. Disease-free survival is shown in Fig. 3. Of the five irradiated patients, three became resectable, achieved a complete resection, and were alive and well at the time of the study's publication (39,58).

Gugliemi et al. have reported an Italian trial in which six children with stage I HBL were treated with surgery alone. There was one postoperative death. The remaining five patients are alive and well with a follow-up of 19 to 36 months. Thirteen patients with localized but unresectable HBL received cisplatin/doxorubicin. Ten had partial responses and eight had radical resections. One patient had minimal change in the tumor but a drop in AFP—this individual also had a radical resection.

TABLE 4. *Results of the Pediatric Intergroup Hepatoma Study (CCG-8881/POG 8945)*

Stage of hepatoblastoma	Cisplatin, vincristine, 5-fluorouracil			Cisplatin, doxorubicin		
	n	Survival	Event-free survival	n	Survival	Event-free survival
I	22	95%	85%	20	95%	95%
II	4	100%	100%	3	100%	100%
III	43	70%	62%	39	65%	61%
IV	23	45%	23%	19	36%	33%

From ref. 65, with permission.

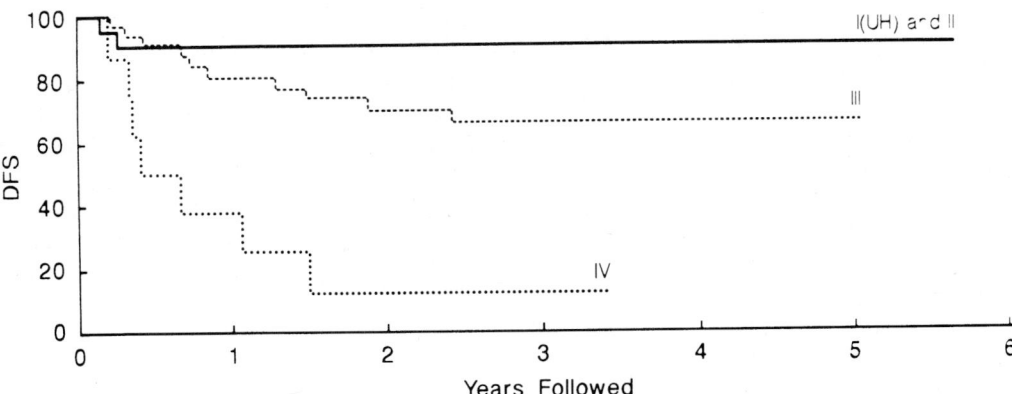

FIG. 3. Disease-free survival for children with hepatoblastoma treated with surgery and cisplatin, vincristine, and 5-fluorouracil in Pediatric Oncology Group Study 8697. (Stage I (UH) ± II, 91 ± 9.2% at 3 yr; stage III, 67 ± 10.8%; stage IV, 12.5 ± 11.7%.) Staging is described in Table 1. UH, unfavorable histology, i.e., fetal and embryonal characteristics. (From ref. 58, with permission. This graph is also found in ref. 39.)

The nine resected patients are free of tumor with a median follow-up of 2 years. Two patients with stage I HCC are alive. Two children with HCC had initial chemotherapy. Neither had significant tumor shrinkage. One of the two is disease-free (52). A SIOP trial following guidelines similar to the Italian study was underway at the time this chapter was written.

The preponderance of the available data indicates that chemotherapy, most often cisplatin and adriamycin, produces a good re-sponse in 70% to 90% of primary HBL (1,2,12,18,61) (Table 5). In view of this data, and because of the frequent conversion by chemotherapy of unresectable disease to resectability, most authorities now use chemotherapy prior to definitive resection in all potentially resectable cases of HBL. Postoperative chemotherapy is also generally given. Epirubicin and carboplatinum are being investigated as alternatives to adriamycin and cisplatin (17).

TABLE 5. *Response rates of unresectable hepatoblastoma to chemotherapy*

Institution or Cooperative group	Regimen	No. of patients	No. of tumor responses	No. of complete tumor resections after preoperative chemotherapy
POG, 1993 (58)	CISDDP/VCR/5FU	33	30	24
CCSG, 1991 (74)	CISDDP/DOXO	33	28	16
SIOP, 1991 (75)	CISDDP/DOXO	8	7	7
Hospital for Sick Children, 1991 (76)	CISDDP/DOXO	15	15	13
M.D. Anderson, 1991 (77)	CISDDP	7	7	6
Italian Pilot Study, 1993 (52)	CISDDP/DOXO	13	10	8
Tagge, 1993 (55)	CISDDP/DOXO + others	15		
Munro, 1994 (49)	CISDDP/DOXO	4	4	4
		128	111 (87%)	86 (67%)

CISDDP, cisplatin; VCR, vincristine; 5 FU, 5-fluorouracil; DOXO, doxorubicin; POG, Pediatric Oncology Group; CCSG, Children's Cancer Study Group; SIOP, International Society of Pediatric Oncology.
Table modified from ref. 52, with permission.

There is clearly a need to develop more effective chemotherapy for anaplastic HBL and HCC. At present, the response of these histologies to chemotherapy is quite poor. HCL, which is often multicentric, can rarely be converted to resectability by up-front chemotherapy (2). It is not clear if there is a difference between the drug-responsiveness of common HCC and that of its FL variant (12). Studies on various combinations of chemotherapy will be hampered by the relatively small number of patients (67).

RADIOTHERAPEUTIC MANAGEMENT

If radiotherapy is administered preoperatively prior to a second-look celiotomy, or postoperatively for residual disease, definition of the liver tumor volume is of paramount importance. It is essential to spare as much normal liver as possible. Therefore, the radiotherapist must carefully examine the diagnostic imaging studies and any available operative reports.

The tumor volume should be delineated and covered by portals with a small margin. In the majority of cases, parallel opposed anterior and posterior fields from a linear accelerator or cobalt-60 machine are appropriate. On occasion, the best treatment plan is a combination of anterior, posterior, and right lateral wedged fields. We have also had occasion to use parallel opposed left anterior oblique/right posterior oblique fields with chemotherapy for treatment preoperatively, and if a fair portion of liver may be spared, then a total dose of 33 to 45 Gy is appropriate. As we described in the previous section concerning POG study 8697, irradiation of an unresectable HBL may convert it to resectability (58). When postoperative irradiation is given for residual disease following a resection, 25 to 45 Gy to a limited area is appropriate for microscopic disease and 35 to 45 Gy is appropriate for bulkier disease.

If radiotherapy is to be administered to the whole liver for advanced tumor, then parallel opposed anterior and posterior fields will al-

most always be indicated. The dose is generally prescribed to the midportion of the liver, and the accepted parameters of liver tolerance to irradiation should not be exceeded. Therefore, with palliative intent for advanced HBL or HCC, 20 to 25 Gy in 2 to 2.5 weeks is reasonable. The treatment of metastasis from HBL or HCC is generally rewarding, and usual palliative doses of irradiation (based on the surrounding normal tissue tolerance) may be used.

For hepatic hemangioma, a dose of 10 to 20 Gy in 1 to 3 weeks has been used; but 4 to 6 Gy seems adequate (36,59,60). In a case report of a child who received postoperative irradiation to convert a mesenchymal hamartoma to resectability, 11 Gy was utilized (68).

Investigational techniques that may have some promise in the treatment of malignant hepatobiliary tumors include intraoperative irradiation, regional hyperthermia in conjunction with intraarterial yttrium-90 microspheres, and iodine-131 antiferritin administered along with chemotherapy (23,36, 69–71). Intraluminal iridium-192 alone and with microwave hyperthermia has been used for the management of malignant biliary obstruction (72,73).

RESULTS

In HBL patients undergoing a complete resection, the probability of survival has been reported to range from 30% to 100%. For those treated with biopsy or incomplete resection, it is 0% to 60% (9,16–18,25,26,28,62, 72). In CCG protocol CCG-81 there was a 70% survival rate for children treated with initially localized and completely excised (stage I) HBL treated with combination chemotherapy. Only 29% of initial stage I patients were alive 3 years after documented recurrence. Results for the Pediatric Intergroup Hepatoma Study are shown in Table 4 and described earlier in this chapter (64,65). The survival rate for early stage HCC was 7 of 7 in the Pediatric Intergroup Hepatoma Study but was close to 10% for stage III to IV disease (64). The FL variant of HCC is more often resectable and curable (16,33).

REFERENCES

References particularly recommended for further reading are indicated by an asterisk.

*1. Habrand J-L, Nehme D, Kalifa C, et al. Is there a place for radiation therapy in the management of hepatoblastoma and hepatocellular carcinomas in children. *Int J Radiat Oncol Biol Phys* 1992;23:525–531.

2. Perilango G, Sinniah D, Evans AE. Liver tumors. In: D'Angio GJ, Sinniah D, Meadows AT, Evans AE, Pritchard J, eds. *Practical pediatric oncology.* New York: Wiley-Liss, 1992:333–337.

*3. Weinberg AG, Finegold MS. Primary hepatic tumors of childhood. *Hum Pathol* 1983;14(6):512–537.

4. Ray BS. Large cavernous hemangioma of the liver. *Ann Surg* 1939;109:373–382.

5. Stringel G, Mercer S. Giant hemangioma in the newborn and infant: complications and management. *Clin Pediatr* 1984;23:498–503.

6. Lack EE, Perez-Atyade AR, Schuster SR. Botryoid rhabdomyosarcoma of the biliary tract: report of five cases with ultrastructural observations and literature review. *Am J Surg Pathol* 1981;5:643–652.

7. Mistry RC, Deshpande RK, Chinoy R, Sampat M, Desai PB. Undifferentiated embryonal sarcoma of the liver in childhood. *Indian J Cancer* 1995;32:175–178.

8. Scheimberg I, Cullinane C, Malone M. Primary hepatic malignant tumor with rhabdoid features. *Am J Surg Pathol* 1996;20(11):1394–1400.

9. Bellani FF, Massimino M. Liver tumors in childhood: epidemiology and clinics. *J Surg Oncol Suppl* 1993;3: 119–121.

10. Malt RA. Surgery for hepatic neoplasms. *N Engl J Med* 1985;313:1591–1596.

11. Novick DM, Deluca SA. Hepatoblastoma. *Am Fam Physician* 1986;33(2):141–142.

12. Greenberg M, Filler RM. Hepatic tumors. In: Pizzo PA, Poplack DG, eds. *Principles and practice of paediatric oncology,* 2nd ed. Philadelphia: JB Lippincott, 1993:697–711.

13. Lack EE, Neave C, Vawter GF. Hepatoblastoma: a clinical and pathologic study of 54 cases. *Am J Surg Pathol* 1982;6:693–705.

14. Schmidt D, Harms D, Lang W. Primary malignant hepatic tumors in childhood. *Virchows Arch* 1985;407: 387–405.

15. Clatworth HW Jr, Schiller M, Grosfeld JL. Primary liver tumors in infancy and childhood: 41 cases variously treated. *Arch Surg* 1974;109:143–147.

16. Farhi DC, Shikes RH, Murari PJ, Silverberg SG. Hepatocellular carcinoma in young people. *Cancer* 1983; 52:1516–1525.

17. Gauthier F, Valayer J, Thai BL, Sinica M, Kalifa C. Hepatoblastoma and hepatocarcinoma in children: analysis of a series of 29 cases. *J Pediatr Surg* 1986;21: 424–429.

18. Pritchard J. Commentary. In: D'Angio GJ, Sinniah D, Meadows AT, Evans AE, Pritchard J, eds. *Practical pediatric oncology.* New York: Wiley-Liss, 1992: 344–345.

19. Quinn JJ, Altman AJ, Robinson HT, Cooke RW, Foster JH. Adriamycin and cisplatin for hepatoblastoma. *Cancer* 1985;56:1926–1929.

20. Smith WL, Franken EA, Mitros FA. Liver tumors in children. *Semin Roentgenol* 1983;18:136–148.

*21. Stocker JT. Hepatoblastoma *Semin Diagn Pathol* 1994; 11(2):136–143.

22. Finegold MS, Weinberg AC. Hepatoblastoma: histologic classification has important prognostic and therapeutic implications. *Pediatr Res* 1983;17(4):233A.

23. Grady ED, McLaren J, Auda SP, McGinley PH. Combination of internal radiation therapy and hyperthermia to treat liver cancer. *South Med J* 1983;76: 1101–1105.

24. Manivel C, Wick MR, Abenoza P, Dehner LP. Teratoid hepatoblastoma: the nosologic dilemma of solid embryonic neoplasms of childhood. *Cancer* 1986;57: 2168–2174.

25. Ablin A, Krailo M, Hass J, et al. Hepatoblastoma and hepatocellular carcinoma in children: a report from the Children's Cancer Study Group (CCG) and the Pediatric Oncology Group (POG). *Med Pediatr Oncol* 1988;16:417.

26. Exelby PR, Filler RM, Grosfeld JL. Liver tumors in children with particular reference to hepatoblastoma and hepatocellular carcinoma: American Academy of Pediatrics Surgical Section Surgery, 1974. *J Pediatr Surg* 1975;10:329–337.

27. Martinez-F LA, Haase GM, Kaep LJ, Akers DR. Rhabdomyosarcoma of the biliary tree: the case for aggressive surgery. *J Pediatr Surg* 1982;17:508–511.

28. Exelby PR, el-Domeri A, Huvos AG, Baehie EJ Jr. Primary malignant tumors of the liver in children. *J Pediatr Surg* 1971;6:272–276.

29. Ternberg JL, Land VJ. Tumors of the alimentary tract. In: Sutow WW, Fernbach DJ, Vietti TJ, eds. *Clinical pediatric oncology.* St. Louis: CV Mosby, 1984:775–785.

30. Mahour GH, Wogo GU, Seigel SE, Isaacs H. Improved survival in infants and children with primary liver tumors. *Am J Surg* 1983;146:236–240.

31. Miller ST, Wollner N, Meyers PA, Exelby P, Jereb B, Miller DR. Primary hepatic or hepatosplenic non-Hodgkin's lymphoma in children. *Cancer* 1983;52: 2285–2288.

32. Norohn R, Gonzeles-Crussi F. Hepatic angiosarcoma in childhood: a case report and review of the literature. *Am J Surg Pathol* 1984;8:683–687.

33. Platt MS, Agamanolis DB, Krill CE Jr, et al. Occult hepatic sinusoid tumor of infancy simulating neuroblastoma. *Cancer* 1983;52:1183–1189.

34. Stocker JT, Ishak KG. Undifferentiated (embryonal) sarcoma of the liver. *Cancer* 1978;42:336–348.

35. Corbella F, Arico N, Podesta AF, Villa A, Beluffi G, Bianchi E. Infantile hepatic hemangioendothelioma treated by radiotherapy. *Pediatr Radiol* 1983;13: 297–300.

36. McKay MJ, Carr PJ, Langlands AO. Treatment of hepatic cavernous hemangioma with radiation therapy: case report and literature review. *Aust N Z J Surg* 1989;59:965–968.

37. Yandza Y, Valayer J. Benign tumors of the liver in children: analysis of a series of 20 cases. *J Pediatr Surg* 1986;21:419–423.

38. Czaja MJ, Goldfarb JP, Cha KC, Biempica L, Morehouse HT, Abelaw A. Bile duct carcinoma in an adolescent. *Am J Gastroenterol* 1985;80:486–489.

*39. Bowman LC, Riely, CA. Management of pediatric liver tumors. *Surg Oncol Clin NA* 1996;5(2):451–459.

40. Ruymann FB, Raney RB Jr, Crist WM, Lawrence W Jr, Lindberg RD, Soule E. Rhabdomyosarcoma of the biliary tree in childhood: a report from the Intergroup Rhabdomyosarcoma Study. *Cancer* 1985;56:575–581.

41. Giacomantonio M, Ein SH, Mancer K, Stephens CA. 30 years of experience with pediatric primary malignant liver tumors. *J Pediatr Surg* 1984;19:523–526.

42. Cohen MD, Bugaieski EM, Haliloglu M, Faught P, Siddiqui AR. Visual presentation of the staging of pediatric tumors. *Radiographics* 1996;16(3):523–545.

43. Miller JH, Weinberg K. Liver and spleen. In: Miller JA, ed. *Imaging and pediatric oncology.* Baltimore: Williams & Wilkins, 1985:164–215.

44. Hypermedia PDQ. Internet Site. Childhood liver cancer. University of Pennsylvania Cancer Center. PDQ Oncolink.upenn.edu.

45. Evans AE, Land VJ, Newton WA, Randolph JG, Sather HN, Tefft M. Combination chemotherapy (vincristine, adriamycin, cyclophosphamide, and 5-fluorouracil) in the treatment of children with malignant hepatoma. *Cancer* 1982;50:821–826.

46. Morita K, Okabe I, Ochino J, et al. The proposed Japanese TNM classification of primary liver carcinoma in infants and children. *Jpn J Clin Oncol* 1983;13:361–370.

47. Reynolds M. Conversion of unresectable to resectable hepatoblastoma and long-term follow-up study. *World J Surg* 1995;19:814–816.

48. Nagasue M, Yakaya H, Chang Y-C, Ogawa Y, Kohno H, Ito A. Active uptake of testosterone by androgen receptors of hepatocellular carcinoma in humans. *Cancer* 1986;57:2162–2167.

49. Munro FD, Azmy AF, Simpson E. Resectability of advanced liver tumours in chidren after combination chemotherapy. *Ann Roy Coll Surg England* 1994;76:253–256.

50. Filler RM, Tefft M, Vawter GF, Maddock C, Mitus A. Hepatic lobectomy in childhood: effects of x-ray and chemotherapy. *J Pediatr Surg* 1969;17(4 Pt 2):233A.

51. Nagaraj HS, Kmetz DR, Leitner C. Rhabdomyosarcoma of the bile ducts. *J Pediatr Surg* 1977;12:1071–1074.

52. Guglielmi M, Perilongo G, Cecchetto G, Rondelli R, Lannio E, Siracusa F. Rationale and results of the international society of pediatric oncology (SIOP) Italian pilot study on childood hepatoma: surgical resection d'emblee or after primary chemotherapy? *J Surg Oncol Suppl* 1993;3:122–126.

53. Von Schweinitz D, Burger D, Mildenberger H. Is laparotomy the first step in treatment of childhood liver tumors?—the experience from the German Cooperative Pediatric live 89. *Eur J Pediatr Surg* 1994;4:82–86.

54. Feusner JH, Krailo MD, Haas JE, et al. Treatment of pulmonary metastases of initial Stage I hepatoblastoma in childhood: report from the Children's Cancer Study Group. *Cancer* 1993;71:859–864.

55. Tagge EP, Tagee DU, Reyes J, et al. Resection, including transplantation for hepatoblastoma and hepatocellular carcinoma. Impact on survival. *J Pediatr Surg* 1992;27:292–296.

56. Superina R, Billik R. Results of liver transplanttaion in children with unresectable liver tumors. *J Pediatr Surg* 1996;31:835–839.

57. Berry CL, Keeling JW. Hepatoblastoma. In: Berry CL, ed. *Pediatric pathology.* Berlin: Springer-Verlag, 1981:660–662.

*58. Douglass EC, Reynolds M, Finegold M, Cantor AB, Glicksman A. Cisplatin, vincristine, and fluorouracil therapy for hepatoblastoma: a pediatric oncology group study. *J Clin Oncol* 1993;11:96–99.

59. Iyer CP, Stanley P, Mahour GH. Hepatic hemangiomas in infants and children: a review of 30 cases. *Am Surg* 1996;62:356–360.

60. Park WC, Phillips R. The role of radiation therapy in the management of hemangiomas of the liver. *JAMA* 1970;212:1496–1498.

61. Douglass EC, Green AA, Wrenn E, Champion J, Shipp M, Pratt CB. Effect of *cis*-platinum (DDP) based chemotherapy in treatment of hepatoblastoma. *Med Pediatr Oncol* 1985;13:187–190.

62. Goladay ES, Mollitt PK, Osteen NP, et al. Conversion to resectability by intra-arterial infusion chemotherapy after failure of systemic chemotherapy. *J Pediatr Surg* 1985;20:715–717.

63. Pazdur R, Bready B, Cangir A. Pediatric hepatic tumors: clinical trials conducted in the United States. *J Surg Oncol* 1993;3(12):127–130.

64. Douglass E, Ortega J, Feusner J, et al. Hepatocelullar carcinoma (HC) in children and adolescents: results from the Pediatric Intergroup Hepatoma Study (CCG 8881/POG 8945). *Proc Am Soc Clin Oncol* 1994;13:A-1439, 420.

65. Ortega JA, Douglas E, Feusner J, et al. A randomized trial of cisplatin (DDP)/vincristine (VCR)/5-flurouracil (5 FU) v. DDP/doxorubicin (DOX) I.V. continuous infusion (CI) for the treatment of hepatoblastoma (HB): results from the pediatric intergroup hepatoma study (CCG-8881/POG 8945). *Proc Am Soc Clin Oncol* 1994;13:A-1421, 416.

*66. Stringer MD, Hennaye ER, Hoowlad ER, et al. Improved outcome for chidren with hepatoblastoma. *Br J Surg* 1995;82:336–391.

67. Yoo HS, Park CH, Suh JH, et al. Radioiodinated fatty acid esters in the management of hepatocellular carcinoma: preliminary findings. *Cancer Chemother Pharmacol* 1989;23[Suppl]:554–558.

68. Strauji MN, Chahen J, Schulman WM, Ziegler MN, Kaap CE. Mesenchymal hamartoma of the liver in infants. *Cancer* 1978;42:2483–2489.

69. Deziel DJ, Kiel KD, Kramer TS, Doolas A, Roseman DL. Intraoperative radiation therapy in biliary tract cancer. *Am Surg* 1988;43:402–407.

70. Leichner PK, Yang NC, Frankel TL, et al. Dosimetry and treatment planning for 90y-labeled antiferritin in hepatoma. *Int J Radiat Oncol Biol Phys* 1988;14:1033–1042.

71. Order SE, Stillwagon GB, Klein JL, et al. Iodine 131 antiferritin, a new treatment modality in hepatoma: a Radiation Therapy Oncology Group Study. *J Clin Oncol* 1985;3:1573–1582.

72. Coughlin CT, Wang TZ, Ryan TP, et al. Interstitial microwave-induced hyperthermia and iridium brachytherapy for the treatment of obstructing biliary carcinomas. *Int J Hyperthermia* 1992;8:157–171.

73. Molt P, Hopfan S, Watson RC, Batet JF, Brennan MF. Intraluminal radiation therapy in the management of

malignant biliary obstruction. *Cancer* 1986;57: 536–544.

*74. Ortega JA, Kraila MD, Haas JE, et al. Effective treatment of unresectable or metastatic hepatoblastoma with cisplatin and continuous infusion doxorubicin chemotherapy: a report from the Children's Cancer Study Group. *J Clin Oncol* 1991;9:2167–2176.

75. Ninane J, Perilongo G, Staten JP, et al. Effectiveness and toxicity of cisplatin and doxorubicin in childhood hepatoblastoma and hepatocellular carcinoma. *Med Pediatr Oncol* 1991;19:199–203.

76. Filler RM, Ehrlich PF, Greenberg PL, et al. Preoperative chemotherapy for hepatoblastoma. *Surgery* 1991; 110:591–596.

77. Black CT, Cangir A, Choroszy M, et al. Marked response to pre-operative high dose cis-platinum in children with unresectable hepatoblastoma. *J Pediatr Surg* 1991;26:1070–1073.

Germ and Stromal Cell Tumors of the Gonads and Extragonadal Germ Cell Tumors

In the human embryo the primordial germ cells are found in the vicinity of the allantoic stalk. From this position the germ cells migrate into the adjoining mesenchyme. The cells then assume positions in the germinal ridges and migrate along these structures. During this migration the cells are surrounded by the epithelium of the developing gonad and develop into the primitive testis or ovary. Germ cell tumors (GCTs) are thought to arise from totipotent primordial germ cells that escape normal organizing influences during development (1). Malignant GCTs occur in fewer than 300 children below the age of 15 years each year in the United States (2,3). GCTs may occur in the ovary, testes, sacrococcygeal region, retroperitoneum, and mediastinal areas. The main histologic types are germinoma, embryonal carcinoma, yolk sac tumor (endodermal sinus tumor, Teilum tumor), malignant mixed germ cell tumors, and malignant teratomas (referred to by some authorities as immature teratomas) (1,4–6) (Fig. 1).

Malignant teratomas may develop anywhere along the pathway of germinal tissue migration. By definition, teratomas are composed of tissues derived from two or three germinal layers (tridermal ancestry): ectoderm, mesoderm, and endoderm. Malignant teratomas are so-named because of foci of endodermal sinus tumor, embryonal carcinoma, germinoma, or choriocarcinoma. There may also be foci of neuroblastoma, nephroblas-

toma, or hepatoblastoma. In general, frank malignancy is identified in approximately 20% of teratomas (1). The distinction needs to be made between immature teratomas with distinct malignant elements, which warrant aggressive adjuvant therapy, and immature teratomas with primitive neuroepithelium, which can be cured with surgery alone.

GENERAL ASPECTS OF CLINICAL PRESENTATION, STAGING, AND WORKUP

There is a bimodal age distribution for GCTs, with a peak in children less than 3 years of age and a second peak in children over 12. The male-to-female ratio is 2:1 (7). Girls predominate in the patient population during the first 3 years of life because of a female predominance in sacrococcygeal tumors. In males there is an association with Klinefelter's syndrome (8,9).

The staging workup should include an assay for alpha-fetoprotein (AFP). AFP is elevated in almost all cases of endodermal sinus tumor and in many other GCT patients (10,11). Successful treatment, whether by surgery, chemotherapy, or radiotherapy, is regularly associated with AFP decline consistent with its half-life of 5 days (7,11,12). AFP falling too slowly, failing to normalize after treatment, or rising generally signifies inadequate tumor response and precedes clinical or

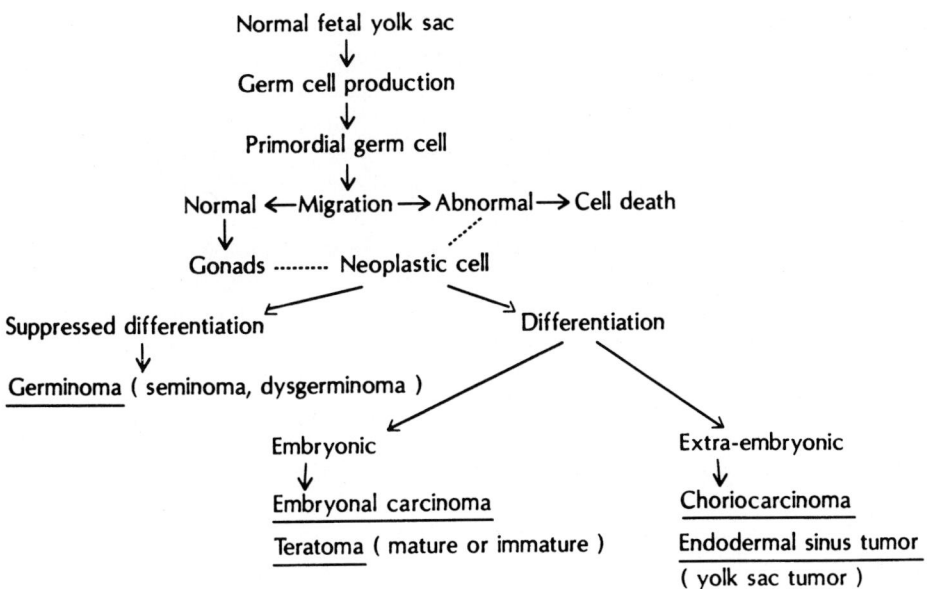

FIG. 1. Classification of germ cell tumors.

radiographic evidence of treatment failure. Human chorionic gonadotropin (HCG) activity is present in some tumors.

Diagnostic imaging of the pelvis and presacral space is best performed with computerized tomography (CT), magnetic resonance imaging (MRI), and sonography (1). CT scanning is useful to assess the presence of pathologic retroperitoneal lymph nodes. Chest CT and bone scan should be used to assess the most likely sites of metastatic disease, including the lungs and bone. Imaging may show GCTs to be cystic, solid, or a combination of both. Sacrococcygeal and ovarian lesions that are predominantly cystic are less likely to be malignant, whereas solid lesions are more likely to be malignant. The correlation, however, is far from perfect. This is particularly important because it argues strongly against using the term *solid teratoma* as the equivalent of *malignant* or *immature teratoma* (1,6,13,14).

Ovary

GCTs account for about two-thirds of malignant ovarian tumors that occur in the first two decades of life (13,15). The histologic types are: dysgerminoma, yolk sac tumor (endodermal sinus), mixed GCTs, embryonal cell tumor, and immature teratoma (16).

In the series by Germa et al. (16) from Barcelona, 46% of childhood ovarian GCTs presented with pain. The ovary descends from the abdomen to the bony pelvis during puberty. For this reason, in younger children and most adolescents the pain will be abdominal rather than pelvic. The long infundibular pedicle in the child is susceptible to torsion (10,16). Other presenting signs and symptoms included an asymptomatic palpable mass (19%), abdominal distention (36%), and, less commonly, menstrual irregularities, malaise, nausea, vomiting, or vaginal bleeding (7,16–18). The stromal Sertoli-Leydig cell tumors may present with defeminization or virilization. Ovarian dysgerminomas are rarely hormonally active or productive of tumor markers. If a patient with an ovarian dysgerminoma is found to have an elevated AFP or signs of hormonal imbalance, there should be a meticulous search of the pathology specimen for elements of other tumor types.

Childhood ovarian GCTs are most often staged according to the FIGO system (Table 1) or the St. Jude Children's Research Hospital (SJCRH) system (Table 2).

Both primary and second-look surgery are used in the treatment of ovarian GCT. The initial surgical procedure should remove as much tumor as possible with a reasonable possibility of retention of fertility. At the time of laparotomy, the entire peritoneal surface should be examined for the presence of metastasis. Particular attention should be paid to the surfaces of the liver and to the inferior surface of the diaphragm (10). The primary tumor and the involved ovary should be removed. Dysgerminoma has a 5% to 10% incidence of bilaterality (15). For childhood ovarian GCT other than dysgerminoma, the probability of bilateral involvement ranges from 0% to 14% (19). The contralateral ovary should, therefore, be biopsied and, if there is no evidence of malignancy, preserved (20). Palpation and biopsy of all suspicious lymph nodes in the pelvic and paraaortic regions should be done. Peritoneal biopsies and washings for cytology are important to complete the surgical staging (21).

The role of second-look laparotomy following chemotherapy for ovarian GCT is controversial. The abdominal exploration is used to establish disease status by visual inspection and biopsies. Many authorities favor second-look surgery as a therapeutic guide; that is, those patients found free of tumor or with only mature teratoma do not require additional chemotherapy. It may be argued, however, that not all patients need second-look surgery. The possibility of a positive second-look operation in the face of a negative physical examination, imaging studies, and negative serum markers is small, and the procedure may not be necessary in such cases (16). The Pediatric Oncology Group (POG) is currently studying this issue.

Ovarian GCTs are lethal malignancies that can kill by early metastasis and rapid invasion of abdominal and pelvic structures. The prognosis of girls with these tumors was poor when treated with operation only, or operation in combination with either radiotherapy or single-agent chemotherapy—except for some cases of dysgerminoma (16). An increasing body of evidence now indicates that postoperative chemotherapy has increased the proba-

TABLE 1. *FIGO staging for primary carcinoma of the ovary[a]*

Stage I: Tumor limited to the ovaries.
Stage IA: Tumor limited to the ovary; no malignant ascites[a] or positive peritoneal washings. No tumor on the external surface, capsule intact.
Stage IB: Tumor limited to both ovaries; no ascites or peritoneal washings. No tumor on the external surface; capsule intact.
Stage IC: Tumor either stage IA or IB, but with malignant ascites, positive peritoneal washings, capsule ruptured, or tumor on ovarian surface.
Stage II: Tumor involving one or both ovaries with pelvic extension.
Stage IIA: Extension and/or implants to the uterus and/or tubes. No malignant cells in ascites or peritoneal washings.
Stage IIB: Extension to other pelvic tissues. Malignant cells in ascites or peritoneal washings.
Stage IIC: Tumor either stage IIA or IIB, but with malignant ascites present or positive peritoneal washings.
Stage III: Tumor involving one or both ovaries, with microscopically confirmed intraperitoneal metastases outside the pelvis and/or regional lymph node metastasis.
Stage IIIA: Microscopic peritoneal metastasis beyond the pelvis.
Stage IIIB: Macroscopic peritoneal metastasis beyond the pelvis 2 cm or less in greatest dimension.
Stage IIIC: Peritoneal metastasis beyond the pelvis more than 2 cm in the greatest dimension and/or regional lymph node metastasis.
Stage IV: Distant metastases.

[a]Ascites is peritoneal effusion that, in the opinion of the surgeon, is pathologic or clearly exceeds normal amounts, or both.
Adapted from ref. 53, with permission.

TABLE 2. *The St. Jude Children's Research Hospital staging system for germ cell tumors*

Stage	Extent of disease
Testicular germ cell tumors	
I:	Limited to one testis (or both), removed by high inguinal orchiectomy; no clinical, radiographic, or histologic evidence of disease beyond the testis; tumor markers normal after appropriate half-life decline (AFP half-life, 5 days; beta-HCG half-life, 16 hours).
II:	Transscrotal biopsy or scrotal orchiectomy, microscopic disease in scrotum or high in spermatic cord (<5 cm from proximal end), retroperitoneal lymph node involvement <2 cm, and/or increased tumor markers after appropriate half-life decline (AFP, 5 days; beta-HCG, 16 hours).
III:	Retroperitoneal lymph node involvement (>2 cm) but no visceral or extraabdominal metastases.
IV:	Visceral abdominal involvement or distant metastases.
Ovarian germ cell tumors	
I:	Limited to one ovary (or both); negative peritoneal washings; no clinical, radiographic, or histologic evidence of disease beyond the ovaries; tumor markers normal after appropriate half-life decline (AFP-half-time, 6 days).
II:	Microscopic residual or microscopic positive lymph nodes; negative peritoneal washings; tumor markers positive or negative.
III:	Gross residual or biopsy only; gross lymph node involvement (>2 cm) but no visceral or extraabdominal involvement; positive peritoneal washings; tumor markers positive or negative.
IV:	Visceral abdominal involvement or distant metastases.
Malignant extragonadal germ cell tumors	
I:	Complete resection at any site, coccygectomy for sacrococcygeal site, negative tumor margins and adjacent lymph nodes (4 weeks post operative); tumor markers negative.
II:	Microscopic residual; microscopic lymph node involvement and/or tumor markers positive.
III:	Gross residual or biopsy only; gross residual lymph nodes (>2 cm); tumor markers positive or negative.
IV:	Visceral abdominal involvement or distant metastases.

bility of survival (6,11,13,16,20,22–26). Active drugs include cisplatin (P), vinblastine (V), bleomycin (B), adriamycin (Ad), actinomycin (A), cyclophosphamide (C), etoposide (E), methotrexate (M), and vincristine (O) (7,27–29). Combinations used include POMB-ACE-PAV, PVB-ACAd, and PEB (2, 11,16).

Radiotherapy appears to be able to maintain local control of ovarian GCT within treated areas for prolonged periods of time. It has never been demonstrated, outside of dysgerminoma, that this improved local control converts into an improvement in survival (14,30). In one study, most patients could not complete the planned course of irradiation because of acute toxicities. Intestinal obstruction and sterilization may result from large-field abdominal radiotherapy (8). Contemporary treatment programs for histologies other than dysgerminoma do not utilize radiotherapy if initial surgery, chemotherapy, and second-look surgery indicate that the child is disease-free (2). Radiotherapy is reserved for residual disease that cannot be resected at sec-

ond operation. The persistent tumor volume, generally with progressive shrinking fields, is irradiated to 40 Gy (2,8,11,16).

Special consideration must be given to an evaluation of treatment options for ovarian dysgerminoma. Radiation therapy was once considered the treatment of choice, much like adult stage I testicular seminoma.

The risk of failure after unilateral oophorectomy for stage IA1 dysgerminoma (no tumor on external surface, capsule intact) has been reported to be 17% to 53%. Most failures that do occur in stage IA1 patients develop in the ipsilateral paraaortic or common iliac lymph nodes and are usually salvaged. Prophylactic irradiation of these areas, however, almost always prevents such failures. With proper pelvic shielding, the risk of radiation-induced ovarian failure and subsequent sterilization is low.

The two principal treatment options in stage IA1 patients are: (a) surgery followed by observation, using radiation only on relapse; and (b) surgery plus prophylactic ipsilateral common iliac plus paraaortic irradiation (15).

To avoid irradiating most girls with ovarian dysgerminoma, the following are the criteria for treatment with unilateral salpingo-oophorectomy alone: (a) unilateral encapsulated tumor (stage IA1); (b) greatest tumor diameter less than 10 cm (although this is not uniformly found to be a prognostic sign); (c) no ascites; (d) no evidence of enlarged or abnormal lymph nodes by palpation, lymphangiogram, biopsy, or CT; (e) well-differentiated pure dysgerminoma; and (f) confidence that the patient will attend regular follow-up appointments. By following these criteria, selected patients may be cured with preservation of fertility (17,18,21,31).

If ovarian dysgerminoma is locally extensive (beyond stage IA1) or bilateral, then chemotherapy or radiotherapy should be administered (2,16,28). When chemotherapy is used, a program such as those previously mentioned for other ovarian GCT histologies is selected. In a series from Germa et al. (16), chemotherapy-induced amenorrhea was reversed in 14 of 15 patients following chemotherapy. Three patients attempted to become pregnant: two had uneventful pregnancies and one had a spontaneous abortion. Whether ovarian failure will ultimately develop in chemotherapy-treated patients remains to be seen, although Mann et al. (11) have stated that "in ovarian dysgerminoma, chemotherapy is preferable to radiotherapy to preserve fertility." The proponents of radiotherapy for ovarian dysgerminoma feel that the indications for radiotherapy are as follows: (a) tumor present on the external surface or tumor rupture (stage IA2, IB2); (b) tumor adhesion or extension in the pelvis (stage II or III); and (c) intraabdominal nodal metastasis detected by biopsy, palpation, lymphangioma, or CT scan (stage III). However, mediastinal/supraclavicular disease (stage IV) or ascites (stage IC or IIC) are indications for chemotherapy. If the extension of tumor is strictly within the ipsilateral pelvis, hemipelvic irradiation has been recommended by Brody (32). In this way, ovarian function may be preserved. Ovarian dysgerminoma, however, may spread throughout the abdomen, and a limited hemipelvic field runs the risk of abdominal tumor recurrence. Whole-abdomen irradiation has, therefore, been recommended as initial treatment by Buskirk et al. (15; also see ref. 21) with a boost to sites of bulk disease.

If ovarian dysgerminoma is treated with radiotherapy rather than chemotherapy, and if disease extends in a nodal drainage pattern through the pelvis and paraaortic nodes, then large fields are required. In the absence of extranodal spread the paraaortic nodes and pelvis are irradiated. Whole-abdominal irradiation is indicated for bulky abdominal nodes or extracapsular extension. The entire abdomen should also be irradiated if there is proven abdominal spread or a high risk of abdominal seeding (positive peritoneal biopsies, tumor rupture). Prophylactic mediastinal irradiation, in the presence of abdominal disease, is rarely done because it compromises the child's tolerance to chemotherapy (15,17,18).

The doses required for dysgerminoma are less than those for other GCTs. Sites that are felt to be clinically uninvolved, but which are being treated prophylactically, receive 20 to 25 Gy in 3 to 4 weeks. Areas of bulk disease are boosted with an additional 10 to 15 Gy. If it is necessary to treat the whole abdomen, then appropriate blocking to the liver and kidneys is required. When re-irradiating for recurrent disease, the possibility of cure is significant and the tolerance of normal tissue to irradiation must be respected (15,17,18,21, 33).

For all histologies of ovarian GCTs combined, the reported probability of survival is on the order of 60% to 98%. Deaths appear, for the most part, to be in stage IV presentations (2,4,11,16,23,28,30,34). The survival of children with ovarian dysgerminoma is 95% to 100% when disease is confined to the pelvis or has limited abdominal involvement (4,28,32). Tumor rupture or extensive metastasis reduces the probability of survival (32). Ovarian stromal and epithelial tumors occur rarely in children. Stromal tumors of the childhood ovary, including juvenile granulosa cell tumors, are often cured by surgical resection alone (35). Surgery and chemotherapy for ovarian epithelial tumors in adolescents follow the same guidelines as those for adults (8,25,36).

Testis

Testicular GCTs generally present as a palpable painless mass or with signs and symptoms that simulate infection, torsion, or posttraumatic hematoma (37). The most common GCT of the testes in children is yolk sac tumor (endodermal sinus) (11,13,37). Less common histologies include embryonal carcinoma, malignant teratoma, and mixed tumor. Testicular GCTs are usually staged by the SJCRH system (Table 2). There is also a British staging system: (I) tumor confined to testes; (II) tumor confined to testes and retroperitoneal/abdominal lymph nodes; (III) supradiaphragmatic nodes (mediastinal and/or supraclavicular); and (IV) extralymphatic spread (liver, lung, bone, brain, skin, etc.) (13). The vast majority of cases, by either system, are stage I at diagnosis. Teenagers may be hesitant to discuss the presence of testicular mass and tend to have more advanced disease at diagnosis (7,10,37).

Most testicular tumors will be suspected prior to surgery. A radical orchiectomy should be performed with high ligation of the spermatic cord. Transscrotal procedures should be avoided because they can spread tumor and alter the protein of lymphatic metastases. If a scrotal biopsy has been done, a hemiscrotectomy is advised (37).

The debate concerning the role of retroperitoneal lymph node dissection in early-stage testicular GCT appears to be resolving in favor of a limited role for the procedure. The older literature indicated that 5% to 33% of children with yolk sac tumors have involved lymph nodes (3,10,38,39). The risk of lymph node metastases is now known to be particularly low (less than 5%) (7). Proponents of retroperitoneal lymph node dissection suggested that it was important in staging and in the removal of small foci of malignant cells and that it possibly improved the chance of cure. Objections to dissection based on loss of

ejaculatory function were obviated by the use of the modified retroperitoneal dissection (37). With the widespread availability of serum tumor marker studies and CT screening, however, it is now clear that the staging node dissection is unnecessary in stage I disease. In children with tumor confined to the testes, where AFP levels normalize within 1 month following orchiectomy and where the chest radiograph and retroperitoneal imaging studies are normal, retroperitoneal lymph node dissection is unnecessary. In one study, 28 patients with stage I testicular yolk sac tumors were treated with radical orchiectomy alone; 86% were cured. The remaining four (14%) relapsed and were rendered free of disease by chemotherapy (40). Both the U.K. Children's Cancer Study Group and the SJCRH series have almost uniform survival for stage I patients treated with radical orchiectomy alone (12,37). There is no difference in disease-free survival between children with stage I disease who undergo retroperitoneal lymph node dissection and those who do not (10,19,40). Retroperitoneal lymph node dissection may still be appropriate for children with either (a) no markers or unknown markers at diagnosis to confirm staging, (b) more aggressive histologies (i.e., embryonal cell), (c) demonstrable moderate-sized nodal metastasis at the time of presentation (i.e., SJCRH stage II), or (d) an elevated AFP following surgery (19,37,38).

Extragonadal

Extragonadal GCTs are usually found in the midline consistent with embryonic patterns of migration. The most common site is the sacrococcygeal, presacral, and buttock region. This is followed by the mediastinal, vaginal, uterine, and prostatic regions. Other reported sites of origin include the neck, retroperitoneum, stomach, orbit, heart, and pericardium.

Sacrococcygeal GCTs may develop early in fetal life. Urinary tract obstruction, compression of the umbilical vessels, and chronic hemorrhage into the tumor and amniotic sac may occur. Prenatal ultrasonography may demonstrate the mass, hydronephrosis, fetal hydrops, or prominent polyhydramnios (1). More than one-half of patients with malignant and benign sacrococcygeal teratomas present to medical attention on the first day of life. These children will frequently have other congenital anomalies such as abnormalities of the genitourinary tract or of the lower vertebral bodies (41).

Approximately 60% to 70% of sacrococcygeal teratomas are unequivocally benign by virtue of the exclusive presence of mature somatic tissue. These lesions in newborns may be cured by surgery. Ten percent to 15% of teratomas are composed of a mixture of embryonic or fetal elements in mature structures along with poorly differentiated embryonic tissue. These lesions constitute a category of indeterminant biologic behavior and are referred to as *immature benign teratomas.* In the surgical treatment of benign and intermediate-grade sacrococcygeal teratomas in infants, every effort must be made to remove the tumor mass. The early, safe, and total extirpation of the tumor and coccyx is necessary. The coccyx should always be removed with the mass because failure to remove the coccyx is associated with a local recurrence rate of 37% (42). Even piecemeal excision of mature and intermediate sacrococcygeal teratomas in infants is rarely associated with local recurrence (25,27,42–44). Only 2% to 10% of sacrococcygeal region tumors are malignant when removed in infants less than 4 months of age. After 4 months of age, the rate of malignancy rises to between 50% and 90% (1,25,42).

A useful classification system for sacrococcygeal GCTs has been developed by the Surgical Section of the American Academy of Pediatrics. In this system, type I tumors are primarily external; type II tumors are dumbbell-shaped with significant external and intrapelvic components; type III tumors have a small external component, with the majority of the lesion extending into the pelvic and abdominal spaces; and type IV tumors occupy the presacral space and have no appreciable external component. The prevalence of malignancy is, as a general rule, lowest in type I tumors and increases as one moves from type II through type IV (1,41).

Preoperative imaging studies help to determine the lesion's type, and they also evaluate whether the lesion is invading adjacent structures rather than displacing them—a suggestion of malignancy. Only a few malignant sacrococcygeal GCTs will be resectable *per primum.* In general, the surgeon will obtain an initial biopsy and chemotherapy will be administered. There is a growing body of evidence documenting complete responses of metastatic as well as primary disease to chemotherapy with long-term survival (2,11,22, 28,45,46). Unresectable tumors have been rendered resectable with long-term survivorship reported. If there is a satisfactory reduction of tumor volume, the tumor may be deemed resectable at a later date (2,42). If a complete response is achieved with surgery and chemotherapy, the probability of local control and cure is quite good (2,11). Active chemotherapeutic agents include the same as those cited for ovarian and testicular GCT.

Mediastinal GCT may be identified as a result of vascular or pulmonary obstructive symptoms or may be found incidentally on a routine chest radiograph. Mediastinal yolk sac (endodermal sinus) tumor almost always occurs in boys between the ages of 15 and 35 years. The tumor will grow rapidly and metastasize early via lymphatic and hematogenous pathways (52). An occasional case has been reported in females (5).

The survival for extragonadal GCT is not as good as for ovarian and testicular lesions. The U.K. Children's Cancer Study Group had an actuarial 48% total survival in 18 sacrococcygeal patients, 100% in four vagina, uterus, and prostate patients, 40% in five thorax primary patients, and 50% in five patients with a variety of other sites (11). The U.S. Children's Cancer Study Group reported 4-year survival and event-free survivals of 48% and 42% for all extragonadal sites combined (2). These results are generally in line with those reported by others (2,4,9,19,22,28,43,45–51).

Radiotherapy is not necessary for those children in whom the tumor has a documented complete response to surgery and chemotherapy (2). The local recurrence rate in this particular set of patients is low. In a study by Flamant et al. (22), the majority of children with nonseminomatous malignant GCT (stages III and IV) did not require radiotherapy when aggressive induction chemotherapy was used as a complement to surgery (22). In 11 of Flamant et al.'s cases failing initial therapy, 9 had a local recurrence as the site of first failure. However, when only a partial response to chemotherapy and surgery is achieved in localized disease, the chance of irradiation achieving local control is only fair. Ablin et al. (2) have described 17 children with GCT of gonadal and extragonadal location who were irradiated for persistent disease following chemotherapy. Radiotherapy failed within the field of treatment in 10 of the 17 cases. The primary site of failure in all seven sacrococcygeal GCTs was at the initial site of tumor. Mann et al. (11) reported irradiating eight patients with GCT in a variety of locations. When obvious disease was present, no sustained responses occurred. There were three survivors who had normal AFP levels at the time of irradiation and who may have been already cured before irradiation. Kersh et al. (17) reviewed the results of radiotherapy in adult and pediatric patients with nonseminoma GCT in the mediastinal, retroperitoneal, and sacrococcygeal regions. Local control was obtained in 2 of 11 patients with mediastinal lesion, 0 of 2 patients with retroperitoneal tumors, and 1 of 4 sacrococcygeal lesions. In summary, the results of radiotherapy for patients with persistent disease following chemotherapy are poor. However, it is also clear that with residual unresected disease following chemotherapy, the risk of regrowth of tumor at the primary site is almost a certainty (42). Therefore, we conclude that radiotherapy is worthy of the effort, albeit with only modest claims for success.

If radiotherapy is used for extragonadal GCT, doses of 45 to 50 Gy are recommended as limited by the tolerance of surrounding normal tissue. The radiotherapy portals will be dictated by the radiographic imaging studies and the surgical exploration. Metastatic lesions may require palliative treatment with local-field irradiation.

REFERENCES

References particularly recommended for further reading are indicated by an asterisk.

1. Wells RG, Sty JR. Imaging of sacrococcygeal germ cell tumors. *Radiographics* 1990;10:701–713.
2. Ablin AR, Krailo MD, Ramsay NKC, et al. Results of treatment of malignant germ cell tumors in 93 children: a report from the Children's Cancer Study Group. *J Clin Oncol* 1991;9:1782–1792.
3. Dehnard LP. Gonadal and extragonadal germ cell neoplasms—teratomas in childhood. In: Feingold M, ed. *Pathology of neoplasia in children and adolescents.* Philadelphia: WB Saunders, 1986:282–312.
4. Brodeur GM, Howarth CB, Pratt CB, Caces J, Hustu HO. Malignant germ cell tumors in 57 children and adolescents. *Cancer* 1981;48:1890–1898.
5. Hawkins EP, Finegold MJ, Hawkins HK, Krischer JP, Starling KA, Weinberg A. Nongerminomatous malignant germ cell tumors in children: a review of 89 cases from the Pediatric Oncology Group, 1971–1984. *Cancer* 1986;58:2579–2584.
6. Slayton RE, Park RC, Silverberg SG, Shingleton H, Creasman WT, Blessing J. Vincristine, dactinomycin, and cyclophosphamide in the treatment of malignant germ cell tumors of the ovary: a gynecologic oncology group study (a final report). *Cancer* 1985;56:243–248.
7. D'Angio GJ. Yolk sac carcinoma. *Med Pediatr Oncol* 1987;15:96–101.
*8. Jereb B, Wollner N, Exelby P. Radiation in multi-disciplinary treatment of children with malignant ovarian tumors. *Cancer* 1979;43:1037–1042.
9. Lack EE, Travis WD, Welch KJ. Retroperitoneal germ cell tumors in childhood: a clinical and pathologic study of 11 cases. *Cancer* 1985;56:602–608.
10. Green DM. The diagnosis and treatment of yolk sac tumors in infants and children. *Cancer Treat Rev* 1983; 10:265–288.
11. Mann JR, Pearson D, Barrett A, Raafat F, Barnes JM, Wallendszus KR. Results of the United Kingdom Children's Cancer Study Group's malignant germ cell tumor studies. *Cancer* 1989;63:1657–1667.
12. Huddart SN, Mann JR, Gornall P, et al. The UK Children's Cancer Study Group: testicular malignant germ cell tumours 1979–1988. *J Pediatr Surg* 1990;25: 406–410.
13. Brammer HM III, Buck JL, Hayes WS, Sheth S, Tavassoli FA. Malignant germ cell tumors of the ovary: radiologic-pathologic correlation. *Radiographics* 1990; 10:715–724.
*14. Cham WC, Wollner N, Exelby P, Clark T, D'Angio GJ. Patterns of extension as a guide to radiation therapy in the management of ovarian neoplasms in children. *Cancer* 1976;37:1443–1448.

*15. Buskirk SJ, Schray MF, Podartz KC, et al. Ovarian dysgerminoma: a restrospective analysis of results of treatment, sites of treatment failure, and radiosensitivity. *Mayo Clin Proc* 1987;62:1149–1157.

16. Germa JR, Izquierdo MA, Segui MA, Climent MA, Ojeda B, Alonso C. Malignant ovarian germ cell tumors: the experience at the Hospital de la Santa Creu i Sant Pau. *Gynecol Oncol* 1992;45:153–159.

17. Kersh CR, Constable WC, Hahn SS, et al. Primary malignant extragonadal germ cell tumors: an analysis of the effect of radiotherapy. *Cancer* 1990;65:2681–2685.

18. Lucraft HH. A review of thirty-three cases of ovarian dysgerminoma emphasizing the role of radiotherapy. *Clin Radiol* 1979;30:585–589.

19. Grosfeld JL, Billmire DF. Teratomas in infancy and childhood. *Curr Prob Cancer* 1985;9:1–53.

20. Red E. Study: save contralateral ovary in girls with ovarian malignancy. *Oncol Times* 1986;8:1–16.

21. Tewfik HH, Tewfik FA, Lataurette HB. A clinical review of seventeen patients with ovarian dysgerminoma. *Int J Radiat Oncol Biol Phys* 1982;8:1705–1709.

22. Flamant F, Schwartz L, Delons E, Caillaud JM, Hartmann O, Lemerle J. Non-seminomatous malignant germ cell tumors in children: multi-drug therapy in stages III and IV. *Cancer* 1984;54:1687–1691.

23. Gershenson DM, Kavanaugh JJ, Copeland LJ, et al. Treatment of malignant non-dysgerminomatous germ cell tumors of the ovary with vinblastine, bleomycin, and *cis*-platinum. *Cancer* 1986;57:1731–1737.

24. Nichols CR, Heerema NA, Palmer C, Loehrer PJ Sr, Williams SD, Einham LH. Klinefelter's syndrome associated with mediastinal germ cell neoplasms. *J Clin Oncol* 1987;5:1290–1294.

25. Noseworthy J, Lack EE, Kozakewich HPW, Vawter GF, Welch KJ. Sacrococcygeal germ cell tumors in childhood: an updated experience with 118 patients. *J Pediatr Surg* 1981;16:358–364.

26. Raney RB, Sinclair L, Uri A, Schnaufer L, Cooper A, Littman P. Malignant ovarian tumors in children and adolescents. *Cancer* 1987;59:1214–1220.

27. Donnellan WA, Swenson O. Benign and malignant sacrococcygeal teratomas. *Surgery* 1968;64:834–846.

28. Etcubanas E, Thompson E, Rao B, Hustu O, Hammond B, Brodeur G. Treatment of childhood germ cell tumors (GCT): results of a prospective study. *Proc ASCO* 1985;4:238.

29. Williams SD, Birch R, Einhorn LH, Irwin L, Greco FA, Loehrer PJ. Treatment of disseminated germ-cell tumors with cisplatin, bleomycin, and either vinblastine or etoposide. *N Engl J Med* 1987;315:1435–1440.

30. Creasman WT, Fedder BF, Hammond CB, Parker RT. Germ cell malignancies of the ovary. *Obstet Gynecol* 1979;53:226–230.

31. Kephart G, Smith JP, Rutledge F, Delclos L. The treatment for dysgerminoma of the ovary. *Cancer* 1978;41:986–990.

32. Brody S. Clinical aspects of dysgerminoma of the ovary. *Acta Radiol* 1961;56:209–230.

33. Lawson AP, Adler GF. Radiotherapy in the treatment of ovarian dysgerminoma. *Int J Radiat Oncol Biol Phys* 1988;14:431–434.

34. Wollner N, Exelby PR, Woodruff M, et al. Malignant ovarian tumors in childhood. Prognosis in relation to initial stage. *Cancer* 1976;37:1953–1964.

35. Vassai G, Falmant F, Caillaud JM, Demeoca F, Nihoul-Fekete C, Lemerle J. Juvenile granulosa cell tumor of the ovary in children: a clinical study of 15 cases. *J Clin Oncol* 1988;6:990–995.

36. Vogelzang NJ, Anderson RW, Kennedy BJ. Successful treatment of mediastinal germ cell/endodermal sinus tumors. *Chest* 1985;88:64–69.

37. Fernandes ET, Etcubanas E, Rao BN, Durnar APM, Thompson EI, Jenkins JJ. Two decades of experience with testicular tumors in children at St. Jude Children's Research Hospital. *J Pediatr Surg* 1989;24:677–682.

38. Duckett J. Testicular tumors in childhood. In: Hays DM, ed. *Pediatric surgical oncology.* Orlando, FL: Grune & Stratton, 1986:189–204.

39. Ise T, Ohtsuka H, Matsumoto K, Sano R. Management of malignant testicular tumors in children. *Cancer* 1976;37:1539–1545.

40. Flamant F, Diez P. Cure of testicular Stage I yolk sac tumor (endodermal sinus tumor) in children by conservative treatment. *Proc ASCO* 1985;4:235.

41. Altman RP, Randolph JG, Lilly JR. Sacrococcygeal teratoma: American Academy of Pediatric Surgical Section Survey—1973. *J Pediatr Surg* 1974;9:389–398.

42. Ein SH, Mancer K, Adeyemi SD. Malignant sacrococcygeal teratoma—endodermal sinus, yolk sac tumor—in infants and children: a 32 year review. *J Pediatr Surg* 1985;20:473–477.

43. Thomas WJ, Kelleher JF, Duval-Arnould B. Successful treatment of metastatic extragonadal endodermal sinus (yolk sac) tumor in childhood. *Cancer* 1981;48:2371–2374.

44. Valdiserri RO, Yunis EJ. Sacrococcygeal teratomas: review of 68 cases. *Cancer* 1981;48:217–221.

45. Cushing BA, Phillippart AI, Brough AJ, Daas L. Extragonadal endodermal sinus tumor in early childhood: treatment response and longterm effects. *Proc ASCO* 1985;4:242.

46. Feun LG, Sampson MK, Stephens RL. Vinblastine (VLB), Bleomycin (BLEO), *cis*-platinum (DDP), and disseminated extragonadal germ cell tumors: a Southwest Oncology Study. *Cancer* 1980;45:2543–2549.

47. Anderson WA, Sabio H, Durso N, Mills SE, Levien M, Underwood PB Jr. Endodermal sinus tumor of the vagina: the role of primary chemotherapy. *Cancer* 1985;56:1025–1027.

48. Atkins J. Malignant ovarian and other germ cell tumors. In: Hays DM, ed. *Pediatric surgical oncology.* Orlando, FL: Grune & Stratton, 1986:123–138.

49. Beddis IR, Noblett H, Mott MG. Effective chemotherapy for metastatic malignant sacrococcygeal tumor. *Med Pediatr Oncol* 1984;12:231–232.

50. Israel A, Bosl GJ, Golbey RB, Whitmore W Jr, Martini N. The results of chemotherapy for extragonadal germ-cell tumors in the cisplatin era: the Memorial Sloan-Kettering Cancer Center experience (1975–1982). *J Clin Oncol* 1985;3:1073–1078.

51. Logothetis CJ, Samuels ML, Selig DE, et al. Chemotherapy of extragonadal germ cell tumors. *J Clin Oncol* 1985;3:316–325.

52. Gooneratne S, Keh P, Streekanth S, Recant W, Talerman A. Anterior mediastinal endodermal sinus (yolk sac) tumor in a female infant. *Cancer* 1985;56:1430–1433.

53. American Joint Committee for Cancer Staging and End Results Reporting. *Manual for staging of cancer,* 4th ed. Philadelphia: JB Lippincott, 1992.

16

Endocrine, Aerodigestive Tract, and Breast Tumors

ENDOCRINE CARCINOMA

Adrenal Cortical Carcinoma

Adrenal cortical carcinoma (ACC) comprises approximately 0.2% of childhood cancer (1–7). The tumor is approximately twice as frequent in girls as in boys. ACC is generally secretory, and *virilization* is the most common sign. There is premature pubic hair, clitiromegaly or phallomegaly, and excessive muscular development. Bone age may be advanced. In *Cushing's syndrome* there is moon facies, plethora, hypertension, striae, weight gain, acne, hirsutism, and an intracapsular fat pad. Children with ACC rarely have pure Cushing's syndrome; most also have some evidence of virilization. *Feminization* or *aldosterone-secreting tumors* are quite rare. Children with ACC may also present with pain or a palpable mass.

Urinary 17-keto- and 17-hydroxycorticosteroids are usually elevated (2). ACC steroid production is generally not influenced by adrenocorticotropic hormone (ACTH) suppression. Ultrasound, computerized tomography (CT), and/or magnetic resonance imaging (MRI) are used for assessing the size and extent of the primary tumor as well as the presence of liver and lymph nodes metastases (8). The primary tumor is usually hypovascular on angiography (5).

Surgical removal of a localized primary ACC is the best hope for cure (9–11). The surgeon will attempt a complete excision of the primary tumor and resectable regional metastases. Meticulous attention must be given to perioperative steroid management. Surgery may also be used to treat resectable abdominal recurrences or localized distant metastases (12).

The distinction between benign and malignant ACC is made on cytologic abnormality, tumor weight, and presence of metastases (13,14). Some lesions will be frankly malignant on microscopic examination. For those of borderline histologic appearance, one should consider resectability, the extent of capsular invasion, adherence to surrounding structures, the presence of aberrant vessels on angiography, tumor size, and the presence or absence of metastases in distinguishing benign from malignant lesions. Well-encapsulated and easily excised tumors may be cured by surgery alone. In the remaining resected but more locally advanced cases, there is a substantial risk of local relapse and distant metastases (5,10,12,15,16).

The role of adjuvant radiotherapy has been described infrequently. Stewart et al. (11) recommended 15 to 30 Gy of whole-abdominal irradiation, with shielding of the contralateral kidney and adrenal, as adjuvant therapy for resected tumors. They administered whole-abdominal irradiation without chemotherapy to four children. There were three survivors, without recurrence of tumor, at 1 to 6 years. One of these children had unresectable tumor invading the inferior vena cava. She was free of tumor at re-exploration following irradiation. Percarpio and Knowlton (17) gave preoperative irradiation to two adults with ACC (50 Gy, 45 Gy). Resection was possible in one individual. Four patients (3 adults and 1 child) received postoperative irradiation for unresectable lesions or for tumor spillage. Three patients recurred in field in 2 to 34 months. One failed outside the field 11 years later. Bradley (1) administered adjuvant external beam radiotherapy to four adults (2300 to 4500 R). One patient is a long-term survivor 15 years after surgery. Magee et al. (13) described 15 patients, including 5 children, 9 of whom had postoperative irradiation. Three of Magee's patients were girls who presented under the age of 2 years with hormonally active tumors and who survived for more than 10 years following gross total tumor resection and 30 Gy of postoperative irradiation in 4 weeks. Two of the three patients died of second malignancies arising in the irradiated field. Markoe et al. (18) have reported 13 patients, including a 9-year-old girl. Local relapse was a frequent contributor to tumor relapse, and the authors argue that, in some cases, local irradiation (50 to 60 Gy) may have contributed to improved local control. Kasperlik-Zaluska et al. gave postoperative irradiation to two patients who survived only 5 and 12 months (19). Zografos et al. briefly mentioned giving radiotherapy to seven patients with inoperable tumors. The results are not explicitly stated (20). The existing data may be used to support the use of adjuvant radiotherapy for gross or microscopic residual disease following surgery. While there is no clear evidence for radiotherapy's usefulness following a gross total tumor resection, a plausible argument may be made for adjuvant irradiation in this situation in view of the poor overall survival statistics and the lack of other adjuvant treatment options (13). The second malignancies in Magee's series are, however, chastening. Palliation of bone pain or soft-tissue masses has been achieved with 30 to 45 Gy in 2 to 6 weeks.

It is not clear if adjuvant chemotherapy is useful following gross total resection of tumor (21). One retrospective study from Poland, however, argues for its benefit (19).

Most authorities feel that chemotherapy is clearly indicated for inoperable, recurrent, and metastatic disease (5,10,12,18,21). Mitotane is considered to be the drug of choice. The drug, an isomer of the insecticide DDD and a chemical congener of the insecticide DDT, has adrenolytic activity. Pooled data shows approximately a 35% response rate (22). Median duration of response is 6 to 7 months (12,21,23). Responses may be more frequent when high serum levels of the drug are achieved. The drug has significant toxicity including anorexia, nausea, vomiting, diarrhea, and CNS toxicity. Aminoglutethimide blocks adrenocortical hormone synthesis. It has been used to decrease signs and symptoms of Cushing's disease along with mitotane (12).

The probability of survival of childhood ACC has been reported to range between 10% and 80% (7,10,11,23,24). The consensus is between 25% and 45%, 5-year survival (22). This wide variation between individual institutions is certainly the result of case selection, quality of steroid management, and treatment policies. The survival of children with resected tumors weighing less than or equal to 160 g appears superior to that of patients with heavier tumors (7).

Pheochromocytoma

Pheochromocytoma is a rare tumor. Approximately 10% of all patients with pheochromocytoma are children (25–27). The tumors may arise in one or both adrenals or in an extraadrenal location. The tumor is responsible for approximately 1% of cases of childhood hypertension, and it typically presents between 8 and 14 years of age (28,29). Familial pheochromocytoma is associated with other endocrine tumors in multiple endocrine neoplasia (MEN) syndromes (30). MEN type II (31) includes familial pheochromocytoma or adrenal medullary hyperplasia, medullary thyroid cancer, and hyperparathyroidism. MEN type III (31) includes pheochromocytoma or adrenal medullary hyperplasia, medullary thyroid cancer, mucosal neuromas, marfanoid habitus, thickened corneal nerves, ganglioneuromata of the alimentary tract and, rarely, hyperparathyroidism (26).

Almost two-thirds of children with pheochromocytoma are boys. The most common presenting signs and symptoms of pheochromocytoma in childhood include sustained hypertension (in contrast to adults, who usually have paroxysmal hypertension), diaphoresis, fatigue, and headache (25,28,32). Convulsions can also occur.

Adrenal medullary pheochromocytomas produce epinephrine and norepinephrine, whereas most extraadrenal pheochromocytomas produce only norepinephrine. Screening studies include urinary levels of epinephrine, norepinephrine, metanephrine, and vanilylmandelic acid (25,29,32). Preoperative tumor imaging is most often accomplished with ultrasound, CT, and/or MRI (25). Examination with iodine-131 metaiodobenzylguanidine (MIBG) scans may be of value in assessing tumor location. MIBG is concentrated in catecolamine-producing cells and, therefore, can be used to image pheochromocytoma and neuroblastoma (1).

The definitive therapy for pheochromocytoma in childhood is surgical. Preoperative and intraoperative adrenergic receptor blockade of catecholamine-induced receptor stimulation is necessary for successful resection. Phenoxybenzomine is the principal drug used (33). Other drugs such as phentolamine, prazosin, nifedipine, labetalal, nitroprusside, propranolol, alpha-methyl-tyrosine, and lidocaine, have been used. During and following tumor resection, blood volume correction (i.e., normal saline, plasma, whole blood) and pressors may be necessary for variable periods of time to maintain the blood pressure (25,34).

Total tumor resection is usually curative (35). Recurrences may develop several years after initial surgery, are usually heralded by recurrent hypertension, and are cured by additional surgery (36).

External beam radiation therapy is effective for palliation of bone, lymph node, brain, and spinal cord metastases (37). High-dose ^{131}I MIBG has been tried for malignant tumors

with only modest success (26,33). In a series of 14 patients with malignant pheochromocytoma, eight partially or completely responded for a median duration of 21 months to cyclophosphamide, vincristine, and DTIC (26,33).

Thyroid Carcinoma

Thyroid carcinoma represents 1% to 1.5% of cancer from all sites in children (24,38–44). The majority of pediatric tumors occur in 15- to 19-year olds (34). The proportion of female to male patients is about 2:1 (34,45,46).

The types of thyroid cancer in children include:

1. *Papillary carcinoma* (70% to 80% of childhood thyroid cancer). These lesions tend to be infiltrative and multicentric (34). Lymphatic metastases occur in one-third to two-thirds of cases. Hematogenous metastases may occur—most commonly to the lungs. A mixed papillary-follicular pattern is common in children and is included with the papillary classification (42).

2. *Follicular carcinoma* (16% to 20%). No papillary elements are present in these tumors. Vascular invasion is common.

3. *Medullary carcinoma* (rare). These tumors develop from neural crest parafollicular or C cells. Medullary carcinoma may arise as part of one of the multiple endocrine neoplasia (MEN) type IIa and IIb syndromes. The tumor is associated with an immunoreactive thyrocalcitonin marker. Missense mutations in the *ret* protooncogene on chromosome 10 are associated with MEN IIA and B. Medullary thyroid cancer is more aggressive than papillary or follicular cancer and can be fatal. For this reason, some authorities are now advocating genetic testing to identify children who will develop MEN IIA or B and then perform prophylactic thyroidectomy (34,47).

4. *Undifferentiated carcinoma* (rare). The undifferentiated carcinoma may contain sheets of small cells with large dark nuclei, spindle cells, or giant cells. The prognosis of undifferentiated carcinoma is quite poor, with

death usually occurring within 6 months of diagnosis (48).

5. *Insular carcinoma* (very rare). The "insular" variant is a type of poorly differentiated cancer intermediate in clinical behavior and morphology between well-differentiated and anaplastic tumors. It is characterized by nests of tumor cells separated from surrounding cells by artifactual clefts. The tumor may behave aggressively (49,50).

The first sign of thyroid cancer in childhood is either a thyroid nodule or a palpable cervical node (39). Several series indicate that if microscopic disease is included 70% to 90% of children with thyroid cancer will have neck node metastases at presentation—a number significantly higher than the incidence in adults (39,42,45,51,52). Approximately 5% to 10% will have distant metastases at presentation (53,54). Most children with thyroid carcinoma are euthyroid. Conventional neck radiographs or xeroradiographs may show laminated thyroid calcifications. Such calcifications should raise the suspicion of the psammoma bodies of papillary carcinoma. Imaging with an iodine radionuclide is of greatest value. A cold area in the thyroid is highly suspicious for carcinoma (39,55).

An accident and resulting fire at the Chernobyl-4 Nuclear Power Plant in the Ukraine on April 26, 1986, lasted for 10 days and burned through the roof of the building containing the 1,000 MWa water-cooled, graphite-moderated reactor. Approximately 40,000,000 to 50,000,000 curies of I-131 was released into the atmosphere—a staggering number when compared, for example, to the 15 to 20 curies released at the Three Mile Island accident in the United States. In addition, large amounts of radioisotopes of cesium, xenon, krypton, and strontium were also released (56,57).

The incidence of thyroid cancer in Belarus and Ukraine began to rise sharply in 1989 to 1990. In adults, the number of new cases ultimately increased two- to three-fold. In children, the incidence rose 20- to 30-fold (56,57). Almost all the new cases in children are papillary tumors (94% to 98%).

Lymph node metastases are common (65%) and lung metastases at presentation are relatively frequent (5%) in those exposed to I-131 from the Chernobyl accident (57,58). The highest incidences of thyroid cancer are roughly correlated with the highest exposures of the population to radioactive iodine. The exact population radiation exposure is unknown due to some uncertainty in radiation dosimetry and patterns of milk consumption—an important source of iodine absorption. Some of the cases of thyroid cancer may be explicable by chronic iodine deficiency in many of the contaminant areas prior to the accident. A thyroid deficient in iodine would have quickly taken up the radioactive isotopes (56,58).

It is generally agreed that surgery is the principal treatment for childhood thyroid cancer (41,59,60). The extent of surgery for the primary tumor and potentially involved lymph nodes, however, is hotly debated. Depending on the situation, there are advocates of subtotal lobectomy, lobectomy and isthmusectomy, and total thyroidectomy. For management of the cervical nodes there are advocates of node picking, advocates of modified and radical neck dissection, and advocates of no node operation. Underlying the surgical controversy is the extent to which subsequent radioactive iodine (RAI) therapy will sterilize residual tumor following surgery (39,45,61). While we cannot do justice to the breadth of data brought to bear in the argument, we can address the broad outlines of the controversy. The advocates of routine total thyroidectomy cite the relatively high frequency of multifocality of the disease, assert a lower incidence of neck relapse with more extensive surgery, and point out that serum thyroglobulin may be used as a tumor marker in follow-up. In addition, there is a high incidence of pulmonary metastases in children. Total thyroidectomy allows early detection of occult metastases with a RAI scan (34). Supporters of more limited surgery argue that intraoperative palpation of the gland is reasonably reliable for determining the extent of resection, that the cure rates are excellent with more limited surgery, and that vocal cord injury and hypoparathyroidism are more frequent with more extensive surgery (42,52,54). Most surgeons would support removal of adjacent, grossly involved nodes at the time of surgery for the primary tumor. Opponents of carrying the node surgery to the extent of a radical neck dissection point out that the type of lymphatic dissection does not predict the risk of tumor recurrence (42) and the efficacy of RAI in controlling metastatic disease from well-differentiated thyroid cancer (42).

Well-differentiated thyroid cancers are usually hormone-dependent. The suppression of thyroid-stimulating hormone (TSH) by the administration of exogenous thyroid hormone is indicated because it decreases the probability of tumor recurrence in higher risk patients (39,47). Exogenous thyroid hormone also ensures that the child remains euthyroid regardless of the extent of the thyroidectomy. The risks of properly supervised long-term administration of thyroid hormone in children are debatable (24,62). Several studies have suggested that long-term thyroid hormone suppression may decrease bone mineral density in children (47).

RAI is taken up by 50% to 80% of well-differentiated thyroid tumors but is taken up by few poorly differentiated malignancies. RAI has the potential for delivering extremely high focal doses of irradiation to ablate thyroid tissue remaining after surgery and to treat neck nodes or distant metastases. RAI will also deliver a small dose of whole-body irradiation. Bone marrow depression is uncommon unless bone metastases are present. Pulmonary fibrosis occurs occasionally when RAI is repeatedly administered for pulmonary metastases. Parotiditis/sialadenitis, nausea, glossalgia, hypogeusia, gastrointestinal discomfort, or thyroiditis rarely occur (38,63,64). Potential long-term complications of RAI have been alleged, with varying degrees of supporting evidence. These include: leukemia, myelosuppression, bladder cancer, salivary cancer, gastric cancer, breast cancer, and infertility. These reported

risks may be attributable to the reported use, in the past, of high, repetitive doses of RAI (53).

Controversy also surrounds certain aspects of the use of RAI following surgery for childhood thyroid cancer. There is little question about the necessity of postsurgical ablation of iodine-131 concentrating tissue in the thyroid bed in the presence of nodal or distant metastatic disease. One wishes to eliminate thyroid tissue that will concentrate iodine-131 so that, subsequently, one can use iodine-131 therapeutically against the metastases (65). There is considerable uncertainty, however, over the use of RAI for the routine ablation of remaining thyroid tissue in patients with well-differentiated thyroid cancer who are not thought to have metastatic disease (63,66). Some would argue that RAI will treat multifocal disease. However, it is not at all clear that RAI will reduce the risk of local tumor failure in postoperative patients treated with thyroid hormone suppression (42,53,66). At present, because of the high incidence of nodal and distant metastases in childhood thyroid cancer, many authorities favor routine RAI thyroid ablation (12,38,45).

While most studies show that children with well-differentiated thyroid cancer have, on average, larger tumors, more extensive local invasion, and more nodal and distant metastases than adults, these young patients have an excellent prognosis. Cancer-related deaths, particularly from papillary carcinoma, are rare (12,67). Survival rates for children in the Mayo Clinic series of thyroid cancer did not differ significantly from those for age-matched population controls at 20, 25, and 30 years (61). There have been no tumor-induced deaths among 100 children in the Memorial Hospital series (median follow-up 20 years), although 35% had tumor recurrence after initial surgery (42). In an extensive literature review, McClellan and Francis reported a tumor recurrence rate of 0% to 39% and a risk of death from disease of 0% to 18% (53).

External beam radiotherapy is used for the locally unresectable tumor that does not take up RAI or is so bulky that RAI would not be able to control it. Neck or mediastinal recurrences of tumors that are bulky and/or do not take up RAI may also be externally irradiated (41,68–71). A minimum tumor dose of 55 to 65 Gy is administered with an anterior photon field, anterior photons plus electrons, or weighted anterior and posterior parallel opposed fields with appropriate spinal blocking. The treatment volume will encompass the neck and upper mediastinum. Gross disease in the neck is not hopeless and may be cured by external beam radiotherapy. Bone or soft-tissue metastases that are not suitable for RAI or do not respond, may be treated for palliation with conventional external beam doses. In the rare situation where chemotherapy is considered, adriamycin is the most active agent.

AERODIGESTIVE TRACT TUMORS

Juvenile Nasopharyngeal Angiofibroma

Juvenile nasopharyngeal angiofibroma (JNA) is a rare tumor that is far more frequent in males than in females—a ratio of 42:1 in the M.D. Anderson series (72–74). The average age at clinical presentation is 14 to 16 years (62,74,75). Arising from the nasopharynx, the lesion may extend to the nasal cavities, the maxillary and sphenoid sinuses, the orbit, the anterior or middle cranial fossae, the infratemporal region, or the pterygopalatine fossa. The lesion is thought to arise from the vascular structures of the basosphenoid region, particularly in the region of the sphenopalatine foramen (76). The histologic appearance of the tumor is characteristic: numerous thin-walled vessels, lined by endothelium and devoid of a complete muscular layer, with interspersed fibroblasts and collagen (Fig. 1). Presenting signs and symptoms include recurrent epistaxis, nasal obstruction, cheek swelling, and facial deformity. Less common are proptosis, hearing loss, headache, mouth breathing, and cranial nerve palsies (77).

JNA are firm, red masses. Superimposed infection may produce secondary surface ulcerations. Axial, coronal, and sagittal CT and MRI are invaluable in demonstrating tumor extent (73,78,79) (Fig. 2). A typical CT pat-

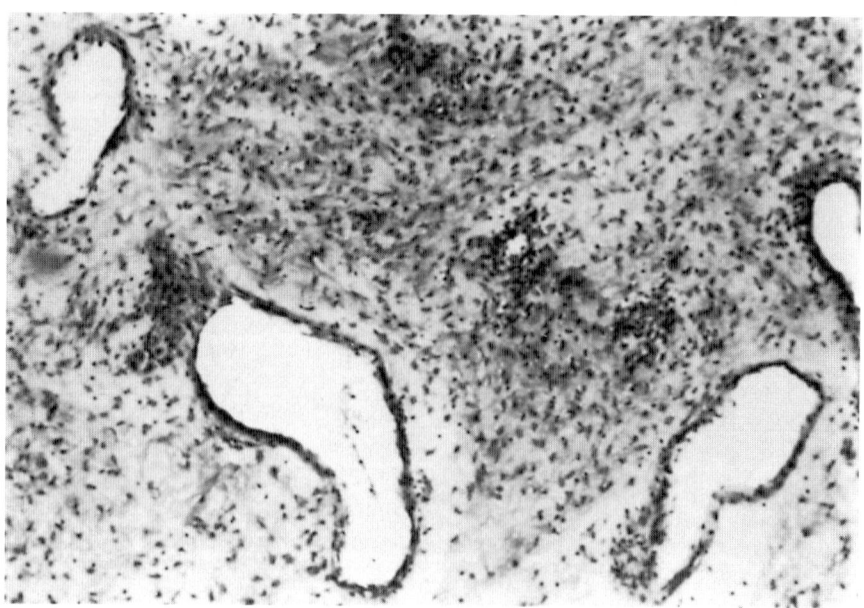

FIG. 1. Juvenile nasopharyngeal angiofibroma with vessels devoid of a complete muscle layer. (From ref. 247, with permission.)

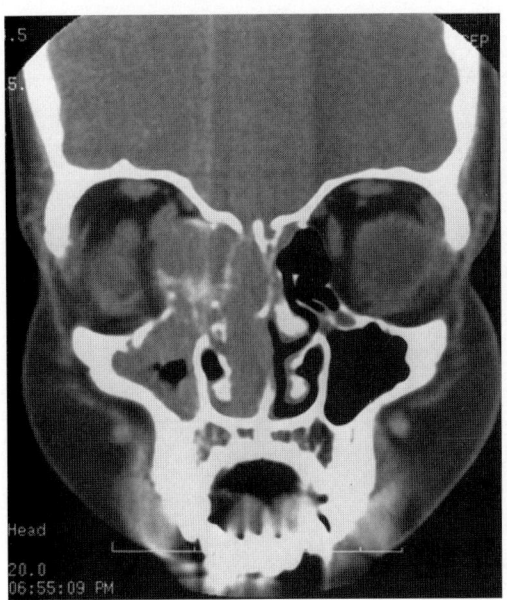 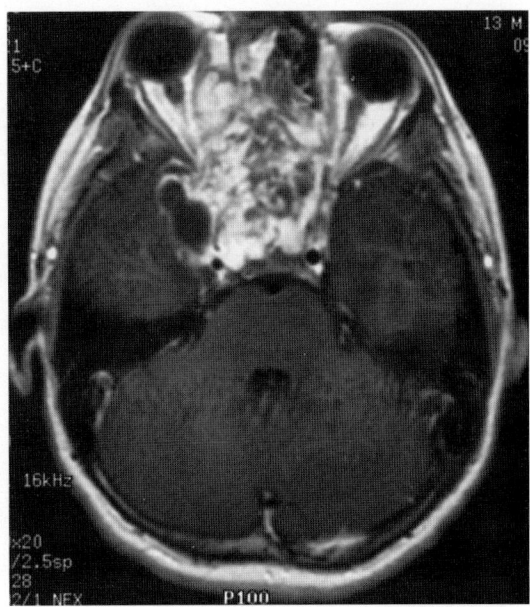

FIG. 2. Coronal CT (left) and axial MRI (right) of a 13-year-old boy with headaches, diplopia, and right proptosis. The mass produced destruction of the ethmoid air cells and superior turbinates, mass effect in the right orbit, compression of the right cavernous sinus, displacement of the right internal carotid artery, and displacement of the pituitary. A biopsy proved the diagnosis of juvenile nasopharyngeal angiofibroma. Three-dimensional treatment planning was used to prepare a four-field non-coplanar external beam radiotherapy treatment technique utilizing rigid head immobilization. A dose of 36 Gy at 2 Gy per fraction was administered. One and one-half years following irradiation the symptoms had significantly improved and the mass was smaller on physical examination and MRI. Shortly thereafter the symptoms recurred and the MRI demonstrated re-growth of the angiofibroma, within and outside the irradiated field. Interferon was administered as an antiangiogenesis agent.

tern of JNA is a contrast-enhancing nasopharyngeal mass with widening of the pterygopalatine fossa. One can also see erosion of the roof of the medial pterygoid plate or indentation of the posterior wall of the maxillary sinus (Holman-Miller sign) (74). The vascular supply may be from the internal maxillary, ascending pharyngeal, or ascending palatine arteries (76). In cases of intracranial extension, blood supply may come from branches of the internal carotid artery (80,81). During angiography a characteristic reticulated pattern is seen in the arterial phase with a subsequent dense blush persisting in the venous phase (73).

The definitive therapies for JNA are surgery and external-beam radiotherapy. Chemotherapy has been used for recurrent lesions that are not amenable to additional surgery or irradiation (74). Other treatments include packings until the tumor undergoes spontaneous regression (a rare occurrence), cryotherapy, electrocoagulation, and implantation of radioisotopes (62,75,78,82–88). Rather than being competitive, surgery and radiotherapy have complementary roles in the management of JNA. As is often the case, proper patient selection is the key. Systems of classification have been proposed by many centers (72,81,89–91) (Table 1). All systems recognize that local infiltration of JNA, particularly into the infratemporal region or within the cranial vault, makes definitive surgery more difficult and dangerous.

The treatment of smaller JNA (i.e., Sessions' stage I to IIA) is generally accepted to be surgical (92). There are several surgical approaches, including transpalatal, lateral rhino-

TABLE 1. *Staging of juvenile nasopharyngeal angiofibroma*

Chandler et al. (58) and Jacobson et al. (81)

Stage I:	Tumor confined to nasopharynx
Stage II:	Extension into nasal cavity and/or sphenoid sinus
Stage III:	Extension into one or more of the following: antrum, ethmoid sinuses, pterygomaxillary and infratemporal fossae, orbit, and/or cheek
Stage IV:	Intracranial extension

Fields et al. (72)

Stage I:	Tumor confined to nasopharynx and/or nasal fossae
Stage II:	Extending into the sphenoid sinus and/or pterygomaxillary fossae
Stage III:	Extending beyond stage II limits into maxillary sinus, ethmoid sinuses, orbits, infratemporal fossae, cheeks, or palate
Stage IV:	Intracranial extension

Sessions et al. (91)

Stage IA:	Limited to posterior nares or nasopharynx
Stage IB:	Extension into one or more paranasal sinuses
Stage IIA:	Minimal spread into pterygopalatine fossa
Stage IIB:	Occupation of the pterygopalatine fossa displacing posterior maxillary wall; possibly erosion into orbit
Stage IIC:	Extension through pterygopalatine fossa into infratemporal fossa or cheek
Stage III:	Intracranial extension

Andrews et al. (89)

Type I:	Tumor limited to the nasopharynx and nasal cavity. Bone destruction negligible or limited to the sphenopalatine foramen
Type II:	Tumor invading the pterygopalatine fossa or the maxillary, ethmoid or sphenoid sinus with bone destruction
Type IIIa:	Tumor invading the infratemporal fossa or orbital region without intracranial involvement
Type IIIb:	Tumor invading the infratemporal fossa or orbit with intracranial extradural (parasellar) involvement
Type IVa:	Intracranial intradural tumor without infiltration of the cavernous sinus, pituitary fossa or optic chiasm
Type IVb:	Intacranial intradural tumor with infiltration of the cavernous sinus, pituitary fossa or optic chiasm

tomy, and craniofacial resection with an infratemporal approach (74,81). Endoscopic resection has also been described (93). Operative blood loss may be as high as 1500 to 3000 mL. Hormone therapy and embolization may be useful preoperative adjuvants. The fact that JNAs are far more common in males than in females, raised the hypothesis that the tumors were related to some imbalance in the pituitary adrenogenital system. Hormone therapy may be useful in an attempt, preoperatively, to decrease tumor vascularity. Preoperative arterioembolization with particles (i.e., gelatin foam or dura mater) or balloons carried out 1 to 2 days before surgery is able to significantly reduce operative blood loss (80). With adequate operative exposure and resection, 70% to 100% of patients need no additional treatment (72,74,76,82).

Intracranial, orbital, or pterygopalatine extension of JNA (Sessions' stages IIB to III) increases the risks of resection (88,92). External beam radiotherapy is best used for the definitive treatment of these advanced cases. Parallel opposed lateral field treatment or two lateral fields with an anterior field will usually be adequate. Inadequate treatment fields are a major course of failure of local control of JNA by irradiation (94). If marginal misses are to be avoided, proper mapping of the tumor volume is crucial, including the intracranial extensions. The pertinent studies (CT, MRI, and angiographic) must be reviewed with care to establish the treatment volume.

A considerable range of external-beam doses have been used. Economou et al. (83) and McGahan et al. (95) have argued, based on retrospective data, that doses greater than 32 to 36 Gy are necessary. Others (78,79,88,94), however, do not support this view and have achieved good results with 30 Gy (Table 2). Most of the available data supports a total dose of 30 to 36 Gy. Intracavitary irradiation has been used (83). Such treatment runs the obvious risks of major bleeding and inadequate coverage of the treatment volume (94).

Nasopharyngeal Carcinoma

Many of the principles established in adult head and neck oncology are applicable to childhood nasopharyngeal carcinoma. It would be a mistake, however, to treat children with this tumor by simply following the guidelines applicable to the treatment of adults. Childhood nasopharyngeal carcinoma has certain peculiar features that affect its presentation, treatment, outcome, and late ill effects.

Two percent to 20% of nasopharyngeal carcinomas (NPCs) occur in individuals younger than 30 years of age. In general, NPC represents less than 1% of all childhood malignant tumors but constitutes 20% to 50% of pediatric malignancies of the nasopharynx (96,97). In children, NPC is a disease of adolescence. In most series there are more boys than girls (98–100). It was noted early in this century that the disease is common among Chinese living in China (98). Hong Kong has the highest documented incidence rate of NPC in the world (101). Among Chinese living outside of China, NPC is less common— although still greater than that of a comparable non-Chinese population. These observations suggest that genetic and environmental factors are important in the development of this neoplasm (102,103). Elevated anti-Epstein-Barr virus (EBV) antibody titers have been found in patients with NPC, and childhood cases of NPC seem to have a closer association with EBV than do adult cases (104). There appears to be a correlation of titer levels with stage at presentation. Treated

TABLE 2. *Radiotherapy for juvenile nasopharyngeal angiofibroma*

Reference	Year of report	Number of cases	Dose range	Local control	Follow-up
Apostol and Frazell (81)	1965	9	3000–3600 rad[a]	6/9 (67%)[b]	1–12 years
Briant et al. (62)	1970[c]	22	30 Gy	17/22 (77%)[d]	1–<3 years
Jereb et al. (85)	1970	66	2000–6000 rad[a]	(>80%) "minimal"	1–<40 years
Ward et al. (88)	1974	4	3000 rad[a]	2/2 (100%)	1–2 years
		2	3000 rad[a]		
Briant et al. (75)	1978[c]	45	3000–3500 rad	35/45 (78%)[e]	2–20 years
Cummings et al. (94)	1984[c]	40	30 Gy	32/40 (80%)[e]	3–26 years
		15	35 Gy	12/15 (80%)[e]	
Benghait (78)	1986	1	30 Gy	1/1 (100%)	9 months
Economou et al. (83)	1988	3	<36 Gy	0/3 (0%)	1–25 years
		11	>36 Gy	11/11 (100%)	
Cuyler (92)	1988	1	36–84 cGy	1/1 (100%)	1 year
McGahan et al. (95)	1989	4	32 Gy	0/4 (0%)	1–14 years
		10	36–46 Gy	10/10 (100%)	
Robinson et al. (77)	1989	10	30–40 Gy	9/10 (90%)	8–141 months
Fields et al. (72)	1990	13[f]	35–52 Gy	11/13 (85%)	29–255 months
Kasper et al. (79)	1993	9[f]	30–35 Gy	9/9 (100%)	3–15 years
Wiatrak et al. (238)	1993	3	36–50.4 Gy	3/3 (100%)	1.7–4.5 years
Ungkanat et al. (74)	1996	2	35–45 Gy	1/2 (50%)	

[a]It is not clear if doses are reported in roentgens or rads. In the Jereb series, some patients received brachytherapy.
[b]Some of the failures may have died of complications while the angiofibroma was controlled.
[c]These series include many of the same patients.
[d]The local control rate is not clear.
[e]Many of the failures are salvaged by additional irradiation or surgery.
[f]Some of these patients had relapses after surgery rather than primary radiotherapy.

patients with no evidence of recurrence have low titers.

Although a variety of malignant tumors arise in the nasopharynx, only squamous cell carcinoma is considered in this section. Classification schemes include dividing the cases into lymphoepithelioma; well to poorly differentiated transitional cell tumors; and keratinizing versus nonkeratinizing. The World Health Organization (WHO) has classified NPC as: WHO-1: well to moderately differentiated squamous, including transitional carcinoma with obvious keratin production; WHO-2: nonkeratinizing carcinoma; WHO-3: undifferentiated carcinoma including lymphoepithelioma with anaplastic, clear cell, and spindle cell variants (97,105). Lymphoepithelioma is characterized by a syncytium of malignant epithelial cells with penetration of the tumor mosaic by lymphocytes. The neoplastic element is epithelial, not lymphocytic (103,106). Most cases of childhood NPC are relatively undifferentiated epidermoid carcinoma (106,107).

The most common symptoms in 50 patients younger than 16 years of age with NPC evaluated at the University of Istanbul, were neck swelling (68%) and nasal symptoms (66%). The clinical examination will disclose cervical lymphadenopathy, a nasopharyngeal mass, and/or cranial nerve palsies (102,108). Metastases to the neck nodes are often bilateral. The route of spread is most commonly to the digastric region and to the anterior and middle cervical nodes of the anterior cervical triangle.

The appropriate diagnostic workup will include (a) cranial CT scanning to assess local tumor extent and base of skull involvement, and (b) an evaluation for distant metastases with chest radiograph and bone scan. In some cases, cranial MRI will also be useful. CT and MRI often demonstrate mucosal thickening of the maxillary antra. This is generally the result of postobstruction inflammation rather than tumor extension (82). In recent years, PET scans have been used to assess questionable neck nodes. The American Joint Committee for Cancer Staging system (AJCC) is generally used for NPC (Table 3), although some Asian authorities prefer the classification proposed by Ho (101). Three recent series of childhood NPC indicate that almost all children have AJCC stage III or IV disease at presentation: Medical College of Georgia, U.S.: 100% stage IV; Northern Israel Oncology Center, Israel: 20% stage III; 80% stage IV; University of Istanbul, Turkey: 87.5% stage IV (96,109,110).

Surgical therapy of the primary tumor is limited to biopsy (111). Tumors of this region are generally regarded as unresectable. The initial diagnostic biopsy may also be obtained from a neck node. Surgical treatment of the neck with a radical neck dissection is appropriate if the primary tumor appears to be controlled and there are persistent neck nodes after neck irradiation, or if tumor recurs in the neck after definitive radiotherapy (18,59,112–114). Many clinicians use planned excision of bulky nodes after an initial treatment with irradiation and chemotherapy. This philosophy is predicated on the view that large aggregates of tumor are unlikely to be controlled by tolerable doses of cytotoxic therapy alone.

Radiation therapy is the principal management of the primary tumor and neck disease. In preparation for radiotherapy, dental evaluation and institution of a vigorous program of dental prophylaxis is necessary. Because portions of the hypothalamic pituitary axis are irradiated, baseline neuroendocrine testing is performed. The inclusion of portions of the auditory apparatus in the beam, as well as the common use of cis-platinum, argues for baseline audiograms.

Precision external beam radiotherapy for childhood NPC calls for a customized face mask stabilization device. A bite block should be considered to move part of the tongue and floor of the mouth away from the beam. The anatomy of the primary tumor volume is established by physical examination and diagnostic imaging studies. As a minimum, the anatomic limits of the nasopharynx are irradiated with a margin. The anatomy of the nasopharynx, pertinent to the design of an external radiotherapy field, is precisely detailed by Professor C. C. Wang:

TABLE 3. *Staging system for carcinoma of the nasopharynx*[a]

Primary tumor

Tis	Carcinoma *in situ*
T1	Tumor limited to one subsite
T2	Tumor invades more than one subsite
T3	Extension into nasal cavity or oropharynx
T4	Invasion of skull, cranial nerve involvement, or both

Nodes

Nx	Regional nodes cannot be assessed
N0	No regional lymph node metastases
N1	Single positive homolateral node 3 cm or less in greatest dimension
N2	Single clinically positive homolateral node more than 3 but not more than 6 cm in diameter or multiple positive homolateral nodes, none more than 6 cm in diameter; or in bilateral or contralateral lymph nodes, none more than 6 cm in greatest dimension
N2A	Single positive homolateral node more than 3 cm but not more than 6 cm in diameter.
N2B	Multiple positive homolateral nodes, none more than 6 cm in diameter
N2C	Metastasis in bilateral or contralateral nodes, none more than 6 cm in diameter
N3	Metastasis in a lymph node more than 6 cm in greatest dimension

Distant metastases

MX	Requirements to assess presence of distant metastases cannot be met
M0	No known distant metastases
M1	Distant metastases

Stage

0	TisN0M0
I	T1N0M0
II	T2N0M0
III	T1–T3, N0–N1, M0
IV	T4, N0–N1, M0 or T1–T4, N2–N3, M0 or T1–T4, N0–N3, M1

[a] From ref. 31, with permission.

Anatomically, the nasopharynx is a cubical chamber that has four walls. The superior and posterior walls are bordered by the base of the skull and floor of the sphenoid sinus, sloping downward continuously to the second cervical vertebra at the level of the uvula. The lateral walls are perforated by the cartilaginous portion of the eustachian tube, which enters the nasopharynx through the sinus of Morgagni. The latter is a gap between the uppermost fibers of the superior pharyngeal constrictor muscle and the base of the skull. The gap is closed by a fascia known as the pharyngobasilar fascia, which is attached to the base of the skull superiorly and passes inferiorly deep to the constrictor muscles. The raised anterior portion of the cartilaginous portion of the eustachian tube is termed the torus tubularis, lying posteriorly to the eustachian tube orifice. The lateral nasopharyngeal recess or the fossa of Rosenmüller lies posterosuperiorly to the torus. The inferior wall of the nasopharynx is the dorsal surface of the soft palate and its posterior portion opens into the oropharynx at the isthmus.

The nasopharyngeal structures are supported by the pharyngobasilar fascia, which is continuous with the foramen lacerum and in close proximity with the eustachian tube and foramina in the base of the skull, including the ovale, spinosum, carotid, jugular, and hypoglossal, which provide routes of direct tumor intracranial extension and access to the carotid canal, middle ear, and petro-occipital suture. Other routes of tumor spread may occur into the nasal cavity anteriorly and the oropharynx posteriorly (105).

Simulation will be facilitated by the use of radiopaque markers on palpable neck nodes and the fleshy outer canthi of the eyes. Younger children will express concern about having lead wires taped to the skin or near the eyes. This is readily dealt with by calm reassurance and demonstration of the technique on a parent or other adult.

The incidence of neck node disease at presentation is 80% to 90%; 50% of cases having bilateral neck involvement (97). Because node disease is so common, radiotherapy is always directed to the primary tumor site and the neck—even if the neck is clinically free of disease. The extent of the radiation dose-response relationship for NPC in children is debatable (115)–particularly in light of the growing use of chemotherapy. In general, if conventional 1.8- to 2-Gy per day fractionation is used, 40 to 50 Gy is delivered to the primary tumor and the upper neck with parallel opposed fields. The clinically uninvolved low anterior neck and paraclavicular region receives 45 to 50 Gy. The field then excludes the spinal cord; and with lateral fields, arcs, or three-field technique, an additional 10 to 25 Gy is given to the primary tumor and palpable nodes (100,116). Some clinicians use a cesium-137 brachytherapy application in an ovoid or a pediatric endotracheal tube for a final boost of 5 to 9 Gy to the primary site. Others use an oscillating iridium-192 in a remote afterloading brachytherapy machine. Bulky neck nodes are boosted with photons or electrons. The final total dose to the primary tumor is 50 to 72 Gy (104,117). The spinal cord dose is limited to less than or equal to 45 to 50 Gy, the brain stem to less than or equal to 45 to 55 Gy; and the optic chiasm to less than or equal to 45 to 55 Gy. Involved neck nodes receive a similar dose to the primary tumor, although, as previously noted, many physicians prefer surgical resection to high-dose boosting of neck nodes (98,108,118–121). Utilizing doses of this size, local tumor control of childhood NPC is excellent (101,104). However, the radiotherapist is well-advised not to be complacent. Inadequate attention to tumor volume mapping and insufficient attention to field and block design in this complex anatomical area can lead to tumor relapse due to a marginal miss (104). On occasion, the patient with local relapse can be salvaged with re-irradiation.

In an attempt to capitalize on the apparent benefits of multiple-fraction-per-day (MFD) irradiation, some clinicians treat adults with advanced NPC with 2 or 3 fraction per day irradiation. Many authorities on adult radiotherapy consider MFD irradiation the "standard of care" for advanced NPC. In the b.i.d. technique, 1.2 to 1.6 Gy is used per fraction. The possibility must be considered that MFD irradiation may provide good local control for childhood NPC with diminution in undesirable late effects. This hypothesis may warrant testing in pilot studies in children.

In Table 4, we summarize the results of treatment of NPC in children. Prognosis appears to be related directly to T stage (116). The N stage is not a significant influence on survival independent of T stage. This is undoubtedly because of the high incidence of neck disease (104). Survival in modern series is 50% to 80%; many of the treatment failures are in distant sites—particularly bone. The incidence of distant failures increases with increasing N stage (104,122). Exceptionally good results with chemotherapy plus irradiation suggest that planned adjuvant chemotherapy, which may be given before, during, and/or after irradiation, may now be indicated in T3 or T4 disease (96,104,107,109,110,115,116,123,124). A randomized prospective trial conducted jointly by several adult oncology cooperative groups, found that progression-free survival was superior for radiotherapy (70 Gy/35 fractions/7 weeks) plus cisplatin and 5-FU to that achieved with radiotherapy alone. Two-year survival was 80% for radiation plus chemotherapy versus 55% for radiation alone ($p = 0.0007$).

By necessity, the radiotherapy fields for NPC will include a portion of the hypothalamic-pituitary axis. Radiotherapy for NPC is associated with decreases, at long-term follow-up, in serum values of growth, follicle-stimulating, and leutinizing hormones as well as prolactin and cortisol levels. The serum TSH level may rise. How often these changes in serum hormone levels are of clinical significance is not clear (98,104). Xerostomia, neck atrophy, and dentition problems are other potential late effects.

Other Nasopharyngeal Neoplasms

A wide variety of neoplasms can arise in, or project into, the nasopharynx. These in-

TABLE 4. *Survival in childhood nasopharyngeal carcinomas*

Year of report (Ref.)	Number of cases	Treatment[a]	Survival		
			T1–T2	Combined	T3–T4
1973 (73)	7	R + Cy		7/7	
1974 (239)	1	R or R-RND		1/1	
1974 (106)	9	R or R + Cy		5/9	
1974 (242)	1	R or R - Ch		0/1	
1976 (108)	10	R or R - Ch	2/2		4/8
1975,1977 (87,103)	7	R or R + RND		4/7	
1977 (142)	22	R	11/22		
1978 (245)	83	R	8/15		20/63
1980 (98)	39	R or R + Ch		45% at 3 yr	
1980 (246)	16	R	2/6		0/10
1980 (247)	25	R	8/12		5/13
1981 (121)	103	R ± Ch	30/41		23/62
1987 (118)	10	R	2/2		2/8
1982 (240)	20	R ± CAV	7/8		1/12
1983 (242)	27	R	8/11		6/16
1984 (243)	17	R	3/9		0/8
1985 (244)	21	R + Ch		10/21	
1986 (248)	10	R		4/10	
	12	R + Ch		9/10	
1986 (249)	18	R ± Ch		7/18	
1987,1988 (116,124)	15 (T3–4)	R		20% 5 yr RFS[b]	
	12 (T3–4)	R + Ch		75% 5 yr RFS[b]	
1988 (100)	67	R		43 (64%) 5 yr	
1989 (104)	27	R ± Ch	9/10		6/17
1989 (107)	7	R + CAV/5FU			7/7
1990 (122)	57	R ± Ch	61%	49%	
1994 (109)	10	R or R + cisDDP/5FU		8/10	
1994 (110)	1 (T1–2)	R or		63% 5 yr DFS[b]	
	9 (T3–4)	R + CAV or R + cisDDP/5FU or R + ABVD or R + cisDDP/5FU/ABVD or R + Bleo/5FU or		54% 10 yr DFS[b]	
1996 (96)	13 (T1–2)	R or		R:47% 10y FFS[b]	
	35 (T3–4)	R + cisDDP/5FU or		R then Ch: 54% 5y FFS[b]	
		R + Bleo/cisDDP/Epi		Ch then R:72% 3y FFS	
1996 (97)	6 Stage IV	R + cisDDP/5FU or R + Cy/cisDDP		83% 5y a[b]	
1997 (115)	1 (T1–2)	R or		4/5	
	4 (T3–4)	R + BACON R + UICC2 or R + UICC/V			

[a]Abbreviations for radiotherapy, surgery, and chemotherapy: R, radiotherapy; Cy, cyclophosphamide; R-RND, radical neck dissection for relapse; Ch, chemotherapy, not otherwise specified; CAV, cyclophosphamide, doxorubicin, vincristine; 5FU, 5-fluorouracil; cisDDP, cisplatin; Bleo, bleomycin; Epi, epirubicin, UICC2, bleomycin, methotrexate, cisplatin, vinblastine; V, vincristine; ABVD, adriamycin, bleomycin, vinblastine, DTIC.
[b]Abbreviations for statistics: RFS, relapse-free survival; DFS, disease-free survival; FFS, failure-free survival.

clude germ cell tumors such as teratomas and, rarely, endodermal sinus tumors (125–128). In addition, there are gliomas, hemangiomas, congenital rhabdomyomas, and hematomas. The radiotherapist may be asked to participate in the management of nasopharyngeal rhabdomyosarcoma, Hodgkin's disease, or non-Hodgkin's lymphoma (129). In addition, nasopharyngeal projections of chordoma or craniopharyngioma may necessitate irradiation. These latter neoplasms are considered in their respective chapters.

Esthesioneuroblastoma/Olfactory Neuroblastoma

Esthesioneuroblastoma (ENB) is a rare tumor of neural crest origin arising from the olfactory epithelium of the superior nasal cavity close to the cribriform plate (130–133). It was first described in the French literature in 1924 as "l'esthesioneuroepitheliome olfactif" (134). The histologic features of the tumor include neuroepithelial cells arranged in pseudorosettes (called *olfactory rosettes* by some), a surrounding stroma of undifferentiated nuclei and fibrillary cords, palisading of neuroepithelial cells around blood vessels, few miotic figures, and interstitial calcification (131,132,135). Tumors may be separated into low and high grade—a distinction that may be of prognostic importance in predicting 5-year survival in the Mayo Clinic series (low vs. high grade, 62% vs. 25%) (136). Some centers find histologic grading of no use (137). The clinical presentation may include nasal obstruction, facial pain, recurrent epistaxis, loss of smell, proptosis, diplopia, lethargy or syncope (105,137).

There is a slight male predominance (131,132,135). The tumor has been reported in all age groups. Elkan et al. found a bimodal age distribution, with peaks in the 11- to 20-year range and the 51- to 60-year range (138).

ENB presents as an intranasal, nasopharyngeal, and/or paranasal soft-tissue mass. The ethmoid and maxillary sinuses are most frequently involved. Bone destruction is common. Intracranial extension of the tumor can occur. Neck node involvement has been reported as ranging from 10% to 50% (130,132,133,135,136). Patients are grouped according to the method of Kadish, Goodman, and Wang (105,135): group A patients have a tumor confined to the nasal cavity, group B patients have a tumor involving the nasal cavity and paranasal sinuses; and group C patients exhibit tumor spread beyond the nasal cavity and paranasal sinuses. A litera-

ture review by Broich et al. found 18% of cases were group A, 32% were group B, and 49% were group C (62). There are several other staging systems in use (137).

The mainstays of therapy are surgery and radiotherapy (Table 5). Group A and B disease has been treated by resection alone. The local recurrence rate, however, is 45% to 100% (135,136,139). Most authorities, therefore, recommend a combination of surgery and radiotherapy for group A disease (except for small low-grade lesions) and, even more strongly, for groups B and C (136).

The surgical procedure usually begins with a lateral rhinotomy followed, as necessary, by maxillectomy, ethmoidectomy, and sphenoidectomy for tumor excision (105). Frequently, a combined otorhinolaryngology/neurosurgical procedure of craniofacial resection is necessary for adequate tumor excision (133,140). In a craniofacial resection a frontal craniotomy is combined with a lateral rhinotomy or midfacial degloving for an en bloc resection, which may include tumor, cribriform plate, olfactory bulbs, medial maxillae, septum, fovea ethmoidalis, ethmoid air cells, and anterior cranial fossa dura. A defect engendered by a dural resection can be repaired with a pericranial flap or fascia grafts. The nasal defect may be repaired with a split-thickness skin graft (137). Unequivocal complete surgical extirpation of ENB is rarely achieved in advanced cases and local tumor control with surgery alone is poor, therefore, the need to combine surgery with irradiation (136). Some authorities favor using radiation postoperatively to allow (a) assessment of surgical margins unimpeded by prior therapy, (b) establishment of sinus drainage, and (c) intraoperative evaluation of tumor anatomy prior to radiotherapy (105,130,135). Proponents of postbiopsy but predefinitive surgery irradiation argue that the tumor is best treated prior to extensive manipulation to improve the resection and that preoperative radiation may decrease wound seeding by tumor (133). Some physicians favor preoperative chemotherapy. Patients who respond well to chemotherapy receive high-dose irradiation—

TABLE 5. *Recent clinical reports concerning the treatment of esthesioneuroblastoma: combined pediatric + adult series*

Year of report	Reporting institution (Ref.)	Number of patients	Kadish stage distribution, if known	Follow-up	Survival
Management with surgical resection alone					
1993	Mayo Clinic (136)	22	A 2 B 10 C 9 D 1	Median is ~7.3 years	5 yr survival 81% 5 yr disease-free survival 68%
Management with major surgical resection + radiation therapy ± chemotherapy					
1993	Mayo Clinic (136)	16	A 0 B 1 C 13 D 2	Median is ~7.3 years	5 yr survival 69% 5 yr disease-free survival 64%
1994	University of Virginia (140)	23 (most received surgery, radiotherapy, and chemotherapy)	A or B 9 C 14	Most have minimum follow-up of 5 years	5 yr survival 89% 10 and 15 yr survival 74%
1994	University Hospital St. Rafael, Leuven, Belgium (250)	2 (neither received chemotherapy in the initial management)	C 2	3 yr, 11.5 yrs	2/2 were disease-free survivors
1996	Christie Hospital, Manchester UK (251)	3	A 1 C 2	Average follow-up is ~2 yrs	2/3 DOD 1/3 NED but died of intercurrent disease
1996	Helsinki University Central Hospital, Finland (252)	11 (2 received chemotherapy)	A 1 B 1 C 9	Median follow-up is 5.25 yrs	5/11 NED 4/11 DOD 1/11 died of intercurrent disease
1996	Baylor University, Houston, TX, USA (137)	9 (No chemotherapy)		6 mo–9 y	5/9 NED
Management with biopsy and radiation therapy ± chemotherapy					
1994	University Hospital St. Rafael, Leuven, Belgium (250)	5 (none received chemotherapy in the initial management)	C 5	6 months to 12 yrs	2/5 NED at 5 yrs; one of the NED survivors died of intercurrent disease at 6 yrs
1996	Christie Hospital, Manchester UK (132)	3 (none received chemotherapy in the initial management)	B 1 C 2	Average follow-up is ~6 yrs	2/3 NED 1/3 AWD
1997	Massachusetts General Hospital, Boston, MA, USA (253)	5 (Etoposide + Cisplatin)	Not stated	~14 mo	This report includes esthesio-neuroblastoma (5 cases) and neuroendocrine carcinoma (4 cases). Most patients responded to initial chemotherapy.

potentially avoiding extensive surgery (141). Both approaches are defensible, and the sparse data do not support one view over the other.

The establishment of local control of ENB appears to require a higher dose of irradiation than is required for neuroblastomas in general. Doses of 50 to 60 Gy at 1.8 to 2 Gy per fraction, in combination with surgery, are generally recommended (105,130,133,136). As with other nasal/nasopharyngeal/paranasal sinus tumors, treatment planning based on sophisticated imaging, computerized dosimetry, and rigid head immobilization is crucial. A commonly used plan involves a heavily weighted anterior field with two lateral wedged fields. The anterior cranial fossa and cribriform plate are included in the field. Careful attention is necessary in order to protect the pituitary, optic chiasm, and globes if the tumor position allows.

Several centers believe there is a role for chemotherapy in ENB. Vincristine plus cyclophosphamide, cisplatin plus 5-fluorouracil, and cisplatin plus etoposide have been given prior to or following surgery and radiotherapy. Tumor responses have been seen, and some retrospective data have been brought to bear, arguing that survival has been favorably influenced (6,141,142). Some patients with relapsed ENB have been successfully treated with high-dose chemotherapy and autologous bone marrow transplantation (140).

It is generally stated that with a risk of cervical nodal disease of 20% in most series, prophylactic neck dissection or irradiation is not indicated (105,135). This proposition may be arguable in children who appear to have more advanced and aggressive disease than their elders (143). Relapse in cervical lymph nodes is frequent (136,140). Recently, the role of elective neck dissection or radiation to the neck in advanced cases has been discussed (137). At the least, radiotherapy fields should be generous and the threshold for biopsy of suspicious neck nodes should be low. Combined adult/pediatric series report a 90% to 96% survival for group A, 80% for group B, and 50% to 80% for group C (105,133,136,139) (Table 5).

Malignancies of the Oral Cavity, Oropharynx, Hypopharynx, and Larynx; Salivary Gland Tumors

Squamous cell carcinoma of the head and neck rarely occurs in children (144,145). Epidermoid cancers constituted only 2.5% of the 388 head and neck cancers in children seen at the Institut Gustave-Roussy from 1975 to 1987 (146). They constituted 5.8% of head and neck tumors seen at Saint Sofia Children's Hospital in Athens (147). Some pediatric cases may be related to smoking, tobacco chewing, or passive smoking. Chronic irritation by dental caries and/or poor oral hygiene may contribute to a malignant change. Other proposed causal factors include oral viral infections, xeroderma pigmentosa (particularly for lip cancer), and a genetic predisposition (i.e., a past history of hereditary retinoblastoma) (148).

Children have been reported to develop squamous cell carcinoma of the lip, floor of the mouth, buccal mucosa, tongue, tonsil, palate, hypopharynx, and larynx (149,150). There is nothing to suggest that the clinical presentation or routes of spread of childhood head and neck cancer differs substantially from adults.

Therapeutic guidelines mimic those for adults. One seeks to control the primary site and the routes of tumor spread in the neck with either surgery, radiotherapy, or both. Considerations for reasonable cosmesis, preservation of swallowing, quality of voice, and the long-term consequences of radiation play a role in the selection of therapy (148–151).

Series of salivary gland tumors in children have been reported by the Memorial Sloan-Kettering Cancer Center in New York and by the M.D. Anderson Cancer Center in Houston (152,153). Pleomorphic adenoma is the most common benign lesion. Of the malignant neoplasms, mucoepidermoid carcinoma is the most common. Acinic cell carcinoma, adenocarcinoma, and adenoid cystic carcinoma have also been reported. These lesions usually present with a mass. The mainstay of therapy is surgical excision (153,154). The indications for radiotherapy include (a) high-grade primary malignancy, (b) cervical metastases, (c) positive margins, (d) gross postoperative residual tumor, (e) aggressive histologic findings such as the perineural invasion typical of adenoid cystic carcinoma, (f) vascular or lymphatic invasion, (g) local extraglandular soft-tissue extension, or (h) inoperability (152).

Facial nerve involvement can occur with parotid neoplasms. In some cases, resection of some branches or the main trunk of the facial nerve may be necessary. Facial nerve grafting may be used to restore deficits. Occult nodal metastases in the neck are rare, and neither elective neck dissection nor irradiation is routinely indicated (152,153). Local tumor control is highly associated with the absence of aggressive features such as nodal metastases, local extraglandular tumor extension, and/or perineural, perivascular, or perilymphatic invasion.

Rhabdomyosarcoma of the larynx may occur in childhood (155). Its management is discussed in Chapter 11. Involvement of the mucosal surfaces of the upper respiratory tract by acquired immune deficiency syndrome (AIDS) associated Kaposi's sarcoma may cause pain, hemorrhage, or airway obstruction (156). Doses of 20 to 25 Gy, in 2 to 2.5 weeks, will often produce a satisfactory response.

Infantile Subglottic Hemangiomas

Infantile subglottic hemangiomas (ISHs) are rare lesions. There is a 2:1 female to male predominance and 80% to 90% present before the age of 6 months. The most common symptoms are respiratory distress (inspiratory stridor), a hoarse cry, cough, dysphagia, cyanosis, emesis, and hemoptysis. Cutaneous hemangiomas occur in 44% to 51% of these patients. The diagnosis is usually made by direct laryngoscopy (69,157,158).

Spontaneous regressions have occurred, but are infrequent. The low rate of spontaneous regression is the impetus for more definitive therapy. Many forms of treatment have been proposed: CO_2 laser, intralesional steroid injection, cryotherapy, systemic steroids, injection of sclerosants, tracheostomy alone or in combination with other treatments, surgical excision, external beam irradiation, and Au^{198} or P^{32} have been used alone or in combination (65,69,157–163).

Tracheostomy and observation for the involution of the hemangioma is considered by many to be the standard of care. A drawback of this therapy is that it may affect speech and language development. Some clinicians advocate the use of the CO_2 laser to remove subglottic hemangiomas. Subglottic stenosis, however, is a recognized possible complication of this approach. Small, circumscribed lesions can be treated by surgical excision. Intralesional steroids as therapy is advocated by some.

Because of concerns about the development of secondary malignancy (particularly thyroid) and deleterious effects of radiation on growth and development of the larynx, radiotherapy is rarely used (150). In 1919, New and Clark (164) applied radium outside the larynx for ISH and reported good results. They reported that radium "is specific for all true vascular growths of the larynx, as well as other parts of the body." Others have also reported treatment with brachytherapy (65,159,160). Using endolaryngeal microsurgical technique, a Au^{198} seed is inserted into a submucosal pocket below and medial to the edge of the true vocal cord. Seed position is checked by a postoperative radiograph or xeroradiogram. Responses occur over 1 to 2 months. Beta ray brachytherapy with P^{32} has also been tried (162).

The cure rate with external radiotherapy used alone or in combination with tracheostomy is approximately 80%. Between 3.5 and 5 Gy at 0.5 to 1.5 Gy per fraction is used (98). Advocates of irradiation point out its generally satisfactory and reliable results and raise concerns of late scarring with laser surgery. When dealing with a life-threatening situation, one should be prepared to use irradiation if other treatment modalities are either inapplicable or unsuccessful (165). Radiotherapy will, however, rarely be used.

Esophagus

Esophageal carcinoma may develop in adolescents—it may arise spontaneously, years following lye ingestion in the setting of Barrett's esophagus, and, in one reported case, in association with Cornelia de Lange syndrome (166–170). Both squamous cell carcinoma and adenocarcinomas have been reported. They are managed similarly to adults (171). The rare case of esophageal sarcoma (leiomyosarcoma, carcinosarcoma, malignant schwannoma) may be treated with pre- or postoperative irradiation (172). Palliative radiotherapy is occasionally necessary for leukemia or secondary or primary lymphomatous infiltration of the esophagus (173,174). Other rare esophageal neoplasms include leiomyoma, desmoid, and teratoma (175–177).

Lung

A variety of rare primary lung and pleural tumors occur in children, including pleuropulmonary blastoma, endobronchial adenomas (carcinoids, cyclindromas, and mucoepidermoid tumors), mesothelioma, mesenchymal sarcoma, branchioalveolar carcinoma, lymphoepithelioma and bronchogenic carcinoma (squamous cell carcinoma, adenocarcinoma, undifferentiated large-cell carcinoma and small cell carcinoma) (34,53,178–190). The most common presenting symptoms are cough, hemoptysis, dyspnea, and fever.

The pleuropulmonary blastoma is a rare primary malignancy of the lung and pleura. It is thought to originate from pluripotent primitive blastermal cells. The tumor contains mesenchymal and epithelial cellular components. It morphologically mimics the embryonal structure of the lung (18,188,191–193). Most cases are initially managed with surgery. The tumors are often large and locally extensive, making complete surgical excision infrequent (192,194). Local recurrence and distant metastases (brain, liver, and bone) are common among patients with tumors larger than 5 cm in diameter (188). Thoracic irradiation has been used for the postoperative treatment of patients with large tumors and/or positive margins (30 to 55 Gy) (194). One should also consider radiotherapy for the treatment of local tumor recurrence, where the situation is grim but not hopeless (188,194). Chemotherapy has shown some promise as adjuvant therapy postoperatively and for preoperative tumor reduction. Drugs utilized include various combinations of actinomycin D, adriamycin, cyclophosphamide, cisplatin, etoposide, and vincristine (195). A case has been reported in which high-dose chemotherapy with autologous blood stem cell transplantation failed to prevent local recurrence of tumor and death (196).

Endobronchial adenomas are usually slow-growing but possess a low-grade malignant potential. The tumors fill and invade the bronchus and produce obstructive symptoms. The mucoepidermoid, carcinoid, and cylindroid adenomas are increasingly malignant, in that order. Cures are possible with complete resection (190,197). Malignant mesotheliomas rarely occur in childhood. There is rarely a history of asbestos exposure in children (180,198). Radiotherapy may be used for palliative treatment or after an attempted resection with close or positive margins.

Bronchogenic carcinoma occurs in children, arising *de novo* as well as associated with cigarette smoking (184,187,197,199).

Stomach

Non-Hodgkin's lymphoma is the most common malignancy of the stomach in childhood (174). Its management is discussed in Chapter 8. Leiomyosarcoma and leiomyoblastoma are, as a group, the second most common gastric malignancies in children (200–202). The average size of a gastric leiomyosarcoma in childhood is 6 to 7 cm in diameter. Infiltration of tumor to adjacent structures, including the liver or nodal metastasis may occur (203). Therapy of gastric leiomyosarcoma begins with surgery. The operative bed and the upper abdomen are frequent sites of tumor recurrence. Postoperative external-beam irradiation is justifiable when there is a particularly high risk of local recurrence created by positive surgical margins or posterior penetration. The efficacy of adjuvant radiotherapy in this setting, however, is not proven.

Gastric adenocarcinoma is rare in children (174,204). It may occur *de novo* or in association with Peutz-Jegher syndromes (190,205). There is epidemiologic evidence that long-standing *Heliobacter pylori* infection and chronic gastritis are involved in the development of a variety of gastric malignancies including adenocarcinomas, lymphomas, and MALT lymphomas. Acquisition of infection in childhood appears to be a risk factor for development of neoplasia as an adult. There is certainly no evidence at present, however, that the treatment of all *H pylori* infected children would influence the risk of gastric malignancy decades later (206). Rhabdomyosarcoma, Hodgkin's disease, malignant teratoma and nerve sheath tumors also may occur in the stomach. (See Chapters 7, 11, and 12.)

Pancreas

Primary neoplasms of the pancreas are rare in childhood. An infantile type of carcinoma of the pancreas, *pancreatoblastoma,* is characterized by well-formed acinair areas along with squamoid corpuscles and zymogen-like granules. Positive staining by periodic-acid-Schiff, alpha-trypsin, and alpha-keratin are common (207). Many cases have been associated with a high level of alpha-fetoprotein (207,208).

Pancreatoblastoma may behave in a relatively indolent fashion. Localized, non-metastatic tumor that can be resected locally without radical pancreatoduadenectomy may be cured (209). In many cases, unfortunately, the tumor is clearly malignant with local invasion, recurrence, and metastasis. In a review from Memorial Sloan-Kettering Cancer Center, 35% of patients presented with metastases and 42% of evaluable patients died of tumor (207).

A resectable tumor without metastases can be treated with surgery alone. If the tumor secretes AFP, this marker can be used along with CT and ultrasound for follow-up. Radiation therapy has been used to render unresectable tumors resectable, to treat local-regional recurrent tumor, and as postoperative therapy for microscopic disease. A dose on the order of 40 to 50 Gy seems appropriate (208,209). We are aware of one patient successfully treated for recurrent tumor with intraoperative radiation (20 Gy) (208).

A variety of chemotherapy programs have been used in an attempt to shrink unresectable tumors, treat metastastic disease, or as adjuvant therapy. Cyclophosphamide, vincristine, 5-fluorouracil, adriamycin, mitomycin-C, cisplatin, VP-16, ifosfamide, actinomycin D, bleomycin, vinblastine, and epirubicin have been used. Cases are so rare that firm statements regarding the indications and specifics of chemotherapy treatment policy are inappropriate (71,114,208–212).

The adult form of pancreatic adenocarcinoma occurs rarely in children. Abdominal pain, weight loss, an increase in abdominal girth, a palpable abdominal mass, and jaundice are usually presenting signs/symptoms (213). Principles of management are similar to those of adults. Children can tolerate extensive pancreatic resection and still grow and develop. Vejchow reported 9 of 37 children (24%) surviving 1 to 10 years following surgery for pancreatic adenocarcinoma (212).

Appendix

Carcinoids are the most frequently occurring neoplasm of the appendix in children (112,190,214,215). Almost all appendiceal carcinoids are incidental findings in specimens removed because of appendicitis or during abdominal surgery. Metastasis of appendiceal carcinoids to lymph nodes occurs in less than 10% of cases. The risk of metastases is related to tumor size and local invasion (215). Adequate surgical excision is the treatment of choice.

Small Bowel

Non-Hodgkin's lymphoma is the most common malignancy of the small intestine in children (126,216) (see Chapter 8). Small intestine adenocarcinoma develops *de novo* or in association with Peutz-Jeghers syndrome (190). Surgery is the initial treatment. Non-fixed jejunal and ileal lesions are usually treated with surgery alone. As a general rule, radiation therapy should not be used for routine adjuvant treatment of small-bowel carcinoma or sarcomas when the primary tumor is in a mobile part of the small bowel. In the retroperitoneal fixed portions of the duodenum, where local recurrence following surgery is a risk, an argument may be made for postoperative irradiation. Unresectable tumors may be treated with palliative irradiation for pain and bleeding. The survival rate for small-bowel adenocarcinoma is poor.

Sarcomas of the small bowel occur in children. They are treated with surgery. Adjuvant radiation therapy is appropriate when there are close or positive surgical margins (217). Small-intestinal carcinoids are treated surgically (214). Palliative radiation therapy may be used for liver metastases.

Large Bowel

Carcinomas of the colon and rectum in childhood present with pain, vomiting, anemia, a palpable mass, hematochezia, diarrhea, and/or constipation (218,219). Because of the lack of specificity of the symptoms and the rarity of the disease (about one case per million children per year), the possibility of a child having colorectal carcinoma is infrequently considered and the interval between clinical complaints and diagnosis is often long (27,143,174,218,220). In Japan, for example, 1 to 3 colon carcinomas are identified annually (219). These tumors may arise *de novo* or may, in children, be associated with one of the polyposis syndromes such as Gardner's syndrome, Turcot's syndrome, and Peutz-Jeghers syndrome. Carcinoma may also arise in the chronically irritated colon of ulcerative colitis (101,221). It is generally felt that when a carcinoma arises in ulcerative colitis, a total colectomy should be performed. Unfortunately, involvement of regional lymph nodes, distant metastases, and inoperability are frequent in children (141,220). The prognosis for young patients with colon cancer is worse than that for adults. In a review of the Japanese literature of carcinoma of the colon in children younger than 15 years of age, 48% of the identified patients were disease-free survivors (219). This finding has been attributed to a delay in diagnosis resulting in more advanced disease (222,223).

Leiomyosarcoma of the colon has been reported in children. It is curable by surgical resection (224).

Breast

A form of breast cancer, occurring in young girls, is referred to as "juvenile secretory carcinoma." The malignant cells are characterized by abundant secretion of mucin and mucopolysaccharide-containing materials (225). Estrogen and progesterone receptors are generally negative (226). Seashore (227) has suggested that local tumor excision alone may be adequate therapy in juvenile secretory carcinoma. Simple and radical mastectomies have also been used (225,226,228,229). The prognosis is excellent, and no radiotherapy or chemotherapy is generally necessary.

Most cases of adenocarcinoma of the breast in children have a histologic appearance and pattern of spread similar to those in adults (99,223,230). Infiltrating ductal, lobular, and medullary carcinoma have been reported in young girls. With the limited amount of data available in children, we would be cautious about varying from the principles of clinical management set by adult oncology (225, 227,231).

There have been case reports of primary non-Hodgkin's lymphoma, rhabdomyosarcoma, adenoid cystic carcinoma, radiation-induced spindle cell sarcoma, and cystosarcoma phylloides of the breast in children (59,

232–237). Reported breast metastasis in children include hepatocarcinoma, non-Hodgkin's lymphoma, rhabdomyosarcoma, Hodgkin's disease, neuroblastoma, and adenocarcinoma (235).

REFERENCES

References particularly recommended for further reading are indicated by an asterisk.

1. Bradley EL III. Primary and adjunctive therapy in carcinoma of the adrenal cortex. *Surg Gynecol Obstet* 1975;141:507–511.
2. Honour JW, Price DA, Grant DB. Virilizing adrenocortical tumors in childhood. *Pediatrics* 1986;78:547.
3. Jones GS, Shah KJ, Mann JR. Adreno-cortical carcinoma in infancy and childhood: a radiological report of ten cases. *Clin Radiol* 1985;36:257–262.
4. Kirkland JL, Kirkland RT. Tumors of the endocrine glands. In: Fernbach DJ, Vietti TJ, eds. *Clinical pediatric oncology,* 4th ed. St. Louis: CV Mosby, 1991:595–610.
5. Linos DA, Vassilopoulos PP, Papadimitrious J, Tountas K. The surgical management of adrenal cortical carcinoma. *Int Surg* 1986;71:104–106.
6. May CA, Garnett WR. Treatment of adrenocortical carcinoma: a case report and review of the literature. *Drug Intell Clin Pharm* 1986;20:24–32.
7. Michalkiewicz EL, Sandrini R, Bugg MF, et al. Clinical characteristics of small functioning adrenocortical tumors in children. *Med Pediatr Oncol* 1997;28;175–178.
8. Petrus LV, Hall RT, Boechat MI, et al. The pediatric patient with suspected adrenal neoplasm: which radiologic test to use? *Med Pediatr Oncol* 1992;20:53–57.
9. Neblett NW, Frexes-Steed M, Scott HW Jr. Experience with adrenocortical neoplasms in childhood. *Am Surg* 1987;53:117–125.
10. Sipio JC, Rohner TJ Jr, Drago JR. Adrenal cortical carcinoma: case report. *J Surg Oncol* 1986;31:52–55.
11. Stewart DR, Morris-Jones PH, Jolleys A. Carcinoma of the adrenal gland in children. *J Pediatr Surg* 1974;9:59–67.
*12. Mazzaferi EL. Treating differentiated thyroid carcinoma: where do we draw the line? *Mayo Clin Proc* 1991;66:105–111.
13. Magee BJ, Gattameneni HR, Pearson D. Adrenal cortical carcinoma: survival after radiotherapy. *Clin Radiol* 1987;38:587–588.
14. Page DL, DeLellis RA, Hough AJ Jr. *Atlas of tumor pathology, second series, fascicle 23. Tumors of the adrenal.* Washington, DC: Armed Forces Institute of Pathology, 1985:203–207.
15. Chrousos GP. Endocrine tumors. In: Pizzo PA, Poplack DG, eds. *Principles and practice of pediatric oncology.* Philadelphia: JB Lippincott, 1989:733–757.
16. Daneman A, Chan HSL, Martin DJ. Adrenal carcinoma and adenoma in children: a review of 17 patients. *Pediatr Radiol* 1983;13:11–18.
17. Percarpio B, Knowlton AH. Radiation therapy for adrenal cortical carcinoma. *Acta Radiol Ther Phys Biol* 1976;15:288–292.
18. Markoe AM, Serber W, Micaily B, Brady LW. Radiation therapy for adjunctive treatment of adrenal cortical carcinoma. *Am J Clin Oncol (CCT)* 1991;14:170–174.
19. Kasperlik-Zaluska AA, Migdalska BM, Zgliczyinski S, Makowska AM. Adrenocortical carcinoma: A clinical study and treatment results of 52 patients. *Cancer* 1995;75:2587–2591.
20. Zografos GC, Driscoll DL, Karakousis CP, Huben RP. Adrenal adenocarcinoma: a review of 53 cases. *J Surg Oncol* 1994;56:160–164.
21. Haak HR, Hermans J, van de Velde CJH, et al. Optimal treatment of adrenocortical carcinoma with mitotane: results in a consecutive series of 96 patients. *Br J Cancer* 1994;69:947–951.
22. Wooten MD, King DK. Adrenal cortical carcinoma: Epidemiology and treatment with mitotane and a review of the literature. *Cancer* 1993;72:3145–3155.
23. Sloan DA, Schwartz ARW, McGrath PC, Kenady DE. Diagnosis and management of adrenal tumors. *Curr Opin Oncol* 1996;8:30–36.
24. Schweisguth O. *Solid tumors in children.* New York: John Wiley & Sons, 1982.
25. Caty MG, Coran AG, Geagen M, Thompson NW. Current diagnosis and treatment of pheochromocytoma in children: experience with 22 consecutive tumors in 14 patients. *Arch Surg* 1990;125:978–981.
26. Gifford RW, Manger WM, Bravo EL. Pheochromocytoma. *Endocrinol Metab Clin North Am* 1994;23:387-404.
27. Ko WS, Lin LH, Chen DF. Carcinoma of the colon in a child. *Acta Paediatr Sin* 1994;36:227–230.
28. Fonkalsrud EW. Pheochromocytoma in childhood. *Prog Pediatr Surg* 1991;26:103–111.
29. Januszewicz P, Wieteska-Klimczak A, Wyszynska T. Pheochromocytoma in children: difficulties in diagnosis and localization. *Clin Exp Hypertens* 1990;A12(4):571–579.
30. Gagel RF, Tashijian AH Jr, Cummings T, et al. The clinical outcome of prospective screening for multiple endocrine neoplasia type 2a: an 18-year experience. *N Engl J Med* 1988;318:478–484.
31. American Joint Committee for Cancer Staging and End Results and End Results Reporting. *Manual for staging of cancer,* 4th ed. Philadelphia: JB Lippincott, 1992.
32. Gakce O, Gakce C, Gunel S, et al. Pheochromocytoma presenting with headache, panic attacks and jaundice in a child. *Headache* 1991;31:473–475.
33. Raum WJ. Pheochromocytoma. *Curr Ther Endocrinol Metab* 1994;5:172–178.
34. Geiger JD, Thompson NW. Thyroid tumors in children *Otolaryngol Clin North Am* 1996;29:711–719.
35. Loh KC, Shlossberg AH, Abbott EC, Salisbury SR, Tan MH. Phaeochromocytoma: a ten-year survey. *Quat J Med* 1997;90:51–60.
36. Ein SH, Shandling B, Wesson D, Filler RM. Recurrent pheochromocytomas in children. *J Pediatr Surg* 1990;25:1063–1065.
37. Yu L, Fleckman AM, Chadha M, Sacks E, Levetan C, Vikram B. Radiation therapy of metastatic pheochromocytoma: case report and review of the literature. *Am J Clin Oncol* 1996;19:389–393.

38. Blahd WH. Treatment of thyroid cancer. *Compr Ther* 1985;11:26–32.
39. Desjardins JG, Bass J, Leboeuf G, et al. A twenty-year experience with thyroid carcinoma in children. *J Pediatr Surg* 1988;23:709–713.
40. Fjalling M, Tisell L, Carlsson S, Hansson G, Lundberg L, Oden A. Benign and malignant thyroid nodules after neck irradiation. *Cancer* 1986;58:1219–1224.
41. Klopp CT, Rosvoll RV, Winship T. Is destructive surgery ever necessary for treatment of thyroid cancer in children? *Ann Surg* 1967;165:745–750.
42. LaQuaglia MP, Corbally MT, Heller G, Exelby PR, Brennan MF. Recurrence and morbidity in differentiated thyroid carcinoma in children. *Surgery* 1988; 104:1149–1156.
43. McWhirter WR, Masel JP. *Paediatric oncology: an illustrated introduction.* Sydney: Williams & Wilkins, 1987:289–294.
44. Winship T, Rosvoll RV. Childhood thyroid carcinoma. *Cancer* 1961;14:734–743.
45. Ceccarelli C, Pacini F, Lippi F, et al. Thyroid cancer in children and adolescents. *Surgery* 1988;104: 1143–1148.
46. Pizzo PA, Horowitz ME, Poplack DG, Hays DM, Kun LE. Solid tumors in childhood. In: DeVita VT Jr, Hellman S, Rosenberg SA, eds. *Cancer: principles and practice of oncology,* 3rd ed. Philadelphia: JB Lippincott, 1989:1652.
*47. McClellan DR, Francis GL. Thyroid cancer in children, pregnant women, and patients with Graves' disease. *Endocrinol Metab Clin North Am* 1996;25:27–49.
48. Shvero J, Gal R, Avidor I, Hadar T, Kessler E. Anaplastic thyroid carcinoma: a clinical histologic and immunohistochemical study. *Cancer* 1988;62:319–325.
49. Flynn SD, Forman BH, Stewart AF, Kinder BK. Poorly differentiated ("insular") carcinoma of the thyroid gland: an aggressive subset of differentiated thyroid neoplasms. *Surgery* 1988;104:963–970.
50. Hassall E, Dimmick JE, Magee JF. Adenocarcinoma in childhood Barrett's esophagus: case documentation and the need for surveillance in children. *J Gastroenterol* 1993;88:282–288.
51. Duffy BJ Jr, Fitzgerald PJ. Thyroid cancer in childhood and adolescence: report of 28 cases. *J Clin Endocrinol* 1950;10:1296–1308.
52. LoGerfo P, Chabot J, Gazetas P. The intraoperative incidence of detectable bilateral and multicentric disease in papillary cancer of the thyroid. *Surgery* 1990;108:958–963.
53. McCann MP, Fu Y, Kay S. Pulmonary blastoma: a light and electron microscopic study. *Cancer* 1976; 38:789–797.
54. Webb AJ, Brewster S, Newington D. Problems in diagnosis and management of goitre in childhood and adolescence. *Br J Surg* 1996;83:1586–1590.
55. Miller JH, DeClerk YA. Orbit, paranasal sinuses, pharynx, thyroid, and soft tissues of the neck. In: Miller JH, ed. *Imaging in pediatric oncology.* Baltimore: Williams & Wilkins, 1985:116–136.
56. Balter M, Children become the first victims of fallout. *Science* 1996;272:357–360.
57. Becker DV, Robbins J, Beebe GW, Bouville AC, Wachholz BW. Childhood thyroid cancer following the Chernobyl accident. *Endocrinol Metab Clin North Am* 1996;25:197–211.
58. Antonelli A, Miccoli P, Derzhitski VE, Panasiuk G, Solovieva N, Baschieri L. Epidemiologic and clinical evaluation of thyroid cancer in children from the Gomel Region (Belarus). *World J Surg* 1996;20: 867–871.
59. Deodhar SD, Joshi S, Khubchandani S. Cystosarcoma phyllodes. *J Postgrad Med* 1989;35:98–103.
60. Ontai S, Straehley CJ. The surgical treatment of well-differentiated carcinoma of the thyroid. *Am Surg* 1985;51:653–657.
61. Zimmerman D, Hay ID, Gough IR, et al. Papillary thyroid carcinoma in children and adults: long-term follow-up of 1039 patients conservatively treated at one institution during three decades. *Surgery* 1988; 104:1157–1166.
62. Briant TDR, Fitzpatrick PJ, Book H. The radiological treatment of juvenile nasopharyngeal angiofibromas. *Ann Otololaryngol* 1970;79:1108–1113.
63. Beirwaites WH. Controversies in the treatment of thyroid cancer: the University of Michigan approach. *Thyroid Today* 1983;6:1–5.
64. Harbert JC. Radioiodine therapy of differentiated thyroid cancer. In: *Nuclear medicine therapy.* New York: Thieme Medical Publishers, 1987:37–89.
65. Holborow CA, Mott TJ. Subglottic haemangioma in infancy. *J Laryngol Otol* 1973;87:1013–1017.
66. Leeper R. Controversies in the treatment of thyroid cancer: the New York Memorial Hospital Approach. *Thyroid Today* 1982;5:1–4.
67. Buckwalter JA, Thomas CG, Freeman JB. Is childhood thyroid cancer a lethal disease? *Ann Surg* 1975; 181:632–639.
68. Sheline GE, Galante M, Lindsay S. Radiation therapy in the control of persistent thyroid cancer. *AJR* 1966; 97:923–930.
69. Shikhani AH, Marsh BR, Jones MM, Holliday MJ. Infantile subglottic hemangiomas: an update. *Ann Otol Rhinol Laryngol* 1986;95:336–347.
70. Smedal MI, Meissner WA. Results of x-ray treatment in undifferentiated carcinoma of the thyroid. *Radiology* 1961;76:927–935.
71. Tubiana M, Locour J, Mannier JP, et al. External radiotherapy and radio-iodine in the treatment of 359 thyroid cancers. *Br J Radiol* 1975;48:894–907.
72. Fields JN, Halverson KJ, Devinein VR, Simpson JR, Perez CA. Juvenile nasopharyngeal angiofibroma: efficacy of radiation therapy. *Radiology* 1990;176: 263–265.
73. Palmer FJ. Preoperative embolisation in the management of juvenile nasopharyngeal angiofibroma. *Australas Radiol* 1989;33:348–350.
74. Ungkanont K, Byers RM, Weber RS, Callender DL, Wolf PF, Helmuth G. Juvenile nasopharyngeal angiofibroma: an update of therapeutic management *Head Neck* 1996;Jan/Feb:60–66.
75. Briant TDR, Fitzpatrick PJ, Berman J. Nasopharyngeal angiofibroma: a twenty year study. *Laryngoscope* 1978;88:1247–1251.
76. Iannetti G, Belli E, DePonte F, Cicconetti A, Delfini R. The surgical approaches to nasopharyngeal angiofibroma. *J Craniomaxillofac Surg* 1994;22:311–316.
77. Robinson ACR, Khoury GG, Ash DV, Daly BD. Evaluation of response following irradiation of juvenile angiofibromas. *Br J Radiol* 1989;62:245–247.
78. Benghait A. Juvenile nasopharyngeal angiofibroma

treated by radiotherapy. *J Laryngol Otol* 1986;100: 351–356.

*79. Kasper ME, Parsons JT, Mancuso AA, et al. Radiation therapy for juvenile angiofibroma: evaluation by CT and MRI, analysis of tumor regression, and selection of patients. *Int J Radiat Oncol Biol Phys* 1993;25:689–694.

80. Garcia-Cervigan E, Bien S, Rufenacht D, et al. Preoperative embolization of nasopharyngeal angiofibromas: report of 58 cases. *Neuroradiology* 1988;30: 556–560.

81. Jacobsson M, Petruson B, Svedsen P, Berthelsen B. Juvenile nasopharyngeal angiofibroma: a report of eighteen cases. *Acta Otolaryngol* 1988;105:132–139.

82. Apostol JV, Frazell EL. Juvenile nasopharyngeal angiofibroma: a clinical study. *Cancer* 1965;18: 869–878.

83. Economou TS, Abemayor E, Ward P. Juvenile nasopharyngeal angiofibroma: an update of the UCLA experience, 1960–1985. *Laryngoscope* 1988;98: 170–178.

84. Gross M, Gutjahr P. Therapy of rhabdomyosarcoma of the larynx. *Int J Pediatr Otorhinolaryngol* 1988; 15:93–97.

85. Jereb B, Anggard A, Baryd I. Juvenile nasopharyngeal angiofibroma: a clinical study of 69 cases. *Acta Radiol (Ther)* 1970;9:302–310.

86. Makek MS, Andrews JC, Fisch U. Malignant transformation of a nasopharyngeal angiofibroma. *Laryngoscope* 1989;99:1088–1092.

87. Snow JB Jr. Neoplasms of the nasopharynx in children. *Otol Clin North Am* 1977;10:11–24.

88. Ward PH, Thompson R, Calcaterra T, Kadin MR. Juvenile angiofibroma: a more rational therapeutic approach based upon clinical and experimental evidence. *Laryngoscope* 1974;84:2181–2194.

89. Andrews C, Fish U, Valavanis A, et al. The surgical management of extensive nasopharyngeal angiofibromas with infratemporal fossa approach *Laryngoscope* 1989;99:429–437.

90. Chandler JR, Goulding R, Moskowitz L, Quencer RM. Nasopharyngeal angiofibromas: staging and management. *Ann Otol Rhinol Laryngol* 1984;93: 322–329

91. Sessions RB, Bryan R, Naclerio R, Alfred B. Radiographic staging of juvenile angiofibroma. *Head Neck Surg* 1981;3:279–183.

92. Cuyler JP. Treatment options for angiofibroma. *J Otolaryngol* 1988;17:214–218.

93. Kamel RH. Transnasal endoscopic surgery in juvenile nasopharyngeal angiofibroma. *J Laryngol Otol* 1996;110:962–968.

*94. Cummings BJ, Blend R, Keane T, et al. Primary radiation therapy for juvenile nasopharyngeal angiofibroma. *Laryngoscope* 1984;94:1599–1605.

95. McGahan RA, Durrance FY, Parke RB Jr, Easley JD, Chau JL. The treatment of advanced juvenile nasopharyngeal angiofibroma. *Int J Radiat Oncol Biol Phys* 1989;17:1067–1072.

96. Ayan I, Altun M. Nasopharyngeal carcinoma in children: retrospective review of 50 patients. *Int J Radiat Oncol Biol Phys* 1996;35:485–492.

97. Werner-Wasik M, Winkler P, Uri A, Goldwwein J. Nasopharyngeal carcinoma in children. *Med Pediatr Oncol* 1996;26:352–358.

98. Counter RT, Linares L, Shaw HJ, Dalley VM. Cancer of the nasopharynx in under 21-year-olds: a review. *Clin Oncol* 1980;6:213–220.

99. Farrow JH, Ashikari H. Breast cancer in young girls. *Surg Clin North Am* 1969;49:261–269.

100. Gin D, Hu Y, Yan J, et al. Analysis of 1379 patients with nasopharyngeal carcinoma treated by radiation. *Cancer* 1988;61:1117–1124.

101. Tsao SY, Shiu WCT. Radiotherapy and chemotherapy for nasopharyngeal carcinoma. *Ear Nose Throat J* 1990;69:272–278.

102. DelBalso AM, Sweeney AT, Kapur S. An unusual cause of facial trismus in a child: report of case. *J Am Dent Assoc* 1986;112:207–209.

103. Snow JB Jr. Carcinoma of the nasopharynx in children. *Ann Otol* 1975;84:817–826.

104. Pao WJ, Hustu OH, Douglass EC, Beckford NS, Kun LE. Pediatric nasopharyngeal carcinoma: long term follow-up of 29 patients. *Int J Radiat Oncol Biol Phys* 1989;17:299–305.

105. Wang CC. *Radiation therapy for head and neck neoplasms,* 3rd ed. Chicago: Wiley-Liss, 1997.

106. Pick T, Maurer HM, McWilliams NB. Lymphoepithelioma in childhood. *J Pediatr* 1974;84:96–100.

107. Kim TH, McLaren J, Alvardo CS, et al. Adjuvant chemotherapy for advanced nasopharyngeal carcinoma in childhood. *Cancer* 1989;63:1922–1926.

108. Fernandez CH, Camgir A, Samaan N, Rivera R. Nasopharyngeal carcinoma in children. *Cancer* 1976; 37:2787–2791.

109. Arush MB, Stein ME, Rosenblatt E, Lavie R, Kuten A. Advanced nasopharyngeal carcinoma in the young: the Northern Israel Oncology Center experience, 1973–1991. *Pediatr Hematol Oncol* 1995;12: 271–276.

110. Martin WD, Shah KJ. Carcinoma of the nasopharynx in young patients. *Int J Radiat Oncol Biol Phys* 1994;28:991–999.

111. Burkey B, Koopman CF, Brunberg J. The use of biopsy in the evaluation of pediatric nasopharyngeal masses. *Int J Pediatr Otorhinolaryngol* 1990;20: 169–179.

112. Gray GF Jr, Wackym PA. Surgical pathology of the vermiform appendix. In: Sommers SC, Rosen PP, Fechner RE, eds. *Pathology annual,* part 2. Norwalk, CT: Appleton-Century-Crofts, 1986:125–144.

113. Hedlund GL, Bisset GS III, Bove KE. Malignant neoplasms arising in cystic hamartomas of the lung in childhood. *Radiology* 1989;173:77–79.

114. Horie A, Yano Y, Kotoo Y, Miwa A. Morphogenesis of pancreatoblastoma, infantile carcinoma of the pancreas: report of two cases. *Cancer* 1977;39:247–254.

115. Strojan P, Benedik MD, Kragelj B, Jereb B. Combined radiation and chemotherapy for advanced undifferentiated nasopharyngeal carcinoma in children. *Med Pediatr Oncol* 1997;28:366–369.

*116. Gasparini M, Lombardi F, Rottoli L, Ballerini E, Marandi F. Improved relapse free survival with combined radiotherapy and chemotherapy in stage T3-T4 nasopharyngeal carcinoma. *J Clin Oncol* 1988;6: 491–494.

117. Moss WT, Brand WN, Baltifora H. *Radiation oncology: rationale, technique, results.* St. Louis: CV Mosby, 1979.

118. Baker SR, McClathey KD. Carcinoma of the na-

sopharynx in childhood. *Otolaryngol Head Neck Surg* 1987;89:555–559.

119. Chatani M, Teshima T, Inoue T, et al. Radiation therapy for nasopharyngeal carcinoma: retrospective review of 105 patients based on a survey of Kansai Cancer Therapist Group. *Cancer* 1986;57:2267–2271.

120. Haghbin M, Kramer S, Patchefsky AS, Prestipino AJ, Diener-West MD. Carcinoma of the nasopharynx: a 25-year study. *Am J Clin Oncol* 1985;8:334–392.

121. Jenkin RDT, Anderson JR, Jereb B, et al. Nasopharyngeal carcinoma—a retrospective review of patients less than thirty years of age: a report from Children's Cancer Study Group. *Cancer* 1981;47:360–366.

*122. Ingersoll L, Woo SY, Donaldson S, et al. Nasopharyngeal carcinoma in the young: a combined M.D. Anderson and Stanford experience. *Int J Radiat Oncol Biol Phys* 1990;19:881–887.

123. Cangir A. Miscellaneous childhood tumors. In: Fernbach DJ, Vietti TJ, eds. *Clinical pediatric oncology,* 4th ed. St. Louis: Mosby-Year Book, 1991:627–645.

124. Gasparini M, Rottoli L, Ballerini E, Lombardi F. Improved RFS in stage T3-T4 nasopharyngeal carcinoma (NPC) of children with radiotherapy (RT) and ADM + VCR + CTX. *Proc Am Soc Clin Oncol* 1987;6:A864.

125. Aughton DJ, Sloan CT, Milad MP, Huang TE, Michael C, Harper C. Nasopharyngeal teratoma ('hairy polyp'), Dandy-Walker malformation, diaphragmatic hernia, and other anomalies in a female infant. *J Med Genet* 1990;27:788–790.

126. Azab MB, Henry-Amar M, Rougier P, et al. Prognostic factors in primary gastrointestinal non-Hodgkin's lymphoma: a multivariate analysis, report of 106 cases, and review of the literature. *Cancer* 1989;64:1208–1217.

127. Har-El G, Zirkin HY, Tovi F, Sidi J. Congenital pleomorphic adenoma of the nasopharynx: report of a case. *J Laryngol Otol* 1985;99:1281–1287.

128. Tischer W, Reddemann H, Herzog P, et al. Experience in surgical treatment of pulmonary and bronchial tumors in childhood. *Prog Pediatr Surg* 1987;21:118–135.

129. Mallouh A. Nasopharyngeal Hodgkin's disease with intracranial extension in a child. *Med Pediatr Oncol* 1989;17:174–177.

130. Lochrin C. Esthesioneuroblastoma. *Med Pediatr Oncol* 1989;17:433–438.

131. Silva EG, Butler JJ, MacKay B, Goepfert H. Neuroblastomas and neuroendocrine carcinomas of the nasal cavity: a proposed new classification. *Cancer* 1982;50:2388–2405.

*132. Slevin NJ, Irwin CJR, Banerjee SS, Gupta NK, Farrington WT. Olfactory neural tumours—the role of external beam radiotherapy. *J Laryngol Otol* 1996;110:1012–1016.

133. Spaulding CA, Kranyak MS, Constable WC, Stewart FM. Esthesioneuroblastoma: a comparison of two treatment errors. *Int J Radiat Oncol Biol Phys* 1988;15:581–590.

134. Berger L, Lue G, Richard D. L'esthesioneuraepitheliome olfactif. *Bull Assoc Franc Etude Cancer* 1924;13:410–421.

135. Kadish S, Goodman M, Wang CC. Olfactory neuroblastoma: a clinical analysis of 17 cases. *Cancer* 1976;37:1571–1576.

136. Foote RL, Morita A, Ebersold MJ, et al. Esthesioneuroblastoma: the role of adjuvant radiotherapy. *Int J Radiat Oncol Biol Phys* 1993;27:835–842.

137. Fordice JO. Esthesioneuroblastoma. Baylor College of Medicine. Bobby R. Alford Dept. of Otorhinolaryngology and communicative sciences. Internet Site. 1996.

138. Elkon D, Hightower SI, Lim ML, Cantrell RW, Constable WC. Esthesioneuroblastoma. *Cancer* 1979;44:1087–1094.

139. Million RR, Cassini NJ. *Management of head and neck cancer: a multidisciplinary approach.* Philadelphia: JB Lippincott, 1984.

*140. Eden BV, Debo RF, Larner JM, et al. Esthesioneuroblastoma. *Cancer* 1994;73:10:2556–2562.

141. Bhattacharyya N, Thornton AF, Joseph MP, Goodman ML, Amrein PC. Successful treatment of esthesioneuroblastoma and neuroendocrine carcinoma with combined chemotherapy and proton radiation. *Arch Otol Head Neck Surg* 1997;123:34–40.

142. Papvasiliou C, Pavaltou M, Pappas J. Nasopharyngeal cancer in patients under the age of thirty years. *Cancer* 1977;40:2312–2316.

143. Hwang EH, Chung WH. Adenocarcinoma of the transverse colon in a child with survival—a case report. *Kyoemi Med J* 1993;34:287–292.

144. Clayton GW. Tumors of the endocrine glands. In: Sutow WW, Fernbach DJ, Vietti TJ, eds. *Clinical pediatric oncology.* St. Louis: CV Mosby, 1984:744–761.

145. Mendez P Jr, Maves MD, Panje WR. Squamous cell carcinoma of the head and neck in patients under 40 years of age. *Arch Otolaryngol* 1985;111:762–764.

146. Schwaab G, Bouzouita K, Janot F, Flamant F, Lubainski B. Les cancers oral de l'enfant repartition histologique et topographique. Indications therapeutiques (a propos de 380 cas IGR 1975–1987). *Bull Cancer* 1989;76:757–762.

147. Rapidis AD, Economidis J, Goumas PD, et al. Tumours of the head and neck in children: a clinicopathological analysis of 1007 cases. *J Craniomaxillofac Surg* 1988;16:279–286.

148. Usenius T, Karja J, Collan Y. Squamous cell carcinoma of the tongue in children. *Cancer* 1987;60:236–239.

149. Moore C. Visceral squamous cancer in children. *Pediatrics* 1958;21:573–581.

150. New GB, Hertz CS. Malignant disease of the face, mouth, pharynx, and larynx in the first three decades of life. *Surg Gynecol Obstet* 1940;70:163–169.

151. Patel DD, Dave RI. Carcinoma of the anterior tongue in adolescence. *Cancer* 1976;37:917–921.

152. Callender DL, Frankenthaler RA, Luna MA, Lee SS, Goepfert H. Salivary neck neoplasms in children. *Arch Otolaryngol Head Neck Surg* 1992;118:474–476.

153. Castro EB, Huvos AG, Strong EW, Foote FW. Tumors of the major salivary glands in children. *Cancer* 1972;29:312–317.

154. Gustafson H, Dahlquist A, Anniko M, Carlson B. Mucoepidermoid carcinoma in a minor salivary gland in childhood. *J Laryngol Otol* 1987;101:1320–1323.

155. Griffin BR, Wishbeck WM, Schaller RT, Benjamin DR. Radiotherapy for locally recurrent infantile pancreatic carcinoma (pancreato-blastoma). *Cancer* 1987;60:1734–1736.

156. Roy TM, Dow FT, Puthuff DL. Upper airway obstruction from AIDS-related Kaposi's sarcoma. *J Emerg Med* 1991;9:23–25.

157. Meeuwis J, Bas CE, Hoeve LJ, vander Voort E. Subglottic hemangiomas in infants: treatment with intralesional corticosteroid injections and intubation. *Int J Pediatr Otorhinolaryngol* 1990;19:145–150.

158. Remacle M, Declaye X, Mayne A. Subglottic hemangia in the infant: contribution of CO_2 laser. *J Laryngol Otol* 1989;103:930–934.

159. Benjamin B. Treatment of infantile subglottic hemangioma with radioactive gold grain. *Ann Otol* 1978;87: 18–21.

160. Benjamin B, Carter P. Congenital laryngeal hemangioma. *Ann Otol Rhinol Laryngol* 1983;92:448–455.

161. Hertzanu Y, Mendelsohn DB, Davidge-Pitts K, Cohen M. Preoperative embolization in paediatric maxillofacial haemangiomas. *J Laryngol Otol* 1985;99: 1089–1095.

162. Mouzard A, Damalain MN, Chassagne D. Intubation tracheale des angiomas sous-glottiques due nourisson brachytherapie locale du ^{32}P. *Intensive Care Med* 1977;3:186.

163. Seid AB, Pransky SM, Kearns DB. The open surgical approach to subglottic hemangioma. *Int J Pediatr Otorhinolaryngol* 1991;22:85–90.

164. New GB, Clark CM. Angiomas of the larynx. Report of three cases. *Ann Otol Rhinol Laryngol* 1919;28: 1025–1037.

165. D'Angio GJ. Pediatric tumors. In: Perez CA, Brady LW, eds. *Principles and practices of radiation oncology.* Philadelphia: JB Lippincott, 1987:1199–1203.

166. DuVall GA, Walden DT. Adenocarcinoma of the esophagus complicating Cornelia de Lange Syndrome. *J Clin Gastroenterol* 1996;22(2):131–133.

167. Hassoun AAK, Hay ID, Goellner JR, Zimmerman D. Insular thyroid carcinoma in adolescents. *Cancer* 1997;79:1044–1048.

168. Hassall E. Barrett's esophagus: new definitions and approaches in children. *J Pediatr Gastroenterol Nutr* 1993;16:345–364.

169. Isolauri J, Markkula H. Lye ingestion and carcinoma of the esophagus. *Acta Chir Scand* 1989;155: 269–271.

170. Wahrendorf J, Chang-Claude J, Liang QS, et al. Precursor lesions of oesphangeal cancer in young people in a high-risk population in China. *Lancet* 1989; 2:1239–1241.

171. Shahi UP, Sundersan D, DaHagupta S, et al. Carcinoma oesophagus in a 14 year old child: report of a case and review of literature. *Trop Gastroenterol* 1989;10:225–228.

172. Perch SJ, Saffen EM, Whittington R, Brooks JJ. Esophageal sarcomas. *J Surg Oncol* 1991;48:194–198.

173. Bolandi L, DeGiorgia R, Santi V, et al. Primary non-Hodgkin's T-cell lymphoma of the esophagus: a case with peculiar endoscopic ultrasonographic pattern. *Dig Dis Sci* 1990;35:1426–1430.

174. Goldthorn JF, Canizaro PC. Gastrointestinal malignancies in infancy, childhood, and adolescence. *Surg Clin North Am* 1986;66:845–861.

175. Bourque MD, Spigland N, Bensoussan AL, et al. Esophageal leiomyoma in children: two case reports and reviews of the literature. *J Pediatr Surg* 1989; 24:1103–1107.

176. Vade A, Nolan J. Posterior mediastinal teratoma involving the esophagus. *Gastrointest Radiol* 1989;14: 106–108.

177. Wolf Y, Katz S, Lax E, Okon E, Schiller M. Dysphagia in a child with aggressive fibromatosis of the esophagus. *J Pediatr Surg* 1989;24:1137–1139.

178. Curcio LD, Cohen JS, Grannis FW, Paz IB, Chilcote R, Weiss LM. Primary lymphoepithelioma-like carcinoma of the lung in a child. *Chest* 1996; 111:250–251.

179. Gonzalez-Crussi F, Wolfson SL, Misugi K, Nakajima T. Peripheral neuroectodermal tumors of the chest wall in childhood. *Cancer* 1984;54:2519–2527.

180. Gruber B, Kron TK, Goldman ME, Matz GJ. Nasopharyngeal angiofibroma in two young children. *Otolaryngol Head Neck Surg* 1985;93:803–806.

181. Kern WH, Stiles QR. Pulmonary blastoma. *J Thorac Cardiovasc Surg* 1976;72:801–808.

182. Kowalski P, Rodziewicz B, Pejcz J. Bilateral bronchioalveolar carcinoma of the lungs in a 7 year old girl treated for Hodgkin's disease. *Tumor* 1989;75: 449–451.

183. Lodge JPA, Hamilton JRL, Walker DR, Bailey CC. Surgical management of thoracic malignancy in childhood: eight years' experience in Leeds. *Ann R Coll Surg Eng* 1988;70:109–112.

184. Niitu Y, Kubota H, Hasegawa S, Horikawa M, Komatsu S. Lung cancer (squamous cell carcinoma) in adolescence. *Am J Dis Child* 1974;127:108–111.

185. Parikh PM, Charak BS, Banavali SD, et al. Treatment of Askin Rosai tumor—need for a more aggressive approach. *J Surg Oncol* 1988;39:126–128.

186. Pettinato G, Manivel JC, Saldana MJ, Peyser J, Dehner LP. Primary bronchopulmonary fibrosarcoma of childhood and adolescence: reassessment of a low grade malignancy. *Hum Pathol* 1989;20:463–471.

187. Sawyer KC, Sawyer RB, Lubchenco AE, McKinnon DA, Hill KA. Fatal primary cancer of the lung in a teenage smoker. *Cancer* 1967;20:451–457.

188. Senac MO Jr, Wood BP, Isaacs H, Weller M. Pulmonary blastoma: a rare childhood malignancy. *Radiology* 1991;179:743–746.

189. Shankwiler RA, Athey PA, Lamki N. Aggressive infantile fibromatosis: pulmonary metastases documented by plain film and computed tomography. *Clin Imag* 1989;13:127–129.

190. Tovar JA, Eizaguirre I, Albert A, Jimenez J. Peutz-Jeghers syndrome in children: report of two cases and review of the literature. *J Pediatr Surg* 1983;18:1–6.

191. Barnard WG. Embryona of lung. *Thorax* 1952;7: 299–301.

192. Koss MN, Hochholzer L, O'Leary T. Pulmonary blastomas. *Cancer* 1991;67:2368–2381.

193. Merriman TE, Beasley SW, Chow CW, Smith PJ, Robertson CF. A rare tumor masquerading as an empyema: pleuropulmonary blastoma. *Pediatr Pulmonol* 1996;28:408–411.

194. Manivel JC, Priest JR, Walterson J, et al. Pleuro-pulmonary blastoma: the so-called pulmonary blastoma of childhood. *Cancer* 1988;62:1516–1526.

195. Ozkaynak MF, Ortega JA, Laug W, Gilsanz V, Isaacs H Jr. Role of chemotherapy in pediatric pulmonary blastoma. *Med Pediatr Oncol* 1990;18:53–56.

196. Schmaltz C, Sauter S, Opitz O, et al. Pleuro-Pulmonary Blastoma: A Case Report and Review of the Literature. *Med Pediatr Oncol* 1995;25:479–484.

197. deParedes CG, Pierce WS, Groff DB, Waldhausen JA. Bronchogenic tumors in children. *Arch Surg* 1970;100:574–576.

198. Fraire AE, Cooper S, Greenberg SD, Buffler P, Langston C. Mesothelioma of childhood. *Cancer* 1988;62:838–847.

199. DeCaro L, Benfield JR. Lung cancer in young persons. *J Thorac Cardiovasc Surg* 1982;83:372–376.

200. Lavin P, Hajdu SI, Foote FW Jr. Gastric and extragastric leiomyosarcomas: clinicopathologic study of 44 cases. *Cancer* 1972;29:305–311.

201. Mahour GH, Isaacs H Jr, Change L. Primary malignant tumors of the stomach in children. *J Pediatr Surg* 1980;15:603–608.

202. Wright JR Jr, Kyriakos M, DeSchryver-Keeskemeti K. Malignant fibrous histiocytomas of the stomach. *Arch Pathol Lab Med* 1988;112:251–258.

203. Jaeger HJ, Schmitz-Stolbrink A, Albrecht M, Mathias K. Gastric leiomyosarcoma in a child. *Eur J Radiol* 1996;23:111–114.

204. Siegel SE, Hays DM, Romansky S, Isaacs H. Carcinoma of the stomach in childhood. *Cancer* 1976;38:1781–1784.

205. Chatura KR, Nadar S, Pulimood S, Mathai D, Matha M. Gastric carcinoma as a complication of dyskeratosis congenita in an adolescent boy. *Dig Dis Sci* 1996;41:2340–2342.

206. Bourque MD, DiLorenzo M, Collin P-P, Russo P, Laberge J-M, Moir C. Malignant small-cell tumor of the thoracopulmonary region: `Askin tumor.' *J Pediatr Surg* 1989;24:1079–1083.

207. Klimstra DS, Wenig BM, Adair CF, Heffess CS. Pancreatoblastoma: a clinicopathologic study and review of the literature. *Am J Surg Pathol* 1995;19:1371–1389.

208. Murakami T, Ueki K, Kawakami H, et al. Pancreatoblastoma: case report and review of treatment in the literature. *Med Pediatr Oncol* 1996;27:193–197.

209. Willnow U, Willberg B, Schwamborn D, Korholz D, Gobel U. Pancreatoblastoma in children case report and review of the literature. *Eur J Pediatr Surg* 1996;6:369–372.

210. Gudea F, Van Limbergen E, Van Den Bogaert. High dose level radiation therapy for local tumour control in esthesioneurblastoma. *Eur J Cancer* 1994:12;1757–1760.

211. Rich RH, Dehner LP, Okinaga K, Deeb LC, Ulstrom RA, Leonard AS. Surgical management of islet–cell adenoma in infancy. *Surgery* 1978;84:519–526.

212. Vejcho S. Carcinoma of the pancreas in childhood: a case report of long term survival. *J Med Assoc Thai* 1993;76:177–183.

213. Tsukimoto I, Watanabe K, Lin J, Nakajima T. Pancreatic carcinoma in children in Japan. *Cancer* 1973;31:1203–1207.

214. Field JL, Adamson LF, Stoeckle HE. Review of carcinoids in children: functioning carcinoid in a 15-year old male. *Pediatrics* 1962;29:953–960.

215. Moertel CG, Weiland LH, Nagorney DM, Dockerty MB. Carcinoid tumor of the appendix: treatment and prognosis. *N Engl J Med* 1987;317:1699–1701.

216. Tharrington CL, Bossen EH. Nasopharyngeal teratomas. *Arch Pathol Lab Med* 1992;116:165–167.

217. Freeman J. Leiomyosarcoma of small bowel: a case report. *J Pediatr Surg* 1979;14:477–478.

218. Takahoshi H, Hansmann M-L. Primary gastrointestinal lymphoma in childhood (up to 18 years of age). *J Cancer Res Clin Oncol* 1990;116:190–196.

219. Yamamoto K, Tanaka T, Kuno K, Amoh Y, Takahashi Y, Murakami H. Carcinoma of the colon in children: case report and review of the Japanese literature. *J Gastroenterol* 1994;29:647–652.

220. Lamego CMB, Tarlani H. Colorectal adenocarcinoma in childhood and adolescence: report of 11 cases and review of the literature. *Pediatr Radiol* 1989;19:504–508.

221. Pratt CB, Rivera G, Shanks E, et al. Colorectal carcinoma in adolescents: implications regarding etiology. *Cancer* 1977;40:2464–2472.

222. Rose RH, Axelrod DM, Aldea PA, Beck AR. Colorectal carcinoma in the young: a case report and review of the literature. *Clin Pediatr* 1988;27:105–108.

223. Umpleby HC, Williamson RC. Large bowel cancer in the young. *Ann Acad Med Singapore* 1987;16:456–461.

224. Nagaya M, Tsuda M, Ishiguro Y. Leiomyosarcoma of the transverse colon in a neonate: a rare case of meconium peritonitis. *J Pediatr Surg* 1989;24:1177–1180.

225. Dugue G, Back G, Molho L, Cordice JW Jr. Breast cancer in the young. *J Natl Med Assoc* 1989;81:1184–1187.

226. Eskelinen M, Vainio J, Tuominen L, Vihko R, Klemi P, Callan Y. Carcinoma of the breast in children. *Z Kinderchir* 1990;45:52–55.

227. Bower R, Bell MJ, Ternberg JL. Management of breast lesions in children and adolescents. *J Surg* 1976;11:337–346.

228. Sears JB, Schlesinger MJ. Carcinoma of the breast in a ten-year old girl: report of a case. *N Engl J Med* 1940;223:760–761.

229. Taguchi T, Suita S, Hirata Y, Ishii E, Ueda K. Carcinoma of the colon in children: a case report and review of 41 Japanese cases. *J Pediatr Gastroenterol Nutr* 1991;12:394–399.

230. Hildreth NG, Shore RE, Dvoretsky PM. The risk of breast cancer after irradiation of the thymus in infancy. *N Engl J Med* 1989;321:1281–1284.

231. Rosenfield NS, Haller JO, Berdon WE. Failure of development of the growing breast after radiation therapy. *Pediatr Radiol* 1989;19:124–127.

232. Blichert-Taft M, Hansen JPH, Hansen OH, Schiadt T. Clinical course of cysto-sarcoma phyllodes related to histologic appearance. *Surg Gynecol Obstet* 1975;140:929–932.

233. El-Ghazawy IM, Singletary SE. Surgical management of primary lymphoma of the breast. *Ann Surg* 1991;214:724–726.

234. Miliauskas JR, Leong AS-Y. Adenoid cystic carcinoma in a juvenile male breast. *Pathology* 1991;23:298–301.

235. Rogers DA, Lobe TE, Rao BN, et al. Breast malignancy in children. *J Pediatr Surg* 1994;24:48–51.

236. Senocak ME, Gagus S, Hicsanmez A, Buyukpamukcu N. Cystosarcoma phylloides in an adolescent female. *Z Kinderchir* 1989;44:253–254.

237. Squire R, Bianchi A, Jakate SM. Radiation-induced sarcoma of the breast in a female adolescent. *Cancer* 1988;60:2444–2447.

238. Wiatrak BJ, Koopmann CF, Turrisi AT. Radiation therapy as an alternative to surgery in the management of

intracranial juvenile nasopharyngeal angiofibroma. *Int J Pediatr Otorhinolaryngol* 1993;28;51–61.

239. Stier J, Huh C, Lapidot A. Squamous carcinoma of nasopharynx in a child. *Bull NY Acad Med* 1974;49: 610–612.

240. Lombardi F, Gasparini M, Gianni C, DeMarie M, Molinari R, Pilotti S. Nasopharyngeal carcinoma in childhood. *Med Pediatr Oncol* 1982;10:243–250.

241. LaNasa JJ, Putney FJ. Nasopharyngeal malignancy in childhood. *South Med J* 1974;67:1363–1364.

242. Castro-Vita, Mendiondo O, Shaw E, et al. Nasopharyngeal carcinoma in second decade of life. *Radiology* 1983;148:253–256.

243. Morales P, Bosch A, Salaverry S, Correa JN, Martinez I. Cancer of nasopharynx in young patients. *J Surg Oncol* 1984;27:181–185.

244. Sarrazin D, Schwaab G, Fontaine F, Kalifa C, Rich J, Archambault R. La radiotherapie des carcinomes nasopharynx chez l'enfant aprages chimotherapie primable. Resultants preliminaires sur 21 cas traites a l'institut Gustave-Roussy entre 1978 et 1981. *Ann Otolaryngol* 1985;175–178.

245. Ellouz R, Cammoun M, Attia RB, Bahi J. Nasopharyngeal carcinoma in children and adolescents in Tunisia: clinical aspects and the paraneoplastic syndrome. In: de The G, ed. *NPC etiology and control.* WHO-IARC science publication no. 20. WHO-IARC. Lyon: International Agency for Research on Cancer, 1978:115–130.

246. Jereb B, Huvos AG, Steinherz P, Unal A. Nasopharyngeal carcinoma in children. Review of 16 cases. *Int J Radiat Oncol Biol Phys* 1980;6:415–421.

247. Berry CL, ed. *Pediatric pathology.* Berlin: Springer-Verlag, 1981.

248. Lobo-Sanahuja F, Garcia I, Carranza A, Camacho A. Treatment and outcome of undifferentiated carcinoma of the nasopharynx in childhood: a 13-year experience. *Med Pediatr Oncol* 1986;14:6–11.

249. Roper RH, Essex-Cater A, Marsen HB, Dixon PF, Campbell RHA. Nasopharyngeal carcinoma in children. *Pediatr Hematol Oncol* 1986;3:143–152.

250. Grundy GW, Miller RW. Malignant mesothelioma in childhood: report of 13 cases. *Cancer* 1972;30: 1216–1218.

*251. Al-Sarraf M, LeBlanc M, Giri PG, et al. Superiority of chemoradiotherapy (CT-RT) v. radiotherapy (RT) in patients (pts) with locally advanced nasopharyngeal cancer (NPC). Preliminary results of intergroup (0099) (SWOG 8892, RTOG 8817, ECOG 2388) randomized study. *Proc ASCO* 1996;15:A-882,313.

252. Jekuen AP, Kairem KJA, Lehtonen HP, Kajanti MJ. Treatment of olfactory neuroblastoma. *Am J Clin Oncol (CCT)* 1996;19(4);375–378.

253. Bhargava R, Winer-Muram, HT, Kauffman WM, Jennings SG, Pratt CB. Chest radiographic features of thoracic metastatic disease in adolescents with colon cancer. *Pediatr Radiol* 1994;24:491–493.

17

Langerhans' Cell Histiocytosis

HISTORICAL BACKGROUND

The diseases formerly grouped under the heading Histiocytosis X are now referred to as *Langerhans' cell histiocytosis* (LCH) (1). Paul Wilhelm Heinrich Langerhans was born in Berlin in 1847. Both his father and his two brothers were physicians. While still an undergraduate student, Langerhans used Cohnheim's gold chloride staining technique to identify a novel nonpigmentary dendritic cell in the epidermis. He described this finding, when he was 21 years old, in an 1868 paper entitled "Uber die Nerven der menschilichen Haut"—On the nerves of the human skin (2). Langerhans' initially regarded these cells as intraepidermal receptors for extracutaneous signals of the nervous system. He later changed his mind and, in 1882, wrote that "my cells are in no way essential for nerve endings" (3). Later in his career, Langerhans described the fine structure of the pancreas in a research project performed under the supervision of Rudolf Virchow. The groups of cells that Langerhans described are now generally referred to as "Islets of Langerhans" in his honor. Langerhans died in 1888, five days before his 41st birthday, of progressive renal degeneration due to tuberculosis (4).

In 1893, Dr. Alfred Hand, Jr., a 25-year-old resident at the Children's Hospital of Philadelphia, reported the case of a 3-year-old boy with a history of great thirst and polyuria ... undersized and puny." At autopsy, he found a lesion in the skull (5):

"A yellow spot about the size of a five-cent piece was noticed near the right parietal eminence. When the skull-cap was removed, this spot was seen on the inner side as well, and the entire thickness of the bone there was soft and movable.... The lymphatic glands...all through the body were greatly enlarged.... The liver and spleen were enlarged and firm, and the former had minute gray nodules in its substance.... Microscopial sections showed nodular masses of small, round-celled infiltration in the liver, spleen, kidneys...."

Hand suspected that he was dealing with a case of tuberculosis. In 1921, he noted the similarity of his original case to ones subsequently reported by Schuller, Christian, and Kay (6). Eventually, the term Hand-Schuller-Christian disease or triad was used to describe a disease occurring in children over 2 years of age. It was characterized by exophthalmos, lesions in the bones of the skull, and diabetes insipidus. The full triad was rarely seen, and the prognosis was relatively good (7–9).

In 1924 and 1933, the pathologist Letterer and pediatrician Siwe described what they perceived to be an entity distinct from Hand-Schuller-Christian disease. *Letterer-Siwe disease* generally occurred in children under the age of 2. The diagnostic criteria included splenomegaly, hepatomegaly, lymphadenopathy, anemia, and a hemorrhagic diathesis. The prognosis was quite poor (6–9).

In 1940, Otani and Ehrlich (10) described a granuloma of bone simulating a primary neoplasm. The *solitary eosinophilic granuloma* was described, eventually, as occurring in children over 2 years of age and characterized by a solitary, usually bony site of involvement. The prognosis was excellent (8,9).

In 1953, the pathologist Lichtenstein argued that eosinophilic granuloma of bone, Letterer-Siwe disease, and Hand-Schuller-Christian disease were related manifestations of a single nosologic entity (6,9). He used the name *Histiocytosis X* to refer to a spectrum of diseases of the mononuclear phagocyte (histiocyte). The "X" was used to refer to the unknown etiology and pathogenesis of the disease or diseases.

DEFINITION, PATHOGENESIS, PATHOLOGY

The Langerhans' cells are a family of related cells characterized by their dendritic morphology and multiple thin membrane projections. They have a high surface concentration of major histocompatibility complex (MHC) class II molecules. The Birbeck granule, a small tennis racket-shaped cytoplasmic organelle containing a central area that appears opaque on electron microscopy, is often found in Langerhans' cells and is diagnostic for LCH (Fig. 1). The function of the Birbeck granule is unknown. In normal anatomy, Langerhans' cells are found in the epidermis and skin appendages, in squamous mucosal epithelium such as the buccal mucosa, vagina, cervix, and esophagus, and in the spleen and lymphatic system. In normal physiology, the Langerhans' cell is involved in presenting antigens introduced via epithelial surfaces to T cells. These cells cooperate with lymphocytes and enable them to carry out their functions of recognition and elimination of antigens (11,12).

LCH cells cause tissue damage by infiltration and excessive production of cytokines and prostaglandins (13). Cells produce excessive amounts of interleukin-1 (IL-1) and prostaglandin E2, which can cause bone resorption through osteoclast activation. IL-1 may cause release of interleukin-2 (IL-2) and gamma interferon from helper-inducer T lymphocytes, leading to the stimulation of other lymphocytes and histiocytes. Tissue injury occurs from the local immune response as the collection of immune cells impairs normal tissue structure and function (14). On microscopic evaluation, the lesions of LCH are found to be consistent with Hand's original description: a pleomorphic infiltrate of lymphocytes, eosinophils, polymorphonuclear leukocytes, and Langerhans' cells (Fig. 2). A more definitive diagnosis is made when electron microscopy shows Birbeck granules or when light microscopy shows that the Langerhans' cells are ATPase-positive, stain for S-100 protein, CD11 and CD14, anti-CD1 marker (also called the T6 surface marker), alpha-D-mannosidase, and bind peanut lectin (13,15–18).

LCH has been traditionally treated by oncologists (6,19). Until recently, the disease was generally not thought to be monoclonal in origin. It was argued that the individual cells do not show atypia and that the disease lacked the usual histologic criteria for malignancy. LCH was, therefore, generally considered to fall within the realm of reactive immunologic disorders or, perhaps, be of infectious origin. Viral and immune causation theories have, however, been largely bereft of supporting evidence. In 1994, Williman et al., provided evidence that LCH is a clonal proliferative disorder. These investigators studied ten lesions from patients with LCH and found that they all contained clonal populations of cells. The proportion of clonal cells corresponded to the proportion of lesional Langerhans-like cells, whether from solitary lesions or extensive multisystem disease. (20,20a) Yu et al. reported similar findings by flow sorting CD1a positive cells from three patients (20b). The hypothesis that LCH arises from somatic mutation of DNA in a normal Langerhans' or precursor cell must be considered (22).

The evidence for a genetic mutation or mutations leading to LCH is circumstantial. Patients with multiorgan LCH are, on average, younger than those with single bone disease. In those rare instances of familial LCH, all the affected members have multiorgan disease. These two observations, reminiscent of the pattern of heritable versus nonheritable retinoblastoma, suggested to Egeler the possibility of LCH's behavior being explicable by

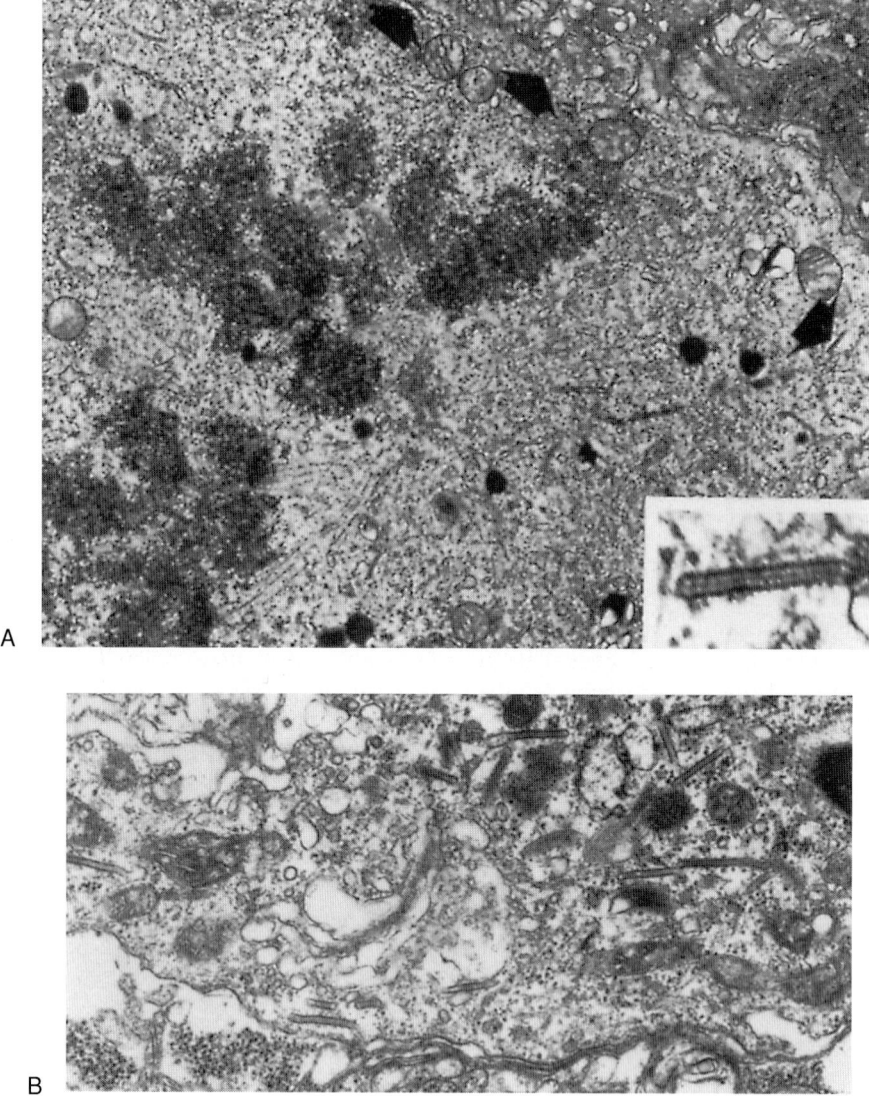

FIG. 1. A: The Birbeck granule is a small rod- or tennis racket-shaped cytoplasmic organelle found in Langerhans' cells. It is diagnostic for LCH. In this transmission electron micrograph (×11,500; inset ×70,100) a granule is shown in the inset and marked by arrows in the larger picture. (From ref. 109, with permission.) **B:** A group of Birbeck granules are seen in the cytoplasm of a normal Langerhans' cell of human epidermis. Some of the granules have a "drumstick" configuration. (×41,600). (From ref. 110, with permission.)

the Knudson's "two hit hypothesis" and a tumor suppressor gene (23,24). (The "two hit" hypothesis is discussed in detail in Chapter 5.)

The distinction between calling LCH malignant or considering it a reactive immuno-logic disorder bears consideration. Classification has significant consequences for how the clinician thinks about and manages the disease. If one carries in their mind the notion that LCH is primarily a malignancy, then ra-

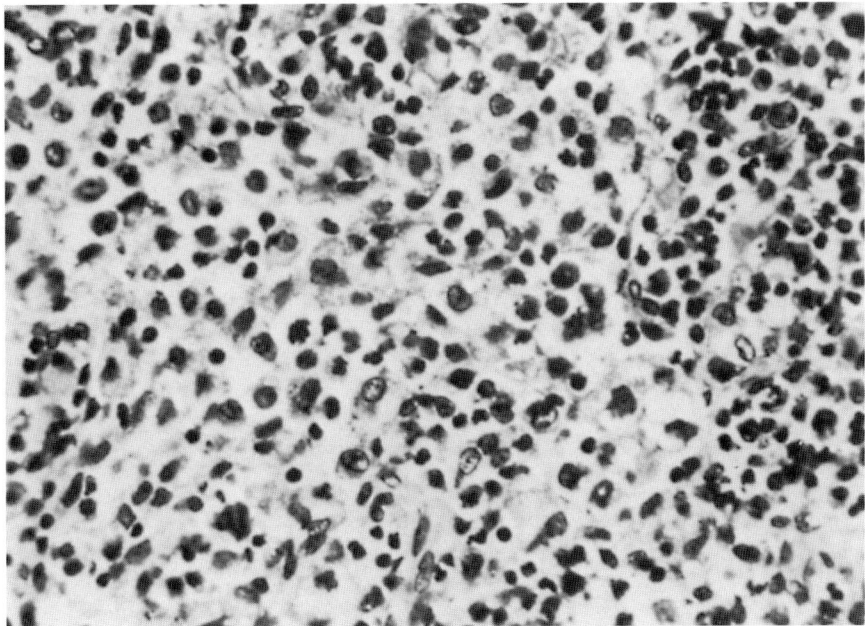

FIG. 2. This pleomorphic infiltrate of LCH in a lymph node includes eosinophils, large mononuclear lymphocytes, and polymorphonuclear leukocytes (hematoxylin and eosin, ×180). (From ref. 111, with permission.)

diation therapy, cytotoxic chemotherapy, and even bone marrow ablation and transplantation seem to be acceptable primary therapies. If, however, one thinks about LCH primarily as a reactive disorder, then one would be prone to use, at least initially, more conservative and less toxic therapies including, in many cases, nothing more than expectant observation. For the clinician, the truth lies partway between these two classifications. Most cases of LCH are not life-threatening and can be managed with minimal therapy. There are a few instances of the disease running a fulminant and fatal course—a situation that calls for an aggressive response.

CLINICAL PRESENTATION, DIAGNOSTIC EVALUATION, AND STAGING

The annual incidence is approximately 0.5 to 2.0 cases per 100,000 children per year. There is a male predominance: ranging from 56% to 66% males (13,16,25–27).

The form of clinical presentation is related to the child's age (Table 1). In children under the age of 2 years, there may be a widespread, seborrheic rash (Fig. 3). The rash is often most pronounced on the scalp and in the groin. Ulceration and secondary skin infection may occur. Involvement of the mastoid and middle ear may present as a chronic draining otitis. The child's parents may have noted the infant to be irritable with a diminished appetite and failure to thrive. Palpable lymphadenopathy may be seen secondary to LCH infiltration. Liver involvement is common in disseminated LCH. Hepatomegaly, elevation of liver enzymes, increased conjugated bilirubin, ascites, edema, and failure to thrive may be attributable to liver disease and/or involvement of the gastrointestinal tract. Diarrhea may be the result of abnormal bile acid metabolism or malabsorption (18,23). Splenomegaly may be accompanied by anemia, leukopenia, and/or thrombocytopenia (23,28–36).

In children older than 2 years, the most common presenting symptoms are related to

TABLE 1. *Presenting signs and symptoms of Langerhans' cell histiocytosis: a summary from the published literature*

Author (Reference) Number of patients	Broadbent (13,99) 30	Selch (68) 56	Sessa (41) 40	Kilpatrick[a] (77) 172	Gadner (61) 78	French Histiocytosis Group (25) 348	Willis (44) 71
Sign or Symptom							
Skin rash	50%	18%	b		53%	37%	13%
Aural Discharge/ Mastoiditis	27%		b	8%		13%	
Bone pain	17%	71%	>25%	62%	74%	79%	82%[d]
Scalp lumps	17%		>28%				
Proptosis	13%						
Failure to thrive	10%		b				
Dyspnea	10%		b		17%	4%	
Lymphadenopathy	7%		b	6%	29%	9%	
Hepatosplenomegaly	3%		b		32% hepatomegaly, 23% splenomegaly	15% liver, 6% spleen	
Spinal cord compression	3%						
Soft-tissue swelling		21%		48%	42%		
Decreased range of limb motion		14%	>8%				
Tooth complaint		9%					
Oral ulcer		9%	3%	3%	13%		
Diabetis insipidus		10%		6%	8%	10%	
Anemia			b		14%[c]		
Fever				11%			
Mediastinal mass					4%		
Gastrointestinal tract findings					13%		

[a]This series consists of 0- to 16-year-old patients with LCH of bone.
[b]This sign/symptom occurred in this series, but its frequency is not specified.
[c]Refers to "bone marrow findings" in this study which, presumably, includes anemia.
[d]82% had bone lesions at diagnosis—not all sites were painful.

bone involvement (Table 2). There is localized pain, with or without an associated soft-tissue mass. Involvement of the orbital bones may cause exophthalmos. LCH may produce premature eruption of the teeth and/or tooth loss because of gum and mandibular disease (37,38). Back pain and loss of vertebral height may be seen. Spinal cord compression is rare but has been reported.

Diabetes insipidus (DI) is the most common complication of central nervous system (CNS) involvement in LCH. The incidence varies, in different reports, from 11% to 50%. MRI may show lesions in the posterior pituitary or the pituitary stalk (39). The mechanism of injury is thought to be either infiltration of the meninges adjacent to the posterior hypothalamic-pituitary axis or direct involvement of the brain. DI is often associated with skull lesions, which may be seen before the DI (40,41). This may be of importance because, if the index of suspicion for DI is high, and it is diagnosed early, then prompt irradiation, in the opinion of some authorities, may reverse or ameliorate the DI. Lung and oral mucous membrane involvement with LCH frequently occurs in patients in which DI develops (42). In a Dutch-German-Austrian study 3 out of 93 patients (3%) with primary localized disease versus 16 of 106 patients (15%) with dissemination of LCH at diagnosis had DI (39). In a series of patients from London's Hospital for Sick Children, DI was more common among children with multisystem disease (12 of 32) than among those with disease apparently confined to bone (3 of 20). Fourteen of the 15 children with DI had bone disease involving the skull. The cumulative

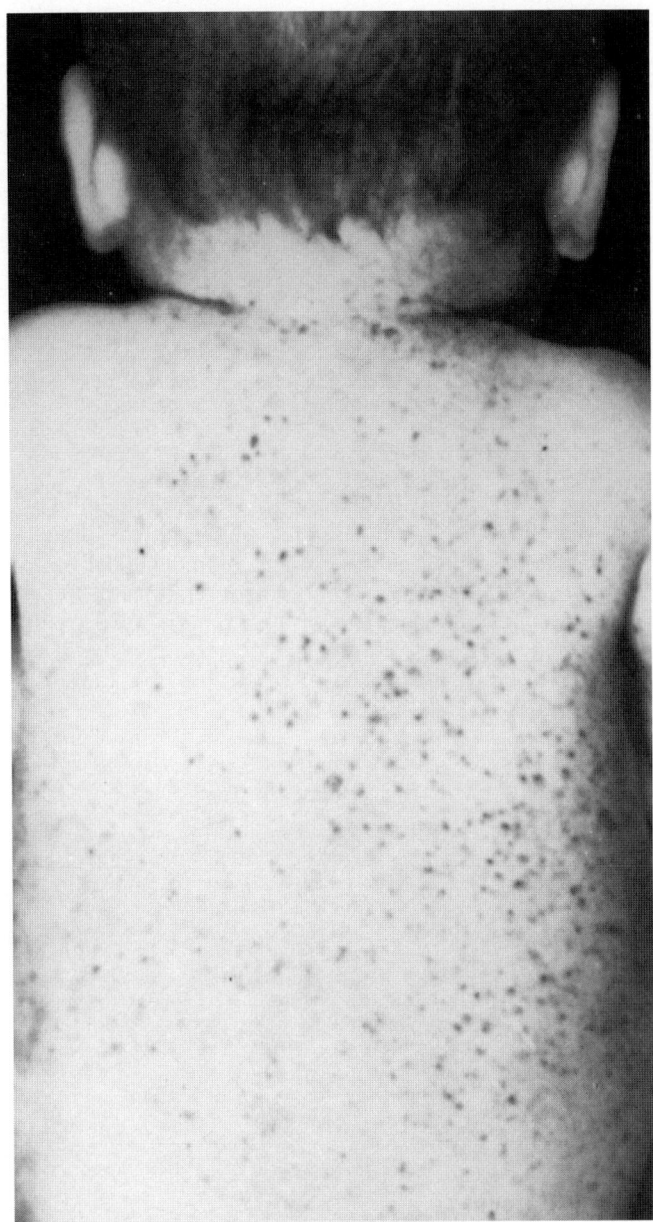

FIG. 3. Truncal rash and hepatosplenomegaly in an infant with LCH. (From ref. 111, with permission.)

risk of the development of DI during the first 4 years after presentation with LCH was 42% (43). In a series from San Francisco, 25% of patients developed DI (44).

Calavarial lesions can have epidural extension. They may extend beneath the dura into the brain parenchyma. In disseminated LCH cerebral involvement may occur (23). CNS involvement with LCH can take several forms. There can be meningeal involvement with formation of large plaques of subdural tumor. There can also be intraparenchymal le-

TABLE 2. *Sites of bone involvement in Langerhans' cell histiocytosis:*
a summary from the published literature

Author (Ref.) Number of patients	Slater (122) 639	Kilpatrick (77) 263	Sessa (121) 40
Bone(s) Involved			
Skull, including mandible	51%	73%	80%
Ribs	14%	16%	38%
Pelvis	13%	18%	20%
Vertebrae	10%	16%	50%
Upper extremity	7%	12%	5%
Lower extremity	18%	33%	30%
Other	9%	20%	15%

The percentages shown represent patients with this/these bone(s) involved/total number of patients in series, *not* patients with this/these bone(s) involved/total number of bony sites involved.

sions. The most common sites for intraparenchymal disease are the hypothalamus and cerebellum. Less common locations are the frontal and temporal lobes (13,45). Occasionally, LCH can first present to medical attention as an isolated, unifocal lesion of the CNS. The hypothalamus is the most common site for this rare situation. In such cases, the diagnosis is made following surgical exploration and biopsy (32,46).

It is clear that LCH has a wide clinical spectrum and can affect many different or-

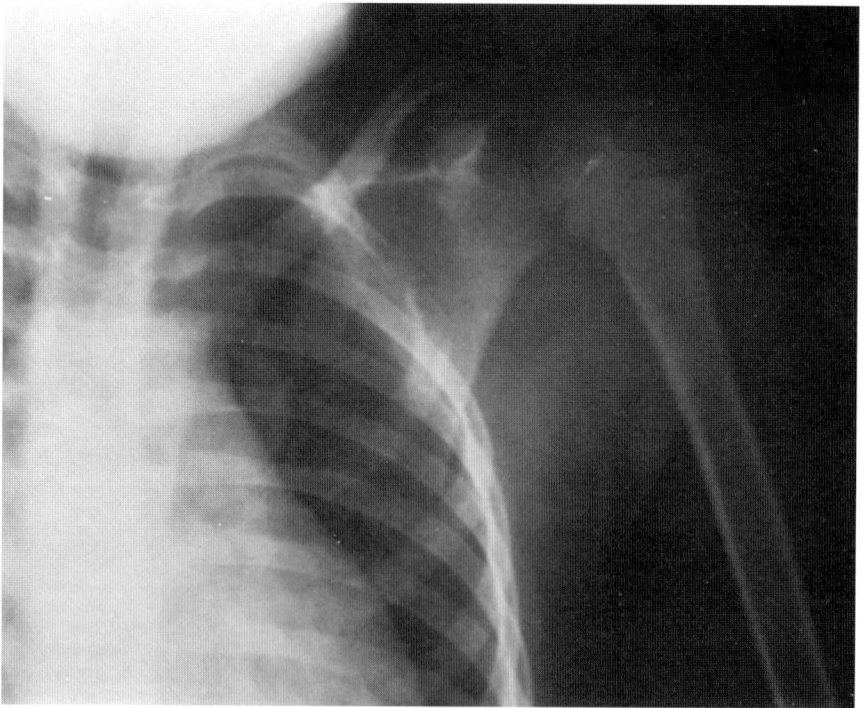

FIG. 4. LCH involving the left second rib in a 5-year-old girl. The lesion was painful. The involved portion of the rib was subtotally resected and was diagnostic of LCH. This localized, unifocal bone lesion was adequately treated with surgery alone. There was no recurrence of LCH.

TABLE 3. *Grouping and staging systems for histiocytosis*

Revised Lahey system (28)

Liver dysfunction is defined as being present if there is hypoprotenemia (<5.5 g/dL total protein and/or <2.5 g/dL of albumin), edema, ascites, or hyperbilirubinemia (total serum bilirubin >1.5 mg/dL).

Lung dysfunction is defined as being present if there is tachypnea, dyspnea, cyanosis, cough, pneumothorax, or pleural effusion.

Hematopoietic dysfunction is defined as existing if there is anemia (hemoglobin <10 g/dL), leukopenia (white blood cell count <4000/mm^3), neutropenia (neutrophil count <1500/mm^3), or thrombocytopenia (platelet count <100,000/mm^3).

A good prognosis is associated with the absence of organ system dysfunction. A poor prognosis is associated with the presence of dysfunction of one or more systems.

Osband et al.'s staging system (58)

Factor	Points
Age at presentation	
>2	0
<2	1
Number of organs involved	
<4	0
>4	1
Presence of liver, lung, or hematopoietic dysfunction defined by Lahey	
No	0
Yes	1

Stage	Total points
I	0
II	1
III	2
IV	3

Grouping system of Lipton (8)

The point scoring system is the same as that of Osband et al. The groupings are, however, slightly different.

Group	Total points
0	Monostotic eospinophilic granuloma
I	0
II	1
III	2
IV	3

Staging system of Greenberger (59)

Stage I	a. Single monostotic bone lesion.
	b. Multiple lesions in one bone or multiple bones.
Stage II	a. Age 24 mo at diagnosis and having one or more of the following organ systems involved: diabetes insipidus; teeth and gingivae; lymph nodes; skin; seborrhea, any site; "mild lung involvement" (i.e., infiltrates seen on chest radiograph without pulmonary symptoms or gross consolidation); bone marrow focally positive.
Stage III	a. Age <24 mo at diagnosis with any of the systems involved in stage II above or:
	b. Age >24 mo with involvement of liver and/or spleen; massive nodal involvement (nodes 5 × 5 × 5 cm in several sites above or below the diaphragm); "honeycomb lung" (major lung involvement in all areas with apparent fibrosis); bone marrow packed.
Stage IV	Spleen >6 cm palpable below costal margin and fever >1 mo with or without any or all of the above systems involved.
Stage V	"Special" monocytosis in peripheral blood >20% of differential cell count, in addition to stage III or stage IV findings.

Southwest Oncology Group risk groups (57)

Organ dysfunction is defined by Lahey's criteria. Patients without organ dysfunction who are over 2 years of age form the good-risk group. The intermediate-risk group are children less than 2 years of age without organ dysfunction. Patients of any age with organ dysfunction are poor risk.

Staging System of the Deutsche Arbeitsgemeinschaft für Leukaemieforschung Trial (39,60,61)

Localized disease—unifocal bone only or skin disease only or solitary lymph node.

Disseminated disease

Group A—Lesions in multiple bones or two lesions in one bone.

Group B—Soft-tissue involvement, ± bone lesions, without organ dysfunction. Bone lesions and a biopsy proven contiguous soft-tissue mass, regional lymph node involvement, or endocrinologic disability, i.e., diabetes insipidus or growth hormone deficiency.

Group C—Dysfunction of the liver, lung, or hematopoietic system.

---

gans. The frequency of presenting symptoms seen by a practitioner will, of course, be a result of the intrinsic nature of LCH but is also likely to be influenced by referral patterns. The diagnosis is generally proven by a biopsy of involved bone, skin, and/or bone marrow. A diagnostic radiograph skeletal survey should be performed to assess the extent of bony involvement (Fig. 4). LCH is one of the few conditions where conventional skeletal surveys are of more value than isotopic bone scans (47,48). In skeletal radiographs, LCH produces a focal area of rarefaction (49–51). The lucent area begins with the medullary cavity and extends to involve the inner table of the cortical bone. MRI may show that the area of bone abnormality is larger than suspected from other studies.

Some clinicians have urged that the term "staging" be abandoned in reference to LCH and replaced with "scoring" the extent of disease. This view reflects a concern that by invoking the notion of "staging" we are reinforcing the view that LCH is a malignancy (6,52,53). This concern does not seem to us to be warranted. LCH has a variable prognosis, and a system of grouping patients by predicted outcome is a valuable guide for the clinician (54). The two clinical extremes of LCH are relatively well-defined. At one extreme is the good-risk group characterized by a unifocal lesion in bone that responds to minimal therapy. At the other extreme, is the poor-risk group less than 2 years of age with organ dysfunction. The intermediate groups of patients are less well-defined. There is no uniformly accepted and applied staging system. The failure to agree on a single system is a result of disagreement concerning the principal prognostic factors. The formal staging systems reflect, to varying degrees, the patient's age, the number and types of anatomic sites involved, and the severity of disease (Table 3).

Lahey and co-workers (28,29,55,56) derived a scoring system based on the number of organ systems involved. A retrospective analysis found a striking difference in survival between those patients with and without organ dysfunction. Of the 50 patients without

organ dysfunction, 33 (66%) responded to chemotherapy and 2 (4%) died. In 33 patients with dysfunction of one or more of the three organ systems, only 11 (33%) responded to chemotherapy and 22 (67%) died.

The Southwest Oncology Group (SWOG) has developed a prognostic group system based on the patient's age and organ dysfunction (57). In an analysis of 155 children, the 6-year probability of survival for good, intermediate, and poor prognostic groups was, respectively, 90%, 66%, and 48%.

Osband et al. (58) derived a staging system based on age at presentation, presence of organ dysfunction, and the number of organs involved. Lipton (31) uses a similar system. Greenberger et al. (59) have proposed a complex staging system based on the patient's age, number of organ systems involved, and severity of organ involvement. The 20-year actuarial survival probability by Greenberger stage is as follows: I, 78%; II, 90%; III, 60%; IV, 0%; and V, 28%.

The staging system of the Deutsche Arbeitsgemeinschaft für Leukaemieforschung simply divides patients into localized and disseminated disease and then subgroups the disseminated disease patients (39,60,61).

The stage distribution of LCH at presentation is almost certainly influenced by referral patterns. A children's hospital is likely to see a higher proportion of advanced disease than a community hospital. In the Children's Hospital of Philadelphia series, 33 of 64 patients (52%) had localized disease at presentation, 22 (34%) had multifocal disease without organ dysfunction, and 9 (14%) had multifocal disease with evidence of organ dysfunction (26). In a series by McLelland et al. of 58 children, 14 (24%) had single-system disease, 22 (38%) had multisystem disease without organ dysfunction, and 22 (38%) had multisystem disease with organ dysfunction (19).

SELECTION OF THERAPY

In many cases LCH can take a relatively indolent course or spontaneously remit. If there is no organ dysfunction or systemic effects threatening the child, it may be possible to use minimal or no therapy. Asymptomatic lesions in older patients with disease confined to one organ system are frequently best managed by observation (6,13,19,52,62). One should carefully balance the risks of treatment against the apparent course of the disease. The potentially toxic effects of therapy should not be engendered unless absolutely necessary (47,62). In Table 4 the authors outline a conservative management strategy for LCH. A detailed discussion of the particulars of therapy follows.

Surgery

Pediatric Oncology Group (POG) Study 8047 evaluated the response rate of LCH bone lesions to incisional or excisional biopsy. The study was open to patients younger than 21 years of age with no more than two bone lesions and no systemic involvement by LCH. Open biopsy was recommended with curet-

tage when possible. Needle biopsy was performed for vertebral lesions, and excision was performed for expendable bone. Surgery proved highly effective, because 20 of 23 lesions (87%) were controlled without local LCH relapse (63).

POG study 8047, in conjunction with other literature, strongly supports the notion that solitary bone lesions may be treated surgically. There is an equal probability of local control with biopsy, curettage, or excision (8,64). A wide excision may be considered in an expendable bone such as the clavicle, ribs, or tip of the scapula. In nonexpendable bone locations, a small, mill-like biopsy instrument will allow a tissue diagnosis and access to the medullary cavity for a curettage. Relative contraindications to curettage are those situations where the procedure would result in loss of function, severe orthopedic deformity, or an extremely poor cosmetic result. A curettage should not be performed at certain locations because of the risk of bone instability:

TABLE 4. *A management strategy for Langerhans' cell histiocytosis*

Stage	Anatomic site of involvement	Symptoms	Recommended options for therapy
Localized disease without organ dysfunction	Bone or soft tissue	None	If the diagnosis is not established, then excisional biopsy (or biopsy and curettage) is diagnostic and therapeutic. If the diagnosis is already established, then expectant observation is appropriate.
Localized disease without organ dysfunction	Bone, soft tissue, or skin	Pain or disruption of function	Disease in noncrucial bone and soft-tissue sites can be managed by biopsy, excision, curettage, or steroid injection. At some sites, such as adjacent to the eye, ear, or spine or in critical weight-bearing bones with the potential to fracture, consider systemic steroids or local irradiation. Symptomatic skin disease may be treated with topical nitrogen mustard, although some authorities prefer systemic therapy.
Multifocal, no organ dysfunction	Any sites	None	Complete absence of symptoms in this situation is rare, but if the child is truly asymptomatic, then expectant observation is appropriate.
Multifocal, with organ dysfunction	Any sites	Fever, weight loss, failure to thrive, local symptoms from bone and soft-tissue lesions.	Begin with high-dose pulse steroids; if this fails, then use single-agent chemotherapy such as vinblastine or etoposide; if this fails, then consider chemotherapy such as vinblastine or etoposide; if this fails, then consider multiagent chemotherapy or cyclosporine.
Multifocal with organ dysfunction	Liver, lung, hematopoietic	Symptoms related to organ dysfunction	Sequence as immediately above. If these fail and the situation is life-threatening, consider bone marrow transplantation.

the axis, atlas, or femoral neck. Gingival curettage may be useful for gum disease (32).

Direct Injection of Steroids

Methylprednisolone or depomedrone may be injected into some bone lesions under fluoroscopic guidance. Because the transient expansion of the medullary cavity causes extreme pain, the procedure should be performed under general anesthesia (Table 5).

One cannot be certain if responses are obtained from the steroids or from the disruption of the microenvironment caused by the needle.

Radiation Therapy

The use of radiation therapy to manage localized bone or soft-tissue LCH is generally decreasing. This trend is attributable, in the authors' opinion, to a better understanding of the prognostic factors predicting the behavior of LCH, an appreciation of the frequency of disease remission following minimally toxic therapy, and concern about the long-term ill effects of radiation—albeit at low doses (18). The complete response rate of solitary LCH in bone to curettage or excision is 70% to 90% (8,63,64). There is no evidence that immediate postoperative irradiation improves on these results. Therefore, postoperative irradia-tion should be reserved for those individuals who have no clinical or radiographic signs of local healing. In addition, radiotherapy is indicated in the following situations: (a) for local relapse following surgery when the relapsed bone is the sole site of recurrent disease; (b) where curettage is not appropriate because of the risk of fracture (i.e., a lytic lesion of the femoral neck; mandibular involvement producing a loose, painful tooth and reluctance to eat) or poor cosmesis (i.e., the orbital bones) (7,65–67); (c) when the potential compromise of critical structures from expansile bone lesions (spinal cord compression, pressure on the globe or optic nerve) demands a reliable and rapid response (47); or (d) for relief of pain (63).

Selch and Parker (68) obtained local control with radiotherapy in 15 of 15 LCH lesions in pediatric patients compared to 29 of 41 (71%) in adults. Bone pain resolved within 4 months in all 40 treated sites. Radiographic healing occurred in 37 of 40 lesions (93%), with long-term control document in 35 (88%). El-Sayed and Brewin (69) found that radiation relieved bone pain symptoms in 14 of 15 cases (93%). Willis et al. achieved uniform in-field control of lesions with radiotherapy in 37 patients (44).

Asymptomatic bone lesions with sclerotic margins will often spontaneously resolve (70). Radiotherapy is usually not necessary in

TABLE 5. *Treatment of localized LCH of bone with intralesional corticosteroid injection*

Reference	Number of patients	Anesthesia requirement: general/local	Speed of relief of pain in weeks	Speed of resolution of bone disease in months	Complete responders/ total number of patients	Complications
Cohen (112)	9	8/1	1	2–4	8/9	None
Scaglietti (113)	9	9/0	<1	2	9/9	None
Nauert (114)	12	10/2	1–2	NS	12/12	None
Ruff (115)	1	1/0	NS	NS	1/1	None
Capana (76)	11	11/0	2	3	11/11	None
Fradis (116)	3	3/0	NS	NS	3/3	None
Wirtschafter (117)	1	1/0	NS	NS	1/1	None
Jones (105)	1	1/0	NS	NS	1/1	Abscess
Kindy-Degnan (118)	1	NS	1	12	1/1	None
Egeler (119)	8	8/0	1–2	3–6	8/8	Osteomyelitis

NS, not stated.
This table is modified from one that appeared in two different papers by Egeler and co-workers (119,119a).

these situations. If the clinician obtains follow-up radiographs of the child with bony LCH, evidence of healing is frequent. Meyer et al. described radiographic "lesion improvement" in 14 out of 15 patients with multifocal LCH (93%) and 7 out of 8 patients with unifocal LCH (88%) (71). A change from nontrabecular to a trabecular pattern, evolution of sclerosis in a nonsclerotic lesion, and loss of distinct margins indicate healing (72). Minimum time from diagnosis to evidence of mild healing was 3 months—although complete resolution often takes considerably longer (21).

Vertebral lesions should be considered as a special situation. Partial or complete collapse (vertebra plana) of a vertebral body may be asymptomatic (Fig. 5). These asymptomatic lesions generally do not require therapy because partial regrowth usually occurs irrespective of treatment. If, however, a vertebral lesion is painful, it may be irradiated (73).

In patients with multifocal LCH or with organ dysfunction, local irradiation also has a place. Lesions that are painful in spite of chemotherapy should be considered for local irradiation. The local recurrence rate for bone lesions treated with chemotherapy alone was

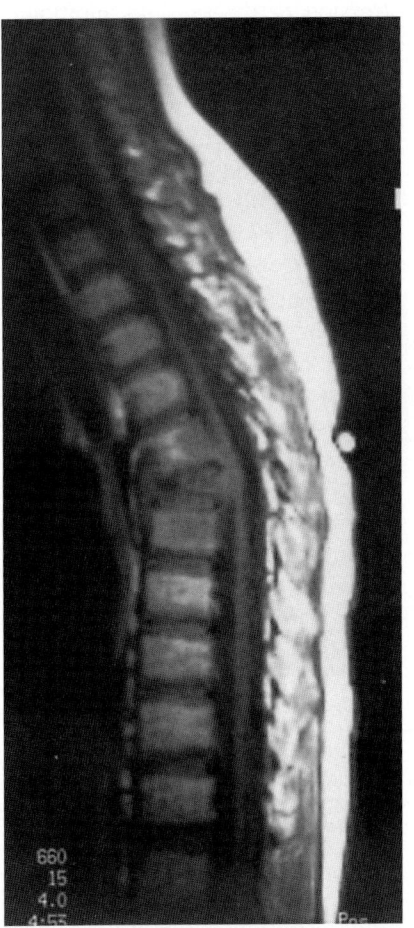
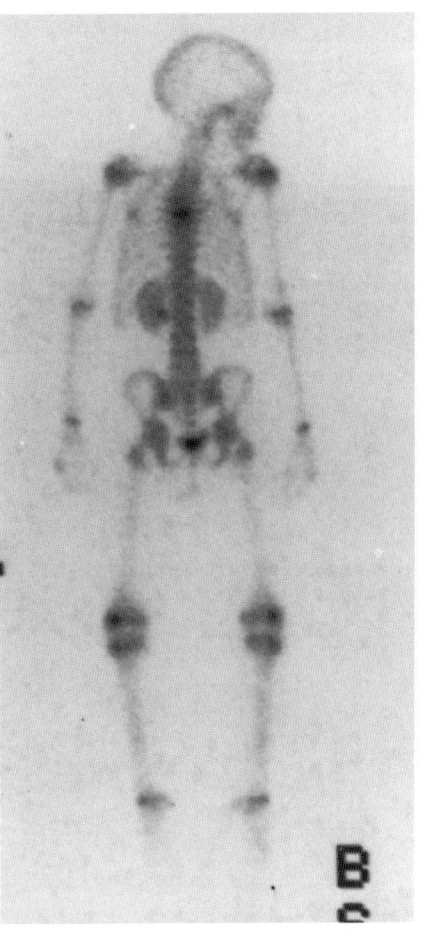

FIG. 5. MRI scan **(A)** and bone scan **(B)** showing complete vertebral collapse (vertebra plana) secondary to LCH, in 1992. No therapy was given beyond a needle biopsy to establish the diagnosis. Pain resolved over a month's time. Typically, healing includes fusion to adjacent vertebrae. The child remained without evidence of recurrent LCH in 1997, 5 years following the initial diagnosis.

5 of 15 cases in one study (74). Disfiguring bone/soft-tissue lesions or those bones at substantial immediate risk for fracture are also appropriate for local radiation therapy. Recalcitrant skin lesions may be treated with electron beam or orthovoltage photon therapy, but this should rarely be necessary in view of the other available agents (47,68).

The value of irradiation for LCH-associated DI is controversial. Greenberger et al. (65) reported 21 patients irradiated for DI. They noted a complete reversal of symptoms in four patients with discontinuation of pitressin for 2, 5, 5, and 25 years. A complete response to irradiation was observed in three of four patients treated within 1 week of the onset of symptoms. Only 1 of 15 patients responded when the duration of symptoms prior to radiotherapy exceeded 2 weeks. Smith et al. (75), however, reported no response in seven patients irradiated for DI. Broadbent and Chu (13) have reported six patients with DI who failed to respond to irradiation. Selch and Parker irradiated two patients with DI 3 months after the onset of symptoms. Neither of these patients responded (76). There were no responses among 7 patients treated with chemotherapy ± irradiation by Willis et al. (44). El-Sayed and Brewin (69) have reported successful radiotherapy of two patients with DI. Grois et al. found that none of five patients treated with 10 Gy of radiotherapy to the pituitary within 1 month of the occurrence of DI was able to decrease the required desmopression dose (39). Some have discounted the value of radiation therapy for DI without contributing additional supporting data to the literature (23,40).

The largest series of DI in LCH has been reported by Minehan et al. and Kilpatrick et al. from the Mayo Clinic. In 45 evaluable patients, the principal findings were as follows: (a) 10 of the 28 (36%) irradiated patients had a complete or partial improvement in their DI, as opposed to none of the 17 nonirradiated patients. (b) Six patients were complete responders, five of whom were irradiated within 14 days of the diagnosis of DI. (c) Seventy-seven percent of all LCH patients with DI had a

non-CNS head and neck site involved with LCH. (d) Computerized tomography (CT) or MRI improvement in a pituitary-hypothalmic mass did not correlate well with improvement in DI. (e) In 12 of the 28 patients (43%), irradiated for DI, growth hormone deficiency or parahypopituitarism developed (42,77). Minehan et al. did a literature review, to which we can add published patients they did not include, to generate an overall response rate of less than 25% of DI to radiation (13,39,42,43,68,77). We feel that radiotherapy is worth a trial in DI if symptoms are of recent onset (approximately 1 week). Others recommend radiotherapy even for long-standing DI in the hope of preventing local progression of disease and additional neuroendocrine dysfunction (47).

Focal LCH involving the brain can be successfully treated with radiotherapy (78). On rare occasions, LCH may diffusely involve the parenchyma of the brain (56). The true incidence of this event is not known. Brain involvement of this sort occurs in the most aggressive form of the disease and is unlikely to be influenced by cranial radiotherapy (5).

A single patient with systemic LCH is reported in the literature as having been treated with hemibody irradiation, vincristine, and prednisone. The patient died of a peripheral neuropathy, and an autopsy revealed no evidence of LCH in irradiated tissues but extensive involvement of unirradiated tissues (79). A multiinstitution trial of hemibody irradiation for LCH was closed after only six patients were accrued. In these patients, hemibody irradiation appeared to be more effective in those patients without sclerotic pulmonary nodules than in those patients with long-standing pulmonary involvement (T.W. Griffin, *personal communication,* 1987). Later in this chapter, we will consider the use of total-body irradiation prior to bone marrow transplantation for LCH.

Chemotherapy

We have previously emphasized that children with solitary LCH of bone or multifocal but single-system disease (usually bone, skin, or lymph nodes) have a good prognosis. Expectant observation or local therapy (surgery, local irradiation, or topical chemotherapy) is appropriate and generally results in a favorable outcome (13,19).

In multifocal LCH the indications for systemic therapy are controversial. Because there is no agreement on the important prognostic factors in LCH, the selection of patients requiring chemotherapy is difficult (80). In some series, age and number of sites of involvement confer a poor prognosis and appear, therefore, to allow selection of patients for systemic treatment (31,59). Chemotherapy is most frequently used in patients with fever, pain, severe involvement of the skin, failure to thrive, or dysfunction of vital organs (18). One should begin with the least toxic agent possible. More toxic agents are indicated if treatment with initial single-agent therapy fails. Unfortunately, the lack of a uniformly applied staging system makes comparison of specific chemotherapy programs difficult.

Of particular interest in considering the therapy of multisystem disease is the study of McClelland et al. (19). Forty-four children with multisystem disease, including 22 with vital organ dysfunction as defined by Lahey, were treated with a conservative philosophy. Five had no treatment, 1 received topical nitrogen mustard only, 2 received radiotherapy alone, and 36 were treated with prednisone. Of these 36, 21 later were given cytotoxic drugs when disease progressed in spite of prednisone. The 2-year mortality rate of the patients in the study by McClelland et al. (36% with organ dysfunction, 0% without) was no different from that of studies using aggressive up-front systemic cytotoxic chemotherapy. The rate of development of DI in the group of McClelland et al. was 36%, which is higher than that in some, but not all, other series. This matter merits additional review (13).

The complete and partial response rate of advanced LCH to prednisone and to a wide variety of single-agent cytotoxic chemothera-peutic agents (chlorambucil, cyclophosphamide, etoposide, vinblastine, vincristine) is between 50% and 100% (13,16,42,44, 81–84) (Table 6). Relapse after initial therapy is frequent (66). There is no evidence that multiagent cytotoxic chemotherapy is superior to the single-agent therapy or steroids. Certainly the toxicity of more aggressive chemotherapy is greater, particularly in infants. If systemic therapy is elected for LCH, then the current consensus view is to begin with high-dose steroids, usually prednisone. If this fails, then most clinicians would opt for either etoposide or vinblastine as a single agent. The toxicity of these drugs may be less than some of the other choices. Third-line therapy would include the variety of combinations shown in Table 6. Because of the immune system abnormalities detected in patients with LCH, calf thymus extract (thymosin) interleukin-2, and cylosporine have been proposed as treatments. Experience with these agents is limited, response rates vary, and responses are often short-lived (14,58,85–88).

Skin involvement is a relatively common component of multisystem LCH in younger children. Skin symptoms may include pruritus, ulceration, purulent exudation, odor, and painful defecation due to anogenital involvement (89). Sheehan et al. (90) have treated 16 patients with symptomatic cutaneous LCH with a topical nitrogen mustard solution made by adding tap water to nitrogen mustard powder and applying it to the skin with a water-color brush. A complete or partial response was obtained in all cases. Mayou et al. (91) successfully treated a case of cutaneous LCH in an adult with oral etoposide. These authors, concerned about the mutagenicity of nitrogen mustard, labeled the topical use of that compound for LCH as "retrogressive."

Restraint and patience must be exercised in the follow-up of LCH patients on chemotherapy. The response to chemotherapy may be slow, and periods of improvement may alternate with relapses. Drug failure may be said to have occurred if there is a progressive systemic deterioration or active

TABLE 6. *Chemotherapy for LCH*[a]

Year	Reporting Institution or group	Therapy	Number of evaluable patients	Combined complete plus partial response rate (%)	Reference
1972	SWCCSG	VCR	6	50	
		VBL	20	55	
		CYC	22	63	64
1974	ALGB	Induction therapy			
		MTX/PRED	17	53 (median remission: 315 d)	
		VCR/PRED	11	64 (median remission: 96 d)	
1975	CCSG	Patients 2 years of age			
		VBL	7	29	
		VBL/PRED	6	83	
		6-MP/PRED	3	33	
1977	SWOG	CYC/VBL/PRED			
			<1 year of age 8	25	
			>1 year of age 17	88	79
1977	SWOG	CYC/vincristine/procarbazine/PRED	<2 years of age 9	56	
1979	CCSG	Chlorambucil	26	27	95
		CYC/VBL/MTX/PRED	16	33	87
1980	SWOG	Chlorambucil	Have received no prior therapy 32	Have received no prior therapy 56	53
			Received prior therapy 13	Received prior therapy 62	
		Chlorambucil/PRED	Have received no prior therapy 8	Have received no prior therapy 75	53
1981	Children's Hospital, Boston	Calf thymus gland extract	17	59	
1983	Institute of Child Health, London	Calf thymus gland extract	17	59	2
		Synthetic thymic hormone	1	0	119
1984	Boston City Hospital	Calf thymus gland extract	3	0	
1988	Italian Cooperative Study	Etoposide	30	57	17
1989	CHOP, Philadelphia	Chlorambucil/VBL/PRED/CYC	18	83	76
		PRED/6-MP/MTX	1	100	
		VBL/PRED/MTX/CYC/6-MP	1	100	
		Steroids	7	100	
		VBL/PRED	1	100	29
			2	100	

TABLE 6. *Continued*

Year	Reporting Institution or group	Therapy	Number of evaluable patients	Combined complete plus partial response rate (%)	Reference
1989	Hospital for Sick Children, London	Etoposide	10	90	13
1991	St. Bartholomew's	Etoposide	1	100	24
1991	Hospital for Sick Children, London	Topical nitrogen mustard	16	100	31
1991	SJCRH	Cyclosporine	3	100	77
1991	Hospital dos Clinas, Brazil	Etoposide	6	84 (3 of 5 responders subsequently relapsed)	114
1991	Vilnius, Lithuania	Etoposide/VBL/PRED/6-MP	17	82	120
1991	University of Pavia, Italy	Cyclosporine	1	100	40
1992	University of Malaysia	Etoposide	6	67 (39% of complete responders relapsed)	71
		Etoposide/PRED	18		
1993	Italian Cooperative Study (AIEOP-CNR-H.X. '83)	Calf Thymic Extract	10	10	106
1993	Italian Cooperative Study (AIEOP-CNR-H.X. '83)	VBL	54	85	106
		ADM	7	71	
		Etoposide	17	88 (These are complete + partial responses + stable disease rates.)	
		VCR/CYC/A/FM/PRED (Poor responders to VBL received ADM. Poor responders to ADM received etoposide. The 4 drug program was utilized for poor prognosis patients.)	11	36	
1994, 1987	Deutsche Arbeitsgemeinschaft fur Leukaemieforschung (DAL-HX 83)	Initial therapy: PRED/VBL/Etoposide/6-MP Continuation therapy: Group A	28	89	60,61
		PRED/VBL Group B	57	91	
		PRED/VBL/Etoposide Group C	21	67	
		PRED/VBL/VP-16/MTX (For definition of groups, see *Table 3*)			
1995	University Hospital of Tokushima, Japan	Interleukin-2	1	1 (PR, short term)	87

ALGB, Acute Leukemia Group B; CCSG, Children's Cancer Study Group; CHOP, Children's Hospital of Philadelphia; CYC, cyclophosphamide; MTX, methotrexate; PRED, prednisone; 6-MP, 6-mercaptopurine; VCR, vincristine; VBL, vinblastine; SJCRH, St. Jude Children's Research Hospital; SWCCSG, Southwest Children's Cancer Study Group; SWOG, Southwest Oncology Group; VBL, vinblastine; PR, Partial response.

437

disease at many sites (35). There is a moderate response rate to therapy with different drugs in patients who have failed initial chemotherapy.

LIVER AND BONE MARROW TRANSPLANTATION

Liver involvement is relatively common in young children with multisystem LCH. The etiology of liver damage in LCH is not well understood. Several mechanisms have been postulated, including: histiocytic and immunocyte proliferation in the portal tracts, which produces biliary damage, fibrosis, and chronic cholestasis; extrahepatic biliary obstruction by lymphadenopathy in the porta hepatis; primary sclerosing cholangitis; and/or iatrogenic injury from chemotherapy, transfusion-related hepatitis, or total parenteral nutrition. In some children, liver failure is the immediate cause of death from LCH. There are a few case reports of successful orthotopic liver transplantations for LCH. These patients did not appear to have active LCH at the time of the transplant. It is tantalizing to speculate that the cyclosporine used for immunosuppression following the transplant may also have an effect against recrudescence of the LCH (14,74,92).

There is a subset of LCH patients with multisystem disease and vital organ dysfunction who fail to respond to all immunologic and conventional chemotherapy (6,52,93). These patients, in a last-ditch effort to effect cure, may be considered for myelobalative and immunosuppressive therapy combined with allogeneic or autologous bone marrow transplantation. The preparative regimen will include some combination of cyclophosphamide, BCNU, and busulfan. Total-body irradiation is also used: 2 to 2.25 Gy per fraction for 6 or 7 daily fractions has been reported, although other regimens are certainly plausible. We are aware of at least ten patients who have received bone marrow transplantation for life-threatening LCH. Eight are alive with tolera-

ble toxicity—one with 12 years of follow-up (25,62,94–96,Ringden).

RADIOTHERAPEUTIC MANAGEMENT

Dose

There is no clear relationship between the dose of irradiation and local control of lesions. Childs and Kennedy (49) reported a series of 12 patients treated with radiotherapy. Their series began with an infant treated in 1927 to 1928 with a radium source. They felt that a dose of approximately 600 roentgens was necessary to control individual lesions. Smith et al. (75) have reported on 89 courses of irradiation administered with 250-kV x-rays or cobalt-60. Less than 1,000 cGy was administered in 92% of the cases, and the local "success" rate was 87%. Three of five sites treated with less than 450 cGy had a local failure, but were salvaged with additional irradiation. Doses higher than 1,000 cGy did not appear to be more effective than doses of 450 to 1000 cGy. Ochsner (51) reported that radiotherapy was effective for bony sites at doses of 600 to 1,000 cGy. Similarly, in a report confined to solitary lesions of the skull, Rawlings and Wilkins (97) noted almost uniformly successful results with doses of 600 to 2,500 cGy. McGaran and Spady (64) had good results with 300 to 3,500 cGy. Caution should be exercised in the interpretation of retrospective dose-response data. The bone dose would obviously be higher from kilovoltage irradiation than from megavoltage treatment. Doses may have been modified based on the extent of disease.

Older retrospective reports of the absence of a dose-response relationship have been confirmed by the more recent reports. Greenberger et al. described 89 patients receiving radiotherapy to 380 fields for control of bone lesions. Between 100 and 2,000 cGy, local control was obtained in 75% of courses (Fig. 6). In a study of 56 irradiated sites, Selch and Parker

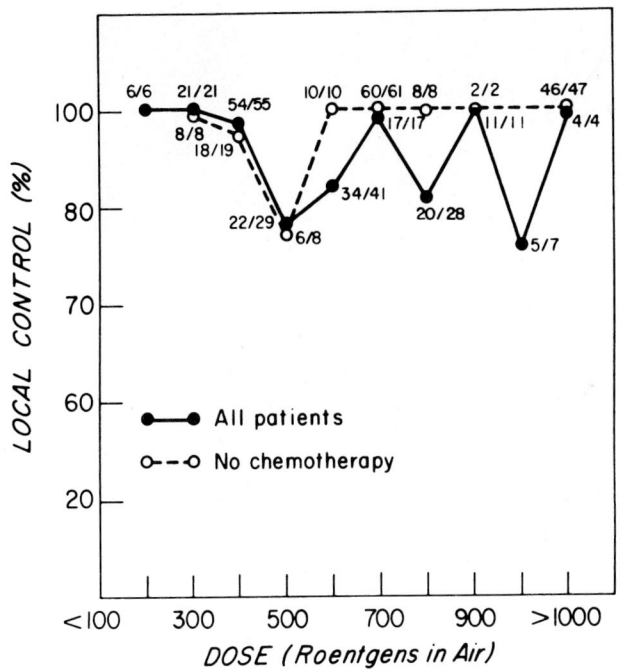

FIG. 6. Local control of bone lesions as a function of dose delivered. (From ref. 65, with permission.)

(68) found no difference in median dose between controlled and relapsed bony sites (9 vs. 10 Gy) or soft-tissue sites (median dose 15 Gy for either controlled or relapsed sites). Overall local control was 82% (Fig. 7). More recent reviews describe the use of total doses of 5 to 35 Gy, with 5 to 10 Gy in 3 to 5 fractions being the favored range (13,16,43,83,98) (Fig. 8). Cassady (47) advises using a total dose of 15 to 20 Gy in patients older than 18 to 20 years of age because of an alleged higher risk of local failure and a lower risk of bone damage by radiation.

For DI, Smith et al. (75) reported no relief in seven patients treated with 500 to 1,830 cGy. Greenberger et al. (65) administered 345 to 1,600 cGy to 21 patients and, as discussed previously, observed a complete response in four patients and a partial response in another four. Minehan et al. (42) reported 3 of 5 cases (60%) of DI responding when treated with more than 15 Gy, as compared to 7 of 23 (30%) treated with less than 15 Gy.

Volume

For treatment of DI, a 5 × 5- to 7 × 7-cm set of parallel opposed fields, arcs, or a three-field technique are usually adequate to cover the hypothalamic-pituitary axis (99,100). Bone lesions should be treated with a field designed to cover the radiographic abnormality with a small margin. In the treatment of skull lesions, we attempt to minimize the dose to the underlying brain by treating with electrons or orthovoltage equipment. If electrons are used, an adjustment for attenuation by compact bone infiltrated by LCH should be made. This is best done by taking density measurements of the involved bone with a cranial CT scan.

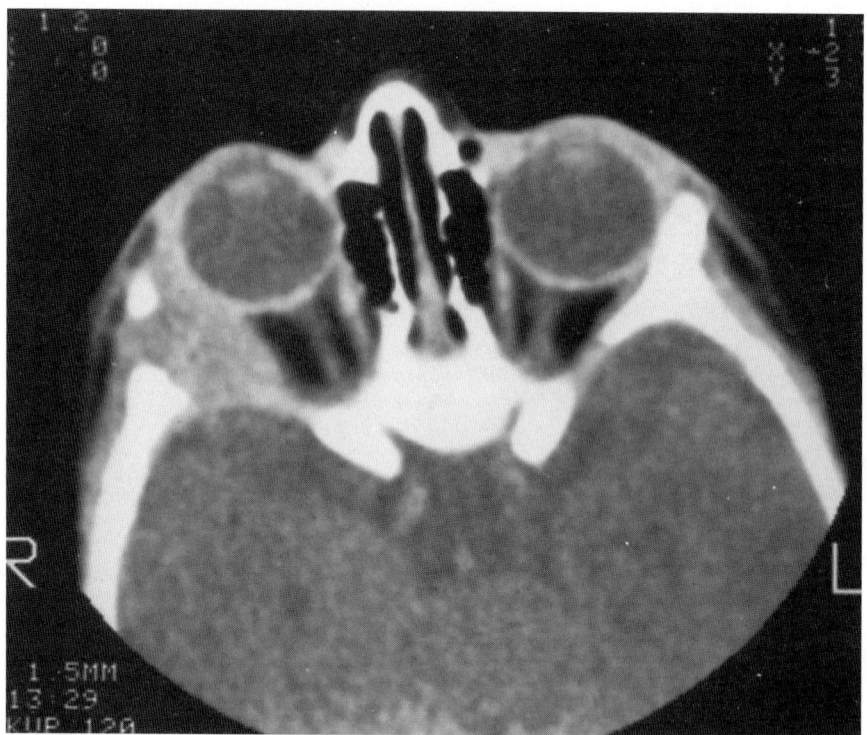

FIG. 7. A 4-month-old white boy developed a seborrheic skin rash with focal areas of ulceration. Skin biopsy showed LCH. No other organ systems were involved. At 6 months of age, proptosis was noted and orbital CT scan demonstrated erosion of the lateral wall of the right orbit by a destructive lesion. Surgery was felt to be ill-advised because of concern over damage to the lateral rectus muscle as well as an unacceptable cosmetic result. Vinblastine and prednisone were administered. Proptosis improved but then subsequently worsened. A total dose of 6 Gy in 4 fractions was administered with a right anterior oblique half-beam-blocked 4-MV photon field with shielding of the lens and two-thirds of the globe in 1984. Vinblastine was continued for 15 months following radiotherapy. The bone lesion healed within 2 months following irradiation. There is no evidence of LCH 11 years following the initial diagnosis.

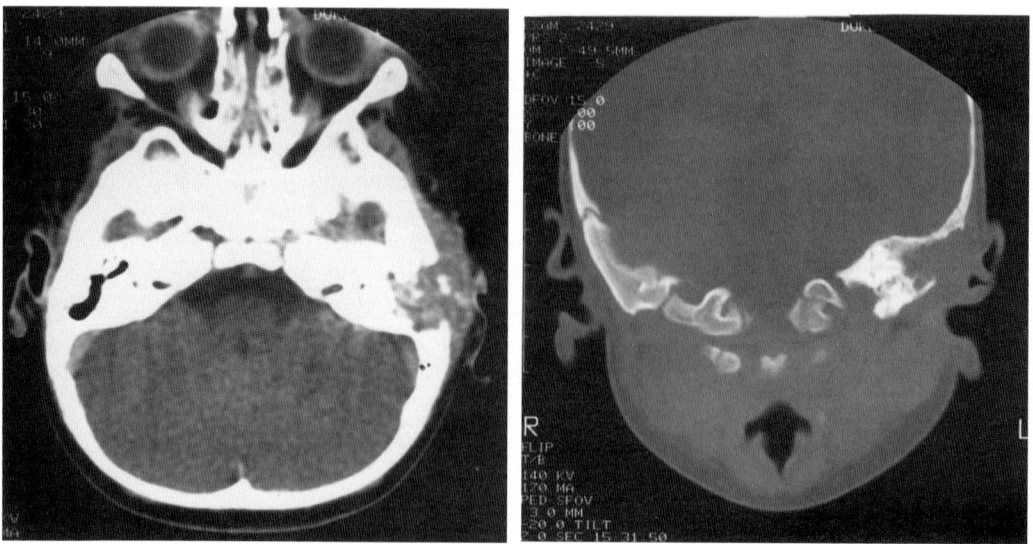

LONG-TERM SEQUELAE OF LCH AND ITS TREATMENT

Because of the low dose of irradiation used, acute side effects of radiotherapy for LCH are rare. It is, however, common to see late sequelae of LCH, most of which may be attributable to the disease and some of which may be attributable to the treatment (7,101,102).

Long-term disabilities are frequent in survivors of LCH. The French Langerhans' Cell Histiocytosis Group reported 320 living patients followed for a median of 39.5 months. The most common sequelae were DI (18%), growth hormone deficiency and short stature (5%), hypothyroidism (2.5%), deafness (2.5%), and vertebra plana/orthopedic sequelae (2.5%) (25). The most common sequelae in the University of California, San Francisco, series were DI (26%), growth failure (20%), sex hormone deficiency (16%), and hearing loss (16%) (44). The 90 children followed by the Italian Cooperative Group had an overall incidence of disease-related disabilities of approximately 48%. These included DI, orthopedic abnormalities, growth defects, tooth loss, chronic hepatitis, exophthalmus, and hearing loss (100). The Southwest Oncology Group has described a significant incidence of neurologic symptoms, intellectual problems, and growth failure (102). McLelland et al. have described orthopedic abnormalities, endocrine dysfunction, hearing deficits, and liver fibrosis as well as DI (19,53). Ransom et al. has indicated, in a study of 15 long-term survivors of LCH, seven had an IQ lower than 89 (103).

The frequency of secondary malignancy following therapy of LCH is uncertain (8,59,102). In a report describing the association between LCH and other malignancies (91 patients), 39 had LCH and lymphoma (Hodgkin's or non-Hodgkin's), 22 had LCH and leukemia, and 30 had LCH and a solid tumor, most commonly lung cancer. Although the leukemias and nonlung solid tumors most commonly occurred years after LCH, most of the lymphomas and lung cancers preceded LCH or were diagnosed concurrently, in a yet unexplained association (104). Affected patients had initially received the following treatment for their LCH: irradiation and chemotherapy, irradiation only, and chlorambucil only (43,60,105). One case of leukemia was seen among 90 patients followed in the Italian Cooperative Group Study (106). One case of leukemia was seen in 51 patients followed more than 3 years at the University of California, San Francisco (44). There were no second malignancies in 106 LCH patients treated in the Dutch-German-Austrian DAL HS-83 Trial (45,87).

Haupt et al. evaluated children with LCH enrolled in three protocols of the Italian Association of Pediatric Hematology/Oncology. These patients received a variety of chemotherapy programs including vinblastine, adriamycin, VP16, vincristine, cyclophosphamide, and prednisone. The median follow-up after entry into the study cohort was 5 years and 5 months. There were three cases of acute nonlymphocytic leukemia (ANLL) all in children who had received VP16. Two had received VP16 alone and one had received VP16 in combination with alkylating agent chemotherapy in combination with other chemotherapy and or irradiation. While the absolute number of patients in this study is small, the occurrence of three episodes of ANLL results in a high simple incidence rate of secondary leukemia (107).

FIG. 8. An 11-year-old white boy presented to medical attention with protrusion of the superior aspect of the left ear. CT scan showed a left mastoid soft-tissue mass with erosion into the temporal bone. Open biopsy made the diagnosis of LCH. In 1987, the child received local irradiation with 12 MeV electrons to a total dose of 6 Gy in 3 fractions. Following irradiation he was treated with vinblastine and prednisone. He remained without evidence of persistent or recurrent LCH 8 years later.

RESULTS

In patients presenting with solitary LCH of bone, close to 100% survival has been reported (26,44,64,65,108). In the presence of organ dysfunction with multisystem disease, survival ranges from 33% to 54%. In its absence, survival ranges from 82% to 96% (13,19,26,28,29,31,56). In the 348 patients reported from 32 French Centers, treated from 1983 to 1993, the 6-year actuarial survival according to the DALHX Staging system was: Localized disease, isolated unifocal or bifocal bone involvement, 100%; soft tissue involvement with or without bone involvement, no organ dysfunction, 90%; liver, lung, or bone marrow dysfunction, 49% (25). In the DAL-HX 83 Trial, children with LCH received chemotherapy according to a complex stratification, summarized in an entry in Table 3. The probability of survival, utilizing the DAL-HX 83 staging system for disseminated disease (see Table 3), was 100% for Group A, 96% for Group B, and 62% for Group C. The 15-year survival rates in the series of Willis et al., by type of initial presentation, was skin disease only, 83%, monostotic disease, 100%; polyostotic disease, 100%, and multisystem disease, 76% (44).

REFERENCES

References particularly recommended for further reading are indicated by an asterisk.

1. D'Angio GJ, Favara BE, Ladisch S. Editorial: toward an understanding of the childhood histiocytoses. *Med Pediatr Oncol* 1986;14:104.
2. Langerhans P. Uber die nerven der menschlichen haut. *Arch Pathol Anatom* 1868;44:325–327.
3. Langerhans P. Berichtigungen (u.a. zu den nervenenden der haut, und nervenfasern im rete.) *Arch Mikrosk Anat* 1882;20:641–643.
4. Egeler RM, Zantinga AR, Coppes MJ. Paul Langerhans Jr. (1847–1888): a short life, yet two eponymic legacies. *Med Pediatr Oncol* 1994;22:129–132.
5. Hand A. Polyuria and tuberculosis. *Arch Pediatr* 1893;10:673–675.
6. Komp DM. Concepts in staging and clinical studies for treatment of Langerhans' cell histiocytosis. *Semin Oncol* 1991;18:18–23.
7. Lanzkowsky P. Histiocytosis X. In: *Pediatric hematology-oncology.* New York: McGraw-Hill, 1980:359–362.
*8. Lieberman PH, Jones CR, Dargeon HWK, Begg CF.

A reappraisal of eosinophilic granuloma of bone, Hand-Schuller-Christian syndrome and Letterer-Siwe syndrome. *Medicine* 1969;48:375–400.
9. Lichtenstein L. Histiocytosis X: integration of eosinophilic granuloma of bone, "Letterer-Siwe disease," and "Schuller-Christian disease" as related manifestations of a single nosologic entity. *Arch Pathol* 1953;56:84–102.
10. Otani E, Ehrlich J. Solitary eosinophilic granuloma of bone simulating primary neoplasm. *Am J Pathol* 1940;16:479–490.
*11. Ishii E, Watanabe S. Biochemistry and biology of the Langerhans' cell. *Hematol Oncol Clin North Am* 1987;1:99–118.
12. Unanue ER. Macrophages, antigen presenting cells, and the phenomena of antigen handling and presentation. In: Paul WE, ed. *Fundamental immunology,* 2nd ed. New York: Raven Press, 1989:95–116.
*13. Broadbent V, Chu AC, Langerhans' cell histiocytosis. In: Plowman PN, Pinkerson CR, eds. *Paediatric oncology: clinical practice and controversies,* second edition. London: Chapman & Hall, 1997;547–560.
14. Mahmoud HH, Wang WC, Murphy SB. Cyclosporine therapy for advanced Langerhans cell histiocytosis. *Blood* 1991;77:721–725.
15. Castleman B, McNeely BU. Case records of the Massachusetts General Hospital, case 17-1970. *N Engl J Med* 1970;282:917–925.
16. Cornelius AS. Histiocytosis. In: D'Angio GJ, Sinniah D, Meadows AT, Evans AE, Pritchard J, eds. *Practical pediatric oncology.* New York: Wiley-Liss, 1992:346–351.
17. Ladisch S, Jaffe ES. The histiocytoses. In: Pizzo PA, Poplack DG, eds. *Principles and practice of pediatric oncology,* 2nd ed. Philadelphia: JB Lippincott, 1993:617–632.
18. Velez-Yanguas MC, Warrier RP. Langerhans' cell histiocytosis. *Orthop Clin North Am* 1996;27:615–623.
*19. McLellan DJ, Broadvent V, Yeomans E, Malone M, Pritchard J. Langerhan's cell histiocytosis: the case for conservative treatment. *Arch Dis Child* 1990;65:301–303.
*20. Willman CL, Busque L, Griffith BB, et al. Langerhans cell histiocytosis (histiocytosis X): a clonal proliferative disease. *N Engl J Med* 1994;331:154–160.
20a. Cotter FE, Pritchard J. Clonality in Langerhan's cell histiocytosis. *BMJ* 1995;310:74–75.
20b. Yu RC, Chu C, Buluwela L, Chu AC. Clonal proliferation of Langerhans cells in Langerhans cell histiocytosis. *Lancet* 1994;343:767–768.
21. Womer RB, Rainey RB, D'Angio GJ. Healing rates of treated and untreated bone lesions in histiocytosis X. *Pediatrics* 1985;76:286–288.
*22. Cotter FE, Pritchard J. Clonality in Langerhans' cell histiocytosis. *BMJ* 1995;310:74–75.
23. Egeler RM, Nesbit ME. Langerhans cell histiocytosis and other disorders of monocyte-histiocyte lineage. *Crit Rev Oncol Hematol* 1995;18:9–35.
24. Knudson AG. Mutation and cancer: statistical study of retinoblastoma. *Proc Natl Acad Sci USA* 1971;68:620–623.
25. French Langerhans' Cell Histiocytosis Study Group. A multicentre retrospective survey of Langerhans' cell histiocytosis. 348 cases observed between 1983 and 1993. *Arch Dis Child* 1996;75:17–24.

*26. Raney RB Jr, D'Angio GJ. Langerhans' cell histiocytosis (histiocytosis X): experience at the Children's Hospital of Philadelphia, 1970–1984. *Med Pediatr Oncol* 1989;17:20–28.

27. Starling KA, Donaldson MH, Haggard ME, Vietti TJ, Sutow WW. Therapy of histiocytosis X with vincristine, vinblastine, and cyclophosphamide. *Am J Dis Child* 1972;123:105–110.

28. Lahey ME. Histiocytosis X—comparison of three treatment regimens. *J Pediatr* 1975;87:179–183.

*29. Lahey ME. Prognostic factors in histiocytosis X. *Am J Pediatr Hematol Oncol* 1981;3:57–60.

30. Lechner W, Ortner A, Thoni A, Schuler G, Mikuz G. Histiocytosis X in gynecology. *Gynecol Oncol* 1983; 15:253–260.

31. Lipton J. The pathogenesis, diagnosis, and treatment of histiocytosis syndromes. *Pediatr Dermatol* 1983; 1:112–120.

32. Pritchard J. Commentary. In: D'Angio GJ, Siniah D, Meadows AT, Evans AE, Pritchard J, eds. *Practical pediatric oncology.* New York: Wiley-Liss, 1992: 352–353.

33. Schweisguth O. *Solid tumors in children.* New York: John Wiley & Sons, 1982:144–156.

34. Simone JV, Cassady JR, Filler RM. Cancers of childhood. In: DeVita VT Jr, Hellman S, Rosenberg SA, eds. *Cancer: principles and practice of oncology.* Philadelphia: JB Lippincott, 1982:1316–1320.

35. Starling KA. Chemotherapy of histiocytosis. *Am J Pediatr Hematol Oncol* 1981;3:157–160.

36. Starling KA, Fernbach DJ. Histiocytosis. In: Sutow WW, Fernback DJ, Vietti TJ, eds. *Clinical pediatric oncology,* 3rd ed. St. Louis: CV Mosby, 1984: 498–515.

37. Dagenais M, Pharoah MJ, Sikorski PA. The radiographic characteristics of histiocytosis X. *Oral Surg Oral Med Oral Pathol* 1992;74:230–236.

38. Filcoma D, Weedleman H, Arceci R, Bebber R, Donnelly M. Pediatric histiocytomas: characterization, prognosis and oral management. *Am J Pediatr Hematol Oncol* 1993;15:226–230.

39. Grois N, Flucher-Wolfram B, Heitger A, Mostbeck GH, Hofmann J, Gadner H. Diabetes insipidus in Langerhans cell histiocytosis: results from the DAL-HX 83 study. *Med Pediatr Oncol* 1995;24: 248–256.

40. Angeli SI, Hoffman HT, Alcalde J, Smith RJH. Langerhans cell histiocytosis of the head and neck in children. *Ann Otol Rhinol Laryngol* 1995;104: 173–180.

41. Sessa S. Sommelet D, Lascombes P, Prevot J. Treatment of Langerhans-cell histiocytosis in children: experience at the Children's Hospital of Nancy. *J Bone Joint Surgery* 1994;76:1513–1525.

*42. Minehan KJ, Chen MG, Zimmerman D, Su JQ, Colby TV, Shaw EG. Radiation therapy for diabetes insipidus caused by Langerhans cell histiocytosis. *Int J Radiat Oncol Biol Phys* 1992;23:519–524.

*43. Dunger DB, Broadbent V, Yeoman E, et al. The frequency and natural history of diabetes insipidus in children with Langerhans' cell histiocytosis. *N Engl J Med* 1989;321:1157–1162.

44. Willis B, Ablin A, Weinberg V, Zager S, Wara WM, Matthay KK. Disease course and late sequelae of Langerhans' cell histiocytosis: 25-year experience at

the University of California, San Francisco. *J Clin Oncol* 1996;14:2073–2082.

45. Hayward J, Packer R, Finlay J. Central nervous system and Langerhans' cell histiocytosis. *Med Pediatr Oncol* 1990;18:325–328.

46. Rube J, Para SDL, Pickren JW. Histiocytosis X with involvement of brain. *Cancer* 1967;20:486–492.

*47. Cassady JR. Current role of radiation therapy in the management of histiocytosis X. *Hematol Oncol Clin North Am* 1987;1:123–130.

48. Gerrard MP, Hendry MM, Eden OB. Comparison of radiographic and scientigraphic assessment of skeletal lesions in histiocytosis X. *Med Pediatr Oncol* 1986;14:113.

49. Childs DS Jr, Kennedy RLJ. Reticuloendotheliosis of children: treatment with roentgen rays. *Radiology* 1951;57:653–661.

50. Miller JH, Shore NA. Histiocytosis. In: Miller JH, ed. *Imaging in pediatric oncology.* Baltimore: Williams & Wilkins, 1985, pp. 461–471.

51. Ochsner SF. Eosinophilic granuloma of bone. Experience with twenty cases. *AJR* 1966;97:719–726.

*52. Komp DM. Therapeutic strategies for Langerhans cell histiocytosis. *J Pediatr* 1991;119:274–275.

53. McLelland J, Pritchard J, Chu AC. Current controversies. *Hematol Oncol Clin North Am* 1987;1:147–162.

54. Chu A, D'Angio GJ, Favara BE, Ladisch S, Nezelof C, Pritchard J. Report and recommendations of the workshop on the childhood histiocytosis: comments and controversies. *Med Pediatr Oncol* 1968;14:116.

55. Lahey ME. Histiocytosis X—comparison of three treatment regimens. *J Pediatr* 1975;87:179–183.

56. Lahey ME, Heyn RM, Newton WA Jr, et al. Histiocytosis X: clinical trial of chlorambucil: a report from Children's Cancer Study Group. *Med Pediatr Oncol* 1979;7:197–203.

57. Komp DM, Herson J, Starling KA, Vichi T, Hvizdala E. A staging system for histiocytosis X: a southwest oncology group study. *Cancer* 1981;47:798–800.

58. Osband ME, Lipton JM, Lavin P, et al. Histiocytosis X: demonstration of abnormal immunity, T-cell histamine H2-receptor deficiency, and successful treatment with thymic extract. *N Engl J Med* 1981;304: 146–153.

*59. Greenberger JS, Crocker AC, Vawter G, Jaffe N, Cassady JR. Results of treatment of 127 patients with systemic histiocytosis (Letterer-Siwe syndrome, Schuller-Christian syndrome and multifocal eosinophilic granuloma). *Medicine* 1981;60: 311–338.

60. Gadner H, Heitger A, Ritter J, et al. Langerhanszell-histiozytose im kindesalter-ergebnisse der DAL-HS 83 studies. *Klin Padiat* 1987;199:173–182.

61. Gadner H, Heitger A, Grois N, Gatterer-Menz I, Ladisch S. Treatment strategy for disseminated Langerhans cell histiocytosis. *Med Pediatr Oncol* 1994;23:72–80.

62. Komp DM. Langerhans cell histiocytosis. *N Engl J Med* 1987;316:747–748.

63. Berry DH, Gresik M, Maybee D, Marcus R. Histiocytosis in bone only. *Med Pediatr Oncol* 1990;18: 292–294.

64. McGaran MH, Spady HA. Eosinophilic granuloma of bone. A study of 28 cases. *J Bone Joint Surg* 1960;42A:979–992.

65. Greenberger JS, Cassady JR, Jaffe N, Vawter G, Crocker AC. Radiation therapy in patients with histiocytosis: management of diabetes insipidus and bone lesions. *Int J Radiat Oncol Biol Phys* 1979;5: 1749–1755.

66. Matus-Ridley M, Raney RB Jr, Thawerani H, Meadows AT. Histiocytosis X in children: patterns of disease and results of treatment. *Med Pediatr Oncol* 1983;11:99–105.

67. Richter MP, D'Angio GJ. The role of radiation therapy in the management of children with histiocytosis X. *Am J Pediatr Hematol Oncol* 1981;3:161–163.

68. Selch MT, Parker RG. Radiation therapy in the management of Langerhans cell histiocytosis. *Med Pediatr Oncol* 1990;18:97–102.

69. El-Sayed S, Brewin TB. Histiocytosis X: does radiotherapy still have a role? *Clin Oncol* 1992;4:27–31.

*70. Sartoris DJ, Parker BR. Histiocytosis X: rate and pattern of resolution of osseous lesions. *Radiology* 1984;152:679–684.

71. Meyer JS, Harty MP, Mahboubi S, et al. Langerhans cell histiocytosis: presentation and evolution of radiologic findings with clinical correlation. *Radiographics* 1995;15:1135–1146.

72. Alexander JE, Seibert JJ, Berry DH, Glasier CM, Williamson SL, Murphy J. Prognostic factors for healing of bone lesions in histiocytosis X. *Pediatr Radiol* 1988;18:326–332.

*73. Kieffer SA, Nesbit ME, D'Angio GJ. Vertebra plane due to histiocytosis X: serial studies. *Acta Radiol* 1969;8:241–250.

74. Concepcion W, Esquivel CO, Terry A, Nakazato P, Garcia-Kennedy R, Houssin D, Cox KL. Liver transplantation in Langerhans' cell histiocytosis (histiocytosis X). *Semin Oncol* 1991;8:24–28.

*75. Smith DG, Nesbit ME Jr, D'Angio GJ, Levitt SH. Histiocytosis X: role of radiation therapy in management with special reference to dose levels employed. *Radiology* 1973;106:419–422.

76. Capana R, Springfield DS, Ruggieri P, et al. Direct cortisone injection in eosinophilic granuloma of bone. *Radiology* 1980;136:289–293.

77. Kilpatrick SE, Wenger DE, Gilchrist GS, Shives TC, Wollan PC, Unni KK. Langerhans' cell histiocytosis (histiocytosis X) of bone. *Cancer* 1995;76:2471–2484.

78. Nezelof C, Barbey S, Gane P, Jaubert F, Rousseau-Merck MF. Histiocytosis X: a proliferation disorder of the Langerhans' cell system. *Med Pediatr Oncol* 1986;14:108–109.

79. Griffin TW. The treatment of advanced histiocytosis X with sequential hemibody irradiation. *Cancer* 1977;39:2435–2436.

80. Berry DH, Gresik MV, Humphrey GB, et al. Natural history of histiocytosis X: a pediatric oncology group study. *Med Pediatr Oncol* 1986;14:1–5.

81. Crocker AC. The histiocytosis syndromes. In: Gellis SS, Kagan BM, eds. *Current pediatric therapy,* 10th ed. Philadelphia: WB Saunders, 1982:661–662.

82. Raney RB Jr. Chemotherapy for children with aggressive fibromatosis and Langerhans' cell histiocytosis. *Clin Orthop* 1991;262:58–63.

83. Savinas A, Rageliene L. Role of chemotherapy in disseminated Langerhans cell histiocytosis. *Med Pediatr Oncol* 1992;20:452.

84. West WO. Velban as treatment for disseminated eosinophilic granuloma of bone: follow-up note after seventeen years. *J Bone Joint Surg Am* 1984;66:1128.

85. Arico M. Cyclosporine therapy for refractory Langerhans' cell histiocytosis. *Blood* 1991;78:3107.

86. Davies EG, Levinsky RJ, Butler M, Broadbent V, Pritchard J, Chessells J. Thymic hormone therapy for histiocytosis X? *N Engl J Med* 1983;309:493–494.

87. Hirose M, Saito S, Yoshimoto T, Kuroda Y. Interleukin-2 therapy of Langerhans cell histiocytosis. *Acta Paediatr* 1995;84:1204–1206.

88. Osband ME, Cohen EB, Shipman DL. Treatment of histiocytosis X with suppression. In: Byrom NA, Hobbs JR, eds. *Thymic factor therapy.* New York: Raven Press, 1984:391–398.

89. Iwatsuki K, Tsugiki M, Yoshizawa N, Takigawa M, Yamada M, Shamoto M. The effect of phototherapies on cutaneous lesions of histiocytosis X in the elderly. *Cancer* 1986;57:1931–1936.

*90. Sheehan MP, Atherton DJ, Broadbent V, Pritchard J. Topical nitrogen mustard: an effective treatment for cutaneous Langerhans cell histiocytosis. *J Pediatr* 1991;119:317–321.

91. Mayou SC, Chu AC, Munro DD, Plowman N. Langerhans-cell histiocytosis—excellent response to etoposide. *Clin Exp Dermatol* 1991;16:292–294.

92. Mahmoud H, Gaber O, Wang W, Whitington G, Vera S, Murphy SB. Successful orthotopic liver transplantation in a child with Langerhans' cell histiocytosis. *Transplantation* 1991;51:278–280.

93. Arceci RJ. Treatment options-commentary. *Br J Cancer* 1994;23[Suppl]:558–560.

94. Conter V, Reciputo A, Arrigo C, Bazzato N, Sala A, Arico M. Bone marrow transplantation for refractory Langerhans' cell histiocytosis. *Haematologica on internet.* Internet site. e mail: aricom@ipv36.unipv.it.

95. Greinix HT, Storb R, Sanders JE, Petersen FB. Marrow transplantation for treatment of multisystem progressive Langerhans' cell histiocytosis. *Bone Marrow Trans* 1992;10:39–44.

*96. Morgan G. Myeloablative therapy and bone marrow transplantation for Langerhans' cell histiocytosis. *Br J Cancer* 1994;23[Suppl]:552–553.

97. Rawlings CE III, Wilkins RH. Solitary eosinophilic granuloma of the skull. *Neurosurgery* 1984;15: 155–161.

98. Komp DM, Silva-Sosa M, Miale T, Sexauer C, Herson J. Evaluation of a MOPP-type regimen in histiocytosis X—a Southwest Oncology Group study. *Cancer Treat Rep* 1977;61:855–859.

99. Broadbent V, Heaf D, Pritchard J, Pincott J. Occult multisystem involvement in histiocytosis X (HX). *Med Pediatr Oncol* 1986;14:113.

100. Ceci A, DeTerlizzi M, Calella R, et al. Etoposide in recurrent childhood Langerhans' cell histiocytosis: an Italian cooperative study. *Cancer* 1988;62: 2528–2531.

101. Jones RO, Pillsbury HC. Histiocytosis X of the head and neck. *Laryngoscope* 1984;94:1031–1035.

*102. Komp DM. Long-term sequelae of histiocytosis X. *Am J Pediatr Hematol Oncol* 1981;5:165–168.

103. Ransom JL, Morris P, John RG, Anderson HR, Murphy SB. Neuropsychological late sequelae of histiocytosis X. *Pediatr Res* 1978;12:47(abst).

104. Egeler RM, Neglia JP, Puccetti DM, Brennan CA, Nesbit ME. The association of Langerhans' cell histi-

ocytosis with malignant neoplasms. *Cancer* 1993;71: 865–874.

105. Jones LR, Toth BB, Cangir A. Treatment for solitary eosinophilic granuloma of the mandible by steroid injection: report of a case. *J Oral Maxillofac Surg* 1989;47:306–309.

106. Ceci A, de Terlizzi M, Colella R, et al. Langerhans cell histiocytosis in childhood: results from the Italian cooperative AIEOP-CR-H.X. '83 study. *Med Pediatr Oncol* 1993;21:259–264.

107. Haupt R, Fears TR, Rosso P, et al. Increased risk of secondary leukemia after single-agent treatment with etoposide for Langerhans' cell histiocytosis. *Pediatr Hematol Oncol* 1994;11:499–507.

108. Waters KD. Miscellaneous tumours. In: Ekert H, ed. *Clinical paediatric hematology and oncology.* Melbourne: Blackwell, 1982:218–221.

109. Favara B, McCarthy RC, Mieraw GW, et al. Histiocytosis X. In: Finegold M, ed. *Pathology of neoplasia in children and adolescents.* Philadelphia: WB Saunders, 1986:126–144.

110. Shelburne JD, Scroggs MW. Ultrastructural alterations in pathologic states. In: Garner A, Klintworth GK, eds. *Pathobiology of ocular disease: a dynamic approach,* part A. New York: Marcel Dekker, 1994:1–62.

111. Berry CL, ed. *Paediatric pathology.* Berlin: Springer-Verlag, 1991.

112. Cohen M, Fornoza J, Cangir A, Murray JA, Wallace S. Direct injection of methylprednisolone sodium succinate in the treatment of solitary eosinophilic granuloma of bone. *Radiology* 1980;136:289–293.

113. Scaglietti O, Marchetti PG, Bartolozzi P. Final results obtained in the treatment of bone cysts with methyl-prednisolone acetate (Depo-Medrol) and a discussion of results achieved in other bone lesions. *Clin Orthop* 1982;165:33–42.

114. Nauert C, Zornoza J, Ayala A, Harle TS. Eosinophilic granuloma of bone: diagnosis and management. *Skeletal Radiol* 1983;10:227–235.

115. Ruff S, Chapman GK, Taylor TKF, Ryan MD. The evolution of eosinophilic granuloma of bone: a case report. *Skeletal Radiol* 1983;10:37–39.

116. Fradia M, Podoshin L, Ben-Davie J, Grishkan A. Eosinophilic granuloma of the temporal bone. *J Larngol Otol* 1985;99:475–479.

117. Wirtschafter JD, Nesbit ME, Anderson P, McClain K. Intralesional methylprednisolone for Langerhans cell histiocytosis of the orbit and cranium. *J Pediatr Opthalm Strabism* 1987;24:194–197.

118. Kindy-Degnan NA, Laflamme P, Duprat G, Allaire GS. Intralesional steroid in the treatment of an orbital eosinophilic granuloma [Letter]. *Arch Opthalmol* 1991;109:617–628.

*119. Egeler RM, Thompson RC Jr, Voute PA, Nesbit Me Jr. Interlesional infiltration of corticosteroids in localized Langerhans cell histiocytosis. *J Pediatr Orthop* 1992;12:811–814.

119a. Egeler RM, Nesbit ME. Langerhans cell histiocytosis and other disorders of monocyte-histiocyte lineage. *Crit Rev Oncol Hematol* 1995;18(1):9–35.

120. Libicher M, Roeren T, Troger J. Localized Langerhans' cell histiocytosis of bone: treatment and follow-up in children. *Pediatr Radiol* 1995;25:S134–137.

121. Sessa S, Sommelet D, Lascombes P, Prevot J. Treatment of Langerhans-cell histiocytosis in children. Experience at the Children's Hospital of Nancy. *J Bone Joint Surg AM* 1994;76(10):1513–1525.

122. Slater JM, Swarm OJ. Eosinophilic granuloma of bone. *Med Pediatr Oncol* 1980;8(2):151–164.

18

Skin Cancer, Hemangioma, and Lymphangioma

Carcinoma of the skin is rare in children. Malignant melanomas occur, but rarely develop before puberty. Basal and squamous cell carcinomas are even less common. Cutaneous hemangiomas frequently occur in children, but radiotherapy is rarely indicated. Lymphangiomas are even more rarely considered for irradiation.

HEMANGIOMAS

Hemangiomas are common developmental vascular abnormalities. They are benign blood vessel tumors and may be encountered in any portion of the body (1–5). In this chapter, we will consider cutaneous, ocular, and vertebral body hemangiomas. Hepatic and subglottic hemangiomas are considered, respectively, in Chapters 14 and 16.

Historically, hemangiomas were divided into three clinical types. Nevus flammeus (port wine stains) are usually located on the face and neck and vary in size and color. Facial nevus flammeus in the cutaneous distribution of cranial nerve V, in association with leptomeningeal angiomas, is referred to as the Sturge-Weber syndrome (6). Nevus vasculosus (strawberry marks) are red and elevated. Angiocavernosum (cavernous hemangioma) were considered lesions of the deep vessels—especially the veins (7–9). Cavernous hemangiomas may be complicated by thrombocytopenia and consumptive coagulopathy (with hypofibrinogenemia) due to platelet seques-

tration within the lesion (Kasabach-Merritt syndrome).

A modern classification of the hemangiomata divides these lesions on the basis of their clinical and histopathologic features as well as their depth and capacity for dynamic growth and involution (10,11). This classification scheme splits the lesions into cellularly dynamic and adynamic lesions (Table 1).

Only 20% of hemangiomas are present at birth. The other 80% arise within the first 8 weeks of life. The natural history of the common juvenile hemangioma is one of increasing size during the first 6 to 9 months of life and then a period of slower growth when size increases parallel to the infant's growth. Involution generally follows at about 10% per year—with complete disappearance of 50% of lesions by 4 or 5 years of age and 90% by 9 years (4,5,7,9,11–14). In most cases, juvenile hemangiomas are best managed by observation. There are some indications for treatment, including: (a) rapid progression of the lesion producing unacceptable symptoms (such as a lid hemangioma, which obstructs vision and produces deprivation amblyopia or other ocular complications); (b) progression of a lesion with ulceration and infection (diaper area lesions are at high risk for ulceration); (c) progression of a lesion with the induction of unacceptable deformity from compression, or overgrowth of an extremity from increased blood flow from a limb he-

TABLE 1. *Classification of hemangiomas and vascular malformations*

By depth	New term	Old term
	Superficial (Involving only the dermis)	Strawberry
	Mixed (Involving the dermis and subcutaneous tissue)	Capillary/Cavernous
	Deep (Involving panniculus and deep structures)	Cavernous
By endothelial turnover rate		
	Normal or low (cellularly adynamic)	*High (cellularly dynamic)*
	Port wine stain	Hemangiomas
	Salmon patch	Capillary or "strawberry"
	Arteriovenous malformations	Mixed capillary/cavernous
	Venous malformations	Cavernous

Modified from refs. 5 and 22, with permission.

mangioma (hemangiomatous gigantism); (d) growth of a lesion in an intertriginous area where it is highly susceptible to trauma, ulceration, and secondary infection; (e) facial lesions producing cosmetic deformity; (f) high output cardiac failure; and (g) life-threatening Kasabach-Merritt syndrome (1,7–9,13, 15–19).

When a decision has been made to treat a hemangioma, one has many options: steroids, therapeutic embolization, vasoligation, cryotherapy, surgical excision, laser therapy, interferon, estrogen compounds, and cyclophosphamide (3,10,13,20,21). In the treatment of hemangiomas, 60% to 80% will respond to steroid therapy (22). Interferon alpha is also frequently effective. Some clinicians utilize it in cases that have failed to respond to steroids. Others consider it first-line therapy (5,23). Resection or arterial ligation is indicated for small lesions in which excision would not lead to significant cosmetic deformity. Surgery is also appropriate for treatment of uncontrolled ulceration, bleeding, or infection, arteriovenous shunts with heart failure, or obstruction of the visual axis (5).

Radiotherapy should only be considered for lesions that have failed to respond to steroids and interferon and that are not appropriate for other modalities of treatment. Significant late effects have been attributed to irradiation of hemangiomas, including scarring, abnormalities of bone growth, and secondary malignancies (3,8,13,15–17). The incidence of cancer after radiotherapy for skin hemangioma has been extensively studied and reported in a series of articles from Sweden (8,15,16,24–27). These articles describe 14,633 to 15,634 children irradiated at the Radiumhemmet, Stockholm, from 1909 to 1959 and 12,055 treated at Sahlgrenska University Hospital, Goteborg, from 1930 to 1965. At the Radiumhemmet, the most common type of treatment was by means of ^{226}Ra applicators (81%) or contact x-ray therapy (less than or equal to 60 KVP, 16%). At Goteborg, ^{226}Ra was used for 99% of the treatments. The median age at treatment was 6 months at Radiumhemmet and 5 months at Goteborg. There is an increased incidence of cancer as well as cancer mortality in these irradiated children when compared to expected rates—a finding given added emphasis by a long follow-up. Significantly increased numbers of cancers were found in the thyroid and, in females, the breast. Reconstructions of the dosimetry of the ^{226}Ra applicators seem to indicate a dose-response relationship. These data may be used to argue strongly against the use of radiotherapy for hemangiomas (8,15,16,24–27).

With the abandonment of ^{226}Ra and the wide availability of electron therapy, some ill effects of radiotherapy conceivably can now be avoided. Nonetheless, it seems prudent that radiotherapy should be avoided in general, and in the region of the breast buds, thyroid, and gonads, in particular.

The response of juvenile capillary hemangioma to external irradiation can be dramatic. In 1946, MacKee and Cipallaro (9) reported that the "results of beta-ray therapy in nevus vasculosus are so striking, so perfect, that they may be placed among the most notable achievements of radiation therapy in the treatment of cutaneous diseases." Furst et al. (8,15,16) reported good results in 88% of treated cases. If radiation is used, the treatment volume should include the visible and palpable lesion with a small margin. When treatment is administered in the region of the eye, appropriate lead shields or lead contact lenses should be used to shield the underlying visual structures. The dose per fraction should be between 150 and 300 cGy. The majority of lesions will respond to 2 or 3 fractions, for a total dose of 300 to 750 cGy. Occasionally, slightly higher doses may be indicated, but the total dose should never exceed 10 to 15 Gy (9,13). By observing these guidelines, regressions will generally occur rapidly and scarring will be minimal.

The radiotherapist will, on rare occasions, be asked to consult in cases of hemangiomas that began in infancy but instead of regressing, slowly enlarged as the child aged. The older child or young adult will present to medical attention with severe deformity and, rarely, hemodynamic compromise or coagulopathy (4,22). A host of other forms of treatment will have been tried and failed before radiotherapy is considered. The response to radiotherapy in these large symptomatic hemangiomas is often gratifying (1,19,28). The lesion should be evaluated by careful physical examination and diagnostic imaging—usually computerized tomography (CT), magnetic resonance imaging (MRI), and/or angiography. The lesion is irradiated with relatively tight margins. Treatment with fractionated continuous or split course radiotherapy at 1.5 to 2 Gy per fraction to a total dose of 30 to 40 Gy is appropriate based on the available dose-response data (28,29) (Fig. 1).

Another special case is the management of orbital hemangiomas. When irradiation of lid lesions is required, care is taken to protect the eye by placing a lead cup or shield behind the lids and against the eye. Superficial x-rays or electrons are then used for treatment. Posterior orbit hemangiomas may be successfully treated with total doses of 12 to 18 Gy using techniques similar to the commonly used lateral beam approach for retinoblastoma (see Chapter 5) (1,13).

Hemangiomas of bone are benign slow-growing tumors, which can be of cavernous or capillary structure. The majority are asymptomatic and are detected on routine radiographs. The hemangioma produces replacement of the normal cancellous bone with thick bony traberculae. On plain radiographs and CT a "honeycomb" or "polka-dot" appearance is characteristic (30,31). The incidence increases with age, and fewer than 10% of all cases occur in the first two decades of life (32). Hemangiomas of the vertebrae may give rise to neurologic symptoms ranging from pain and tenderness to severe spinal cord compression. The pathophysiology of these lesions include: (a) ballooning of the vertebrae with narrowing and deformation of the spinal canal; (b) extension of the hemangioma into the epidural space; and, rarely, (c) vertebral compression fracture. While asymptomatic vertebral hemangiomas do not require treatment, intervention is required for significant pain or for paresis or paraplegia. Laminectomy is recommended by some for rapid-onset cord compression but is hazardous because of the risk of severe hemorrhage. Catheter emobilization of feeder vessels has been successful but runs the risk of vascular catastrophe (31). External-beam irradiation, 20 to 30 Gy in 2 to 3 weeks with single or multiple fields, given as the sole treatment or postoperatively will relieve symptoms in the majority of cases. The CT scan, particularly with intraspinal contrast, will allow delineation of the lesion for treatment planning (2,8,30, 32–34).

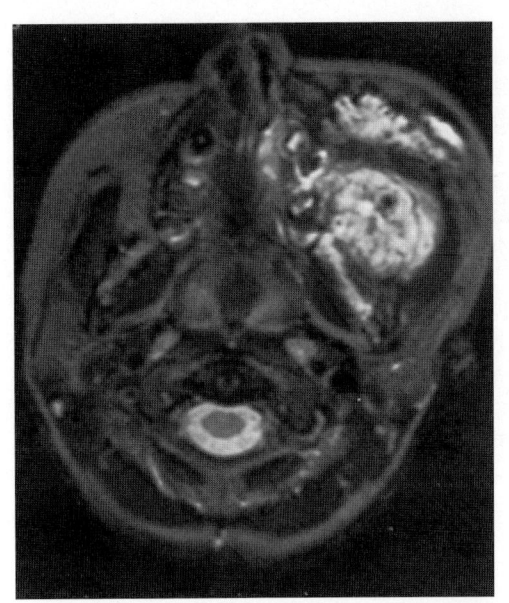

A

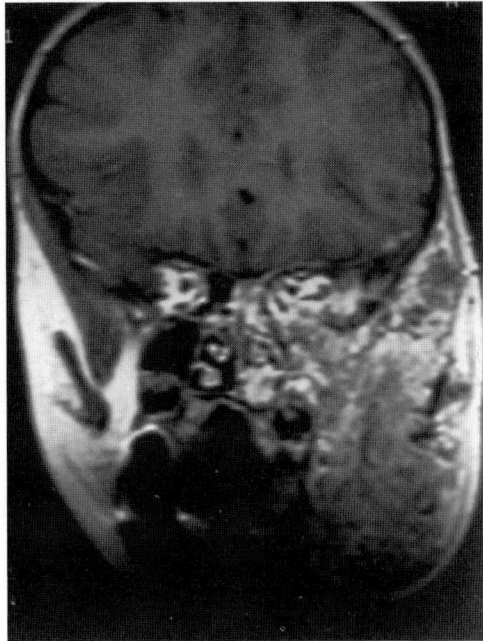

B

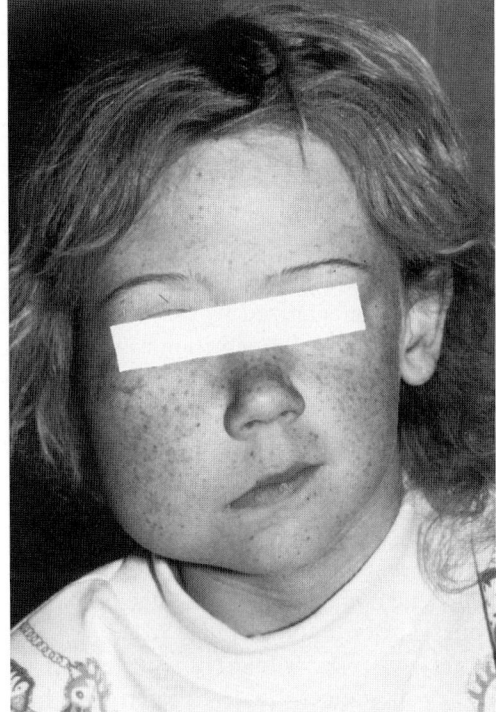

C

FIG. 1. A and **B**: This hemangioma grew from birth until, when the child was 8-years old, there was significant facial deformity and bleeding from the intraoral component of the lesion. There was a moderate response following a split course of irradiation to a total dose of 45 Gy. **C**: Disease remains stable 6.5 years following irradiation.

LYMPHANGIOMA

Lymphangiomas are usually first noted in infancy and can cause symptoms in the neonate, young child, or adult. They can occur throughout the body but are preponderant in the neck. They may infiltrate the tongue or the floor of the mouth, causing deformity, pain associated with frequent infections, and obstruction of the aerodigestive passages. Spontaneous regression of these lesions is rare (35,36).

Lymphangiomas are composed of dilated lymph vessels, the walls of which consist of endothelial cells and fibrous tissues (37). Four distinct forms have been described. These include *capillary lymphangiomas,* an uncommon lesion that may have the appearance of an ordinary wart or group of small vesicles. These lesions consist of a network of spaces formed by small- and medium-sized lymphatic vessels. *Cavernous lymphangiomas* occur in the skin and subcutaneous tissue, salivary glands, and lips. These are diffuse, spongy masses often with indistinct margins. They consist of multiple dilated lymph channels that are lined with either single or multiple layers of endothelial cells. *Cystic hygromas* are the most frequent of the lymphangiomas. They are composed of cysts that are from a few millimeters to several centimeters in diameter. These cysts compress surrounding tissues while small vessels coarse over their walls. Finally, *lymphangeal hemangiomas* consist of a combination of blood- and lymph-containing channels. While these lesions are quite similar to cavernous lymphangiomas, they also contain some spaces filled with erythrocytes and are, therefore, presumed to be in direct communication with the vascular system (35,37,38).

Surgical excision is the best therapy for lymphangiomas, although this may be difficult in certain situations and may require more than one surgical procedure (38). Sclerosing agents have, in the past, been deemed unsatisfactory. Tanigawa et al. (38) suggests treating unresectable lesions with bleomycin in a microsphere-in-oil emulsion. Radiation therapy is rarely used. Dose inhomogeneity and the risk of infection have discouraged radiotherapists from utilizing interstitial irradiation. Some dramatic responses of neck, chest, and mesenteric lymphangioma to external-beam irradiation have been reported in the literature (39–42). One must be cautious, however, because physicians are more likely to report their therapeutic successes rather than their failures (37).

Fractionated irradiation to a total dose of 15 to 30 Gy has been utilized bearing in mind the known risks of radiation to the head and neck, including inhibition of bone growth and soft tissue development as well as the risk of induction of thyroid cancer.

BASAL AND SQUAMOUS CELL CARCINOMAS

Basal and squamous cell skin cancers are infrequently diagnosed in children (43,44). When they do occur in childhood, there is usually a predisposition to skin cancer—that is, basal cell nevus syndrome (BCNS) or xeroderma pigmentosa. They have also been reported as arising in a nevus sebaceous (45), following cranial irradiation for acute lymphoblastic leukemia (46), and following thorium X treatment of a hemangioma (47). BCNS is characterized by the occurrence of multiple basal cell epitheliomas, a positive family history for the syndrome, keratocysts of the jaw, epidermal cyst and hamartoma formation, palmar and plantar pits, skeletal abnormalities, and oculoneurologic abnormalities (29). The basal cell epitheliomas that occur and require treatment develop on the face, neck, and trunk. Patients may be treated with chemotherapy, immunotherapy, electrodesiccation, cryotherapy, Moh's chemosurgery, or primary surgery with reconstruction of the defect. Some children have been treated with radiotherapy, although this treatment is generally reserved for adults.

BCNS may provide a unique example of the genetic-environmental interaction for the production of malignancies. Several patients have been reported with BCNS who have also developed medulloblastoma in early childhood. In each survivor, multiple basal cell epitheliomas have developed within 6 months to 3 years of craniospinal irradiation. These skin cancers develop at an age distinctly earlier and in a distribution unlike that of family members with BCNS. The distribution of basal cell epitheliomas corresponds to the radiotherapy ports. The development of multiple cutaneous skin cancers has not been generally reported in the general population of long-term survivors in medulloblastoma (48). This unusual illustration of multi-hit mutagenesis may suggest that radiotherapy for skin epitheliomas is relatively contraindicated in young children with BCNS.

Xeroderma pigmentosa (XP) is an autosomally dominant inherited disease. The clinical manifestations occur primarily on sun-exposed skin that develops abnormal pigmentation and multiple malignant tumors. Areflexia, mental retardation, and other neurologic abnormalities are associated with XP. The biochemical defect appears to be a relatively poor ability to repair ultraviolet-induced DNA damage. Basal cell and squamous cell carcinomas of the skin may develop in patients with XP. These carcinomas are usually treated with the standard techniques of electrodesiccation, curettage, surgery, cryosurgery, or chemosurgery. Because ionizing radiation damage to XP cells is repaired normally, there is no theoretical objection to radiotherapy treatment of tumors if indicated. Situations where radiotherapy will be appropriate, however, are quite rare (49).

At St. Jude Children's Research Hospital (SJCRH), eight children with skin carcinomas were seen from 1962 to 1986. In four patients, basal cell epitheliomas developed in previously irradiated fields (acute lymphoblastic leukemia, Hodgkin's disease, neuroblastoma). There was a fifth case with BCNS. The three patients treated for squamous cell carcinoma had a prior diagnosis of XP (49–52).

From 1971 to 1991, seven cases of basal cell carcinoma and three cases of squamous cell carcinoma were encountered at the National Institute of Pediatrics in Mexico City (43). Five of the 7 children with basal cell carcinoma had XP, one had BCNS, and one developed in a previous radiotherapy field. One of the 3 patients with squamous cell carcinoma also had XP.

MALIGNANT MELANOMA

The incidence of malignant melanoma before the age of 15 years is estimated to be 1 to 2 per million population in the United States and United Kingdom and 4 per million in Australia. Fewer than 1% of all malignant melanomas are seen in children and adolescents (6,11,14,22,53–57). Childhood melanoma in Australia is higher than that reported in other series—accounting for 3.3% of all pediatric neoplasms. This is presumably associated with excessive UV exposure (22).

At least five factors are worthy of particular consideration in the etiology of malignant melanoma in children: large congenital nevocytic nevi (LCNN), dysplastic nevus syndrome (DNS), immunosuppression, transplacental malignant melanoma, and XP.

LCNN are defined as congenital nevi 20 cm or more in diameter (58). They may occur anywhere on the body and include the so-called "bathing trunks" nevi. There is controversy in the literature regarding the relative risk of malignant melanoma arising in LCNN, with lifetime risks ranging from 2% to 31% (56,58,59). Familial DNS is an autosomal dominant trait characterized by unusual nevi at risk for developing melanoma. XP patients are at significant risk for developing melanoma for reasons described previously in this chapter. The influence of immunosuppression on the development of melanoma is evidenced by the increased risk of the malignancy in genetically transmitted immunodeficiency syndromes as well as following iatrogenic immunosuppression (56). There are rare reports of transplacental transmission of metastatic melanoma from mother to child (16,56,60). The infant usually has disseminated disease at birth and the prognosis is poor.

Childhood melanoma may be staged with the following system: stage I, localized disease; stage II, regional lymph node involvement; stage III, distant metastatic disease (60). Three important factors should be considered in evaluating stage I patients: the presence of local ulceration, Clark's level of invasion, and Breslow's depth of invasion. All three have been shown to be important prognostic indicators in childhood melanoma (55) (Table 2). In children, metastatic disease is rare in lesions less than 1.5 mm thick (22). It is important to distinguish malignant melanoma from the *juvenile melanoma* or *nevi of large spindle* and/or *epithelioid cells* or *Spitz nevi*. Melanoma was believed to have a benign course in children (54). In 1948, Dr. Sophie Spitz, a pathologist at New York's Memorial Hospital, described 12 of 13 children who were long-term survivors of this peculiar "benign" childhood melanoma (61). Spitz nevi are usually symmetrical, small, exhibit epithelial hyperplasia, contain clefts between nests of melanocytes and epidermis, exhibit maturation of melanocytes, and contain dull pink epidermal globutes called Kamino bodies (62,63).

The inclusion of benign Spitz nevi cases in pediatric malignant melanoma series results in an overdiagnosis of melanoma and an underestimate of its associated mortality rate (56). Series of pediatric patients with malignant melanoma that exclude the benign Spitz nevi cases, indicate that survival rates are similar to those of adults. There were 85 patients younger than 18 years of age with malignant melanoma among the 8,635 patients registered with the Duke Melanoma Clinic (1%)

(53,56). Fifty-nine percent of the patients had the superficial spreading histologic type, and 20% of the remaining patients were Clark's level III or IV. There was no difference in the actuarial survival rate between adult and juvenile stage I patients (Fig. 2).

The standard treatment for localized malignant melanoma is a wide local excision. In certain situations, a skin graft may be required to close the resulting defect (64,65). The role of elective node dissection of clinically uninvolved regional lymph nodes is a subject of debate. It is clear that not all patients are candidates for elective lymph node dissection. However, for patients with melanomas greater than 0.75 mm thick, the proper initial extent of surgery is debatable (51). The arguments in favor of elective node dissection include staging, detecting microscopic disease, and providing treatment of occult metastatic disease if present—therefore, reducing tumor burden as well as removing a potential source of future metastases (60). There may be a survival benefit to lymph node dissection for intermediate-to-thick lesions. In trunk locations, however, it may be difficult to determine the draining nodal site(s). The arguments against lymph node dissection include the fact that many patients will be found to have no nodal involvement, the high morbidity of the procedure, and the lack of benefits attendant to the operation in randomized trials (51).

Recently, many surgeons have adopted a staged procedure to select patients for lymph node dissection. The first lymph node that drains the primary tumor is called the sentinel lymph node (SLN). It may be localized with

TABLE 2. *Classification of the primary lesion in malignant melanoma*

Clark's et al.'s "levels" (72)	Breslow's "thickness" (64)
Level I: All tumor cells above the basement membrane	Using an ocular micrometer, measure
Level II: Tumor cells into the papillary but not reticular dermis	maximal thickness of lesion from granular
Level III: Tumor of the papillary/reticular dermis interface	cell layer to deepest point of lesion. If the
Level IV: Neoplastic cells into the collagen bundles of the	lesion is ulcerated, measure from the ulcer
reticular dermis	base over the deepest point of the lesion
Level V: Invasion of subcutaneous tissue	(i.e., <0.76 mm, 0.76–1.50 mm, >1.50 mm).

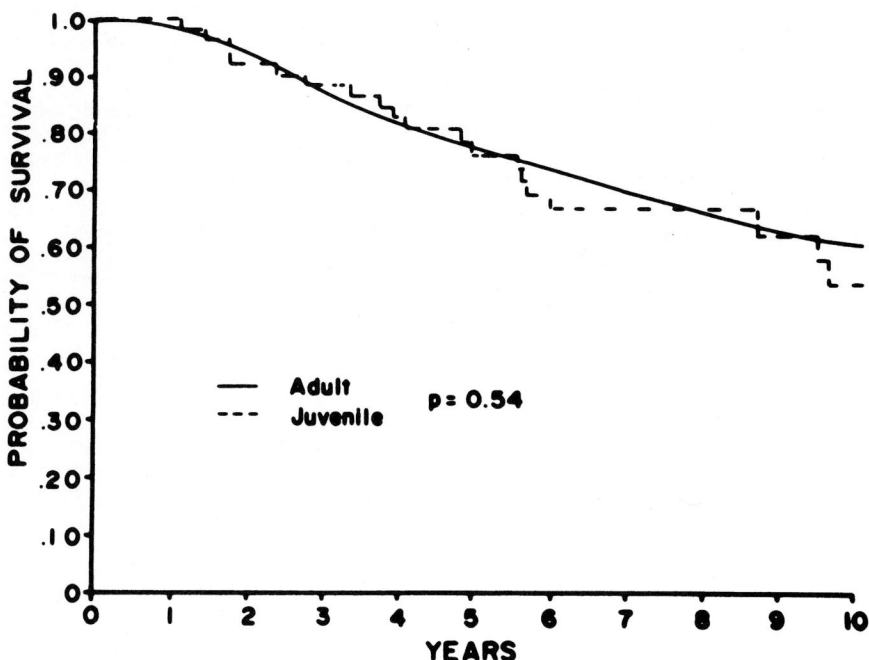

FIG. 2. Actuarial survival rates of the adult and juvenile stage I patients registered at the Duke University Melanoma Clinic. Of 18 pediatric patients who were disease-free for more than 7 years, 12 (67%) ultimately developed recurrent disease—including 5 patients who recurred more than 13 years after the initial diagnosis. Late recurrences indicate that patients must be carefully followed for a lifetime. (From ref. 56, with permission.)

vital blue dye and/or radial lymphoscintigraphy with a gamma probe. Subsequently, a directed selective lymphadenectomy may be performed to remove the SLN. Elective full lymph node dissections are reserved for those patients with metastatic disease in the SLN (51).

In the SJCRH series of 33 children treated from 1967 to 1988, there were no tumor-related deaths in children with thin melanomas (Clark's level I to II, Breslow thickness less than 1.5 mm) (55,60,66,67). Ten of 22 patients with lesions 1.55 mm or greater in thickness are alive without tumor. Twenty-four patients 16 years of age or younger with malignant melanoma were reviewed at St. Thomas' Hospital, London, from 1981 to 1993. Three of three patients with tumors 1.2 mm or smaller are alive without tumor whereas 3 of 19 children with tumors 1.6 mm or larger are alive but suffered local or nodal

relapse, 1 died of tumor, and 15 are event-free survivors (59).

There is some published evidence supporting the use of cyclophosphamide, vincristine, and dactinomycin for relapsed and/or metastatic disease. SJCRH has reported a complete/partial response in 8 of 18 patients (44%) (55,60). Dacarbazine as a single agent and melphalan with hyperthermic isolated limb perfusion are also active (50,68).

Radiotherapy is reasonably effective for the symptomatic palliation of metastases (69). Radiobiologic interest had been focused on the possibility that, at a cellular level, malignant melanoma is truly "radioresistant" (70). A survey of D_q values (shoulder width) of various mammalian cell lines suggests that a typical value for D_q is about 90 cGy. Observations from several investigators, however, suggest that malignant melanoma, grown in culture, has a particularly broad-shoulder survival curve with low linear energy transfer (LET) radiation with a D_q in excess of 200 cGy. These data reinforced an opinion that malignant melanoma was relatively radioresistant but might be more responsive to relatively high doses per fraction. In a review of several retrospective studies on fraction size and response in malignant melanoma in adults, the response probability when a fraction size was less than 400 cGy was 49% while the response when fraction size was greater than 600 cGy was 85% (71). These statistics excluded bone metastases where responses were approximately equivalent for small and large fractions. In a prospective trial of patients 15-years old or older with measurable lesions of malignant melanoma randomized between 4 fractions of 8 Gy on days 0, 7, 14, and 21 versus 20 fractions of 2.5 Gy, 5 days per week; on consecutive treatment days, there was approximately a 60% combined complete and partial response rate in 126 patients, with no difference between the two fractionation schemes. Stratification by tumor size (greater than or less than 5 cm) or tumor site (soft tissue/skin, nodal, other) also failed to show any difference between the 8 Gy and 2.5 Gy per fraction programs (69). If one relies on the data from retrospective studies, it would seem reasonable to use large fraction sizes in the palliation of malignant melanoma at sites other than bone when the problems of late ill effects of irradiation are less worrisome. The recent prospective trial suggests that more conventional palliative fractionation is equally reasonable in certain palliative situations where there is a significant probability of a long-term survival.

REFERENCES

References particularly recommended for further reading are indicated by an asterisk.

1. Dutton SC, Plowman PN. Paediatric haemangiomas: the role of radiotherapy. *Br J Radiol* 1991;64:261–269.
2. Eisenstein S, Spira F, Browde S, Lewer AL, Grabler CM. The treatment of symptomatic vertebral hemangioma by radiotherapy: a case report. *Spine* 1986;11: 640–642.
3. Enjairas O, Riche MC, Merland JJ, Escande JP. Man-

4. Morelli JG. Hemangiomas and vascular malformations. *Pediatr Ann* 1996;25:91–96.
5. Ricketts RR, Hatley RM, Corden BJ, Sabio H, Howell CG. Interferon-alpha 2a for the treatment of complex hemangiomas of infancy and childhood. *Ann Surg* 1994;219:605–614.
6. Paller AS. The Sturge-Weber syndrome. *Pediatr Dermatol* 1987;4:300–304.
7. Braun-Falco O, Goldschmidt H, Lukacs S. *Dermatologic radiotherapy.* New York: Springer-Verlag, 1976.
*8. Furst CJ, Lundell M, Holm LE. Radiation therapy of hemangiomas, 1909–1959. A report based on 50 years of clinical practice at Radiumhemmet, Stockholm. *Acta Oncol* 1987;26:33–36.
9. MacKee GM, Cipallaro AC. *X-rays and radium in the treatment of diseases of the skin.* Philadelphia: Lea & Febiger, 1946:513–521.
10. Hurvitz CH, Alkalay AL, Sloninsky L, Kallus M, Pomerance JJ. Cyclophosphamide therapy in life-threatening vascular tumors. *J Pediatr* 1986;109: 360–363.
11. Pasyk KA. Classification and clinical and histopathological features of hemangiomas and other vascular malformations. In: Ryan TJ, Cherry GW, eds. *Vascular birthmarks: pathogenesis and management.* Oxford: Oxford University Press, 1987:1–55.
12. Akyuz C, Yaris N, Kutluk MT, Buyukpanukcu M. Benign vascular tumors and vascular malformations in childhood: a retrospective analysis of 1127 cases. *Turk J Pediatr* 1997;39(4):435–445.
13. Markoe AM, Brady LW, Grant GD, Shields JA, Augsburger JJ. Radiation therapy of the ocular disease. In: Perez CA, Brady LW, eds. *Principles and practice of radiation oncology.* Philadelphia: JB Lippincott, 1987: 453–454.
14. Persky MS. Congenital vascular lesions of the head and neck. *Laryngoscope* 1986;96:1002–1015.
*15. Furst CJ, Lundell M, Holm L-E, Silfversward C. Cancer incidence after radiotherapy for skin hemangioma: a retrospective cohort study in Sweden. *Natl Cancer Inst* 1988;80:1387–1392.
*16. Furst CJ, Silfversward C, Holm L-E. Mortality in a cohort of radiation treated childhood skin hemangiomas. *Acta Oncol* 1989;28:789–794.
17. Lenarsky C. Etiology of childhood malignancy. In: Lanzkowsky P. *Pediatric oncology: a treatise for the clinician.* New York: McGraw-Hill, 1983:1–12.
18. Plowman PN, Harnett AN. Radiotherapy in benign orbital disease. I. complicated ocular angiomas. *Br J Ophthalmol* 1988;72:286–288.
*19. Schild SE, Buskirk SJ, Frick LM, Cupps RE. Radiotherapy for large symptomatic hemangiomas. *Int J Radiat Oncol Biol Phys* 1991;21:729–735.
20. Trout HH. Management of patients with hemangiomas and arteriovernous malformations. *Surg Clin North Am* 1986;66:333–338.
21. White CW, Sandheimer HM, Crouch EC, Wilson H, Fan LL. Treatment of pulmonary hemangiomatosis with recombinant interferon alfa-2a. *N Engl J Med* 1989;320:1197–1200.
22. McWhirter WR, Dobson C, Ring I. Childhood cancer in Australia, *Int J Cancer* 1996;65:34–38.
23. Illum N, Karlsmark T, Svejgaard F, Ullman S, Yssing

M. Ulcerated haemangioma successfully treated with interferon alfa-2a and topical granulocyte-macrophage colony-stimulating factor. *Dermatol* 1995;191: 315–317.

24. Lindberg S, Karlsson P, Arvidsson B, Holmberg E, Lundberg LM, Wallgran A. Cancer incidence after radiotherapy for skin haemangioma during infancy. *Acta Oncol* 1995;34:735–740.

25. Lundell M, Hakulinen T, Holm L-E. Thyroid cancer after radiotherapy for skin hemangioma in infancy. *Radiat Res* 1994;140:334–339.

26. Lundell M, Holm L-E. Risk of solid tumors after irradiation in infancy. *Acta Oncol* 1995;34:727–734.

27. Lundell M, Mattson A, Hakulinen T, Holm L-E. Breast cancer after radiotherapy for skin hemangioma in infancy. *Radiat Res* 1996;145:225–230.

28. Sealy B, Barry L, Buret E, et al. Cavernous hemangioma of the head and neck in the adult. *J R Soc Med* 1989;82:198–202.

29. Southwick GJ, Schwartz RA. The basal cell nevus syndrome: disasters occurring among a series of 36 patients. *Cancer* 1979;44:2294–2305.

30. Jeleniewski-Rudyk A. Treatment of vertebral hemangiomas. *Pol Rev Radiol Nucl Med* 1967;31:155–160.

31. Raco A, Ciappetta P, Artico M, Salvati M, Guidetti G, Guglielmi G. Vertebral hemangiomas with cord compression: the role of embolization in five cases. *Surg Neurol* 1990;34:164–168.

32. Unni KK, Irvius JC, Beabaul JW. Hemangioma, hemangiopericytoma, and hemangioendothelioma (angiosarcoma) of bone. *Cancer* 1971;27:1403–1414.

33. Lindquist I. Vertebral hemangioma with compression of the spinal cord. *Acta Radiol* 1951;35:400–406.

34. McAllister VL, Kendall BE, Bull JWD. Symptomatic vertebral hemangiomas. *Brain* 1975;98:71–80.

*35. Gordon RF, Parkin JL. Lymphangioma of the head and neck. *Ear Nose Throat J* 1982;61:338–342.

36. Saija M, Munro IR, Mancer K. Lymphangioma: a long-term follow-up study. *Plast Reconstr Surg* 1975;56:642–651.

37. Holmes GW, Hawes LE. Radiation treatment of lymphangioma. *AJR* 1943;49:799–802.

38. Tanigawa N, Shimatsuya T, Takahashi K, et al. Treatment of cystic hygroma and lymphangioma with the use of bleomycin fat emulsion. *Cancer* 1987;60:741–749.

39. Dajee H, Woodhouse R. Lymphangiomatosis of the mediastinum with chylothorax and chylopericardium: role of radiation treatment. *J Thorac Cardiovasc Surg* 1994;108:594–595.

40. Ikemura K, Hidaka H, Fujiwara T, Ohkuma R, Terashinma H. A case of cystic lymphangioma extending from the neck to the tongue. *J Craniomaxofac Surg* 1987;15:369–371.

41. Johnson DW, Klazynski PT, Gordon WH, Russell DA. Mediastinal lymphangioma and chylothorax: the role of radiotherapy. *Ann Thorac Surg* 1986;41:325–328.

42. Tai PTH, Jewell LD. Case report: mesenteric mixed haemangioma and lymphangioma; report of a case with 10 year follow-up after radiation treatment. *Br J Radiol* 1995;68:657–661.

43. de la Luz Orozco-Cavarrubias M, Tamoyo-Sanchez L, Duran-McKinster C, Ridaura C, Ruiz-Maldonada R. Malignant cutaneous tumors in children: twenty years of experience at a large pediatric hospital. *J Am Acad Dermatol* 1994;30:243–249.

44. Hay WE. Nonmelanoma skin carcinoma in Albuquerque, New Mexico: experience of a major health care provider. *Cancer* 1996;77:2489–2495.

45. Hughes JR, O'Donnell PJ, Pembroke AC. Basal cell carcinoma arising in a naevus sebaceous in a 5 year old girl. *Clin Exp Dermatol* 1995;20:177.

46. Yoshihara T, Ikuta H, Hibi S, Todo S, Imashuku S. Second cutaneous neoplasms after acute lymphoblastic leukemia in childhood. *Int J Hematol* 1993;59:67–71.

47. Scerri L, Navaratnam AE. Basal cell carcinoma presenting as a delayed complication of thorium X used for treating congenital hemangioma. *J Am Acad Dermatol* 1994;31:796–797.

48. Strong LC. Genetic and environmental interactions. *Cancer* 1977;40:1861–1866.

49. Robbins JH, Kraemer KH, Lutzner MA, Festoff BW, Coon HG. Xeroderma pigmentosum: an inherited disease with sun sensitivity, multiple cutaneous neoplasms, and abnormal DNA repair. *Ann Intern Med* 1974;80:221–248.

50. Baas PC, Hoekstra HJ, Koops HS, Oosterhuis WJ, Vander Weele LT. Hyperthermic isolated regional perfusion in the treatment of extremity melanoma in children and adolescents. *Cancer* 1989;63:199–203.

51. Ablertini JJ, Cruse CW, Rapaport D, et al. Intraoperative radial lymphoscintigraphy improves sentinel lymph node identification for patients with melanoma. *Ann Surg* 1996;223:217–224.

52. Pratt CB, George SL, Green AA, Fields LA, Dodge RK. Carcinomas in children: clinical and demographic characteristics. *Cancer* 1988;61:1046–1050.

53. Davidoff AM, Cirrincione C, Seigler HF. Malignant melanoma in children. *Ann Surg Oncol* 1994;1: 278–282.

54. Nassan A, Al-Nafussi A, Quaba A. Cutaneous malignant melanoma in children and adolescents in Scotland 1979–1991. *Plast Reconstr Surg* 1996;98:442–446.

55. Rao BN, Hayes FA, Prah CB, et al. Malignant melanoma in children: its management and prognosis. *J Pediatr Surg* 1990;25:198–203.

*56. Reintgen DS, Vollmer R, Seigler HF. Juvenile malignant melanoma. *Surg Gynecol Obstet* 1989;168:249–253.

57. Swerdlow AJ. Epidemiology of cutaneous malignant melanoma. *Clin Oncol* 1984;3:407–437.

58. Gari LM, Rivers JK, Kopf AW. Melanomas arising in large congenital nevocytic nevi: a prospective study. *Pediatr Dermatol* 1988;5:151–158.

59. Handerfield-Jones SE, Smith NP. Malignant melanoma in childhood. *Br J Dermatol* 1996;134:607–616.

60. Pratt CB, Palmer MK, Thatcher N, Croutha D. Malignant melanoma in children and adolescents. *Cancer* 1981;47:392–397.

61. Spitz S. Melanomas of childhood. *Am J Pathol* 1948; 24:591–609.

62. Barnhill RL, Flotte TJ, Fleischli M, Perez-Atayde A. Cutaneous melanoma and atypical spitz tumors in childhood. *Cancer* 1995;76:1833–1845.

63. Helm KF, Schwartz RA, Janniger CK. Juvenile melanoma (Spitz nevus). *Cutis* 1996;57:35–39.

64. Breslow A. Tumor thickness, level of invasion and node of dissection in stage I cutaneous melanoma. *Ann Surg* 1975;182:572–575.

65. Horgan K, Lawlor D, Corcoran N, Prendiville JB. Prepubertal melanoma. *J Pediatr Surg* 1987;22:1039–1040.

66. Hayes FA, Green AA. Malignant melanoma in child-

hood: clinical course and response to chemotherapy. *J Clin Oncol* 1984;2:1229–1238.

67. Roth ME, Grant-Kels JM, Kuhn K, Greenberg RD, Hurwitz S. Melanoma in children. *J Am Acad Dermatol* 1990;22:265–274.

68. Boodie AW Jr, Cangir A. Adjuvant and neoadjuvant chemotherapy with dacarbazine in high-risk childhood melanoma. *Cancer* 1987;60:1720–1723.

69. Sause WT, Cooper JS, Rush S, et al. Fraction size in external beam radiation therapy in the treatment of melanoma. *Int J Radiat Oncol Biol Phys* 1990;20: 429–432.

70. Dewey DL. The radiosensitivity of melanoma cells in culture. *Br J Radiol* 1971;44:816–817.

71. Habeshaw T, Wheldon TE. Malignant melanoma: the role of radiotherapy. *Clin Oncol* 1984;3:571–596.

72. Clark WH Jr, Fram L, Bernardino EA, Mihm MC. The histogenesis and biologic behavior of primary human malignant melanomas of the skin. *Cancer Res* 1969; 29:705–726.

19

Late Effects of Cancer Treatment

The use of radiation therapy (RT) in the management of childhood cancer must be determined, in part, by a knowledge of the late effects of radiation on normal tissues. As more children with cancer survive following therapy, the obligation grows for the oncologist to critically assess the adverse effects of therapy on the physical, intellectual, and emotional development of children. The impact of death due to treatment complications on overall survival and the increase in its relative importance with the increasing survival of children with cancer, is demonstrated by data from St. Jude Children's Research Hospital (1) (Fig. 1).

"Late effects" have their onset months or years following the cessation of treatment. This implies that therapeutic decisions intended to obviate late effects can only be based on the probability, not the certainty, that such events affect the interplay of therapy, patient, and tumor factors. Therapy factors include the total and fractional dose of irradiation, dose rate, overall treatment time, machine energy, treatment volume (2), dose distribution, and the use of other therapies (surgery, chemotherapy, radiosensitizers and protectors). Patient factors include the child's developmental status, genetic predisposition, inherent tissue sensitivities and capacity for normal tissue repair, underlying disease or abnormalities (structural and functional), and compensating mechanisms (i.e., the presence of an unirradiated second kidney). Tumor factors include direct tissue effects (such as extent of invasion), systemic effects of tumor-induced organ dysfunction or chemical secretion, and indirect mechanical effects (e.g., hydronephrosis).

Determining the frequency and pathogenesis of late effects is difficult for several reasons: (a) the patient must be a long-term survivor to manifest late effects; (b) the numbers of affected and unaffected patients must be known in order to assign a probability risk; (c) dramatic late effects are recognized by most physicians, more subtle or subclinical damage receives little attention; (d) the use of combined modality therapy, as well as the latent period resulting in the development of late effects, makes it difficult to unequivocally assign blame to any single therapy; (e) the influence of complicating factors is difficult to identify such as other illnesses or genetic abnormalities.

In rapidly proliferating tissues, cell kill is expressed clinically as an acute injury. Tissues in which cells are postmitotic and fully differentiated were previously thought to be relatively resistant to chemotherapy. It is now known that drug action is so diverse that such assessments are inaccurate. For example, Adriamycin affects mature cardiac myocytes by cell membrane or DNA binding, producing cell damage even when cell replication is not occurring (3). It is clear that cell injury may occur, depending on the chemotherapeutic agent, at different levels of cell cycle activity or cell differentiation. The effect of chemotherapeutic insult may not necessarily be expressed as frank cell injury. It may be expressed as a depletion of stem cell reserve or as loss of the normal mitotic potential of reserve stem cells.

Radiation damage is produced by some combination of parenchymal cell loss and injury to the underlying vasculature (4,5). Initial tissue recovery is due mainly to parenchymal

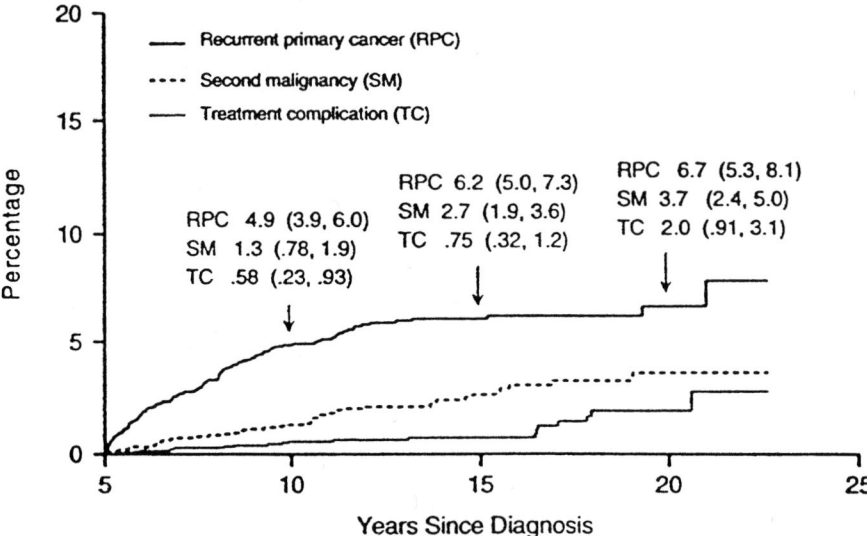

FIG. 1. Cumulative incidence (percentage) for mortality from recurrence, second malignancy, and nonneoplastic treatment complication for childhood cancer patients treated between 1971 and 1983 who survived at least 5 years. (From ref. 1, with permission.)

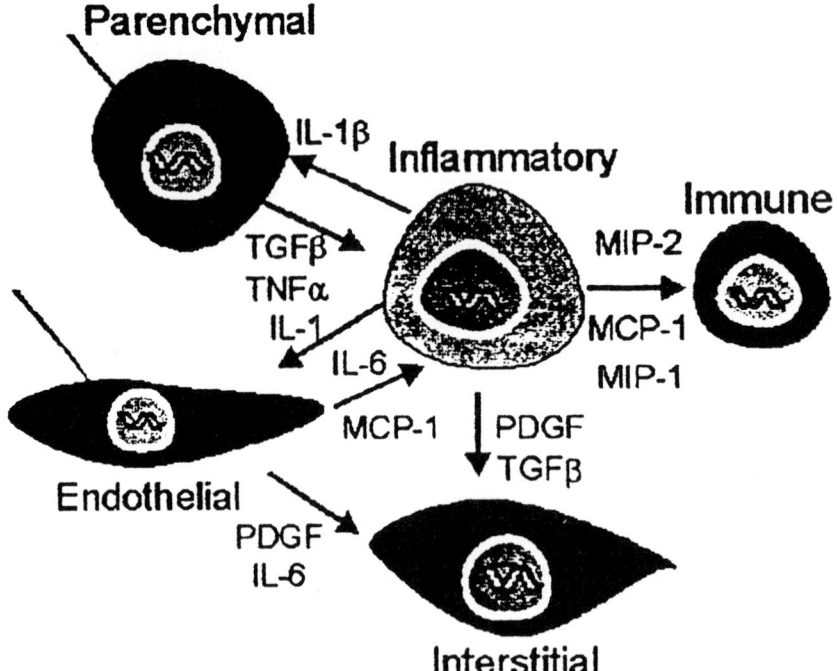

FIG. 2. Cell-cell interaction and control of gene expression by cytokines, chemokines, and growth factors in radiation injury. (From ref. 6, with permission.)

cell repopulation. The progressive component of damage is the arteriocapillary fibrosis, which predominates in the late irreparable injury and accentuates the cellular depletion of the parenchyma. It is the vascular changes that follow irradiation, but not chemotherapy, that partially account for the differences in late effects of the two modes of treatment. The distribution of late radiation damage reflects primarily vascular injury and cannot be explained simply as an indirect effect of parenchymal cell loss. Devastating late effects of radiation or of radiation and chemotherapy can occur in both rapidly and slowly proliferating normal tissues without a clinically recognizable acute phase because of this vascular injury.

Advances in molecular biophysiology have provided insights into the responses of normal tissues to chemotherapeutic and radiation injury. The classic concept of a single target cell that can explain the dynamic sequence of events leading to organ damage is supplanted by that of multiple cell systems interacting. Moreover, the acute and late phases of adverse effects are actually manifestations of an ongoing sequence of events due to autocrine, paracrine, and endocrine messages that occur immediately after injury to a variety of cells: epithelial, endothelial, fibroblasts, and inflammatory. As schematized in Fig. 2, a variety of growth and inhibitory factors are released, specific cell receptors are altered, and the resulting signals received by these receptors are translated into postreceptor cytoplasmic, nuclear, and interstitial events. The importance of this is that interventions are possible that can upregulate or downregulate cytokine responses, leading to a modulation of the toxic reaction (6).

EFFECTS OF CHEMOTHERAPY AND RT ON NORMAL TISSUE

Late effects have been reported in patients who received seemingly "safe doses" of

TABLE 1. *Tolerance doses TD$_5$–TD$_{50}$ (fractionated dose, whole or partial organ)[a]*

Target cell	Complication end point	Dose range (Gy) TD$_5$–TD$_{50}$
Range: 2 to 10 Gy		
Lymphoid and lymphocytes	Lymphopenia	2–10
Testes spermatogonia	Sterility	1–2
Ovarian oocytes	Sterility	6–10
Diseased bone marrow (CLL or multiple myeloma)	Severe leukopenia and thrombocytopenia	3–5
Range: 10 to 20 Gy		
Lens	Cataract	6–12
Bone marrow stem cell	Acute aplasia	15–20
Range: 20 to 30 Gy		
Kidney: renal glomeruli	Arterionephrosclerosis	23–28
Lung: type II: VCTS	Pneumonitis/fibrosis	20–30
Range: 30 to 40 Gy		
Liver central veins	Hepatopathy	35–40
Bone marrow	Hypoplasia	25–35
Range: 40 to 50 Gy		
Heart/whole organ	Pericarditis and pancarditis	43–50
Bone marrow microenvironments	Permanent aplasia	45–50
Range: 50 to 75 Gy		
Gastrointestinal	Infarction necrosis	50–55
Heart/partial organ	Cardiomyopathy	55–65
Spinal cord	Myelopathy	50–60
Brain	Encephalopathy	54–70
Mucosa (UAD)	Ulcer	65–75
Rectum	Ulcer	65–75
Bladder	Ulcer	65–75
Mature bones	Fracture	65–70

VCTS, vasculoconnective tissue systems; UAD, upper aerodigestive tract.
[a]Modified from ref. 328, with permission.

chemotherapy and radiotherapy, below the generally accepted threshold levels for either of the two when used alone. One must be circumspect in accepting "tolerance doses" for normal tissues and organs in the combined treatment modality era. Untoward reactions can occur at unexpected time intervals and in an unpredictable fashion. Chemotherapy acts predominantly on the cellular parenchymal component, whereas radiation acts on the microcirculatory system and parenchymal cells. In rapid renewal systems, the same stem cell population is affected and the increased acute toxicity of both modes can usually be reduced by applying them sequentially. In slow renewal tissues, the additive ill effects of drugs and radiation are often related to entirely different target cell populations in the same organ system. Late effects may not be avoidable because chemotherapy, whenever applied, can result in additional stem cell kill and lead to expression of subclinical radiation effects. Therefore, the tolerance doses of fractionated RT, listed in Table 1 (6), might be lower in the setting of chemotherapy, as well as in children of younger age (discussed in the following section).

INFLUENCE OF THE DEVELOPMENTAL STAGE OF THE TARGET ORGAN ON ITS SENSITIVITY TO THERAPY

The potential for the development of debilitating effects in normal tissues is related to the cellular activity and maturation within the tissue under consideration. In children, a mosaic of different tissues are developing at different rates and in different temporal sequences. The vulnerability of tissues to adverse effects is increased during the periods of rapid proliferation, whereas in adults the same tissues are in a mature steady state with slow cell renewal kinetics (7,8). Immature pediatric tissue contains cells that are initially totipotent, then multipotent, and eventually unipotent. At this final stage they are either resting or actively proliferating, with or without differentiation, into specialized tissues or organs. Inherent within this development sequence are critical time points of exquisite vulnerability to therapy. Adding to the complexity is the fact that some slow renewal systems can become active if challenged or stimulated. Therefore, recognition of the various stages of cellular development in pediatric tissues is vital to determining the potential for late effects. Traditionally, radiation doses in children are modified by age—but without specific recognition of the periods of active proliferation, differentiation, and eventual maturation of one organ or tissue as it differs from another. When does a pediatric tissue or organ become similar to an adult tissue or organ? This is a major question that must be addressed in order to predict the sensitivity to late effects (7,8).

The growth of any given tissue follows one of four general developmental patterns (9,10) (Fig. 3). The first is commonly recognized skeletal pattern with peak growth rates in the early postnatal period and during puberty. The organs of circulation and digestion also follow this pattern. The second is the neural type, characterized by a rapid postnatal growth that slows in late infancy and ceases in adolescence. The respiratory and renal organs tend to follow this pattern. The third is the genital pattern, which shows little change during early life but shows rapid development just before and coincident with puberty. The sequence is followed by breast tissue, testes, and ovaries. The fourth pattern is the lymphoid type, characterized by a gradual evolution and involution to the time of puberty. Identification of these different rates and ages at which each tissue matures is necessary for determining its radiosensitivity. In addition, recognition of the mechanism of organ growth—that is, an increase in the size of cells (hypertrophy) as opposed to the number of cells (proliferation)—allows better identification of relative radiosensitivity, because organs that only hypertrophy are less vulnerable to functional disturbance by irradiation.

The late effects of therapy in a number of organ systems will be examined.

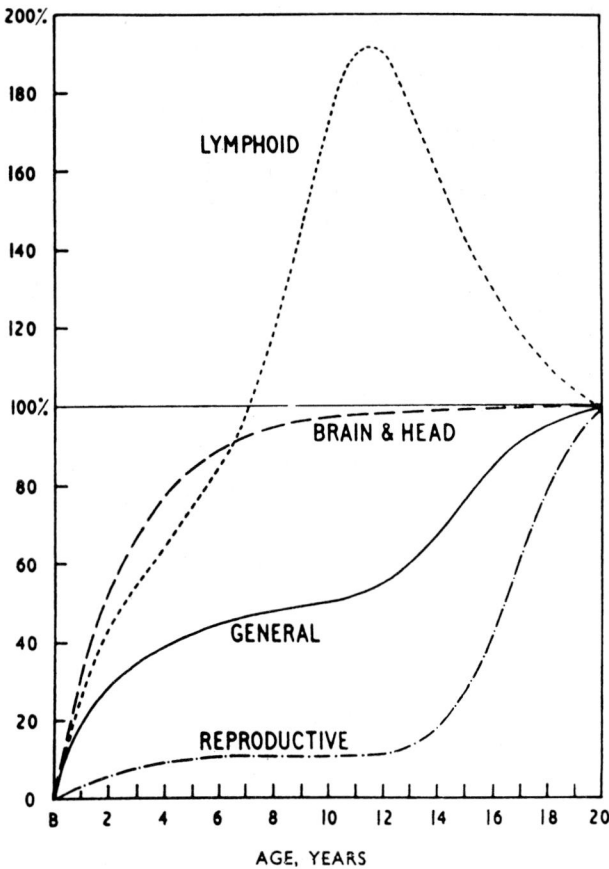

FIG. 3. Growth curves of different tissues. (From refs. 9, 323, with permission.)

BONE

It has long been established that bone growth can be impaired by radiation. As in so many areas of scientific inquiry, we are indebted to animal research for developing the foundation of our understanding of radiation's effects on bone growth. In 1903, Perthes (11) reported that chickens irradiated to one wing had retarded growth of that wing compared to the unirradiated side. In 1906, Forsterling (12) noted gross impairment of growth after irradiation of one-half the body of a rabbit. Studies in the albino rat and dog, conducted between 1940 and 1947 by a variety of investigators, showed that some epiphyseal growth retardation could be produced at a threshold dose of 400 to 600 R. Complete growth inhibition occurred at 1,200 R or more (13–15). Highly instructive experiments were reported by Arkin and Simon (16) in 1950. The rabbit vertebral column was exposed to an inhomogeneous radiation dose by unilateral implantation of radon seeds as well as by external-beam treatment. When the animals were sacrificed, the vertebral bodies were wedge-shaped. There was an absence of cartilaginous columns on the irradiated side. The zones of temporary calcification were acellular (17).

Pathophysiology

The pathophysiology of radiation injury to growing bone is probably attributable to damage to the chondroblasts (14,18,19). Single doses of 2 to 20 Gy inhibit proliferation of cartilage cells, thereby decreasing cellularity and causing disarray of the cellular columns within the growth plate (20). The resulting retarded bone growth is attributed to this loss of proliferating cells in the growth plate, the decreased ability of surviving cells to synthesize matrix, and/or the production of an abnormal matrix that fails to calcify.

The effects of radiation on growing bone have been summarized by Rubin and co-workers (7,8,21). (a) Epiphyseal irradiation, to a sufficient dose, causes an arrest of chondrogenesis; (b) metaphyseal irradiation results in a failure of absorptive processes in calcified bone and cartilage; and (c) diaphyseal irradiation produces an alteration in periosteal activity, which causes abnormal bone modeling. Therefore, the location of a radiotherapy field on a long bone can significantly influence the nature and severity of the subsequent deformity.

By identifying the location of the most rapidly growing epiphyseal plate of a given bone, we may infer the extent of growth stunting produced by placement of a radiotherapy field. In the femur, approximately 30% of growth comes from the proximal epiphysis and 70% from the distal. In the tibia, 60% of growth is from the proximal epiphysis and 40% is from the distal, whereas in the humerus, 80% is derived from the proximal and 20% is derived from the distal (8,14,18,22,23).

Clinical Manifestations

Clinically, radiation's effects on growing bone may be most simply characterized as shortening of long bones (i.e., femur, tibia, humerus) or hypoplasia of flat bones (i.e., ilium). The crucial factors influencing the ultimate height of the patient may be inferred from the data previously presented: (a) the radiation total dose and dose per fraction; (b) the energy, dose distribution, and absorptive properties of the beam(s); (c) which bone(s) are irradiated and which epiphyseal plate(s) are encompassed; (d) the age at the time of irradiation—implying that the amount of growth already obtained is important in judging ultimate outcome; (e) the influence of other toxins on growth, such as exogenous

steroids and cytotoxic chemotherapy; and (f) the patient's genetic constitution (14,18,24). In 1952, Neuhauser et al. (15) demonstrated that patients treated when less than 2-years old and with doses greater than 2,000 R suffered the most pronounced vertebral body deformities. Doses less than 1,000 R produced no radiographically detectable bone damage, and 1,000 to 2,000 R produced growth arrest lines but no change in vertebral contour (15). Probert and Parker (25) measured the standing and sitting heights of children irradiated for Hodgkin's disease, medulloblastoma, and acute lymphoblastic leukemia (ALL). The reduction in sitting height was related to the dose of vertebral irradiation and was also age-dependent. The greatest retardation of spinal growth occurred in children irradiated during the periods of most active growth (under 6 years of age and during puberty) and at doses greater than 35 Gy.

Recent data on 124 children treated at Stanford University Medical Center for Hodgkin's disease, demonstrate the relationship of RT dose and age (26). Patients who received greater than 33 Gy demonstrated a statistically significant height impairment irrespective of age group, but most dramatic for the prepubertal group who had a mean loss of final attained stature of 7% to 8% or approximately 13 cm. Patients receiving less than 33 Gy demonstrated significant impairment in standing and sitting height for the prepubertal age group only (Fig. 4). In a study by Mauch et al. (27) of children treated for Hodgkin's disease, 42 patients treated with 36 to 44 Gy were followed 2.5 years or more. Six of seven (86%) children irradiated at 3 to 8 years of age and 10 of 16 (63%) children irradiated at 9 to 12 years of age had sitting heights of at least 1 SD below the mean. In contrast, children treated between the ages of 13 and 16 years had normal sitting heights. There was no discernible increase in these abnormalities with continued follow-up.

A considerable body of knowledge has been developed concerning loss of height following childhood irradiation. The pediatric radiation oncologist will counsel the young

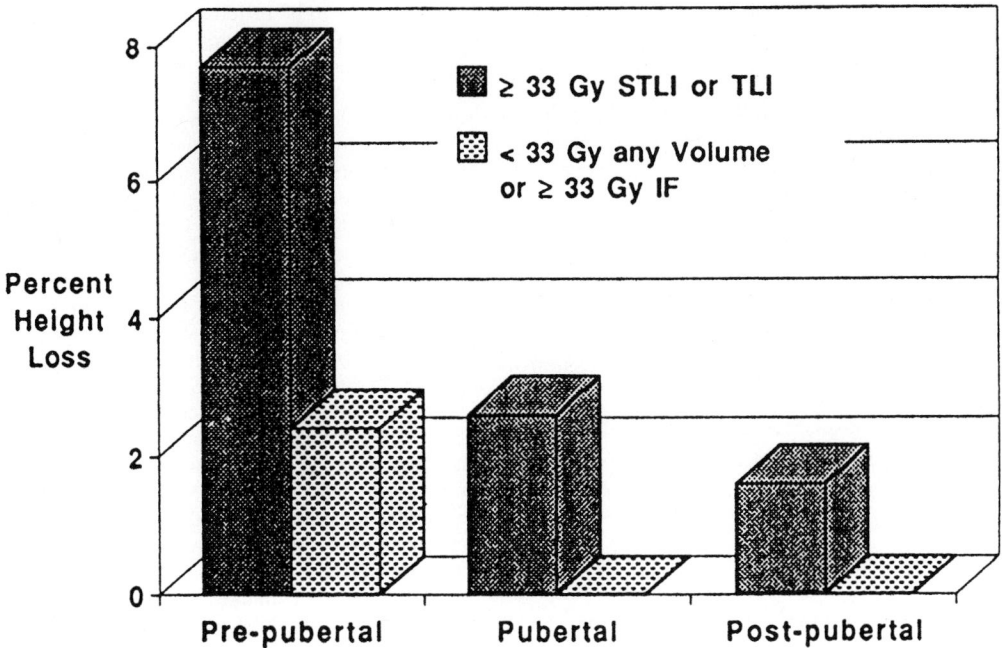

FIG. 4. Relative height impairment for six groups according to age at treatment and radiation dose/volume. (From ref. 26, with permission.)

patient's parents about decreased sitting or standing height and/or limb length discrepancy following radiotherapy. Parents will frequently respond, "But how short will my child be?" To such a question, an answer couched in terms of standard deviations from the mean is generally unsatisfactory. Silber et al. (28) have attempted to address this problem with a mathematical model to predict adult stature following treatment of cancer in childhood. An estimate of ideal adult stature (IAS) in the absence of cancer treatment is made based on anthropomorphic data from a normal population. By using the subject's sex, age, stature, weight, and the statures of the subject's mother and father, a prediction can be made of the ultimate IAS following growth. Silber et al. (28) found that a model that included dose of irradiation, the vertical distance of the spine irradiated, whether or not the femoral heads or acetabula were irradiated, and sex was highly predictive of the ultimate adult height ($R^2 = 0.74$, multiple correlation coefficient). The model, however, was only consti-

tuted from 49 patients. Donaldson (19) was unable to confirm the model's efficacy in two of three cases. Additional refinements of mathematical predictive models are eagerly awaited.

Scoliosis and kyphosis are frequent consequences of spinal or flank irradiation. In Probert's series (29), 4 of 29 (14%) patients treated for Hodgkin's disease or medulloblastoma with doses greater than 35 Gy became scoliotic. A greater frequency might have been observed with longer follow-up into the adolescent growth spurt. Asymmetric spinal growth has most frequently been seen following irradiation for Wilms' tumor and neuroblastoma, where there has been flank surgery (e.g., nephrectomy) and radiation (16,30). The types of deformities observed included a lateral flexion curve, concave to the side of the primary tumor, and a rotary scoliosis (17). Of 81 Wilms' tumor patients reported by Riseborough et al. (30), 57 (70.4%) developed scoliosis, including 19 with concomitant kyphosis. An additional two children developed pure kyphosis. Seventy-four of these patients were treated with orthovoltage radiation to doses as high as 61 Gy, with a mean dose of 32 Gy. It was postulated that the higher differential energy absorption in bone with the use of orthovoltage irradiation caused greater structural damage than megavoltage energies. The mean curve in the 57 scoliotic patients was 20° (range 5° to 67°). The 14 patients with curves greater than 25° received a mean dose of 36 Gy, as compared to 32 Gy for children with the lesser curves. The most significant progression of scoliosis occurred with the adolescent growth spurt, irrespective of the age at the time of irradiation. Eighteen of the 43 patients with curves less than 15° had not yet entered puberty. When scoliosis did develop, the curves became rigid early, presumably due to the tethering effect of the adjacent fibrotic soft tissues. Scoliosis has developed following doses as low as 25 Gy when patients were followed for many years past puberty. Table 2 summarizes several series, providing guidance to tolerance doses. Asymmetric irradiation of the vertebrae seemed to promote the development of rotary scoliosis and lateral flexion curvature. These late effects in humans seemed to recapitulate the early studies in animal models: an inhomogeneous dose across a growth plate may lead to curvature of bone growth (17). Some clinicians articulate this principle as follows: "It is better to arrest a growth plate than partially irradiate it and cause a curvature." Neuhauser et al. (15) stated it well:

If the spine is to be included in the field of irradiation in a growing child, as it must in the paraspinal neuroblastomas, the fields should be so arranged that the spine receives uniform intensity of irradiation throughout the course of therapy. It is for this reason that we prefer true anteroposterior portals. Lateral and tangential ports may give sufficient variation in intensity of radiation to the epiphyseal plates of the spine to produce scoliosis by the irregular advance of the epiphyses.

Caution should also be exercised in the treatment of unilateral intra-abdominal tumors of childhood. If therapy is limited to one-half of the abdomen, it would seem advisable to bring the ports slightly beyond the midline, so that the entire transverse diameter of the spine is included, receiving irradiation of fairly uniform intensity. If the entire abdomen requires treatment and it must be subdivided into quadrant, caution should be exercised in avoiding quadruple cross-firing of the spine producing a so-called "hot spot" in the region of the first or second lumbar vertebrae.

Longer follow-up of patients who have entered puberty will be necessary to confirm the impression in some series that the degree of scoliosis plateaus while kyphosis progresses during adolescence.

Slipped femoral capital epiphysis is a clinically significant adverse effect observed in patients following irritation of the femoral head (31–34). There is a threshold dose of 25 Gy for this complication. It occurred in about 50% of children irradiated at less than 4 years of age (7 of 15), as compared to only 1 of 21, 5- to 15-year-olds (Fig. 5). The mechanism of

TABLE 2. *Scoliosis and kyphosis after radiation therapy for Wilms' tumor*[a]

Series	RT dose range (Gy)[b]	Scoliosis			Patients with kyphosis (%)	Comments
		Number of patients	Patients (%)	Curvature (degrees)		
Riseborough et al. (30)	29–62 (30.1)	81	70	5–67	26	Scoliosis increases after higher doses
Oliver et al. (329)	20–45	21	67	5–45	14	Flank atrophy in 100%
Heaston et al. (330)	25–42 (35)	25	80	<5–17	48	Scoliosis in 100% of patients reaching puberty

RT, radiation therapy.
[a]Modified from ref. 331, with permission.
[b]Numbers in parentheses indicate means.

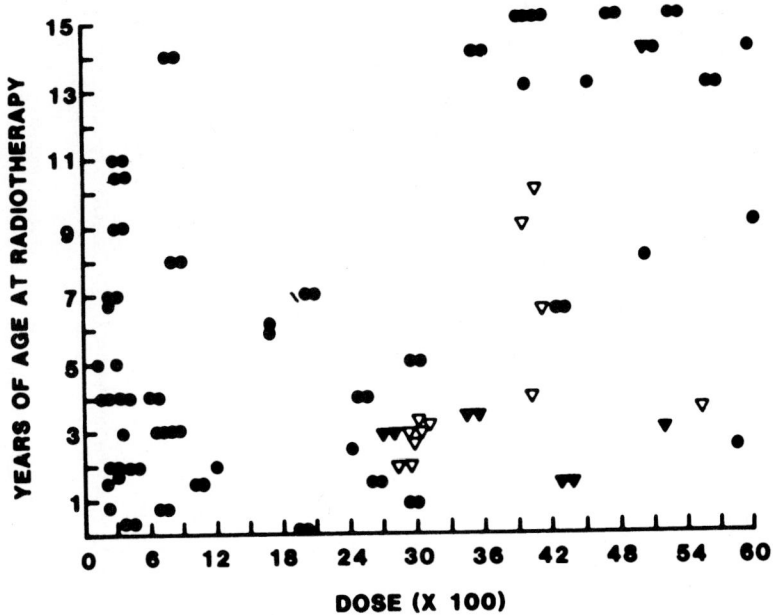

FIG. 5. The relationship of radiation dose and age in the production of slipped capital femoral plates in the study population (closed triangles) and from other reports (open triangles) (refs. 31, 34, 324). Normal epiphyseal plates are the closed circles. (From ref. 33, with permission.)

femoral capital epiphyseal plate slippage is postulated to be a radiation-induced delay in maturation of the epiphyseal plate with disruption of normal calcification and bone matrix deposition. This renders the plate weak and prone to slippage due to shearing stress at the tilted femoral line (14). When the femoral heads are shielded during irradiation, the frequency of this complication is small. Only 1 of 179 children treated for Hodgkin's disease at Stanford were affected, though the number of children who received pelvic irradiation is not stated (19,22,23).

Avascular necrosis of the femoral or humeral heads can occur 2 to 3 years following irradiation (32). It is most frequently reported following combined radiation and chemotherapy as in the treatment of Hodgkin's and non-Hodgkin's lymphoma. The etiology of this complication is unclear but may be related to the combined use of steroids and irradiation. Libshitz and Edeikin (35) reported necrosis in 16 of 44 children receiving 30 to 60 Gy to the femoral heads. This

complication was bilateral in 4 of 5 cases who received irradiation to both hips. This debilitating injury is fortunately rare when the femoral and humeral heads are shielded and/or when lower irradiation doses are used (14,18). Of interest is recent information on the occurrence of osteonecrosis in children treated for acute lymphoblastic leukemia. Finnish investigators found magnetic resonance imaging (MRI) evidence of osteonecrosis in 9 of 28 imaged children, and this was symptomatic in 4. This finding was attributed to the intensive dexamethasone component of therapy (36).

A variety of other skeletal abnormalities can be seen after irradiation. These include: sternal deformity (hypoplasia, asymmetry, pectus excavatum, pectus carinatum) (37); hypoplasia of the iliac bones or lower ribs; cartilaginous exostoses (38); osteochondromata (17); hypoplasia of the mandible; deformity of orbital, maxillary, nasal, or temporal bone (17,39); and lower extremity abnormalities such as acetabular dysplasia, coxa vara, hip

TABLE 3. *Evaluation of patients at risk for late effects: musculoskeletal*[a]

Late effects	Causative treatment			Signs and symptoms	Screening and diagnostic tests	Management and intervention
	Chemotherapy	Radiation	Surgery			
Muscular hypoplasia		>20 Gy (growing child) Younger children more sensitive	Muscle loss or resection	Asymmetry of muscle mass when compared with untreated area Decreased range of motion Stiffness and pain in affected area (uncommon)	Careful comparison and measurement of irradiated and unirradiated areas Range of motion	Prevention: good exercise program, range of motion, muscle strengthening
Spinal abnormalities: Scoliosis Kyphosis Lordosis Decreased sitting height		For young children, RT to hemiabdomen or spine (especially hemivertebral) 10 Gy (minimal effect) >20 Gy (clinically notable defect)	Laminectomy	Back pain Hip pain Uneven shoulder height Rib humps or flares Deviation from vertical curve Gait abnormalities	Standing and sitting height at each visit and plot on chart (stadiometer); During puberty examine spine q 3–6 months until growth is completed and then q 1–2 yr; Spinal films baseline during puberty, then prn curvature (COBB technique to measure curvature)	Refer to orthopedist if any curvature is noted, especially during a period of rapid growth
Length discrepancy		>20 Gy		Lower back pain, limp, hip pain, discrepancy in muscle mass and length when compared with untreated extremity, scoliosis	Annual measurement of treated and untreated limb (completely undressed patient to assure accurate measurements) Radiograph baseline to assess remaining epiphyseal growth Radiographs annually during periods of rapid growth	Contralateral epiphysiodesis Limb-shortening procedures
Pathological fracture		>40 Gy	Biopsy	Pain, edema, ecchymosis	Baseline radiograph of treated area to assess bone integrity, then prn symptoms	Prevention Consider limitation of activities (e.g., contact sports) Surgical repair of fracture; may require internal fixation
Osteonecrosis	Steroids	>40–50 Gy (more common in adults)		Pain in affected joint, limp	Radiograph, CT scan prn symptoms	Symptomatic care Joint replacement
Osteocartilaginous exostoses		RT		Painless lump/mass noted in the field of radiation	Radiograph baseline and prn growth of lesion	Resection for cosmetic/functional reasons, Counsel regarding 10% incidence of malignant degeneration
Slipped capitofemoral epiphysis	High-dose steroids	>25 Gy (at young age)		Pain in effected hip, limp, abnormal gait	Radiograph baseline to assess integrity of the treated joint(s), then prn symptoms	Refer to orthopedist for surgical intervention

RT, radiation therapy; CT, computed tomography.
[a]From ref. 44, with permission.

dislocation, and leg shortening (40,41). Roentgenographic abnormalities can be seen in the long bones of children treated with chemotherapy alone. From this we may infer that chemotherapy may produce bone injury as well as accentuate the effects of radiotherapy (40). Skeletal undermineralization (osteoporosis) leading to fractures may occur with methotrexate (42) or corticosteroids (43).

Table 3 reviews several musculoskeletal late effects with respect to causative treatments, signs and symptoms, screening and diagnostic tests, and management and intervention (44).

NEUROENDOCRINE

Hypothalamic-pituitary (H-P) irradiation may produce neuroendocrine abnormalities. The effects of cranial irradiation on growth hormone (GH) production and release are worthy of detailed consideration.

Pathophysiology

GH is secreted episodically by the anterior pituitary gland. Growth-hormone-releasing hormone (GHRH), produced in the hypothalamus, stimulates GH production, whereas the hypothalamic neuropeptide somatostatin excretes an inhibitory effect. In the liver and other tissues, circulating GH stimulates the production of insulin-like growth factor 1 (IGF-1, also called somatomedin-C), which promotes cell proliferation and protein synthesis. GH is secreted in bursts throughout the day and night. A simple and reliable test for GH reserve is not yet available. Current technology relies on a variety of provocative agents capable of stimulating GH release to assess GH reserve. These agents include insulin-induced hypoglycemia, intravenous arginine hydrochloride, oral L-Dopa, and oral clonidine (45,46). The anatomic site of the radiation injury that produces GH deficiency is probably the hypothalamus. Both Lannering and Albertsson-Wikland (47) and Blacklay et al. (48) have studied children who are GH-deficient following irradiation to the H-P axis.

Most demonstrate a prompt rise in GH following administration of GHRH. This implies that GH deficiency in the irradiated patient may be the result of disturbances in the hypothalamic production of GHRH. This finding is supported by a study of GH-deficient brain tumor patients who had been irradiated to the posterior fossa. Although the pituitary gland had been excluded from the treatment field, the ventromedian nucleus of the hypothalamus, which is thought to be the site of GHRH, was included (49,50).

Clinical Manifestations

Having considered the anatomic site of radiation's damage to GH production, we may turn our attention to the frequency of the ill effect, the dose-response relationship, and the time interval between therapy and the onset of the deficiency. The limited data available indicate that (a) 60% to 80% of irradiated pediatric brain tumor patients will ultimately have impaired serum GH response to provocative stimulation; (b) there is a positive dose-response relationship with a threshold of 18 to 25 Gy [as used for treatment of subclinical central nervous system (CNS) leukemia]; and (c) the higher the radiation dose, the earlier the GH deficiency will occur after treatment (51–59).

Relevant data concerning postirradiation GH deficiency in children treated for brain tumors include the study of Duffner et al. (53). These investigators evaluated endocrinologic function in 11 children. The children received 24 to 54.4 Gy to the hypothalamus and 39.1 to 54 Gy to the pituitary gland for brain tumors remote from the H-P axis. GH secretion was normal in the 7 patients assessed prior to therapy, but deficient in 2 of 7 patients 3 months following irradiation, in 9 of 11 patients 6 months following irradiation, and in 7 of 8 patients 12 months following irradiation. The permanence of GH deficiency following high-dose irradiation is suggested by the finding of GH deficiency in 10 of 12 patients (83%) tested 1 to 8 years following irradiation (51,52).

Brauner et al. (60) have prospectively studied GH levels in 27 children irradiated for medulloblastoma, ependymoma, and head and neck sarcomas. The H-P dose ranged from 31 to 55 Gy. Some patients also received chemotherapy. Sixteen of the 27 patients (59%) were GH-deficient 2 years following radiotherapy. At the 2-year follow-up, the children who received craniospinal irradiation had a mean height 1.46 ± 0.4 SD below the mean, whereas those receiving cranial irradiation only were, on average, 0.15 ± 0.18 SD short. Therefore, most of the growth retardation appears attributable to lack of spinal growth. Spinal irradiation may, of course, have a profound effect on spinal growth. The younger the age at which a child's spine is irradiated, the greater the subsequent skeletal disproportion (28).

Precocious puberty has been reported in some children receiving cranial irradiation, but almost exclusively in females receiving 24 Gy or more (61). Shalet et al. (45) have shown that the age of pubertal onset is positively correlated with the age at the time of cranial irradiation (Fig. 6). The impact of early puberty in a child with radiation-associated GH deficiency is significant (45,51,53,54). If one delays GH therapy for 1 or 2 years following brain irradiation to avoid the risk of tumor relapse, and if precocious puberty occurs, there may be little time left to administer efficacious GH therapy.

If the diagnosis of GH deficiency is made, synthetic GH may be administered. Such treatment allows children to maintain the postirradiation growth percentile. "Catch-up" growth to the preradiotherapy percentile, however, is unusual (19,45,46,51,62,63).

The frequency of chemical and clinically manifested GH deficiency following prophylactic cranial irradiation in children with acute lymphoblastic leukemia (ALL) is more complicated than for brain tumors because the doses used are at the threshold for hypothalamic injury. A graphic depiction of the RT

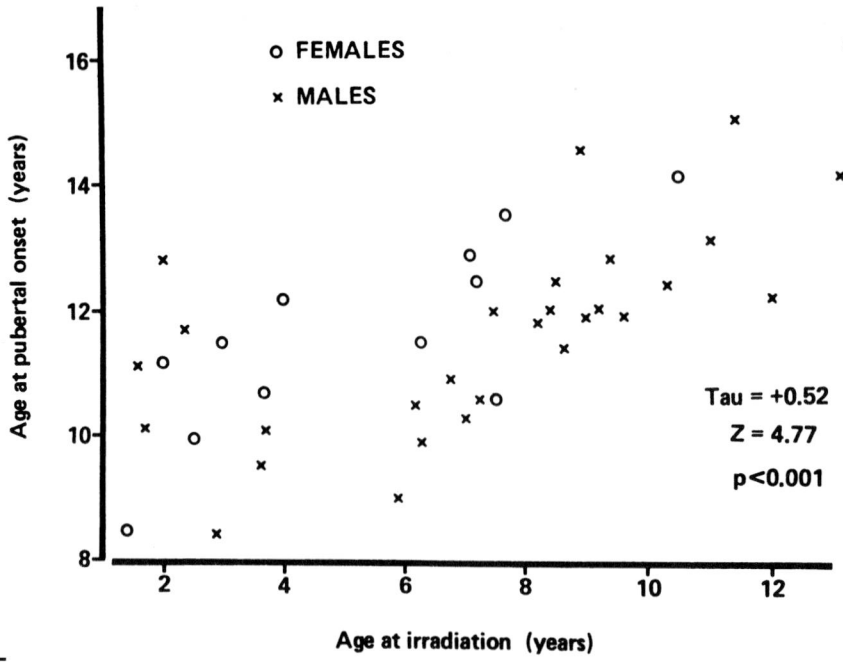

FIG. 6. The relationship between age at the time of cranial/craniospinal irradiation and age of pubertal onset. (From ref. 45, with permission.)

dose dependency of GH deficiency is shown in Fig. 7, which represents stimulated GH responses in 121 children treated with cranial RT for ALL or total-body irradiation (TBI) (64). Girls may be somewhat more sensitive than boys, and chemotherapy alone has an effect on growth. Data from Sklar on 127 children (68 female) demonstrate that girls under age 4 years with ALL prophylaxed with 24 Gy had the greatest loss in height, but significant decrements also occurred in those prophylaxed with 18 Gy and, importantly, even in those treated for ALL without any RT (Fig. 8). The mean age at treatment was 6.4 years, and at testing it was 18.3 years (65). Other investigators have found that children treated for ALL without RT recover from subnormal growth by 5 years posttherapy, but patients numbers in these series are much smaller (51,52,66,67).

Important historic data include that reported in 1976 by Shalet et al. (56) who demonstrated a relationship between radiation to the H-P region and GH response to provocative testing in children with ALL. Fourteen of 17 (82%) children receiving 25 Gy in 2 to 2.5 weeks had abnormal GH responses but normal growth velocity, serum somatomedin activity, and bone age when measured within 2 years of irradiation. This suggested that, perhaps, the normal physiologic requirement of GH was being met (45). Interestingly, only 1 of 9 (11%) children who received 24 Gy in 20 fractions over 4 weeks had an impaired GH response. It is possible that the lower dose per fraction produced fewer late ill effects (51,54). In 1981, Voorhes et al. (68) described H-P function in 93 children who received CNS prophylaxis with intrathecal methotrexate (IT MTX) alone, IT

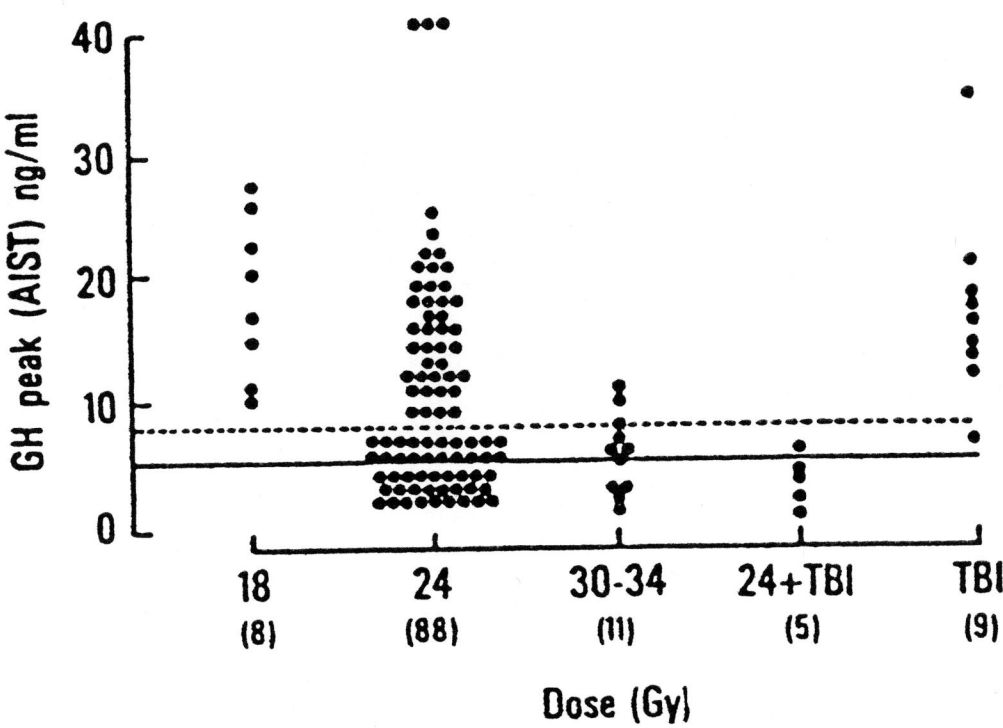

FIG. 7. The growth hormone (GH) responses to a combined arginine-insulin stimulation test in 121 children treated with cranial irradiation. The TBI groups received 10 Gy in a single exposure. The dotted (8 ng/mL) and the solid (5 ng/mL) lines represent the values in partial and complete GH deficiency. (From ref. 64, with permission.)

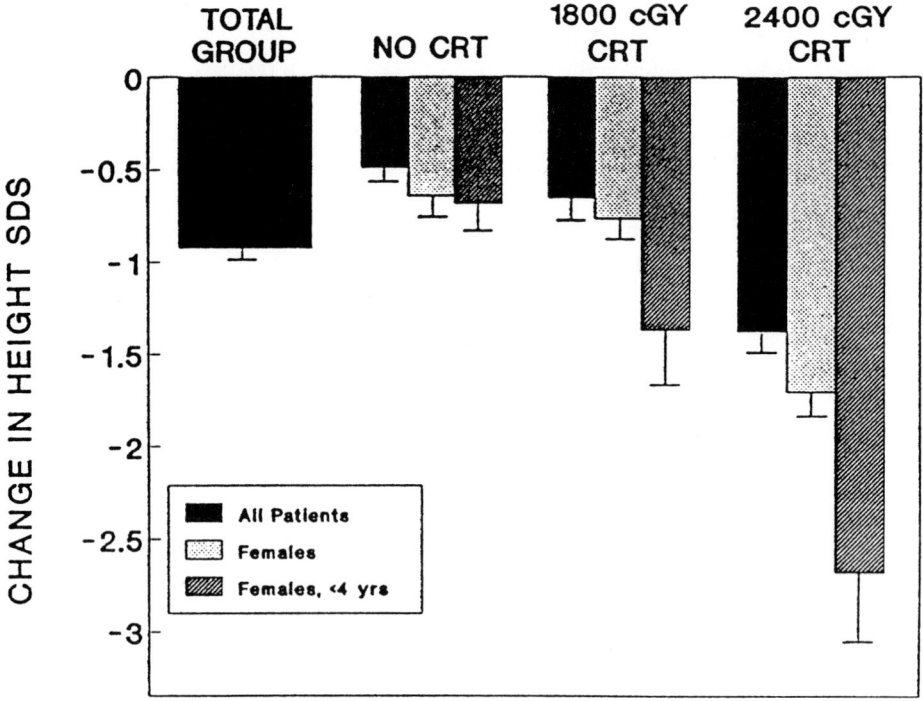

FIG. 8. Change in mean height standard deviation score (SDS) (mean ± SEM) from diagnosis to final height for selected patient groups for each treatment regimen. (From ref. 65, with permission.)

MTX plus 24 Gy cranial irradiation, and IT MTX plus intravenous (IV) intermediate-dose MTX. Eleven patients had subnormal GH responses to arginine-insulin stimulation. There were no differences among the three groups with regard to long-term linear thyroid-stimulating hormone (TSH), adrenocortico-tropic hormone (ACTH), or follicle-stimulating hormone-luteinizing hormone (FSH-LH) secretion, and 60% were prepubertal and still receiving chemotherapy at the time of evaluation. Other reports, however, buttress the Shalet report in describing a high frequency of chemical abnormality. In 1987, Kirk et al. (69) described 77 children treated for ALL who received 24 Gy prophylactic cranial irradiation. Thirty of 46 (65%) had partial or complete GH deficiency, and all 34 tested for pulsatile GH secretion were abnormal. Height for age fell by more than 1 standard deviation (SD) in 32% of children studied 6 years after diagnosis, and in 71% 6 years after diagnosis.

Sixteen ALL survivors were studied at Children's Hospital of Los Angeles. All had received 18 to 24 Gy of cranial irradiation. Eleven of the 16 (69%) were GH-deficient (70). Overall, the most severe growth disturbances occur in children irradiated before age 4 years and who have tall parents. Summary data for children with ALL indicate that the final height is 0.17 to 1.41 SD (1SD = 7–8 cm) for males and 0.52 to 1.65 SD for females, and about 30% are 2 SD below normal after 24 Gy or more (67,71).

Pediatric radiation oncologists have been evaluating the efficacy as well as the cognitive and neuroendocrine late effects of 18 versus 24 Gy of prophylactic cranial irradiation in the management of ALL. In 1988, Blatt et al. (72) reported an evaluation of pulsatile GH secretion in children treated with the two different doses. Those children treated with 18 Gy had normal GH secretion—superior to those treated with 24 Gy. In 1992, Shalet et al. (45)

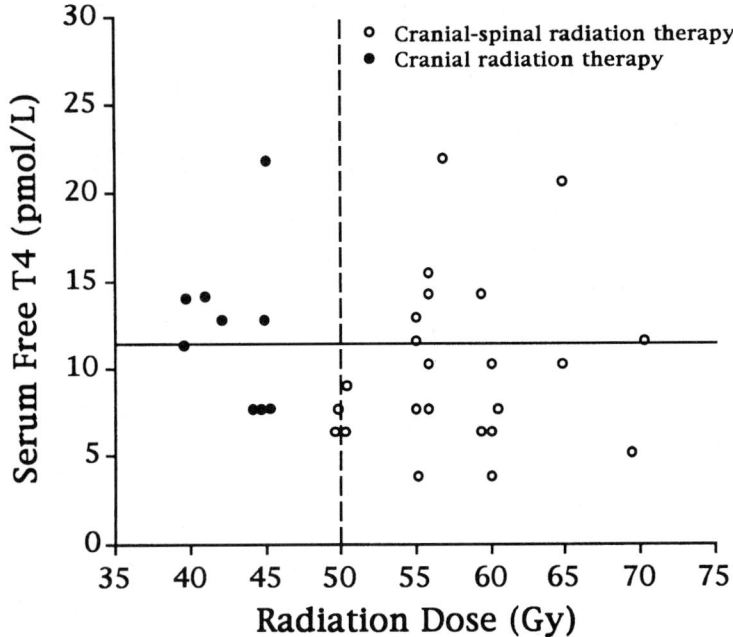

FIG. 9. Serum free T4 concentrations in patients with brain tumors treated with cranial radiation (open circles) or craniospinal radiation (solid circles) as a function of the dose of radiation. The dashed line is arbitrarily placed at a dose of 50 Gy and the solid line indicates the lower limit of serum free T4 concentrations in normal subjects. (Modified from ref. 74, with permission.)

TABLE 4. *Type and frequency of hormonal abnormalities in 32 patients who received cranial or craniospinal radiation*[a]

	Patient number (percent)		
Variable	Cranial RT ($n=23$)	Craniospinal RT ($n=9$)	All patients ($n=32$)
Type of abnormality			
Thyroid	17 (74)	5 (56)	22 (69)
Gonadal[b]	11 (65)	3 (50)	14 (61)
Prolactin	12 (52)	4 (44)	16 (50)
Adrenal[b]	12 (55)	1 (11)	13 (42)
Number of abnormalities			
0	1 (4)	2 (22)	3 (9)
1	5 (22)	4 (44)	9 (28)
2	7 (30)	1 (11)	8 (25)
3	7 (30)	1 (11)	8 (25)
4	3 (13)	1 (11)	4 (12)

RT, radiation therapy.
[a]From ref. 74, with permission.
[b]Gonadal abnormalities were not evaluated in nine prepubertal and pubertal patients (6 who received cranial radiation, and 3 who received craniospinal radiation). Adrenal abnormalities were not evaluated in one patient who received cranial radiation.

TABLE 5. *Evaluation of patients at risk for late effects: neuroendocrine* [a]

Late effects	Causative treatment			Signs and symptoms	Screening and diagnostic tests	Management and intervention
	Chemotherapy	Radiation	Surgery			
Growth hormone deficiency		>18 Gy to H/P axis	Tumor in region of H/P axis	"Falling off" of growth curve Inadequate growth velocity Inadequate pubertal growth spurt	Annual stadiometer height (q 6 mo at age 9–12 yr) Growth curve Bone age at 9 yr, then q yr to puberty (Insulin stimulation test and pulsatile GH analysis)	Growth hormone therapy Delay puberty with GnRH agonist
ACTH deficiency		>40 Gy to H/P axis	Tumor in region of H/P axis	Muscular weakness, Anorexia, Nausea, Weight loss, Dehydration, Hypotension, Abdominal pain, Increased pigmentation (skin, buccal mucosa)	Cortisol (a.m.) baseline, prn symptoms (Insulin-hypoglycemia; metapyrone stimulation tests)	Hydrocortisone
TRH deficiency		>40 Gy H/P axis	Tumor in region of H/P axis	Hoarseness, Fatigue, Weight gain, Dry skin, Cold intolerance, Dry brittle hair, Alopecia, Constipation, Lethargy, Poor linear growth, Menstrual irregularities, Pubertal delay, Bradycardia, Hypotension	Free T$_4$, T$_3$, TSH baseline, q 3–5 yr	Hormone replacement with thyroxine Anticipatory guidance regarding symptoms of hypothyroidism
Precocious puberty (especially females)		>20 Gy to H/P axis	Tumor in region of H/P axis	Early growth spurt False catch-up Premature sexual maturation: Female: Breast development and pubic hair before 8 yr and menses before 9 yr. Male: Testicular/penile growth and pubic hair before 9–9.5 yr	Height, growth curve q yr Bone age q 2 yr until mature (LH, FSH, estradiol or testosterone) (Pelvic ultrasound, GnRH-stimulation testing)	GnRH agonist

472

TABLE 5. *Continued*

Late effects	Causative treatment			Signs and symptoms	Screening and diagnostic tests	Management and intervention
	Chemotherapy	Radiation	Surgery			
Gonadotropin deficiency: Male		>40 Gy to hypothalamic region	Tumor in region of hypothalamus	Delayed/arrested/absent pubertal development: Lack of or diminished: pubic and axillary hair, penile and testicular enlargement, voice change, body odor, acne Testicular atrophy (softer and smaller) Failure to impregnate	LH, testosterone q 3–5 yr (GnRH testing)	Testosterone replacement
Gonadotropin deficiency: Female:		>40 Gy to hypothalamic region	Tumor in region of hypothalamus	Delayed/arrested/absent pubertal development including: breasts, female escutcheon, female habitus, vaginal estrogen effect, body odor, acne Changes in duration, frequency, and character of menstruation (less cramping) Estrogen deficiency: hot flashes, vaginal dryness, dyspareunia, low libido Infertility: If not on birth control pills	Tanner stage LH, FSH, estradiol q 3–5 yr GnRH-stimulation tests	Anticipatory guidance regarding symptoms of estrogen deficiency Hormone replacement Early intervention may prevent osteoporosis Atherosclerosis
Hyperprolactinemia		>40 Gy H/P axis	Tumor in region of hypothalamus	Female: Menstrual irregularities Loss of libido Infertility Galactorrhea Hot flashes Osteopenia Male: Loss of libido Impotence Infertility	Prolactin-level baseline, then prn symptoms	Dopamine agonist (bromocriptine)

ACTH, adrenocorticotropic hormone; FSH, follicular-stimulating hormone; GH, growth hormone; GnRH, gonadotropin releasing hormone; H/P, hypothalamic-pituitary; LH, luteinizing hormone; T_3, triiodothyronine; T_4, thyroxine; TRH, thyrotropin-releasing hormone; TSH, thyroid-stimulating hormone.
[a]From ref. 44, with permission.

evaluated the 24-hour GH secretion in 19 ALL children who had received 18 Gy, comparing pubertal children with prepubertal ones. For those children who had received 18 Gy prior to puberty, growth and GH secretion was attenuated during puberty. It was also of interest that GH secretion was not different in the prepubertal irradiated ALL cases when compared with controls. Shalet et al. concluded, therefore, that the lowered doses of cranial irradiation for ALL produced no change in prepubertal GH secretion in most children but that GH secretion during puberty was attenuated in a significant proportion of cases.

Deficiencies of H-P hormones other than GH have been described following irradiation. Samaan et al. (73) described 110 patients treated for nasopharyngeal or paranasal sinus carcinoma where more than 60 Gy was typically administered, and they found deficiencies in 83%. Twenty-seven percent had thyroid abnormalities, attributed to hypothalamic injury in one-third of the patients and pituitary injury in the remainder. Cortisol deficiency attributable to hypothalamic injury also occurred in 27% of patients. Abnormalities of prolactin and LH were noted in 39% and 30%, respectively. Tan and Kunaratman (58) and Perry-Keene et al. (55) described panhypopituitarism in three patients who received more than 60 Gy to the pituitary. Constine et al. (74) documented non-GH abnormalities in 32 patients (20 children and 12 adults) treated with irradiation for brain tumors not involving the H-P region. Fifteen of 23 patients (65%) who received cranial irradiation only (40 to 70 Gy with mean dose 53.6 Gy to the H-P axis) had low free T4 levels due to hypothalamic or pituitary injury (Fig. 9). Seven of 10 (70%) females who were postpubertal when studied had oligomenorrhea, and 40% to 50% had low LH and estradiol. Because GnRH stimulation testing was generally normal, these patients may have an abnormal pulsatile release of LH, a possibility that is under investigation. Despite their functional and chemical abnormalities, most of the children (80%) demonstrated normal sexual development. In addition, 30% of 20 children

had an elevated prolactin, 15% had an abnormally low metyrapone test, and 1 had panhypopituitarism. Several children in this study first became abnormal as long as 5 years after irradiation. Overall, only 3 of 32 patients had no endocrine abnormalities, which demonstrates that a high frequency of clinical or subclinical (chemical) H-P injury exists in patients who are irradiated for brain tumors (Table 4). The team treating clival tumors with protons of the Harvard Cyclotron Laboratory evaluated 14 patients, aged 16 to 65 years, for endocrine abnormalities following a median of 67.6 cobalt gray equivalent to the pituitary. Four of the 14 developed endocrine dysfunction at up to 5 years 8 months follow-up. All four had more than one abnormality, including hypothyroidism, gonadotropin abnormality, corticotropin abnormality, and elevated prolactin (75).

A summary of neuroendocrine complications of therapy, the relationship to dose, diagnostic studies, and interventions are provided in Table 5 (44).

THYROID

Radiation-induced thyroid neoplasms are considered in Chapter 20. In this section, we will review the effects of therapeutic irradiation on the endocrine function of the thyroid. The thyroid may be directly irradiated in the treatment of (a) childhood head and neck cancers such as rhabdomyosarcoma, nasopharyngeal lymphoepithelioma, and squamous cell carcinoma, and (b) a variety of aerodigestive tract tumors. Irradiation of upper thoracic tumors may also encompass the thyroid as well as the mantle field of Hodgkin's disease. A photon spinal field utilized during craniospinal irradiation for brain and spinal tumors and for leukemia will provide some dose to the thyroid.

Pathophysiology

The thyroid gland is the largest pure endocrine gland and is located between the thyroid cartilage and third or fourth tracheal cartilages. It is comprised of follicles filled with colloid and lined by follicular cells, which trap iodide. The glycoprotein, thyroglobulin, is a major component of the colloid, and participates in the formation and storage of thyroid hormones. The primary, hormonally active iodothyronines, triiodothyronine (T3) and thyroxine (T4) are largely bound to plasma proteins when released by the gland. Thyroxine-binding globulin is the major transport protein, and only a small percentage of unbound T3 and T4 is available for activity. The pituitary hormone, thyroid stimulating hormone (TSH) regulates synthesis and release of T3 and T4. TSH secretion is stimulated by the hypothalamic hormone, thyrotropin release hormone (TRH), and inhibited by the circulating free thyroid hormones (76,77). The pathophysiology of radiation-induced thyroid dysfunction is not precisely defined. Direct radiation damage to the thyroid follicular cells, the thyroid vasculature, or the supporting stroma may occur. Less likely mechanisms that, however, could be contributory include the induction by irradiation of an immunologic reaction, or damage from the iodine load administered during lymphangiography (LAG). Support for the latter is based on the observation that radioiodine will induce hypothyroidism in patients with autoimmune thyroiditis (78). Histopathologic changes in an irradiated thyroid gland include progressive obliteration of the fine vasculature, degeneration of follicular cells and follicles, atrophy of the stroma, and, less commonly, lymphocytic infiltration (7,79,80). Because radiation damage is dependent on the degree of mitotic activity and the thyroid of a developing child grows in parallel with body growth, this gland might be expected to show an age-related degree of injury and repair.

Hypothyroidism

The legion of symptoms include cold intolerance, constipation, inordinate weight gain, dry skin, brittle hair, menorrhagia or spotting, muscle cramps or generalized muscle weakness, and slowed mentation. Signs include a round puffy face, slow speech, hoarseness, hypokinesia, delayed relaxation of deep tendon reflexes, periorbital or peripheral edema, and pleural or pericardial effusions (81,82). In addition to the classic signs and symptoms of hypo- or hyperthyroidism, patients who present with pleural or pericardial effusions, cardiac arrhythmias, or hypercholesterolemia after cervical or mantle irradiation should also be evaluated for thyroid dysfunction (77).

The incidence of radiation-induced hypothyroidism may be significantly influenced by a variety of methodological factors. "Clinical hypothyroidism" may be defined as the clinical symptoms of hypothyroidism associated with an elevation in basal TSH levels, increased TSH response to TRH, and depressed levels of T4 and T3 parameters. "Subclinical hypothyroidism" may be defined as an elevation of the basal TSH level and an increased TSH response to TRH, but with normal T3 and T4 parameters with no clinical symptoms of hypothyroidism (83). One can readily see that the reported clinical incidence of hypothyroidism following irradiation of the gland may be affected by which laboratory tests the investigator used (i.e., T3 and T4 alone vs. these parameters plus a TSH assessment), by how carefully the clinical symptoms of thyroid dysfunction are pursued (i.e., the degree to which the nonspecific complaint of "being tired" is evaluated by the physician or reported by the patient), and by the frequency with which the patient is evaluated in the posttreatment period. It is also possible, as we shall consider, that the frequency of hypothyroidism following irradiation is affected by the interval since the radiotherapy was given, the dose administered, the nature of the underlying malignant disease, and the age of the patient at the time of radiotherapy (13, 83–92).

Patients with Hodgkin's disease (HD) and non-Hodgkin's lymphoma constitute the larger part of the population for the late effects of RT on thyroid function (93). A variable incidence of hypothyroidism following radiotherapy has been reported. Although variable, the incidence appears significant and is worthy of more detailed study. Most of the available clinical studies are retrospective. Few patients have been subject to detailed baseline thyroid function testing followed by prospective evaluation, in long-term survivors, of the endocrine outcome of treatment (83,91,92). Consequently, if an elevated serum TSH concentration is the determinant, then 4% to 79% of patients become affected (77,81,83,84,87,92–97). A study by Hancock et al. (93) of 1,677 children and adults with Hodgkin's disease irradiated to the thyroid showed that the actuarial risk at 26 years for overt or subclinical hypothyroidism was 47% (Table 6). Although the peak incidence occurred at 2 to 3 years, and one-half the risk was manifested within 5 years, some patients developed hypothyroidism as long as 20 years after therapy. In most reports, the incidence of overt clinical hypothyroidism is approximately one-fourth the incidence of subclinical (compensated) hypothyroidism. Some patients may demonstrate a spontaneous recov-

ery of thyroid function, as indicated by a report by Constine et al. in which 20 of 75 (27%) affected patients normalized (84). Data from St Jude Children's Research Hospital are supportive. Twenty-nine of 85 children developed abnormal thyroid function tests (34%), and 8 patients spontaneously recovered (28%) (98). Data from adult patients with head and neck epithelial cancers indicate that the incidence of hypothyroidism is dramatically increased if radiotherapy is combined with surgical treatment of the cancer, which included partial thyroidectomy (90). In a similar vein, some have speculated that the rare patient in whom the primary malignancy (such as a lymphoma) has infiltrated the thyroid and destroyed some of its function may be at greater risk of a "treatment-associated" induced hypothyroidism.

Radiation dose is the most relevant parameter in predicting the likelihood of hypothyroidism. In the assessment of dose, however, radiation technique must be considered. A differential anterior versus posterior field

TABLE 6. *Thyroid disease after treatment of Hodgkin's disease[a]*

Disease	Percent of patients	Actuarial risk (%)		Time to occurrence	
		20 yrs	26 yrs	Median	Range
≥1 Thyroid diseases	573[b]	50.0	63.0	4.6	0.2–25.6
	570	52.0	67.0	4.6	0.2–25.6
Hypothyroidism	513[b]	41.0	44.0	4.0	0.2–23.7
	512	43.0	47.0	4.0	0.2–23.7
Graves' disease[c]	34[b]	3.1	3.1	4.8	0.1–17.6
	32	3.3	3.3	4.8	0.1–17.6
Ophthalmopathy[c]	21	—	—	—	—
Silent thyroiditis	6	0.6	0.6	3.7	0.8–15.3
Hashimoto's thyroiditis	4	0.7	0.7	7.9	3.5–15.2
Thyroidectomy	26	6.6	26.6	14.0	1.5–25.6
Thyroid cancer	6	1.7	1.7	13.3	9.0–18.9
Benign adenoma	10	—	—	12.0	1.5–25.6
Adenomatous nodule	6	—	—	17.4	12.7–24.4
Multinodular goiter	4	—	—	14.8	10.8–19.4
Clinically benign nodule	12	3.3	5.1	12.6	2.4–22.6
Clinically benign cyst	4	0.7	0.7	8.1	1.6–16.7
Multinodular goiter[d]	2	0.5	0.5	13.8	10.5–17.0

[a]Modified from ref. 93, with permission.

[b]Refers to the 1,787 patients at risk; the remainder refer to the 1,677 patients who underwent irradiation of the thyroid region.

[c]Thirty of the 34 patients who had been given a diagnosis of Graves' disease had hyperthyroidism; ophthalmopathy developed in three patients during a period of hypothyroidism and in one patient during a period of euthyroidism.

[d]Identified by clinical examination.

weighting may have been used, cervical blocks may have been introduced during treatment, specific thyroid blocks may have been used, and anterior "beam spoilers" to increase the superficial dose from high-energy linear accelerators may have been in place. All these factors may affect the actual dose the thyroid received and may have not been reflected in the midplane central axis dose reported (91,92,99). An increasing incidence of hypothyroidism above threshold doses of 20 to 30 Gy have been reported (84,94,100). Constine et al. (85) noted thyroid abnormalities in 4 of 24 children (17%) who received mantle irradiation of 26 Gy or less, and in 74 of 95 children (78%) who received greater than 26 Gy; the relationship of basal TSH to radiation dose was significant ($p < 0.001$). In a report by Bhatia et al., the relative risk of hypothyroidism increased by 1.02 per Gy, $p < 0.001$ (94). The latent interval to hypothyroidism and the relationship to radiation dose is shown in Fig. 10.

Other factors may affect risk for radiation-induced hypothyroidism. The influence of young age at the time of RT is unclear because most young children are treated with lower dose radiation in combination with chemotherapy (84,87,93,94). In Hancock's report, the incidence of hypothyroidism rose from 15% for patients treated before 5 years of age (usually with reduced RT doses) to 39% for those irradiated between 15 and 20 years of age. The incidence declined gradually during advancing adulthood (93). Prior to age 16 years, RT dose was the predominant

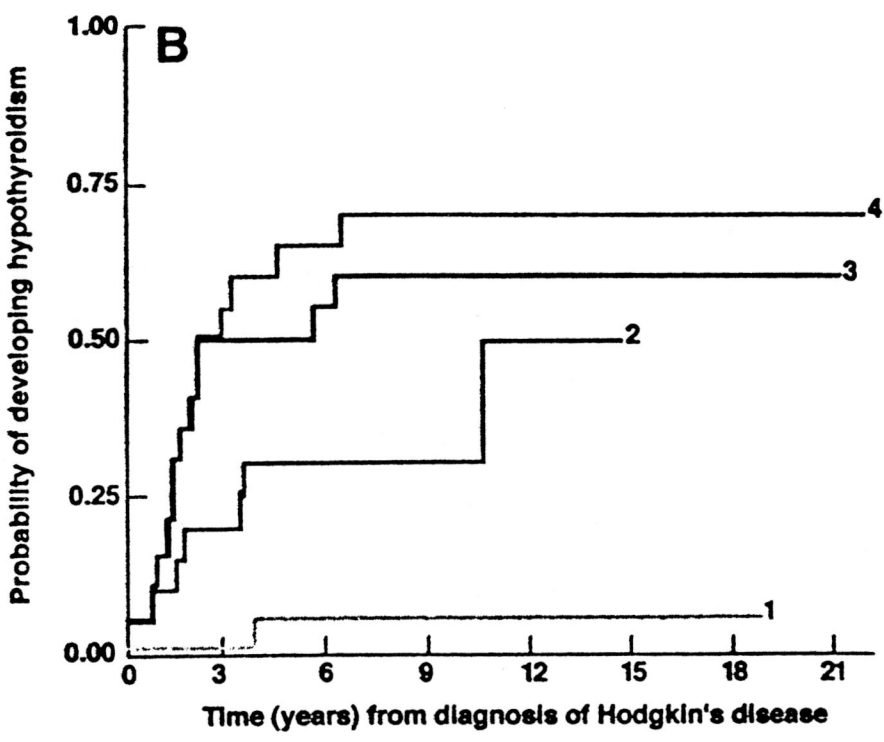

FIG. 10. Actuarial risk of hypothyroidism in 89 children treated for Hodgkin's disease. Curve 1 represents the risk in 13 children who did not undergo irradiation to the thyroid, curve 2 the risk in 10 children who received less than 30 Gy, curve 3 the risk in 26 children who received between 30 and 45 Gy and curve 4 the risk in 40 children who received greater than 45 Gy ($p = 0.002$). (From ref. 94, with permission.)

determinant of risk, whereas female gender and chemotherapy were additional risk factors in older patients. In Constine's study age did not affect the incidence of hypothyroidism but was weakly correlated with the degree of abnormality as suggested by higher serum TSH concentrations in adolescents compared with younger children (84). Such an age effect could reflect the greater sensitivity of the thyroid gland in rapidly growing pubertal children compared to preadolescents (8,21). The iodine load from LAG may be a causal factor in the hypothyroidism observed in patients who are irradiated for Hodgkin's disease. There is a low but greater than expected incidence of hypothyroidism in patients having LAG without neck irradiation. In some reviews, thyroid function was more likely to be abnormal in patients irradiated soon after LAG and mantle irradiation (83, 92,101). For example, in patients treated for HD at the Fox Chase Cancer Center, biochemical hypothyroidism occurred in 42% of patients at 5 years if they had a LAG, compared with 28% for patients without a LAG (101). However, no influence of LAG on thyroid dysfunction was noted in several other studies (27,83,92,94,97,98,102).

The frequency of primary hypothyroidism following irradiation to the spinal axis in the course of treating CNS tumors has not been as well studied. Ogilvy-Stuart et al. (103) evaluated 85 children and found a 32% incidence of compensated hypothyroidism. Constine et al. (74,85) evaluated eight children treated with 4- to 10-MV photon irradiation to the spinal axis (mean dose 30 Gy). Three demonstrated primary thyroid injury with low free T4 (FT4) and an exaggerated TSH response to TRH. Oberfield et al. (104) studied 36 patients following craniospinal irradiation for medulloblastoma. Many of the patients also received chemotherapy. Abnormal thyroid function as ascertained by TRH stimulation testing and/or TSH, T3, and T4 levels was identified in 21 cases (58%). The definition of thyroid dysfunction was apparently broad. Livesey and Brook (105) have reported that 69% of their population who received spinal

irradiation and chemotherapy had elevated TSH levels.

Patients undergoing bone marrow transplantation who receive TBI are also at risk for thyroid injury. Sklar et al. (106) found that a single dose of 7.5 Gy caused a decrease in T4 in 9% of patients and an elevated TSH in 35%.

Thyroid abnormalities have been observed among long-term survivors of ALL. Robison et al. (107) collected data on 175 survivors first evaluated 7 years after diagnosis. Seventeen (10%) had thyroid function abnormalities, including 5 with primary hypothyroidism and 11 with compensated hypothyroidism. Eight in the latter group became euthyroid without replacement therapy. No significant association was observed between hypothyroidism and the radiation fields (cranial versus craniospinal), dose (18 Gy vs. 24 Gy), duration of chemotherapy (3 vs. 5 years), or age at the time of irradiation.

It is not clear whether or not chemotherapy influences the incidence of radiation-associated thyroid dysfunction. The available data are limited and conflicting (91,92). In any event, one would have to be particularly cautious in interpreting such data. If radiotherapy dose influences the risk of subsequent thyroid injury and if patients treated with combined modality therapy had, on average, lower radiation doses, then the uncritical observer might conclude the chemotherapy had a "protective" effect when, in fact, all one would be observing is a radiation dose response (83). The influence of chemotherapy on the development of thyroid dysfunction among Hodgkin's disease patients appears to be negligible in most reports (84,87,94,108).

Hyperthyroidism

Thyrotoxicosis may occur following mantle or cervical irradiation for HD. In Hancock's report (93), approximately 2% of patients ($n = 34$) developed Graves' disease. Almost all had a diffuse goiter, high FT4, low TSH, and increased thyroid uptake of radioiodine. One-half of these patients developed infiltrative

TABLE 7. Evaluation of patients at risk for late effects: thyroid[a]

Late effects	Causative treatment			Signs and symptoms	Screening and diagnostic tests	Management and intervention
	Chemotherapy	Radiation	Surgery			
Overt hypothyroidism (Elevated TSH, decreased T_4)		>20 Gy to the neck, cervical spine >7.5 Gy TBI (total body irradiation)	Partial or complete thyroidectomy	Hoarseness, fatigue, weight gain, dry skin, cold intolerance, dry brittle hair, alopecia, constipation, lethargy, poor linear growth, menstrual irregularities, pubertal delay, bradycardia, hypotension	Free T_4, TSH annually up to 10 years postradiation or if symptomatic. Plot on growth chart	Thyroxine replacement. Anticipatory guidance regarding symptoms of hyperthyroidism/hypothyroidism
Compensated hypothyroidism (Elevated TSH, normal T_4)		Same as *Overt hypothyroidism*	Same as *Overt hypothyroidism*	Asymptomatic	Same as *Overt hypothyroidism*	Thyroxine to suppress gland activity
Thyroid nodules		Same as *Overt hypothyroidism*		Same as *Overt hypothyroidism*	Same as *Overt hypothyroidism*. Physical exam. Ultrasound for technetium^{99}m scan baseline and then prn symptoms	Thyroid scan. Biopsy/resection
Hyperthyroidism Decreased TSH, elevated T_4		Same as *Overt hypothyroidism*		Nervousness, tremors, heat intolerance, weight loss, insomnia, increased appetite, diarrhea, moist skin, tachycardia, exophthalmus, goiter	Same as *Thyroid nodules*. T_3, antithyroglobulin, antimicrosomal antibody baseline, then prn symptoms	Refer to endocrinologist. PTU, Propranol ^{131}I. Thyroidectomy

[a]From ref. 44, with permission.
Ifos, Ifosfamide; LH, luteinizing hormone; PCB, procarbazine; PTU, propylthiouracil; T_3, triiodothyronine; T_4, thyroxine; TBI, total body irradiation; TSH, thyroid-stimulating hormone.

ophthalmopathy, as did an additional four patients who did not have overt hyperthyroidism. The relative risk for Graves' disease was 7.2 to 20.4. Six patients developed silent thyroiditis characterized by transient mild symptoms of thyrotoxicosis, an increased serum FT4 and low TSH, no thyroid enlargement or tenderness, and low thyroid uptake of radioiodine (109). All of these patients subsequently developed hypothyroidism.

Thyroid Enlargement

Diffuse, symmetric enlargement of the thyroid gland with a normal or low serum FT4, representing Hashimoto's thyroiditis, is reported but rare after external irradiation (93). However, it is unclear as to whether a causal relationship exists. Some have speculated that irradiation of the gland liberates compounds that set off the autoimmune response (83,92,102).

Detection and Screening

Laboratory screening evaluations for asymptomatic patients should include serum concentrations of TSH and thyroxine (usually free T4) tests. The measurement of free T4 rather than other tests (usually total T4 by radioimmunoassay) is recommended because the former is not affected by changes in binding proteins. Because the latent interval to the development of abnormality can be prolonged, systematic clinical and laboratory evaluation should be performed yearly. Although some patients with normal serum free T4 and TSH concentrations might show an exaggerated TSH response to provocative testing with TRH, the clinical significance of this finding is unclear. In patients with clinical and laboratory findings suggestive of thyrotoxicosis, radioiodine uptake aids in distinguishing Graves' disease (increased uptake) from silent thyroiditis (diminished uptake) (77,82). Measurements of serum antimicrosomal, antithyroglobulin, and thyroid stimulating antibodies can assist in confirming Graves'; abnormalities in asymptomatic pa-

tients are again of uncertain clinical significance.

Management

Patients with uncompensated hypothyroidism (low serum concentration of thyroxine) clearly require thyroid replacement therapy. Patients with elevated serum concentrations of TSH but normal thyroxine are treated with thyroid replacement therapy in most institutions. The rationale for this approach is that subclinical hypothyroidism may evolve into overt hypothyroidism, and prolonged TSH stimulation of an irradiated thyroid gland may increase the risk for carcinoma (82,84,92,93,110). In support of this approach is that thyroid hormone replacement reduces the risk for recurrent cancer after thyroidectomy or an irradiated gland (111). For patients with overt hypothyroidism, thyroxine replacement should be gradual to avoid the rare occurrence of cardiovascular overload (82). Approaches to decrease the risk of thyroid injury in the setting of RT for Hodgkin's disease have included shielding the gland from irradiation (99), and administering thyroxine before irradiation (112). The former approach places patients at risk for shielding of involved cervical lymph nodes, and the latter did not prevent subsequent hypothyroidism. Therefore, these approaches are not recommended.

Table 7 reviews several thyroid late effects with respect to causative treatments, signs and symptoms, screening and diagnostic tests, and management and intervention (44).

OVARY

Radiation and chemotherapy can cause transitory or permanent effects on reproductive capacity, endocrine integrity, and sexual function. The concerns of survivors range from their functional status to consequences on the health of their offspring. The complexity of defining these sequelae stems from the differential dose-dependent effects caused by different chemotherapy agents, RT, and their combination. Injury to the ovaries can cause both sterilization and suppressed hormone production because of the relationship of the latter to the presence of ova and maturation of the primary follicle (113). Therefore, affected patients can have impaired development of secondary sexual characteristics, menstrual irregularities including amenorrhea, and symptoms associated with menopause such as hot flashes, loss of libido, and osteoporosis (114–117).

Pathophysiology

The ovary produces oocytes and secretes steroid hormones. Active mitosis of oogonia occurs during fetal life, reaching a peak of 6 million at 5 months after conception, dropping to 2 million at birth, with only 100,000 present at puberty (118,119). The cortices of the ovaries harbor the follicles within connective tissue. The follicles arise from the germinal epithelium, which covers the free surface of the ovary. Through involution, atresia, and, to a much lesser extent, ovulation, the follicles disappear entirely at menopause. Hypothalamic gonadotropin releasing hormone (GnRH) surges in late childhood to initiate puberty. GnRH stimulates release of the pituitary gonadotrophs which orchestrate follicular maturation (follicle-stimulating hormone, FSH) and ovarian luteinization (luteinizing hormone, LH). With sexual maturity comes the 28-day cycle with an estrogen-dependent midcycle surge of FSH/LH. After ovulation, the corpus luteum forms and produces progesterone, estradiol, and 17- hydroxyprogesterone, and the resultant endometrial changes. Without chorionic gonadotropin from a conceptus, the corpus luteum is exhausted and progesterone and estrogen fall. As FSH increases, the endometrium sloughs (menstruation). The normal premenopausal ovary, $4 \times 3 \times 2$ cm in size, contains degenerating ova, and follicles in varying stages of maturity. Ovarian hormones have critical physiologic effects on other organs, including maturation and maintenance of the breasts and vagina, bone mineralization, integrity of the cardiovascular system, and libido. With depletion of oocytes

by radiation, chemotherapy, or aging, the ovaries undergo atresia, and menstruation and estrogen production cease.

Radiation causes a decrease in the number of small follicles, impaired follicular maturation, cortical fibrosis, and atrophy, generalized hypoplasia, and hyalinization of the capsule. These effects are more direct and indirect through vascular sclerosis (80). Alkylating chemotherapeutic agents affect the resting oocyte in a dose-dependent, cell–cycle-independent manner. Thecal cells and ova are depleted, as are the primordial follicles, resulting in arrest of follicular maturation and decreased estrogen secretion. Because girls treated prior to puberty have a greater complement of ova than do older women, ovarian function is relatively more resistant to RT in younger girls.

Clinical Manifestations

The dose of radiation that will ablate ovarian function depends on the patient's stage of development, and whether the dose is fractionated. Data from Ash summarized the effect of fractionated RT on ovarian function in women of reproductive age (120) (Table 8). However, after single fractions, temporary sterility can occur with ovarian doses of 1.7 to 6.4 Gy, and permanent sterility after 3.2 to 10 Gy (121). Wallace reviewed data to estimate an LD50 of 600 cGy for the oocyte (122). Shalet et al. (117) studied 18 females who received 20 to 30 Gy over 25 to 44 days for nongonadal tumors. All 16 who received whole-abdominal irradiation had evidence of ovarian failure. Twelve patients who were older than 13 years of age had amenorrhea. All patients had an elevated FSH and low estradiol. Serum LH was elevated in 15 patients (83%) and was higher in older girls than in those less than 11 years of age. A study of ovarian morphology following abdominal irradiation indicated that follicle growth was significantly inhibited and the number of oocytes reduced by doses on the order 20 Gy (123). Stillman et al. (124) studied girls less than 17 years of age who were treated with 12 to 15 Gy, and they confirmed the relationship

TABLE 8. *Effect of fractionated irradiation on ovarian function in women of reproductive age*[a]

Minimum Ovarian Dose in Gy[b]	Effect
0.6	No deleterious effect
1.5	No deleterious effect in most young women. Some risk of sterilization especially in women age >40
2.5–5.0	Variable. Age 15–40 yrs: 30–40% sterilized permanently. Aged >40: >90% sterilized permanently
5–8	Variable. Age 15–40 yrs: 50–70% sterilized permanently, temporary amenorrhea in some of remainder
>8	100% permanently sterilized

[a]Modified from ref. 120, with permission.
[b]No attempt has been made to allow for variation in mode of fractionation.

between ovarian failure and radiation dose. Ovarian failure occurred in 17 of 25 girls (68%) whose ovaries received the full irradiation dose. Five of 35 girls (14%) with at least one ovary at the edge of the abdominal treatment volume (estimated dose 0.9 to 10 Gy with a mean of 2.9 Gy) experienced ovarian failure. None of 34 girls who received an estimated ovarian dose of 0.5 to 1.5 Gy (mean 0.54 Gy), by having at least one ovary outside the treatment volume, had ovarian failure. It is possible that direct or scattered irradiation from the spinal component of craniospinal irradiation may produce ovarian damage (122,125,126).

To shield the ovaries from direct irradiation during, for example, pelvic irradiation from Hodgkin's disease, an oophoropexy may be performed at the time of staging laparotomy or as a separate procedure. Typically, the ovaries are moved to a midline position in front of or behind the uterus. Alternately, they may be moved laterally to the iliac wings, which is particularly helpful for young girls or adolescents undergoing cranial spinal irradiation for brain tumors. The ovaries should be marked by the surgeon with clips that can later by identified by a simulator film. Central pelvic blocking at the time of "inverted Y" field will prevent direct irradiation, although scatter dose and transmitted dose will be inevitable. Medial or lateral transposition of the ovaries results in ovarian doses of 8% to 10% and 4% to 5%, respectively, of the pelvic dose (127–129). For most patients this will be compatible with preservation of fertility, although there may be temporary amenorrhea. In a review of Hodgkin's disease treated at Stanford University Medical Center, 11 of 11 girls less than 13 years of age treated with upper abdominal radiation and 7 of 7 treated to the pelvis with midline ovarian blocking retained ovarian function. Among women between the ages of 13 and 40 years who were treated with total lymphoid irradiation (TLI) to 30 to 40 Gy, 18 of 19 retained ovarian functions. Thirteen (68%) did have temporary amenorrhea lasting up to 4 years, and 6 (32%) had menopausal symptoms. Of 10 patients in the older age group who had a potential for becoming pregnant, 7 women had 11 pregnancies with 9 normal births and 2 therapeutic abortions (22,128). For patients treated with subtotal nodal irradiation with the inferior border of the field at L5/S1, or S1/S2, the ovarian dose is calculated to be 2% to 8% of the nodal dose, depending on technique, and, therefore, less than 3 to 4 Gy (130,131). As documented in a recent report from Stanford, such patients should not have radiation-induced menopause (130).

Sklar et al. (132) has documented amenorrhea and the failure to develop secondary sexual characteristics in prepubertal girls who received 10 Gy TBI, and ovarian failure in all pubertal women, of whom 50% had menopausal symptoms.

Cyclophosphamide, nitrogen mustard, vinblastine, and busulfan are capable of causing ovarian dysfunction (113,133,134). The age of the patient, the dose of chemotherapy, and the combined use of irradiation are all relevant to

TABLE 9. *Evaluation of patients at risk for late effects: ovarian*[a]

Late effects	Causative treatment			Signs and symptoms	Screening and diagnostic tests	Management and intervention
	Chemotherapy	Radiation	Surgery			
Ovarian failure	CPM, PCB, Bus, BCNU, CCNU, Ifos	4–12 Gy Tolerance decreases with increasing age	Oophorectomy or oophoropexy	Delayed/arrested/absent pubertal development including: Breasts, Female escutcheon, Female habitus, Vaginal estrogen effect, Development of body odor and acne Changes in duration, frequency, and character of menses (cramping) Estrogen deficiency: Hot flashes, Vaginal dryness, Dyspareunia, Low libido, Infertility	Tanner stage LH, FSH, estradiol: 1) Age 12 yrs 2) Failure of pubertal development 3) Baseline when fully mature 4) prn symptoms Assess basal body temperature (midcycle elevation suggests ovulation) (DHEAs for failure of development)	Hormone replacement (estrogen), Anticipatory guidance regarding symptoms of estrogen deficiency and early menopause, Alternate strategies for parenting, early intervention (hormone replacement may prevent: osteoporosis, atherosclerosis)

BCNU, 1, 3-Bis[2 chloroethyl-1 nitrosoureal]; Bus, busulfan; CCNU, 1, -[2-Chloroethyl-3-cyclohexyl- 1 -nitrosourea]; CPM, cyclophosphamide; DHEA, dehydroepiandrosterone; FSH, follicular-stimulating hormone; Ifos, Ifosfamide; LH, luteinizing hormone; PCB, procarbazine.
[a]From ref. 63, with permission.

the potential for ovarian injury. For example, prepubertal girls are apparently more resistant to large cumulative doses of cyclophosphamide than are adults (135). Chapman et al. (115) documented chemotherapy-induced ovarian failure in 84% of women older than 30 years, as compared to 31% in women under that age, at the time of therapy. In a review by Horning et al. (133), women between the ages of 13 and 40 years who received MOP(P) (nitrogen mustard, vincristine, procarbazine, prednisone) or PAVe (procarbazine, L-phenyl-alanine mustard, vinblastine) noted irregular menses. Amenorrhea occurred in 15%. In those patients who, in addition, received pelvic irradiation, 28% had irregular menses and 52% had amenorrhea. Among the women treated with chemotherapy alone, 10 pregnancies occurred in 8 women, resulting in 6 normal births, 1 premature birth, and 3 therapeutic abortions. Among those receiving combined radiation and chemotherapy, 7 pregnancies occurred among 5 women, resulting in 6 normal births, 1 premature birth, and 1 child with a low-birth weight. In Donaldson and Kaplan's review (22) of children treated for Hodgkin's disease with combined chemotherapy and irradiation, 22 of 25 (88%) retained normal menses. In a recent review of available data by Green (113), younger women commonly maintained fertility following MOPP chemotherapy, regardless of the number of cycles administered. Some chemotherapy combinations, such as MVPP (nitrogen mustard, vinblastine, procarbazine, prednisone), are more likely to cause ovarian failure (113).

Table 9 reviews several ovarian late effects with respect to causative treatments, signs and symptoms, screening and diagnostic tests, and management and intervention (44).

TESTES

Germ cell integrity, Leydig and Sertoli cell functioning, and the neuromuscular control of ejaculation are vulnerable to cancer therapy. While fertility and hormone production are closely related in the ovary due to their dependence on the ova and primary follicle, these functions are somewhat discrepant in the testes due to the differential sensitivity of the spermatogonia and Leydig cells to cytotoxic therapy. Therefore, the effects of surgery, radiation, and chemotherapy must be considered in the context of various specific functions.

Pathophysiology

Spermatogenesis, or the process of formation of spermatozoa from immature germ cells, takes place in the seminiferous epithelium within the tubules. The least differentiated germ cells, the spermatogonia, divide to form spermatocytes. These cells, immediately after formation, undergo meiosis to form spermatids, which then metamorphose into motile spermatozoa. This process may take up to 74 days (136). A constant supply of germ cell precursors is essential to the continuous production of spermatozoa, which are then transported through the lumen of the seminiferous tubules into the epididymis where they are stored. Leydig cells are the primary androgen-secreting cells, and account for at least 75% of the total testosterone produced by the normal adult male (137). Normal secretion of luteinizing hormone (LH) by the pituitary gland is essential for Leydig cell function; LH levels rise if inadequate androgen is produced. The physiologic role of FSH in spermatogenesis is to trigger an event in the immature testis that is essential for the completion of spermiogenesis. FSH levels rise if such spermatid differentiation is compromised. Once the process of spermatogenesis is established, it will proceed continuously as long as the supply of testosterone is available. Testosterone also stimulates the development of male secondary sex characteristics and, through negative feedback, pituitary LH secretion. Measurement of testosterone production by the testis is, therefore, of major significance in the evaluation of testicular function. However, because intact Leydig cell function is required for normal spermatogenesis, these measurements may not be necessary when sperm production is determined to be normal (136).

Clinical Manifestations

There can be no question that radiation can cause infertility. The testes can be irradiated directly, by scattered irradiation, or by dose transmitted through shielding blocks. Because the spermatogonia are exquisitely sensitive to radiation, even small doses can produce measurable damage. Depression of sperm counts is discernible at doses as low as 15 cGy. This decrease in sperm counts may evolve over a term of 3 to 6 weeks following irradiation, and, depending on the dose, recovery may take 1 to 3 years. Complete sterilization may occur with fractionated irradiation to a dose of 1 to 2 Gy (138). Spermatocytes generally fail to complete maturation division at doses of 2 to 3 Gy and are visibly damaged after 4 to 6 Gy with resulting azoospermia. Higher doses are necessary to damage spermatids when compared to the more sensitive spermatocytes. This sensitivity is convincingly demonstrated by Heller (139), who documented changes in sperm counts in men after various single doses of irradiation. Oligospermia occurred after a dose as low as 0.5 Gy. Recovery to normal cell counts required 9 to 18 months after doses lower than 1 Gy, 30 months after 2 to 3 Gy, and 5 or more years after 4 to 6 Gy. At the highest doses, permanent sterility is frequent. At lower doses, this reduced sperm count is seen 60 to 80 days after exposure, which is the time that maturation would otherwise be complete (139).

A variety of studies have shown that multiple small fractions of radiation are more toxic to spermatogenesis than a large, single fraction. This has been termed the "reverse fractionation effect." It is the result of the extreme radiosensitivity of the testicular germinal epithelium, the small number of stem cells, and rapid cell turnover (138,139). Table 10 summarizes the fractionated dose-related effect on spermatogenesis as well as Leydig cell function (120).

Several studies have addressed the effects of testicular irradiation on spermatogenesis in children. These studies have utilized semen analysis as well as measurement of the FSH level. Although FSH is usually elevated in the setting of impaired spermatogenesis, the correlation is not perfect. The threshold dose of irradiation that will damage the germinal epithelium in childhood is unknown. Some information was provided by Shalet et al. (56) in a study of 10 men treated as boys for nephroblastoma. After scattered irradiation doses of 2.7 to 9.8 Gy in 20 fractions, 8 (80%) had oligospermia or azoospermia and 7 (70%) had an elevated FSH. When patients are treated for Hodgkin's disease, the scattered dose to the testes from a mantle or paraaortic field is negligible. However, when the pelvis is treated, the calculated dose depends on the relative location of the testes to the inguinal field, with doses ranging from 3% to 10% without a specially designed testes shield, and less than 1% with such a shield. Therefore, less than 1 to 2 Gy is delivered or scattered with well-designed shielding, and this dose can be even additionally reduced with use of multileaf collimation. That is, the transmitted dose through the leaves is less than through cut blocks. The available data on males treated for Hodgkin's disease suggest that fertility is either maintained or only transiently depressed. Twenty boys treated for Hodgkin's disease were studied by a group from Stanford University (129). Five of the boys were prepubescent at the time of diagnosis and treatment. Eight of the children were treated for Hodgkin's disease with radiotherapy alone: 1 received no pelvic irradiation, whereas the other 7 received 31.2 to 44.74 Gy. Four of the boys, 3 of whom received pelvic irradiation, subsequently have fathered children 3 to 19 years following radiotherapy. Three had azoospermia 10 to 15 years after irradiation, and one other child had testicular atrophy at biopsy 1 year after irradiation. Five additional boys had received chemotherapy and 20 to 44 Gy of pelvic irradiation at 8 to 15 years of age. Four were azoospermic 3 to 10 years later. One had fathered a child.

Castillo et al. (140) evaluated semen analyses of several late-pubertal/young-adult males (15- to 20-years old) who received 12 Gy of testicular irradiation and chemotherapy for

TABLE 10. *Effect of fractionated testicular irradiation on spermatogenesis and Leydig cell function*[a]

Testicular dose in Gy	Effect on spermatogenesis	Effect on Leydig cell function
<0.1	No effect	No effect
0.1–0.3	Temporary oligospermia. Complete recovery by 12 mos	No effect
0.3–0.5	Temporary oligo-azoospermia at 4–12 mos after RT 100% recovery by 48 mos	Variable
0.5–1.0	>90% temporary oligo-azoospermia for 3–17 mos after RT Recovery beginning at 8–26 mos	Transient rise in FSH with eventual normalization
1–2	100% azoospermia from 2 mos to at least 9 mos Recovery beginning at 11–20 mos with return of sperm counts at 30 mos	Transient rise in FSH & LH
2–3	100% azoospermia beginning at 1–2 mos Some will suffer permanent azoospermia, others show recovery starting at 12–14 mos Reduced testicular volume	Prolonged rise in FSH with some recovery Slight increase in LH No change in testosterone
3–4	100% azoospermia No recovery observed up to 40 mos All have reduced testicular volume	Permanent elevation in FSH Transient rise in LH Reduced testosterone response to HCG stimulation
12	Permanent azoospermia Reduced testicular volume	Elevated FSH & LH Low testosterone Decreased or absent testosterone response to HCG stimulation Testosterone replacement may be needed to ensure pubertal changes
>24	Permanent azoospermia Reduced testicular volume	Effects more severe and profound than at 12 Gy Prepubertal testes appear more sensitive to the effects of radiation Replacement hormone treatment probably needed in all prepubertal cases

FSH, Follicle-stimulating hormone; HCG, human chorionic gonadotropin; LH, luteinizing hormone; RT, radiation therapy.

[a]Modified from ref. 113, with permission.

ALL. Testicular irradiation had been administered when the patients were 5- to 12-years old, and all were azoospermic. Sklar et al. (141) has evaluated the effects of scattered testicular irradiation from craniospinal irradiation (CSI) and CSI with extended abdominal fields, which included the testes in 34 children with ALL. Twenty-three patients had received CSI with an estimated gonadal dose of 36 to 300 cGy. Eleven had received the extended abdominal field with a gonadal dose of 12 Gy. All patients also received chemotherapy. In an attempt to separate out the effect of the scattered irradiation from the CSI, a third group of children were studied who have received chemotherapy and cranial irradiation only. FSH elevations occurred in 50% of the CSI/abdominal irradiation group, 10% of the CSI group, and none of the cranial irradiation group ($p = 0.005$). Abnormal decreases in testicular volumes were also related to radiation fields, with the highest incidence (50%) occurring in the CSI/abdominal irradiation group.

The limited data available indicate that chemical changes in Leydig cell function are observable following direct testicular irradiation. Shalet et al. (142) studied 11 boys irradiated with 24 Gy in 12 to 16 fractions for a testicular relapse of ALL. Abnormalities of gonadotropin secretion consistent with testicular damage were seen in nine (82%) of the boys. The mechanism for the increase in FSH is not entirely clear, but it is inversely proportional to the loss of germ cells within the seminiferous tubules. Blatt et al. (143) examined seven boys irradiated with 24 Gy for ALL involving the testes. Three of the four who had bilateral involvement demonstrated delayed sexual maturation in addition to elevated FSH and LH levels and low testosterone levels. Brauner et al. (144) studied 12 boys for 10 months to 8.5 years following direct testicular irradiation for the treatment of ALL. Basal testosterone levels were normal in the five prepubertal children, and LH levels were normal in 4 of the 5. Three of the five, however, had a decreased testosterone response to human chorionic gonadotropin (HCG) stimulation. Of the 7 postpubertal children, 3 had low basal testosterone levels and 6 had elevated basal LH levels. Five had diminished response to HCG stimulation. A follow-up study (145) enlarged the patient population to 21 boys who had received 24 Gy of testicular irradiation and who were followed up, on average, 3.8 years following irradiation. Basal testosterone levels were normal in the 12 prepubertal males. Basal LH levels were normal in nine and increased in three. Plasma testosterone response to HCG was diminished in 10 and normal in 2. There were nine pubertal patients. Basal testosterone levels were normal in three and diminished in six. Response of testosterone to HCG was normal in two and diminished in seven. There was a correlation between age and response to HCG stimulation ($r = 0.46$). Fig. 11 depicts the relationship of radiation dose to testosterone production as gleaned from several reports (137).

The germinal epithelium of the prepubertal testes is susceptible to damage produced by several chemotherapeutic agents including cyclophosphamide, nitrogen mustard, and procarbazine. Testicular biopsies following chemotherapy have demonstrated aplasia of the germinal epithelium. The effects are almost certainly dose-related (146). Azoospermia is consistently induced with a cumulative dose of 18 g of cyclophosphamide in men. Several reports in men indicate that permanent sterility is produced in the majority of men treated with programs including nitrogen mustard or cyclophosphamide for lymphoma (147–149). There may be a slightly decreased sensitivity to chemotherapy-induced gonadal toxicity in the prepubertal testis compared with the adult testis, but irreversible azoospermia can still occur after the use of alkylating agents. The effects of most agents are dose-related, which is well-demonstrated for MOPP chemotherapy where 2 cycles are less likely to cause azoospermia than 6 cycles (150,151). Reports are variable on the recovery of sperm numbers, with ranges from 0% to 50% reported (152,153). The latent interval can be as long as 10 years (153). Although full recovery of sperm numbers is much less common, pregnancies may be obtained with severe oligospermia. The relationship between FSH levels and sperm recovery is inconsistent (153).

The prepubertal state cannot be considered completely protective of the male gonads. In a report by Sherins et al. (154) of 13 pubertal boys treated with MOPP, 9 (69%) demonstrated gynecomastia and had evidence of germinal aplasia on testicular biopsy. FSH and LH levels were increased, testosterone levels were decreased, and prolactin and estrogen levels were normal. Other data demonstrate that 6 or more cycles of MOPP will sterilize 90% of males, whereas 3 or fewer cycles will cause oligospermia in 25% (151). While FSH and LH levels are often increased, testosterone usually remains normal. Some degree of recovery of sperm occurs in 10% to 25% of patients (perhaps more after fewer cycles) and may take as long as 2 to 5 years, though recovery is rare if it has not occurred in that interval (149,151, 155–157). While LH (and testosterone if affected) often normalizes, FSH may remain elevated even in males who demonstrate recovery of sperm counts (157). Children treated with chemotherapy may demonstrate normal gonadotropins in childhood but may exhibit an evolving pattern of abnormality after puberty (158,159). In recent years, the chemotherapy program ABVD (adriamycin, bleomycin, vinblastine, and dacarbazine) has been offered as an alternative to MOPP. Available data support the assertion that the long-term risk of sterility

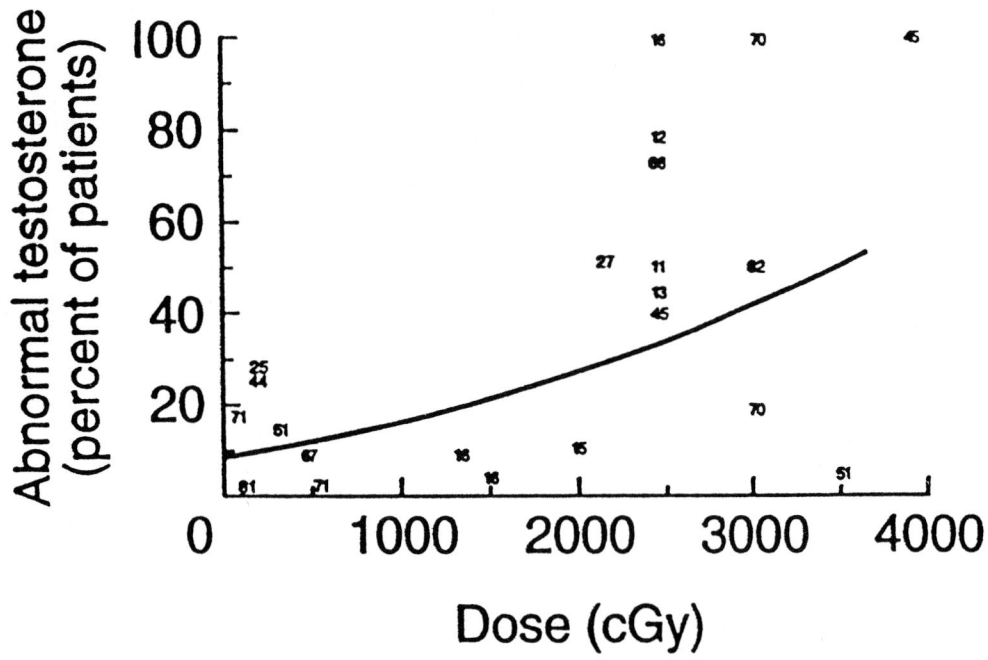

FIG. 11. Percent of patients with an abnormal testosterone value plotted against the stated dose of radiation to the testicles. The curve shows the best fit (extrapolated from the values by logistic regression). Refer to Fig. 3. of ref. 137 for references from which data was obtained. (From ref. 137, with permission.)

induction is less in males treated with ABVD than in those treated with MOPP (147,160). Other types of combination chemotherapy may be compatible with continued gonadal function. Boys with ALL treated with conventional therapy (prednisone, vincristine, methotrexate, 6-mercaptopurine) may progress normally through puberty with appropriate levels of FSH, LH, and testosterone and eventually normal levels of motile sperm (161). In one study of boys treated for ALL, biopsies showed that the percentage of seminiferous tubules containing identifiable spermatogonia was frequently low. Almost all patients had normal testosterone responses to HCG, suggesting that the Leydig cell function was at least compensated. The effects of various chemotherapeutic regimens on fertility was reviewed by Green (113) (Table 11).

With the growing use of bone marrow transplantation for the treatment of malignant and nonmalignant diseases, the effects of the

TABLE 11. *Frequency of azoospermia following completion of combination chemotherapy[a]*

Treatment regimen	Frequency of azoospermia (patient numbers)	
MOPP	75%	(42/56)
M(O/V)PP, COPP	87%	(5/6)
MVPP	86%	(132/154)
COPP	100%	(106/106)
ChlVPP	100%	(11/11)
ChlVPP/EAV	95%	(21/22)
ABVD	0%	(0/13)

ABVD, Adriamycin, bleomycin, vincristine, dacarbazine, COPP, cyclophosphamide, vincristine, procarbazine, prednisone; ChlVPP, chlorambucil, vincristine, prednisone, procarbazine; EAV, etoposide, adriamycin, vincristine; M(O/V)PP, nitrogen mustard, (vincristine/vinblastine), procarbazine, prednisone.

[a]From ref. 113, with permission.

TABLE 12. *Evaluation of patients at risk for late effects: testicular*[a]

Late effects	Causative treatment			Signs and symptoms	Screening and diagnostic tests	Management and intervention
	Chemotherapy	Radiation	Surgery			
Germ cell damage: Oligospermia/ azoospermia	CPM, HN₂, CCNU/BCNU, PCB, Ifos	>1–6 Gy	Orchiectomy or surgical manipulation	Testicular atrophy (softer and smaller), failure to impregnate	Tanner stage, inquire regarding previous sperm banking, determine testicular size and consistency LH, FSH, testosterone: 1) For failure of pubertal development 2) Baseline when sexually mature 3) For failure to impregnate (repeat q 3 yr for possible recovery) Analysis of sperm at maturity or for failure to impregnate (repeat q 3–5 yrs to assess recovery)	Instruct on testicular self-examination Anticipatory guidance regarding germ-cell damage Infertility counseling Alternate strategies for fathering
Leydig cell damage: Testosterone deficiency	CPM VP-16	>24 Gy to the testes (direct or scattered from pelvis)	Orchiectomy	Delayed/arrested/absent pubertal development, Pubic and axillary hair (female hair pattern), Lack of penile and testicular enlargement, voice change, body odor and acne, testicular atrophy (softer & smaller)	LH and testosterone at: Age 13 years Failure of pubertal development Baseline, if sexually mature Changes in libido or sexual performance	Testosterone replacement Anticipatory guidance regarding testosterone deficiency

BCNU, 1, 3-Bis[2 chloroethyl-1 nitrosourea]; CCNU, 1, -[2-Chloroethyl-3-cyclohexyl- 1 -nitrosourea]; CPM, cyclophosphamide; FSH, follicular-stimulating hormone; HN₂, nitrogen mustard; Ifos, ifosfamide; LH, luteinizing hormone; PCB, procarbazine; VP-16, etoposide.
[a]From ref. 44, with permission.

transplantation preoperative regimen on the reproduction is of considerable interest. High doses of alkylating agents are often used in the treatment program. After 200 mg/kg of cyclophosphamide and marrow transplantation for aplastic anemia, 18 prepubertal boys who were 2 to 13 years of age at the time of transplantation were evaluated, on average, 9 years after transplant. All the boys over 13 years of age have shown normal progression through puberty and have demonstrated normal LH, FSH, and testosterone levels. In eight patients who have undergone semen analysis, 2 are azoospermic and 6 are normal. Another population of prepubertal boys who received either TBI or TBI plus testicular irradiation have been studied. All the boys who received TBI plus additional testicular irradiation of 18 to 24 Gy have delayed development and elevated FSH and LH levels with diminished testosterone levels. The majority of those who received TBI alone have normal LH levels with elevated FSH (143,146,162).

The available data concerning irradiation of the testes indicate that radiation can produce profound depression of spermatogenesis, including permanent azoospermia. This can occur whether a child is pre- or postpubertal at the time of irradiation. Suppression of Leydig cell function is more pronounced at 24 Gy than at 12 Gy. Ill effects of radiation on Leydig cells are manifested in postpubertal and prepubertal males, although the ultimate severity of the injury is a direct function of younger age at the time of radiotherapy (138).

Many postpubertal cancer patients will have depressed sperm quantity or quality (percent motility, velocity, morphology) prior to RT or chemotherapy. Marmor et al. (163) documented abnormal spermatoanalysis in 19 of 57 (33%) Hodgkin's disease patients prior to therapy. Patients with advanced stage disease or "B" symptoms may have more pronounced abnormalities. Other studies have also documented that a significant portion of cancer patients have impaired semen quality, rendering them unfit for semen cryopreservation before administration of any toxic therapy (157,164–166). These sperm abnormalities have been attributed to the effects of stress, surgical trauma, fever, or the effect of systemic illness or pituitary hormone production (138). Nevertheless, many patients have normal sperm parameters prior to therapy, and these patients should be encouraged to cryopreserve semen (165).

Current efforts to protect patients from chemotherapy or radiation-induced damage to spermatogenesis involve eliminating those agents known to damage spermatogenesis, and optimizing testicular shielding from irradiation. Work in an animal model demonstrates that pretreatment with testosterone and estradiol, which reversibly inhibits the completion of spermatogenesis, protects spermatogonial stem cells from procarbazine and radiation (167). Testing such a strategy in patients may be worthwhile.

Table 12 reviews several testicular late effects with respect to causative treatments, signs and symptoms, screening and diagnostic tests, and management and intervention (44).

OFFSPRING

Many survivors of childhood cancer previously treated with cytotoxic therapy will remain fertile. The clinic needs to consider if treatment causes hereditary damage in patients; that is, does chemotherapy or radiotherapy cause cancer or genetic disease in the offspring of cancer survivors, or mutational events without clinical significance (162, 168)? As previously noted in the discussion of ovarian function, women treated for Hodgkin's disease with radiation or chemotherapy are capable of conceiving normal children. In a study by Horning et al. (133), neither fetal stage nor birth defects were seen. In a study concerning the outcome of pregnancy among survivors of Wilms' tumors, 99 patients treated between 1931 and 1979 carried or sired 191 singleton pregnancies of at least 20-week duration. Among the 114 pregnancies in women who received abdominal irradiation, 70% resulted in normal babies, 15% resulted in low-birth weight babies, and 15% resulted in prenatal deaths. Compared to the general population, the excess risk for death and low-birth weight was 7.9 and 4.0, respectively. The male patients sired normal offspring except in two cases (169,170).

The etiology for the increased frequency of perinatal deaths, premature births, and low-birth weight infants is not known. It probably relates to the abdominal irradiation causing somatic rather than germinal abnormalities such as a shortened trunk, fibrosis of the abdomen or uterine musculature, or a relatively decreased pelvic girth (30). A decrease in abdominal or uterine distensibility might result in the preterm delivery of low-birth weight babies or even malformed children. Uterine vascular insufficiency may also be a contributing factor (171,172).

In a study of survivors of Hodgkin's disease treated with radiation, chemotherapy, or both, the frequency of pregnancy was somewhat reduced. This reduction was greater for the partners of male patients than it was for female patients. However, there was no apparent increase in complications of pregnancy, spontaneous abortions, or congenital abnormalities compared with the general population (173).

Mulvihill and Byrne (168,174) have published an extensive literature review of the outcomes of pregnancy of patients who had cancer as a child or young adult, finished therapy, and later began a pregnancy. Over 844 cancer patients or survivors, nearly four-fifths women, initiated 1,761 recognized pregnancies. Of 1,389 liveborn outcomes, only 4% had a major birth defect—a statistic that matches the population rate for such malformations. The same authors have described a large-scale study of the National Cancer Institute to evaluate pregnancy outcomes in long-term survivors of childhood and adolescent cancers. There did not appear to be an overall excess risk of cancer in offspring of cancer survivors except for that attributable to known hereditary syndromes. There was also no increase in the risk of genetic disease. There is also no evidence of an increased risk of cancer in the offspring of survivors of the Japanese atomic bombings. This finding holds true even if the analysis is confined to so-called "germ-line" cancers such as Wilms' tumor (136).

While there is undoubtedly laboratory evidence that radiation and certain forms of chemotherapy are teratogenic, there is no persuasive clinical evidence of an increased likelihood of malignancies arising in the offspring of survivors of cancer and its therapy (123,128,147,161,168,174).

CENTRAL NERVOUS SYSTEM

Pathophysiology

The brain develops rapidly in the first 3 years of life and very little after age 6. This growth is due to an increase in the size, but not the number, of neurons. Axonal growth, dendritic arborization, and synaptogenesis are most active at this time (175). If maturation is judged by the degree of myelinization, then most regions are well developed by the second year but are not complete until puberty (176). Radiation injury would be expected to be profound during the early years. The essential radiation insult in radiation injury to the CNS is a demyelinating lesion with focal or diffuse areas of white matter necrosis (177–179). In the first weeks following irradiation, early demyelinating changes are generally restricted to scattered astrocytic or microglial reactions with occasional perivascular collections of mononuclear cells. Subsequently, neural tissue begins to break down with the appearance of regions of myelin destruction, proliferative and degenerative changes in glial cells, and vascular changes including endothelial cell loss, proliferation, capillary occlusion, degeneration, and hemorrhagic exudates. When a critical mass of capillary endothelial cells fails, then vasogenic edema develops in response to the loss of essential support of dependent neurons reflecting cerebral cortical atrophy. Intracerebral calcifications are sometimes present and presumably represent lesions of mineralizing microangiopathy.

The basic mechanisms underlying the pathologic changes are not precisely known for any particular syndrome of irradiation damage. The three most commonly proposed mechanisms may act alone or in combination. The *vascular mechanism* acknowledges that the endothelial cell is essential for patency of the microcirculation. This cell is radiosensitive, and damage is expressed as cell death or endothelial hyperplasia. Because endothelial cell turnover is slow, injury based on these cells occurs over a prolonged time interval. The evolution of hyalin degeneration and obliterating sclerosis of the arterioles produces areas of complete and incomplete necrosis (180). The *clonogenic death of glial cells mechanism* postulates a radiation-induced reproductive death of the slowly reproducing oligodendrocyte. The oligodendrocyte maintains myelin. These cells show a decrease in numbers within weeks following irradiation. Damage in individual nerve fibers can be demonstrated quantitatively by electron microscopy as early as 2 weeks after irradiation and preceding vascular damage (181). Effects on myelin synthesis and maintenance may be especially important in childhood because myelogenesis is most active in the first year of life. The ultimate result is demyelination. Radiation-induced endothelial cell death followed by vascular occlusion will also promote necrosis (182). The *allergic mechanism* of pathologic change in the brain following irradiation argues that the lesions of delayed radiation necrosis sometimes consist of disseminated plaques of demyelination with central necrosis and occasional petechial hemorrhage. In the patent blood vessels that remain, there may be perivascular cuffing with lymphocytes and plasma cells. The postulated autoimmune mechanism is that an antigen is produced by the reaction of ionizing irradiation with the oligodendromyelin complex. This antigen, subsequently, would stimulate the accumulation of inflammatory cells (180). One cannot prove that a single hypothesis explains delayed radiation necrosis, and it is possible that the pathophysiology is explicable by some combination of the three mechanisms. The classic findings of radiation-induced necrosis of the CNS are (a) large areas of confluent, coagulative necrosis of the

white matter and deep layers of the cortex; (b) the vascular changes of fibrinoid necrosis or fibrin incontinence; (c) atypia or absence of endothelial cells; (d) vascular thickening; (e) telangiectasis; and (f) vascular proliferation (177,180,182). When radiation necrosis occurs at a distance from the neoplasm—as might occur, for example, following large doses of radiation to extracranial lesions such as one on the scalp—the diagnosis is readily acceptable if the histologic findings are present. More controversial, however, is the diagnosis of radiation necrosis in an area adjacent to a parenchymal brain tumor where the differential diagnosis includes (a) therapeutic necrosis of the tumor induced by treatment, and (b) spontaneous tumor necrosis. It may be true that areas adjacent to a tumor are more susceptible to radiation necrosis because of the preexisting tissue injury (177, 180,182). The diagnosis usually rests on (a) the characteristic vascular findings such as fibrinoid necrosis, and (b) the absence of the characteristic changes of tumor such as the proliferative microvascular changes of glioblastoma multiforme (182). It is quite important to make the diagnosis of radiation necrosis in the treated patient. One wishes to avoid the clinical trap of calling a posttreatment mass with symptoms *recurrent tumor* rather than *radiation necrosis*. A patient might receive "salvage" chemotherapy or re-irradiation for "recurrence" when, in fact, necrosis was the underlying diagnosis. If the symptoms of necrosis spontaneously improved, as they sometimes do, then a patient might be erroneously scored as a "chemotherapy responder."

The contemporary pediatric radiation oncologist has a variety of imaging tools at their disposal to aid in the diagnosis of radiation necrosis. Computerized tomography (CT) of the brain will show either regions of low density without mass effect or contrast enhancement, a localized low-density contrast-enhancing mass, or diffuse lesions of varying density without mass effect but with occasional enhancement. Such lesions will develop months to years following therapy. MRI will show prolonged T1 and T2 relaxation times (183). Positron emission tomography (PET) is particularly promising. Labeled glucose is utilized. Hypermetabolic areas, using glucose, are more likely to represent proliferating tumor. Hypometabolic areas, devoid of glucose utilization, are more likely to be representative of radiation necrosis. No imaging modality, however, is infallible, and the clinician can only rely on biopsy to make the diagnosis—with the caution that even biopsy can be misleading because of the possibility of sampling error (66,182).

Clinical Manifestations

Necrosis

The incidence of radiation necrosis following therapeutic doses is uncertain. Quoted incidence data range from 0.1% to 5% after doses of 50 to 60 Gy fractionated over 5 to 6 weeks (49,178–180). The variability in the data is the result of (a) the uncertainty, in some studies, concerning the denominator; (b) the long time delay until the occurrence of necrosis; (c) the lack of histologic confirmation in many surviving patients; and (d) the absence of postmortem data in patients who succumb.

The clinical signs and symptoms of radiation necrosis are headache and mass effect. Surgical debulking is performed when possible and is often therapeutic (13,49,50). Corticosteroid may offer transient relief (184). Anecdotal reports exist of the benefits of anticoagulation with heparin or warfarin compounds (50–52,66,180).

Necrotizing Leukoencephalopathy and Mineralizing Microangiopathy

Leukoencephalopathy is a late complication of cranial irradiation and chemotherapy, particularly IV and IT MTX. The histologic appearance is of multifocal white matter destruction, especially in the centrum semiovale and periventricular regions, with loss of myelin and oligodendrocytes. Hypodense areas emerge in the white matter, and there is cerebral atrophy, an increase in the sulcal width, and enlargement of the ventricles. Mineralizing microangiopathy can occur which will be visualized, on CT scanning, as intracerebral calcification (50,52,66,183). The clinical features include lethargy, seizures, spasticity, paresis, and ataxia. The multifactorial etiology and risk for leukoencephalopathy has been studied in ALL survivors. As shown in Fig. 12, radiation and

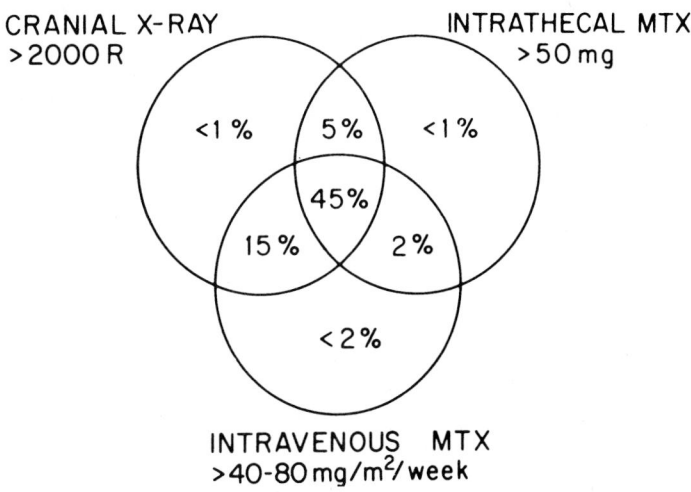

FIG. 12. Approximate risks of leukoencephalopathy. (From ref. 185, with permission.)

MTX appear to be contributing factors (185). Of interest is a report from the German Late Effects Working Group, which documented CT/MR evidence of atrophy, leukoencephalopathy, calcification or gray matter changes in approximately 50% of children treated for ALL (186). The frequency and severity of abnormalities was greater in children treated with cranial RT and MTX than in those treated with MTX alone. It is worth emphasizing that the situation is decidedly worse in children who have CNS involvement with ALL. In these situations, the presence of leukemia can alter the cerebrospinal clearance of MTX and heighten the risk of injury.

Neuropsychologic and Intellectual Deficits

Cranial irradiation of children may have significant adverse effects on intelligence, learning, and social-emotional adjustment (50–52,187,188). Follow-up studies of children receiving prophylactic CNS therapy for leukemia, therapy for CNS involvement with leukemia (at presentation or at relapse), or therapy for a brain tumor have helped elucidate the extent and nature of the problem. Studies of brain tumor patients must deal with the confounding variables of CNS injury by the tumor, seizures and their therapy, increased intracranial pressure, and surgery. In general, the leukemic patients receiving prophylactic CNS therapy do not have many of these problems and may provide a less complex situation to assess radiation's effects (51,52). In leukemic and brain tumor patients, however, the use of chemotherapy and the impact of the illness on body image and school attendance may complicate the issue.

Whole-brain irradiation has been extensively utilized for prophylactic CNS treatment of childhood leukemia. The effects of such treatment on subsequent intellectual function has been studied in considerable detail. The review of the literature that follows is selective—concentrating on those findings that are of clinical import and are supported by the bulk of the data. The tools by which we measure intelligence are varied. The "intelligence scale" or "intelligence quotient" (IQ) generally is reported as three values. The verbal IQ measures performance on vocabulary, general fund of information, and reasoning. The "performance" IQ assesses visual-spatial tasks such as puzzle assembly, block construction, visual memory, and nonverbal reasoning. The "full-scale" IQ combines verbal and performance scores (189). We may also evaluate children with achievement tests of skills such as spelling or arithmetic, as well as with questionnaires designed to ascertain social-emotional functioning (187,188). School performance and the need for special schooling is another way of attempting to quantitate intellectual performance. All of these tools have been used to assess the effects of radiation, chemotherapy, and surgery on children.

In 1984, Rowland et al. (190) described 104 leukemic children in continuous complete remission and without CNS leukemia. The children had received either IT MTX, IT MTX plus IV MTX, or cranial radiation for CNS prophylaxis. Most children were found to be functioning within the normal intelligence range. The irradiated children did have relatively lower IQ and achievement test results. In 1985, Copeland et al. (191) similarly found radiation-associated depression in performance and full-scale IQ. In 1986, Williams and Davis (192) reviewed 28 published articles that attempted to demonstrate the effects of cranial irradiation or chemotherapy on CNS. They were unable to unequivocally implicate any single method of CNS prophylaxis as being most closely associated with mental deficits. Among the methodological problems identified with prior studies are (a) lack of random assignment to groups, (b) failure to control for confounding influences such as severity of illness or parents' educational status, and (c) sufficient follow-up (193).

In 1991, Halberg et al. (189) from the University of California, San Francisco, described 19 ALL patients who received 24 Gy cranial irradiation at 2 Gy per fraction, 16 patients who received 18 Gy at 1.8 Gy per fraction, and 12 other oncology patients (generally Wilms' tumor) who served as controls to account for the disruptive effect of severe childhood illness. All the leukemic patients received IT MTX, but none received high-dose IV MTX. The mean IQ and achievement test scores were within normal range for all three groups. When detailed analysis was performed, the investigators found that there were lower IQ scores in the 24-Gy group (full-scale IQ: 24 Gy, 94; 18 Gy, 110; control, 106; $p < 0.1$) and that more children treated to 24 Gy had IQs less than 85. Eight of nine irradiated children with IQs lower than 90 were irradiated before age 5. Waber and co-workers (194) from Boston's Children's Hospital evaluated a stratified, randomized group of ALL patients who had received 18 versus 28 Gy and some of whom had also been randomized to low-dose versus high-dose IV MTX. In multivariate analysis, IQs were significantly lower in females and in those who received high-dose MTX. The higher dose of cranial irradiation may have been associated with impairment of verbal memory and coding. Excluding the high-dose MTX group, most children had IQs in the normal range irrespective of radiation dose. This group has more recently analyzed 66 patients on a successor protocol that involved treatment with and without 18 Gy cranial RT, and randomization to conventional dose or high-dose MTX with leucovorin rescue. Results were consistent with the earlier study; the combination of high-dose MTX, RT, and female sex were associated with IQ declines, and the most consistent impairments were in verbal memory and coding. Cranial RT (CRT) was not independently associated with impaired cognition (195). Mulhern et al. evaluated children treated for ALL at St. Jude Children's Research Hospital and noted that the mean full scale, verbal and performance IQs for patient groups treated with IT MTX/CRT (18 or 24 Gy) or high-dose MTX were within normal limits for the general population; however, significant declines (more than 15 points) had occurred in 22% to 30% of individual children regardless of treatment. No difference was seen among the various CNS treatment approaches (196) (Fig. 13). In a review of this subject, Waber and Tarbell point

out that more current treatment approaches are less likely to cause cognitive damage, though young female patients remain at highest risk, and particularly when treated with cranial irradiation and high-dose MTX (197). Controversy regarding the role of RT in impairing neurocognition will continue, largely due to differences in the radiation doses and drugs used in various protocols, and different endpoints. For example, in contrast to the mentioned data is a multiinstitutional report on 110 survivors of childhood ALL in which patients were treated with CRT (24 Gy) and IT MTX, or intermediate dose MTX and IT-MTX (Cancer and Leukemic Groups B[CALGB] protocol); the former group had significantly poorer academic achievement, poorer self-images, and greater psychologic stress (198). In summary, prophylactic cranial irradiation of 24 Gy at 2 Gy per fraction in the treatment of ALL can produce diminution in IQ and achievement tests. IQ drops may be on the order of 8 to 10 points (i.e., median of normals of 100 down to 90 to 92). A drop of this magnitude results in children being at the lower end of the normal range (189). Learning disabilities most commonly manifested are memory (especially short-term) deficits, difficulty in acquiring new knowledge, and decreased speed of mental processing (199). Ill effects are more severe the younger the child is at the time of irradiation and, perhaps, in females (50,192,200–202) (Fig. 14). Some studies suggest that the undesirable consequences of 18 Gy are less than 24 Gy, but the data on this point are not definitive (189,194,202,203). It is appropriate to point out that the combination of IT MTX plus high-dose IV MTX, without irradiation, may produce memory impairment (203).

Children who suffer a CNS relapse of ALL and receive IT chemotherapy and CSI are at risk for leukemia, radiation, and drug-associated injury to cognition. Kumar et al. (201) prospectively studied 11 long-term survivors of a CNS relapse of ALL treated with CSI (24 Gy cranium, 15 Gy spine) and systemic and IT chemotherapy. Full-scale IQ did not fall significantly in children 4 years of age or

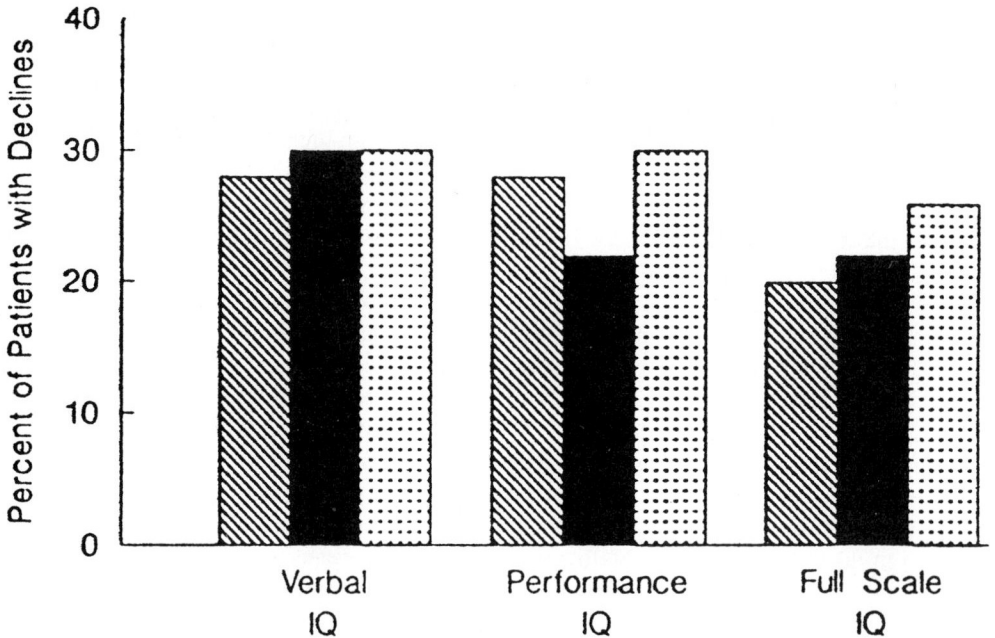

FIG. 13. Percentage of patients in the MTX (diagonal line bar), 18-Gy (solid bar), and 24-Gy (dotted bar) groups with clinically significant decline (≥ 15 points) of Verbal, Performance, or Full Scale IQ from first to most recent testing. (From ref. 196, with permission.)

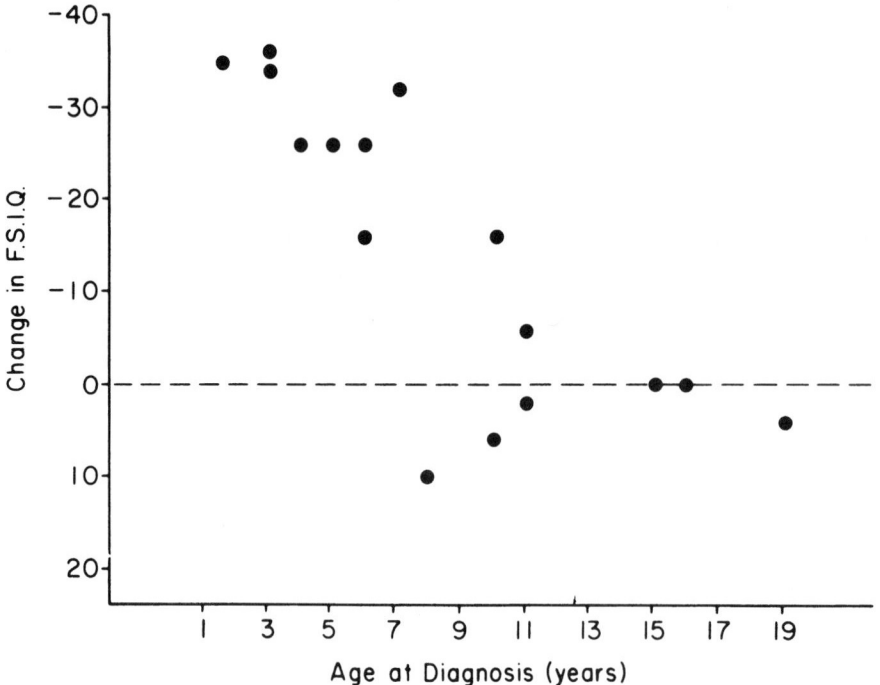

FIG. 14. This scattergram shows the correlation between changes in IQ and patient age at the time of irradiation in a population of children with brain tumors. (From ref. 205, with permission.)

older. The combination of young age at diagnoses and low initial IQ was predictive of a low IQ following treatment.

Children irradiated for brain tumors are well documented to experience adverse neurocognitive effects. Older studies that reported a relatively high functional level in most (70% to 80%) children following cranial irradiation for brain tumors utilized simple clinician-scored performance scales (188,204). More detailed assessment of IQ, achievement tests, learning ability, and school performance suggests a far less favorable outcome. The results of a variety of studies are summarized in Table 13. It is worth emphasizing several important points concerning these studies: (a) as in ALL, ill effects are more severe the younger the age at the time of treatment; (b) undesirable effects may be more likely with higher doses of irradiation and whole-brain, as opposed to limited-field, treatment; (c) particularly in the very young (under the age of 5), IQ drops may worsen as the time interval from treatment increases; (d) the practical implications of lowered IQs include an increased demand for special schooling and educational resources; (e) when one evaluates patients with posterior

fossa tumors treated with surgery alone (cerebellar astrocytoma) compared to surgery plus irradiation (medulloblastoma), the ill effects of radiation are demonstrable; (f) the presence of hydrocephalus at diagnosis does not correlate with intellectual outcome; (g) tumor location may help predict outcome, patients with hemispheric and hypothalamic tumors have worse sequelae than patients with infratentorial tumors (49,51,52,66,175,187,188,198,205).

Chemotherapy may contribute to radiation-associated injuries to cognition. Leukemic involvement of the CNS, intracranial bleeding, or solid tumor obstruction of cerebrospinal fluid (CSF) outflow may affect the clearance of IT MTX. Transependymal flow of the drug into the surrounding brain parenchyma may produce a greater chance of leukoencephalopathy. MTX also appears to be more injurious when administered after irradiation rather than before (49,51,52).

Irradiation of the brain of children can result in the "somnolence syndrome." This syndrome was first described by Druckmann (206) in 1929 in children who were irradiated for ringworm of the scalp. The syndrome has its onset from 4 to 8 weeks following irradia-

TABLE 13. *Neurocognitive effects of cranial radiotherapy for brain tumors*

Authors/reference	Year	Number of patients	Outcome
Hirsh et al. (332)	1979	28	12% had IQs >90, 31% had IQs <70, 93% had behavior disturbances.
Raimondi and Tomita (333)	1979	18	46% had IQs <70.
Spunberg et al. (334)	1981	14	42% were retarded.
Danoff et al. (49)	1982	38	17% had IQs <70, 56% had IQs >90, 37% had emotional difficulties.
Duffner et al. (335)	1983	10	50% had IQs <80, 20% had IQs >90, 4 of 5 with IQs >80 were learning-disabled.
Kun et al. (188)	1983	30	The number with IQ <90 is in excess of the distribution normally expected. 53% with supratentorial tumors or posterior fossa tumors requiring whole-brain RT had test results significantly below normal.
Ellenberg et al. (337)	1987	73	Ages at the time of treatment and whole-brain RT were associated with increased cognitive deficits.
Packer et al. (338)	1988	28	Mean IQ was 96 (range 50–120).
Packer et al. (205)	1989	18[a]	Children ≤7 years of age at diagnosis had a mean decline in IQ of 25 points at 2 years.
Packer et al. (336)	1992	17	No significant IQ drop in older children.

RT, radiation therapy.
[a]Full-scale IQ and academic performance was worse in the irradiated group than in 14 children with brain tumors in similar sites who were not irradiated.

tion and is characterized by drowsiness, nausea, irritability, anorexia, apathy, and/or dizziness. The majority of children reported to have developed this syndrome were irradiated for ALL, although it can occur after treatment of a brain tumor. The incidence may be as high as 40% to 60% of cases (50,180,207). Rarely, a previously resolved neurologic deficit may reappear for a short time. This should not be confused with recurrent malignancy. The somnolence syndrome will resolve spontaneously, but the administration of corticosteroid will hasten recovery. Arterial cerebrovasculopathy is an infrequent occurrence, almost always described following irradiation to the parasellar region, primarily in children. Single or multiple vessel narrowing or obliteration results in typical stroke deficits (208).

Myelopathy

The spectrum of radiation injuries to the spinal cord includes transient and irreversible syndromes (180). A rapidly evolving permanent paralysis can rarely be seen. This is presumed to result from an acute infarction of the cord. A more common form of radiation injury to the cord was first described by the French neurologist Lhermitte as a sign of multiple sclerosis. The so-called "Lhermitte's sign" or "Lhermitte's symptom" consists of an electric shock-like sensation that radiates down the spine and, frequently, into the limbs (209). The location of the sensation can change with time. The symptoms may be precipitated by flexion of the neck, walking on a hard surface, sitting on a hard surface, or other forms of physical exertion. The syndrome generally occurs a few months after spinal irradiation. The incidence after mantle irradiation for Hodgkin's disease may be on the order of 10% to 15% (210). The mechanism is thought to be transient demyelinization, although detailed human pathologic studies are lacking. There are no known CT or MRI correlations.

Chronic progressive radiation myelitis (CPRM) is rare. Intramedullary vascular damage that progresses to hemorrhagic necrosis or infarction is the likely mechanism, although extensive demyelination which progresses to white matter necrosis is an alternative explanation. The initial symptoms, generally subtle, are usually paresthesias and sensory changes (including diminished temperature sensation or proprioception), which start 9 to 15 months following therapy and progress over the subsequent year (102). Much longer intervals to initial symptomatology have occasionally been seen. Because a definitive diagnosis of myelitis requires pathology, which cannot be obtained except at autopsy, the diagnosis rests on supportive information. The neurologic lesion must be within the irradiated volume. Recurrent or metastatic tumor must be ruled out. CSF protein may be elevated, and myelography can demonstrate cord swelling or atrophy. MRI and CT provide additional supportive information.

The frequency of CPRM and radiation dose causing this event are poorly defined. This is due to the diagnostic difficulties and the variety of radiation techniques (with uncertain dosimetries). A review by Wara et al. (211) suggests that 42 Gy in 25 fractions carries a 1% risk, 45 Gy a 5% risk, and 61 Gy a 50% risk. Cohen and Creditor's data indicate the 5% risk to be at 49 Gy (2). Data from Marcus and William (212) suggest that the cervical cord may be more tolerant to radiation than previously presumed when 1.8- to 1.9-Gy fractional doses are used; of 324 patients treated to doses of 55 Gy or less, no cases of myelitis were seen. A review by Schultheiss et al. (102) supports this and suggests that the 5% incidence of myelopathy, at least in adults, probably requires total doses of 57 to 61 Gy. However, a lower tolerance in children might exist.

An increased risk of myelopathy is associated with higher individual fraction sizes, shorter overall treatment time, higher total doses, and long lengths of the cord treated (especially more than 10 cm) (83). Children may be more sensitive to CPRM, developing it after lower radiation doses and with shorter latency periods (102). Actinomycin D may decrease the dose threshold (213).

TABLE 14. *Evaluation of patients at risk for late effects: central nervous system*[a]

Late effects	Causative treatment			Signs and symptoms	Screening and diagnostic tests	Management and intervention
	Chemotherapy	Radiation	Surgery			
Neurocognitive deficit	High-dose IV MTX IT MTX	>18 Gy	Resection of CNS tumor	Difficulty with: reading, language, verbal and nonverbal memory, arithmetic, receptive and expressive language, decreased speed of mental processing, attention deficit, decreased IQ, behavior problems, poor school attendance, poor hand–eye coordination	Neurocognitive testing: psychoeducational neuropsychologic	Psychoeducation assistance
Leukoencephalopathy	MTX: IT or IV IT ara-C	>18 Gy (with MTX)		Seizures, neurologic impairment, compare with premorbid status	CT/MR scan baseline, PRN symptoms	Symptom management: muscle relaxant, anticonvulsants, physical therapy, occupational therapy
Focal necrosis	MTX: IT or high-dose IV BCNU, CDDP	>50 Gy (especially with >2 Gy daily fraction) >60 Gy	Resection of tumor	Headaches, nausea, seizures, papilledema, hemiparesis/other focal findings, speech, learning, and memory deficits	CT/MR scan baseline, prn symptoms PET or SPECT scan	Steroid therapy, debulking of necrotic tissue
Large-vessel stroke				Headache, seizures, hemiparesis, aphasia, focal neurologic findings	CT scan/MRI Arteriogram	Determined by specific neurologic impairment
Blindness	Intraarterial BCNU, CDDP	RT (optic nerve chiasm, occipital lobe)	Resection of tumor	Progressive visual loss	Ophthalmic evaluation visual-evoked response	Visual aids
Ototoxicity	CDDP	>50 Gy (middle/inner ear)		Abnormal speech development, hearing	Audiogram baseline prn symptoms	Speech therapy, hearing aid
Myelitis		>45–50 Gy	Spinal cord surgery	Paresis, spasticity, altered sensation, loss of sphincter control	MRI	Steroids, physical therapy, occupational therapy

BCNU, 1, 3-Bis[2 chloroethyl-1 nitrosourea]; CDDP, cisplatin; CT, computed tomography; IV, intravenous; IT, intrathecal; MRI, magnetic resonance imaging; MTX, methotrexate; PET, positron emission tomography; RT, radiation therapy; SPECT, single photon emission computed tomography.
[a]From ref. 44, with permission.

Table 14 reviews several CNS late effects with respect to causative treatments, signs and symptoms, screening and diagnostic tests, and management and intervention (44).

KIDNEY

Pathophysiology

The progression of renal dysfunction following irradiation is grouped into three periods (7). The acute period (up to 6 months) is rarely symptomatic, and a decreased glomerular filtration rate may be present. In the subacute period (6 to 12 months) the signs and symptoms include dyspnea on exertion, headaches, ankle edema, lassitude, anemia, hypertension, albuminuria, papilledema, elevated blood urea, and urinary abnormalities (granular and hyalin casts, red blood cells). Death might occur from chronic uremia or left ventricular failure, pulmonary edema, pleural effusion, and hepatic congestion. In the chronic period (generally after 18 months) either benign or malignant hypertension is seen, depending on the severity of the renal insult. Chronic radiation nephropathy in its mildest forms may not be diagnosed until 10 to 14 years following therapy. Abnormalities may include only proteinuria and azotemia with urinary casts and mild or no hypertension. A contracted renal size (mild atrophy) is seen on intravenous pyelogram (IVP). When chronic nephropathy is severe, death may result.

The pathologic process is a progressive arteriolonephrosclerosis. The lesion involves the microvasculature with injury to the intercellular connections between the renal capillary and arterioles. There is degeneration and sclerosis of these arterioles with narrowing or occlusion of the lumen and secondary degeneration of dependent structures (glomeruli, tubules). Associated changes in connective tissue include a thickened basement membrane, increased interstitial connective tissue, hyalinization, and fibrosis. Decreased perfusion of the kidney can occur with capillary and venous thrombosis and, eventually, necrosis. Withers et al. (214) (also see ref. 215),

have used animal data to argue for a different pathogenesis with the essential lesion involving the tubules with secondary loss of nephrons and parenchymal cell depletion.

Clinical Manifestations

Abdominal irradiation for Wilms' tumor, neuroblastoma, non-Hodgkin's lymphoma, and Hodgkin's disease have all been associated with renal damage (216). The severity of the effect of radiation is related to dose. While there is a significant risk of renal damage with doses in excess of 25 Gy to both kidneys, lower doses of radiation can be toxic to a child's kidney—particularly in the infant and/or when chemotherapy is also administered (217,218). In the second National Wilms' Tumor Study (NWTS) (220), 47 children received whole-abdominal irradiation and, therefore, had the remaining kidney irradiated. Three children (6%) exhibited transient elevations of blood urea nitrogen (BUN) and blood pressure. These patients received 12, 15, and 18 Gy. Prevention of nephropathy is accomplished by keeping renal doses below 20 Gy in 1.5- to 2.0-Gy fractions (Table 15). Postnephrectomy irradiation, as in Wilms' tumor, inhibits hypertrophy of the remaining kidney. Of note is a report regarding renal failure in children treated on NWTS 1–4. As expected, children with unilateral Wilms' tumor and a normal contralateral kidney have a low incidence of failure. However, the incidence of renal failure in bilateral Wilms' tumor was 16.4% for NWTS-1 and 2, 9.9% for NWTS-3, and 3.8% for NWTS-4. Most af-

TABLE 15. *Renal function in long-term survival of Wilms' tumor following irradiation[a]*

Radiation dose (Gy)	Number of patients	Number (%) with decreased creatinine clearance[b]
<12	70	13 (19)
12–24	27	9 (33)
>24	11	8 (73)
Total	108	30 (28)

[a]From ref. 339, with permission.
[b]Creatinine clearance <54 mL/min/m²

fected patients had undergone bilateral nephrectomy for persistent or recurrent tumor; radiation nephritis was uncommonly implicated as a cause of nephrectomy (221).

The renal arteries and the superior pole of the left kidney are frequently irradiated in Hodgkin's disease. Hypertension is rare (less than 2% of patients), but renal scanning shows decreased activity in the upper pole of the left kidney in up to 38% of patients (216).

Dose-volume histograms of renal radiation correlated with various renal function endpoints will be necessary for accurate determination of functional tolerance levels. In a review by Cassady of several reports, he determined a threshold dose of approximately 15 Gy delivered with conventional fractionation (in the absence of interactive drugs and underlying renal disease) as a reasonable estimate, while doses of more than 25 to 30 Gy to the total renal mass are likely to eliminate useful renal function in patients followed for

sufficiently long periods of time (222) (Fig. 15).

Late renal dysfunction has been documented following TBI prior to bone marrow transplantation for childhood malignancies. Tarbell et al. (223) reported a 35% incidence in children with ALL and a 71% incidence in children with neuroblastoma who received fractionated TBI (12 to 14 Gy over 3 to 4 days). All patients had anemia, hematuria, and elevated BUN and creatine levels. Renal biopsies in two patients showed changes consistent with radiation nephropathy or hemolytic uremic syndrome. The onset of renal dysfunction following TBI is 3 to 6 months. Therefore, the time course is similar to that of classically described radiation nephritis. While Tarbell et al.(223) found that renal injury occurs at a relatively young age, Lonnerholm et al. (224) found an 18% incidence of renal dysfunction in autografted children without an apparent age effect. The risk for injury may

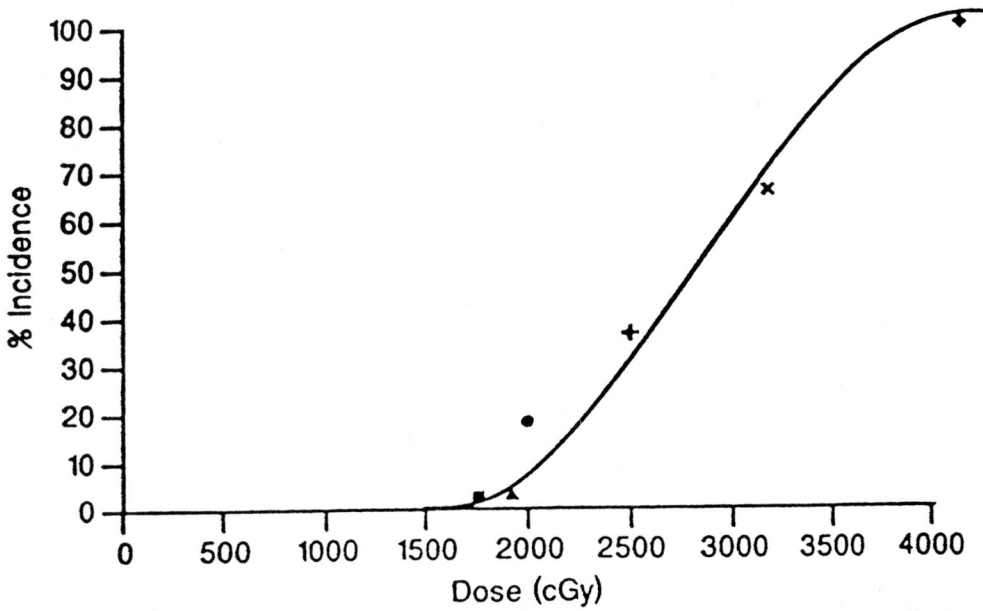

FIG. 15. Radiation dose-response curve for the occurrence of symptomatic radiation nephropathy generated from data presented in several reports. An approximate threshold dose of 15 Gy (conventional fractionation) is seen and a plateau is noted beyond doses of 30 Gy. (Modified from ref. 222, with permission.)

TABLE 16. *Evaluation of patients at risk for late effects: genitourinary[a]*

Late effects	Causative treatment			Signs and symptoms	Screening and diagnostic tests	Management and intervention
	Chemotherapy	Radiation	Surgery			
Glomerular dysfunction	CDDP			Asymptomatic or fatigue, poor linear growth, anemia, oliguria	Annual: Blood pressure, height, weight, hemoglobin/hematocrit, urinalysis, creatinine, BUN, creatinine clearance baseline and q 3 yr	Low-protein diet, Dialysis, Renal transplant
Hypoplastic kidney/renal arteriosclerosis		20–30 Gy 10–15 Gy with chemotherapy		Fatigue, poor linear growth, hypertension, headache, edema (ankle, pulmonary), albuminuria, urinary casts, hepatomegaly	Same as Glomerular dysfunction	Same as Glomerular dysfunction
Tubular dysfunction	CDDP Ifos			Seizures ($\downarrow$Mg, weakness ($\downarrow$PO$_4$), glycosuria, poor linear growth	Same as Glomerular dysfunction, and Mg, PO$_4$ (24 h urine for Ca, PO$_4$)	Mg supplement, PO$_4$ supplement
Nephrotic syndrome		20–30 Gy		Proteinuria, edema	Urinalysis q yr, Blood pressure q yr, (Serum protein, albumin, Cr, BUN) (24 hr urine for protein, Cr)	Low-salt diet, diuretics
Bladder: fibrosis or hypoplasia (reduced bladder capacity)	CPM Ifos	>30 Gy prepubertal >50 Gy postpubertal		Urgency, frequency, dysuria, incontinence (nocturia), pelvic hypoplasia	Urinalysis q yr (cystoscopy, IVP/US: volumetrics)	Exercises to increase bladder capacity, surgical referral
Hemorrhagic cystitis	CPM Ifos	RT enhances chemotherapy effect		Hematuria, frequency, urgency, dysuria, bladder tenderness	Urinalysis q yr to R/O UTI, renal calculi (cystoscopy if hematuria on 2 exams)	Transfusion, antispasmotics, Formalin, counsel regarding risk of bladder cancer
Prostate		40–60 Gy (lower doses inhibit development; higher doses cause atrophy)		Decreased volume of seminal fluid, hypoplastic or atrophied prostate	Examination of prostate gland, semen analysis × 1 (ultrasound)	Counsel regarding possible infertility due to inadequate seminal fluid, monitor prostate (exam, ? prostate-specific antigen)
Vagina: fibrosis/diminished growth	(Act-D, Doxo enhance RT effect)	>40 Gy		Painful intercourse, vaginal bleeding, small vaginal vault	Pelvic exam (possibly under anesthesia) baseline, during puberty and prn symptoms	Dilations, reconstructive surgery, potential need for cesarean section
Uterus: fibrosis/decreased growth		>20 Gy (prepubertal) >40–50 Gy (postpubertal)		Multiple spontaneous abortions, low birthweight infants, small uterus	Pelvic, baseline, puberty, then annually	? Endometrial biopsy, counsel regarding pregnancy
Ureter: fibrosis		>50–60 Gy		Frequent UTIs, pelvic hypoplasia, hydronephrosis	Urinalysis q yr (urethrogram)	UTI prophylaxis
Urethra: strictures		>50 Gy	GU	Frequent UTIs, dysuria, stream abnormalities	Urinalysis q yr (voiding cystogram)	UTI prophylaxis, surgical intervention

Act-D, actinomycin D; BUN, blood urea nitrogen; Ca, calcium; CDDP, cisplatin; CPM, cyclophosphamide; Cr, creatinine; Doxo, doxorubicin; GU, genitourinary; Ifos, ifosfamide; IVP, intravenous pyelogram; Mg, magnesium; PO$_4$, phosphate; R/O, rule out; RT, radiation therapy; US, ultrasound; UTI, urinary tract infection.
[a]From ref. 44, with permission.

be increased when TBI is administered on t.i.d. schedule when the interfraction intervals are less than 5 to 6 hours (N. Tarbell, *personal communication,* 1996). Some radiotherapists use partial transmission blocks over the kidneys to slightly reduce the renal dose and, consequently, the risk of renal injury. Not only does high-dose chemotherapy along with TBI increase the risk of renal injury, but conditioning regimens using chemotherapy alone (depending on the agents) may cause greater dysfunction than TBI regimens (225). Of interest is that proximal tubular dysfunction is more commonly abnormal than distal tubular function.

Table 16 reviews several renal late effects with respect to causative treatments, signs and symptoms, screening and diagnostic tests, and management and intervention (44).

LUNGS

The target cells for pulmonary injury are type I and II pneumocytes, fibrocytes, endothelial cells, and macrophages (7,8,226). Several pulmonary radiation syndromes occur in the child. Acute pneumonitis and chronic fibrosis result from injury to the type II pneumocytes and endothelial cells. Chronic respiratory limitations result from impairment in the development of new alveoli or from impairment of growth of established ones. Limitations of a different character result from a reduction in growth of the muscle, cartilage, and bone that form the thoracic cage.

Pathophysiology

The acute reactions of radiation pulmonary injury, known as the "exudative" phase, can be detected within 24 hours of irradiation. It is signified by intraalveolar edema and exudation of proteinaceous material into the alveoli, impairing gas exchange. Infiltration by inflammatory cells and desquamation of epithelial cells from the alveolar walls occur. A "proliferative" phase occurs between 2 and 6 months with accumulation of type II alveolar cells and protein leakage into the alveolar spaces. Interstitial edema organizes into collagen fibrils, leading to the thickening of the alveolar septa and a clinical pneumonitis. Injury to the type II pneumocyte, with resultant changes in the surfactant system (and thus alveolar surface tension and compliance) and in the endothelial cell and capillary permeability, causes these changes (227,228). After 6 months the "fibrotic" phase occurs. Alveolar septa become fibrotic and thickened by bundles of elastic fibers, forming the basis for chronic respiratory injury. Eventually, the alveoli collapse and are obliterated by connective tissue. Capillaries are lost, replaced, and then recanalized. The target cells that trigger this process are less clearly established but include the septal fibrocyte and endothelial cell (229).

Clinical Manifestations

Acute pneumonitis usually occurs 3 to 6 months after the start of irradiation. The symptoms include fever, congestion, a hacking but eventually productive cough, dyspnea, chest tightness, and pleuritic pain. Signs are initially absent, but consolidation and pleural fluid or a friction rub may be detected. If a large enough volume (greater than 75%) of lung is treated to doses in excess of 45 Gy, then cor pulmonale and death can occur. Surviving patients experience a protracted phase that slowly resolves. Lung function abnormalities are generally not detected for 4 to 8 weeks following completion of irradiation. Restrictive changes with volume loss occur, accompanied by a fall in diffusion capacity with mild arterial hypoxemia. Hypoperfusion of the irradiated area and decreased lung compliance can be demonstrated. The earliest radiographic changes (1 to 3 months after therapy) are a diffuse infiltrate corresponding to the radiation field with volume loss.

Chronic fibrosis is seen months to years following therapy, but most changes are apparent by 1 to 2 years. Most patients are asymptomatic, but chronic respiratory impairment with dyspnea, orthopnea, cyanosis, or cor pulmonale may occur. Maximum breathing capacity and tidal volume decrease. Chest radiographs show linear streaking that may extend outside of the irradiated field. Regional contraction, pleural thickening, and tenting of the diaphragm occur. The hilum may retract, with resulting compensatory hyperinflation of adjacent lung. CT and perfusion scans have been used to demonstrate and quantitate these changes (230–232).

Radiation Dose and Volume Parameters

Table 17 shows the risk for pneumonitis with or without actinomycin D. The estimated dose causing death in 5% of patients receiving whole-lung irradiation was 26.5 Gy in 20 fractions, and in 50% was 30.5 Gy in 20 fractions (233). Doses of 25 Gy in 20 fractions *without* actinomycin and 15 Gy *with* actinomycin are generally safe.

In the modern management of pediatric malignancies, radiotherapy is often given in combination with chemotherapy. It is important to take note of the fact that many chemotherapeutic agents either induce lung damage on their own or potentiate the damaging effects of radiation on the lung. As pointed out in the previous paragraph, actinomycin D accentuates the incidence of radiation pneumonitis. Bleomycin, cyclophosphamide, and, to a lesser extent, vincristine also enhance the damaging effects of thoracic irradiation (232). Although 500 units of bleomycin without irradiation can cause death in 1% to 2% of patients, as little as 30 units can be fatal in the presence of irradiation. Chemotherapy can also reactivate latent radiation damage (230,232,234). Table 18 lists several agents and their associated pulmonary syndromes (235,236).

Bone marrow transplantation with TBI as a component of the conditioning regimen is associated with acute pneumonitis and chronic pulmonary fibrosis. Fryer et al. (227) and Keane et al. (237) analyzed the relationship between single doses of irradiation to the whole lung and resulting fatal pneumonitis. After correcting for an increased lung transmission of 15% to 20%, a dose-response relationship was generated. Lethal pneumonitis was seen in 5% of patients after 8.2 Gy, 50% after 9.3 Gy, and 90% after 11 Gy. A difference of 2 Gy could thus change mortality from 0% to 50%, which emphasizes the importance of correcting for lung density. Increasing the dose rate from 0.1 to 0.5 Gy per minute increased the frequency of injury from 50% to 90%. TBI for bone marrow transplantation is associated with acute and sometimes fatal pneumonitis, and also chronic pulmonary compromise (238). The risk for acute pneumonitis increases from 5% after autologous transplantation, to 20% after allogeneic. The use of fractionated and low-dose rate regimens may decrease the risk.

The risk of chronic obstructive lung disease following allogeneic bone marrow transplantation in children was assessed by investigators at British Columbia's Children's Hospital (239). Various conditioning regimens were used, including TBI (various doses, and usually a single fraction) in 41 of the 65 patients (61%). The diagnosis was based on clinical findings (cough, wheezing, dyspnea), pulmonary function tests, lung biopsy and CT. About 20% of children developed obstructive lung disease (Fig. 16), and the risk was asso-

TABLE 17. *Risk of radiation pneumonitis*[a]

Total dose (Gy)	% affected post-RT (% affected post-RT & actinomycin)			
	5 Fx	10 Fx	20 Fx	30 Fx
10.0	0 (0)	0 (0)	0 (0)	0 (0)
12.5	0 (80)	0 (0)	0 (0)	0 (0)
15.0	60 (100)	0 (15)	0 (10)	0 (10)
20.0	100 (100)	20 (99)	0 (10)	0 (10)
30.0	100 (100)	100 (100)	85 (100)	1 (95)

Fx, fraction; RT, radiation therapy.
[a]Modified from ref. 233, with permission.

TABLE 18. *Chemotherapeutic agents associated with pulmonary toxicity[a]*

Drug (or group)	Syndromes	Dose response	Risk factors
Bleomycin	Pneumonitis/fibrosis (Hypersensitivity pneum)[b]	Yes	Age, O_2 renal insufficiency, RT, CT
Methotrexate	Hypersensitivity pneum Pneumonitis/fibrosis (Pulmonary edema)[c]	No	RT
Mitomycin	Pneumonitis/fibrosis (Pulmonary edema)	No	Anesthesia, RT, Velban
Nitrosoureas	Pneumonitis/fibrosis (Pulmonary edema)	Yes	Cyclophosphamide
Alkylating agents	Pneumonitis/fibrosis (Pulmonary edema)	No	RT, Nitrosureas
Cytosine Arabinoside	Pulmonary edema	Yes	
Vinca alkaloids	Bronchospasm Pneumonitis/fibrosis	No	Mitomycin, infants
Procarbazine	Hypersensitivity pneum	No	
Doxorubicin	Pneumonitis/fibrosis	Yes	RT, Infants
Dactinomycin	Pneumonitis/fibrosis	Yes	RT, Infants

CT, chemotherapy; RT, radiation therapy;
[a]From ref. 236, with permission.
[b]Parentheses indicate less commonly associated syndrome.
[c]Noncardiogenic pulmonary edema.

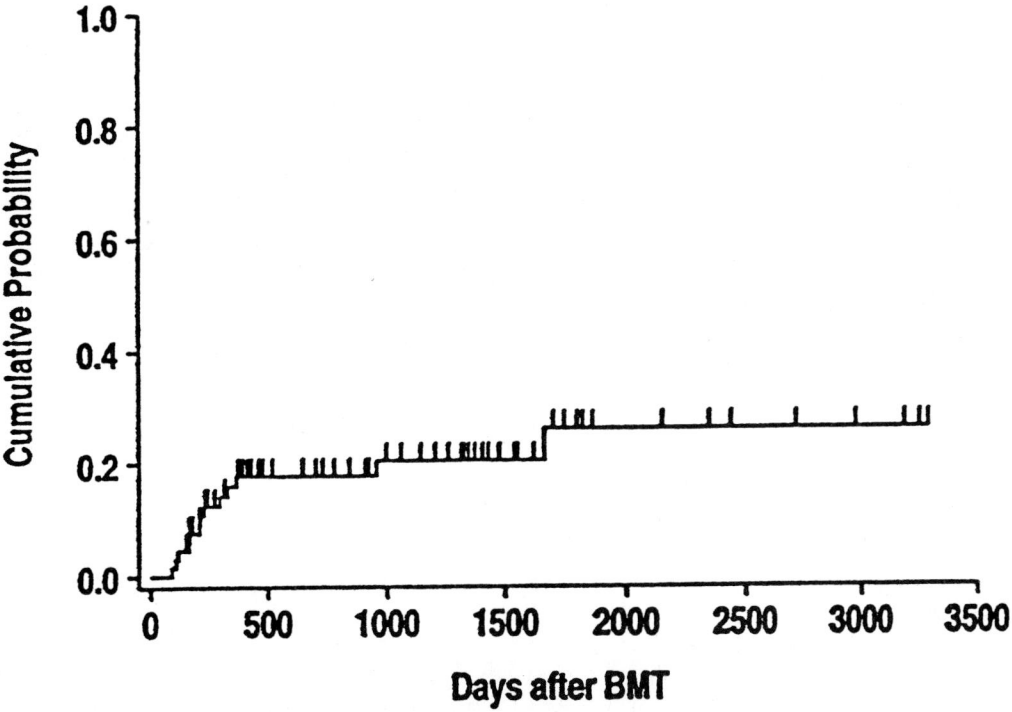

FIG. 16. Cumulative incidence for the development of obstructive lung disease (OLD). Onset of OLD was measured in a time-dependent manner using a Kaplan-Meier curve and is represented to 3,200 days after bone marrow transplant. (From ref. 239, with permission.)

TABLE 19. *Evaluation of patients at risk for late effects: pulmonary*[a]

| Late effects | Causative treatment | | | Signs and symptoms | Screening and diagnostic tests | Management and intervention |
	Chemotherapy	Radiation	Surgery			
Pulmonary fibrosis	Bleo, CCNU, BCNU, (CPM), (MTX), (Mitomycin), (Vinca alkaloids)	Pulmonary RT >15–20 Gy Risk increases with dose, larger volume irradiated, and younger age		Fatigue, cough, dyspnea on exertion, reduced exercise tolerance, orthopnea, cyanosis, finger clubbing, rales, Cor pulmonale	Baseline CXR and O_2 saturation, PFT including DLCO, then q 3–5 yr or prn	Consider pulmonary evaluation, steroid therapy Prevention: avoidance of smoking, avoidance of infections: influenza vaccine, pneumovax After bleomycin: avoid FiO_2 >30% intraoperatively and postoperatively Avoid excessive hydration

BCNU, 1,3-Bis [2 chloroethyl-1 nitrosourea]; Bleo, bleomycin; CCNU, 1, -[2-Chloroethyl-3-cyclohexyl- 1 -nitrosourea]; CPM, cyclophosphamide; CXR, chest radiography; DLCO, diffusing capacity for carbon monoxide; FiO_2, fractional inspired oxygen; MTX, methotrexate; PFT, pulmonary function test; RT, radiation therapy.
[a]From ref. 44, with permission.

ciated with chronic and acute graft-versus-host disease, either mismatched related or matched unrelated donors, and donor age. TBI was not a risk factor. Autologous BMT is rarely associated with chronic clinically significant ventilatory dysfunction (240).

Changes in lung function in children treated to the whole lung for metastatic Wilms' tumor have been reported. A dose of 12 to 14 Gy reduced total lung capacity and vital capacity to about 70% of predicted values, and even lower if the patient had undergone thoracotomy (232,234,241). Following 35- to 40-Gy mantle irradiation for Hodgkin's disease, pneumonitis has been documented in 5% of patients. Lowering the radiation dose to 15 to 25 Gy essentially eliminates this complication. Therapy with corticosteroids decreases symptomatology but must be withdrawn slowly (242).

Table 19 reviews several renal late effects with respect to causative treatments, signs and symptoms, screening and diagnostic tests, and management and intervention (44).

DIGESTIVE TRACT

The esophagus, stomach, and small and large intestines are irradiated in a variety of pediatric malignancies. While primary tumors of these organs are rare in childhood, they may be incidentally irradiated in the treatment of Hodgkin's and non-Hodgkin's lymphoma, Wilms' tumor, neuroblastoma, soft-tissue sarcomas, and bone tumors.

The direct effect of digestive tract irradiation is loss of regenerating cells lining the gut. Radiation damage of the fine vasculature of the digestive tract may progress to obliterative vasculitis with the ultimate development of ischemia (243,244). Acute radiation injury results from the depletion of normally proliferating cell, mucosal sloughing, villi shortening, and subsequent inflammatory infiltration and edema. The patient may suffer from odynophagia, dysphagia, abdominal pain, and/or diarrhea, depending on the site irradiated. Malabsorption of nutrients and decreased bile salt reabsorption can produce a nutritional wasting state (244). Such nutritional compromise must be treated with the utmost seriousness because it can lead to life-threatening risks of organ failure and, in the long run, severely impair the ability to administer adequate anticancer treatment. The clinician's threshold for the use of vigorous enteral or parenteral nutrition should be low.

Late radiation injury to the digestive tract is attributable to vascular injury. As the radiation vasculopathy progresses to obliteration, necrosis, ulceration, stenosis, or perforation may result (244,245). Late radiation enteropathy is characterized by malabsorption, pain, and recurrent episodes of bowel obstruction, as well as perforation, infection, and death. The onset is generally 6 to 24 months after the conclusion of radiotherapy. Donaldson et al. (246) evaluated 44 children who received abdominal irradiation for lymphoma, Wilms' tumor, or other malignancies. Eleven percent of the entire population and 36% of the long-term survivors developed bowel obstruction. Contributing factors included prior abdominal surgery, the use of concurrent actinomycin D, and very young age. In general, fractionated doses of 20 to 30 Gy can be delivered to the small bowel without significant long-term morbidity. Doses greater than 45 Gy, however, place the child at risk of low-term small bowel injury. The use of chemotherapy may modify these dose limits downwards. Portions of the esophagus, stomach, and large bowel appear to be able to tolerate slightly higher doses.

The prevention and management of radiation digestive tract injury relies, foremost, on the exclusion of normal tissues from the treatment beam whenever possible. For the esophagus, stomach, and large bowel, this usually relies on beam direction planning and patient positioning. For the mobile portions of the small bowel, the clinician will also evaluate (a) the prone versus supine position; (b) the use of compression, tilt tables, and false table tops; (c) surgical placement of omental slings and absorbable mesh; and (d) other techniques. The patient with acute radiation enteropathy may be helped by symptomatic interventions such as topical anesthetics for esophagitis, antidiarrheal agents, antispasmodics, antiemetics, bile salt binding agents, and an elemental or lactose-free diet (246). Medical therapy for late-onset radiation enteritis is unsatisfactory and has relied on intermittent steroids, Azulfidine, parenteral nutrition, and other supportive care. Surgical resection of damaged and/or obstructed bowel may be used, but there is a relatively high incidence of anastomotic dehiscence, operative mortality, and reobstruction (244).

The clinical signs and symptoms of radiation hepatitis include abdominal pain, increased girth, ascites, weight gain, jaundice, and elevation of liver enzymes—especially alkaline phosphatase (247,248). Severe thrombocytopenia can be seen, most commonly in children who have also been treated with actinomycin D (249). The clinical and laboratory expression of hepatic injury in terms of its time to expression and association with irradiation with or without chemotherapy is outlined in Table 20 (250).

In the acute phase of radiation injury (within 3 months of radiation), the liver is hyperemic and enlarged in the treated area (249,251). Dilatation and sinusoidal congestion accompanied by atrophy around the central vein of the lobule may be seen. As the chronic phase evolves (more than 3 months after treatment), characteristic central vein lesions develop. The lumen progressively narrows due to fibrotic changes involving the intima, leading to increasing sinusoidal congestion and liver cell atrophy. Inflammatory exudate is uniformly absent. After 6 months, and up to 6 years following irradiation, the distance between the central vein and portal space decreases, indicating the atrophy of hepatocytes. Nodules of regeneration are rare. Central veins become small and inconspicuous, and lobules are distorted or collapsed. Concentric fibrosis in the portal spaces around the portal veins occurs. This pathologic picture has been classified as *veno-occlusive disease* (VOD). Preliminary experimental evidence suggests that increased hepatic concentration of transforming growth factor $\beta 1$ in response to radiation injury may be important in the pathogenesis of radiation hepatitis (252).

In a series by Ingold et al. (249), no cases of radiation-induced liver disease occurred below a dose of 25 Gy, whereas 21% and 42% of patients had abnormalities following 30 to 36 Gy and 38 to 42 Gy, respectively. Tefft et al. (253) studied changes in hepatic function in children treated to varying portions of the liver for Wilms' tumor, neuroblastoma, or hepatoma. Fractionated doses to 12 to 25 Gy caused abnormal liver function tests and radionuclide scans in 50% of patients, 25 to 35 Gy caused abnormalities in 63%, and greater than 35 Gy was toxic in 86%. Children may

TABLE 20. *Comparison of radiation-induced liver disease and combined modality-induced liver disease*[a]

Clinical feature	Radiation-induced liver disease	Combined modality liver disease
Time to presentation after treatment	2–16 wk (typically 4–8 wk)	1–4 wk (typically 1–2 wk)
Signs/symptoms		
Jaundice	+	++++
Weight gain	+++	++++
RUQ pain	+	+++
Hepatomegaly	++	+++
Ascites	++++	++
Encephalopathy	+/–	++
Laboratory findings		
Increased bilirubin	+	++++
Increased AST	++	++++
Increased alkaline phosphatase	++++	+++
Outcome	10–20% mortality	30–50% mortality

AST, aspartate amino transferase; RUQ, right upper quadrant.
[a]From ref. 250, with permission.

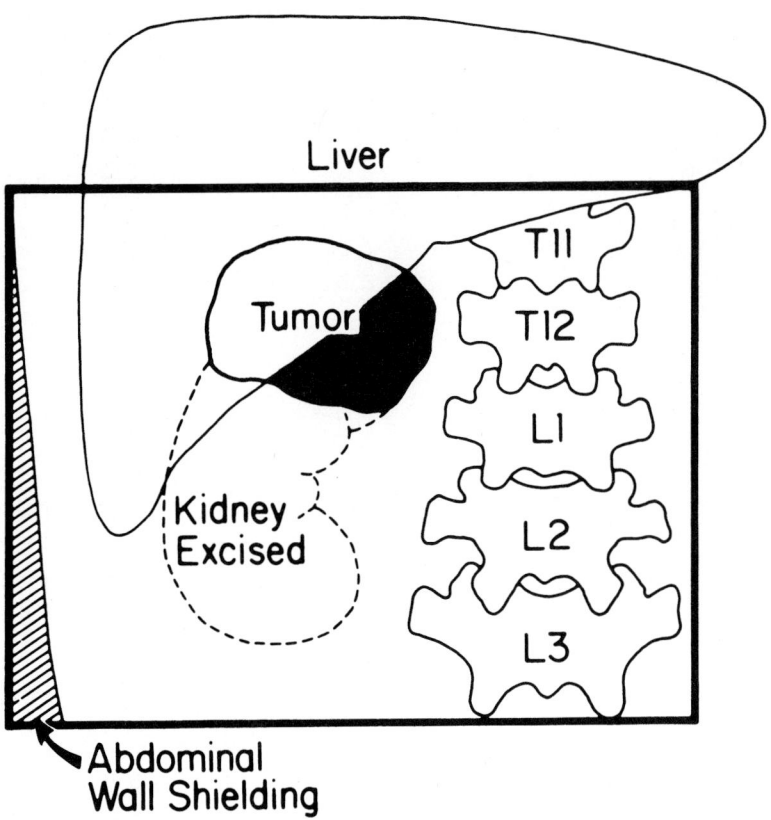

FIG. 17. A typical flank portal for Wilms' tumor arising from the right upper pole of the kidney will encompass a significant portion of the liver. The patient will be at increased risk for liver injury. (From ref. 220, with permission.)

be more sensitive to injury than adults, particularly in the setting of actinomycin D. Severe hepatitis has been seen after doses as low as 20 Gy with actinomycin D. The regenerating liver (e.g., after partial hepatectomy) appears to be even less tolerant to irradiation. Recent data concerning hepatic injury in childhood cancer treatment come from the second National Wilms' Tumor Study (220). Sixteen out of 303 patients (5.3%) had liver toxicity. The injury was manifest as thrombocytopenia, hepatomegaly, ascites, and, in four cases, hepatic failure. The doses of radiation to portions of the liver ranged from less than 15 Gy to over 30 Gy. It was interesting to note that 8.6% of patients receiving right-flank or whole-abdominal irradiation exhibited toxicity, as opposed to 2% of patients receiving left-flank irradiation ($p = 0.01$) (Fig. 17). All

TABLE 21. *Chemotherapeutic agents producing hepatic toxicity[a]*

Drug	Effect
Nitrosoureas	
BCNU	Elevated liver enzymes
CCNU	Elevated liver enzymes
Streptozotocin	Elevated liver enzymes
Antimetabolites	
Methotrexate	Fibrosis, cirrhosis
6-mercaptopurine	Cholestasis, necrosis
Azathioprine	Cholestasis, necrosis
Cytosine arabinoside	Elevated liver enzymes
Antibiotics	
Mithramycin	Acute necrosis
Enzymes	
L-asparaginase	Fatty metamorphosis

BCNU, 1, 3-Bis [2 chloroethyl-1 nitrosourea]; CCNU, 1, -[2-Chloroethyl-3-cyclohexyl- 1 -nitrosourea].
[a]From ref. 255, with permission.

TABLE 22. *Evaluation of patients at risk for late effects: gastrointestinal/liver*

Late effects	Causative treatment			Signs and symptoms	Screening and diagnostic tests	Management and intervention
	Chemotherapy	Radiation	Surgery			
Enteritis	Act-D, Doxo, enhance RT effect	>40 Gy	Abdominal surgery enhances RT effect	Abdominal pain, diarrhea, decreased stool bulk, emesis, weight loss, poor linear growth	Height and weight q yr, stool guaiac q yr, CBC with MCV q yr, total protein & albumin q 3–5 yr, (Absorption tests, vitamin B$_{12}$ level, and contrast studies)	Dietary management, refer to gastroenterologist
Adhesions		RT enhances effect	Laparotomy	Abdominal pain, bilious vomiting, hyperactive bowel sounds	Abdominal radiograph	NPO, gastric suction, adhesion lysis
Fibrosis: esophagus (stricture)	Doxo and Act-D (RT enhancers)	>40–50 Gy	Abdomen	Dysphagia, weight loss, poor linear growth	Height and weight q yr, CBC q yr, (BA swallow/endoscopy prn)	Esophageal dilation Antireflux surgery
Fibrosis: small intestines		>40 Gy	Abdomen	Abdominal pain, constipation, diarrhea, weight loss, obstruction	Height and weight q yr, CBC with MCV q yr, serum protein & albumin q 3–5 yr, (Upper GI, small bowel biopsy)	High-fiber diet, decompression, resection, balloon dilation
Fibrosis: large intestine, colon		>40 Gy	Abdomen	Abdominal colic, rectal pain, constipation, melena, weight loss, obstruction	Height and weight q yr, rectal exam, stool guaiac q yr, lower GI, colonoscopy, sigmoidoscopy	Stool softeners, high-fiber diet
Hepatic fibrosis/cirrhosis	MTX Act-D 6MP 6-TG	>30 Gy	Massive resection	Itching, jaundice, spider nevi, bruising portal hypertension: esophageal varices, hemorrhoids, hematemesis encephalopathy	Height and weight q yr, CBC, retic, platelets q yr, LFTs q 2–5 yr (hepatic screen) (liver biopsy) (endoscopy)	Hepatitis screen (hepatitis A, B, C/CMV), diuretics, liver transplant, varices: sclerosis, vascular shunting

Act-D, actinomycin D; BA, barium swallow; CBC, complete blood count; Doxo, doxorubicin; GI, gastrointestinal; LFT, liver function tests; MCV, mean corpuscle volume; NPO, nothing by mouth; RT, radiation therapy; 6-MP, 6-mercapto-purine; 6-TG, 6-thioguanine.

[a]From ref. 44, with permission.

the patients received chemotherapy in accordance with study guidelines, including vincristine, actinomycin D, and, in some patients, Adriamycin. The volume of liver irradiated influences tolerance to dose. New developments in three-dimensional organ imaging, in combination with the available clinical data, allow reasonable predictions of the probability of liver injury as a function of radiation dose. In the absence of chemotherapy, 30 Gy of whole-liver irradiation involves a significant risk of radiation hepatitis. In the presence of chemotherapy used for the treatment of childhood malignancy, most authorities are hesitant to treat the whole organ to more than 12 to 15 Gy—except, perhaps, in desperate situations such as that produced by marginally resectable primary hepatic tumors (see Chapter 14). The changes induced in the liver by radiation may be imaged by scintillation nuclear medicine scanning (which will show a cold area), CT, or MRI (248,254).

Several chemotherapeutic agents used to treat ALL, lymphoma, and other pediatric cancers can cause a hepatopathy similar to that seen following radiation (255) (Table 21). Severe damage is uncommon, although diffuse hepatocellular necrosis and fatty replacement can occur. In contrast to irradiation, the drug acts directly on the hepatocyte. Of particular interest is a report from the Intergroup Rhabdomyosarcoma Study Group (IRS) on the occurrence of VOD in children treated with vincristine, actinomycin D, and cyclophosphamide. Ten patients, or 1.2% of 821 patients, treated according to IRS IV had evidence of VOD. This incidence was greater than in previous studies and considered to be associated with an escalation of the cyclophosphamide dose in IRS-IV (256).

VOD is an uncommon but severe complication of TBI administered in preparation for bone marrow transplantation. It can occur following single doses as low as 7.5 Gy (247).

Table 22 reviews several gastrointestinal/hepatic effects with respect to causative treatments, signs and symptoms, screening and diagnostic tests, and management and intervention (44).

EYE

The eye is composed of several tissues that vary greatly in their radiosensitivity. Acute reactions include iridocyclitis, keratitis, conjunctivitis, and blepharitis. Delayed reactions, which generally occur after 6 months, include retinopathy, optic neuropathy, lacrimal gland atrophy or duct stenosis, glaucoma resulting from iridocyclitis, cataract, corneal vascularization and scarring, conjunctival telangiectasia, and eyelid atrophy with entropion or ectropion.

Retina

Radiation retinopathy is characterized by a slowly progressive microangiopathy, which may result in macular edema, capillary nonperfusion, retinal and disc neovascularization, vitreous hemorrhage, and traction retinal detachment. The microangiopathic changes may appear 6 months to 3 years following therapy (257). Visual loss is painless unless neovascular glaucoma develops. Using 1.8 to 2 Gy per fraction, the threshold for injury is 46 Gy, although the frequency is rare below doses of 50 to 60 Gy. As fraction size increases to 2.5 Gy or more, the frequency of injury increases (258). It is important to note that certain chemotherapeutic agents can cause retinal toxicity, and the risk is increased in children with impaired renal function who thereby accumulate drug (259).

Lacrimal Apparatus

Radiation may cause scarring of the canaliculi and puncta, ectropion of one punctum, failure of the lacrimal pump secondary to decreased eyelid mobility, and reflex lacrimation associated with ectropion, entropion, or conjunctival keratinization (257). Secondary symptoms can develop within months and be fully developed by 1 year. The patient may suffer from excess tearing, a foreign-body sensation, and photophobia secondary to corneal epithelial damage. When injury is severe, corneal ulceration, opacification, and vascularization

TABLE 23. *Evaluation of patients at risk for late effects: eye*[a]

Late effects	Causative treatment			Signs and symptoms	Screening and diagnostic tests	Management and intervention
	Chemotherapy	Radiation	Surgery			
Lacrimal glands: decreased tear production	5FU	>50 Gy		Dry, irritated red eye, foreign-body sensation, positive fluorescein staining	Penlight/slit lamp exam, fluorescein staining	Tear replacement, occlude lacrimal puncta, education regarding avoiding rubbing lids when puncta plug is intact
Lacrimal duct: fibrosis	5FU	>50 Gy		Tearing	Ophthalmic exam	Dilation of duct
Eyelids: ulceration		>50 Gy		Blepharitis, bleeding/crusted lesion, previous infections	Physical exam	Topical/oral steroids, skin balm
telangiectasia		>50 Gy		Enlarged, tortuous blood vessels Pigmentary changes	Slit lamp/penlight exam, open and closed eyelid exam	Teach: lid hygiene, radio-sensitizing drugs, UV protection Avoid trauma, harsh soaps and lotions
Conjunctiva: necrosis scarring subconjunctival, hemorrhage		Radioactive plaque therapy >50 Gy >45 Gy		Dry, irritated eye, foreign-body sensation, irregular rough conjunctival surface, telangiectasia Irritated eye, foreign-body sensation, dry, irregular conjunctival surface	Slit lamp/penlight exam, fluorescein stain	Steroids/antibiotic drops, tear replacement (resolves spontaneously) patching
Sclera: thinning		>50 Gy		May be asymptomatic, dry eyes, foreign-body sensation, grey, charred, blue sclera	Slit lamp/penlight exam	Antibiotic drops, avoid trauma, protective glasses
Cornea: ulceration		>45 Gy		Pain, foreign-body sensation, decreased VA, photosensitivity	Slit lamp/penlight exam, fluorescein staining	Tear replacement, Antibiotics, soft bandages, soft contact lens, surgery, ophthalmology

TABLE 23. *Continued*

Late effects	Causative treatment			Signs and symptoms	Screening and diagnostic tests	Management and intervention
	Chemotherapy	Radiation	Surgery			
Neovascularization		>50 Gy		Increased tearing, increased vessels surrounding edge of cornea	Slit lamp exam	Same as *Ulceration*
Keratinization		>50 Gy		Decreased corneal sensation, photosensitivity, fluorescein staining	Slit lamp exam, fluorescein stain	
Edema		>40 Gy		Decreased visual acuity, hazy cornea	Penlight/slit lamp exam: white, opaque cornea	
Lens: Cataract	Steroids (incidence varies with dose)	>8 Gy (single dose) >10–15 Gy (fractionated)		Decreased visual acuity, opaque lens	Direct ophthalmoscopic exam, decreased red reflex, slit lamp/penlight exam: opaque lens	Prevention by shielding during treatment, surgical removal, educate regarding UV protection
Iris: neovascularization		>50 Gy		May be asymptomatic, new blood vessels in iris (rubeosis), blood in anterior chamber, different colored irises	Slit lamp/penlight exam	Steroid drops
Secondary glaucoma		>50 Gy		Eye pain, headache, nausea/vomiting, decreased peripheral vision, increased IOP	Measure ocular pressure	Beta blocker drops, Atropine, Diamox
Atrophy				Decreased iris stroma at pupillary margin	Slit lamp/penlight exam	photocoagulation
Retina:				Blanched white cotton specs, decreased visual acuity, decreased visual field, blurred vision (central or peripheral)	Visual acuity, visual field (confrontation computerized or Amslergrid), direct and indirect ophthalmoscope exam, fundus photography	Steroids, photocoagulation, education regarding avoiding ASA and bleeding precautions
Infarction		>50 Gy				
Exudates		>50 Gy				
Hemorrhage		>50 Gy		Blood vessels: yellow fluid, bleeding, thin, incompetent vessels, tortuous, enlarged vessels		
Telangiectasia		>50 Gy				
Neovascularization		>50 Gy				
Macular edema (VA and VF)		>50 Gy		Blister of fluid in the macula		
Optic neuropathy		>50 Gy	Tumor resection	Pale optic disc, abnormal pupillary responses	Visual evaluation	Visual aids

ASA, aspirin; 5FU, 5-fluorouracil; IOP, intraocular pressure; UV, ultraviolet light; VA, visual acuity; VF, visual field.
aFrom ref. 44, with permission.

513

sufficient to cause visual loss occur. The frequency of injury is rare at doses below 45 Gy and common above 60 Gy (260).

Lens

Low-dose irradiation damages the germinal zone of the epithelium on the equator of the lens. The radiation-induced cataract is a central, posterior subcapsular opacity, which appears as a dot at the posterior pole of the lens. As the cataract enlarges, small vacuoles and granules appear around it. With continued enlargement, the opacity develops a relatively clear center, giving it a doughnut-shaped appearance (257). This progresses to the anterior pole, and the cortex then becomes opaque. Merriam and Focht (261) reported an evaluation of the dose-response relationship in 1957. After single doses of 200 R, abnormalities were detected but were not clinically significant until doses in excess of 400 to 500 R. With fractionated irradiation, a 60% frequency (progressive in one-half) was seen after 750 to 950 R, whereas 100% was seen after 1,150 R. Other investigators (262) have suggested a threshold for damage of about 2,000 R. Reevaluation of the atomic bomb survivor data suggests a 20% to 40% incidence of radiation cataract following a single eye dose of 5 Gy mixed photons/neutrons (263). The interval to abnormality in various studies is 2 to 3 years, but ranges from 6 months to 35 years depending on dose. Cataracts are seen after TBI for bone marrow transplantation, and data exist suggesting that fractionation and dose rate are relevant to outcome. Deeg et al. (264) reported that 80% of patients were affected after a single dose of 10 Gy, but only 19% after fractionated regimens to 12 to 15 Gy. In a report from France on 494 patients undergoing TBI, high instantaneous dose rate (greater than or equal to 9 cGy/min) was identified as the main risk factor for cataractogenesis (265).

Radiation-induced cataracts are one of the reported complications of retinoblastoma treatment. One might think, based on first principles, that an unblocked anterior beam for all or part of the treatment, as opposed to an angled lateral "lens-sparing" setup, would have a higher incidence of cataract formation. This hypothesis, however, is not supported by the data, and cataracts may occur after either technique (266,267). This is almost certainly due to the fact that variations in daily setup make complete lens-sparing unlikely with most lateral approaches. If a radiation-induced cataract causes visual impairment in the retinoblastoma patient, it may be removed. Persistent tumor is a contraindication to cataract removal. Final visual acuity following cataract removal depends on the presence or absence of macular tumor, the existence of radiation-induced keratopathy or retinopathy, severe amblyopia, a history of rhegmatogenous retinal detachment, and tumor control. In the absence of negative factors, visual acuity following cataract removal would be expected to be in the 20/20 to 20/50 range (268).

Optic Nerve

Injury to the distal nerve end produces ischemic optic neuropathy, whereas more proximal injury produces retrobulbar optic neuropathy. These are potentially blinding complications. The peak onset is 1 to 2 years, manifested by visual field deficits or central scotoma (269).

Lid

Rounding of the lid margins are not seen below 40 Gy, and ectropion is uncommon below 50 to 60 Gy. The eyelash is usually spared by anterior megavoltage beams so that it may remain partially intact (257).

Orbit

When young children are treated with either orbital irradiation or enucleation, as for retinoblastoma, orbital development can be impaired. In fact, the impact of these two treatments are not significantly different (270). For children undergoing enucleation, a prosthesis (implanted orbital sphere) is necessary for orbital development, and small implants more commonly result in small orbital volumes.

Table 23 reviews several late effects involving the eye with respect to causative treatments, signs and symptoms, screening and diagnostic tests, and management and intervention (44).

HEARING

The auditory apparatus may be irradiated during the treatment of brain tumors, aerodigestive tract malignancies, soft-tissue sarcomas, and lymphoma. Fractionated doses of more than 50 Gy can produce permanent changes in the temporal bone and adjacent soft tissues, including empty lacunae in the bone, resorption, absent marrow, and replacement by fibrous tissue. Temporal bone osteoradionecrosis is extremely rare with modern pediatric radiotherapy technique. Radiation changes in the external auditory canal may in-

clude thickening of the epithelium overlying the tympanic membrane, atrophic ceruminous glands, and absent hair follicles. The combination of abnormal epithelium of the external auditory canal and bacterial overgrowth can, on occasion, produce a persistent otitis externa requiring the use of wicks, otic antibiotics, and otic steroid preparations (271).

Cranial irradiation alone rarely has a significant effect on hearing. The hearing loss produced by cisplatin (CDDP), however, is related to dose and inversely related to age and can be significant. CDDP hearing loss is characteristically high frequency, bilaterally symmetrical, and irreversible. The combination of radiation and CDDP may produce a significant worsening of hearing than would the drug used alone in patients who receive the drug after irradiation. The administration of preradiotherapy CDDP does not seem to

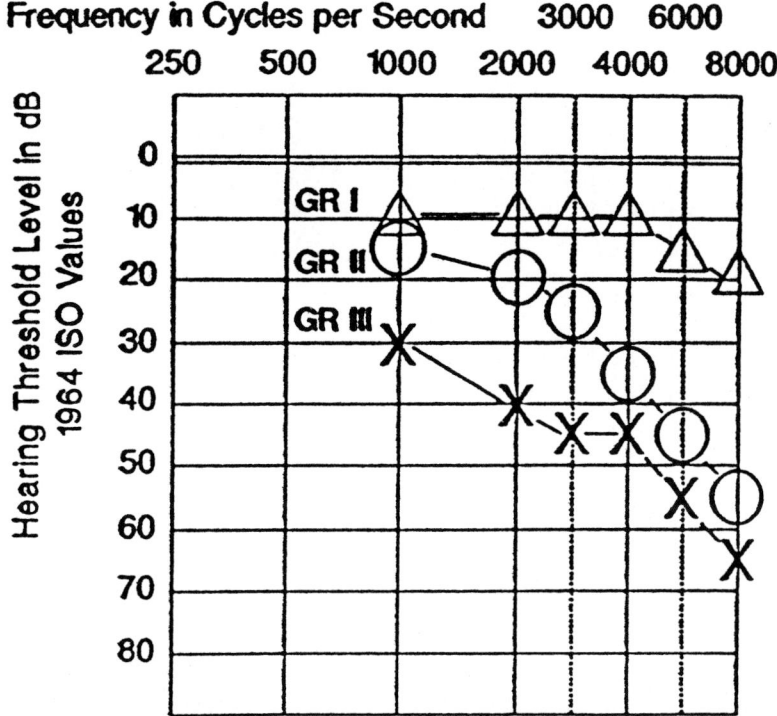

FIG. 18. Mean hearing thresholds for three groups of brain tumor patients. Group I (GRI—triangles) received cranial irradiation only; Group II (GRII—circles) received CDDP; Group III (GRIII—x) received cranial irradiation then CDDP. (From ref. 272, with permission.)

TABLE 24. *Evaluation of patients at risk for late effects: ear*

| Late effects | Causative treatment | | | Signs and symptoms | Screening and diagnostic tests | Management and intervention |
	Chemotherapy	Radiation	Surgery			
Chronic otitis		≥40–50 Gy		Dryness and thickening of canal and tympanic membrane, conductive hearing loss, perforation of tympanic membrane	Otoscopic exam, audiometry	Antibiotic therapy, decongestants, myringotomy, PE tubes, preferential seating in school, amplification
Sensorineural hearing loss	Cisplatin	≥40–50 Gy Cranial RT enhances the platinum effect		High frequency hearing loss (bilateral), tinnitus, vertigo	Conventional pure tone audiogram baseline and then q 2–3 yr Bilateral, symmetrical, irreversible	Preferential seating in school, amplification
Decreased production of cerumen		≥30–40 Gy		Hard and encrusted cerumen in canal Hearing impairment Otitis externa	Examination of canal	Periodic cleaning ear canal, Cerumen-loosening agents, otitic drops for otitis externa Keep ear dry: ear plugs, drying solution
Chondritis Chondronecrosis		≥50 Gy ≥60 Gy		Cauliflower ear	Inspection of auricle	Antibiotics, surgical repair (reconstruction may be hampered by poor blood supply)

PE, pressure equalization; RT, radiation therapy.
[a]From ref. 44, with permission.

be as toxic to hearing, and one might speculate that radiation causes some changes in the auditory apparatus, which renders the child more susceptible to the drug's effects (272) (Fig. 18). Of note is that bone marrow transplantation for children with brain tumors, when cisplatin or carboplatin-based regimens are used, is associated with significant hearing loss (273). Hearing loss in the pediatric cancer patient is a problem worthy of detailed attention, because it may lead to additional difficulties with communication, speech and language acquisition, and development of learning skills. The judicious use of amplification and other hearing aids is well-advised.

Table 24 reviews several late effects involving the ear with respect to causative treatments, signs and symptoms, screening and diagnostic tests, and management and intervention (44).

BONE MARROW

The hematopoietic progenitor cells and their offspring are cradled on a stroma of endothelial cells, adventitial cells, fibroblasts, macrophages, and fat cells. Mechanisms of marrow-induced failure include direct killing of hematopoietic progenitor cells, accessory cells (e.g., lymphocytes and monocytes), damage to the stroma and microcirculation, and disturbance of hematopoietic growth and regulatory factors (274,275).

The bone marrow is extremely sensitive to irradiation, to the degree that some injury is produced by any fractional dose. Irradiated bone marrow becomes hypocellular. There is destruction of fine vasculature followed by fatty marrow replacement of the normal hematopoietic marrow (276–278). If the radiation dose is sufficiently high, destruction of the sinusoidal circulation precludes migration of hematopoietic cells from distant nonirradiated sites. The radiation dose causing permanent local marrow aplasia has been assessed by several investigators using techniques of

bone marrow aspiration, scanning with ^{99M}Tc-S, ^{52}Fe, or ^{111}In as tracers, or MRI (276,277, 279,280). Following 40 Gy fractionated irradiation, 85% of irradiated sites will show a return of activity in 2 years; in 55% of those areas, recovery will become complete. Conversely, single doses of 20 Gy to localized regions can produce permanent aplasia. Radiation-induced changes in bone marrow may be detected by increased signal intensity on MRI due to the decreased T1 relaxation time of the increased fatty marrow content. MRI findings support those of nuclear medicine scanning and bone marrow aspiration studies—namely, that doses of up to 40 Gy, to limited areas, do not preclude repopulation of the irradiated marrow in the years following treatment (278). Doses in excess of 50 Gy seem to produce irreversible depletion of myeloid tissue (281).

The regenerative capacity of the bone marrow is dependent on the volume irradiated (282). Following irradiation to less than 25% of the bone marrow, the unexposed portion is stimulated and successful in compensating for hematopoietic demands, and the treated portion may never regenerate. When larger volumes (greater than 50%) are irradiated, the unexposed bone marrow is not adequate to meet the body's demands. Consequently, the paradoxical phenomenon of in-field regeneration is seen 2 to 5 years later, and extension of bone marrow activity into previously quiescent long bones is seen within 1 to 2 years.

Differences between children and adults in the response of the bone marrow to irradiation relate primarily to the differing extent of active bone marrow at different ages (283). In the immediate postnatal period, conversion from active red to fatty yellow marrow begins and is first evident in the extremities. This conversion progresses from peripheral (appendicular) toward the central (axial) skeleton, and from diaphyseal to metaphyseal in individual long bones (Fig. 19). Beyond these changes in active bone marrow volume, some investigators have suggested that younger

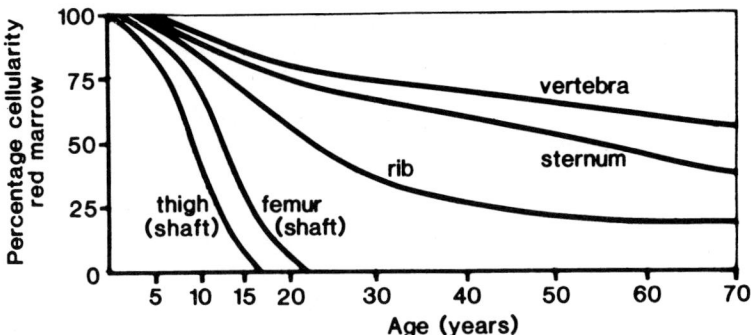

FIG. 19. The relative amount of red and yellow bone marrow in different anatomic sites as a function of age. (From ref. 326, with permission. Modified from ref. 327.)

people have a greater regenerative capacity for as yet unexplained reasons (280,282). The self-renewal capacity or numbers of stem cells might simply be greater in youth.

The acute and chronic effects of chemotherapeutic agents on the hematopoietic compartment has been reviewed (275) and will not be detailed in this section. However, radiation oncologists must be familiar with the acute myelosuppressive effects of various drugs, and this is summarized in Table 25.

TEETH AND SALIVARY GLANDS

Radiation-induced damage to developing teeth causes cosmetic and functional difficulties throughout life. The age of the child at the time of therapy and the radiation dose determine the consequences. Teeth begin to develop from the dental lamina 6 weeks after conception. The crowns of deciduous incisors are fully formed at birth. Calcification begins 3 to 5 months after birth in the central in-

TABLE 25. *Antineoplastic drug category/agent with their relative degree and duration of myelosuppression*[a]

Drug or drug class	Myelosuppression		
	Degree of suppression[b]	Nadir (d)	Time to marrow recovery (d)
Anthracycline	III	6–13	21–24
Vinca alkaloids	I–II	4–9	7–21
Mustard alkylator	III	7–14	28
Antifolates	III	7–14	14–21
Antipyrimidines	III	7–14	22–24
Antipurines	II	7–14	14–21
Podophyllotoxins	II	5–14	22–28
Alkylators	II	10–21	18–40
Nitrosoureas	III	26–60	35–85
Miscellaneous[c]			
Busulphan	III	11–30	24–54
Cisplatin	I	14	21
Dacarbazine	III	21–28	28–35
Hydroxyurea	II	7	14–21
Mithramycin	I	5–10	10–18
Mitomycin	II	28–42	42–56
Procarbazine	II	25–36	35–50
Razoxane	II	11–16	12–25

[a]Modified from ref. 275, with permission.
[b]I, mild; II, moderate; III, severe (based on common dose schedules).
[c]Agents differing from their class of compounds.

cisors, canines, and first molars; by 1 year in the maxillary lateral incisors; and by 2.5 years in premolars. By the end of the third year, the whole deciduous dentition is developed (284).

Developing teeth are irradiated in the course of treating head and neck sarcomas, Hodgkin's disease, neuroblastoma, retinoblastoma, and potential or established CNS leukemia, as well as during TBI for bone marrow transplantation. The defects that occur include (a) destruction of the tooth germ causing tooth agenesis, (b) stunted growth of the whole tooth or its root, (c) impaction, (d) incomplete calcification, (e) premature closures of apices, (f) premature eruption, (g) tapering roots with apical constriction, (h) delayed development, and (i) caries (284,285). Maxillofacial abnormalities include trismus, abnormal occlusal relationships, and facial deformities. Tooth defects are most severe before histodifferentiation and incremental calcification of the tooth buds, and the extent of damage is not apparent until the teeth erupt.

Doses of 20 to 40 Gy can cause root shortening or abnormal curvature, dwarfism, and hypocalcification. Studies of children treated for head and neck sarcomas with 40 to 60 Gy document abnormalities in greater than 85% of patients. In a study of 68 long-term survivors of childhood cancer, Jaffe et al. (39) found that 82% of patients receiving maxillofacial radiation exhibited dental abnormalities. Children treated with 18 to 30 Gy for leukemia are less frequently affected, with about 40% showing root or crown abnormalities of the maxillary first molars. Of note, however, is that chemotherapy alone for the treatment of leukemia can cause shortening (by 63% to 84%) and thinning of the premolar roots. This could be due to direct inhibiting effects of chemotherapy, altered marrow milieu due to leukemic involvement, or systemic factors altering growth. Radiographic abnor-

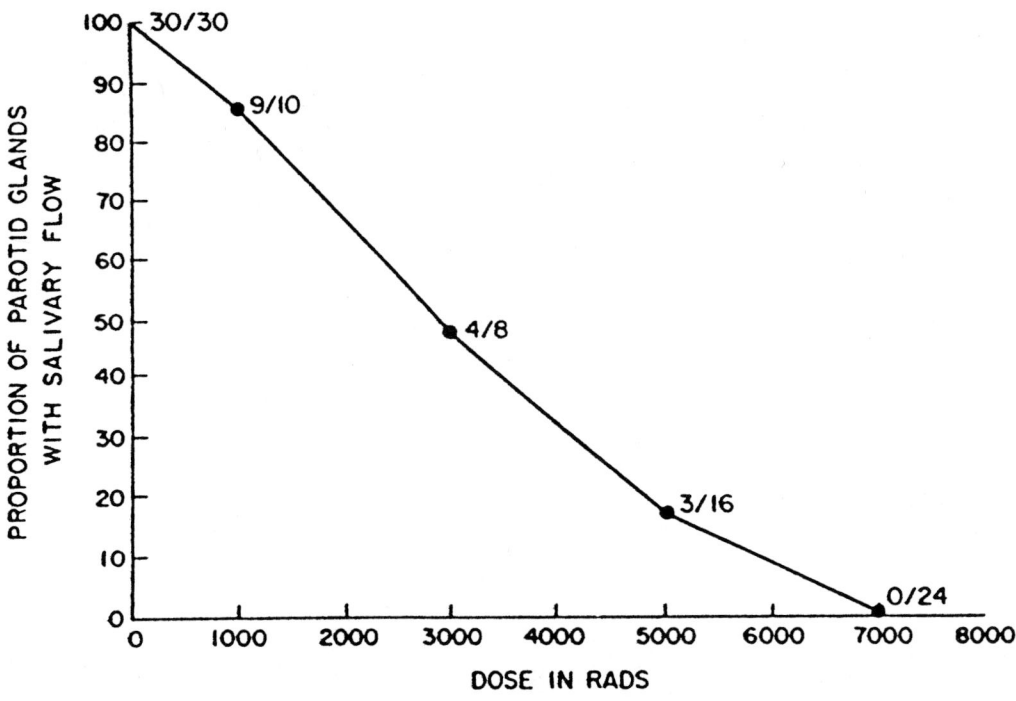

FIG. 20. Proportion of unirradiated and irradiated parotid gland with measurable salivary flow as a function of radiation dose. (From ref. 292, with permission.)

TABLE 26. *Evaluation of patients at risk for late effects: teeth[a]*

Late effects	Causative treatment			Signs and symptoms	Screening and diagnostic tests	Management and intervention
	Chemotherapy	Radiation	Surgery			
Xerostomia (decreased salivary gland function)		>40 Gy and >50% of gland must be radiated		Decreased salivary flow, dry mouth, altered taste perception, dental decay, Candida (thrush)	Dental examination, salivary flow studies, attention to early caries, periodontal disease	Encourage meticulous oral hygiene, Saliva substitution, Prophylactic fluoride, dietary counseling regarding avoiding fermentable carbohydrates, Nystatin for oral candidiasis, Pilocarpine
Abnormal tooth and root development	(VCR, Act-D, CPM, 6MP, PCZ, HN₂)	Generally ≥ 10 Gy can destroy developing roots		Enamel appears pale, teeth appear small, uneven, malocclusion	Dental exam q 6 mos with attention to early caries, periodontal disease, and gingivitis Panorex/bite-wing radiographs baseline (age 5–6)	Careful evaluation prior to tooth extraction, endodontics, and orthodontics Fluoride Antibiotics prn risk of infection (e.g., trauma)

ACT-D, actinomycin D; CPM, cyclophosphamide; HN₂, nitrogen mustard; PCZ, procarbazine; VCR, vincristine; 6-MP, 6-mercaptopurine.
[a]From ref. 44, with permission.

malities are common after radiotherapy for leukemia and sarcoma (39,286,287).

When 10 Gy of TBI is administered for bone marrow transplantation, impaired root development resulting in short, V-shaped roots is found in all patients, whereas microdontia, enamel hypoplasia, and premature apical closure are found in 30% to 50% (288). These effects seem to result from irradiation, not chemotherapy.

Salivary gland irradiation causes a qualitative and quantitative change in salivary flow. When salivary glands are irradiated, acinar cells are destroyed and replaced by ductal remnants and loose connective tissue (289,290). Such damage is evident after 20 Gy of fractionated irradiation. Salivary flow rate drops rapidly during a course of fractionated irradiation. Postradiotherapy xerostomia is irreversible if all major salivary glands are treated with doses of 50 to 60 Gy (289,290). Stimulated and nonstimulated salivary flow are primarily due to the parotid and submandibular glands. In Fromm's study of children treated for head and neck sarcomas, about 40% of parotid glands had absent secretions, and these patients received the highest radiation dose (mean 51 Gy) (286). Patients treated with less than 40 Gy were not affected. Among patients treated for Hodgkin's disease with 40 Gy to regions including the submandibular glands, flow rate reductions of about 55% have been documented (291). The radiation dose-effect of radiation on parotid salivary flow is seen in Fig. 20 (292). In normal saliva, cariogenesis is diminished by salivary antimicrobial substances. Radiation-induced changes in salivary pH and quantity produce a highly cariogenic microflora along with a decrease in protective salivary electrolytes and immunoproteins (289,290). In addition, the pediatric cancer patient is often on a high-carbohydrate diet due to parental indulgence and/or to maintain adequate calorie intake (285). These circumstances render the patient highly susceptible to radiation-induced caries.

Excellent oral hygiene and attentive dental care are the keys to dealing with radiation's effects on teeth and salivation in children. *Prior* to radiation and chemotherapy a dental evaluation is indicated. As possible foci of infection, loose exfoliating primary teeth and orthodontic appliances should be removed (285). The daily use of topical fluoride can dramatically reduce the frequency of radiation caries in the treated patient (290,293). Xerostomia is palliatively treated with saliva substitutes and sialagogues (289). Data support the efficacy of pilocarpine in improving saliva production and relieving symptoms of xerostomia, with minor risks that are predominantly limited to sweating (294).

Table 26 reviews several dental/salivary late effects with respect to causative treatments, signs and symptoms, screening and diagnostic tests, and management and intervention (44).

CARDIAC

The functional and structural complexity of the heart is monitored by the variety of radiation injuries that can occur: (a) acute pericarditis during radiation (rare and associated with juxtapericardial cancer); (b) delayed pericarditis that can present abruptly or as chronic pericardial effusion; (c) pancarditis that includes pericardial and myocardial fibrosis with or without endocardial fibroelastosis (only after large doses); (d) myopathy in the absence of significant pericardial disease; (e) coronary artery disease (uncommon), usually involving the left anterior descending artery; (f) functionally valvular injury; and (g) conduction defects (see Table 27). The hallmark of these injuries histologically is fibrosis in the interstitium with normal-appearing myocytes and capillary and arterial narrowing (295).

Several parameters must be considered in the evaluation of these injuries, including: (a) relative weighting of the radiation portals and, therefore, the amount of radiation delivered to different depths of the heart; (b) the presence of juxtapericardial tumor; (c) the volume and specific areas of the heart irradiated; (d) the total and fractional irradiation dose; (e) the

TABLE 27. *Nonfatal cardiac diagnosis among 635 patients treated for Hodgkin's disease (HD)
during childhood and adolescence[a]*

Diagnosis	Number	(%)	Interval from radiation (yrs)	
			Mean	Range
Acute myocardial infarction[b]	3	(0.5)	12	6.2–19.8
Coronary artery disease requiring revascularization[b]	3	(0.5)	21	18.0–23.8
Pericardiectomy for constrictive pericarditis	12	(1.9)	7	0.8–16.8
Acute pericarditis during HD therapy	8	(1.3)	—	—
Acute pericarditis after HD therapy	30	(4.7)	6	0.3–18.0
Pericarditis following corticosteroid withdrawal	2	(0.3)	11	6.7–14.8
Valvular heart surgery[c]	3	(0.5)	18	15.0–21.3
Heart murmur	26	(4.1)	14	1.1–27.5
Mitral valve prolapse	3	(0.5)	6	4.0–9.3
Valvular disease before HD	6	(0.9)	—	—
Recurrent congestive heart failure/cardiomyopathy	3	(0.5)	13	5.3–22.3
Electrocardiographic abnormalities/arrhythmia[d]	4	(0.6)	15	1.5–23.8
Persistent tachycardia from vagus injury	3	(0.5)	—	—
Total	106	(16.7)	—	—

[a]From ref. 302, with permission.

[b]One status post cardiac transplantation for ischemic cardiomyopathy; one status post left ventricular aneurysmectomy and left anterior descending artery bypass.

[c]Coronary revascularization performed with aortic valve replacement in two patients.

[d]Includes two patients with bundle branch block: one patient with pacemaker for complete heart block, one patient with paroxysmal atrial tachycardia.

presence of other risk factors in each individual patient such as age, weight, blood pressure, family history, lipoprotein levels, and habits such as smoking; and (f) the use of specific chemotherapeutic agents. Specific data on drug-related cardiotoxicity is presented under "myocardiopathy."

Pericarditis

Delayed acute pericarditis can be symptomatically occult or present suddenly with fever, dyspnea, pleuritic chest pain, friction rub, ST and T wave changes, and decreased QRS voltage (296–298). Up to 30% of patients treated for Hodgkin's disease with a mean midplane heart dose of 46 Gy will be affected (299,300). With equally weighted anterior and posterior fields and the use of subcarinal blocking, the frequency decreases to 2.5% (27). A report by Stewart et al. (297) on 25 patients who developed cardiac damage, primarily pericarditis, shows the relevance of radiation dose and cardiac volume to the type of injury. The onset of delayed

acute pericarditis averages 6 months, and 92% of effusions occur within 12 months. Although the effusion usually resolves in 1 to 10 months, it may persist for years. Up to 50% of patients will develop some degree of tamponade (paradoxical pulse, Kussmaul's sign) occasionally requiring a pericardiocentesis. Chronic effusive-constrictive pericarditis develops in 10% to 15% of patients and may require pericardectomy. Pericardectomy is a high-risk procedure in this setting because of the coexistence of other types of radiation-induced damage such as fibrosis of the myocardium and lung, coronary artery and valvular disease, impaired chest wall healing, and the patient's general condition (301). However, in a report by Hancock et al. (302), which described cardiac morbidity in children treated for Hodgkin's disease, the actuarial risk of requiring pericardiectomy was 4% at 17 years (occurring only in children treated with higher radiation doses), and most patients improved following surgery. It is noteworthy that constriction may present 5 to 50 years following irradiation with no antecedent acute disease (296,298,303). Diuretics are sometimes necessary to control peripheral edema or ascites.

Pancarditis

Pancarditis is rare and severe and probably requires doses of at least 60 Gy (297,298). Intractable congestive heart failure can result. Restrictive hemodynamics are demonstrated by catheterization.

Myocardiopathy

Myocardiopathy is highly potentiated by Adriamycin, but occurs in its absence (27,304). An autopsy study of patients who were treated with at least 35 Gy, many with anterior-only portals (mean dose of 56 Gy to anterior heart surface), showed myocardial fibrosis in 50%, fibrous thickening of the mural endocardium in 75%, and pericardial thickening in over 90% (3,301). Right ventricular end-diastolic function may also be reduced by up to 25% in asymptomatic patients (305,306). Ejection fractions may be decreased in up to 33%. However, with modern radiation techniques and appropriate cardiac blocking, measures of cardiac function including left ventricular ejection fraction (LVEF) and peak filling rate (PFR) in patients irradiated to portions of the heart are commonly preserved. This was demonstrated by Constine et al. who assessed 50 asymptomatic survivors of Hodgkin's disease treated with mean central cardiac RT doses of 35.1 Gy (range 18.5 to 47.5 Gy). The mean LVEF and PFR were normal, and 2 (4%) and 8 (16%) of patients, respectively, had low test results (307).

Although a discussion of the late cardiotoxic effects of anthracycline administration will not be presented in depth, its importance and frequency must be emphasized. Doxorubicin has been most extensively studied, and its cardiotoxicity is often progressive and disabling. Lipshultz et al. assessed 120 children and adults who received cumulative doses of 244 to 550 mg/m^2 of doxorubicin at a mean of 8.1

years after therapy, and their findings indicate the spectrum of abnormalities that might occur (308). All echocardiographic measurements were abnormal at follow-up a minimum of 2 years after therapy, with more frequent and severe abnormalities in female patients (Fig. 21). In multivariate analysis, female sex and a higher drug dose were associated with depressed contractility (measured as stress-velocity index). A higher rate of drug administrated was associated with increased afterload (measured as end-systolic wall stress), left ventricular dilatation, and depressed left ventricular function. Higher cumulative drug dose was associated with depressed left ventricular function. Younger age at diagnosis was associated with reduced left-ventricular wall thickness and mass, and increased afterload. Finally, a longer time since completion of drug therapy was associated with reduced left-ventricular wall thickness and increased afterload. Data from the Pediatric Oncology Group (POG) are also revealing. The incidence of clinical cardiotoxicity was determined in 6,493 children who had received anthracycline on POG protocols (309). Types of cardiotoxicity and its frequency was as follows: congestive heart failure not due to other causes—58 patients, abnormal measurements of cardiac function that prompted discontinuation of therapy—43 patients, and sudden death from presumed cardiac causes—5 patients. Relative risks (RR) included cumulative dose greater than or equal to 550 mg/m^2 (RR = 5.2), maximal individual dose greater than 50 mg/m^2 (RR = 2.8), female sex (RR = 1.9), black race (RR = 1.7), presence of trisomy 21 (RR = 3.4), and exposure to amsacrine (RR = 2.6). Cardiotoxicity within 1 year after the completion of anthracycline treatment represented 89.5% of cases. The relationship of several other chemotherapeutic agents, such as cyclophosphamide, busulfan, 5-fluorouracil, paclitaxel, etc., has been reviewed (310).

Assessment of the cardiovascular complications of bone marrow transplantation will assume greater importance with the increasing number of children undergoing this therapy. In

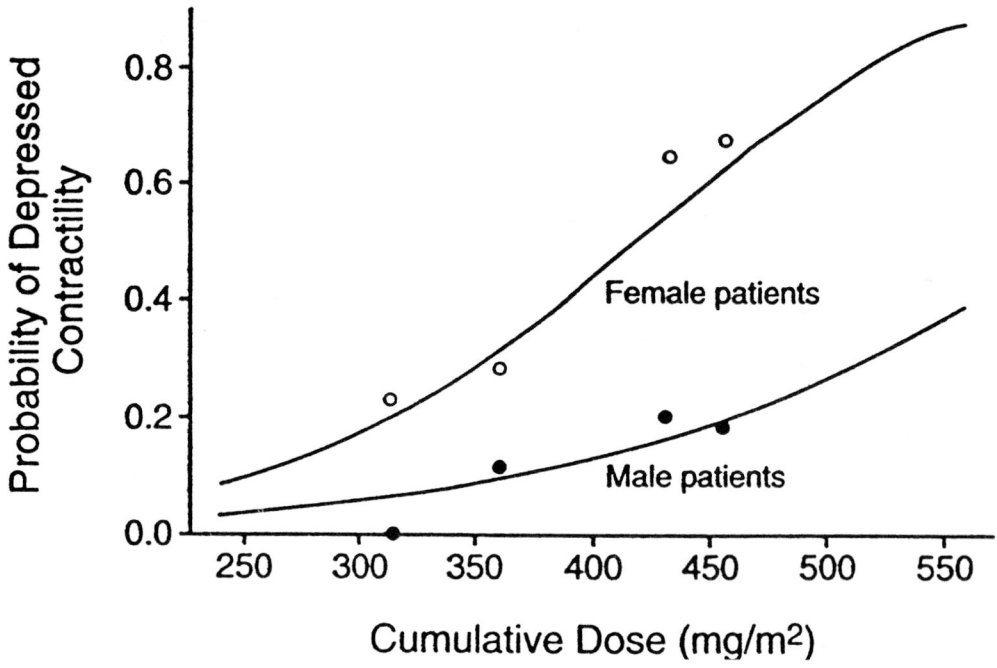

FIG. 21. Probability of depressed contractility as a function of the cumulative dose of doxorubicin in female and male patients. (From ref. 308, with permission.)

a report from the University of Minnesota on 63 transplanted children, 74% of children old enough to undergo treadmill exercise testing had a borderline or abnormal response to exercise, and 12.7% of patients had symptomatic cardiovascular abnormalities (311). The preparative regimen included TBI in slightly more than one-half the patients, but this was independently associated with outcome.

Valvular Disease

Fibrous valvular endocardial thickening occurs in 80% of autopsied patients treated with high radiation doses. The mitral, aortic, and tricuspid valves are most frequently affected (312). While such valvular lesions are relatively frequent, they rarely evolve into symptomatic valvular disease. In some patients, the radiation-induced cellular injury to the valvular endocardium, combined with chronic pressure-related trauma, may eventually lead to valvular deformity resulting in

stenosis or insufficiency. Carlson et al. (312) have collected 35 cases of radiation-associated valvular disease. In a report by Hancock et al. (302) on 635 children treated for Hodgkin's disease, two patients died of valvular disease, and three others have undergone aortic (two patients) or mitral (one patient) valve replacement. A contribution of mediastinal irradiation to significant or accelerated valvular disease could not be clearly determined. Unfortunately, in another report, valve replacement in such patients is infrequently successful and operative mortality is high (66%) (313).

Arrhythmia

High-degree atrioventricular (AV) conduction abnormalities are rarely seen and have been attributed to fibrosis of the AV node conducting branches (314). In one series, all patients with radiation-associated AV block had received more than 40 Gy to the chest, with a median time to development of the block of 14 years (315).

Coronary Artery Disease

As the population of cured childhood cancer patients ages and becomes exposed to the risk factors for coronary artery disease (CAD) such as smoking, obesity, hypertension, diabetes, and elevated cholesterol, it is possible that excess morbidity and mortality from ischemic heart disease may occur if radiotherapy and/or chemotherapy accelerates atherosclerosis (316). Radiotherapy can lead to ischemic heart disease via endothelial damage and obliteration of the microvasculature as well as by accelerated atherosclerosis of large vessels.

The manner in which thoracic irradiation is administered may significantly affect the inci-

dence of radiation-associated CAD. Mantle irradiation utilizing only a single anterior beam or an anteriorly weighted pair of opposed beams, or treating only one field per day, may significantly increase the cardiac dose. The cardiac dose and the risk of CAD may also be influenced by the extent of cardiac blocking via left ventricle and subcarinal blocks, the radiation dose per fraction, and the total dose. However, it is important to note that the proximal coronary arteries, which are commonly the site of obstruction, are not shielded with routine cardiac blocking (317) (Fig. 22). Data from the University of Rochester demonstrated that the site of coronary artery stenosis in patients irradiated for Hodgkin's disease was most commonly in the proximal coronary arteries, and this was no different than that which would be found in

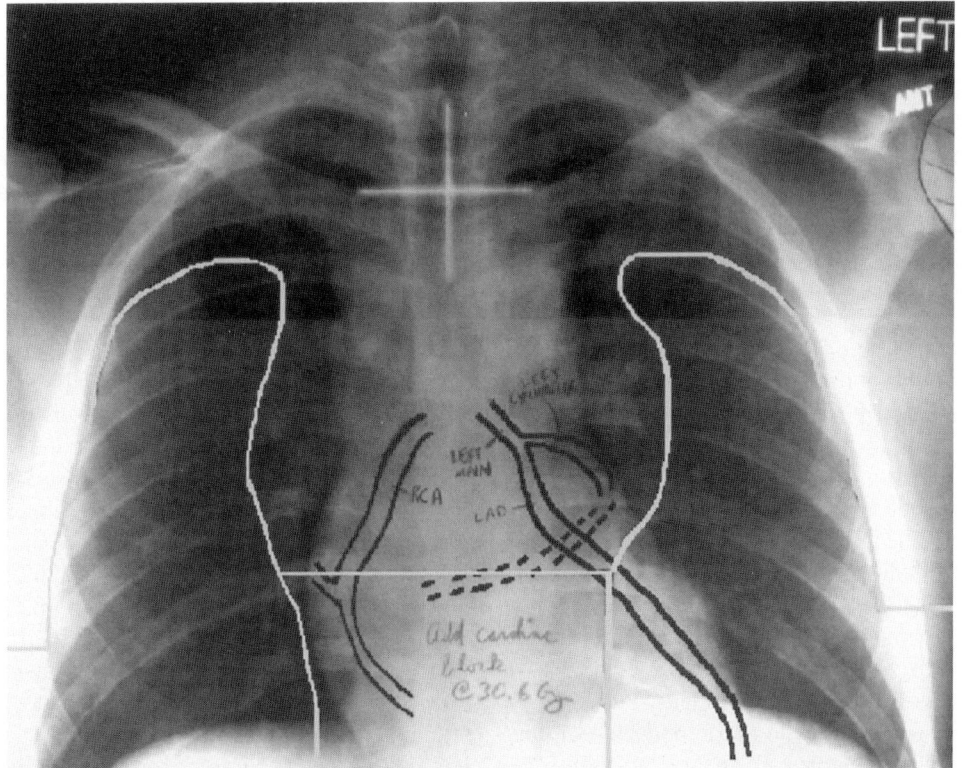

FIG. 22. Location of the coronary vessels (dark lines) on a standard mantle field is illustrated. The blocks are outlined in white. (From ref. 317, with permission.)

the general population. More specifically, the left main and the proximal portions of the left anterior descending and right coronary arteries are most commonly involved (317). Retrospective reviews that indicate an association between chest irradiation and CAD may reflect the ill-advisable nature of older forms of radiotherapy and, therefore, only serve to be of historical interest to the modern pediatric radiation oncologist (296,318).

Conflicting data have been reported concerning the incidence of cardiac failure, myocardial infarction (MI), and CAD in the long-term follow-up of adults and adolescents treated with radiotherapy for Hodgkin's disease. The Institut Gustave-Roussy reported 13 MIs in 499 mantle-irradiated patients (10-year cumulative incidence of 30%) but observed no MIs in 138 patients who received no irradiation ($p < 0.05$). The long-term follow-up of Hodgkin's disease patients treated in the clinical trials of the European Organization for Treatment and Research on Cancer (EORTC) showed a strong association between mediastinal irradiation and MI as well as death from cardiac failure (318). These data are buttressed by an autopsy study of 16 Hodgkin's disease patients under 35 years of age who received 35 Gy to the heart with anterior weighted radiation techniques. The irradiated patients had significantly more coronary artery narrowing than did matched controls, most frequently involving the proximal portion of the arteries. The media and adventitia were thickened or replaced by fibrotic tissue, either diffusely or focally. Bizarre fibroblasts, hyalinization, intimal thickening with collagen, endothelial cells, and histiocytes are seen (305).

Among the retrospective series evaluating the incidence of CAD following heart irradiation of adults and adolescents, one can readily find data indicating that moderate- to low-dose irradiation does not exacerbate the risk of MI or cardiac death. Hancock et al. (300) at Stanford found that in Hodgkin's disease patients irradiated with more modern radiotherapeutic techniques, there was no significant difference in MI mortality when compared to that in age- and sex-matched controls. Mauch,

Tarbell, and colleagues (319) at the Harvard-Joint Center for Radiation Therapy also found no increase in the incidence of MIs in irradiated Hodgkin's disease patients when compared to matched controls. Of interest is data from the University of Rochester that assessed the risk of CAD in survivors of Hodgkin's disease and also the prevalence of cardiac risk factors. While the risk of cardiac death was elevated at 2.8 (3.1 for males and 1.8 for females), other risk factors were more common than in the general population; among patients, 72% smoked, 72% were male, 78% had hypercholesterolemia, 61% were obese, 28% had a positive family history, 33% had hypertension, and 6% had diabetes (317). This suggests that RT is one of several risk factors for CAD in patients treated for Hodgkin's disease.

Data are accumulating on radiation-associated CAD specific to children. Among 635 children treated (< 21 years of age) at Stanford for Hodgkin's disease, 12 patients have died of cardiac disease (relative risk 29.6), including seven deaths from acute MI (relative risk 41.5). Deaths only occurred in children treated with 42 to 45 Gy (fraction size 1.5 to 2.75 Gy to anterior and posterior fields on alternate days). Among children treated with 15 to 26 Gy, none developed carditis (22,302). Another series of 28 children treated with 30 Gy (average dose) showed pericardial thickening in 43% but no functional abnormalities (299). Using a battery of tests, one may detect and quantitate cardiopulmonary abnormalities in children. We are aware of two studies that have taken this approach. Among 12 patients treated at the Mayo Clinic with 19.5 to 55 Gy (median dose 35 Gy) for Hodgkin's disease, 33% had abnormal echocardiograms and 50% had abnormal exercise studies (315). A team at the Children's Hospital of Helsinki (219) studied 21 patients who had received, as children, thoracic irradiation for a variety of malignancies. Many also received chemotherapy. The testing battery included electrocardiography (ECG), chest radiograph, echocardiography, auscultation, stress testing, and pulmonary function studies. Fourteen of the 21 patients (67%), followed up 11

TABLE 28. *Evaluation of patients at risk for late effects: cardiac*[a]

| Late effects | Causative treatment | | | Signs and symptoms | Screening and diagnostic tests | Management and intervention |
	Chemotherapy	Radiation	Surgery			
Cardiomyopathy	Anthracycline >300 mg/m² >200 mg/m² and RT to mediastinum High-dose CTX (BMT) (Possibly Ifos)	>35 Gy >25 Gy and Anthracyclines		Fatigue, cough, dyspnea on exertion, peripheral edema, hypertension, tachypnea/rales, tachycardia, cardiomegaly (S3/S4), hepatomegaly, syncope, palpitations, arrhythmias	EKG, ECHO/RNA and CXR baselines, q 2–5 yr (depending on risk factors) Holter monitor and exercise testing baseline, prn symptoms and after high cumulative anthracycline dose (> 300 mg/m²)	Diuretics, digoxin, afterload reduction, antiarrhythmics, cardiac transplant, education regarding risks of: isometric exercises; alcohol consumption; drug use; smoking; pregnancy; anesthesia
Valvular damage (mitral/tricuspid aortic)		>40 Gy		Weakness, cough, dyspnea on exertion, new murmur, pulsating liver	ECHO and CXR (baseline), q 3–5 yr then prn symptoms	Penicillin prophylaxis for surgery/dental procedures
Pericardial damage		>35 Gy		Fatigue, dyspnea on exertion, chest pain, cyanosis, ascites, peripheral edema, hypotension, friction rub, muffled heart sounds, venous distension, pulsus paradoxus	ECG (ST-T changes, decreased voltage), ECHO, CXR baseline, q 3–5 yr	Pericardial stripping
Coronary artery disease		>30 Gy		Chest pain on exertion (radiates to arm/neck), dyspnea, diaphoresis, pallor, hypotension, arrhythmias	EKG q 3 yrs Stress test (consider thallium scintigraphy) baseline, q 3–5 yr or prn symptoms	Diuretics, cardiac medications, low-sodium, low-fat diet, conditioning regimens

BMT, bone marrow transplant; CTX, cyclophosphamide; CXR, chest radiograph; ECHO, echocardiogram; ECG, electrocardiogram; Ifos, ifosfamide; RNA, radionuclear angiography; RT, radiation therapy.
[a]From ref. 44, with permission.

to 27 years after radiotherapy, had at least one abnormal test—but in only one case did these abnormalities appear to be of clinical impact. It seems safe to conclude that cardiac radiation using sophisticated treatment planning and careful blocking to doses of up to 25 Gy is generally safe, and 40 Gy may be administered to small cardiac regions. We cannot exclude the possibility, however, that longer follow-up of patients treated in the modern era will reveal an unexpected frequency of cardiac-related difficulties.

Anthracyclines and high-dose cyclophosphamide can damage the heart. Adriamycin cardiotoxicity is dose- and age-dependent (320). Although heart failure has been documented at cumulative doses of less than 200 mg/m², doses of less than 550 mg/m² are generally well-tolerated in the absence of cardiac irradiation. No more than 300 mg/m² should be given in the presence of cardiac irradiation, which also should not exceed doses of 25 Gy (304).

Cardiac dysfunction (defined as posterior wall stress and pathologic Q wave on ECG) has been described in children treated with spinal irradiation (313). This was presumed to arise from the asymmetric distribution of radiation to a growing heart.

Finally, cardiac complications following bone marrow transplantation may occur, with arrhythmias, pericarditis, and myopathies predominating. High-dose cyclophosphamide is clearly a causative agent. TBI is a secondary contributing factor (321,322).

Table 28 reviews several cardiac late effects with respect to causative treatments, signs and symptoms, screening and diagnostic tests, and management and intervention (44).

REFERENCES

For additional information on organ specific normal tissue damage following radiation, chemotherapy, and surgery, see:

Green DM, D'Angio GJ, eds. *Late effects of treatment for childhood cancer.* New York: Wiley-Liss, 1992.

Rubin P, Constine LS, Fajardo LF, Phillips TL, Wasserman TH. (eds) Late effects of normal tissues (LENT) consensus conference, including RTOG/EORTC SOMA scales. *Int J Radiat Oncl Biol Phys* 1995;31:1035–1367.

Rubin P, Constine L, Williams J. Late effects of cancer treatment: radiation and drug toxicity. In: Perez C, Brady L, eds. *Principles and practice of radiation oncology.* Philadelphia: Lippincott–Raven Publishers, 1998:155–211.

Schwartz C, Hobbie W, Constine L, Ruccione K, eds. *Survivors of childhood cancer: assessment and management.* St. Louis: Mosby, 1994.

References particularly recommended for further reading are indicated by an asterisk.

*1. Hudson M, Jones D, Boyett J, et al. Late mortality of long-term survivors of childhood cancer. *J Clin Oncol* 1997;15:2205–2213.

*2. Cohen L, Creditor M. Iso-effect tables for tolerance of irradiated normal human tissues. *Int J Radiat Oncol Biol Phys* 1983;9:233–241.

3. Bristow MR, Mason JW, Billingham ME, et al. Doxorubicin cardiomyopathy: evaluations by phonocardiology, endomyocardial biopsy, and cardiac catheterization. *Ann Intern Med* 1978;88:168–175.

*4. Casarett GW. Similarities and contrasts between radiation and time pathology. In: Strehler B, ed. *Advances in gerontological research.* New York: Academic Press, 1964:109–163.

5. Casarett GW. Aging. In: Vaeth JM, ed. *Frontiers of radiation therapy and oncology,* vol 6. New York: S. Karger, 1972:479–485.

*6. Rubin P, Constine L, Williams J. Late effects of cancer treatment: radiation and drug toxicity. In: Perez C, Brady L, eds. *Principles and practice of radiation oncology.* Philadelphia: Lippincott-Raven Publishers, 1998:155–211.

*7. Rubin P, Cassarett GW. *Clinical radiation pathology,* vols. I and II, Philadelphia: WB Saunders, 1968.

*8. Rubin P, Van Houtte P, Constine L. Radiation sensitivity and organ tolerances in pediatric oncology: a new hypothesis. *Front Radiat Ther Oncol* 1982;16: 62–82.

9. Tanner JM. *Growth at adolescence.* Oxford: Blackwell Scientific Publications, 1962.

10. Tanner JM. Physical growth and development. In: Forfar JO, Arneil GCY, eds. *Textbook for pediatrics.* Edinburgh: Churchill Livingston, 1978:249–304.

11. Perthes G. Uber deb ein fluss der roentgenstrahlen auf epitheliale gewebe. insbesandere aus des carcinom. *Arch Klin Chir* 1903;51:955–1000.

12. Forsterling K. Uber allgemeine und partielle washstums storungen nach kurz davenden rontgen bestrahlungen von saugethieren. *Arch Klin Chir* 1906; 81:506.

*13. D'Angio GJ. An overview and historical perspective of late effects of treatment of childhood cancer. In: Green DM, D'Angio GJ, eds. *Late effects of treatment for childhood cancer.* New York: Wiley-Liss, 1992:1–6.

14. Dalinka MK, Mazzea V. Complications of radiation therapy. *Crit Rev Diagn Imag* 1984;23:236–267.

*15. Neuhauser EBD, Wittenborg MH, Berman CZ, et al. Irradiation effects of roentgen therapy on the growing spine. *Radiol* 1952;59:637–650.

16. Arkin AM, Simon N. Radiation scoliosis: an experimental study. *J Bone Joint Surg* 1950;32A:396–401.

17. Rutherford H, Dodd GD. Complications of radiation

therapy; growing bone. *Semin Roentgenol* 1974;9: 15–27.

18. Dawson WB. Growth impairment following radiotherapy in childhood. *Clin Radiol* 1968;19:241–256.

*19. Donaldson SS. Effects of irradiation on skeletal growth and development. In: Green DM, D'Angio GJ, eds. *Late effects of treatment for childhood cancer*. New York: Wiley-Liss, 1992:63–70.

20. Blackburn J, Wells AB. Radiation damage to growing bone; the effect of x-ray doses of 100-1000 rads on mouse tibiae and knee joints. *Br J Radiol* 1963;36: 505–513.

*21. Rubin P. The Franz Buschke lecture: late effects of chemotherapy and radiation therapy. A new hypothesis. *Int J Radiat Oncol Biol Phys* 1984;10:5–34.

22. Donaldson SS, Kaplan HS. Complications of treatment of Hodgkin's disease in children. *Cancer Treat Rep* 1982;66:977–989.

23. Donaldson SS, Kleeberg P, Cox R. Growth abnormalities associated with radiation in children with Hodgkin's disease. *Proc Am Soc Clin Oncol* 1988;7: 224(abst).

24. Slanina J, Mueshoff K, Rahner T, et al. Long term side effects of irradiated patients with Hodgkin's disease. *Int J Radiat Oncol Biol Phys* 199;2:1–19.

25. Probert JC, Parker BP. The effects of radiation therapy on bone growth. *Radiol* 1975;114:155–162.

*26. Willman K, Cox R, Donaldson S. Radiation induced height impairment in pediatric Hodgkin's disease. *Int J Radiat Oncol Biol Phys* 1994;28:85–92.

27. Mauch PM, Weinstein H, Batnick L, et al. An evaluation of long-term survival and treatment complications in children with Hodgkin's disease. *Cancer* 1983;51:925–932.

*28. Silber JH, Littman PS, Meadows AT. Stature loss following irradiation for childhood cancer. *J Clin Oncol* 1990;8:304–312.

*29. Probert JC, Parker BR, Kaplan HS. Growth retardation in children after megavoltage irradiation of the spine. *Cancer* 1973;32:634–639.

*30. Riseborough EJ, Grabias SL, Burton RI, et al. Skeletal alterations following irradiation for Wilms' tumor. *J Bone Joint Surg* 1976;58A:526–536.

31. Chapman JA, Deakin DP, Green JH. Slipped upper femoral epiphysis after radiotherapy. *J Bone Joint Surg* 1980;62B:337–339.

32. Prosnitz LR, Lawson JP, Friedlaender GE, et al. Avascular necrosis of bone in Hodgkin's disease patients with combined modality therapy. *Cancer* 1981;47: 2793–2797.

*33. Silverman CL, Thomas PR, McAlister WH, et al. Slipped femoral capital epiphysis in irradiated children: dose, volume, and age relationships. *Int J Radiat Oncol Biol Phys* 1981;7:1357–1363.

34. Wolf EL, Berdon WE, Cassady JR, et al. Slipped capital femoral epiphysis as a sequela to childhood irradiation for malignant tumors. *Radiology* 1977;125: 781–784.

*35. Libshitz A, Edeikin BS. Radiotherapy changes of the pediatric hip. *AJR* 1981;137:585–588.

36. Ojala AE, Lanning FP, Paakko E, et al. Osteonecrosis in children treated for acute lymphoblastic leukemia: a magnetic resonance imaging study after treatment. *Med Pediatr Oncol* 1997;29:260–265.

37. Morris LL, Cassady JR, Jaffe N. Sternal changes following mediastinal irradiation for childhood Hodgkin's disease. *Radiology* 1975;115:701.

38. Murphys FD, Blount WP. Cartilaginous exostoses following irradiation. *J Bone Joint Surg* 1981;44: 662–668.

*39. Jaffe N, Toth BB, Hoar RE, et al. Dental and maxillofacial abnormalities in long-term survivors of childhood cancer: effects of treatment with chemotherapy and radiation to the head and neck. *Pediatrics* 1984;73:816–823.

*40. Goldwein JW. Effects of radiation therapy on skeleton growth in childhood. *Clin Orthop* 1991;262: 101–107.

41. Katzman H, Waugh T, Berdon W. Skeletal changes following irradiation of childhood tumors. *J Bone Joint Surg* 1969;51:825.

42. Nesbit M, Krivit W, Heyn R. Acute and chronic effects of methotrexate on hepatic, pulmonary and skeletal systems. *Cancer* 1976;37:1048.

43. Rimsza ME. Complications of corticosteroid therapy. *Am J Dis Child* 1978;132:806–810.

44. Constine LS, Hobbie W, Schwartz C. Facilitated assessment of chronic treatment by symptom and organ systems. In: Schwartz C, Hobbie W, Constine L, et al., eds. *Survivors of childhood cancer, assessment and management*. St. Louis: Mosby, 1994:21–80.

*45. Shalet SM, Ogilvy-Stuart AL, Crowne EC, et al. Indications for human growth hormone treatment of radiation-induced growth hormone deficiency. In: Green DM, D'Angio GJ, eds. *Late effects of treatment for childhood cancer*. New York: Wiley-Liss, 1992:71–79.

*46. Sklar CA. Physiology of growth hormone production and release. In: Green DM, D'Angio GJ, eds. *Late effects of treatment for childhood cancer*. New York: Wiley-Liss, 1992:49–54.

47. Lannering B, Albertsson-Wikland K. Growth hormone release in children after cranial irradiation. *Hormone Res* 1987;27:13–22.

48. Blacklay A, Grossman A, Ross RJM, et al. Cranial irradiation for cerebral and nasopharyngeal tumours in children: evidence for the production of a hypothalamic defect in growth hormone release. *J Endocr* 1986;108:25–29.

49. Danoff BF, Cowchock S, Marquette C, et al. Assessment of the long-term effects of primary radiation therapy for brain tumors in children. *Cancer* 1982; 49:1580–1586.

50. Dropcha EJ. Central nervous system injury by therapeutic irradiation. *Neurol Clin* 1991;9:969–988.

*51. Duffner PK, Cohen ME. The long-term effects of central nervous system therapy on children with brain tumors. *Neurol Clin* 1991;9:479–495.

52. Duffner PK, Cohen ME. Long-term consequences of CNS treatment for childhood cancer. part II: clinical consequences. *Pediatr Neurol* 1991;7:237–242.

53. Duffner PK, Cohen ME, Anderson SW, et al. Longterm effects of treatment on endocrine function in children with brain tumors. *Ann Neurol* 1983;14: 528–532.

54. Duffner PK, Cohen ME, Voorhess ML, et al. Long term effects of cranial irradiation on endocrine function in children with brain tumors. *Cancer* 1985;56: 2189–2193.

55. Perry-Keene DA, Connelly JF, Young RA, et al. Hy-

pothalamic hypopituitarism following external radiotherapy for tumours distant from the adenohypophysis. *Clin Endocrinol* 1976;5:373–380.

56. Shalet SM, Beardwell CG, Pearson D, et al. The effects of varying doses of cerebral irradiation on growth hormone production in childhood. *Clin Endocrinol* 1976;5:287–290.

*57. Sklar C. Neuroendocrine complications of cancer therapy. In: Schwartz C, Hobbie W, Constine L, et al., eds. *Survivors of childhood cancer, assessment and management*. St. Louis: Mosby, 1994:97–110.

58. Tan BC, Kunaratman N. Hypopituitary dwarfism following radiotherapy for nasopharyngeal carcinoma. *Clin Radiol* 1966;17:302–304.

59. Wara WM, Richards GE, Grumbach MM, et al. Hypopituitarism after irradiation in children. *Int J Radiat Oncol Biol Phys* 1977;2:549–552.

60. Brauner R, Rappaport R, Prevot C, et al. A prospective study of the development of growth hormone deficiency in children given cranial irradiation and its relation to natural growth. *J Clin Endocrinol Metab* 1989;68:346–351.

61. Leiper AD, Stanhope R, Kitching P, et al. Precocious and premature puberty associated with treatment of acute lymphoblastic leukemia. *Arch Dis Child* 1987; 62:1107–1112.

62. DiGeorge AM. The endocrine system. In: Behrman RE, Kliegman RM, Nelson WE, et al., eds. *Nelson textbook of pediatrics*. Philadelphia: WB Saunders, 1992:1397–1472.

63. Thorner MO, Reschke J, Chitwood J, et al. Acceleration of growth in two children treated with human growth hormone-releasing factor. *N Engl J Med* 1985;312:4–9.

64. Rappaport R, Brauner R. Growth and endocrine disorders secondary to cranial irradiation. *Pediatr Res* 1989;25:561–567.

*65. Sklar C, Mertens A, Walter A, et al. Final height after treatment for childhood acute lymphoblastic leukemia: comparison of no cranial irradiation with 1800 and 2499 centigrays of cranial irradiation. *J Pediatr* 1993;123:59–64.

66. Cohen ME, Duffner PK. Long-term consequences of CNS treatment for childhood cancer. part I: pathologic consequences and potential for oncogenesis. *Pediatr Neurol* 1991;7:157–163.

67. Hobhen-Koelega A, van Doorn J, Hahlen K, et al. Long-term effects of treatment for acute lymphoblastic leukemia with and without cranial irradiation on growth and puberty: a comparative study. *Pediatr Res* 1993;33:577–582.

68. Voorhes ML, Brecher ML, Glicksman AS. Hypothalamic-pituitary function of children with acute lymphocytic leukemia after three forms of central nervous system prophylaxis: a retrospective study. *Cancer* 1986;57:1287–1291.

69. Kirk JA, Raghapathy P, Stevens MM, et al. Growth failure and growth-hormone deficiency after treatment for acute lymphoblastic leukemia. *Lancet* 1987; 1:190–193.

70. Costin G. Effects of low-dose cranial radiation on growth hormone secretory dynamics and hypothalamic-pituitary function. *Am J Dis Child* 1988;142: 847–852.

71. Romshe C, Zipf W, Miser A, et al. Evaluation of growth hormone release and human growth hormone treatment in children with cranial irradiation-associated short stature. *J Pediatr* 1984;104:177–181.

72. Blatt J, Lee P, Suttnes J, et al. Pulsatile growth hormone secretion in children with acute lymphoblastic leukemia after 1800 cGy cranial radiation. *Int Radiat Oncol Biol* 1988;15:1001–1006.

73. Samaan NA, Vieto R, Schultz PN, et al. Hypothalamic pituitary and thyroid dysfunction after radiotherapy to the head and neck. *Int J Radiat Oncol Biol Phys* 1982;8:1857–1867.

*74. Constine L, Woolf P, Cann D, et al. Hypothalamic-pituitary dysfunction after radiation for brain tumors. *N Engl J Med* 1993;328:87–94.

75. Slater JD, Austin-Seymour M, Munzenrider J, et al. Endocrine function following high dose proton therapy for tumors of the upper clivus. *Int J Radiat Oncol Biol Phys* 1988;15:607–611.

76. Capen CC. Anatomy, comparative anatomy, and histology of the thyroid. In: Braverman LE, Utiger RD, eds. *Werner and Ingbar's the thyroid*. Philadelphia: Lippincott, 1991;22–40.

*77. Hancock S, McDougall I, Constine L. Thyroid abnormalities after therapeutic external radiation. *Int J Radiat Oncol Biol Phys* 1995;31:1165–1170.

78. Braverman LE, Ingbar SH, Vagenakis AG, et al. Enhanced susceptibility to iodide myxedema in patients with Hashimoto's disease. *J Clin Endocrinol Metab* 1971;32:515–521.

79. Carr RF, Livolsi VA. Morphologic changes in the thyroid after irradiation for Hodgkin's and non-Hodgkin's lymphoma. *Cancer* 1989;64:825–829.

*80. Fajardo LF. *Pathology of radiation injury*. New York: Masson Publishers, 1982.

81. Glatstein E, McHardy-Young S, Brast N, et al. Alterations in serum thyrotropin (TSH) and thyroid function following radiotherapy in patients with malignant lymphoma. *J Clin Endocrinol Metab* 1971;32: 833–841.

82. McDougall IR. *Thyroid disease in clinical practice*. London: Chapman & Hall Medical, 1992:304–324.

83. Feyerabend T, Kapp B, Richter E, et al. Incidence of hypothyroidism after irradiation of the neck with special reference to lymphoma patients: a retrospective and prospective analysis. *Acta Oncol* 1990;29: 597–602.

*84. Constine LS, Donaldson SS, McDougall IR, et al. Thyroid dysfunction after radiotherapy in children with Hodgkin's disease. *Cancer* 1984;53:878–883.

85. Constine LS, Rubin P, Woolf PD, et al. Hyperprolactinemia and hypothyroidism following cytotoxic therapy for central nervous system malignancies. *J Clin Oncol* 1987;5:1841–1851.

*86. D'Angio Ged. Delayed consequences of cancer therapy: proven and potential. *Cancer* 1976;37:999–1013.

87. Devney RB, Sklar CA, Nesbit ME,Jr., et al. Serial thyroid function measurements in children with Hodgkin's disease. *J Pediatr* 1984;105:223–229.

88. Fjalling M, Tisell LE, Carlsson S, et al. Benign and malignant thyroid nodules after neck irradiation. *Cancer* 1986;58:1219–1224.

89. Fleming ID, Black TL, Thompson EI, et al. Thyroid dysfunction and neoplasia in children receiving neck irradiation for cancer. *Cancer* 1985;55:1190–1194.

90. Liening DA, Duncan NO, Blackeslee DB, et al. Hy-

pothyroidism following radiotherapy for head and neck cancer. *Otolaryngol Head Neck Surg* 1990;103: 10–13.

91. Schimpff SC, Diggs CH, Wiswell JG. Radiation-related thyroid dysfunctions: implications for the treatment of Hodgkin's disease. *JAMA* 1980;245:46–49.

92. Schimpff SC, Diggs CH, Wiswell JG, et al. Radiation-related thyroid dysfunction: implications for the treatment of Hodgkin's disease. *Ann Intern Med* 1980;92:91–98.

*93. Hancock S, Cox R, McDougall I. Thyroid diseases after treatment of Hodgkin's disease. *N Engl J Med* 1991;325:599–605.

*94. Bhatia S, Ramsay N, Bantle J, et al. Thyroid abnormalities after therapy for Hodgkin's disease in childhood. *Oncologist* 1996;1:62–67.

95. Constine L, Schwartz C. The thyroid gland. In: Schwartz C, Hobbie W, Constine L, et al., eds. *Survivors of childhood cancer, assessment and management*. St. Louis: Mosby, 1994:151–158.

96. Fuks Z, Glatsten E, Marsa GW, et al. Long-term effects of external radiation on the pituitary and thyroid glands. *Cancer* 1976;37:1152–1161.

97. Nelson DF, Reddy KV, O'Mara RE, et al. Thyroid abnormalities following neck irradiation for Hodgkin's disease. *Cancer* 1978;42:2553–2562.

98. Hudson M, Greenwald C, Thompson E. Efficacy and toxicity of multiagent chemotherapy and low-dose involved-field radiotherapy in children and adolescents with Hodgkin's disease. *J Clin Oncol* 1993;11: 100–108.

99. Marcial-Vega VA, Order SE, Lastner G, et al. Prevention of hypothyroidism related to mantle irradiation for Hodgkin's disease: preoperative photon study. *Int J Radiat Oncol Biol Phys* 1990;18:613–618.

100. Wilhelm KR, Schulz-Wendtland R. Auswirkuhg der Berstrahlung van mund-, rachem-, und larynxtumaren auf die schilddv. auusen funktion. *Strahlentherapie* 1988;164:270–277.

101. Fein D, Hanlon A, Corn B, et al. The influence of lymphangiography on the development of hypothyroidism in patients irradiated for Hodgkin's disease. *Int J Radiat Oncol Biol Phys* 1996;36:13–18.

102. Schultheiss TE, Higgins EM, EL-Mahdi HM. The latent period in radiation myelopathy. *Int J Radiat Oncol Biol Phys* 1984;10:1109–1115.

103. Ogilvy-Stuart A, Shalet S, Gattamamenti H. Thyroid function after treatment of brain tumors in children. *J Pediatr* 1991;119:733–737.

104. Oberfield SE, Sklar C, Allen J, et al. Thyroid and gonadal function and growth of long-term survivors of medulloblastoma/PNET. In: Green DM, D'Angio GJ, eds. *Late effects of treatment for childhood cancer*. New York: Wiley-Liss, 1992:55–62.

105. Livesey EA, Brook CGD. Thyroid dysfunction after radiotherapy and chemotherapy of brain tumors. *Arch Dis Child* 1989;64:593–595.

106. Sklar CA, Kim TH, Ramsay NKC. Thyroid dysfunction among long-term survivors of bone marrow transplantation. *Am J Med* 1982;73:688–694.

107. Robison LL, Nesbit ME, Sathes HN, et al. Thyroid abnormalities in long-term survivors of childhood acute lymphoblastic leukemia. *Pediatr Res* 1985;19: 266A(abst).

108. Sutcliffe SB, Chapman R, Wrigley PF. Cyclical combination chemotherapy and thyroid function in patients with advanced Hodgkin's disease. *Med Pediatr Oncol* 1981;9:439–448.

109. Petersen M, Keeling CA, McDougall IR. Hyperthyroidism with low radioiodine uptake after head and neck irradiation for Hodgkin's disease. *J Nucl Med* 1989;30:255–257.

110. DeGroot LJ. Clinical review 2: Diagnostic approach and management of patients exposed to irradiation to the thyroid. *J Clin Endocrinol Metabol* 1989;69: 925–928.

111. Schneider AB, Recant W, Pinsky SM, et al. Radiation-induced thyroid carcinoma: Clinical course and results of therapy in 296 patients. *Ann Intern Med* 1986;105:405–412.

112. Bantle JP, Lee CKK, Levitt SH. Thyroxine administration during radiation therapy to the neck does not prevent subsequent thyroid dysfunction. *Int J Radiat Oncol Biol Phys* 1985;11:1999–2002.

*113. Green DM. Fertility and pregnancy outcome after treatment for cancer in childhood or adolescence. *Oncologist* 1997;2:171–179.

114. Chapman RM, Sutcliffe SB. Protection of ovarian function by oral contraceptives in women receiving chemotherapy for Hodgkin's disease. *Blood* 1981;58: 849–851.

*115. Chapman RM, Sutcliffe SB, Malpas JS. Cytotoxic-induced ovarian failure in women with Hodgkin's disease. I. Hormone function. *JAMA* 1979;242: 1877–1881.

*116. Chapman RM, Sutcliffe SB, Malpas JS. Cytotoxic-induced ovarian failure in women with Hodgkin's disease. II. Effects on sexual function. *JAMA* 1979;242: 1882–1884.

117. Shalet SM, Beardwell CG, Jacobs HS, et al. Ovarian failure following abdominal irradiation in childhood. *Br J Cancer* 1976;33:655–658.

118. Jones WH III. Cyclic histology and cytology of the genital tract. In: Jones HW III, Wentz AC, Burnett LS, eds. *Novak's textbook of gynecology*. Baltimore: Williams & Wilkins, 1988.

*119. Torano A, Halperin E, Leventhal B. The ovary. In: Schwartz C, Hobbie W, Constine L, et al., eds. *Survivors of childhood cancer, assessment and management*. St. Louis: Mosby, 1994:213–224.

*120. Ash P. The influence of radiation on fertility in man. *Br J Radiol* 1980;53:271–278.

*121. Lushbaugh CC, Casarett GW. The effects of gonadal irradiation in clinical radiation therapy: a review. *Cancer* 1976;37:1111–1120.

122. Wallace WHB, Shalet SM, Hendry JH, et al. Ovarian failure following abdominal irradiation in childhood: the radiosensitivity of the human oocyte. *Br J Radiol* 1989;62:995–998.

123. Himelstein-Braw R, Peters H, Faber M. Influence of irradiation and chemotherapy on the ovaries of children with abdominal tumors. *Br J Cancer* 1977;36: 269–275.

124. Stillman RJ, Schinfeld JS, Schiff I, et al. Ovarian failure in long-term survivors of childhood malignancy. *Am J Obstet Gynecol* 1981;139:62–66.

125. Halperin EC. Concerning the spinal component of the craniospinal irradiation field for central nervous system malignancies. *Int J Radiat Oncol Biol Phys* 1993;26:357–362.

126. Wallace WHB, Shalet SM, Crowne EC, et al. Ovarian failure following abdominal irradiation in childhood: natural history and prognosis. *Clin Oncol* 1989;1: 75–79.

*127. Haie-Meder C, Mlika-Cabanne N, Michel G, et al. Radiotherapy after ovarian transposition: ovarian function and fertility preservation. *Int J Radiat Oncol Biol Phys* 1993;25:419–424.

*128. LeFloch O, Donaldson SS, Kaplan HS. Pregnancy following oophoropexy and total nodal irradiation in women with Hodgkin's disease. *Cancer* 1976;38: 2263–2268.

129. Sy Ortin TT, Shastak CA, Donaldson SS. Gonadal status and reproductive function following treatment for Hodgkin's diseases in childhood: the Stanford experience. *Int J Rad Oncol Biol Phys* 1990;19: 873–880.

*130. Madsen B, Giudice L, Donaldson S. Radiation-induced premature menopause: a misconception. *Int J Radiat Oncol Biol Phys* 1995;32:1461–1464.

131. Niroomand-Rad A, Cumberlin R. Measured dose to ovaries and testes from Hodgkin's fields and determination of genetically significant dose. *Int J Radiat Oncol Biol Phys* 1993;25:745–751.

132. Sklar CA, Kim TH, Williamson JF, et al. Ovarian function after successful bone marrow transplantation in post-menarchal females. *Med Pediatr Oncol* 1983;11:361–364.

*133. Horning WJ, Hoppe RT, Kaplan HS, et al. Female reproductive potential after treatment for Hodgkin's disease. *N Engl J Med* 1981;304:1377–1382.

134. Mackie E, Radford M, Shalet S. Gonadal function following chemotherapy for childhood Hodgkin's disease. *Med Pediatr Oncol* 1996;27:24–28.

135. Lange B, Littman P. Management of Hodgkin's disease in children and adolescents. *Cancer* 1983;51: 1371–1377.

*136. Leventhal B, Halperin E, Torano A. The testes. In: Schwartz C, Hobbie W, Constine L, et al, eds. *Survivors of childhood cancer, assessment and management.* St. Louis: Mosby, 1994:225–244.

*137. Izard M. Leydig cell function and radiation: a review of the literature. *Radiother Oncol* 1995;34:1–8.

138. Griffin JE, Wilson JD. Disorders of the testes and the male reproductive tract. In: Wilson JD, Foster DW, eds. *Williams textbook of endocrinology.* Philadelphia: WB Saunders, 1992:799–852.

*139. Heller GC. Effects on the germinal epithelium in radiobiological factors in manned space flight. In: Langham WH, ed. *NRC Publication 1487.* Washington, D.C.: National Academy of Sciences, National Research Council, 1967;124–133.

140. Castillo LA, Craft AW, Kernahan J, et al. Gonadal function after 12-Gy testicular irradiation in childhood acute lymphoblastic leukemia. *Med Pediatr Oncol* 1990;185–189, 1990.

141. Sklar CA, Robison LL, Nesbit ME, et al. Effects of radiation on testicular fundtion in long-term survivors of childhood acute lymphoblastic leukemia: a report from the Children's Cancer Study Group. *J Clin Oncol* 1987;8:1981–1987.

142. Shalet SM, Horner A, Akrned SR, et al. Leydig cell damage after testicular irradiation for acute lymphoblastic leukemia. *Med Pediatr Oncol* 1985;13: 65–68.

143. Blatt J, Sherins RJ, Niebrugge D, et al. Leydig cell function in boys following treatment for testicular relapse of acute lymphoblastic leukemia. *J Clin Oncol* 1985;3:1227–1231.

*144. Brauner R, Czernichow P, Cramer P, et al. Leydig-cell function after direct testicular irradiation for acute lymphoblastic leukemia. *N Engl J Med* 1983;309: 25–28.

145. Brauner R, Catlabiano P, Rappaport R, et al. Leydig cell insufficiency after testicular irradiation for acute lymphoblastic leukemia. *Horm Res* 1988;30: 111–114.

*146. Sanders JE. Effects of bone marrow transplantation on reproductive function. In: Green DM, D'Angio GJ, eds. *Late effects of treatment for childhood cancer.* New York: Wiley-Liss, 1992:95–102.

147. Averette HE, Baike GM, Jarrell MA. Effects of cancer chemotherapy on gonadal function and reproductive capacity. *CA Cancer J Clin* 1990;40:199–209.

148. Clayton PE, Shalet SM, Price DA, et al. Testicular damage after chemotherapy for childhood brain tumors. *J Pediatr* 1988;112:922–926.

149. Fairley KF, Barrie JU, Johnson W. Sterility and testicular atrophy related to cyclophosphamide therapy. *Lancet* 1972;1:568–569.

150. Braumswig J, Heimes U, Heiermann E, et al. The effects of different cumulative doses of chemotherapy on testicular function. Results in 75 patients treated for Hodgkin's disease during childhood or adolescence. *Cancer* 1990;65:1298–1302.

*151. da Cunha M, Meistrich M, Fuller L, et al. Recovery of spermatogenesis after treatment for Hodgkin's disease: limiting dose of MOPP chemotherapy. *J Clin Oncol* 1984;2:571–577.

152. Heikens J, Behrendt H, Adriaanse R, et al. Irreversible gonadal damage in male survivors of Pediatric Hodgkin's disease. *Cancer* 1996;78:2020–2024.

153. Marmor D, Duyck F. Male reproductive potential after MOPP therapy for Hodgkin's disease: a long-term survey. *Andologia* 1995;27:99–106.

154. Sherins RJ, Olweny CLM, Ziegler JL. Gynecomastia and gonadal dysfunction in adolescent boys treated with combination chemotherapy for Hodgkin's disease. *N Engl J Med* 1978;299:12–16.

155. Cox JD. The testicle. In: Moss WT, Cox JD, eds. *Radiation oncology: rationale, technique, results.* St. Louis: CV Mosby, 1989:468–486.

156. Etteldorf JN, West CD, Pitcock JA, et al. Gonadal function, testicular histology and meiosis following cyclophosphamide therapy in patients with nephrotic syndrome. *J Pediatr* 1974;88:206–212.

157. Viviani S, Ragni G, Santoro A, et al. Testicular dysfunction in Hodgkin's disease before and after treatment. *Eur J Cancer* 1991;27:1389–1392.

158. Shalet SM, Hann IM, Lendon M, et al. Testicular function after combination chemotherapy for acute lymphoblastic leukemia. *Arch Dis Child* 1981;56: 275–278.

159. Whitehead E, Shalet SM, Morris-Jones PH, et al. Gonadal function after combination chemotherapy for Hodgkin's disease in childhood. *Arch Dis Child* 1982;47:287–291.

160. Kulkarni S, Sastry P, Saikia T, et al. Gonadal function following ABVD therapy for Hodgkin's disease. *Am J Clin Oncol* 1997;20:354–357.

161. Aubier F, Flamant F, Brauner R, et al. Male gonadal function after chemotherapy for solid tumors in childhood. *J Clin Oncol* 1989;7:304–309.

162. Blatt J, Mulvihill JJ, Ziegler JL, et al. Pregnancy outcome following cancer chemotherapy. *Am J Med* 1980;69:828–832.

*163. Marmor D, Elefant E, Danchez C, et al. Semen analysis in Hodgkin's disease before the onset of treatment. *Cancer* 1987;57:1986–1987.

164. Bracken RB, Smith KD. Is semen cryopreservation helpful in testicular cancer? *Urology* 1990;15:581–583.

165. Shekarriz M, Tolentino M, Ayzman I, et al. Cryopreservation and semen quality in patients with Hodgkin's disease. *Cancer* 1995;72:2732–2736.

166. Sherins RJ, Mulvihill JJ. Gonadal dysfunction. In: DeVita VT,Jr., Hellman S, Rosenberg SA, eds. *Cancer: principles and practice of oncology*. Philadelphia: JB Lippincott, 1989:2170–2180.

167. Kurdoglu B, Wilson G, Parchuri N, et al. Protection from radiation-induced damage to spermatogenesis by hormone treatment. *Radiat Res* 1994;139:97–102.

*168. Mulvihill JJ, Byrne J. Offspring of long-term survivors of childhood cancer. *Clin Oncol* 1985;4:334–343.

169. Green DM, Fine WE, Li FP. Offspring of patients treated for unilateral Wilms' tumor in childhood. *Cancer* 1982;49:2285–2288.

170. Li FP, Gimbrere K, Gelber RD, et al. Outcome of pregnancy in survivors in Wilms' tumor. *JAMA* 1987;257:216–219.

171. Holmes GE, Holmes FF. Pregnancy outcome of patients treated for Hodgkin's disease. *Cancer* 1978;41:1317–1322.

172. Hopewell JW. The importance of vascular damage in the development of late radiation effects in normal tissues. In: Meyn RE, Withers HR, eds. *Radiation biology in cancer research*. New York: Raven Press, 1980:449–459.

173. Aisner J, Wiernik P, Pearl P. Pregnancy outcome in patients treated for Hodgkin's disease. *J Clin Oncol* 1993;11:507–512.

*174. Mulvihill JJ, Byrne J. Genetic counseling for the cancer survivor: Possible germ cell effects of cancer therapy. In: Green DM, D'Angio GJ, eds. *Late effects of treatment for childhood cancer*. New York: Wiley-Liss, 1992:113–120.

175. Packer RJ, Meadows AT, Rocke LB, et al. Long-term sequelae of cancer treatment of the central nervous system in childhood. *Med Pediatr Oncol* 1987;15:241–253.

176. Dobbing J, Sands J. The quantitative growth and development of the human brain. *Arch Dis Child* 1963;48:757–767.

177. Halperin EC, Burger PC. Conventional external beam radiotherapy for central nervous system malignancies. *Neurol Clin* 1985;3:867–882.

178. Marks JE, Wong J. The risk of cerebral radionecrosis in relation to dose, time, and fractionation. A follow-up study. *Prog Exp Tumor Res* 1985;29:210–218.

179. Martins AN, Johnston JS, Henry MJ, et al. Delayed radiation necrosis of the brain. *J Neurosurg* 1977;47:336–345.

180. Anscher MS, Green DM, Kneece SM, et al. Radiation injury of the brain and spinal cord. In: Wilkins RH, Rengachary SS, eds. *Neurosurgery update II: vascular, spinal, pediatric and function neurosurgery*. New York: McGraw-Hill, 1991:42–49.

181. Van der Kogel A. Mechanisms of late radiation injury in the spinal cord. In: Meyh RE, Withers HR, eds. *Radiation biology in cancer research*. New York: Raven Press, 1980:461–473.

182. Burger PC, Scheithauer B, Vogel FS. *Surgical pathology of the nervous system and its coverings*. New York: Churchill Livingstone, 1991:229–236.

183. Constine LS, Konski A, Ekholm S, et al. Adverse effects of brain irradiation correlated with MR and CT imaging. *Int J Radiat Oncol Biol Phys* 1988;15:319–330.

184. Woo E, Lam K, Yu Y, et al. Cerebral radionecrosis: Is surgery necessary? *J Neurol Neurosurg Psychiatry* 1982;50:1407–1414.

*185. Griffin TW. White matter necrosis, microangiopathy and intellectual abilities in survivors of childhood leukemia. Association with central nervous system irradiation and methotrexate therapy. In: Gilbert HA, Kagan AR, eds. *Radiation damage to the nervous system*. New York: Raven Press, 1980:155–174.

186. Hertzberg H, Huk W, Ueberall M, et al. CNS late effects after ALL therapy in childhood. Part I: neuroradiological findings in long-term survivors of childhood ALL. *Med Pediatr Oncol* 1997;28:387–400.

*187. Jannoun L. Are cognitive and educational development affected by the age at which prophylactic therapy is given in acute lymphoblastic leukemia? *Arch Dis Child* 1983;58:955–958.

*188. Kun LE, Mulhern RK, Crisco JJ. Quality of life in children treated for brain tumors, intellectual, emotional and academic function. *J Neurosurg* 1983;58:1–6.

189. Halberg FE, Kramer JH, Moore IM, et al. Prophylactic cranial irradiation dose effects on late cognitive function in children treated for acute lymphoblastic leukemia. *Int J Radiat Oncol Biol Phys* 1991;22:13–16.

190. Rowland JH, Glidewell OJ, Sibley RF, et al. Effects of different forms of central nervous system prophylaxis on neuropsychologic function in childhood leukemia. *J Clin Oncol* 1984;2:1327–1335.

191. Copeland DR, Fletcher JM, Pfefferbaum-Levine B, et al. Psychological sequelae of childhood cancer in long-term survivors. *Pediatrics* 1985;75:745–753.

192. Williams JM, Davis KS. Central nervous system prophylactic treatment for childhood leukemia neuropsychological outcome studies. *Cancer Treat Rev* 1986;13:113–127.

193. Prince MT, Souheaver GT, Berry DH. Neuropsychological effects of irradiation and chemotherapy treatments upon children with acute lymphoblastic leukemia: a case study of monozygotic twins. *Neurotoxicology* 1988;9:341–349.

194. Waber DP, Tarbell NJ, Kahn CM, et al. The relationship of sex and treatment modality to neuropsychologic outcome in childhood acute lymphoblastic leukemia. *J Clin Oncol* 1992;10:810–817.

195. Waber D, Tarbell N, Fairclough D, et al. Cognitive sequelae of treatment in childhood acute lymphoblastic leukemia: cranial radiation requires an accomplice. *J Clin Oncol* 1995;13:2490–2496.

*196. Mulhern RK, Fairclough D, Ochs J. A prospective

comparion of neuropsychologic performance of children surviving leukemia who received 18-Gy, 24-Gy, or no cranial irradiation. *J Clin Oncol* 1991;9: 1348–1356.

*197. Waber D, Tarbell N. Toxicity of CNS prophylaxis for childhood leukemia. *Oncology* 1997;11:259–264.

198. Syndikus I, Tait D, Ashley S, et al. Long-term follow-up of young children with brain tumors after irradiation. *Int J Radiat Oncol Biol Phys* 1994;30: 781–787.

*199. Mulhern R, Hancock J, Fairclough D. Neuropsychological status of children treated with brain tumors: a critical review and integrated analysis. *Med Pediatr Oncol* 1992;20:181–191.

200. Bleyer A, Robinson L, Fallovollita J, et al. Influence of age, sex and concurrent intrathecal methotrexate therapy on intellectual function after cranial irradiation during childhood. *Pediatr Hematol Oncol* 1990; 7:329–338.

201. Kumar P, Kun LE, Rivera GK, et al. A prospective neuropsychological evaluation of children treated with additional chemotherapy and craniospinal irradiation (CSI) following isolated central nervous system (CNS) relapse in acute lymphoblastic leukemia (ALL). *Int J Radiat Oncol Biol Phys* 1993;27:134 (abst).

202. Meadows AT, Gordon J, Massari DJ, et al. Declines in IQ scores and cognitive dysfunctions in children with acute lymphocytic leukemia treated with irradiation. *Lancet* 1981;2:1015–1018.

*203. Mulhern R, Wasserman A, Fairclough D, et al. Memory function in disease-free survivors of childhood acute lymphocytic leukemia given CNS prophylaxis with or without 1800 cGy cranial irradiation. *J Clin Oncol* 1988;6:315–320.

204. Bloom HJC, Wallace ENJ, Henk JM. The treatment and prognosis of medulloblastoma in children: a study of 82 verified cases. *AJR* 1969;105:43–62.

205. Packer RJ, Sutton LA, Atkins TE, et al. A prospective study of cognitive function in children receiving whole-brain radiotherapy and chemotherapy: 2-year results. *J Neurosurg* 1989;70:707–713.

206. Druckmann A. Schlafsucht als Folge der rontgenbestrahlung: beitrag zur strahlenempfindlichkeit des genirns. *Strohlenther Onkol* 1929;33:382–384.

207. Eiser C. Intellectual abilities among survivors of childhood leukemia as a function of CNS irradiation. *Arch Dis Child* 1978;53:391–395.

208. Mitchell W. Stroke at a late sequela of cranial irradiation for childhood brain tumors. *J Child Neurol* 1991;6:128–133.

209. Jones AM. Transient radiation myelopathy (with reference to Lhermitte's sign of electrical paresthesia). *Br J Radiol* 1964;37:727–744.

210. Kaplan HS. *Hodgkin's disease.* Cambridge: Harvard University Press, 1800.

211. Wara W, Phillips T, Sheline G, et al. Radiation tolerance of the spinal cord. *Cancer* 1975;35:1558–1562.

*212. Marcus R, William R. The incidence of myelitis after irradiation of the cervical spinal cord. *Int J Radiat Oncol Biol Phys* 1990;19:3–8.

213. Littman P, Rosenstock J, Bailey C. Radiation myelitis following craniospinal irradiation with concurrent actinomycin D therapy. *Med Pediatr Oncol* 1978;5: 145–151.

214. Withers R, Mason K, Thames H. Late radiation response of kidney assayed by tubule-cell survival. *Br J Radiol* 1986;59:587–595.

215. McGill CW, Holder TM, Smith TH, et al. Postradiation renovascular hypertension. *J Pediatr Surg* 1979; 14:831–833.

216. LeBourgeois JP, Meignan M, Parmentier C, et al. Renal consequences of irradiation of the spleen in lymphoma patients. *Br J Radiol* 1979;52:56–60.

217. Kim T, Somerville P, Freeman C. Unilateral radiation nephropathy—the long-term significance. *Int J Radiat Oncol Biol Phys* 1984;10:2053–2059.

*218. Kunkler P, Farr R, Luxton R. The unit of renal tolerance to x-rays. *Br J Radiol* 1952;25:190–201.

219. Makinen L, Makipernaa A, Rautanen J, et al. Long-term cardiac sequelae after treatment of malignant tumors with radiotherapy or cytostatics in childhood. *Cancer* 1990;65:1913–1917.

220. Thomas PRM, Tefft M, D'Angio GJ, et al. Acute toxicities associated with radiation in the second National Wilms' Tumor Study. *J Clin Oncol* 1988;6: 1694–1698.

221. Ritchey M, Green D, Thomas P, et al. Renal failure in Wilms' tumor patients: a report from the National Wilms' Tumor Study Group. *Med Pediatr Oncol* 1996;26:75–80.

*222. Cassady JR. Clinical radiation nephropathy. *Int J Radiat Oncol Biol Phys* 1995;31:1249–1256.

*223. Tarbell N, Guinan E, Neimeyer C, et al. Late onset of renal dysfunction in survivors of bone marrow transplantation. *Int J Radiat Oncol Biol Phys* 1988;15: 99–104.

224. Lonnerholm G, Carlson K, Bratteby LE, et al. Renal function after autologous bone marrow transplantation. *Bone Marrow Trans* 1991;8:129–134.

225. Patzer L, Hempel L, Ringelmann F, et al. Renal function after conditioning therapy for bone marrow transplantation in childhood. *Med Pediatr Oncol* 1997;28:274–283.

226. Rubin P, Finkelstein JN, Siemann DW, et al. Predictive biochemical assays for late radiation effects. *Int J Radiat Oncol Biol Phys* 1986;12:469–476.

227. Fryer CJH, Fitzpatrick PJ, Rider WD, et al. Radiation pneumonitis: experience following a large single dose of radiation. *Int J Radiat Oncol Biol Phys* 1978; 4:931–936.

228. Gross NJ. Experimental radiation pneumonitis. IV: Leakage of circulatory proteins onto the alveolar surface. *J Lab Clin Med* 1980;95:19–31.

229. Rosenkrans WA, Penny DP. Cell-cell matrix interactions in induced lung injury: III. Long term effects of X-irradiation on basal laminar proteoglycans. *Anat Rec* 1986;215:127–133.

230. Littman P, Meadows AT, Polgar G, et al. Pulmonary function in survivors of Wilms' tumor. *Cancer* 1976; 37:2773–2776.

231. Mah K, van Dyke J. Quantitative measurements of changes on human lung density following irradiation. *Radiother Oncol* 1988;11:169–179.

232. McDonald S, Rubin P, Maasilta P. Response of normal lung to irradiation tolerance doses/tolerance volumes in pulmonary radiation syndromes. *Front Radiat Ther Oncol* 1989;23:255–276.

233. Phillips T. Pulmonary section—cardiorespiratory workshops. *Cancer Clin Trials* 1981;3:45–52.

*234. Wara WM, Phillips TL, Margolis LW, et al. Radiation pneumonitis: a new approach to the derivation of time-dose factors. *Cancer* 1973;32:547–552.

*235. Cooper J, Zitnik R, Matthay R. Mechanisms of drug-induced pulmonary disease. *Annu Rev Med* 1988;39: 395–404.

*236. McDonald S, Rubin P, Phillips T, et al. Injury to the lung from cancer therapy: clinical syndromes, measurable endpoints, and potential scoring systems. *Int J Radiat Oncol Biol Phys* 1995;31:1187–1203.

237. Keane T, van Dyke J, Rider W. Idiopathic interstitial pneumonia following bone marrow transplantation: the relationship with total body irradiation. *Int J Radiat Oncol Biol Phys* 1981;7:1365–1370.

238. Champlin R, Gale R. The early complications of bone marrow transplantation. *Semin Hematol* 1984;12: 101–108.

239. Schultz KR, Green GJ, Wensley D, et al. Obstructive lung disease in children after allogeneic bone marrow transplantation. *Blood* 1994;84:3212–3220.

*240. Carlson K, Backlund L, Smedmyr B, et al. Pulmonary function and complications subsequent to autologous bone marrow transplantation. *Bone Marrow Trans* 1994;14:805–811.

241. Wohl MEB, Griscom NT, Traggis DG, et al. Effects of therapeutic irradiation delivered in early childhood upon subsequent lung function. *Pediatrics* 1975;55: 507–516.

242. Castellino R, Glatstein E, Turbow M, et al. Latent radiation injury of lungs or heart activated by steroid withdrawal. *Ann Intern Med* 1974;80:593–599.

243. Chowhan NM. Injurious effects of radiation on the esophagus. *Am J Gastroenterol* 1990;85:115–120.

244. Sher ME, Bauer J. Radiation induced enteropathy. *Am J Gastroenterol* 1990;85:121–128.

245. Churnratanakul S, Wirzba G, Lam T, et al. Radiation and the small intestine. Future perspectives for preventive therapy. *Dig Dis* 1990;8:45–60.

*246. Donaldson SS, Jundt S, Ricour C, et al. Radiation enteritis in children. *Cancer* 1975;35:1167–1178.

*247. Woods W, Dehner L, Nesbit M, et al. Fetal veno-occlusive disease of the liver following high dose chemotherapy, irradiation and bone marrow transplantation. *Am J Med* 1998;60:285–290.

248. Yankelevitz DF, Knapp PH, Henschke CI, et al. MR appearance of radiation hepatitis. *Clin Imag* 1992;16: 89–92.

249. Ingold JA, Reed GB, Kaplan HS, et al. Radiation hepatitis. *AJR* 1963;93:200–208.

*250. Lawrence T, Robertson J, Ansher M, et al. Hepatic toxicity resulting from cancer treatment. *Int J Radiat Oncol Biol Phys* 1995;31:1237–1248.

*251. Fajardo L, Colby T. Pathogenesis of veno-occlusive liver disease after irradiation. *Arch Pathol Lab Med* 1980;104:584–588.

252. Anscher MS, Crocker IR, Jirtle RL. Transforming growth factor-B1 expression in irradiated liver. *Radiat Res* 1990;122:77–85.

253. Tefft M, Mitus A, Das L, et al. Irradiation of the liver in children: review of experience in the acute and chronic phases, and in the intact normal and partially resected. *AJR* 1990;108:365–385.

254. Lawrence TS, Ten Haken RK, Kessler ML, et al. The use of 3-D dose volume analysis to predict radiation hepatitis. *Int J Radiat Oncol Biol Phys* 1992;23:781–788.

255. Perry M. Hepatotoxicity of chemotherapeutic agents. *Semin Oncol* 1982;9:65–74.

256. Ortega J, Donaldson S, Percy S, et al. Venoocclusive disease of the liver after chemotherapy with vincristine, actinomycin D, and cyclophosphamide for the treatment of rhabdomyosarcoma. A report of the Intergroup Rhabdomyosarcoma Study Group. *Cancer* 1997;79:2435–2439.

*257. Nanda SK, Schachat AP. Ocular complications following radiation therapy to the orbit. In: Green DM, D'Angio GJ, eds. *Late effects of treatment for childhood cancer.* New York: Wiley-Liss, 1992:11–22.

*258. Wara W, Irvine A, Neger R, et al. Radiation retinopathy. *Int J Radiat Oncol Biol Phys* 1979;5:81–83.

259. Hilliard L, Berkow R, Watterson J, et al. Retinal toxicity associated with cisplatin and etoposide in pediatric patients. *Med Pediatr Oncol* 1997;28:310–313.

260. Parsons J, Fitzgerald C, Hood C, et al. The effects of irradiation of the eye and optic nerve. *Int J Radiat Oncol Biol Phys* 1983;9:609–622.

261. Merriam G, Focht E. Radiation dose to the lens in treatment of tumors of the eye and adjacent structures: possibilities of cataract formation. *Radiology* 1958;71:357–369.

*262. Britten M, Halman K, Meredith W. Radiation cataract—new evidence on radiation dosage to the lens. *Br J Radiol* 1966;39:612–617.

263. Otake M, Schull WJ. A review of forty-five years study of Hiroshima and Nagasaki atomic bomb survivors radiation cataract. *J Radiat Res* 1991;32: 283–293.

*264. Deeg H, Flournoy N, Sullivan K, et al. Cataracts after total body irradiation and marrow transplantation: a sparing effect of dose fractionation. *Int J Radiat Oncol Biol Phys* 1984;10:957–964.

*265. Belkacemi Y, Ozsahin M, Pene F, et al. Cataractogenesis after total body irradiation. *Int J Radiat Oncol Biol Phys* 1996;35:53–60.

266. Foote RL, Garretson BR, Schomberg PJ, et al. External beam irradiation for retinoblastoma: patterns of failure and dose-response analysis. *Int J Radiat Oncol Biol Phys* 1989;16:823–830.

267. McCormick B, Ellsworth R, Abramson D, et al. Results of external beam radiation for children with retinoblastoma: a comparison of two techniques. *J Pediatr Ophthalmol Strabismus* 1989;26:239–243.

268. Brooks HL,Jr., Meyer D, Shields JA, et al. Removal of radiation-induced cataracts in patients treated for retinoblastoma. *Arch Ophthalmol* 1990;108: 1701–1708.

269. Kline L, Kim J, Ceballos R. Radiation optic neuropathy. *Ophthalmol* 1985;92:1118–1126.

*270. Kaste S, Chen G, Fontanesi J, et al. Orbital development in long-term survivors of retinoblastoma. *J Clin Oncol* 1997;15:1183–1189.

271. Adler M, Hawke M, Bergern G, et al. Radiation effects on the external auditory canal. *J Otolaryngol* 1985;14:226–232.

*272. McHaney V, Kavnar E, Meyer W, et al. Effects of radiation therapy and chemotherapy on hearing. In: Green DM, D'Angio GJ, eds. *Late effects of treatment for childhood cancer.* New York: Wiley-Liss, 1992:7–10.

273. Freilich R, Kraus D, Budnick A, et al. Hearing loss in children treated with cisplatin and carboplatin-based

high-dose chemotherapy with autologous bone marrow rescue. *Med Pediatr Oncol* 1996;26:95–100.

274. Hendry J. The cellular basis of long-term marrow injury after irradiation. *Radiother Oncol* 1985;3: 331–338.

*275. Mauch P, Constine L, Greenberger J, et al. Hematopoietic stem cell compartment: acute and late effects of radiation therapy and chemotherapy. *Int J Radiat Oncol Biol Phys* 1995;31:1319–1339.

276. Storb R, Deeg HJ, Applebaum FR, et al. Total-body irradiation in bone marrow transplantation. In: Browne D, et al., eds. *Treatment of Radiation Injuries*. New York: Plenum Press, 1990:29–33.

277. Sykes M, Chu F, Savel H, et al. The effects of varying dosages of irradiation upon sternal marrow regeneration. *Radiology* 1964;83:1084–1087.

278. Yankelevitz DF, Henschke CI, Knapp PH, et al. Effect of radiation therapy on thoracic and lumbar bone marrow: evaluation with MR imaging. *AJR* 1992; 157:87–92.

279. Parmentier C, Morardet N, Tubiana M. Late effects of human bone marrow after extended field radiotherapy. *Int J Radiat Oncol Biol Phys* 1983;9:1301–1311.

280. Rubin P, Scarantino C. The bone marrow organ: the critical structure in radiation-drug interaction. *Int J Radiat Oncol Biol Phys* 1978;4:3–23.

281. Casamassima F, Ruggkiero C, Carmaella D, et al. Hematopoietic bone marrow recovery after radiation therapy: MRI evaluation. *Blood* 1989;73:1677–1681.

282. Sachs E, Goris M, Glatstein E, et al. Bone marrow regeneration following large field irradiation. Influence of volume, age, dose and time. *Cancer* 1978;42: 1057–1065.

283. Cristy M. Active bone marrow distribution as a function of age in humans. *Phys Med Biol* 1981;26: 389–400.

284. Maguire A, Craft A, Evans R, et al. The long-term effects of treatment on the dental condition of children surviving malignant disease. *Cancer* 1987;60: 2570–2575.

285. Best JD. The dentist and the pediatric oncology patient. *NY State Dent J* 1990;56:29–30.

286. Fromm M, Littman P, Raney B, et al. Late effects after treatment of twenty children with soft tissue sarcomas of the head and neck. *Cancer* 1986;57:2070–2076.

287. Kaste S, Hopkins K, Crom D, et al. Dental abnormalities in children treated for acute lymphoblastic leukemia. *Leukemia* 1997;11:792–796.

288. Dahllof G, Barr M, Balme P, et al. Disturbances in dental development after total body irradiation in bone marrow transplant recipients. *Oral Surg Oral Med Oral Pathol* 1988;65:41–44.

289. Makkonen T, Nordman E. Estimation of long-term salivary gland damage induced before the onset of treatment. *Cancer* 1987;57:1986–1987.

290. Maxymiw WG, Wood RE. The role of dentistry in head and neck radiation therapy. *Can Dent Assoc J* 1988;55:193–198.

291. Bucker J, Fleming T, Fuller L, et al. Preliminary observations on the effect of mantle field radiotherapy on salivary flow rates in patients with Hodgkin's disease. *J Dent Res* 1988;6:518–521.

292. Marks J, Davis C, Gottsman V, et al. The effects of radiation on parotid salivary function. *Int J Radiat Oncol Biol Phys* 1981;7:1013–1019.

293. Myers RE, Mitchell DL. Fluoride for the head and neck radiation patient. *Mil Med* 1988;153:411–413.

294. Johnson J, Ferretti G, Nethery J, et al. Oral pilocarpine for post-irradiation xerostomia in patients with head and neck cancer. *N Engl J Med* 1993; 329:390–395.

295. Fajardo L, Stewart J. Human and experimental observations. In: Bristow M, ed. *Drug-induced heart disease*. Amsterdam: Elsevier/North-Holland, 1980: 241–260.

296. Applefeld MM. The late appearance of chronic pericardial disease in patients treated by radiotherapy for Hodgkin's disease. *Ann Intern Med* 1981;94: 338–341.

297. Stewart J, Cohen K, Fajardo L, et al. Radiation-induced heart disease: a study of twenty-five patients. *Radiology* 1967;89:302–310.

*298. Stewart JR, Fajardo LF. Radiation-induced heart disease: an update. *Prog Cardiovasc Dis* 1984;27: 173–194.

299. Green D, Gingell R, Pearce J, et al. The effect of mediastinal irradiation on cardiac function of patients treated during childhood and adolescence for Hodgkin's disease. *J Clin Oncol* 1987;5:239–245.

300. Hancock SL, Hoppe RT, Horning SJ, et al. Intercurrent death after Hodgkin's disease therapy in radiotherapy and adjuvant MOPP trials. *Ann Intern Med* 1988;109:183–189.

301. Ni Y, von Segesser LK, Turina M. Futility of pericardiectomy for post-irradiation constrictive pericarditis? *Ann Thorac Surg* 1990;49:445–448.

*302. Hancock SL, Donaldson S, Hoppe RT. Cardiac disease following treatment of Hodgkin's disease in children and adolescents. *J Clin Oncol* 1993;11:1208–1215.

303. Byhardt R, Brace K, Ruckdeschel J. Dose and treatment factors in radiation-related pericardial effusion associated with the mantle technique for Hodgkin's disease. *Cancer* 1975;35:795–802.

*304. LaMonte CS, Yeh S, Straus D. Long-term follow-up of cardiac function in patients with Hodgkin's disease treated with mediastinal irradiation and combination chemotherapy including doxorubicin. *Cancer Treat Rep 1986* 1998;70:439–444.

305. Brosius FC,III, Waller BF, Roberts WC. Radiation heart disease. Analysis of 16 young (aged 15-33 years) necropsy patients who received over 3.500 rads to the heart. *Am J Med* 1981;70:519–530.

306. Burns RJ, Bar-Shlomo B, Druck M. Detection of radiation cardiomyopathy by gated radionuclide angiography. *Am J Med* 1983;74:297–302.

307. Constine L, Schwartz R, Savage D, et al. Cardiac function, perfusion, and morbidity in irradiated long-term survivors of Hodgkin's disease. *Int J Radiat Oncol Biol Phys* 1997;39:897–906.

*308. Lipshultz SE, Lipsitz SR, Mone SM, et al. Female sex and higher drug dose as risk factors for late cardiotoxic effects of doxorubicin therapy for childhood cancer. *N Eng J Med* 1995;332:1738–1743.

*309. Krischer J, Epstein S, Cuthbertson D, et al. Clinical cardiotoxicity following anthracycline treatment for childhood cancer: the Pediatric Oncology Group experience. *J Clin Oncol* 1997;15:1544–1552.

*310. Fishman W, Yee H, Keefe D, et al. Cardiovascular toxicity with cancer chemotherapy. Current problems in cancer. *Curr Probl Cancer* 1997;21:301–360.

311. Eames G, Crosson J, Steinberger J, et al. Cardiovascular function in children following bone marrow transplant: a cross-sectional study. *Bone Marrow Trans* 1997;19:61–66.

*312. Carlson RG, Mayfield WR, Norman S, et al. Radiation-associated valvular disease. *Chest* 1991;99: 538–545.

313. Jakachi R, Goldwein J, Larsen R, et al. Cardiac dysfunction following spinal irradiation during childhood. *J Clin Oncol* 1993;11:1033–1038.

314. Cohen SI, Bharati S, Glass J, et al. Radiotherapy as a cause of complete atrioventricular block as Hodgkin's disease: an electrophysiological-pathological correlation. *Arch Intern Med* 1981;141:676–679.

315. Kadota R, Burgert E, Driscoll D, et al. Cardiopulmonary function in long-term survivors of childhood Hodgkin's lymphoma: a pilot study. *Mayo Clin Proc* 1988;63:362–367.

*316. Corn BW, Tract BJ, Goodman RL. Irradiation-related ischemic heart disease. *J Clin Oncol* 1990;8:741–750.

*317. King V, Constine LS, Clark D, et al. Symptomatic coronary artery disease after mantle irradiation for Hodgkin's disease. *Int J Radiat Oncol Biol Phys* 1996;36:881–889.

318. Cosset JM, Henry-Amar M, Meerwaldt JH. Long-term toxicity of early stages of Hodgkin's disease therapy: the EORTC experience. *Ann Oncol* 1991;2:77–82.

319. Mauch P, Tarbell N, Weinstein H, et al. Stage IA and IIA supradiaphragmatic Hodgkin's disease: prognostic factors in surgically staged patients treated with mantle and para-aortic irradiation. *J Clin Oncol* 1988;6:1576–1583.

320. Van Hoff DD, Layard MW, Basa P, et al. Risk factors for doxorubicin-induced congestive heart failure. *Ann Intern Med* 1979;91:710–717.

321. Cazin B, Gorin N, Laporte J, et al. Cardiac complications after bone marrow transplantation. *Cancer* 1986;57:2061–2069.

322. Constine L, Rubin P. Morbidity of combined chemotherapy and radiotherapy. In: Plowman DN, McElwain T, Meadows A, eds. *Complications of cancer management survey.* London: Butterworth Heinemann, 1991:13–26.

323. Harris JM, Jackson CM, Patterson DG. *The measurement of man.* Minneapolis: University of Minnesota Press, 1930.

324. Ryan BR, Walters TR. Slipped capital femoral epiphysis following radiotherapy and chemotherapy. *Med Pediatr Oncol* 1979;6:279–283.

325. Kricun ME. Red-yellow marrow conversion: its effect on the location of some solitary bone lesions. *Skeletal Radiol* 1985;14:10–19.

326. Custer RP, Ahlfedt FE. Studies on the structure and function of bone marrow. *J Lab Clin Med* 1932; 17:960–962.

*327. Rubin P. Law and order of radiation sensitivity. Absolute versus relative. *Front Radiat Ther Oncol* 1989; 23:7–40.

328. Oliver JH, Gluck G, Gledhill RB, et al. Musculoskeletal deformities following treatment of the central nervous system in childhood. *Med Pediatr Oncol* 1978;15:241–253.

329. Heaston DK, Libshitz HI, Chan RC. Skeletal effects of megavoltage irradiation in survivors of Wilms' tumor. *AJR* 1979;133:389–395.

330. Green DM. *Diagnosis and management of malignant solid tumors in infants and children.* Boston: Martinus Nijhoff, 1985:476–492.

331. Hirsh J, Renier D, Czernechow P. Medulloblastoma in childhood: survival and functional results. *Acta Neurochir* 1979;48:1–15.

332. Raimondi AJ, Tomita T. Advantages of total resection of medulloblastoma and disadvantages of full head postoperative radiation therapy. *Childs Brain* 1979;5: 50–59.

333. Spunberg JJ, Chang CH, Goldman M, et al. Quality of long term survival following irradiation for intracranial tumors in children under the age of two. *Int J Radiat Oncol Biol Phys* 1981;7:727–736.

334. Duffner PK, Cohen ME, Thomas PRM. Late effects of treatment on the intelligence of children with posterior fossa tumors. *Cancer* 1983;51:233–237.

*335. Packer RJ, Radcliffe J, Glauser TA. Prospective evaluation of neuropsychological function in chldren treated for medulloblastoma. In: Green DM, D'Angio GJ, eds. *Late effects of treatment for childhood cancer.* New York: Wiley-Liss, 1992:41–48.

336. Ellenberg L, McComb JG, Siegel SE, et al. Factors affecting intellectual outcome in pediatric brain tumor patients. *Neurosurgery* 1987;21:638–644.

337. Packer RJ, Sposto R, Atkins TE, et al. Quality of life for children with primitive neuroectodermal tumors/medulloblastoma of the posterior fossa. *Pediatr Neurosci* 1988;13:169–175.

*338. Mitus A, Tefft M, Fellers F. Long-term follow-up of renal functions of 108 children who underwent nephrectomy for malignant disease. *Pediatrics* 1969;44: 912–921.

20

Secondary Tumors

Children are susceptible to radiation and chemotherapy-induced cancer (1). Children who develop one malignancy have a 6- to 15-fold increased risk of developing a second cancer when compared to age-matched populations (2–8). The percentage of children treated for one cancer who develop these second malignant neoplasms (SMN) is reported to range from 3% to 12% by age 25. About 68% of all SMNs are found in the field of the original radiation therapy (1,5,6,9–12).

CLASSIC CARCINOGENESIS

The foundations of our understanding of carcinogenesis may be traced to the work of Rous and Kidd (13), Mottram (14), and Berenblum and Shubik (15). Rous and Kidd (13) "initiated" a cancer by applying tar to the ear of a rabbit. Subsequent wounding of the area "promoted" the development of neoplasms along the edge of the wound. Mottram (14) confirmed this pattern by showing that treatment of murine skin with the carcinogen benzpyrene, followed by the irritant croton oil, resulted in a much higher incidence of skin cancer than did treatment with the carcinogen alone. Berenblum and Shubik (15) and, later, Boutwell (16) codified this pattern into the notion that the direct administration of a carcinogen (*initiation* or the *precarcinogenic action*) followed by repeated applications of a second agent (*promotion)* could lead to neoplastic transformation.

The third event in carcinogenesis is *progression* where the dysplastic cell line develops a full complement of characteristics that constitute malignancy. Progression involves the development of *clonogenicity* characterized by cellular evolution of the "precancerous" lesion to malignancy. *Invasiveness* then follows the development of an increasing cellular growth rate, autonomy, and ability to invade and metastasize.

In a more contemporary understanding, carcinogenesis occurs when an agent (i.e., hereditary factors, viruses, chemical and environmental toxic agents, radiation, and other physical agents) injures the DNA of a target gene. Replication of this mutant cell provides the descendants that form a tumor. It is also possible that the mutation affects cellular DNA repair proteins, which lead to a hypermutable state (17,18). Initiation may be understood as the first event where DNA is damaged to a degree beyond the ability for repair by the cell. This cell then has a new phenotype and behavior pattern.

CONTEMPORARY UNDERSTANDING OF CARCINOGENESIS

Two general types of genes lead to neoplastic transformation. The first is the "proto-oncogene," which codes for cellular signaling components that play a role in controlling normal growth and differentiation (17). The ability of proto-oncogenes to participate in neoplastic transformation arises from the fact that the protein products of these genes are crucial relays in the elaborate biochemical circuitry that governs vertebrate cells (19).

There are several general categories of proto-oncogenes. These include growth factor receptors acting via a tyrosine specific protein kinase pathway, GTP binding proteins, membrane/cytoskeletal associated tyrosine specific kinases, extra cellular growth factors, serine/threonine specific protein kinases, and steroid-type growth factor receptors (Fig. 1). Therefore, products of the proto-oncogene may include polypeptide hormones acting upon the cell surface, receptors for these hormones, proteins that convey signals from the cell surface to its depths, and chemicals that affect nuclear functions.

The second category of genes involved in carcinogenesis are called tumor suppressor genes (20). These genes act to restrain cell growth. Carcinogenesis could be the result of inactivation of a tumor suppressor gene, eliminating its growth-suppressing function. This could allow unbridled cell growth and neoplastic transformation.

There has been much interest in tumor suppressor genes in childhood cancer. This interest has, initially, focused on the RB1 gene and its relation to retinoblastoma and osteogenic sarcoma and is now expanding to a variety of other malignancies (21,22). In late G_1 or early S phase the RB1 protein (pRB) becomes progressively more phosphorylated at multiple sites. The enzymes that carry out these phosphorylation reactions are cyclin-dependent kinases, which are activated by complex formation with cyclins A, D, and/or E and regulate cell cycle events. The level of pRB phosphorylation remains high until late in M phase

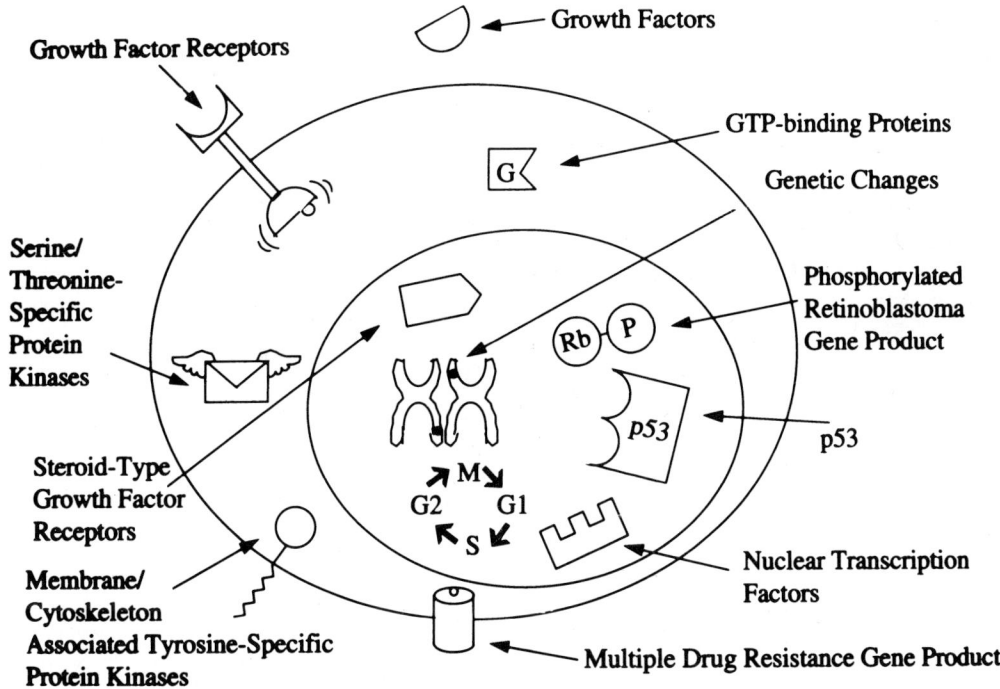

FIG. 1. Proto-oncogenes and tumor suppressor genes can influence the conversion of a benign cell into a malignant one. There are several types of proto-oncogenes. These include growth factor receptors GTP binding proteins, tyrosine specific kinases, extracellular growth factors, serine/threonine specific protein kinases, and steroid-type growth factor receptors. Tumor suppressor gene products, such as pRB or p53, act to restrain cell growth. Carcinogenesis could be the result of cellular proliferation by proto-oncogenes or loss of the restraint of cell growth by tumor suppressor genes. (The concept for this figure is derived from Varmus H, Weinberg RA. *Genes and the biology of cancer.* New York: Scientific American Library, 1993:98.)

when a phosphatase removes these posttranslational modifications. The pRB is again underphosphorylated in G_o/G_1. These periodic phosphorylation and dephosphorylation reactions are believed to modulate pRB's physical and functional interaction with a variety of cellular targets.

In resting cells (G_0) or cells in early G_1 pRB can be found in a complex with a cellular transcription factor called E2F. In general, transcription factors are proteins that, by binding to a specific DNA sequence adjacent to the genes they regulate, promote the expression of particular genes. E2F contributes to the activation of a constellation of genes encoding S-phase functions required for the synthesis of DNA. When complexed to pRB, E2F gene-mediated transcriptional activation does not occur. Therefore, RB1 function in part by its sequestration of E2F in G_1 (23,24).

The p53 gene is another tumor suppressor gene that has provoked interest among those studying childhood cancer. p53 has been shown to be mutated in many histologic types of cancer (20,21,23,24). In various cell lines p53 has been shown to inhibit proliferation, promote differentiation, enable cells to arrest their growth following exposure to certain DNA damaging agents, and mediate apoptosis (23,24).

The mechanism through which p53 exerts its growth-suppressive function is under vigorous investigation. Much of the available evidence suggests that p53 acts as a transcriptional activator or a transcription factor (23,24). Some sequence-specific DNA binding has shown that p53 may also function as a transcription factor by interacting with other DNA-bound proteins, therefore, affecting their activity. Several transcriptional target genes for p53 have now been identified—with the assumption that such genes are likely to mediate the growth-suppressive properties attributed to p53 (23,24).

p21 is one of the most important mediators of p53's actions. The suppression of cell growth by p53 may be related to activating the expression of p21. p53, as a transcription factor, induces p21, which, in turn, inhibits cyclin-cyclin dependent kinases. As an inhibitor of cyclin-dependent kinases, p21 prevents phosphorylation of pRB and, hence, the expression of genes needed for replication.

Apoptosis, or programmed cell death, is an important biological consequence of exposure to ionizing radiation and other DNA-damaging agents. Initial reports of radiation-induced apoptosis emphasized the importance of p53 in this cellular response. Cell cycle arrest after irradiation at the G_1 checkpoint requires the expression of p53 in some cell lines. In tumor cells that undergo p53-dependent apoptosis, it seems that one of the functions of p53 is to screen for damaged DNA. In the presence of damaged DNA, wild-type p53 facilitates cell cycle arrest and DNA repair. Therefore, it prevents the cell with damaged DNA from undergoing any proliferation (25). One might speculate that p53-negative cells that sustain radio-chemotherapeutic damage would exhibit a diminished capacity to detect and respond to such damage. The damaged DNA could, consequently, be duplicated. If a lethal mutation had occurred from radio-chemotherapeutic damage, then the cell would die. If, however, a sublethal mutation had occurred, it is possible that a lack of p53 might allow amplification of the injured DNA and result in a cancer (23,24).

A pervasive dogma in cancer research is that carcinogenesis is a multistage process. As previously described, the classic description of this process involved the concepts of *initiation, promotion,* and *progression*. More recent models involve multiple chromosomal changes in a variety of genes as growth-stimulating oncogenes are activated and tumor suppressor genes inactivated. How is it possible that exposure to a course of therapeutic radiation can result in mutations at the multiplicity of genetic loci necessary to produce a secondary cancer?

One possibility is that a protracted course of radiation will induce sufficient mutations to produce all, or most, of the steps necessary to produce a second cancer. For this to be true, ionizing radiation would need to be capable of producing point mutations to activate proto-oncogenes and point mutations and deletions to inactivate tumor suppressor genes. Radiation would produce cancer by the instantaneous creation of initiated cells (26). Because radiation is relatively ineffective at causing point mutations but extremely effective at causing large deletions, inactivation of tumor suppressor genes such as p53 are likely to be an important mechanism of radiation carcinogenesis (27,28). Cell lines derived from primary thyroid tumors, rendered capable of tumor formation in athymic nude mice by radiation, express p53 mutations (29). The cell initiated by radiation may undergo clonal expansion with subsequent promotion. Once a malignant cell is generated, it gives rise to a tumor after some lag period.

It is also possible that radiation, in addition to inactivating tumor suppressor genes, may generate a malignant diathesis by other subtle mechanisms. For example, a mutation in the gene(s) responsible for DNA mismatch repair could lead to defective repair phenotype. In this way, multiple mutations may derive from a radiation-induced mutation in a repair system (27,28). Radiation, in this postulated mechanism, causes persistent genomic instability resulting in a high rate of spontaneous mutations including those associated with a malignant phenotype (30).

RADIATION CARCINOGENESIS

There are several highly illustrative and oft-quoted episodes of human radiation carcinogenesis. These include, but are not limited to the following:

1. Individuals treated with radiotherapy for ankylosing spondylitis have been carefully followed to ascertain the risk of tumor induction by irradiation. The study population consists of 14,554 patients treated with x-irradiation between 1935 and 1954. With follow-up exceeding 35 years in many patients, the ratio of observed to expected deaths from leukemia is 3.17. The relative risk was at its highest 2.5 to 4.9 years after treatment. The greatest risk was for the induction of acute myeloid leukemia. Mortality from colon cancer, which is associated with spondylitis through a common association with ulcerative colitis, was increased by 30% in irradiated patients. Mortality for neoplasms other than leukemia or colon cancer was increased by 28% (31).

2. Classic studies documenting the fact that diagnostic radiographs of the abdomen and pelvis of a pregnant woman could induce cancer in her child were derived from data collected by the Oxford Survey of Childhood Cancer (OSCC). Each child known to have died in England, Wales, and Scotland was coupled with another living child of the same sex ("the matched control") born in the same district with a similar birth date. By questioning the children's mothers, information was obtained concerning prenatal exposure to diagnostic radiographs. Clinical records were reviewed for data concerning exposure. The odds ratio for cancer strongly suggests that prenatal radiographs increased the risk of malignancy. For the 4-year birth cohort 1947 to 1953, the odds ratio was 1.62 (90% CI 1.4 to 1.87), and for 1958 to 1961 it was 1.23 (90% CI 1.05 to 1.44) (32).

3. Among the myriad problems encountered following the founding of the State of Israel in 1948, was the medical care of large numbers of emigrants. X-ray-induced epilation was used in over 10,000 children to eradicate tinea capitis. This therapy entailed direct irradiation of the scalp, skull, and brain as well as scattered irradiation of the thyroid. Long-term follow-up studies disclose an increased incidence of benign and malignant brain, skin, salivary gland, and thyroid tumors in these individuals (33).

4. Atomic bombs were dropped on Hiroshima and Nagasaki in August 1945. Radiation-related risks among the bomb survivors have been analyzed by a dosimetry system that attempts to account for a survivor's distance from the bomb epicenter, attenuation of radiation by shielding by houses and the body, posture at the time of explosion, orientation (Was the victim facing toward or away from the hypocenter?), and the person's age. Dose estimates have been periodically modified—par-

ticularly because of reevaluation of the neutron dose in the Hiroshima bombing. It is established that the incidence of leukemia is increased among atomic bomb survivors. The time interval between irradiation and the appearance of a malignancy is referred to as the latent period. The latent period for leukemia was short. The increased risk appeared 1 to 3 years after the bombing and peaked at 6 to 7 years. There is also a dose-related increase for cancers of the esophagus, stomach, colon, lung, breast, ovary, thyroid, urinary tract, and multiple myeloma. With the exception of leukemia, the excess risk is manifest only after the exposed individual reaches the age at which the cancer is normally prone to develop. Most radiation-induced cancers do not develop until the irradiated persons reach the age when the type of tumor in question occurs spontaneously. This implies that age-dependent factors influence the expression of the disease. Radiation effects were significantly influenced by the individual's age at the time of the bomb-

ing. The relative risk (RR) of neoplasia is higher for survivors who were young at the time of radiation exposure (1,34–39) (Fig. 2).

Studies have been done concerning the mortality and morbidity from malignancies with onset before 20 years of age in relation to parental atomic bomb radiation exposure. No increased incidence is discernible. When analysis is confined to tumors where there is a strong possibility that a parental germ-line mutation is a predisposing factor (i.e., retinoblastoma followed by sarcoma, Wilms' tumor), there is still no association seen (37).

5. Occupational exposure to ionizing radiation is a well-known carcinogen. Uranium miners suffered an excess of lung cancer due to the inhalation of radon gas, and workers who painted the luminous radium dials on watch faces developed bone sarcomas because of the habit of shaping the paint brush in the mouth and ingesting bone-seeking radium.

6. Thorotrast was used as a contrast medium in diagnostic radiology, particularly

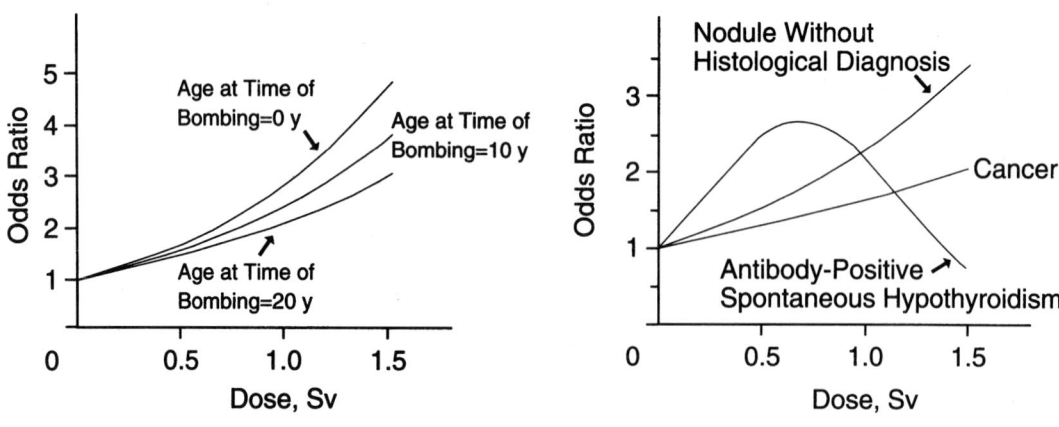

FIG. 2. A team from the Radiation Effects Research Foundation, Nagasaki, Japan, evaluated data from 2,587 individuals exposed to radiation from the Nagasaki atomic bomb blast in 1945 and who underwent physical examinations between October 1984 and April 1987. **A:** The odds ratio for the presence of a solid thyroid nodule in women exposed to radiation from the bomb at 0, 10, and 20 years of age, as a function of radiation dose, shows a progressive increase in prevalence as a function of radiation dose—as well as an effect of age at the time of exposure. The nodules included thyroid cancers as well as adenomas. **B:** The odds ratio for the prevalence of a nodule without histological diagnosis in women, cancer, and antibody positive spontaneous hypothyroidism, where the prevalence is adjusted for sex and age at the time of the bombing (cancer) and for age at the time of the bombing (hypothyroidism) is shown in this figure. The development of nodules and cancer rises with increasing dose. (From ref. 151, with permission.)

angiography, from the 1930s to the 1950s. Thorotrast is a colloidal suspension of the alpha emitter thorium dioxide. Taken up by macrophages, such as those lining hepatic sinusoids, the compound was associated with the late development of angiosarcoma (40).

7. Women with tuberculosis, who were repetitively fluoroscoped for monitoring of induced pneumothorax, have an elevated incidence of breast cancer (28).

8. Nuclear power plant accidents have been responsible for the injection of radionuclides into the atmosphere. In 1979, a partial core meltdown in a reactor at Three Mile Island power station near Harrisburg, Pennsylvania released 1×10^{12} Becquerels (Bq). The Chernobyl nuclear power plant accident of April 26, 1986, led to widespread radionuclide contamination and the release of 2×10^{18} Bq (41). The accident and the observed increase in the incidence of thyroid cancer in Belarus and Ukraine are described in detail in Chapter 16. No increase in common childhood leukemia has been documented so far. There may, however, be an increase in infant leukemia for those children who were exposed *in utero* (42).

INDUCED THYROID CANCER AS AN ILLUSTRATION OF THERAPEUTIC RADIATION CARCINOGENESIS

The RR of neoplasm induction by irradiation varies considerably among tissues. The risk is strongly dependent on the organ irradiated, the age of the patient at the time of radiation, and the delivered dose. Organs particularly sensitive to radiation-induced cancer include the thyroid, bone marrow, colon, stomach, and lung. In addition, different tissues have their maximum susceptibility at different ages (36,43).

The thyroid is particularly susceptible to the development of neoplasia as well as changes in thyroid function following neck irradiation. In 1950, Duffy and Fitzgerald (44) reported that 10 of 28 children treated for thyroid carcinoma at Memorial Sloan-Kettering Cancer Center had been irradiated during infancy for

an "enlarged thymus." In 1961, Winship and Rosvoll (45) reported that 38% of all children with thyroid carcinoma were known to have received therapeutic irradiation in infancy or early childhood for "thymic enlargement," tonsillar and adenoidal hypertrophy, hemangiomas, nevi, acne, eczema, and cervical tubercular adenitis. Fjalling et al. (46) have followed 444 persons who received radiotherapy for cervical tuberculous adenitis. Seventeen percent ultimately underwent surgery for benign thyroid nodules, and 6% underwent for thyroid carcinoma. The latency period for carcinoma ranged from 14 to 62 years. There was a positive correlation between absorbed radiation dose and the probability of developing a benign or malignant thyroid nodule. Fleming et al. (47) reviewed a series of 298 patients treated at St. Jude Children's Research Hospital with neck irradiation for childhood cancer and followed for at least 5 years free of recurrent tumor. Two patients developed follicular adenomas, 2 developed thyroid carcinoma, 1 had a colloid goiter, and 2 are being followed with undiagnosed thyroid nodules. Schneider et al. (48,49) have evaluated 2,958 of 5,379 patients who received head and neck irradiation at Michael Reese Hospital in Chicago between 1939 and 1962. Thyroid tumors were diagnosed in 37% (1,108 patients). Of 848 patients with surgically treated nodules, 35% had thyroid cancer and 65% had benign nodules. Numerous other reports have confirmed the increased incidence of thyroid neoplasia in irradiated individuals (5,6,10,11,33,48–51). Representative incidence figures for thyroid nodules are 6% for malignant and 8% to 12% for benign lesions following lower-dose (less than 15 Gy) external-beam irradiation.

In a report from the Late Effects Study Group of 9,170 patients who had survived more than 2 years after diagnosis of a cancer in childhood, the risk for thyroid cancer was increased 53-fold (52). The risk was associated with increasing radiation dose and time from treatment. Sixty-eight percent of the cancers arose directly within the radiation field, and all of the thyroid glands had received at least 1 Gy (via scatter for some patients). In a study by Hancock et al. (53) of 1,677 patients with Hodgkin's disease, the risk for developing thyroid cancer was increased 15.6-fold, occurring 9 to 18 years after therapy.

PRINCIPLES CHARACTERIZING RADIATION-INDUCED CANCER

Several principles characterize radiation-induced cancer (54–56):

1. A variety of histologic types of neoplasms can be induced by irradiation. These cancers are, at present, indistinguishable morphologically from naturally occurring cancers. The identification of a "radiation signature" in tumors would be important in the evaluation of SMNs. There is evidence that radiation produces a different spectrum of mutations than other genotoxic agents. If these mutations could be discerned and characterized, then one could clearly identify radiation-induced tumors and understand, more completely, the radiation dose-response relationship for induced tumors. "Molecular forensics" may, in this manner, affect our understanding of attributable risk (57).

2. Low linear energy transfer (LET) radiation (gamma ray, x-ray) is generally less efficient in inducing tumors than high LET radiation. In a murine hepatocarcinogenesis model, for example, neutron irradiation produced a greater incidence of hepatomas than did gamma irradiation (58). Low LET radiation appears to become less effective at carcinogenesis per centigray as the dose falls, whereas high LET radiation (neutrons, alpha particles) does not (36). With low LET irradiation there is less tumor induction when the dose is fractionated or administered at low-dose rates, implying that repair of carcinogenic damage is occurring. With high LET irradiation, the radiobiological effect is higher at low doses. The effectiveness of high LET radiation is not diminished and may be increased by dose fractionation or protraction (59).

3. Comparison of the frequency of SMN in different centers suggests that orthovoltage therapy is more likely to be carcinogenic than megavoltage therapy (7,56,60). This may be dose-related: By delivering a higher dose to bone, orthovoltage irradiation may increase the risk of an SMN of bone. The increased risk may also be related to the long follow-up available for orthovoltage patients (see point 9).

4. While every tissue in the body is at risk for radiation cancer induction, sensitivity varies according to the tissue. For example, the thyroid gland and breast are sensitive to cancer induction after low radiation doses; lymphoid tissue, lung, and liver require moderate doses; and bone requires higher doses. The relationship between dose and response may vary according to the induced tumor. Cancer risk from radiation may be given per unit dose (Gy or cGy) or per unit dose equivalent (Sievert) where a "quality factor" (Q) is used to take account of the varying biological effectiveness of different radiation (e.g., for a gamma ray $Q = 1$, whereas for a neutron $Q = 20$). Therefore, dose in Sievert (Sv) = dose in Gy $\times$ (Q). Detailed literature reviews indicate that the cancer mortality risk for the general population after whole-body exposure is 1×10^{-4} to 4×10^{-4} per person-cGy. Pooled results of various partial-body exposures give an estimated risk of 1×10^{-4} to 4×10^{-4} per person-cGy (4×10^2 Sv^1). The risk based on incidence is about twice that for mortality (1,36). Leukemia data can be fit by a curvilinear dose-response model, whereas skin cancer appears to have a threshold dose-response function, and breast data fit a linear no-threshold model.

5. The relation of irradiation dose to carcinogenesis is not clearly known. Data are only available for high doses. Evaluation of risks for low doses is of practical concern. In the absence of measurement, extrapolation is used to predict the risk at low doses (59).

6. SMN may also be induced by agents other than radiation (chemotherapy, environmental exposures, hereditary disposition). The low-dose radiation dose-response curve could be influenced by these confounding factors to produce a result that is the sum of two inde-

pendent rates or may be greater than simple addition would indicate. A variety of chemotherapeutic agents, especially alkylators, are known to be carcinogenic, and they may be additive or synergistic with radiation (61–64). Immunosuppressive agents clearly influence the propensity for tumor induction, as is seen in the setting of organ transplantation (65).

7. A large denominator of irradiated patients is necessary to calculate a radiation carcinogenesis risk with reasonable accuracy.

8. Latent periods vary according to the induced tumor. At least two patterns of latent periods for radiation-induced cancer have been described. The first, exemplified by the risk of leukemia in atomic bomb survivors, consists of an early wave-like pulse of increased risk followed by a gradual decline to baseline levels. The second, more typical of solid tumors, is an increase in RR of SMN over many years, which remains constant over time thereafter. The latter pattern suggests that a multievent pattern of carcinogenesis is involved where the initiating initial event (radiation) is followed by promoting events (i.e., smoking, alcohol, environmental exposures) over many years (66). Regardless of the age at the time of exposure, radiation-induced solid tumors often occur later in life at the same times as spontaneous tumors of the same type (1,27,67). Long latent periods complicate the study of radiation-induced cancer, because the presence of other carcinogens or disease processes may not be well-documented.

9. It follows, from point 8, that the duration of follow-up for any study population influences the frequency of tumors seen.

10. It is unclear whether the risk of tumor development following exposure is simply an absolute increase that is proportional to the radiation dose, or a relative increase that builds on an underlying spontaneous risk (greater for some individuals) of developing a malignancy.

11. Age is a critical factor in determining radiation risk. In children, the most frequently observed second cancers occur in tissues undergoing rapid proliferation such as bone and thyroid. An actively proliferating tissue may

be more susceptible to malignant transformation in any single cell because of the increased number of cell divisions. This might explain the higher frequency of secondary bone tumors in children as compared to adults (5,68). Childhood cancer survivors are prone to develop leukemias or sarcomas, whereas secondarily induced embryonal tumors are rare. Some cancers tend to aggregate in families, with specific constellations of tumor types observed (e.g., adenocarcinomas or sarcomas) (69,70). Some inherited syndromes clearly predispose patients to the development of second tumors (71). Patients with the nevoid basal cell carcinoma syndrome who are irradiated for medulloblastoma develop skin cancers in the irradiated fields 6 months to 3 years later (see Chapter 18.) Children with ataxia-telangiectasia may be more prone to irradiation-induced malignancies.

SECONDARY TUMORS IN SURVIVORS OF CHILDHOOD MALIGNANCY

Several large series and dozens of smaller reports document the frequency of SMN in childhood cancer survivors. A major series comes from the Late Effects Study Group (LESG) (5,6,9–12,72). Three hundred and eight secondary malignancies occurred in 353 children (Table 1). The most common first tumor was retinoblastoma (16%), followed by Hodgkin's disease (14%), soft-tissue sarcoma (12%), and Wilms' tumor (11%). Approximately two-thirds of the SMN are associated with prior radiotherapy. For bone sarcomas, a clear dose-response relationship was noted, with RRs ranging from 6 after 10 to 30 Gy to 21 for 40 to 60 Gy, and 38 for more than 60 Gy. There also appears to be an alkylating agent dose-response curve for leukemia as an SMN. Increasing doses of procarbazine, nitrogen mustard, cyclophosphamide, chlorambucil, and CCNU were associated with progressively increasing RRs of induced leukemia. The interval between tumors ranged from less than 1 month to 34 years, with a median of 10 years for patients whose SMN developed in irradiated fields and 5

TABLE 1. *Distribution of first and second malignant neoplasms in the Late Effects Study Group*

First neoplasm			Second, third, and fourth neoplasms		
				RT-associated	No RT
Retinoblastoma	52	17%	Bone sarcomas	52	15
Hodgkin's disease	40	14%	Soft-tissue sarcomas	43	16
Soft tissue sarcoma	40	14%	Leukemia/lymphoma	36	23
Wilms' tumor	36	12%	Skin cancer	19	11[a]
Brain tumor	31	11%	Brain tumors	13	15
Neuroblastoma	28	9%	Thyroid cancer	24	2
Bone sarcomas	18	6%	Breast	9	4
Leukemias	13	4%	Others	12	12
Non-Hodgkins Lymphoma	12	4%			
Other	22	9%			
Total	292			208	98

Modified from ref. 11, with permission.
[a]RT status unknown for some patients.

years for those unassociated with radiotherapy. In most reports the likelihood of developing an SMN increases with time from treatment of the first tumor.

The Childhood Cancer Research Group in Oxford has examined the risk of a second primary tumor in about 10,000 children (3,71). The cumulative risk of a second primary tumor by 25 years following a 3-year survival was $3.7 \pm 0.8\%$. Exclusive of retinoblastoma, this is a risk of 4.5 times that expected. The increased risk following surgery alone was 3.9, following radiotherapy alone 5.6, and after both radiotherapy and chemotherapy 9.3 (Table 2). About 75% of SMN following radiotherapy arose in or at the edge of the irradiated tissues. Bone tumors were more likely to occur after doses of 50 Gy or more. The Oxford Study found an excess of second primary tumors occurring in bone, thyroid, connective tissue, digestive tract, central nervous system (CNS), and leukemia (Table 3). There seems to be an increase in the number of leukemias as second primary tumors in recent

years. This may be related to the increased use of cytotoxic chemotherapy (Table 4).

The German Registry of Childhood malignancies, established in 1980, has recorded 329 patients with SMN. The registry data is summarized in Table 5. The most common primary/secondary tumor combinations were acute lymphoblastic leukemia (ALL)/CNS tumor (9% of all SMN), CNS tumor/CNS tumor (6%), retinoblastoma/osteosarcoma (5%), ALL/acute nonlymphoblastic leukemia (ANLL) (3%), ALL/Hodgkin's disease (3%) (73).

A cohort study of 13,175 3-year survivors of childhood cancer in Great Britain diagnosed between 1940 and 1983 identified 55 subsequent bone cancers. The percentage of 3-year survivors developing a bone cancer as an SMN was 0.9% (Table 6). Retinoblastoma patients and Ewing's sarcoma patients were at particularly high risk. The risk of bone cancer increased substantially with increasing doses of radiation and alkylating agents (74).

The frequency and type of SMN varies according to the primary malignancy.

TABLE 2. *Risk of SMN for 3-year survivors of childhood cancer—except retinoblastoma: the association with treatment observed in the Oxford Study*

Treatment follow-up (yrs)	n	Mean follow-up (yrs)	SMN	Percentage of SMN by specified time from 3-yr survival
Surgery	1495	9.5	10	$1.6 \pm 0.9\%$ (20 yrs)
Radiotherapy	2668	9.8	40	$2.7 \pm 0.8\%$ (20 yrs)
Radiotherapy and chemotherapy	2699	3.8	11	$0.6 \pm 0.7\%$ (10 yrs)

Data were taken from refs. 3, 71.

TABLE 3. *Relative risk of SMN among 9,279 3-yr survivors of childhood cancer in the Oxford Study—except retinoblastoma*

SMN	n	Observed/expected
All sites	50[a]	4.5
Bone	10	17.7
Thyroid	3	16
Connective tissue	5	14.4
Digestive	7	9.5
CNS	10	6.8
Leukemia	6	3.8
Breast	2	2.3
Genitourinary	4	1.9

[a]The site is not specified in three cases.
Data were taken from refs. 3, 71.

Retinoblastoma

In familial retinoblastoma the affected child inherits the mutant, loss-of-function tumor suppressor gene from one parent. A somatic mutation occurs in a normal allele inherited from the other parent. It appears that the frequency of the second mutational event is high. In sporadic retinoblastoma, two mutational events occur in the tumor suppressor genes of both alleles. The existence of the retinoblastoma gene (RB-1) abnormality seems to create a malignant diathesis so that children with heritable retinoblastoma develop bilateral, multifocal retinoblastoma in infancy and are at risk for SMN later in life (20,75). A variety of different tumors contain inactivated RB alleles; these tumors include sporadic sarcomas, sarcomas arising as SMN in familial retinoblastoma patients, and some cases of adult bladder, breast, and small-cell lung cancer (20,76). The occurrence of second nonocular malignancies in patients successfully treated for retinoblastoma has been recognized for several decades (77). Retinoblastoma accounts for not more than 3% of pediatric malignancies, but 16% of childhood SMNs registered by the LESG occurred in children with the initial diagnosis of retinoblastoma (5,6,10,11).

The incidence of SMN in heritable retinoblastoma (bilateral cases or unilateral cases with a positive family history) for irradiated patients in a 1984 evaluation of the Cornell/Columbia series was 20% at 10 years, 50% at 20 years, and 90% at 30 years. For patients who received no radiotherapy or who developed SMN outside of the radiation fields, the corresponding incidences were 10%, 30%, and 68% (78,79). Draper et al. (80) reported cumulative risks of SMN of 4% and 8% at 12 and 18 years, whereas Smith et al. (81,82) found SMN cumulative risks of 6% at 10 years, 19% at 20 years, and 38% at 30 years. Tucker et al. (64) found an SMN risk of 14% at 20 years.

A comprehensive evaluation of SMN in retinoblastoma patients was published in 1993 by Eng et al. (83), and was expanded and updated by Wong et al. in 1997 (84). A total of 1,804 retinoblastoma patients from Columbia-Presbyterian Hospital, New York Hospital-Cornell Medical Center, Massachusetts General Hospital, Massachusetts Eye and Ear Infirmary, Children's Hospital of Boston, and the Dana–Farber Cancer Institute were reviewed—including patients treated as early as 1914. The

TABLE 4. *Cross-tabulation of first and second tumors in the Oxford Study*

Second	Osteosarcoma	CNS	Skin	Leukemia	Soft-tissue sarcoma	Carcinoma	Lymphoma	Other	Total
First tumor diagnosed before 1969									
CNS	1	12	7	1	6	7	1	2	37
Retinoblastoma	16	5	3	0	5	5	0	2	36
Acute leukemia	0	0	0	0	0	0	0	0	0
Wilms'	2	0	2	1	2	5	1	0	13
Hodgkin's	1	1	2	0	0	1	1	0	6
Non-Hodgkin's	0	0	0	0	0	1	0	0	1
Other	2	4	5	1	1	8	0	7	28
Total	22	22	19	3	14	27	3	11	121

From refs. 3, 71, with permission.

TABLE 5. *Second malignant neoplasms in the German Registry of Childhood Malignancies*

Primary tumor		Secondary tumor	
ALL	29%	CNS tumor	20%
CNS tumor	12%	ANLL	13%
Retinoblastoma	9%	Osteosarcoma	11%
Hodgkin's Disease	8%	Soft-tissue sarcoma	6%
Rhabdomyosarcoma	5%	Non-Hodgkin's lymphoma	5%

From ref. 73, with permission.

most common SMN were bone sarcomas, soft-tissue sarcomas, melanoma, and nasal cavity tumors. The RR for development of a second tumor was much higher among patients with hereditary retinoblastoma (RR = 30) than among those with nonhereditary disease (RR = 1.6). At 50 years of follow-up, the cumulative incidence for all second neoplasms was $51 \pm 6.2\%$ for the hereditary group and $5 \pm 3.0\%$ for the nonhereditary group. Among bilateral retinoblastoma patients, cumulative mortality from second neoplasms at 40 years follow-up was 30% for irradiated patients versus 6% for those who did not receive irradiation. Significant excess mortality was found for (a) SMN of bone, connective tissue, and brain, (b) malignant melanoma, and (c) benign neoplasm of the brain and meninges.

The literature gives only slight attention to the role chemotherapy plays in the induction of SMN in retinoblastoma survivors. Draper, Sanders, and Kingston of the Childhood Cancer Research Group of the United Kingdom reviewed the records of children with retinoblastoma from cancer registries and hospitals in England, Scotland, and Wales from 1962 to 1977 and identified 882 patients. Thirty patients developed SMN. The estimated incidence rate of SMN 12 years after diagnosis of retinoblastoma was 4.2% for children treated with radiotherapy plus chemotherapy versus 2.9% for those not given chemotherapy. The rates for SMN outside the radiation field (and including patients who received no radiation) was 4.6% with chemotherapy versus 1.0% without. The overall difference in the incidence of SMN for patients with and without chemotherapy was significant ($p < 0.05$) by one-tailed test (67). In a subsequent study, which included retinoblastoma patients and those with other primary tumors, the risk of secondary bone malignancies was correlated with the extent of exposure to alkylating agents (74).

TABLE 6. *Risk of development of a secondary bone cancer by the type of first cancer: a cohort study using population data from the National Registry of Childhood Cancer, United Kingdom*

First cancer	% with bone cancer by 20 yrs from 3-yr survival
Retinoblastoma	3.5%
Heritable retinoblastoma	7.2%
Nonheritable retinoblastoma	0.3%
All childhood cancers except retinoblastoma	0.5%
Leukemia	0.1%
Hodgkin's disease	0.5%
Non-Hodgkin's disease	0.4%
CNS tumors	0.2%
Wilms' tumor	0.9%
Ewing's sarcoma of bone	5.4%
Other malignant bone cancers	2.4%
Soft-tissue sarcomas	0.9%
Other nonretinoblastoma cancers	0.9%
All childhood cancers	0.9%

From ref. 74, with permission.

The available evidence indicates an extraordinarily increased risk of SMN in heritable retinoblastoma with exacerbation, by radiation and chemotherapy, of the malignant diathesis (3,8,80,85). The risk of SMN in retinoblastoma is additionally considered in Chapter 5. The reader is directed to that chapter with particular attention to figures that demonstrate the cumulative risk of SMN.

Ewing's Sarcoma

Bone sarcoma is the most common SMN in survivors of Ewing's sarcoma (86). There is substantial variation in the data concerning RR of SMN in survivors of Ewing's sarcoma (8,22,70,81,82,87,88). The cumulative incidence of an SMN in a population of 266 survivors of Ewing's sarcoma was 5% at 10 years and 9% at 20 years postinitial diagnosis. The most common SMNs were osteosarcoma (5 of 16), soft-tissue sarcoma (5 of 16), and leukemia (2 of 16) (89,90) (Tables 7 and 8).

Occasional cases of breast cancer have developed years after elective whole-lung irradiation of children with osteogenic or Ewing's sarcoma. As previously noted, female breast tissue in children is particularly susceptible to the carcinogenic effects of radiation (91).

Soft-Tissue Sarcoma

The local managment of soft-tissue sarcomas in children generally involves surgery and frequently includes radiotherapy. Multi-

TABLE 7. *Relationship between treatment factors and the risk of second malignant neoplasms in Ewing's sarcoma*

Feature	p	
	All second malignancies	Secondary sarcomas
Exposure to cyclophosphamide	0.17	0.63
Doxorubicin	0.055	0.35
Dactinomycin	0.28	0.56
Alkylating agents	0.21	0.73
Radiation dose	0.043	0.002

From ref. 89, 90, with permission.

TABLE 8. *Risk of a secondary sarcoma in Ewing's sarcoma patients as a function of radiation dose to the primary tumor*

Radiation dose	Secondary sarcoma cases per 10,000 person-years	20-yr cumulative incidence
0–47.99 Gy	0	0
48–59.99 Gy	24.9	5%
≥60 Gy	131	22%

From ref. 89, 90, with permission.

agent chemotherapy is administered for the treatment of rhabdomyosarcoma and Adriamycin-containing programs are administered for nonrhabdomyosarcoma soft-tissue sarcomas. It is not surprising that SMN may follow such treatment. Twenty SMNs were identified from the population of children treated at M.D. Anderson Cancer Center, Houston, for primary soft-tissue sarcoma from 1961 to 1990 (92). The details of the primary tumors and SMN are shown in Table 9.

Wilms' Tumor

The incidence of SMN has been investigated for patients enrolled in SIOP Wilms' tumor studies 1, 2, 5, and 6. The RR was 4.15

TABLE 9. *Second malignant neoplasms following treatment of soft-tissue sarcomas at M.D. Anderson Cancer Center[a]*

Primary tumors	Second tumors with latent period of 1–33 yrs
Rhabdomyosarcoma 14 (70%)	Osteosarcoma 5[b]
Fibrosarcoma 3 (15%)	Primary brain tumors 3
Synovial sarcoma 2 (10%)	Leukemia 2
Angiosarcoma 1 (5%)	Soft tissue sarcoma 3
	Breast cancer 1
	Testicular cancer 1
	Thyroid cancer 1
	Neuroblastoma 1
	Lymphoma 1
	Renal cell carcinoma 1
	Chondrosarcoma 1[b]

From ref. 92, with permission.
[a]4 treated with surgery alone, 3 with surgery + chemotherapy, 3 with surgery + radiotherapy, 10 with surgery + chemotherapy + radiotherapy.
[b]4 of these 6 tumors developed in the radiotherapy field.

for SMN with a 15-year cumulative incidence of SMN of 0.65% (93). A National Wilms' Tumor Study review found that the observed expected RR ratio for SMN in Wilms' tumor survivors was 8.4. Children who received Adriamycin 35 Gy or more of irradiation had a RR ratio of 36.3 (94). Hawkins et al. (71,74) reported cumulative risks of 3% to 6% for SMN at 20 years following therapy. The majority of SMNs occur within an irradiated field. In patients receiving radiotherapy but no chemotherapy, the RR of SMN is 12 (3,60,71). The LESG reported a higher overall RR of 24, with most SMNs seen in the thyroid gland, bone, connective tissue, gastrointestinal tract, CNS, or bone marrow (leukemia) (10,95). Children with bilateral Wilms' tumor, certain congenital anomalies, or histologic variants may have an even higher risk. Two of six patients with bilateral disease were affected in one report (14,96). Breast cancer and colonic adenocarcinoma have been the subject of specific reports (17,43, 97,98).

Leukemia

Five, 10, and 15 years after the diagnosis of ALL, the risk of SMN is 0.3%, 1.5%, and 2.5%, respectively. Among the SMNs are CNS tumors (particularly in patients treated with cranial irradiation), lymphomas, AML (particularly in patients treated with etoposide), thyroid cancer, and Ewing's sarcoma (63,51,99,100). In the Children's Cancer Study Group report, all the CNS SMNs occurred in patients who had received cranial irradiation, and about one-half of the non-CNS SMNs occurred in previously irradiated fields. In a series of 9,720 children treated for ALL, 24 developed CNS SMN after cranial irradiation (101,102). Of 1,705 children treated at St. Jude Children's Research Hospital for newly diagnosed ALL, 15 developed brain tumors 4.7 to 25 years after radiotherapy (103).

The occurrence of an SMN in the ALL patient may depend on other factors besides therapy. Associations between childhood CNS tumors and hematopoietic neoplasms have been reported; for example, there is an increased risk of hematopoietic neoplasms among siblings of medulloblastoma and other CNS tumor patients. Because older ALL protocols used cranial irradiation more frequently than did recent protocols, there is a longer duration of follow-up for irradiated patients and, therefore, probably a higher incidence of SMN (3,86,102,104,105). The median time to development of a CNS tumor following the diagnosis of ALL is 6 years. In contrast, brain SMNs in patients irradiated for tinea capitis, CNS tumors, and vascular nevi usually occur more than 10 years after exposure (1,106).

Hodgkin's Disease

Dramatic advances in the treatment of pediatric Hodgkin's disease over the past 40 years have resulted in many long-term survivors. The actuarial 10-year survival rate in early-stage disease is 85% to 97%, and in advanced-stage disease it is 70% to 90%. Ironically, however, the cure of Hodgkin's disease is a hollow victory for many who subsequently develop an SMN, which is frequently fatal, or at least associated with morbidity. In 1989, the Late Effects Study Group (LESG) estimated that the cumulative probability of an SMN 20 years following the diagnosis of Hodgkin's disease was 16% for developing a solid tumor and 4% for leukemia (68). The data from the Late Effects Study Group assessment of SMN following treatment for Hodgkin's disease has been published several times (5,6,9–12,72). A 1996 report extended the median follow-up for the study cohort from 7 to 11.4 years and increased the size of the cohort from 979 to 1,380 patients. The SMN included 56 solid tumors, 26 leukemias, and 6 non-Hodgkin's lymphomas. Breast cancer was the most common solid tumor, occurring in 17 patients. Table 10 shows the observed cases/expected cases ratio for the various SMN. There were significantly elevated RRs for all cancers combined, for leukemia, non-Hodgkin's lymphoma, breast,

TABLE 10. *The observed cases to expected cases ratio of second cancers in survivors of childhood Hodgkin's disease in the Late Effects Study Group Cohort*

	Cohort
Type or Site of Second Cancer	Observed Cases to Expected Cases Ratio
All second malignant neoplasms	18.1
Leukemia	78.3
Acute myelogenous leukemia	321.3
Non-Hodgkin's lymphoma	20.9
All solid tumors	11.8
Breast cancer (cohort only includes women)	75.3
Thyroid cancer	32.7
Bone tumors	24.6
Brain tumors	10.5
Colorectal cancer	38.9
Gastric carcinoma	121.3

Modified from ref. 9, with permission.

thyroid, bone, brain, colorectal, and gastric cancers. While radiation did not appear to play a role in the development of leukemia as an SMN (Table 11), radiation was implicated in the development of solid tumors and non-Hodgkin's lymphoma. Of the 17 breast cancer, 16 appeared within or at the margin of a radiation field. Multivariate analysis showed that age of over 10 years at the time of diagnosis of Hodgkin's disease was independently associated with increased risk of breast cancer as was increasing dose of radiation (compared with a radiation dose of less than 20 Gy, the RR of 20 to 40 Gy was 5.9 and for greater than 40 Gy it was 23.7) (9). The risk of leukemia/lymphoma was significantly greater

($p = 0.004$) in patients treated with alkylating agents (Fig. 3).

At the Children's Hospital of Boston, Dana–Farber Cancer Institute, and Harvard Joint Center for Radiation Therapy, 191 patients 16 years of age or younger were followed. Seventeen patients developed SMN including: gastric, 3; breast, 4; thyroid, 1; tonsil, 1; tongue, 1; sarcoma, 1; lung mesothelioma, 1; skin, 3; leukemia, 1; and non-Hodgkin's lymphoma, 1. All the solid tumors arose within or next to radiation fields. The cumulative incidence of SMN (excluding two cases of basal cell carcinoma) at 15 years was 5% in male and 24% in female patients. The use of chemotherapy and female sex were signifi-

TABLE 11. *Risk of second cancers according to the type of treatment of Hodgkin's disease in the Late Effects Study Group Cohort*

Type of cancer and treatment	Cumluative probability of occurrence at 15 yrs
Leukemia	
Radiation	0%
Chemotherapy	7.9%
Radiation + chemotherapy	3.4%
Non-Hodgkin's lymphoma	
Radiation	0.4%
Chemotherapy	0%
Radiation + chemotherapy	0.9%
Solid tumors	
Radiation	3.3%
Chemotherapy	2.9%
Radiation + chemotherapy	4.6%

Modified from ref. 9, with permission.

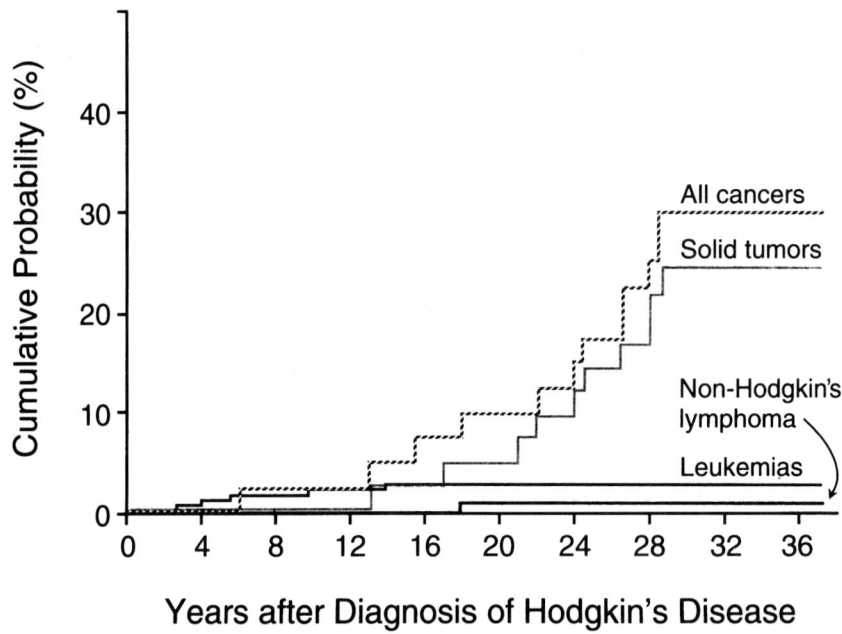

FIG. 3. Cumulative probability of second malignant neoplasms in 1,380 children younger than 16 years of age when their Hodgkin's disease was diagnosed and who received their primary treatment between 1955 and 1986. The median follow-up for the cohort is 11.4 years. (From ref. 9, with permission.)

cant risk factors for SMN in multivariate analysis (107).

Four hundred seventy-eight Hodgkin's disease patients were treated with chemotherapy, RT, or a combination thereof over a 35-year span (1954 to 1989) at the University of Rochester Cancer Center. The status of 97% of patients was established through chart review and/or telephone contact, and 30% of these patients have been followed for greater than 15 years. Observed-to-expected incidence ratios (OER) were calculated using age and sex-adjusted incidence rates from the NCI SEER data for 1973 to 1988. Forty-eight patients developed an SMN for a crude incidence of 10% with a significant OER of 4.47. In patients that received any RT, 75% of the SMN occurred within or near (2 cm) the radiation portal. SMN OER was most elevated between 5 to 10 years and 15 to 20 years following diagnosis. When analyzed by treatment groups, SMN OER was significantly elevated in the RT and RT plus multiagent

chemotherapy groups. The median survival for the entire Hodgkin's disease population was 22.1 years. The median survival following the diagnosis of SMN was 1.5 years.

A subset of patients who were treated as children was evaluated separately. One-hundred fifty six children (less than 20 years old) were treated for Hodgkin's disease between 1954 to 1989, and 151 had their status determined by documentation of death, follow-up examination within the past 15 months, or telephone contact. Treatment strategies have varied, but included radiotherapy alone (33.8%), combined RT and chemotherapy (60.9%), and chemotherapy alone (5.3%). Nine patients have developed SMN at a mean time of 13.1 years (range 6.5 to 29.3 years); 4 of these SMNs occurred at over 18 years after Hodgkin's disease diagnosis. The SMNs included thyroid carcinoma, 2; sarcoma, 2; meningioma, 1; spinal cord astrocytoma, 1; breast cancer, 1; non-Hodgkin's lymphoma, 1; and acute myelogenous leukemia, 1. Eight of the 9 affected patients were female, and their observed to expected risk was 17.4 (vs. 3.04 for males). Four SMNs developed in the RT field, 2 at its margin (<2cm), 1 outside of the field, and for 2 this was nonapplicable. Two SMNs occurred after RT alone, and 7 after RT plus chemotherapy.

Medical records of 499 Hodgkin's disease patients treated between 1962 and 1993 at St. Jude Children's Research Hospital were reviewed with a median follow up of 9 years. The majority of patients were treated with combined radiation and chemotherapy, while 123 received radiation alone, and 30 received chemotherapy only. Twenty-five patients developed a second malignancy (19 solid tumors, 4 ANLL, 1 non-Hodgkin's lymphoma, and 1 chronic myeloid leukemia). Twenty-three out of the 25 SMNs occurred in the 10 years of age or older group, suggesting a higher risk among adolescents treated for Hodgkin's disease. In addition, SMNs were more common among females, even when breast cancer was excluded ($p = 0.007$), and in those patients treated for recurrent Hodgkin's disease ($p = 0.02$). There was no difference between the treatment modalities for radiation alone, chemotherapy only, and the combined therapy groups (107a).

Essentially, all children who develop secondary leukemia die, as do approximately 50% of those developing non-Hodgkin's lymphoma. Although children who develop secondary solid tumors are more curable, substantial morbidity can ensue. Overall, the risk of death from an SMN surpasses the risk for death from Hodgkin's disease in subgroups of patients (108,109).

The three major categories of SMNs following Hodgkin's disease are acute leukemia (25%), non-Hodgkin's lymphoma (17%), and solid tumors (58%) (57,78,110). In the LESG report, the RR of leukemia and non-Hodgkin's lymphoma stabilized at 4% at 17 years; however, the cumulative incidence of solid tumors progressively increased with time (111). The risk of leukemia is predominantly within the first 10 years of initial therapy. In contrast, most solid tumors occur after

10 years though few reports provide follow-up data exceeding 10 to 15 years (112–115). Consequently, a minimum 20-year follow-up is necessary to accurately assess the true incidence of solid tumors. Most reports on SMNs, including those from the LESG, suffer from bias or selectivity in the patients from whom data is captured in that many patients are lost to follow-up. Other weaknesses in most reports include the limited number of patients studied, and uncertainty or a lack of information on treatment specifics including radiation volumes and doses, and chemotherapeutic agents, doses, and schedules.

Specific characteristics of SMNs following Hodgkin's disease are now discussed.

Acute Leukemia

Secondary hematological malignancies present as acute nonlymphoblastic leukemias (ANLL) or myelodysplastic syndromes that confer an almost uniformly fatal outcome. In 1972, Arseneau et al. (54) reported the occurrence of ANLL following treatment for Hodgkin's disease. Subsequently, many studies have shown that the overall 10-year cumulative incidence rates range from 1.5% to 10%. In addition, the overall risk of leukemia varied from 0.5% to 2.0% per year during the first 10 years following treatment and plateaued thereafter.

The type and intensity of Hodgkin's disease therapy are relevant to the development of ANLL. RT in isolation does not appear to be leukemogenic (116,117). The International Database on Hodgkin's Disease (IDHD) demonstrated that the cumulative risk of leukemia following radiation therapy (RT) alone was approximately 0.4% (113). However, in patients treated with MOPP (mechlorethamine, vincristine, procarbazine, and prednisone) chemotherapy only the RR was 2.2, ($p < 0.05$), and in patients treated with combined modality therapy (CMT) the RR was 17.1 ($p < 0.001$). Blayney and co-workers (55) at the National Cancer Institute showed that 11 out of 12 patients developing ANLL had received CMT. In contrast, the British National Lymphoma Investigation showed no differences in the cumulative incidence rates between patients receiving chemotherapy alone as compared to patients treated with CMT (118). Several studies involving large populations with Hodgkin's disease showed no significant differences in the risk of leukemia among patients treated with chemotherapy only or CMT (116,119,120), whereas other reports indicate the converse (110,121). Any additional risk in these reports may be a consequence of the cumulative effects of the extent (volume and dose) of RT, duration and doses of chemotherapy, and the numbers and types of salvage regimens, rather than specific leukemogenic effects of radiotherapy.

Human and animal studies demonstrate that alkylating agents such as those contained in MOPP, MVPP (vinblastine is substituted for vincristine), and nitrosourea-containing combinations are frequently associated with secondary leukemias. Moreover, mechlorethamine has been implicated as a major leukemogenic agent. Van Leeuwen and colleagues (116) showed an increased risk of leukemia when more than 6 cycles of MOPP were administered in comparison to 6 cycles or less. Accordingly, Schellong et al. (122) from the German-Austrian Pediatric Hodgkin's Disease Group, have used chemoradiation without mechlorethamine since 1978, and observed only 5 cases of secondary hematological malignancies in 667 patients with an estimated cumulative risk at 15 years of 1.1% (95% CI, 0.0 to 2.2). In addition, the bone marrow damage induced by MOPP, which can cause a prolonged or chronic thrombocytopenia, may also be associated with an increased risk of leukemia. In comparison, the ABVD (Adriamycin, bleomycin, vinblastine, and dacarbazine) chemotherapeutic regimen has a low leukemic potential (116,123). Valagussa and co-workers (124) showed that in 15 years after treatment for Hodgkin's disease, only one case of leukemia developed following ABVD and RT with a cumulative risk of 0.7% versus a 9.5% risk after MOPP and RT ($p = 0.04$).

In addition to treatment modalities, two other factors have been associated with an increased risk of hematological malignancy, specifically, age at diagnosis of Hodgkin's disease and splenectomy. Patients older than 40 years of age are at increased risk for developing leukemia, as supported by the IDHD, which showed RRs of 2.5 for 40 to 49 years ($p < 0.01$), 3.99 for 50 to 59 years ($p < 0.001$), and 4.49 for 60 years and older ($p < 0.001$) (113).

The relationship of splenectomy to secondary ANLL remains controversial (113, 116,120,125,126). Van Leeuwen and colleagues (127) reported a higher frequency of leukemia in splenectomized patients with RRs ranging from 1.3 to 14. However, this wide variation suggests that other modifying risk factors may be involved. Moreover, it has been postulated that asplenia may have an integral role on tumor immuno-surveillance. Nevertheless, the original and updated LESG reports showed that splenectomy was not a significant risk variable for SMNs (9,68).

Non-Hodgkin's Lymphoma

The cumulative risk for secondary non-Hodgkin's lymphoma (NHL) following treatment for Hodgkin's disease varies between 1.1% and 2.1% at 15 years (9,112,117). In the updated LESG report, the risk plateaued at 1.1% (RR 20.9), and the only significant independent risk factor was the amount of alkylating agent used (9). In contrast to secondary acute leukemia, NHL is more commonly curable, although 4 of 6 affected children in the LESG report died of NHL. Other risk factors associated with the development of NHL include older age at treatment, male gender, and the use of CMT. Mauch et al. (115) observed an increased absolute excess risk of greater than 3-fold for patients over 40 years of age, a 3.1-fold greater risk for men, and a 1.5-fold elevated risk for patients receiving CMT. Although the mechanism remains unknown, the pathogenesis for developing secondary NHL may be related to the altered immunocompetence associated with Hodgkin's disease and its treatment, because NHL commonly occurs in immunodeficient patients associated with organ transplantation, genetic etiologies, or HIV infection (128).

Solid Tumors

Secondary solid tumors comprise over 50% of SMNs following the treatment for Hodgkin's disease. The interval from therapy is prolonged at 10 to 15 years, and the potential for survival is greater than for either secondary ANLL or NHL. Breast cancer is most common, followed by thyroid, skin, bone, brain, and gastrointestinal cancers. However, all histologic subtypes have been reported. In the IDHD, the risk of solid cancers continued to persist and increase after 20 years (113). The Late Effects Study Group estimated that the cumulative probability was 16% for developing a solid cancer 20 years after the diagnosis of Hodgkin's disease, and only 10 of 56 affected patients (18%) died of the secondary solid tumor (and 7 additional patients died of an accident) (68). Few studies report greater than 15 year follow-up data, and the relationship between age, gender, treatment and the risk for solid tumors requires additional study. Available data does suggest a preponderance of females, likely due to the high frequency of breast cancer, and an association with older age and CMT.

Breast Cancer

Historically, an elevated risk of breast cancer has been reported in women exposed to radiation from atomic bomb explosions, multiple chest radiographs, and treatment of postpartum mastitis (129–131). Several large cohort series have reported RRs of breast cancer ranging from 1.5 to 2.1 in women receiving mantle irradiation for Hodgkin's disease (19,54,112). The Stanford experience, involving 885 patients, revealed a 4-fold increased risk for developing breast carcinoma and a 5-fold increased risk of mortality (108). The majority of breast cancers were infiltrating ductal carcinomas occurring within or at the margin of the radiation fields. Age at the time of treatment was associated with an increased risk; women who were irradiated before the age of 20 years had a 33-fold increased risk in comparison to no excess risk in women older than 30 years of age receiving treatment. Additionally, a higher risk was associated with a longer time interval from treatment with the most dramatic risk increases seen in women with greater than 15 years of follow-up. In addition, the RR within 15 years of treatment was 6.3 for women treated with MOPP and RT as compared to an RR of 0.8 in patients undergoing RT alone. After 15 years, the risks were equivalent for the combined treatment group and the radiation only groups.

Bhatia and colleagues (9), found that the women in their cohort had a 75 times greater risk of breast cancer than the general population with an estimated cumulative risk approximating 35% at 40 years of age. However, the results of this study have been criticized for bias or selectivity in patient follow-up and for overestimating the risk of breast cancer by using standardized incidence ratios and RR measurements. Accordingly, when utilizing standardized incidence ratios, the low incidence of cancers in a specified age group for the study group and the general population must be kept in the proper perspective (108,132). For example, the average risk of developing breast cancer between 20 to 30 years of age is 0.04%. However, if the RR for breast cancer in a woman treated for Hodgkin's disease is 39, then the absolute risk is actually 39 × 0.04%, or 1.6%, which is comparable to the risk in an average 45-year-old woman. Assessing absolute and RR in the correct context becomes increasingly important when cancers occur late during the follow-up period and long-term surveillance is not achieved. Consequently, any single event may magnify a percent change. In an editorial on this report, Donaldson and Hancock (133) calculated the absolute risk, or annual excess risk, for the same cohort of patients and found that the incidence of breast cancer was significantly lower than reported. Subsequently, in an editorial reply, Bhatia et al. (9) analyzed the absolute risk of their patients and found risk estimates of 1.6% and 3.2% at 15 and 30 years, respectively.

Proliferating breast tissue in adolescent and young women is most sensitive to the ionizing effects of radiation. Previous studies have indicated that radiation-related breast cancer is greatest after treatment during the pubescent years (10- to 14-years old) (134,135). Moreover, there usually is a 15- to 20-year latency period before breast carcinoma appears, suggesting the necessary long-term follow-up needed to delineate secondary breast cancer. Additionally, other well-known risk factors including family history, age at first pregnancy, onset of menarche/menopause, and exogenous estrogen use must be considered before accurately assessing breast cancer risk.

Lung Cancer

The incidence of lung cancer has been routinely reported in virtually all studies of SMN (68,111,113,118,134). The RRs commonly range from 2.6% to 7.7%. Consistently, the development of lung cancer occurred in patients older than 40 years of age who had a history of cigarette smoking and mantle irradiation. The clear increase in risk of lung cancer over time suggests radiation-related carcinogenesis. This is additionally supported by a report by Kaldor et al. (134) who observed that higher lung irradiation doses were associated with a high risk for lung cancer. In addition, they found that the RR for developing lung cancer was 1.0% for patients receiving RT alone, 1.9% for chemotherapy alone, and 0.5% for combined modality therapy. They attributed the lower risk in the combined modality therapy group to fewer cycles of chemotherapy administered, although decreased RT doses in this patient group may also be significant.

Thyroid Cancer

An increased risk of thyroid cancer has been observed in patients receiving mantle or cervical radiation. The RRs range from 2.4 to 16 (109,113). Age at RT is a well-known risk factor for developing thyroid cancer; the risk is 68 times greater for children treated for Hodgkin's disease as compared to a 16-fold risk among adults. Additionally, increasing RT doses are associated with an increased risk. Because most children are currently treated with lower RT doses for Hodgkin's disease than in previous eras, the risk for thyroid cancer may be diminished. The relationship between thyroid replacement therapy for patients with radiation-induced hypothyroidism might be expected to mitigate the risk for the development of thyroid cancer. One hundred fifty-three children with Hodgkin's disease received therapeutic neck irradiation at St. Jude Children's Research Hospital and were followed for thyroid neoplasia. There were 5 cases of thyroid neoplasms (3%): 2 carcinomas, 2 colloid nodules, and 2 unbiopsied nodules (41). Twenty-one pediatric Hodgkin's disease patients were followed at M.D. Anderson Hospital for 50 to 276 months. While many of these patients had abnormal thyroid ultrasounds (11 of 21), no thyroid SMNs were found (136).

Gastrointestinal Cancer

Several reports have observed moderately increased frequencies of gastrointestinal (GI) cancers while others have not (68,111, 113,137). In a meta-analysis involving 10,472 patients, Boivin et al. (111) showed an RR of 1.8 (95% CI, 1.4 to 2.7) for digestive tract cancers. Regarding site specificity, the British National Lymphoma Investigation (118) reported an RR of 1.3% for gastric carcinomas. Similarly, the Norwegian Cancer Registry (112) and the Netherlands Cancer Registry (118) showed risks for stomach cancers of 2.0 and 1.6, respectively. The risk for pancreatic cancer was 1.7%. The International Database on Hodgkin's Disease reported RRs for small intestine cancers of 9.6% for males, but the risk for females was not elevated (113). However, the significantly high risk of small intestine cancer may reflect the extremely low incidence of these malignancies in the general population. Risks for colon cancer have been reported by the British National Lymphoma Investigation, the International Database on Hodgkin's Disease, and the Netherlands Cancer Registry as 3.2%, 2.5%, and 1.9%, respectively.

In a recent study from Stanford involving 2,441 patients, Birdwell et al. (138) showed that the greatest risk for GI cancer was in the younger age at the time of treatment group (less than 45 years old). Risk was significantly increased within 10 years of treatment for Hodgkin's disease, and was the highest after 20 years. GI sites at the highest risks included the stomach, small intestine, and pancreas. Moreover, patients treated with combined modality therapy for Hodgkin's disease were at modestly elevated risk for secondary digestive tract cancers. This increased risk following combined treatment was noted regardless of whether initial treatment was combined modality therapy or RT alone followed by chemotherapy for relapse. The risk was not increased after chemotherapy or radiotherapy alone.

NEUROBLASTOMA

Thirteen children with POG stage C neuroblastoma were treated at Duke University Medical Center from 1960 to 1995. Two of the three patients followed for over 20 years developed SMN—a dermatofibrosarcoma and an undifferentiated sarcoma. One SMN was clearly in the radiotherapy field and one possibly in the field (139). The Late Effects Study Group data on SMN in 28 neuroblastoma patients included 11 bone and soft-tissue sarcomas (39%), 7 thyroid cancers, 5 leukemias or lymphomas, and 5 other histologies (11).

OSTEOSARCOMA

Because the survival rates for osteosarcoma patients have improved in recent years, it is not surprising that there is a growing cohort of patients susceptible to the development of SMN. In the St. Jude Children's Research Hospital series, the 10-year cumulative incidence of SMN was 2% for patients with localized osteosarcoma and 8% for those who presented with metastatic disease. The SMN included malignant fibrous histiocytoma, melanoma, glioblastoma multiforme, chondrosarcoma, breast cancer, colorectal cancer, and gastric carcinoma. None of the patients who developed SMN had received prior radiotherapy (140).

RADIATION-INDUCED SARCOMA

The distinction between radiation-induced sarcoma (RIS) and a second primary neoplasm must be clear, particularly in view of the frequency of SMNs in children with certain underlying genetic disorders (5,6,10,11, 141). It is well established that internal and external irradiation can induce bone sarcoma in humans and animals (19). The first major review of this subject was by Cahan et al. (142) in 1948. They established the following criteria of a RIS: (a) the RIS must have arisen in an irradiated field; (b) a sufficient latent period, preferably longer than 4 years, must have elapsed; (c) the RIS must be histologically proven; (d) if the RIS is a bone sarcoma, then the bones must have been normal (metabolically, genetically, etc.) prior to radiotherapy. An update of the Cahan's series of radiation-induced osteogenic sarcomas is available. The series now includes 66 patients. Of particular interest are the 42 patients in whom the bone had been normal at the time of irradiation. The median radiation dose was 45 Gy with a range of 25 to 110 Gy. The latent period was, on average, 10.5 years (143,144).

The most common RIS are osteogenic sarcoma, fibrosarcoma, malignant fibrous histiocytoma, and chondrosarcoma. Although an exact dose-response relationship has not been defined, available data for bone sarcomas suggest that a dose-response gradient does exist. Eighty-three percent of RIS of bone occurred within the treatment field, 9.1% occurred within 5 cm of the field, and 7.3% occurred more than 5 cm from the field (68). Alkylating agents are significantly associated with the development of induced sarcomas, after adjusting for radiation exposure (5,6,10,11). Most RIS are diagnosed at an advanced stage and high grade. They frequently occur in areas where radical surgery is difficult or impossible. The results of therapy are, therefore, discouraging, because patients also respond poorly to chemotherapy. Only 1% to 2% are apparently cured, and the average survival is generally 1 to 2 years (range 0.5 to 12 years) (82,85,145–147).

CONDITIONS PREDISPOSING TO THE DEVELOPMENT OF SMN

Several conditions are associated with a high predisposition for tumor induction. Neurofibromatosis (NF) was a frequent predisposing condition in the LESG patients (6,11). Not only are NF patients predisposed to cancer in general, but their tissues may be unusually sensitive to radiation mutagenesis (148). Nevoid basal cell syndrome and ataxia-telangiectasia patients are also at increased risk. The Li Fraumeni syndrome (LFS) is a rare familial cancer syndrome characterized by a high incidence of sarcomas, premenopausal breast cancer, and other neoplasms (brain tumors, leukemia, adrenocortical carcinoma). Germline mutations of p53 have been identified in some families with LFS. The syndrome has an autosomal dominant inheritance pattern (92).

A case-control study from the Institut Gustave Roussy, France, assessed the possible effect on the risk of SMN of unknown genetic factors. The investigators compared the number of relatives of children with SMN with early-onset cancer (i.e., cancer at 45 years of age or less) versus the number of such relatives in pediatric cancer survivors without SMN. The 15-year cumulative incidence of SMN was 2.8% for children without a family history of early onset cancer and 11.7% for children with two or more family members with early onset cancer. Follow-up of childhood cancer survivors should be especially vigilant when a predisposing family history exists (149,150).

REFERENCES

References particularly recommended for further reading are marked by an asterisk.

1. Richardson RB. Past and revised estimates for cancer induced by irradiation and their influence on dose limits. *Br J Radiol* 1990;63:235–245.
2. Fraser MC, Tucker MA. Second malignancies following cancer therapy. *Semin Oncol Nurs* 1989;5:43–55.
3. Hawkins M, Draper G, Kingston J. Incidence of second primary tumors among childhood cancer survivors. *Br J Cancer* 1987;56:339–347.
4. Jaffe N. Late sequelae of cancer and cancer therapy. In: Fernbach DJ, Vietti TJ, eds. *Clinical pediatric oncology.* St. Louis: CV Mosby, 1991:647–674.
5. Meadows AT. Second malignant neoplasms. *Clin Oncol* 1985;4:247–261.
6. Meadows AT, D'Angio GJ, Mike V, et al. Patterns of second malignant neoplasms in children. *Cancer* 1977;40:1903–1911.
7. Potish R, Dehner L, Haselow R, Kim T, Levitt S, Nesbit M. The incidence of second neoplasms following megavoltage radiation for pediatric tumors. *Cancer* 1985;56:1534–1537.
8. Tucker M, D'Angio G, Boice J, et al. Bone sarcomas linked to radiotherapy and chemotherapy in children. *N Engl J Med* 1987;317:588–593.
*9. Bhatia S, Robison LL, Oberlin O, et al. Breast cancer and other second neoplasms after childhood Hodgkin's disease. *N Engl J Med* 1996;334:745–751.
10. Meadows AT. Risk factors for second malignant neoplasms: report from the Late Effects Study Group. *Bull Cancer* 1988;75:125–130.
11. Meadows AT, Baum E, Fossati-Bellani F, et al. Second malignant neoplasms in children: an update from the Late Effects Study Group. *J Clin Oncol* 1985;3:532–538.
12. Meadows AT, Obringer AC, Lansberg P, Marrero O, Lemerle J. Risk of second malignant neoplasms (SMN) in childhood Hodgkin's disease (HD). *Proc Am Assoc Cancer Res* 1985;26:187.
13. Rous R, Kidd JG. Conditional neoplasms and subthreshold neoplastic states. *J Exp Med* 1941;73:365–390.
14. Mottram JC. A developing factor in experimental blastogenesis. *J Pathol Bacteriol* 1944;56:181–187.
15. Berenblum I, Shubik P. A new quantitative approach to the study of the stages of chemical carcinogenesis in the mouse's skin. *Br J Cancer* 1947;1:383–391.
16. Boutwell RK. Some biological aspects of skin carcinogenesis. *Prog Exp Tumor Res* 1964;4:207–250.
17. Farber E. Cancer development and its natural history: a cancer prevention perspective. *Cancer* 1988;62:1676–1679.
18. Weinstein I. The origins of human cancer: molecular mechanisms of carcinogenesis and their implications for cancer prevention and treatment—twenty-seventh GHA Clowes Memorial Award Lecture. *Cancer Res* 1988;48:4135–4143.
19. Boice J. Cancer following medical irradiation. *Cancer* 1981;47:1081–1090.
20. Marshall CJ. Tumor suppressor genes. *Cell* 1991;64:313–326.

*21. Cavenee WK, White RL. The genetic basis of cancer. *Scientific American* 1995 March:72–79.

22. Constine LS, Marcus R, Halperin EC. Molecular biology and the future of therapy for childhood rhabdomyosarcoma. *Int J Radiat Oncol Biol Phys* 1995; 32:1245–1249.

*23. Levine AJ. The genetic origins of neoplasia. *JAMA* 1995;273:592.

*24. Levine AJ. Tumor suppressor genes. *Scientific American Science and Medicine* 1995 January/February 28–37.

25. Hartwell LH, Kastan MB. Cell cycle control and cancer. *Science* 1994;266:1821–1828.

26. Kai M, Luebeck EG, Moolgavkar SH. Analysis of the incidence of solid cancer among atomic bomb survivors using a two-stage model of carcinogenesis. *Radiat Res* 1997;148:348–358.

*27. Hall EJ. What will molecular biology contribute to our understanding of radiation-induced cell kiling and carcinogenesis? *Int J Radiat Biol* 1997;71: 667–674.

28. Hall EJ. *Radiobiology for the radiologist,* 4th edition. Philadelphia: JB Lippincott, 1994:323–350.

29. Riches A, Herceg Z, Wang H, et al. Radiation-induced carcinogenesis: studies using human epithelial cell lines. *Radiat Oncol Invest* 1997;5:139–143.

30. Trott K-R. Radiation and cancer. *Eur J Can Prev* 1996;5:377–378.

31. Darby SC, Dall R, Gill SK, Smith PG. Long-term mortality after a single treatment course with x-rays in patients treated for ankylosing spondylitis. *Br J Cancer* 1987;55:179–190.

32. Mole RH. Childhood cancer after prenatal exposure to diagnostic x-ray examinations in Britain. *Br J Cancer* 1990;62:152–168.

33. Pizarello DJ, Roses DF, Newall J, Barish RJ. The carcinogenicity of radiation therapy. *Surg Gynecol Obstet* 1984;159:189–200.

34. Boivin J, Hutchison G. Second cancers after treatment for Hodgkin's disease: a review. In: Boice J, Fraumeni J, eds. *Radiation carcinogenesis: epidemiology and biological significance.* New York: Raven Press, 1984:181–198.

35. Coleman CN. Adverse effects of cancer therapy: risk of second neoplasms. *Am J Pediatr Hematol Oncol* 1982;4:103–111.

36. Kohn HI, Fry RJM. Radiation carcinogenesis. *N Engl J Med* 1984;310:504–511.

37. Neel JV, Schull WJ, Awa AA, et al. The children of parents exposed to atomic bombs: estimates of the genetic doubling dose of radiation for humans. *Am J Hum Genet* 1990;46:1053–1072.

38. Pitot HC. The natural history of neoplastic development in initiation and promotion. In: *Fundamentals of oncology,* 3rd ed. New York: Marcel Dekker, 1986: 34–73, 139–162.

39. Shimizu Y, Schull WJ, Kafa H. Cancer risk among atomic bomb survivors: the RERF lifespan study. *JAMA* 1990;264:601–604.

40. Alison M, Sarraf M. *Understanding cancer: from basic science to clinical practice.* Cambridge: Cambridge University Press, 1997:37–57.

41. Choppin GR, Liljenzin J-O, Rydberg J. *Radiochemistry and nuclear chemistry* Oxford: Butlerworth-Heinemann Ltd., 1995.

42. Petridou E, Trichopoulos D, Dessypris N, et al. Infant leukaemia after *in utero* exposure to radiation from Chernobyl. *Nature* 1996;382;352–353.

43. Farber E, Sarma D. Biology of disease: hepatocarcinogenesis: a dynamic cellular perspective. *Lab Invest* 1987;56:4–22.

44. Duffy BJ Jr, Fitzgerald PJ. Thyroid cancer in childhood and adolescence: report of 28 cases. *J Clin Endocrinol* 1950;10:1296–1308.

45. Winship T, Rosvoll RV. Childhood thyroid carcinoma. *Cancer* 1961;14:734–743.

46. Fjalling M, Tisell L, Carlsson S, Hansson G, Lundberg L, Oden A. Benign and malignant thyroid nodules after neck irradiation. *Cancer* 1986;58: 1219–1224.

47. Fleming ID, Black TL, Thompson EI, Pratt C, Rao B, Husto O. Thyroid dysfunction and neoplasia in children receiving neck irradiation for cancer. *Cancer* 1985;55:1190–1194.

48. Schneider A, Recant W, Pinsky S, Ryo U, Bekerman C, Shore-Freedman E. Radiation-induced thyroid carcinoma. *Ann Intern Med* 1986;105:405–412.

49. Schneider AB, Shore-Freedman E, Ryo UY, Bekerman C, Favus M, Pinsky S. Radiation-induced tumors of the head and neck following childhood irradiation: prospective studies. *Medicine* 1985;64:1–15.

50. Auguste LJ, Sako K. Radiation and thyroid carcinoma: radiotherapy, head and neck regions, thyroid carcinoma. *Head Neck Surg* 1985;7:217–224.

51. Suit H, DuBois W. The importance of optimal treatment planning in radiation therapy. *Int J Radiat Oncol Biol Phys* 1991;21:1471–1478.

52. Tucker M, Jones P, Boice J, et al. Therapeutic radiation at a young age is linked to secondary thyroid cancer. *Cancer Res* 1991;51:2885–2888.

*53. Hancock S, Cox R, McDougall I. Thyroid disease after treatment of Hodgkin's disease. *N Engl J Med* 1991;325:594–605.

54. Arseneau JC, Sponzo RW, Levin DL, et al. Nonlymphomatous malignant tumors complicating Hodgkin's disease. Possible association with intensive therapy. *N Engl J Med* 1972;307:965–971.

55. Blayney D, Longo D, Young R, et al. Decreasing risk of leukemia with prolonged follow up after chemotherapy and radiotherapy for Hodgkin's disease. *N Engl J Med* 1987;316:710–717.

56. Haselow RE, Nesbit M, Dehner LP, Khan FM, McHugh R, Levitt SH. Second neoplasms following megavoltage radiation in a pediatric population. *Cancer* 1978;42:1185–1191.

57. Anonymous. Report on a workshop to examine methods to arrive at risk estimates for radiation-induced cancer in the human based on laboratory data. *Radiat Res* 1993;135:434–437.

58. Wiley AL Jr, Vogel HH Jr, Clifton KH. The effect of variations in LET and cell cycle on radiation hepatocarcinogenesis. *Radiat Res* 1973;54:284–293.

59. Okey AB, Harper PA, Grant DM, Hill RP. Chemical and radiation carcinogenesis. In: Tannock I, Hill R, eds., *The basic science of oncology,* third edition. New York: McGraw-Hill, 1998:166–196.

60. Li FP, Cassady JR, Jaffe N. Risk of second tumors in survivors of childhood cancer. *Cancer* 1975;35: 1230–1235.

61. deVathaire F, Francois P, Hill C, et al. Role of radio-

therapy and chemotherapy in the risk of second malignant neoplasms after cancer in childhood. *Br J Cancer* 1989;59:792–796.

62. Harris C. The carcinogenicity of anticancer drugs: a hazard of man. *Cancer* 1976;37:1014–1023.

63. Ruymann FB, Mosijczuk AD, Sayers RL. Hepatoma in a child with methotrexate-induced hepatic fibrosis. *JAMA* 1977;238:2631–2633.

64. Tucker MA, Meadows AT, Boice JD, Hoover RN, Fraumeni JF. Cancer risk following treatment of childhood cancer. In: Boice JD, Fraumeni JF, eds. *Progress in Cancer Research and Therapy, Vol. 26: Radiation carcinogenesis: epidemiology and biological significance.* New York: Raven Press, 1984:211–224.

65. Matas A, Hertel B, Rosai J. Post transplant malignant lymphoma, distinctive morphologic features. *Am J Med* 1976;61:716–720.

66. Land CE. Temporal distributions of risk for radiation-induced cancers. *J Chron Dis* 1987;40[Suppl 2]: 45S–57S.

67. Ebbsen P, Villadsen JH, Langkjer ST, Bjerring P. Susceptibility to carcinogenic effect of irradiation: relationship to age at time of exposure. *Acta Radiol Oncol* 1984;23:141–145.

68. Tucker M, Coleman C, Cox R, Varghese A, Rosenberg S. Risk of second cancers after treatment for Hodgkin's disease. *N Engl J Med* 1988;318:76–81.

69. Fraumeni J. Clinical patterns of familial cancer. In: Mulvihill J, Miller R, Fraumeni J, eds. *Progress in Cancer Research and Therapy, Vol. 3: Genetics of human cancer.* New York: Raven Press, 1977:223–234.

70. Strong LC, Stene M, Norsted TL. Cancer in survivors of childhood soft tissue sarcoma and their relatives. *J Natl Cancer Inst* 1987;79:1213–1220.

71. Hawkins MM. Second primary tumors following radiotherapy for childhood cancer. *Int J Radiat Oncol Biol Phys* 1990;19:1297–1301.

72. Meadows A, Obringer A, Marrero O, et al. Second malignant neoplasms following childhood Hodgkin's disease: treatment and splenectomy as risk factors. *Med Pediatr Oncol* 1989;17:477–484.

73. Kaatsch P, Michaelis J. Zweitmalignome nach malignen Erkrankungen im Kindesalter. *Klin Padiatr* 1995; 207:158–163.

*74. Hawkins MM, Wilson LMK, Burton HS, et al. Radiotherapy, alkylating agents, and risk of bone cancer after childhood cancer. *J Natl Cancer Inst* 1996;88: 270–278.

75. Benedict WF, Xu H-J, Takahashi R. The retinoblastoma gene: its role in human malignancies. *Cancer Invest* 1980;8:535–540.

76. Hensen M, Koufas A, Gallie B, et al. Osteosarcoma and retinoblastoma: a shared chromosomal mechanism revealing recessive predisposition. *Proc Natl Acad Sci USA* 1985;86:6216–6220.

77. Reese A, Merriam G, Martin H. Treatment of bilateral retinoblastoma by irradiation and surgery: report on fifteen year results. *Am J Ophthalmol* 1949;32: 175–190.

78. Abramson DH, Ellsworth RM, Kitchin FD, Tung G. Second nonocular tumors in retinoblastoma survivors. *Ophthalmology* 1984;91:1351–1355.

79. Abramson DH, Ronner HJ, Ellsworth RM. Second tumors in non-irradiated bilateral retinoblastoma. *Am J Ophthalmol* 1979;87:624–627.

*80. Draper G, Sanders B, Kingston J. Second primary neoplasms in patients with retinoblastoma. *Br J Cancer* 1986;53:661–671.

81. Smith LM, Donaldson SS. Incidence and management of secondary malignancies in patients with retinoblastoma and Ewing's sarcoma. *Oncology* 1991;5:135–148.

82. Smith LM, Donaldson SS, Egbert PR, Link MP, Bagshaw MA. Aggressive management of secondary primary tumors in survivors of hereditary retinoblastoma. *Int J Radiol Oncol Biol Phys* 1989;17:449–505.

*83. Eng D, Li FP, Abramson DH, et al. Mortality from second tumors among long-term survivors of retinoblastoma. *J Natl Cancer Inst* 1993;85:1121–1128.

*84. Wong FL, Boice JD Jr, Abramson DH, et al. Cancer incidence after retinoblastoma: radiation dose and sarcoma risk. *JAMA* 1997;278:1262–1267.

85. Roarty JD, McLean IW, Zimmerman LE. Incidence of second neoplasms in patients with bilateral retinoblastoma. *Ophthalmology* 1988;95:1583–1587.

86. Malone M, Lumley H, Erdohazi M. Astrocytoma as a second malignancy in patients with acute lymphoblastic leukemia. *Cancer* 1986;57:1979–1985.

87. Cole LJ, Nowell PC. Radiation carcinogenesis: the sequence of events. *Science* 1965;150:1782–1786.

88. Kun LE. The article reviewed. *Oncology* 1991;5: 147–148.

89. Dunst J. Sekkundarmalignomebei Ewing-Sarkom-Patienten. *Strahlanther Onkol* 1997;173:338–339.

*90. Kuttesch JF, Wexler LH, Marcus RB, et al. Second malignancies after Ewing's sarcoma: radiation dose-dependency of secondary sarcomas. *J Clin Oncol* 1996;14:2818–2825.

91. Ivins JC, Taylor WF, Wald LE. Elective whole-lung irradiation in osteosarcoma treatment: appearance of bilateral breast cancer in two long-term survivors. *Skeletal Radiol* 1987;16:133–135.

92. Rich DC, Corpron CA, Smith MB, Blaack CT, Lally KP, Androssy RJ. Second malignant neoplasms in children after treatment of soft tissue sarcoma. *J Pediatr Surg* 1997;32:369–372.

93. Carli M, Frascella E, Toumade MF, et al. Second malignant neoplasms in patients treated on SIOP Wilms' tumor studies and trials 1, 2, 5, and 6. *Med Pediatr Oncol* 1997;29:239–244.

94. Breslow NE, Takashima JR, Whittam JA, et al. Second malignant neoplasms following treatment for Wilms' tumor: a report from the Wilms' Tumor Study Group. *J Clin Oncol* 1995;13:1851–1859.

95. Sabio H, Teja K, Elkon D, Shaw A. Adenocarcinoma of the colon following the treatment of Wilms' tumor. *J Pediatr* 1979;95:424–426.

96. Mulvihill J. Genetic repertory of human neoplasia. In: Mulvihill J, Miller R, Fraumeni J, eds. *Progress in Cancer Research and Therapy, Vol. 3: Genetics of human cancer.* New York: Raven Press, 1977:137–144.

97. Knudson AG. The genetics of childhood cancer. *Bull Cancer* 1988;75:135–138.

98. Li FP, Corkery J, Vawter G, Fine W, Sallan SE. Breast carcinoma after cancer therapy in childhood. *Cancer* 1983;51:521–523.

99. Shen SC, Yunis JG. Leiomyosarcoma developing in a child during remission of leukemia. *J Pediatr* 1976;89:780–782.

100. Tavassoli FA, Lynch RG. Occult adenocarcinoma of

the pancreas in a 17 year old patient with immuno-suppressed leukemia. *Gastroenterology* 1976;66: 1054–1057.

101. Antillon F, Kaste SC, Jenkins JJ, et al. Primitive neuroectodermal tumor of bone as a second malignant neoplasm in a child previously treated for acute lymphoblastic leukemia. *J Pediatr Hematol Oncol* 1997;19:473–476.

*102. Neglia JP, Meadows AT, Robison LL, et al. Second malignant neoplasms after acute lymphoblastic leukemia in childhood. *N Engl J Med* 1991;325: 1330–1336.

103. Pui CH, Ribeiro RC, Hancock ML, et al. Acute myeloid leukemia in children treated with epidophyllotoxins for acute lymphoblastic leukemias. *N Engl J Med* 1991;325:1682–1687.

104. Farwell J, Flanner JT. Cancer in relatives of children with central nervous system neoplasms. *N Engl J Med* 1984;311:749–753.

105. Rimm I, Li F, Tarbell N, Winston K, Sallan S. Brain tumors after cranial irradiation for childhood acute lymphoblastic leukemia. *Cancer* 1987;59:1506–1508.

106. Fontana M, Stanton C, Pompili A, et al. Late multifocal gliomas in adolescents previously treated for acute lymphoblastic leukemia. *Cancer* 1987;60: 1510–1518.

107. Tang TT, Holcenberg JS, Duck SC, et al. Thyroid carcinoma following treatment for acute lymphoblastic leukemia. *Cancer* 1980;46:1572–1576.

107a. Beaty O, Hudson M, Greenwald C, et al. Subsequent malignancies in children and adolescents after treatment for Hodgkin's disease. *J Clin Oncol* 1995;13: 603–609.

108. Hancock SL, Tucker MA, Hoppe RT. Breast cancer after treatment of Hodgkin's disease. *J Natl Cancer Inst* 1993;85:25–31.

109. Hancock SL, Cox RS, McDougall IR. Thyroid diseases after treatment of Hodgkin's disease. *N Engl J Med* 1991;325:599–605.

110. Andrieu JM, Ifrah N, Payen C, Fermanian J, Coscas Y, Flandrin G. Increased risk of secondary acute non-lymphocytic leukemia after extended-field radiation therapy combined with MOPP chemotherapy for Hodgkin's disease. *J Clin Oncol* 1990;8:1148–1154.

111. Boivin JF, Hutchison GB, Zauber AG, et al. Incidence of second cancers in patients treated for Hodgkin's disease [see comments]. *J Natl Cancer Inst* 1995;87: 732–741.

112. Abrahamsen JF, Andersen A, Hannisdal E, et al. Second malignancies after treatment of Hodgkin's disease: the influence of treatment, follow-up time, and age. *J Clin Oncol* 1993;11:255–261.

113. Henry-Amar, M. Second cancer after the treatment for Hodgkin's disease: a report from the International Database on Hodgkin's Disease. *Ann Oncol* 1992;3 [Suppl 4]:117–128.

114. Kaldor JM, Day NE, Band P, et al. Second malignancies following testicular cancer, ovarian cancer and Hodgkin's disease: an international collaborative study among cancer registries. *Int J Cancer* 1987;39: 571–585.

115. Mauch PM, Kalish LA, Marcus KC, et al. Second malignancies after treatment for laparotomy staged IA-IIIB Hodgkin's disease: long-term analysis of risk factors and outcome *Blood* 1996;87:3625–3632.

116. van Leeuwen FE, Chorus AM, van den Belt-Dusebout AW, et al. Leukemia risk following Hodgkin's disease: relation to cumulative dose of alkylating agents, treatment with teniposide combinations, number of episodes of chemotherapy, and bone marrow damage. *J Clin Oncol* 1994;12:1063–1073.

117. Swerdlow AJ, Douglas AJ, Vaughan Hudson B, MacLennan KA. Risk of second primary cancer after Hodgkin's disease in patients in the British National Lymphoma Investigation: relationships to host factors, histology and stage of Hodgkin's disease, and splenectomy. *Br J Cancer* 1993;68:1006–1011.

118. Devereux S, Selassie TG, Vaughan G, Hudson B, Linch DC. Leukaemia complicating treatment for Hodgkin's disease: the experience of the British National Lymphoma Investigation. *BMJ* 1990;301: 1077–1080.

119. Devereux S. Therapy associated leukaemia. *Blood Rev* 1991;5:138–145.

120. Kaldor JM, Day NE, Clarke EA, et al. Leukemia following Hodgkin's disease. *N Engl J Med* 1990;322: 7–13.

121. van der Velden JW, van Putten WL, Guinee VF, et al. Subsequent development of acute non-lymphocytic leukemia in patients treated for Hodgkin's disease. *Int J Cancer* 1988;42:252–255.

122. Schellong G, Riepenhausen M, Creutzig U, et al. Low risk of secondary leukemias after chemotherapy without mechlorethamine in childhood Hodgkin's disease. German-Austrian Pediatric Hodgkin's Disease Group. *J Clin Oncol* 1997;15:2247–2253.

123. Biti G, Cellai E, Magrini SM, Papi MG, Ponticelli P, Boddi V. Second solid tumors and leukemia after treatment for Hodgkin's disease: an analysis of 1121 patients from a single institution. *Int J Radiat Oncol Biol Phys* 1994;29:25–31.

124. Valagussa P, Santoro A, Fossati-Bellani F, Banfi A, Bonadonna G. Second acute leukemia and other malignancies following treatment for Hodgkin's disease. *J Clin Oncol* 1986;4:830–837.

125. Dietrich PY, Henry-Amar M, Cosset JM, Bodis S, Bosq J, Hayat M. Second primary cancers in patients continuously disease-free from Hodgkin's disease: a protective role for the spleen? *Blood* 1994;84: 1209–1215.

126. Tura S, Fiacchini M, Zinzani PL, Brusamolino E, Gobbi PG. Splenectomy and the increasing risk of secondary acute leukemia in Hodgkin's disease. *J Clin Oncol* 1993;11:925–930.

127. van Leeuwen FE, Somers R, Hart A. Splenectomy in Hodgkin's disease and second leukemia. *Lancet* 1982;2:210–211.

128. Zarate-Osorno A, Medeiros LJ, Longo DL, Jaffe ES. Non-Hodgkin's lymphomas arising in patients successfully treated for Hodgkin's disease. A clinical, histologic, and immunophenotypic study of 14 cases. *Am J Surg Pathol* 1992;16:885–895.

129. Baral E, Larsson LE, Mattsson B. Breast cancer following irradiation of the breast. *Cancer* 1977;40: 2905–2910.

130. Miller AB, Howe GR, Sherman JP, et al. Mortality from breast cancer after irradiation during fluoroscopic examinations in patients beeing treated for tuberculosis. *N Engl J Med* 1989;321:1285–1289.

131. Shore RE, Hildreth N, Woodard E, Dvoretsky P,

Hempelmann L, Pasternack B. Breast cancer among women given x-ray therapy for acute postpartum mastitis. *J Natl Cancer Inst* 1986;77:689–696.

132. Mauch P, Henry-Amar M. International Database on Hodgkin's Disease: a cooperative effort to determine treatment outcome. *Ann Oncol* 1992;3[Suppl 4]: 59–61.

133. Donaldson SS, Hancock SL. Second cancers after Hodgkin's disease in childhood. *N Engl J Med* 1996; 334:792–794.

134. Kaldor JM. Day NE, Bell J, et, al. Lung cancer following Hodgkin's disease: a case-control study. *Int J Cancer* 1992;52:677–681.

135. Shapiro CL, Mauch PM. Radiation-associated breast cancer after Hodgkin's disease: risks and screening in perspective. *J Clin Oncol* 1992;10:1662–1665.

136. Sullivan M, Ried H, Boren H, Lewis E. Noninvasive (ultrasound) screening for thyroid abnormalities in 21 survivors of Hodgkin's disease. *Proc Am Soc Clin Oncol* 1986;5:1996.

137. Swerdlow AJ. Risk of second cancers after treatment for Hodgkin's disease. *N Engl J Med* 1988;318:76–81.

138. Birdwell SH, Hancock SL, Varghese A, Cox RS, Hoppe RT. Gastrointestinal cancer after treatment of Hodgkin's disease. *Int J Radiat Oncol Biol Phys* 1997;37:67–73.

139. Halperin EC. Long term results of therapy for stage C neuroblastoma. *J Surg Oncol* 1996;63:172–178.

140. Pratt CB, Meyer WH, Luo X, et al. Second malignant neoplasms occuring in survivors of osteosarcoma. *Cancer* 1997;80:960–965.

141. Robinson E, Neugat A, Wylie P. Clinical aspects of postirradiation sarcomas. *J Natl Cancer Inst* 1988; 80:233–240.

142. Cahan WG, Woodard HQ, Higinbotham ND, Stewart FW, Coley BL. Sarcoma arising in irradiated bone: report of eleven cases. *Cancer* 1948;1:3–29.

143. Huvos AG, Woodard HQ. Postradiation sarcomas of bone. *Health Phys* 1988;55:631–636.

144. Huvos AG, Woodard HQ, Cahan WG, et al. Postradiation osteogenic sarcoma of bone and soft tissue. *Cancer* 1985;55:1244–1255.

145. Halperin EC, Greenberg H, Suit H. Sarcoma of bone and soft tissue following Hodgkin's disease. *Cancer* 1984;53:232–236.

146. Mike V, Meadows AT, D'Angio GJ. Incidence of second malignant neoplasms in children: results of an international study. *Lancet* 1982;2:1326–1331.

147. Weatherby R, Dahlin D, Childs D, et al. Post-radiation sarcoma of bone. Review of 78 Mayo Clinic cases. *Mayo Clin Proc* 1981;56:294–306.

148. Hafex M, Sharaf L, El-Nabi SMA, El-Wehedy G. Evidence of chromosomal instability in neurofibromatosis. *Cancer* 1985;55:2434–2436.

149. Kony SJ, de Vathaire F, Champret A, et al. Radiation and genetic factors in the risk of second malignant neoplasms after a first cancer in childhood. *Lancet* 1997;350:91–95.

150. Nagataki S, Shibata Y, Inoue S, Yokoyama N, Izumi M, Shimaaka K. Thyroid diseases among atomic bomb survivors in Nagasaki *JAMA* 1994;272: 364–370.

21

Anesthesia for External-Beam Radiotherapy

In collaboration with Scott R. Schulman, M.D.

Departments of Anesthesiology and Pediatrics, Duke University Medical Center, Durham,
North Carolina 27710.

Considering the awesome aspect of the therapy machines together with the fact that no one may be with the patient during the period of irradiation, it is surprising that the great majority submit to the complete course of therapy with little or no restraint and no sedation. . . . In a small number of patients in the infant-to-toddler age group of 1 1/2 to 5 years of age, patient co-operation may be impossible to obtain...complete immobility of the patient is absolutely essential for the accuracy and success of treatment. . . . Sedation of the patient becomes virtually a sine qua non.

Harrison and Bennet (1) made these observations over 30 years ago. Their classic article entitled "Radiotherapy Without Tears" marked the first published report describing anesthesia for radiotherapy in children. The problem of inadequate sedation prompted the authors (1) to develop

> . . . the following simple method of anesthesia for radiotherapy of infants. . . . The method is applicable when the anesthetist must remain outside the treatment room, and consists of the insufflation of nitrous oxide, oxygen and halothane through the side-arm of the oropharyngeal airway.

Thirty years of progress in anesthesiology have validated not only Harrison and Bennet's observation, but also their solution to the problem of providing anesthesia for radiotherapy. This chapter will review issues in the sedation of children with an emphasis on monitoring the anesthetized child in the radiotherapy suite, develop a model of the "ideal" anesthetic for pediatric radiotherapy, explore anesthetic options for radiotherapy, and discuss the implications of the child's underlying disease that impact on the anesthetic choice.

FREQUENCY OF ANESTHESIA FOR PEDIATRIC RADIOTHERAPY

When possible, children should be irradiated without anesthesia. Confidence building measures and play therapy are to be used to achieve patient stability and reproducible treatment. When these techniques fail, however, anesthesia must be utilized.

The frequency of anesthesia utilization, as a function of patient age at the initiation of external beam radiation therapy in the Duke University Medical Center pediatric radiotherapy population, is shown in Table 1. For very young children (3 years of age or younger) anesthesia is almost always required. After approximately 5 years of age, however, anesthesia will be rarely required.

TABLE 1. *Frequency of a child receiving external beam radiation therapy and requiring anesthesia as a function of age at initiation of irradiation*

Age (yrs)	Total number of patients receiving external beam radiation therapy under anesthesia	Total number of patients receiving external beam radiation therapy	Percentage of patients requiring anesthesia
0–≤1	25	26	96%
1–≤2	24	27	89%
2–≤3	30	35	86%
3–≤4	20	41	49%
4–≤5	16	44	36%
5–≤6	4	38	11%
6–≤7	2	28	7%
7–≤16	2	273	0.7%
	123	512	

From ref. 21, with permission.

GOALS OF ANESTHESIA FOR RADIOTHERAPY

In order to accomplish the twin goals of irradiating the treatment volume while sparing healthy tissue, control of patient movement must be precise and absolute. How are these goals achieved in children? The approach varies depending on the institutional resources. Conscious or deep sedation is used in some centers, whereas general anesthesia is used in others. Regardless of the institutional practice, there is no substitute for vigilant monitoring and prompt intervention by individuals skilled in the detection and management of complications associated with the administration of sedative drugs to infants and children.

Anesthesiologists are increasingly asked to provide care outside the traditional operating room setting, such as in the radiotherapy suite (2). This is appropriate, because the specialty has unique expertise in patient evaluation and selection, appropriate monitoring, and the ability to respond immediately to any complication of therapy. Drug selection and a comprehensive approach to the care of the child, which includes preanesthetic evaluation, postanesthetic care, and the provision of up-to-date NPO guidelines, are hallmarks of the anesthesiologist.

A prolonged fast prior to the induction of general anesthesia is no longer necessary. Infants, children, and adolescents can safely drink clear liquids (e.g., apple juice, water, popsicles) or (if applicable) breast milk until

TABLE 2. *Goals for ideal anesthesia for out-patient pediatric radiation therapy*

(1) Assurance of immobility
(2) Rapid and smooth onset of effect with sedation, hypnosis, amnesia, and analgesia adequate for relatively non-painful radiation therapy procedures, along with a sufficient degree of muscle relaxation
(3) Brief duration of action
(4) Not painful to administer
(5) Prompt recovery without post-procedure ill side-effects but with residual analgesia and antiemetic effects during recovery
(6) Minimal interference with eating, drinking, and playing
(7) Safe to administer repeatedly
(8) Avoidance of tolerance to the anesthetic agent(s) (tachyphylaxis)
(9) Maintenance of a patent airway in a variety of body positions
(10) Absence of side effects such as cardiovascular instability, respiratory depression, spontaneous movements, excitatory activity
(11) The anesthetic program selected is cost-effective.

Modified from refs. 9, 31, with permission.

3 hours prior to induction. Milk and solid food should be withheld for 4 to 6 hours for infants less than 6 months of age, for 6 hours for toddlers 6 months to 3 years of age, and for 8 hours for children older than 3 years of age.

The goals of anesthesia for pediatric radiotherapy are listed in Table 2. There are several options that, to a greater or lesser degree, accomplish the listed goals. There are no prospective, randomized studies in the setting of pediatric radiotherapy that demonstrate the superiority of one technique of general anesthesia over another.

INHALED ANESTHETICS

The medically controlled state characterized by loss of consciousness, amnesia, analgesia, and muscle relaxation is known as *general anesthesia.* General anesthesia guarantees immobility. The state of general anesthesia includes the loss of protective airway reflexes, along with the ability to independently maintain a patent airway.

Several general anesthetic options exist for radiotherapy. The anesthesiologist individualizes therapy based on data obtained from the patient's history, physical and laboratory examination, and discussions with the child, parents, and radiation oncologist. The physical limitations of the radiotherapy suite (such as the presence of an air exhaust system so that volatile anesthetic agents can be used) are also important in devising the anesthetic plan.

General anesthesia is accomplished with either inhaled agents (Table 3) or intravenous agents (e.g., barbiturates, ketamine, propofol). The first report of anesthesia for pediatric radiotherapy used halothane. Halothane is a halogenated hydrocarbon volatile anesthetic first introduced for clinical use in 1956. Halothane has a long history of safe effective use in pediatric patients. It has superior induction characteristics compared to isoflurane and enflurane, rapidly producing an anesthetic state when inhaled with minimal airway complications such as coughing and laryngospasm. It is delivered by mask to the child

TABLE 3. *Inhalation anesthetic agents commonly used in pediatric radiation therapy*

Sevoflurane CFH_2-O-CH$(CF_3)_2$
Nitrous Oxide N_2O
Isoflurane CF_2H-O-CClH-CF_3
Enflurane CF_2H-O-CFCl-CF_2H
Halothane CF_3-CClBrH
Desflurane CF_3H-O-CFH-CF_3

and is painless to administer. Halothane has been demonstrated to be superior to isoflurane and enflurane in children with malignancies for diagnostic and therapeutic procedures (3). For anesthesia outside the operating room Wolfe and Rao, "after considerable experimentation with various IV, intramuscular, and inhalation anesthetics, with and without intubation," recommended inhalation induction with halothane and nitrous oxide/oxygen and maintenance of anesthesia with halothane and oxygen without intubation (4). Halothane depresses respiration and cardiovascular function in a dose-dependent fashion. At doses used for radiotherapy, these effects are negligible. Spontaneous respiration is typical with halothane anesthesia.

Sevoflurane is a new, disubstituted methyl ethyl ether inhalation anesthetic that, in the opinion of some anesthesiologists, rivals halothane as the anesthetic of choice for infants and children (5). Sevoflurane has minimal pungency compared to halothane and may be more readily tolerated by children. Its lower solubility permits a more precise control over the delivery of anesthesia and a more rapid induction of and recovery from anesthesia. Sevoflurane also seems to have a lower respiratory irritant capacity than halothane and produces less coughing and breath holding than some other inhaled agents. Sevoflurane does, however, present some difficulties compared to other inhalation agents. The drug is susceptible to degradation by the carbon dioxide absorbent soda lime used in rebreathing circuits in anesthesia machines. At low fresh gas flow rates (less than 2 liters/min) this interaction between sevoflurane and soda lime can result in the production of a metabolite known as compound A. Compound A can be nephrotoxic in rats. The clinical significance of this observation in humans is questionable, as well-designed studies have failed to demonstrate clinically significant nephrotoxicity in children or adults receiving sevoflurane. This is particularly true for pediatric radiotherapy because the duration of exposure is exceedingly short. A potential drawback of sevoflurane is its cost. It is relatively expensive compared to other agents (6–9). All volatile anesthetics are commonly used in conjunction with nitrous oxide.

Inhalation anesthesia is frequently complicated by upper airway obstruction. Airway obstruction is often exacerbated in radiation therapy by the position of the patient. Positioning frequently requires immobilization of the child's head in a shell, which can impede airway patency when an insufflation technique is used. This obstruction is re-

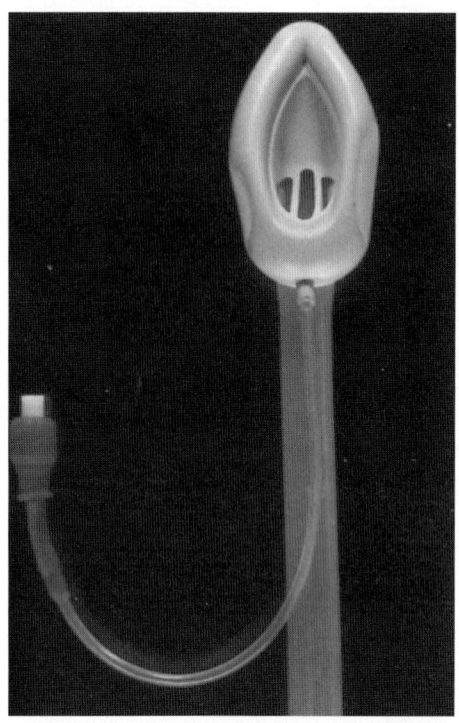

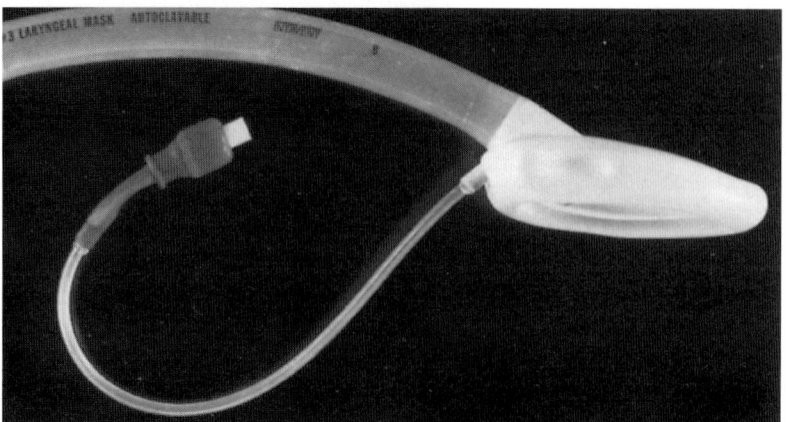

FIG. 1. The laryngeal mask airway is a silicon tube. The distal end of the tube has an elliptical-shaped cuff that, when correctly inserted and inflated, forms a low-pressure seal around the larynx and allows for spontaneous ventilation without the need for endotracheal intubation. (Photographed by permission of Gensia, Inc. San Diego, CA)

lieved with either an oro- or nasopharyngeal airway or a laryngeal mask airway. Although endotracheal intubation may be necessary in a small proportion of patients presenting for radiotherapy, it is preferable to avoid this technique because repeated laryngoscopy and intubation carry with them the risk of airway edema and trauma to the laryngeal structures.

An exciting new anesthetic adjunct for airway management during pediatric radiotherapy is the laryngeal mask airway (LMA). The LMA (Fig. 1) is a silicone tube, the distal end of which has an elliptical-shaped cuff that, when correctly inserted and inflated, forms a low-pressure seal around the larynx and allows for spontaneous ventilation in a variety of body positions without the need for endotracheal intubation. The LMA, therefore, provides all the advantages of endotracheal intubation—that is, a guaranteed patent airway without the disadvantages of repeated laryngoscopy and intubation. The LMA has been used for radiotherapy in children as young as 3 weeks of age. Grebenik et al. (10) reported the use of the LMA for pediatric radiotherapy in 25 children who received over 300 anesthetics. They observed no complications directly related to the use of the LMA. Morris and Marjot (10a) reported one case of posterior pharyngeal wall edema that corresponded to the area of contact between the posterior surface of the LMA and the oropharynx in a child repeatedly anesthetized with an LMA for radiotherapy (10a). Moylan and Luce reported over 2,500 anesthetics given to 145 children with a LMA over a 4-year period of time for radiotherapy. They raise the concern that a prone position for radiotherapy with the neck partially flexed can produce kinking of the LMA with the possibility of airway obstruction. A new reinforced LMA may help alleviate this problem (11,12).

In summary, general inhalation anesthesia has many features that make it an attractive technique for pediatric radiotherapy. Onset is rapid, depth is easily controllable, it is relatively pleasant to administer, recovery is rapid, the incidence of nausea and vomiting due to the anesthetic is low, and the airway is well-preserved. This time-honored technique is widely used.

INTRAVENOUS ANESTHETICS

Intravenous anesthesia is also a popular and effective technique for pediatric radiotherapy. Intravenous anesthesia relies on either intermittent or continuous infusion of anesthetic agent into a peripheral or central vein in order to maintain a therapeutic concentration (13). Although not a new concept (sodium thiopental was administered by continuous drip as early as 1944), the advent of newer, short-acting anesthetic drugs, better equipment for infusing these drugs, and an improved understanding of pharmacokinetics in pediatric patients has led to a resurgence of interest in this technique. Postulated advantages of intravenous anesthesia include fewer peaks and troughs in serum concentration of drug providing a steady-state serum concentration. Proponents of intravenous anesthesia contend that provision of this steady-state concentration results in a more rapid induction of, and emergence from, anesthesia when compared to inhaled anesthetics.

There is an extensive body of experience with ketamine in the radiotherapy suite (14–16). Since its release in the early 1970s, this dissociative anesthetic has been widely used for radiation therapy in children. Ketamine produces excellent analgesia and amnesia of relatively short duration. Ketamine is easy to administer (it can be given intramuscularly if there is no intravenous access), and an anesthesia machine is not required when ketamine is used. Ketamine is felt to better preserve respiration and airway patency compared to inhaled anesthetics. One series (17) described a child with a pharyngeal tumor who experienced airway obstruction with halothane anesthesia. When ketamine was substituted for halothane, the patient had an uneventful anesthetic, which resulted in satisfactory conditions for radiotherapy.

Ketamine is not a panacea. There are several caveats to its use. Ketamine has ocular effects that have implications for radiotherapy. The onset of ketamine anesthesia is frequently accompanied by nystagmus (more commonly horizontal than vertical). Nystagmus with ketamine is usually transient; however, if it persists, it may be impossible to utilize a hanging lens block in an anterior field for the treatment of retinoblastoma. Ketamine can also produce involuntary movement of other muscle groups (jerking), which is undesirable in pediatric radiotherapy. Ketamine raises blood pressure and heart rate. Its use in the setting of increased intracranial pressure (ICP) is contraindicated because it causes ICP to increase.

Although ketamine generally preserves respiratory drive and airway patency, apnea can occur after an intravenous bolus dose. In addition, it is a potent sialogogue, and copious secretions frequently accompany its use. Secretions can cause airway obstruction. Ketamine also sensitizes the airway to irritable stimuli, and reflex laryngeal closure (laryngospasm) often occurs. A drying agent such as atropine or glycopyrrolate should be given in conjunction with ketamine.

Finally, emergence from ketamine anesthesia is frequently characterized by hallucinations and nightmares. The incidence of emergence reactions due to ketamine ranges from 10% to 30% in adult patients. Emergence reactions with ketamine are much less common in children than in adults. The reason for this difference is not known. Whatever the mechanism, the occurrence of these emergence reactions can be attenuated if a benzodiazepine such as diazepam or midazolam is used.

Benzodiazepines such as diazepam (Valium) and midazolam (Versed) are infrequently used as the sole agents for radiotherapy in children. Valium is painful to administer when given intravenously, and its duration of action exceeds the duration of most radiotherapy sessions. Versed is short-acting and not painful when given intravenously, but when used by itself does not produce satisfactory sedation for radiotherapy. A plateau in sedative effect frequently accompanies its use so that additional dosing does not produce the desired clinical effect. The release of flumazenil (Mazicon), a benzodiazepine antagonist (the "Narcan" of benzodiazepines), may improve the margin of safety for benzodiazepines. In the event that a patient receives a relative overdose or demonstrates an exaggerated clinical effect, the drug can be displaced from its receptor by flumazenil and the untoward effects can be reversed.

Barbiturates are sedative-hypnotic drugs that depress the activity of the central nervous system (CNS). These drugs produce sleep within seconds of intravenous administration. Awakening is rapid and occurs by redistribution of the drug from the CNS. Barbiturates are given as an intravenous bolus or as a bolus followed by a continuous infusion. Short-acting barbiturates thiopental (Pentothal) and methohexital (Brevital) have been well-utilized in pediatric radiotherapy (18,19). Side effects include apnea, hiccoughs, laryngospasm, and paradoxical CNS excitation. Some radiotherapists utilize droperidol, a butyrophenone derivative with pharmacologic actions similar to those of haloperidol and phenothiazines, generally followed by pentobarbital for intravenous anesthesia.

Narcotic analgesics produce sedation as a side effect. Other side effects of opiates include respiratory depression, nausea, vomiting, and tolerance with repeated administration. These side effects of narcotics make opiate anesthesia undesirable for radiotherapy. Radiotherapy is not a painful procedure; narcotics should not be necessary.

Opiate use in pediatric radiotherapy is additionally limited by the pharmacokinetic profile of many drugs in this class. Opiates such as meperidine and morphine have long half-lives, which make them unsuitable for short procedures such as radiation therapy. Newer potent synthetic opioids such as fentanyl, sufentanil, alfentanil and remifentanil may have a role, but that role is a limited one due to their ability to depress respiration, cause chest wall rigidity, and to produce tolerance. Mixed opiate agonist-antagonists such as nalbuphine (Nubain) and butorphanol (Stadol) are touted as producing sedation and analgesia with less respiratory depression (plateau effect). These agonist-antagonists may be useful adjuncts in anesthesia for radiotherapy.

Propofol (Diprivan) is an intravenous anesthetic that has hypnotic-sedative properties. Propofol is an alkyl phenol derivative, which is insoluble in water. The active ingredient in propofol, 2,6-diisopropylphenol, is formulated in an emulsion of soybean oil, glycerol, and egg lecithin. This formulation gives it a milky-white appearance. It is a highly lipid-soluble compound and, therefore, has a rapid distribution into the CNS and a rapid elimination. This rapid elimination has made it a popular anesthetic agent for day surgery and/or short procedures. It can be given via a central venous line or a peripheral intravenous catheter (20,21). When given peripherally, pain on injection is a frequent accompaniment. This pain can be attenuated by administering the drug with lidocaine. Propofol has been used by anesthesiologists in pediatric radiotherapy. It is given as an intermittent bolus or as a bolus followed by continuous infusion. Awakening is rapid, and the incidence of side effects is low. When administered as a rapid intravenous bolus, apnea and hypotension are common. However, when the dose is fractionated and administered slowly, spontaneous respiration and blood pressure are preserved. Propofol appears to possess antiemetic properties, which additionally add to its appeal.

A lipid-based anesthetic agent such as propofol can support rapid microbial growth at room temperature. Bennett et al. have documented the association of propofol with postoperative infections. This appears to be associated with lapse in aseptic techniques (20). A significant anesthesia-associated complication of external beam radiation therapy in children is the central venous access line-associated sepsis. Eleven of 74 children with a central venous line at Duke University Medical Center, receiving radiotherapy, developed proven sepsis (15%) with fever and a positive blood culture drawn through the central line. Out of these 11 children, 8 had received prior chemotherapy (73%). Six of the 11 had been anesthestized with propofol (55%), 4 with a short acting barbiturate induction plus inhalation anesthetic (36%), and one with inhalation anesthesia alone (9%). The pathogens cultivated from these 11 individuals included staphylococcus, bacillus, streptococcus, enterobacter, and candida (21).

There are four potential sources for central venous access colonization producing sepsis: the skin insertion site, the catheter hub, hematogenous seeding of the catheter, and infusate contamination such as might be caused by propofol (22). In the setting of anesthesia for pediatric external beam radiotherapy, one is concerned about the possible contamination of the catheter by repeated use by the anesthesiologist. It is well known that there is a high incidence of central venous line sepsis in a variety of high-risk settings including patients receiving chemotherapy, total parenteral nutrition, burn unit patients, and the intensive care unit (21). The risk of sepsis with repeated catheter use, in such settings, ranges from 5% to 29%. Therefore, one should not be surprised by the occasional case of sepsis in the child receiving repeated accession of the central venous line for anesthesia for radiotherapy.

MONITORING

Unrecognized hypoventilation is the primary cause of morbidity and mortality in pediatric anesthesia (20). The respiratory depressant effects of many anesthetic agents combined with the propensity for airway obstruction as a consequence of positioning for radiotherapy make anesthesia for pediatric radiotherapy a risky proposition. The need to be physically removed from the patient during the delivery of radiation adds to the challenge of adequate monitoring.

What constitutes appropriate monitoring for children receiving sedatives and general anesthetics? The American Academy of Pediatrics Section on Anesthesiology (23) and the American Society of Anesthesiologists (24) have published guidelines. The latter organization, in their standards for basic intraoperative monitoring, state:

> During all anesthetics, the patient's oxygenation, ventilation, circulation and temperature shall be continually evaluated. Qualified anesthesia personnel shall be present in the room throughout the conduct of all general anesthetics, regional anesthetics and monitored anesthesia care. In the event there is a direct known hazard, e.g., radiation, to the anesthesia personnel which might require intermittent remote observation of the patient, some provision for monitoring the patient must be made.

Provisions made for monitoring in radiotherapy suites include closed-circuit television screens on which are displayed the patient and the monitors of oxygenation, ventilation, circulation and temperature, and leaded glass windows through which the patient and monitors can be viewed while the radiation treatment is delivered (Fig. 2).

Early reports of anesthesia for radiotherapy relied on visual inspection of patient color as a monitor of adequacy of oxygenation. However, the unreliability of direct observation for the detection of cyanosis has long been known (25). Pulse oximetry is an accurate, noninvasive, continuous measure of arterial oxygen saturation. A pulse oximeter is an optical sensor that measures the concentration of oxyhemoglobin. Oximeters work according to the Beer-Lambert law, which states that (a) when a parallel beam of light falls on a semitransparent homogeneous substance, the intensity of the transmitted light decreases exponentially as distance through the substance increases, and (b) if a parallel beam of light is transmitted a known distance through a clear solution with a dissolved solute, the intensity of the transmitted light decreases exponentially as the concentration of solute increases. In clinical practice, pulse oximeters measure

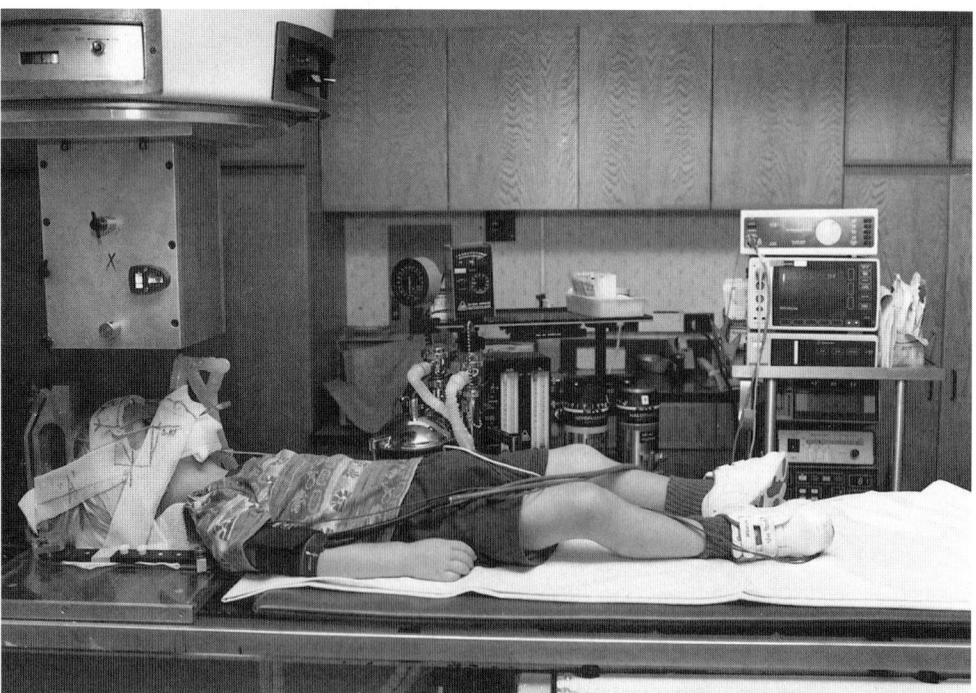

FIG. 2. The anesthetized child is monitored, in the accelerator vault, with ECG, pulse oximetry, and capnometry. Note that the gas delivery mask is well integrated into the radiotherapy head stabilization device.

red and infrared light transmitted through tissue beds such as a finger, earlobe, or nose. The utility of pulse oximetry in the detection of cyanosis in children has been demonstrated in large randomized controlled clinical trials (26). Pulse oximetry is now a monitoring standard in anesthesia practice.

How is ventilation best monitored? The first report of anesthesia for radiotherapy utilized "continual visual observation of the thorax and abdomen" combined with a wisp of cotton placed over the mouth. The cotton fibers moved in and out with inspiration and expiration, respectively, and served as an "amplifier" of air movement. Amplifiers are necessary because the anesthesiologist cannot be physically present while radiation therapy is being delivered. Several amplifiers of ventilation have been described for use in radiotherapy. Visual amplifiers that have been suggested include: (a) attaching a cotton-tipped applicator to the thorax and observing via a closed circuit television monitor the excursions of the cotton tip with inspiration and expiration and (b) placing a light box on the patient's abdomen or chest and observing on the television monitor the movement of the light bulb with each respiratory cycle. Aural amplifiers allow the anesthesiologist to hear the patient's breath sounds while physically removed from the treatment area. An esophageal or precordial stethoscope can be connected to an audio amplifier, and the output can be heard on a speaker or earphone.

Observation of the movements of the reservoir breathing bag by the anesthesiologist is an excellent monitor of gas exchange. This technique is applicable to those patients anesthetized with inhalational agents whose tracheas are intubated, those who have a LMA in place, or those who have a simple face mask applied over the nose and mouth. If the breathing bag cannot easily be seen on the closed circuit monitor or through the leaded glass window, its movements can be amplified by constructing a stick made of tongue blades. One end of the stick is attached to the neck of the breathing bag with a piece of tape, and a 10-cm flag of white paper is placed at the opposite end of the stick. This long lever arm greatly accentuates the movements of the breathing bag and serves as an amplifier of ventilation.

The "gold standard" for assessing ventilation is capnometry. Capnometry is the quantitative measurement of the partial pressure of carbon dioxide (CO_2) produced by the patient during the ventilatory cycle. Capnography is the continuous graphic display of CO_2 concentration as a function of time. End-tidal CO_2 analysis is a means of assessing alveolar ventilation, airway patency, and the functioning of the breathing circuit and ventilator. End-tidal CO_2 monitoring has been shown to be an effective monitor in pediatric anesthesia (25), capable of the early detection of many potentially life-threatening events such as apnea, bronchospasm, and disconnections in the breathing circuit.

The adequacy of circulatory function during the administration of anesthesia is assessed by continuous display of the electrocardiogram (ECG) and by measurement of blood pressure. Noninvasive, automated oscillometric blood pressure determination (DINAMAP, Criti Kom, Inc, Tampa FL) is readily available and uniquely suited for remote monitoring of blood pressure. The displays of ECG and DINAMAP are viewed indirectly on the closed circuit monitor or directly through a leaded glass window if the radiotherapy suite is so equipped (Figs. 3 and 4).

In the Duke series of anesthesia for pediatric radiation therapy, the most frequently used monitoring techniques were ECG (95%), monitoring of blood pressure via manual aneroid sphygmomanometer (71%), blood pressure monitoring via an automated, noninvasive oscillometric device (DINAMAP) (15%), pulse oximetry (93%), capnometry (55%), and monitoring of the fraction inspired oxygen via polarigraphic electrode placed in the inspired gas limb in the anesthesia circuit (57%). In most patients, multiple monitoring techniques were utilized (21).

In summary, standards for monitoring anesthetized children have been published. These standards and guidelines are intended

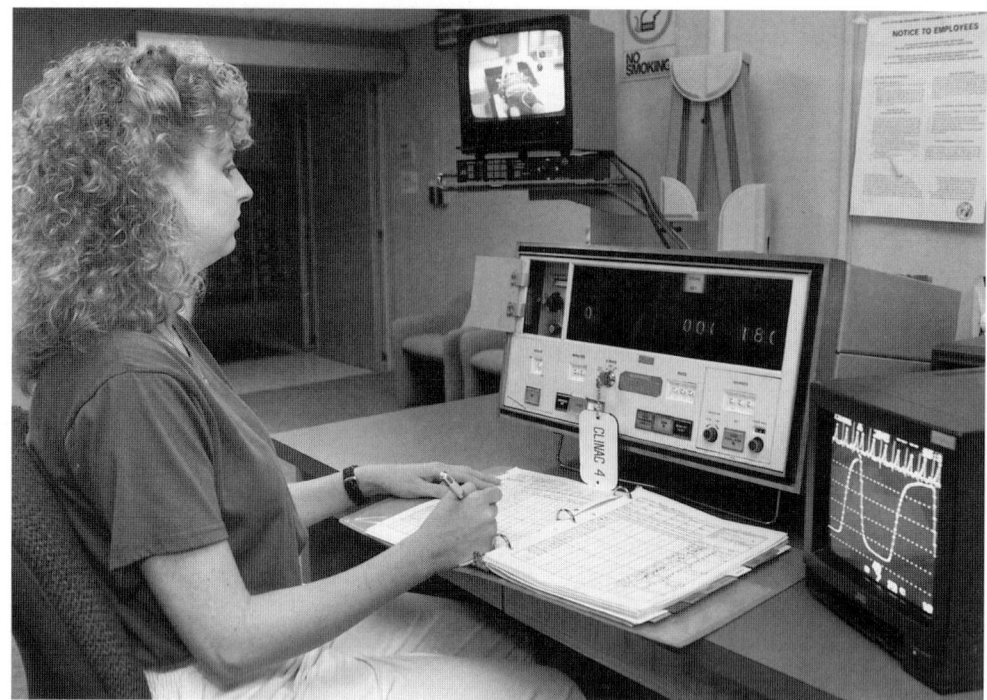

FIG. 3. Monitoring, immediately outside the treatment room, is accomplished with a video screen displaying the child, an intercom system for audio, and a monitor displaying the ECG, respiratory wave, and FiO₂.

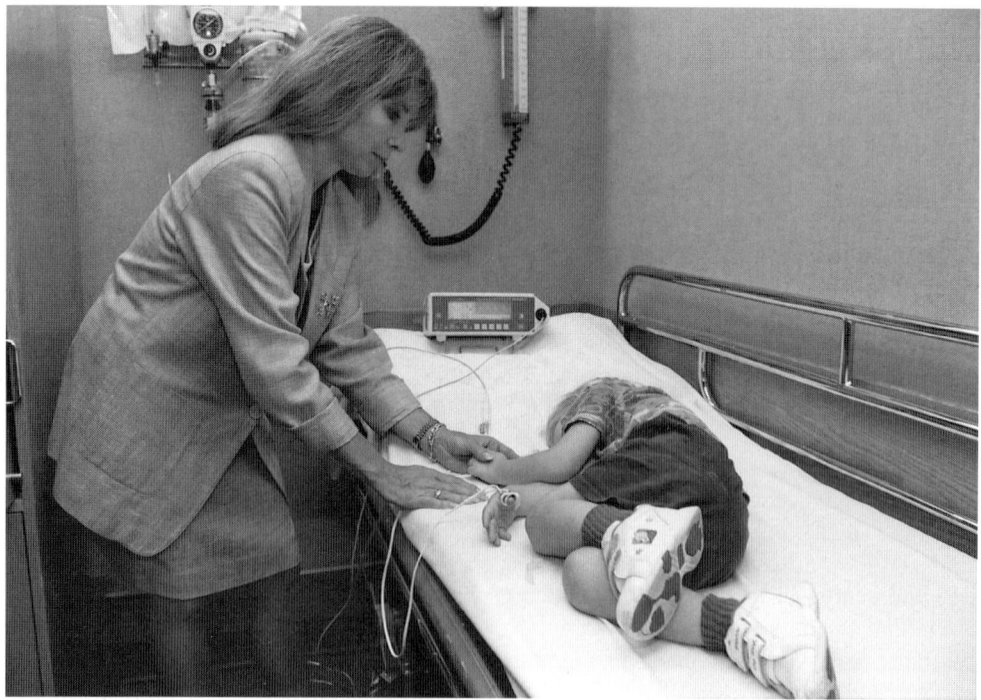

FIG. 4. The anesthesiologist is at the bedside in the recovery area in the radiotherapy department. Oxygen, suction, and pulse oximetry monitoring are immediately available.

to promote high-quality care. No matter how rigorous the adherence to these recommendations, it is impossible to guarantee specific patient outcomes. The provision of anesthesia for radiotherapy carries with it the additional challenge of remote monitoring of patients whose airways may be compromised not only by their underlying disease, but also by the constraints of positioning for the procedure.

ANESTHETIC IMPLICATIONS OF UNDERLYING DISEASE

Radiotherapy is utilized to treat several different pediatric malignancies. In the Duke series, the diagnoses leading to treatment with external beam radiotherapy under anesthesia for primary CNS tumor (28%), retinoblastoma (26%), neuroblastoma (18%), acute leukemia (9%), rhabdomyosarcoma (7%), Wilms' tumor (5%), Langerhans' cell histiocytosis (4%), and other (3%) (21). It is not surprising that the diagnoses leading to radiotherapy under anesthesia differ somewhat from the most frequent diagnoses of cancer in childhood. Leukemia is a relatively infrequent indication for radiotherapy under anesthesia because it is, in general, a malignancy of older children and the role of radiation therapy is limited. Diseases associated with younger age children in which radiotherapy is more frequently used dominate the list (21). Many of these malignancies have implications for the pediatric anesthesiologist. Children with supratentorial brain tumors can have increased ICP. Management of anesthesia for patients with increased ICP includes the avoidance of drugs that can raise ICP, such as ketamine. Anesthetic techniques that result in elevations in arterial CO_2 tension can produce intracranial hypertension by increasing cerebral blood flow.

Some neuroblastomas secrete catecholamines, and systemic hypertension can be seen in this patient population. Blood pressure elevations are associated with abdominal palpation. This problem is rare in pediatric radiotherapy because the tumor is not manipulated.

Wilms' tumors are often massive and can impair ventilation by increasing intraabdominal pressure. An occasional child with a Wilms' tumor will undergo endotracheal intubation for respiratory failure prior to presenting to the radiation oncologist for radiotherapy. These tumors can also extend into the inferior vena cava and renal vein, producing renovascular distortion and systemic hypertension.

Children with Hodgkin's disease, non-Hodgkin's lymphomas, and T-cell acute lymphoblastic leukemia can present with anterior mediastinal masses. These masses can produce tracheal compression and impair ventilation. They can also produce superior vena cava syndrome by compression of the great veins. Some patients with anterior mediastinal masses are referred to the pediatric radiation oncologist for external-beam therapy prior to tissue biopsy. Radiation therapy prior to tissue biopsy is recommended in some of these patients because the induction of anesthesia in some patients with anterior mediastinal masses can be fatal. Death on induction of general anesthesia in these patients is due to either (a) the inability to ventilate because of airway compression, or (b) the inability of the heart to circulate blood due to tumor encroachment on the right heart or pulmonary circulation (5). Prospective identification of children with anterior mediastinal masses who are at risk for cardiorespiratory collapse on induction of general anesthesia involves a thorough history and physical examination aimed at eliciting signs and symptoms of airway and/or cardiovascular impairment. Laboratory studies useful in assessing preanesthetic risk include a chest radiograph, computerized tomography (CT) scan, and upright and supine flow-volume loops. The pediatric radiotherapist may be referred those patients with anterior mediastinal masses for whom the risks of general anesthesia are felt to outweigh the benefits of obtaining tissue prior to the institution of therapy. These patients should not receive anesthesia or sedation.

In addition to these considerations, the pediatric anesthesiologist must consider the associated implications of the treatment of malignancy in children. These implications include the cardiac, hematologic, pulmonary, immunologic, and neurologic impairments due to chemotherapy in children (27).

Anemia is one of the most common problems in children with cancer. Anemia decreases oxygen delivery to the tissues. Oxygen delivery is the product of the arterial oxygen content and the cardiac index. If oxygen delivery to the tissues is inadequate, organ system failure occurs. The minimum acceptable hemoglobin value in anesthetized children is unknown. Hemoglobin values as low as 7 g/dL may be adequate if the patient has normal cardiovascular compensatory mechanisms. However, many patients cannot compensate for low levels of hemoglobin because they have chemotherapy-induced myocardial dysfunction.

Cardiac toxicity is most notably due to the anthracycline antibiotic chemotherapeutic agents doxorubicin (Adriamycin) and daunorubicin. These drugs have both an acute and chronic effect. Acute toxicity manifests as rhythm and conduction disturbances such as supraventricular tachycardia, ventricular ectopic beats, and heart block. Chronic toxicity manifests as a cardiomyopathy which can progress to left ventricular failure in 2% to 10% of patients. Factors that increase the risk of anthracycline cardiotoxicity include doses in excess of 550 mg/m^2, age younger than 1 year, concurrent use of other chemotherapeutic agents such as cyclophosphamide and cisplatin, and a history of mediastinal irradiation.

Pulmonary toxicity occurs in 5% to 10% of patients treated with the antibiotic chemotherapeutic agent bleomycin. Bleomycin produces interstitial pulmonary fibrosis, which results in restrictive lung disease. The damage is thought to be produced by oxygen free radical formation. The role of exogenous oxygen in promoting the pulmonary toxicity of bleomycin is controversial. However, it is prudent to avoid inspired oxygen concentrations in excess of 28% when anesthetizing patients who have been treated with bleomycin, provided that they maintain satisfactory levels of arterial oxygen tension.

On rare occasions, the child requiring anesthesia for radiotherapy will have received a prior course of irradiation to the head and neck or lungs. These children may be at somewhat higher risk for laryngeal edema following instrumentation of the airway for anesthesia and/or difficulties maintaining oxygenation. The anesthesiologist must be aware of the potential for problems of this sort (28–30).

REFERENCES

References particularly recommended for further reading are indicated by an asterisk.

*1. Harrison GG, Bennet MB. Radiotherapy without tears. *Br J Anaesth* 1963;35:720–721.
2. Hall S. Anesthesia outside the OR: the pediatric patient. In: *Refresher course lectures.* Park Ridge, IL: American Society of Anesthesiology, 1992;212:1–7.
3. Fisher DM, Robinson S, Brett CM, et al. Comparison of enflurane, halothane, and isoflurane for diagnostic and therapeutic procedures in children with malignancies. *Anesthesiology* 1985;63:647–650.
4. Wolfe TM, Rao CC. Anesthesia outside the operating room. *Semin Pediatr Surg* 1992;1:81–87.
5. Keon TP. Death on induction of anesthesia for cervical node biopsy. *Anesthesiology* 1981;55:471–472.
6. Eger EI II. New inhaled anesthetics. *Anesthesiology* 1994;80:906–922.
7. Eger EI II. New inhaled anesthetics. *Intern Anesthesiol Clin* 1995;33:61–80.
8. Lerman J. Sevoflurane in pediatric anesthesia. *Anesth Analg* 1995;81:S4–10.
9. Smith I, Nathanson MH, White PF. The role of sevoflurane in outpatient anesthesia. *Anesth Analg* 1995;81:S67–72.
*10. Grebenik CR, Ferguson C, White A. The laryngeal mask airway in pediatric radiotherapy. *Anesthesiology* 1990;72:474–477.
10a. Morris GN, Marjot R. Laryngeal mask airway performance: effect of cuff deflation during anaesthesia. *Br J Anaesth* 1996;76(3):456–458.
11. Moylan SL, Luce MA. The reinforced laryngeal mask airway in paediatric radiotherapy. *Br J Anaesth* 1993;71:172.
12. Wilson IG. The laryngeal mask airway in paediatric practice. *Br J Anaesth* 1993;70:124–125.
13. Jacobs JR, Reves JG, Glass PSA. Rationale and technique for continuous infusions in anesthesia. *Int Anesth Clin* 1991;29:23–38.
14. Amberg HL, Gordon G. Low-dose intramuscular ketamine for pediatric radiotherapy: a case report. *Anesth Analg* 1976;55:92–94.
15. Bennett JA, Bullimore JA. The use of ketamine hydrochloride anesthesia for radiotherapy in young children. *Br J Anaesth* 1973;45:197–201.
16. Edge WG, Morgan M. Ketamine and paediatric radiotherapy. *Anaesth Intensive Care* 1977;5:153–156.
17. Cronin MM, Bousfield JD, Hewett EB, et al. Ketamine

anaesthesia for radiotherapy in small children. *Anaesthesia* 1972;27:135–142.

*18. Menache L, Eifel PJ, Kennamer DL, Belli JA. Twice-daily anesthesia in infants receiving hyperfractionated irradiation. *Int J Radiat Oncol Biol Phys* 1990;18:625–629.

19. Murray WJ, Murray MJ. Anesthesia for twice-daily infant irradiation [Letter]. *Int J Radiat Oncol Biol Phys* 1991;20:909.

20. Bennett SN, McNeil MM, Bland LA, et al. Postoperative infections traced to contamination of an intravenous anesthetic propofol. *N Engl J Med* 1996;333:147–154.

*21. Fortney JT, Halperin EC, Hertz CM, Schulman SR. One hundred forty one consecutive cases of anesthesia for pediatric external beam radiation therapy. 1998 (*submitted*).

22. Daghistani DH, Horn M, Rodriguez Z, Schoenike S, Toledano S. Prevention of indwelling central venous catheter sepsis. *Med Pediatr Oncol* 1996;26:405–408.

23. Committee on Drugs. Guidelines for monitoring and management of pediatric patients during and after sedation for diagnostic and therapeutic procedures. *Pediatrics* 1992;89:1110–1115.

24. American Society of Anesthesiologists. Standards for basic intraoperative monitoring. *Directory of Members* 1993;58:709–710.

25. Comroe JH Jr, Botelho S. The reliability of cyanosis in the recognition of arterial hypoxemia. *Am J Med Sci* 1947;214:1–6.

26. Cote CJ, Goldstein EA, Cote MA, et al. A single blind study of pulse oximetry in children. *Anesthesiology* 1988;68:184–188.

*27. Tobias JD. Special considerations for the pediatric oncology patient. In: Berry FA, Steward DJ, eds. *Pediatrics for the anesthesiologist.* New York: Churchill Livingstone, 1993:287–303.

28. Ginsberg RJ. Surgical considerations after preoperative treatment. *Lung Cancer* 1994;10[Suppl 1]:S213–217.

29. Mark RJ, Bailet JW, Poen J, et al. Postirradiation sarcoma of the head and neck. *Cancer* 1993;72:887–893.

30. Mendel P, Anaes FC, Bristow A. New methods of dealing with the complications of panendoscopy. *J Larngol Otol* 1992;106:903–904.

*31. Glauber DT, Audenaert SM. Anesthesia for children undergoing craniospinal radiotherapy. *Anesthesiology* 1987;67:701–803.

22

Stabilization and Immobilization Devices

Throughout this book, we have emphasized the balance that must be struck by the pediatric radiation oncologist: Administer a sufficient radiation dose to achieve the desired goal of tumor control while not giving a dose that is so high as to engender an unacceptable risk of complications. For many tumors the clinically relevant dose-response curve is sigmoidal in shape and quite steep (1). A small variation in dose can significantly influence the chance of tumor control and the risk of complications. Errors in dose prescription can be the result of physician error. Physician error is best dealt with by training, education, and peer review.

Another source of error is in treatment planning and administration. We can determine the location of the target volume with computerized tomography, magnetic resonance imaging, positron emission tomography, and plain radiography. Computer technology allows three-dimensional tumor volume reconstruction and beam planning. Most patients undergo treatment planning and beam confirmation with a simulator. The linear accelerators used in clinical practice provide beams with sharply defined edges. A skilled dosimetrist can generate treatment plans using combinations of photons and electrons, wedges, beam weighting, and compensators (2,3). All this effort and skill can be for naught, however, if the patient is not holding still or is not put in a reproducible and comfortable position at each treatment ses-

sion. For the anxious child, positioning and stabilization is often the weakest link in the chain of treatment planning and implementation (2,4,5). Quality radiotherapy demands that a daily setup accuracy of a few millimeters be ensured (6–8). For the youngest patients, anesthesia will be required—a topic we reviewed in Chapter 21. In this chapter we will consider, in detail, psychological, educational, and mechanical aids for patient immobilization.

PSYCHOLOGICAL PREPARATION AND PATIENT/FAMILY EDUCATION

Before beginning radiotherapy, many children will have undergone multiple venipunctures, lumbar punctures, bone marrow biopsies, surgery, and chemotherapy. Therefore, the child will frequently be fearful of any attempt to be immobilized. This conditioned and understandable response is best dealt with by patience and understanding. Several strategies can be used to deal with fear. First and foremost, the physician must establish rapport and ensure the confidence of the child's parents. Before the radiation oncologist ever met the child, throughout the treatment, and for long after the treatment concludes, it will be the parents who are the child's primary reference point. It is presumptuous to think that after a few brief meetings the radiotherapist can create such a strong relationship with the child as to ensure cooperation with treatment.

This is not to say that the therapist should neglect efforts to have a good relationship with the child—of course, they should. It is to say, however, that if the child's parents feel comfortable with the plan for treatment and express confidence in the presence of the child, then more than one-half of the battle is won. The therapy team should provide the parents with a tour of the radiotherapy department, a chance to see and touch the equipment, adequate time to meet the personnel involved in their child's case, and an unhurried time to ask questions and have them answered. It is often advisable to conduct this initial visit without the patient present so that conversation is not inhibited. The child must also be given a tour of the department and meet everyone involved in their case. The radiotherapist should be willing to demonstrate simulation and treatment on a favorite doll or stuffed animal toy (9). An unhurried atmosphere, pleasant background music, patience, and positive reinforcement when the child cooperates are important.

Many pediatric inpatient services benefit from the expertise of trained play (or recreation) therapists. These individuals should be made completely familiar with the routines of pediatric radiotherapy. They are often valuable allies in making a child more at ease in the therapy area. Special toy radiotherapy machines, art activities, and acting through the planned treatment are techniques used by play therapists to prepare a child for treatment.

Many children and parents are accustomed to receiving information from television. To meet this need, the physician may now turn to specially prepared and commercially available videotapes describing external-beam radiotherapy. Some of these videotapes are professionally made and utilize animation and professional actors. They can convey a significant amount of information in a short time. Some departments make it a routine to show instructional video tapes to most children and families. In addition, patient-education printed material is available for distribution. These include special coloring books about radiotherapy, pamphlets with cartoon-like drawings describing treatment, as well as more mature material for teenagers and parents. Some departments utilize desktop printing, photographs, and loose-leaf binders to construct "homemade" patient education material.

The widespread availability of computers has created a new world of opportunity for patients to educate themselves about cancer treatment. It is not unusual for a family to have "surfed" the World Wide Web for information about a particular tumor or to have participated in a "chat room" or "bulletin board" in cyberspace about their medical problems. Many pediatric oncology centers, comprehensive cancer centers, and radiation oncology departments have Web site homepages that go into considerable detail about personnel and available protocols. Families may also learn about cancer treatment via the services accessed through toll-free telephone numbers of the National Cancer Institute and patient advocacy groups.

THE IDEAL MECHANICAL AID

Mechanical immobilization of the awake pediatric radiotherapy patient is an adjunct to patient education and psychological preparation, not a substitute for it. The ideal mechanical aid to patient positioning will meet the following goals. (a) The child must feel comfortable and secure. There must be no danger of falling. (b) The device must satisfy the radiotherapy treatment plan regarding patient position for correct geographical irradiation. (c) The setup should be quick and easy for the technologist. (d) The body part treated should be rendered immobile. (e) The position of the body part should be reproducible for daily treatment. (f) Construction of the device should be reasonably quick. It should not be difficult to train technologists, dosimetrists, and physicians in the procedure. (g) The stabilization device should not adversely affect beam buildup and backscatter characteristics. (h) The system should be economical. (i) If anesthesia is being utilized, the device must not interfere with the establishment of a se-

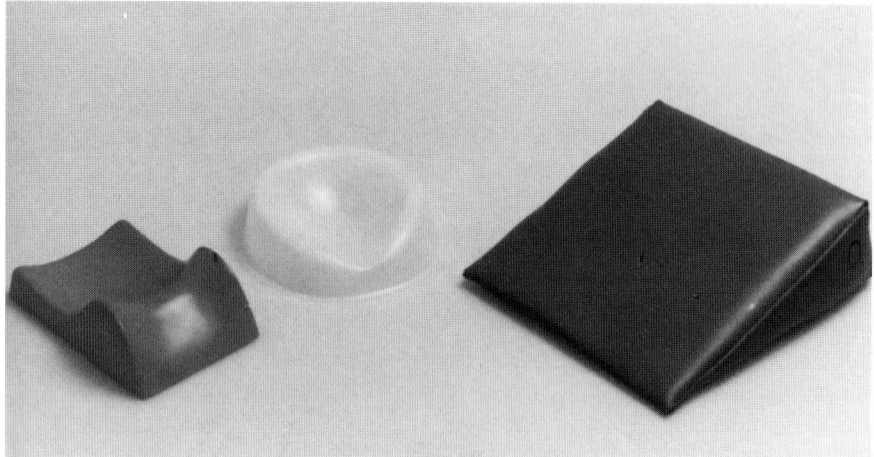

FIG. 1. Supine head supports.

cure airway, intravenous access, and the use of monitoring equipment (3,10,11a–11c).

Several immobilization systems meet these criteria to varying degrees. There is, however, no perfect system. Techniques vary widely between institutions. The skilled radiation oncologist should be knowledgeable about several techniques so they may be used as the situation demands.

STANDARD ACCESSORY DEVICES

There are a large number of commercially available radiotherapy accessories for patient stabilization. These devices have the advantage of being relatively inexpensive and reusable. They have the disadvantage of never being customized to the individual patient and providing relatively poor immobilization (2,12–14).

The plastic head holder provides stability for the head when the patient is supine. The device, called a "doggie dish" because of its resemblance to a pet's feeding bowl, is available in several sizes. Firm head and neck supports are also available in various sizes for supine treatment (Figs. 1 to 3). The "Duncan headrest" and "Osborne fixed-angle head holder" are head stabilizers for prone treatment. These plastic devices have a foam-rubber padding and disposable paper liners.

There are openings for the eyes, nose, and mouth (13).

A simple head holder may be constructed by suspending a vinyl or cloth sheet between two metal bars (14,15). The head may be positioned prone, supine, or lateral. Vertical adjustment may be done by a gear crank. Some institutions have mounted head holders at the end of the treatment couch to allow prone positioning of the head for craniospinal irradiation (CSI).

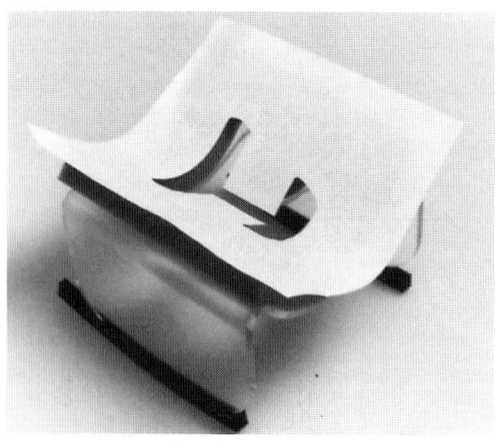

FIG. 2. A prone headrest.

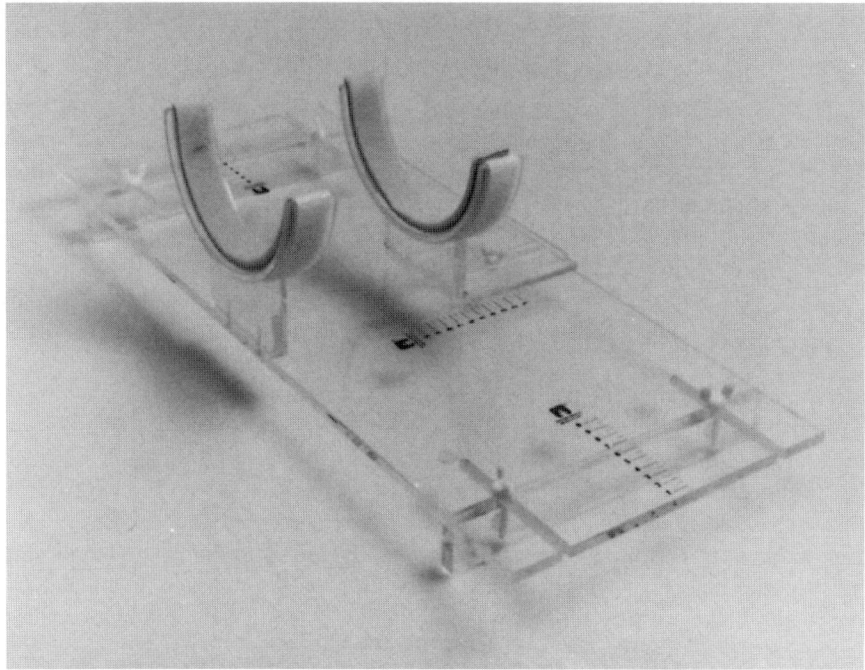

FIG. 3. A commercially available adjustable head support.

Many linear accelerator couches are quite narrow and do not provide a comfortable resting place for a child's arms or legs. Plexiglas, plastic, or wooden sheets or boards may be used to widen the couch. These may be anchored by placing them, in part, under the child's body (12).

Every pediatric radiotherapy unit should be equipped with (a) an assortment of canvas or other fabric straps to attach to the treatment couch, and (b) small sandbags. These cannot be used to restrain an uncooperative child or, by themselves, ensure a reproducible treatment setup. They can, however, be used to good effect as an extra measure of safety against rolling or falling.

THE BITE BLOCK

Bite blocks are utilized in head and neck radiotherapy to stabilize the child's jaw so that the same mouth position is reproduced at each treatment session, to deflect or depress the tongue away from the hard palate during irra-

diation of the nasopharyngeal or hard palate areas, and to fill the natural airspace of the mouth (16,17). A bite impression can be made in the radiation oncology department with rapidly setting dental material on a plastic bite plate of the sort used in dentistry (1,14,16). It is the custom, in some departments, to place the barrel of a hypodermic syringe in the middle of the dental impression to provide an additional airway for the patient. Other departments embed tongue depressors in the modeling compound to provide extra pressure on the back of the tongue.

Some pediatric dentists have training in sophisticated techniques for making full and partial mouth impressions. These impressions can be adopted to create snugly fitting and elegant bite blocks.

If the bite block is used as the sole patient-positioning device, the block is fixed to a calibrated arm that is, in turn, fixed to the treatment couch. Simulation and treatment are done with the arm in the same position each day. Stability is dependent on the willingness of the child to accept the dental impression in the mouth and bite down firmly. If the bite block is to be used in conjunction with a thermal plastic head stabilization device, then it is important to prepare the thermal plastic with the bite block already in place. Only in this way can one be assured that the plastic mold will fit snugly around the facial contour as it is distorted by the bite block.

THERMAL PLASTICS

A custom-made contoured thermal plastic device is often useful for immobilization. Thermal plastics are used by orthopedic surgeons for splints and casts and are commercially available from several suppliers (8,15,18–21). The plastic comes in perforated sheets that soften and become malleable when heated to 160°F to 180°F (70°C to 80°C) in a hot water bath. The material's stickiness and elasticity hold it in place during molding. A working time of 5 to 7 minutes allows shaping of the cast without reheating. The material bonds to itself readily so strips of the plastic can be crossed to create a firmer cast (18). The body part is usually covered in clear plastic wrap, with holes for the nose and mouth. A shower cap may be used to protect the hair instead of clear plastic wrap. Some children will be more comfortable if a gauze pad is placed over bony prominences of the skull to alleviate pressure. Once the casting material has been softened in warm water, the entire sheet or individual plastic strips are applied. The plastic is smoothed and contoured to approximate the body surface. As the plastic cools, it hardens in 7 to 10 minutes but retains the new shape. The new cast may be clamped or screwed to a wooden or plastic board on the treatment couch. The perforations in the plastic allow air circulation and a partial view of patient anatomy. Setup marks may be drawn directly on the cast (Figs. 4 to 6). Stretched thermoplastic causes a slight increase in the radiation surface dose from 6 or 18 MV photons (4).

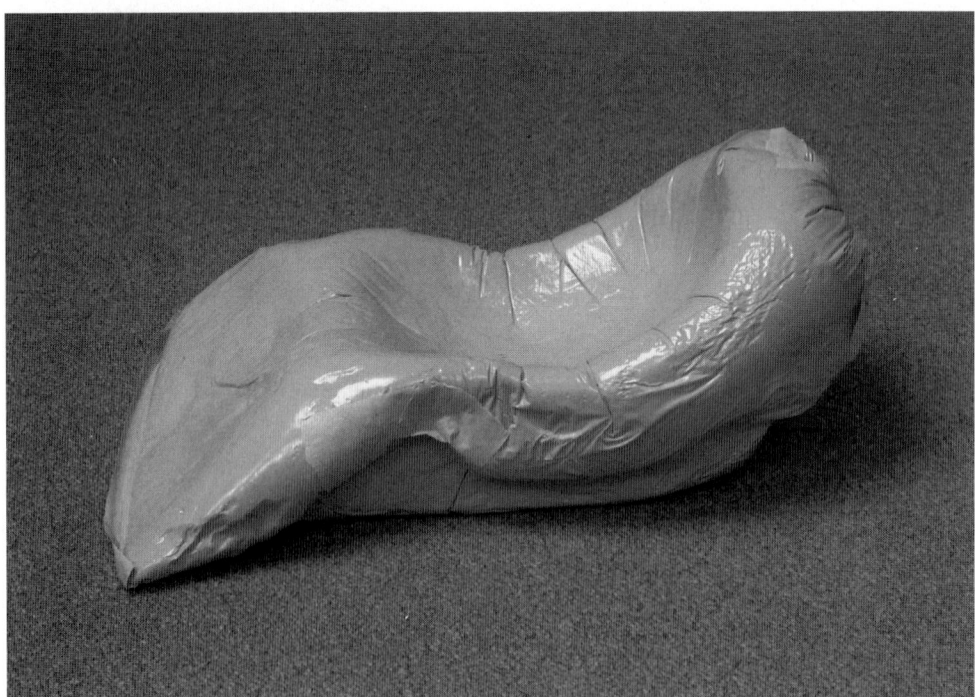

FIG. 4. A polyurethane foam mold of the head and neck in supine position provides stability and reproducable head position. This is combined with a thermoplastic head holder to create a tight fit and a stable patient (see Figs. 5 and 6).

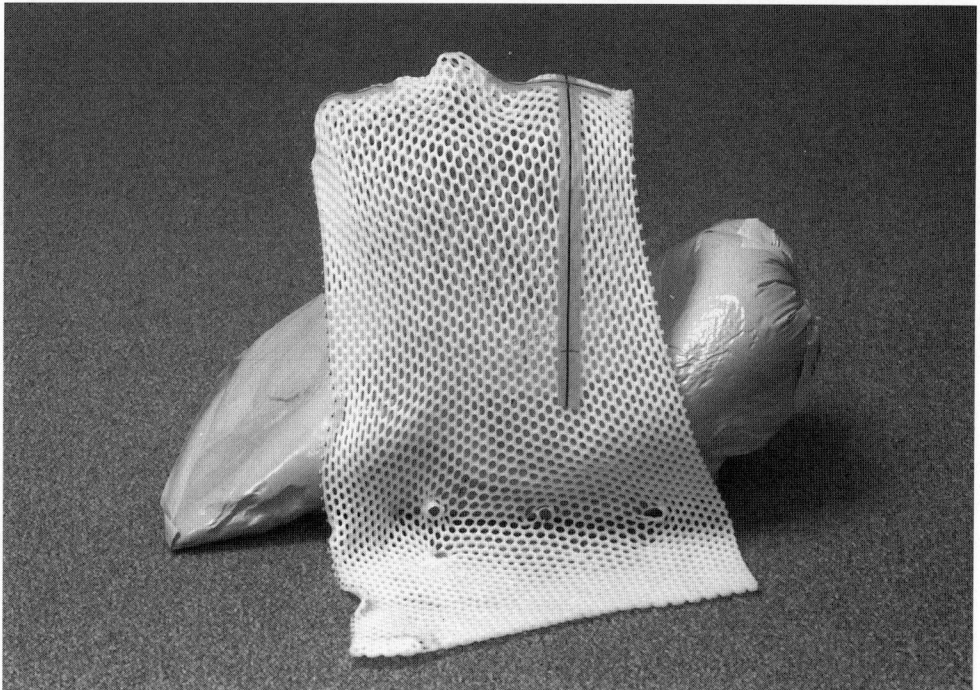

FIG. 5. A thermoplastic head holder made of a single sheet, combined with a polyurethane foam mold of the head and neck will provide the stability needed for three-dimensional conformal therapy of a brain tumor.

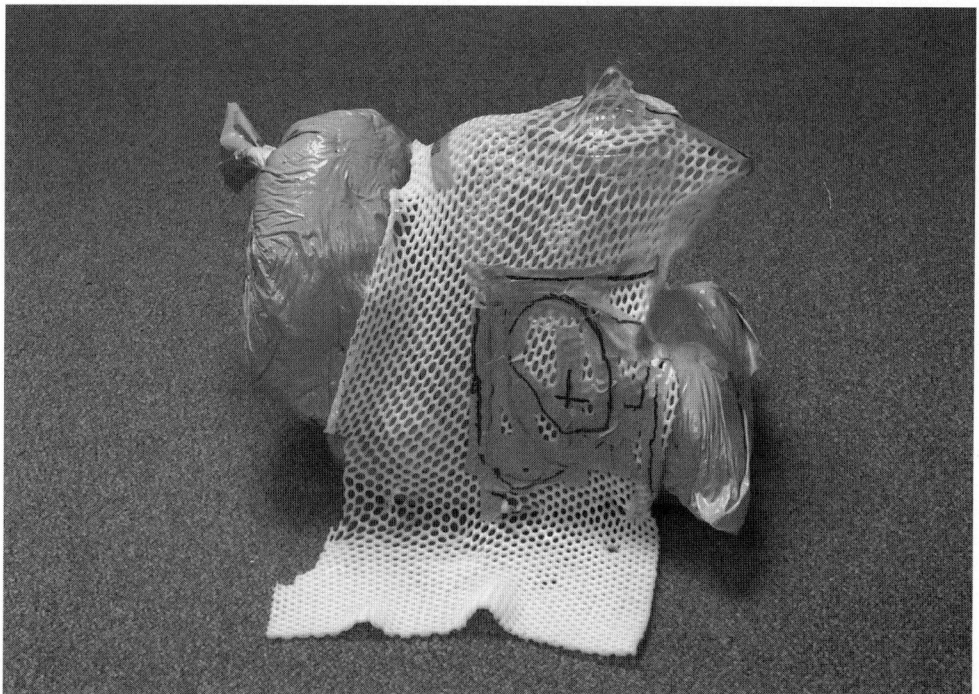

FIG. 6. This thermoplastic head holder and polyurethane foam mold of the back of the head and neck was created for treatment of child with posterior fossa ependymoma. The child required anesthesia for daily treatment. Note how the anesthesiologist's gas mask was built into the head holder for daily use. The markings on the mask, for laser alignment and port marks, may be drawn on tape placed on the mask.

The use of steroids, weight loss or gain, or edema during the course of radiation can render a thermoplastic head holder ill fitting. Often fabrication of a new head holder will be necessary. Sometimes the problem can be addressed by spot heating the problem area with a heat gun until pliable. When the plastic's temperature is tolerable to the touch, the head holder is revised (22).

If the child is to be irradiated under anesthesia, the thermal plastic head holder can be fabricated with the gas mask or CO_2 monitor as integral parts of the immobilizer. The anesthesiologist and radiation oncologist must mutually agree on the head position and degree of neck extension to facilitate radiotherapy as well as anesthesia airway management.

PLASTER OF PARIS

Plaster of Paris is a fine white powder that is prepared from gypsum. Plaster bandages are particularly useful for radiotherapy purposes. The bandage consists of a mesh impregnated with plaster powder. The bandage is immersed in water, the excess water is squeezed out, and the material is ready for molding (2,11,12). An exothermic reaction occurs as the material solidifies. Heat is produced, and one must take care lest a child be burned.

In order to make a cast, the body part to be immobilized is covered with stockinette or other soft lining for protection. Alternatively, one may coat the area with petroleum jelly. The plaster of Paris strips are applied in sufficient number to provide structural stability. The cast may be removed when partially dry and then allowed to harden. Casts may be reinforced, cut out, or drawn on as required.

Plaster casts are useful for CSI, whole-body casting for immobilization of young children, and head immobilization (2,23,24) (Fig. 7). They may be used in conjunction with vacuum-molded thermoplastics (22). Plaster casts can achieve excellent immobilization, but their production is time consuming (25). At least one department utilizes a

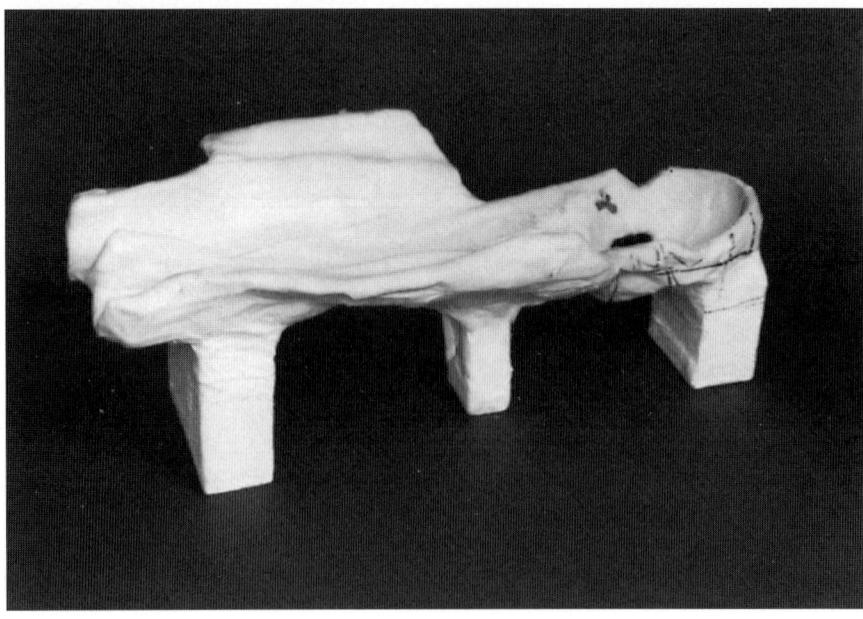

FIG. 7. A plaster of Paris cast for prone treatment with craniospinal irradiation. These casts have been abandoned by some institutions and replaced with polyurethane foam devices or thermoplastic prone face masks.

product that consists of sheets of plaster-soaked bandage sandwiched between cotton flannel and polyurethane foam. The flannel adds to the cast's structural strength when soaked with the plaster. The foam is in contact with the patient (3). The material becomes pliable when wet and is used in the same manner as the plaster bandage strips described previously.

LIGHTCAST

Lightcast is an orthopedic casting product that is rarely used in radiation therapy. It consists of a resin-coated mesh (2,26). Stockinette or plastic wrap is placed over the area to be immobilized. The flexible mesh is then applied and molded into body crevices. The material dries and hardens under ultraviolet light. When wet, the material has an unpleasant odor.

VACUUM-MOLDED THERMOPLASTICS

Several types of clear plastics are available in flat sheets that may be used for the construction of clear, rigid immobilization devices (2,11,16,22,27,28). The initial step in the construction of these devices is the preparation of a plaster mold. The body part of interest is molded with plaster bandages. The plaster impression is allowed to dry, and then the ends are closed off to form a container for plaster casting. Plaster of Paris powder is mixed with water to a creamy consistency, and the impression is filled. After the casting has been allowed to dry, the impression bandages are peeled off, leaving a model of the body part. The plaster model is then placed in a vacuum molding machine that heats the clear plastic sheet and, with the aid of a vacuum, draws the plastic tightly over the cast (2,16,27,29). The plastic becomes hard when cool. Some technical skill is required when using the vacuum-molding machine to avoid wasting the plastic material, tearing the plastic as it molds, or wrapping the plastic too far around the model—locking the plastic on the plaster.

When the plastic mold is completed, it may be fitted to the body part and attached to the treatment couch. Visibility is excellent, and one may draw directly on the plastic.

POLYURETHANE FOAMS

A commercially available system for the creation of a polyurethane mold, Alpha Cradle and Alpha Cradle Mold Maker (Smithers Medical Products, Inc., Akron, OH, USA), is a popular way to immobilize for pediatric radiotherapy (2,9,20). The body part to be immobilized is placed on a polystyrene bag that is filled with chemicals. The chemical reaction that occurs generates an expanding polyurethane foam. The foam fills the bag and molds around the body part. Various frames may be used with this system for thorax, abdominal, or limb immobilization. Styrofoam sheets, 0.75 inch to 1 inch thick, may be placed inside the bag to be incorporated into the expanding foam and add structural strength to the device. After the chemical reaction is initiated by mixing the chemicals one has 4 to 5 minutes to position the patient. The child must remain motionless for approximately 15 minutes as the immobilizer hardens and cools (Figs. 4 to 6, and 8). The exothermic chemical reaction generates temperatures that do not exceed 105.7°F. This degree of heat may be uncomfortable for some children. A sheet of paper on the bag usually allows enough heat displacement for comfort without interfering with molding.

In the treatment of abdominal/pelvic malignancies, such as neuroblastoma, Wilms' tumor, retroperitoneal sarcoma, and lymphoma, it is generally desirable to avoid, to the extent possible, bowel irradiation. A variety of techniques have been used to exclude bowel from the treatment field. A prone position, the use of a full bladder to displace bowel, and compression devices all have proponents. A polyurethane mold and reinforcing styrofoam sheets can be used to construct a "belly board" to exclude bowel from the treatment field. The child is simulated prone, with small bowel contrast. The polyurethane mold is

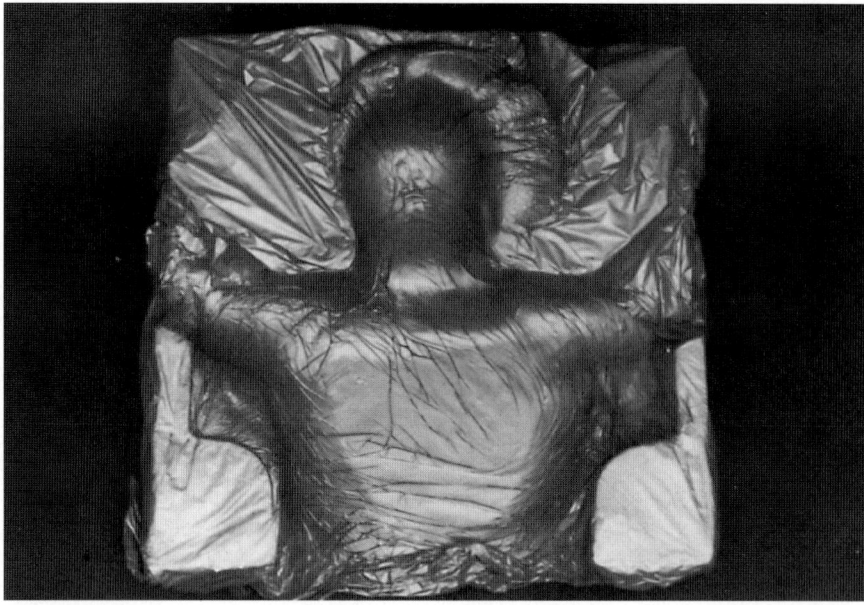

FIG. 8. A polyurethane foam mold for supine Hodgkin's disease mantle therapy.

made so that the hips are slightly elevated to allow gravity to pull the mobile bowel out of the pelvis. A hole is cut in the center of the board so that the abdomen falls slightly into the opening. By this means, a lateral field can be constructed that may exclude bowel. If the simulation is conducted with small bowel contrast, the degree of bowel protection can be documented (12,30).

The Alpha Cradle system has a density of 0.03 gm per cm^3 (31). For Co^{60}, 6MV, and 18 MV photon beams the presence of an Alpha Cradle will increase the surface dose. The magnitude of the increase is a function of the thickness of the transited cradle and the energy of the beam (4,31). The authors of this book have occasionally noticed an increase in skin reactions in skin irradiated through an Alpha Cradle.

Polyurethane casts are relatively expensive. Mixing and pouring the chemicals requires speed and dexterity. Gases are produced during foam production and dust is generated if the cast is cut for modification. Measures should be taken for fume exhaustion and chemical and dust containment (25). Although there are drawbacks, reproducible positioning is relatively easily achieved with these cradles (28,32).

VACUUM BAGS

Vacuum bags or pillows are used by a few institutions (VacFix™ is one such commercial system, S & S Par Scientific Inc., 1101 Linwood St., Brooklyn, NY 11208). These systems consist of a bag filled with styrofoam or plastic beads. The patient lays on the bag in the treatment position. Air is evacuated from the bag through a valve. This conforms the bag to the body. The shape is retained throughout the course of treatment.

A vacuum bag immobilizer can be created in a few minutes, it can be adjusted after forming, and it can be reused for several patients (Fig. 9). The surface dose, for a beam passing through the bag, is increased. This could, conceivably, increase the skin reaction

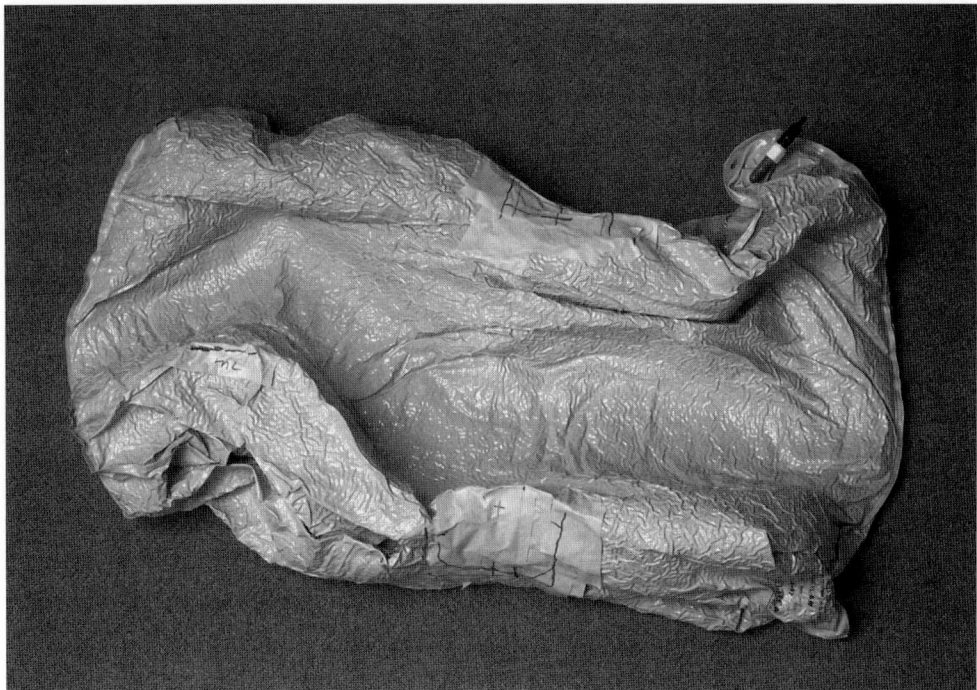

FIG. 9. This vacuum bag was created for the treatment of a 5-year-old girl with retroperitoneal embryonal rhabdomyosarcoma. The child was positioned in a right lateral decubitus position to allow small bowel to fall away from the treatment area. The mold held her in a stable and reproducible position each day. Treatment setup marks are drawn on tape on the device.

to radiation (31). Reproducibility of setup with the system is quite good (25).

SWADDLING

Swaddling with blankets, tape, or sandbagging continue to have their proponents. Other departments use cardboard cutouts in an attempt to reproduce the daily patient-beam alignment (2). Such techniques are inexpensive but provide poor immobilization and are not easily reproducible.

REFERENCES

References particularly recommended for further reading are indicated by an asterisk.

1. Hauskins LA, Thompson RW. Patient positioning device for external beam radiation therapy of the head and neck. *Radiology* 1973;106:706.
*2. Bentel GC, Nelson CE, Noell KT. *Treatment planning and dose calculation in radiation oncology.* Elmsford, NY: Pergamon, 1989:58–67.
3. Goldson AL, Young J Jr, Espinoza MC, Henschke UK. Simple but sophisticated immobilization casts. *Int J Radiat Oncol Biol Phys* 1978;4:1105–1106.
4. Klein EE, Purdy JA. Entrance and exit dose, regions for a Clinac-2100C. *Int J Radiat Oncol Biol Phys* 1993;27:429–435.
5. Williamson TJ. Improving the reproducibility of lateral portal placement. *Int J Radiat Oncol Biol Phys* 1979;5:407–409.
6. Hendrickson FR. Precision in radiation oncology. *Int J Radiat Oncol Biol Phys* 1982;8:311–312.
7. Van Arsdale ED, Greenlaw RH. Formalized immobilization and localization in radiotherapy. *Radiology* 1971;99:697–698.
8. Verhey LJ, Goitein M, McNulty P, Munzenrider JE, Suit H. Precise positioning of patients for radiation therapy. *Int J Radiat Oncol Biol Phys* 1982;8:289–294.
9. Donaldson SS, Shastak CA, Samuels SI. Technical and practical considerations in the radiotherapy of children. *Front Radiat Ther Oncol* 1987;21:256–269.
10. Doppke KP. Treatment simulation organization. In: Write AE, Boyer AL, eds. *Advances in radiation therapy treatment planning.* New York: American Institute of Physics, 1983:131–137.
11. Watkins DMB. Patient positioning. In: *Radiation therapy mold technology: principles and design.* Toronto: Pergamon Press, 1981:7–18.
11a. Watkins DMB. The preparation of a larynx shell. In: *Radiation therapy mold technology: principles and design.* Toronto: Pergamon Press, 1981:19–32.

11b. Watkins DMB. Appendix I: Technical considerations of some of the more commonly used impression, casting and molding materials. In: *Radiation therapy mold technology: principles and design.* Toronto: Pergamon Press, 1981:127–131.

11c. Watkins DMB. Appendix II: Photographs and constructional details of accessory equipment and positioning devices. In: *Radiation therapy mold technology: principles and design.* Toronto: Pergamon Press, 1981:132–137.

*12. Bentel GC. The treatment preparation process–I: target localization, treatment uncertainties, and patient immobilization. In: *Radiation therapy planning, second edition.* New York: McGraw-Hill, 1996;162–218.

13. The Duncan Headrest: Product information. M-G Equipment Company, Inc., St. Paul, MN, USA.

14. Sampiere VA, Khan FM, Delclos L. Treatment aids for external beam radiotherapy. In: Levitt SH, Tapley N, eds. *Technological basis of radiation therapy: practical clinical applications.* Philadelphia: Lea & Febiger, 1984:13–37.

15. Levitt SH. *Treatment aids for external beam radiotherapy.* Department of Therapeutic Radiology, University of Minnesota, Minneapolis, 1974.

16. Pointon RCS, Studd D. Mould room practice. In: Pointon RCS, ed. *The radiotherapy of malignant disease,* 2nd ed. Berlin: Springer-Verlag, 1991:81–109.

17. van der Geijn J, Harrington FS, Lichter AS, Glatstein E. Simplified bite block immobilization of the head. *Radiology* 1983;149:851.

18. Barish RJ, Lerch IA. Patient immobilization with a low-temperature splint/brace material. *Radiology* 1978;127:548.

19. Gerber RL, Marks JE, Purdy JA. The use of thermal plastics for immobilization of patients during radiotherapy. *Int J Radiat Oncol Biol Phys* 1982;8:1461–1462.

20. Thermoplastic splinting material: Product information. M&N Consultants, Inc., Chapel Hill, NC, USA.

21. Product information. WFR/Aquaplast Co., Wycoff, NJ, USA.

22. Sorensen NE, Sell A. Immobilization, compensation and field shaping in megavolt therapy. *Acta Radiol Ther Phys Biol* 1972;11:129–134.

23. Mallion WE, White DR. Immobilization of the head in radiotherapy. *Br J Radiol* 1968;41:236.

24. Paterson R. *The treatment of malignant disease by radiotherapy.* London: Edward Arnold, 1963:150–166.

25. Jakosben A, Iversen P, Gadeberg C, Hansen JL, Hjelm-Hansen M. A new system for patient fixation in radiotherapy. *Radiother Oncol* 1987;8:145–151.

26. Lewinsky BS, Walton R. Lightcast: an aid to planning, treatment and immobilization in radiotherapy and research. *Int J Radiat Oncol Biol Phys* 1976;1:1011–1015.

27. Devereux C, Grundy G, Littman P. Plastic molds for patient immobilization. *Int J Radiat Oncol Biol Phys* 1976;1:553–557.

28. Light KL. Immobilization and treatment of patients receiving radiation therapy for extremity soft-tissue sarcoma. *Med Dosim* 1992;17:135–139.

29. Dickens CW. A machine for moulding thermoplastics. *Br J Radiol* 1960;33:64–65.

30. Shanahan TG, Menta MP, Bergelrud KL, et al. Minimization of small bowel volume within treatment fields utilizing customized "belly boards." *Int J Radiat Oncol Biol Phys* 1990;19:469–476.

31. Johnson MW, Griggs MA, Sharma SC. A comparison of surface doses for two immobilizing systems. *Med Dosim* 1995;20:191–194.

32. Gosselin M, Benk V, Charron F, Podgorsak EB, Evans MDC. Postoperative radiotherapy for chondrosarcoma of the L1 vertebral body: a case report. *Med Dosim* 1994;19:217–222.

Subject Index

References followed by "f" indicate figures; those followed by "t" denote tables

A

Abdomen
  neuroblastoma metastasis to, 196t
  Wilms' tumor metastasis to, 363–364, 366
ABVD regimen
  adverse effects of, 216–217
  for Hodgkin's disease, 216
  leukemic potential, 553
  MOPP regimen and, combined therapy, 217
  testicular effects, 487–488
ACOP regimen, 237
Actinomycin D
  hepatitis and, 509
  for optic pathway tumors, 50
  pneumonitis risk and, 504
  pulmonary toxicity associated with, 505t
Acute lymphoblastic leukemia
  age of onset, 10
  B-cell lineage, 10–11
  central nervous system involvement
    description of, 12–17
    neuropsychologic deficits associated with, 495, 497
    radiotherapy for, 13–19
  chromosomal translocations and, 11
  clinical presentation of, 12–13
  cranial irradiation effects, 470–471
  frequency of, 10
  genetic disorders and, 10
  growth hormone deficiency, 468–469
  lymphoblastic lymphoma and, similarities between, 235
  ophthalmic manifestations of, 12–13
  pathophysiology of, 10
  secondary gliomas and, 39–40
  secondary malignant neoplasms associated with, 550
  subgroups, 12t
  T-cell, 11, 573
  in testes, 22–23
  thyroid gland abnormalities associated with, 478
  treatment of
    bone marrow transplantation, 18, 26–27
    radiotherapy. See Radiotherapy, acute lymphoblastic leukemia

Acute lymphocytic leukemia, 2t–3t
Acute myelogenous leukemia
  bone marrow transplantation for, 25–26
  central nervous system involvement in, 24
  chromosomal abnormalities, 23
  incidence of, 10, 23
  subtypes of, 23, 24t
  treatment of, 24
Acute nonlymphoblastic leukemia, 552–553
Adenocarcinoma
  bile duct, 375–376, 378
  of breast, 414
  gastric, 413
  pancreatic, 413
Adrenal cortical carcinoma, 395–396
Adrenocorticotropic hormone deficiency, treatment late effects related to, 472t
Adriamycin
  bleomycin, vinblastine, and dacarbazine regimen. See ABVD regimen
  secondary malignant neoplasms associated with, 550
  treatment-related late effects of
    myocardiopathy, 523, 574
    tissue, 457
Adverse effects
  of chemotherapy. See Chemotherapy, late effects of
  of radiotherapy. See Radiotherapy, late effects of
Aerodigestive tract tumors
  esthesioneuroblastoma, 408–410, 409t
  infantile subglottic hemangiomas, 411
  juvenile nasopharyngeal angiofibroma. See Juvenile nasopharyngeal angiofibroma
  nasopharyngeal carcinoma. See Nasopharyngeal carcinoma
ALL. See Acute lymphoblastic leukemia
Alpha-fetoprotein
  germ cell tumors, 386
  pineal region tumors, 68
  primary malignant liver tumors, 373
Alveolar soft part sarcomas, 322
Amenorrhea, from irradiation, 482
AML. See Acute myelogenous leukemia

Anaplastic astrocytoma, 58
Anemia
  anesthetic considerations, 574
  aplastic. *See* Aplastic anemia
  Fanconi's. *See* Fanconi's anemia
Anesthesia, for radiotherapy
  disease-specific considerations
    mediastinal masses, 573
    neuroblastomas, 573
    Wilms' tumors, 573
  frequency of, 563, 564t
  general
    agents for, 565–566
    airway obstruction, 566–567
    description of, 565
    laryngeal mask airway, 566f, 567
  goals of, 564t, 564–565
  intravenous
    barbiturates, 568
    benzodiazepines, 568
    description of, 567
    ketamine use, 567–568
    opiates, 568–569
  monitoring
    capnometry, 571
    equipment for, 570
    guidelines for, 569–570
    pulse oximetry, 570–571
    techniques for, 571–573, 572f
  thermal plastic head holder use during, 582
Angiocavernosum, 446
Angiofibroma. *See* Juvenile nasopharyngeal
  angiofibroma
ANLL. *See* Acute nonlymphoblastic leukemia
Anthracycline
  for acute myelogenous leukemia, 24
  cardiotoxicity associated with, 523–524, 528,
    574
Antiferritin antibody, 228
Aplasia of bone marrow, radiation-induced, 517
Aplastic anemia
  bone marrow transplantation for, 27–28
  characteristics of, 27
Apoptosis, 540
Appendix, carcinoids of, 413
Arrhythmias, secondary to radiotherapy, 525
Arteriocapillary fibrosis, 459
Arteriography, for non-rhabdomyosarcoma soft-
  tissue sarcomas, 323
Arteriolonephrosclerosis, 500
Askin's tumor, 248, 261
Astrocytomas
  anaplastic, 58
  cerebellar. *See* Cerebellar astrocytoma
  diencephalic
    description of, 40–42
    in infants and young children, 56–57
  fibrillary, 40

  gemistocytic, 40
  high-grade, 114
  Holocord, 114
  incidence of, 2t
  juvenile pilocytic. *See* Juvenile pilocytic
    astrocytoma
  pleomorphic xanthoastrocytoma, 40
  protoplasmic, 40
  spinal cord, 113–114, 117–118
  subependymal giant cell, 40
  treatment of
    chemotherapy, 45
    radiotherapy, 42–43, 45–47, 118–119
    results, 47
    surgery, 42
    survival rates, 119
Atypical teratoid/rhaboid tumors
  definition of, 55
  in infants and young children, 60
Autologous bone marrow transplantation
  for acute lymphoblastic leukemia, 18
  definition of, 25t
  for neuroblastomas, 191
  for non-Hodgkin's lymphoma, 240t
Azoospermia, 487–488, 490

B

Barbiturates, for anesthesia, 568
Basal cell nevus syndrome (BCNS), 450–451,
  545
Beckwith-Wiedemann syndrome, 345
Berlin—Franfurt—Munster regimen, 13
Bile duct adenocarcinoma, 375–376, 378
Birbeck granule, 423, 424f
Bite block, 579–580
Bladder
  late treatment effects, 502t
  rhabdomyosarcoma of, treatment approaches
    for, 305–309, 306t–307t
Bleomycin, pulmonary toxicity associated with,
  505t, 574
Blood, placental, 28
Bone
  Ewing's sarcoma metastasis to, 261–262
  hemangiomas of, 448
  Langerhans' cell histiocytosis involvement in,
    428t
  neuroblastoma metastasis to, 196t
  radiation-induced effects on growth of
    clinical manifestations, 462–465, 467
    historical descriptions, 461
    kyphosis, 463–464
    loss of height, 462–463
    pathophysiology of, 461–462
    scoliosis, 463–464
  Wilms' tumor-related effects on, 368
Bone marrow
  chemotherapy-induced late effects, 518

neuroblastoma metastasis to, 170–173, 196t
non-Hodgkin's lymphoma involvement, 236
radiation-induced late effects
   aplasia, 517
   in children vs. adults, 517–518, 518f
   regenerative capacity, 517
Bone marrow transplantation
  allogeneic, 25t, 28
  autologous, 18, 25t, 191, 240t
  cardiac complications secondary to, 528
  clinical uses
    acute lymphoblastic leukemia, 18, 26–27
    acute myelogenous leukemia, 25–26
    aplastic anemia, 27–28
    Ewing's sarcoma, 262
    Fanconi's anemia, 27, 27f
    Hodgkin's disease recurrence/relapse, 219–222
    Langerhans' cell histiocytosis, 438
    neuroblastoma, 187–189, 188t, 191
    non-Hodgkin's lymphoma recurrence/relapse, 240, 240t, 242
  description of, 24–25
  preoperative regimens for
    cyclophosphamide, 28
    description of, 25
    hearing-related effects, 517
    testes-related effects, 488, 490
    total body irradiation. *See* Total body irradiation, as preoperative regimen for bone marrow transplantation
  terms associated with, 25t
Bone sarcoma, 549
Brachytherapy
  for non-rhabdomyosarcoma soft-tissue sarcoma, 332–334
  for Wilms' tumor, 364
Brain, 491
Brainstem gliomas. *See also* Pontine tumors
  diagnostic tests, 97–98
  diffusely infiltrating pontine glioma, 97
  dorsally exophytic "benign," 98
  gender predilection, 96
  illustration of, 97f
  incidence of, 96
  signs and symptoms of, 96–97
  treatment of
    chemotherapy, 100–101
    radiotherapy. *See* Radiotherapy, brainstem glioma
    surgery, 100
  types of, 96
Brain tumors. *See also* specific tumor
  etiology of, 39–40
  incidence of, 38t
  in infants
    description of, 55–56

radiotherapy. *See* Radiotherapy, brain tumor
  sign and symptoms of, 55
  surgery for, 56–57
  survival rates, 55–56
  neurocognitive effects, 497, 497t
  in posterior fossa. *See* specific tumor
  WHO classification of, 38t
  in young children, 55–60
Breast cancer
  adenocarcinoma, 414
  radiation-related, 554–555
  secondary, in Hodgkin's disease patients, 554–555
  whole-lung irradiation and, 549
Bronchogenic carcinoma, 412
Burkitt's lymphoma
  characteristics of, 235–236
  chemotherapeutic treatment of, 237, 239
  Epstein-Barr virus involvement in, 233
  incidence of, 2t
  staging of, 235t

C
Cade technique, for osteosarcoma, 271, 274, 274t
Cancer. *See also* Carcinoma
  breast
    adenocarcinoma, 414
    radiation-related, 554–555
    secondary, in Hodgkin's disease patients, 554–555
    whole-lung irradiation and, 549
  effect of site of care on, 7–8
  gastrointestinal, 556–557
  incidence of, 1–2, 4–5
  lung
    description of, 412
    radiation-related, 555
  mortality rates, 3–4
  radiation-induced
    latent periods, 545
    organs susceptible to, 543
    patient age and, 545
    principles of, 544–545
    of thyroid gland, 543–544
  skin. *See* Skin cancer
  survival rate increases, 3
  trends in, 3
  in United States, 2–3
  worldwide incidence of, 1–3
Cancer center
  effect on survival rates, 7–8
  requirements for, 7t
Capillary lymphangioma, 450
Capnometry, 571
Carboplatin, for optic pathway tumors, 50

Carcinogenesis
    multievent pattern of, 545
    pathophysiology of, 538
    radiation, 541–543. *See also* Cancer,
        radiation-induced
Carcinoma. *See also* Cancer
    adrenal cortical, 395–396
    bronchogenic, 412
    esophageal, 412
    incidence of, 2t
    squamous cell
        description of, 450–451
        of head and neck region, 410
    thyroid. *See* Thyroid gland, carcinoma of
Cardiac system, treatment-related late effects of
    arrhythmia, 525
    coronary artery disease, 525–528, 527t
    myocardiopathy, 523–524, 524f
    overview, 521–522, 522t
    pancarditis, 523
    pericarditis, 522–523, 527t
    valvular disease, 524, 527t
Cardiomyopathy, secondary to chemotherapy
        and radiotherapy, 523–524, 524f
Cataracts, radiation-induced
    description of, 513t, 514
    retinoblastoma therapy, 156
Catecholamines
    metabolism of, 172f
    neuroblastomas and, 172
Cavernous lymphangioma, 450
CCNU regimen
    for brainstem tumors, 100
    for medulloblastoma, 86
CDDP. *See* Cisplatin
Cell kill, 457
Central nervous system
    in acute lymphoblastic leukemia
        pathogenesis, 12–18
    in acute myelogenous leukemia pathogenesis,
        24
    non-Hodgkin's lymphoma involvement,
        236–237, 239–240
    radiation-induced late effects of
        intellectual deficits, 494–498
        mechanisms of, 492
        mineralizing microangiopathy, 493–494
        necrosis, 492–493
        necrotizing leukoencephalopathy, 493, 493f
        neuropsychologic deficits, 494–498
        pathophysiology, 491–492
        patient evaluation, 499t
    tumors
        embryonal. *See* Embryonal central nervous
            system tumors
        etiology of, 39–40
        incidence of, 38t
        WHO classification of, 38t, 82

Cerebellar astrocytomas
    age of onset, 111
    clinical presentation of, 111
    description of, 111
    high-grade, treatment approaches for, 113
    juvenile pilocytic astrocytoma. *See* Juvenile
        pilocytic astrocytoma
    signs and symptoms of, 111
    treatment of
        chemotherapy, 112
        radiotherapy. *See* Radiotherapy, cerebellar
            astrocytoma
        results, 113
        surgery, 112
Cerebral neuroblastoma, 61
Cervix, rhabdomyosarcoma of, 311
Charged particle therapy, for osteosarcoma, 283
Chemotherapy. *See also* specific agent or
        regimen
    clinical uses
        acute lymphoblastic leukemia, 13, 17
        acute myelogenous leukemia, 24
        adrenal cortical carcinoma, 396
        brainstem tumors, 100–101
        cerebellar astrocytomas, 112
        embryonal CNS tumors, 62
        ependymomas, 107–108
        esthesioneuroblastoma, 410
        Ewing's sarcoma, 253–256
        germ cell tumors, 69–70
        Langerhans' cell histiocytosis, 434–438,
            436t–437t
        low-grade gliomas, 45
        malignant gliomas, 53–54, 57
        medulloblastoma, 86–87
        neuroblastoma, 186, 190–191
        non-rhabdomyosarcoma soft-tissue
            sarcomas, 327–331
        oligodendroglioma, 51
        optic pathway tumors, 49–50
        osteosarcoma, 279–280
        pineal region tumors, 69–70
        pontine tumors, 100
        primary malignant liver tumors, 377,
            379–382
        retinoblastoma, 147, 148t–149t, 150
        rhabdomyosarcoma, 289
        Wilms' tumor, 362
    disadvantages of, 218–219
    late effects of
        bone marrow, 518
        central nervous system, 499t
        cognitive deficits, 497
        germ cells, 489t
        hearing, 515–517, 516t
        hepatopathy, 511
        hepatotoxicity, 509t
        kidney, 502t

leukoencephalopathy, 493–494, 499t
Leydig cells, 489t
musculoskeletal system, 466t
myocardiopathy, 523–524, 524f
osteonecrosis, 466t
ovarian dysfunction, 483t, 484
pneumonitis, 504
pulmonary toxicity, 505t
slipped capital femoral epiphysis, 466t
testes, 487, 489t
tissue, 460
tooth and root development, 519, 520t
myelosuppression caused by, 518t
secondary malignant neoplasms induced
using, 544–545
Chest, neuroblastoma metastasis to, 196t
Chlorambucil vinblastine, procarbazine,
prednisone (CHlVPP) regimen, for
Hodgkin's disease, 219
CHOP regimen, 237
Choroid plexus tumors, 55
Chronic fibrosis, 503
Chronic obstructive lung disease, 504, 505f, 507
Chronic progressive radiation myelitis, 498
Cisplatin, hearing-related effects of, 515–517,
516t
Clear cell sarcoma, of kidney, 347
Cognition, chemotherapy effects on, 497
COMP regimen, 237, 240
Computerized tomography, diagnostic uses of
desmoid tumors, 338
Ewing's sarcoma, 248, 248f
germ cell tumors, 387
Hodgkin's disease, 210
neuroblastoma, 170
non-rhabdomyosarcoma soft-tissue sarcomas,
323, 324f
osteosarcomas, 267
primary malignant liver tumors, 376
retinoblastoma, 131
Wilms' tumor, 348
Conjunctiva, radiation-induced late effects of,
512t
Cornea, radiation-induced late effects of, 512t
Coronary artery disease, secondary to
radiotherapy
clinical studies of, 526, 528
factors that affect, 525–526
pathophysiology of, 525
Corticosteroids, for diffusely infiltrating
brainstem gliomas, 103
CPRM. See Chronic progressive radiation
myelitis
Cranial irradiation. See also Radiotherapy
for central nervous system leukemia, 18–19
growth hormone production and release
effects
clinical manifestations, 467–474

deficiency, 470
pathophysiology, 467
patient evaluation, 472t–473t
precocious puberty effects, 468
hearing-related effects of, 515–517, 516t
for non-Hodgkin's lymphoma involvement in
central nervous system, 240
prophylactic, 16, 19, 22
Craniopharyngioma
adamantinous, 63
anatomic site of, 63, 64f
clinical manifestations of, 63
description of, 63
imaging diagnosis of, 38
squamous cell, 63
treatment approaches
outcomes, 65, 65t
radiotherapy, 66
surgery, 63–65
Craniospinal irradiation. See also Spinal
irradiation
clinical uses
embryonal CNS tumors, 62–63
medulloblastomas, 87, 89–93
parameningeal rhabdomyosarcoma, 312
spinal cord tumors, 118
trilateral retinoblastoma, 151
plaster of Paris use for, 582–583
testicular effects, 486
CrI. See Cranial irradiation
Cryotherapy, for retinoblastoma, 136
CSI. See Craniospinal irradiation
Cure, definition of, 5–6
Cushing's syndrome, 395
Cyclophosphamide
in CHOP regimen, 237
in COMP regimen, 237
heart damage and, 528
ovarian dysfunction and, 482–483
secondary malignant neoplasms and, 155
Cyclosporine A, for retinoblastoma, 150
Cystic hygroma, 450
Cytokines, in Hodgkin's disease pathology, 204
Cytosine arabinoside, pulmonary toxicity
associated with, 505t

D

Dacarbazine, 279
Dactinomycin. See Actinomycin D
Desmoid tumors
description of, 336
illustration of, 336f
treatment of, 336, 338
Diabetes insipidus
description of, 64
Langerhans' cell histiocytosis and
description of, 426
irradiation therapy, 434

Diabetes insipidus (*contd.*)
    radiotherapy, 439
Diazepam, 568
Diencephalic astrocytoma
    description of, 40–42
    in infants and young children, 56–57
Diffuse large B-cell lymphoma, 236
Diffusely infiltrating pontine glioma
    incidence of, 96
    radiotherapy for, 100–101, 103
Digestive tract, radiation-induced injury
    bowel obstruction, 507
    enteropathy, 507
    obliterative vasculitis, 507
    patient evaluation, 510t
    preventive approaches, 507–508
Diprivan. *See* Propofol
DNS. *See* Dysplastic nevus syndrome
Dorsally exophytic "benign" brainstem tumor
    description of, 98
    treatment approaches
        radiotherapy, 100
        surgery, 99
Doxorubicin, treatment-related late effects of
    cardiotoxicity, 523
    pulmonary toxicity, 505t
Dumbbell tumors
    description of, 113
    treatment of, 182–183
Dysembryoblastic neuroepithelial tumors, 51
Dysgerminoma
    description of, 388
    treatment of, 390
Dysplastic nevus syndrome, 451

E
EBV. *See* Epstein-Barr virus
Elephantiasis, radiation-induced, 332
Embryonal central nervous system tumors
    age of onset, 60
    radiotherapy for, 62–63
    WHO classification of, 38t, 60
ENB. *See* Esthesioneuroblastoma
Endobronchial adenomas, 412
Endocrine carcinoma
    adrenal cortical carcinoma, 395–396
    pheochromocytoma, 396–397
    thyroid carcinoma. *See* Thyroid gland,
        carcinoma of
Enteritis, radiation-induced, 510t
Enteropathy, radiation-induced, 507
Enucleation
    developmental impairments secondary to, 514
    for retinoblastoma, 134–135
Ependymoblastoma
    characteristics of, 60–61
    description of, 104–105
Ependymoma

    age of onset, 105
    classification of, 104–105
    clinical presentation of, 105–106
    craniospinal *See*ding, 108
    gender predilection, 105
    histologic features of, 104
    illustration of, 105f–106f
    incidence of, 2t, 104
    infratentorial, 109t
    intracranial, 108t
    myxopapillary, 104, 115, 116f
    signs and symptoms of, 105–106
    spinal cord, 113–115, 118
    subarachnoid dissemination, 111
    supratentorial, 104
    survival rates, 105, 119
    treatment of
        chemotherapy, 107–108
        outcomes, 55
        radiotherapy. *See* Radiotherapy,
          ependymoma
        results, 111
        surgery, 106–107
Epithelioid sarcoma, 322
Epstein-Barr virus
    in Hodgkin's disease pathogenesis, 205
    non-Hodgkin's lymphoma and, 233
    Reed-Sternberg cells and, 204
Esophageal carcinoma, 412
Esthesioneuroblastoma, 408–410, 409t
Ewing's sarcoma
    Askin's tumor and, 248, 261
    chromosomal abnormalities associated with,
        247
    clinical presentation of, 247–250
    diagnosis of
        evaluation, 247–248
        patient age at, 245
    extraosseous
        chemotherapy for, 328
        description of, 295, 323
    gender predilection, 245
    historical descriptions of, 245, 246f
    imaging studies, 248
    incidence of, 2t–3t, 245
    metastases
        description of, 248–249
        radiotherapy for, 261–262
    pathology of, 245–247
    pelvic, 249f
    primitive neuroectodermal tumors and,
        comparison between, 245–247
    prognostic factors, 250, 251t
    recurrence of, 256–257
    secondary malignant neoplasms associated
        with, 263, 549
    tibial, 250f
    treatment of

chemotherapy, 253–256
combined therapy, 252–253
cure rates, 262–263
local control approaches, 251–252
radiotherapy. *See* Radiotherapy, Ewing's
sarcoma
side effects, 262–263
surgery, 251t, 252–253
survival rates, 262–263
total body irradiation, 262
Exenteration, for retinoblastoma, 135
Extraneural disease, medulloblastoma and, 83
Extraosseous Ewing's sarcoma, 295
Eye
anatomy of, 511
radiation-induced late effects
eyelids, 512t, 514
lacrimal apparatus, 511, 514
lens, 513t, 514
optic nerve, 514
orbit, 514–515
patient evaluation, 512t–513t
retina, 511, 513t
Eyelids, radiation-induced late effects on, 512t,
514

F
Family education, regarding treatment, 576–577
Fanconi's anemia
bone marrow transplantation for, 27, 27f
description of, 27
Ferritin, neuroblastoma cell growth and, 177
Fibromyxoid sarcoma, characteristics of, 322
Fibrosarcoma
adult-type, 322
characteristics of, 322
congenital, 322
incidence of, 2t
Fibrosis
arteriocapillary, 459
chronic, 503
pulmonary, 506t
radiation-induced, 510t
Flumazenil, 568
Follicular carcinoma, 397
Fourth ventricle
ependymomas, 106
medulloblastoma infiltration in, 82

G
Ganglioglioma, 114–115
Ganglioma, 51
Ganglioside GD2, 179
Gastric adenocarcinoma, 413
Gastrointestinal system
cancer of, 556–557
radiation-induced injury
bowel obstruction, 507

enteropathy, 507
obliterative vasculitis, 507
patient evaluation, 510t
preventive approaches, 507–508
GCT. *See* Germ cells, tumors
General anesthesia, for radiotherapy
agents for, 565–566
airway obstruction, 566–567
description of, 565
laryngeal mask airway, 566f, 567
Genitourinary system, late treatment effects, 502t
Germ cells
radiation-induced effects, 489t
tumors
age distribution for, 386
chemotherapy for, 69–70
classification of, 387f
description of, 68
diagnostic workup, 386–387
extragonadal, 391–393
gender predilection, 386
histiotypes, 67
histologic types of, 386
incidence of, 2t, 386
intracranial, 67, 68t
mediastinal, 393
of ovary, 387–391
radiotherapy for, 69–71
results, 71
sacrococcygeal, 391–392
staging of, 386–387
suprasellar, 67
surgery, 68–69
testicular, 391
Giant cell astrocytoma, subependymal, 39
Gliomas. *See* Brainstem gliomas; Low-grade
gliomas; Malignant gliomas
Gliomatosis cerebri, 40
GNRH. *See* Growth-hormone-releasing hormone
Gonadotropin hormone deficiency, treatment
late effects related to, 473t
Gonadotropin releasing hormone, 481
Graft-versus-host disease, 25t
Graft-versus-leukemia effect, 25t
Growth hormone, cranial irradiation effects on
production and release of
clinical manifestations, 467–474
deficiency, 470
pathophysiology, 467
patient evaluation, 472t–473t
precocious puberty effects, 468
Growth-hormone-releasing hormone, 467

H
Halothane, 565
Head holder
description of, 578, 578f
thermal plastic type, 581f

Head supports, 578, 578f
Hearing
    chemotherapy-induced late effects, 515–517,
        516t
    radiation-induced late effects, 515–517,
        516t
Heart. *See* Cardiac system
Hemangioma
    of bone, 448
    cavernous, 446
    classification of, 446, 447t
    clinical presentation of, 446
    description of, 446
    illustration of, 449f
    infantile subglottic, 411
    of liver, 379, 382
    lymphangial, 450
    orbital, 448
    treatment of
        indications, 446–447
        methods, 447
        radiotherapy, 447–448
    of vertebrae, 448
Hemangiopericytoma, 322
Hepatic carcinoma, 2t
Hepatitis, radiation, 508
Hepatoblastoma
    anaplastic, 382
    classification of, 373–374
    incidence of, 2t
    metastatic, 379
    survival rates, 382
    unresectable, response to chemotherapy,
        381t
Hepatocellular carcinoma, 374–375, 382
Hepatomegaly, stage IV-S neuroblastoma-
        induced
    description of, 190
    radiotherapy for, 192, 194
Hepatotoxicity, from Wilms' tumor therapy,
        368
Hereditary effects, of radiotherapy, 490–491
Histiocytosis X. *See* Langerhans' cell
        histiocytosis
Histocompatibility complex, 25t
Hodgkin's disease
    in adolescents vs. children, 208–209
    anesthetic considerations, 573
    biology of, 203–205
    classification of, 206–209, 207t, 208f
    clinical presentation of, 205
    diagnosis of
        criteria, 205–206
        evaluation for, 209–212
    epidemiology of, 205
    future investigations, 227–228
    gender predilection, 205
    genetic influences, 205

historical descriptions of, 203
imaging studies of, 210
incidence of, 2t–3t
interrelationships with other lymphomas,
        208t
lymphocyte depleted, 208
lymphocyte predominant, 204, 207
mixed cellularity, 204, 207
nodular lymphocyte predominant, 205–207
nodular sclerosing, 208
pathogenetic model of, 204
prognostic factors, 212–213
Reed-Sternberg cell in, 203–204, 206
refractory/relapsed
    chemotherapy, 220
    involved field radiation therapy, 221–222
    radiotherapy, 220–221
    typical onset of, 219
secondary malignant neoplasms associated
        with
    acute leukemia, 552–553
    breast cancer, 554–555
    clinical studies of, 551–552
    description of, 550–551
    gastrointestinal cancer, 556–557
    lung cancer, 555
    non-Hodgkin's lymphoma, 554
    solid tumors, 554
    survival rates, 550–551
    thyroid cancer, 555–556
signs and symptoms of, 204–205
splenic involvement of, 210
staging of
    Cotswold, 206t
    description of, 209
    surgical, 211–212
treatment of
    cardiovascular-related late effects,
        521–522, 522t, 526–528, 527t
    chemotherapy, 218–219
    children vs. adults, 213
    clinical studies, 214t–215t, 217
    combined therapy, 216–217
    guidelines, 216t
    hematopoietic stem cell rescue, 220
    radiotherapy. *See* Radiotherapy, Hodgkin's
        disease
    recommendations, 219
    results, 224–226
    survival rates, 4t, 224–226
Hyperfractionated radiotherapy, for brainstem
        gliomas, 102
Hyperprolactinemia, treatment late effects
        related to, 473t
Hyperthermia
    laser, for retinoblastoma, 136
    for non-rhabdomyosarcoma soft-tissue
        sarcomas, 335

Hyperthyroidism, radiation-induced, 478–480, 479t
Hypothalamic tumors
    illustration of, 44f–45f
    treatment outcomes, 47
Hypothyroidism, radiation-induced
    chemotherapy and, 478
    disease states, 475–476
    factors that affect, 475
    management of, 480
    radiation dose and, 476–477
    risk factors, 477–478
    signs and symptoms of, 475
    spinal axis irradiation and, 478

I

Imaging modalities. *See* specific imaging modality
Immobilization devices. *See also* Stabilization devices
    lightcast, 583
    plaster of Paris, 582–583
    polyurethane foam molds, 583–584
    swaddling, 585
    thermal plastic types, 581f, 5820–582
    vacuum bags, 585, 585f
    vacuum-molded thermoplastics, 583
Infantile subglottic hemangiomas, 411
Infertility, radiation-induced, 485–486
Insular carcinoma, 398
International Neuroblastoma Staging System, 173, 190, 196t
Intravenous anesthesia, for radiotherapy
    agents for
        barbiturates, 568
        benzodiazepines, 568
        ketamine, 567–568
        opiates, 568–569
    description of, 567
    sepsis, 569
Involved field radiation therapy, for Hodgkin's disease, 221–222
Iris, radiation-induced late effects of, 513t
ISH. *See* Infantile subglottic hemangioma

J

Juvenile capillary hemangioma, 448
Juvenile nasopharyngeal angiofibroma
    histologic features of, 400, 400f
    imaging studies of, 400, 401f
    incidence of, 400
    signs and symptoms of, 400
    staging of, 401, 402t
    treatment of
        chemotherapy, 401
        hormone therapy, 402
        radiotherapy, 402–403, 403t
        surgery, 401–402

Juvenile pilocytic astrocytoma
    central nervous system involvement, 111
    characteristics of, 40–41, 111
    description of, 40
    magnetic resonance imaging of, 115
    posttherapy survival rates, 42–43
    radiotherapy for, 45–46
    surgical therapy for, 42
Juvenile secretory carcinoma, 414

K

Karnofsky performance scale, 6
Kasabach-Merritt syndrome, 446
Ketamine, 567–568
Kidney
    clear cell sarcoma of, 347
    irradiation of, during neuroblastoma radiotherapy, 195
    radiation-induced dysfunction
        clinical manifestations, 500–501, 503
        pathophysiology of, 500
        patient evaluation, 502t
    radiotherapeutic considerations for, 223
    rhabdoid tumor of, 347
    Wilms' tumor effects, 368
Kyphosis, 463–464

L

Lacrimal gland
    radiation-induced late effects, 511, 514
    retinoblastoma-induced abnormalities of, 158–159
Lactate dehydrogenase, neuroblastoma and, 178
Li-Fraumeni familial tumor syndrome, 39, 320
Langerhans' cell histiocytosis
    bone involvement in, 428t
    central nervous system involvement, 426
    definition of, 423
    diabetes insipidus associated with
        description of, 426
        irradiation therapy, 434
        radiotherapy, 439
    disseminated, 427–428
    genetic involvement in, 423–424
    grouping of, 429t, 430
    historical background of, 422–423
    incidence of, 425
    long-term sequelae of, 441, 439
    multisystem, 435
    pathogenesis of, 423–425
    pathology of, 423
    sign and symptoms of, 425–426, 426t, 427f
    staging of, 429t, 430
    treatment approaches
        bone marrow transplantation, 438
        chemotherapy, 434–438, 436t–437t
        liver transplantation, 438
        protocol, 431t

Langerhans' cell histiocytosis, treatment
    approaches (*contd.*)
    radiotherapy. *See* Radiotherapy,
        Langerhans' cell histiocytosis
    results, 442
    secondary malignancy after, 441
    steroid injection, 432, 432t
    surgery, 431–432
    vertebral effects, 433, 433f
Lansky play–performance scale, 7
Laparotomy, staging, 211
Large bowel, neoplasms of, 414
Large congenital nevocytic nevi, 451
Large mediastinal adenopathy, 209, 226
Laryngeal edema, 574
Laryngeal mask airway, 566f, 567
Laser hyperthermia, for retinoblastoma, 136
Late effects
    of chemotherapy. *See* Chemotherapy, late
        effects of
    of radiotherapy. *See* Radiotherapy, late effects
        of
LCH. *See* Langerhans' cell histiocytosis
LCNN. *See* Large congenital nevocytic nevi
Leiomyoblastoma, of stomach, 412
Leiomyosarcoma
    characteristics of, 322
    of large bowel, 414
    of stomach, 412
Lens of eye, radiation-induced late effects of,
        513t, 514
Leukemia
    acute lymphoblastic. *See* Acute lymphoblastic
        leukemia
    acute myelogenous. *See* Acute myelogenous
        leukemia
    in Hodgkin's disease patients posttreatment,
        552–553
    incidence of, 2t, 10
    meningeal, 18, 22
    overt central nervous system, 17–18
    pediatric forms of, 10
    secondary malignant neoplasms associated
        with, 550
    T cell, 11, 16
    testicular
        in acute lymphoblastic leukemic patients,
            22–23, 29, 31
        description of, 22–23
        treatment of, 23
Leukocoria
    definition of, 130
    in retinoblastoma, 130
Leukoencephalopathy, 493
Leukostasis, in cerebral blood vessels, 18
Leydig cells
    chemotherapy-induced effects, 489t
    function of, 484

radiation-induced effects
    description of, 485, 486t
    patient evaluation, 489t
L'Hermitte's sign, 498
Lids. *See* Eyelids
Lightcast, 583
Liposarcomas, 322
Liver
    chemotherapy and radiotherapy combined
        therapy effects, 508t
    radiation injury to, 508
    transplantation
        for Langerhans' cell histiocytosis, 438
        for primary malignant liver tumors, 378
    tumors of
        benign, 375
        primary malignant. *See* Primary malignant
            liver tumor
LMA. *See* Large mediastinal adenopathy;
        Laryngeal mask airway
Low-grade gliomas. *See also* specific glioma
    treatment approaches
        chemotherapy, 45, 100
        in infants, 56–57
        radiation therapy, 42–43, 45–47
        results, 47
        surgery, 42
    types of, 40–42
Lung
    chemotherapeutic-induced toxicities
        anesthetic considerations, 574
        types of, 505t
    Ewing's sarcoma metastasis to, 261
    non-rhabdomyosarcoma soft-tissue sarcoma
        metastasis to, 326
    osteosarcoma metastasis to
        description of, 271
        illustration of, 272f–273f
        whole-lung irradiation for, 275–279,
            276t–277t
    radiation-induced late effects of
        chronic fibrosis, 503
        description of, 503
        dose parameters, 504, 507
        pathophysiology of, 503
        patient evaluation, 506t
        pneumonitis, 503
        signs and symptoms, 503
        volume parameters, 504, 507
    thyroid carcinoma metastasis to, 398
    Wilms' tumor metastasis to, 348, 365–366,
        507
Lung cancer
    description of, 412
    radiation-related, 555
Lymphangial hemangiomas, 450
Lymphangiogram, for Hodgkin's disease, 210
Lymphangioma, 450

Lymph nodes
    dissection, for malignant melanoma, 452–453
    neuroblastoma metastasis to, 196t
    rhabdomyosarcoma metastasis to, 299t, 301
    thyroid carcinoma metastasis to, 398
Lymphocyte and histiocytic cell, 205–206
Lymphoma
    Burkitt's
        characteristics of, 235–236
        chemotherapeutic treatment of, 237, 239
        Epstein-Barr virus involvement in, 233
        incidence of, 2t
        staging of, 235t
    incidence of, 2t–3t
    non-Burkitt's, 237, 239
    non-Hodgkin's. *See* Non-Hodgkin's
        lymphoma
    precursor B-lymphoblastic, 235
    precursor T-lymphoblastic, 235

M

MADDOC regimen, 191
Magnetic resonance imaging, diagnostic uses of
    brainstem tumors, 97
    desmoid tumors, 338
    ependymomas, 105
    Ewing's sarcoma, 248
    Hodgkin's disease, 210
    neuroblastoma, 170
    osteosarcoma, 267
    primary malignant liver tumors, 376
    spinal cord neoplasms, 115
    Wilms' tumor, 348
Malignant fibrous histiocytoma, 320, 322
Malignant gliomas
    in cerebellum, 111
    clinical presentation of, 52
    description of, 51–52
    illustration of, 53f
    subarachnoid dissemination, 111
    treatment approaches
        chemotherapy, 53–54
        in infants and young children, 57, 58f
        radiotherapy. *See* Radiotherapy, malignant
            glioma
        results, 55
        surgery, 52
Malignant melanoma
    benign Spitz nevi and, 452
    etiologic factors, 451
    incidence of, 451
    metastases, 453–454
    staging of, 452
    treatment of
        lymph node dissection, 452–453
        radiotherapy, 453–454
Malignant mesenchymoma, characteristics of,
    322

Mandible, osteosarcoma involvement of,
    275
Mantle irradiation
    cardiac dose received and, correlation
        between, 525
    complications associated with, 226–227
    thyroid cancer and, 555–556
    volume considerations, 222
Marrow purging, definition of, 25t
Maxilla, osteosarcoma involvement of, 275
Medullary carcinoma, 397
Medulloblastoma
    age of onset, 82
    anatomic sites of, 82
    gender predilection of, 82
    histologic features of, 82
    historical descriptions of, 80, 82
    illustration of, 81f
    incidence of, 2t
    metastasis of, 82–83
    outcomes, 55, 57, 95t
    signs and symptoms of, 82
    staging of, 83–84, 84t
    subarachnoid dissemination, 82–83
    treatment of
        chemotherapy, 57–58, 86–87
        radiotherapy. *See* Radiotherapy,
            medulloblastoma
        results, 93, 95
        surgery, 84–85, 85t
Medulloepithelioma, 60
Melanoma. *See* Malignant melanoma
MEN. *See* Multiple endocrine neoplasia
Meningeal leukemia, 18, 22
Meningioma, radiation-induced, 39–40
Mesoblastic nephroma, 345–346
Metaiodobenzylguanidine, for neuroblastomas,
    170, 195–196
Metastases
    hepatoblastoma, 379
    malignant melanoma, 453–454
    medulloblastoma, 82–83
    neuroblastoma
        description of, 169
        palliative intent, 190
        sites of involvement, 192, 196t
    osteosarcomas
        anatomic sites of, 271
        description of, 267
        to lung, 271, 272f–273f
        surgical treatment, 271
    rhabdomyosarcoma
        anatomic sites of, 294
        chemotherapy for, 315
        incidence of, 315
        lymph nodes, 299t
        whole-lung irradiation for, 275–279,
            276t–277t, 348, 363, 366, 379

Metastases (*contd.*)
  Wilms' tumor
    abdomen, 363–364
    pulmonary, 348, 507
    treatment of, 365–366
Methohexital, 568
Methotrexate
  for acute lymphoblastic leukemia, 13–16
  mineralizing microangiopathy and, 493–494
  pulmonary toxicity associated with, 505t
Midazolam, 568
Midbrain tumor
  tectal plate, 98
  tegmental, 98
Mineralizing microangiopathy, 493–494
Mitomycin, pulmonary toxicity associated with, 505t
MOPP regimen
  ABVD regimen and, combined therapy, 217
  breast cancer and, 554–555
  for Hodgkin's disease, 203, 216
  for medulloblastoma, 86
Moya Moya syndrome, 49
MTX. *See* Methotrexate
Multicellular tumor spheroids, 192
Multiple endocrine neoplasia, 396
Multiple midline germinomas, 67–68
Musculoskeletal system, radiotherapy-induced injury, 465–467, 466t
Myelopathy, 498, 499t, 500
Myocardial infarction, secondary to radiotherapy, 526–528, 527t
Myocardiopathy, secondary to chemotherapy, 523–524, 524f
Myogenesis, 292
Myxopapillary ependymomas, 104, 115, 116f

N

Nasopharyngeal carcinoma
  age of onset, 403
  bilateral, 406
  classification of, 404
  diagnostic workup, 404
  pathology of, 403–404
  signs and symptoms of, 404
  treatment of
    radiotherapy, 404–406
    surgery, 404
    survival rates, 407t
Nasopharyngeal rhabdomyosarcoma, 312
Nasopharynx, 405
Neck region
  rhabdomyosarcoma of, 313
  squamous cell carcinoma of, 410
Necrosis, radiation-induced, 492–493
Necrotizing leukoencephalopathy, 493, 493f
Neoplasms. *See* specific neoplasm

Nephrectomy, for Wilms' tumor
  description of, 362
  renal effects, 368
Nephrogenic rests, 346
Nerve growth factor receptor pathway, role in neuroblastoma pathogenesis, 166
Neuroblastoma
  anatomic sites of, 166f, 169
  anesthetic considerations, 573
  biology of, 163, 166–167
  bone marrow involvement, 170–172
  catecholamine abnormalities and, 172
  chemotherapy for
    description of, 190–191
    intermediate risk disease, 186
  clinical presentation of, 169–170
  complications of, 194–195
  cytogenetic analysis of, 166–167
  diagnosis of
    criteria, 172–173
    evaluation for, 170–172
    patient age, 163, 175
  epidemiology of, 163
  etiology of, 166
  future investigations of, 195–196
  high-risk
    bone marrow transplantation, 187–189, 188t
    treatment options, 187
  histopathologic classification of, 168t, 169
  historical descriptions of, 163, 164f–165f
  incidence of, 163, 180
  intermediate risk, treatment options for, 185–187
  liver involvement, 170
  localized, treatment options for, 181–183
  low-risk
    survival rates for, 184t
    treatment options for, 183
  metastatic
    description of, 169
    palliative intent, 190
    sites of involvement, 192, 196t
  mortality rates, 163
  olfactory, 408–410
  pathologic features of, 168–169
  prognostic factors
    age at diagnosis, 175
    biologic, 177–179
    clinical, 173, 175, 177
    stage of disease, 175, 176f
  radiotherapy for
    description of, 183
    dose, 192–194
    techniques, 194
    volume, 192
  results, 194
  screening for, 179–181
  secondary malignant neoplasms, 557

signs and symptoms of, 169
spinal abnormalities associated with, 194–195
stage IV-S, 190
staging of, 173, 174t, 176t, 196t
subtypes of, 175t
surgical therapy for, 181–183
survival rates, 4t
Neurocytomas, 51
Neurofibromatosis, 558
etiology of, 39
optic pathway tumors and, 47
Neurogenic sarcoma, characteristics of, 322
Neuron-specific enolase, neuroblastoma and, 177–178
Neutron therapy
for non-rhabdomyosarcoma soft-tissue sarcomas, 335
for osteosarcoma, 282
Nevus flammeus, 446
Nevus vasculosus, 446
Nitrogen mustard, vincristine, procarbazine, and prednisone regimen. See MOPP regimen
Nitrosoureas, pulmonary toxicity associated with, 505t
N-myc amplification
in neuroblastoma diagnosis, 167–168, 178
in rhabdomyosarcoma pathogenesis, 292–293
Nodular renal blastema, 346
Non-Burkitt's lymphoma, 237, 239
Non-Hodgkin's lymphoma
anesthetic considerations, 573
bone marrow involvement, 236
central nervous system involvement, 236–237, 239–240
in children vs. adults, 233
clinical presentation of, 233–234
diagnostic evaluation, 234
epidemiology of, 233
etiology of, 233
histologic categories of, 233
incidence of, 2t–3t
large-cell, 234t, 237
lymphoblastic, 234t
prognostic factors
description of, 236–237
event-free survival and, correlation between, 241t
secondary, in Hodgkin's disease patients, 554
of small bowel, 414
small noncleaved, 234t
staging of, 234–235, 235t
of stomach, 412
treatment of
autologous bone marrow transplantation, 240t
chemotherapy, 237–239, 238t
radiotherapy, 239–240

results, 241–242
survival rates, 4t, 238t, 242
Non-rhabdomyosarcoma soft-tissue sarcomas
clinical presentation, 323
incidence of, 320
metastasis of, pulmonary, 326
outcome estimations, 325
pathology of, 320–323
staging of, 323, 325
treatment of
chemotherapy, 327–331
hyperthermia, 335
neutrons, 335
radiotherapy. See Radiotherapy, non-rhabdomyosarcoma soft-tissue sarcoma
results, 335–336, 337t
surgery, 325–326
types of, 321t. See also specific type
workup for, 323
NPC. See Nasopharyngeal carcinoma

O
Oligodendroglioma
characteristics of, 114–115
incidence of, 50
survival rates, 51
treatment approaches, 50–51
Oncogenes, 128
Opiate agents, for anesthetic use, 568–569
Optic chiasm tumor, 44f
Optic neuropathy, secondary to radiotherapy, 513t
Optic pathway tumors
etiology of, 47–48
illustration of, 48f
incidence of, 47
neurofibromatosis and, 47
treatment approaches
chemotherapy, 49–50
radiotherapy, 49–50
surgery, 48–49
Orbit
developmental retardation, secondary to retinoblastoma, 156–158
hemangiomas of, 448
radiation-induced late effects of, 514–515
rhabdomyosarcoma, 293, 313–314
Osteogenic sarcoma, whole-lung irradiation for, 279
Osteonecrosis, 465
Osteosarcoma
anatomic sites of, 268f
breast cancer risk and, 279
classification of, 267–268, 269t
diagnostic evaluation of, 267–268
incidence of, 2t–3t, 267, 268f
metastatic
anatomic sites of, 271
description of, 267

Osteosarcoma, metastatic (*contd.*)
　to lung, 271, 272f–273f
　surgical treatment, 271
　retinoblastoma gene role in pathogenesis of, 267
　secondary malignant neoplasms, 557
　sign and symptoms of, 267
　staging of, 268–269, 269t
　treatment of
　　Cade technique, 271, 274, 274t
　　chemotherapy, 279–280
　　local management approaches, 269–271
　　photon irradiation, 275
　　radiotherapy. *See* Radiotherapy, osteosarcoma
　　surgery, 269–271
Ovary
　anatomy of, 481
　chemotherapy-induced effects, 483t, 484
　function of, 481
　germ cell tumors of
　　prognosis of, 388
　　radiotherapy for, 389
　　signs and symptoms of, 387–388
　　staging of, 388t–389t, 388–389
　　surgical therapy, 389–390
　　treatment of, 388
　radiation-induced effects
　　clinical manifestations, 481–482, 484
　　description of, 480–481
　　long-term sequelae, 481
　　pathophysiology of, 481
　　patient evaluation, 483t
　　preventive measures, 482

P
p53
　abnormalities of
　　Li-Fraumeni familial tumor syndrome and, 39
　　in rhabdomyosarcoma pathogenesis, 293
　apoptosis, 540
　growth-suppressive actions, 540
　p21 mediation of, 540
Pancarditis, secondary to radiotherapy, 523
Pancreatic adenocarcinoma, 413
Pancreatoblastoma, 413
Papillary carcinoma, 397
Paraaortic irradiation, side effects of, 227
Parinaud's syndrome, 67
Parotid gland neoplasms, 411
Patient education, regarding treatment, 576–577
PCV regimen, for oligodendroglioma, 51
Pediatric cancer center
　effect on survival rates, 7–8
　requirements for, 7t
Pelvis
　Ewing's sarcoma metastasis to, 249f, 260

radiotherapeutic considerations for, 223
Pericarditis, secondary to radiotherapy, 522–523, 527t
P-glycoprotein, 179
Pheochromocytoma, 396–397
Photocoagulation, for retinoblastoma, 135–136
Photon irradiation, for osteosarcoma, 275
Pineal region tumors
　treatment approaches
　　chemotherapy, 69–70
　　description of, 68
　　radiotherapy, 69–71
　　results, 71
　　surgery, 68–69
　types of, 66–68
Pineoblastoma
　characteristics of, 61
　description of, 67
　illustration of, 61f
　in infants and young children, 60
Pineocytoma, 67
Placental blood transplantation, 28
Plaster of Paris, 582–583
Pleocytosis, acute lymphoblastic leukemia and, 12
Pleomorphic xanthoastrocytoma, 40
Pleuropulmonary blastoma, 412
PMLT. *See* Primary malignant liver tumor
PNET. *See* Primitive neuroectodermal tumor
Pneumonitis, 504
Polyurethane foam molds, for patient immobilization, 583–584
Pontine tumors. *See also* Brainstem gliomas
　clinical presentation of, 98
　signs and symptoms of, 96–97
　treatment of
　　chemotherapy, 100
　　radiotherapy, 101
　　results, 104
　　surgery, 99–100
Positron emission tomography, of non-rhabdomyosarcoma soft-tissue sarcomas, 323, 324f
Posterior fossa
　anatomy of, 80
　tumors of. *See* specific tumor
pRB, 129
Precursor B-lymphoblastic lymphoma, 235
Precursor T-lymphoblastic lymphoma, 235
Prednisone
　in ChlVPP regimen, 219
　in MOPP regimen. *See* MOPP regimen
Primary malignant liver tumors
　alpha-fetoprotein tests for, 376
　clinical presentation of, 373–376
　geographic predilection, 373
　hepatoblastoma. *See* Hepatoblastoma
　hepatocellular carcinoma, 374–375, 382

incidence of, 373
staging of, 376–377
treatment of
chemotherapy, 377, 379–382
radiotherapy, 378–379, 382
results, 382
surgery, 377–378
Primitive neuroectodermal tumors
characteristics of, 323
chromosomal abnormalities, 247
composition of, 60
definition of, 60
Ewing's sarcoma and, comparison between,
245–247
tumors classified as, 80
Primitive polar spongioblastoma, 60
Procarbazine, 505t
Propofol, 569
Prostate
radiation-induced late effects, 502t
rhabdomyosarcoma of, treatment approaches
for, 309
Proto-oncogenes
in cellular growth, 128
description of, 538
in neoplastic transformation, 538–539, 539f
in rhabdomyosarcoma pathogenesis, 292–293
in tumor formation, 128
types of, 538–539, 539f
Psychological preparations, 576–577
Pulmonary fibrosis, 506t
Pulse oximetry, 570–571

Q

Quality of life, quantitative measurement of,
6–7

R

Radiation-induced elephantiasis, 332
Radiation-induced sarcoma, 557–558
Radioactive iodine, for thyroid carcinoma,
398–399
Radioactive plaques, for retinoblastoma, 136–138
Radioisotopes, for osteosarcomas, 284
Radionuclide bone scan
of non-rhabdomyosarcoma soft-tissue
sarcomas, 323
of Wilms' tumor, 349
Radiotherapy. *See also* Cranial irradiation;
Craniospinal irradiation
acute lymphoblastic leukemia
central nervous system involvement, 13–19
dose, 22
equipment, 22
leukostasis, 18
volume, 18–21
adrenal cortical carcinoma, 395
anesthesia for. *See* Anesthesia

astrocytomas, 45–47
brainstem gliomas
delivery, 103–104
description of, 100
dose, 101–103
technique, 103
volume, 101
brain tumors
description of, 7
dose, 59
technique, 59
volume, 59
cerebellar astrocytomas
clinical studies of, 112
indications, 112
chemotherapy and, combined approach using
gastrointestinal cancer associated with,
556–557
Hodgkin's disease, 216–217
liver effects, 508t
craniopharyngioma, 66
ependymomas
clinical studies of, 107
delivery, 109
description of, 107
dose, 109
technique, 109
volume, 108–109
esthesioneuroblastoma, 408, 410
Ewing's sarcoma
dose, 257–259
metastatic disease, 261–262
secondary malignant neoplasms associated
with, 549
technique, 259–260
volume, 256–257
germ cell tumors
description of, 69–71
extragonadal, 392–393
ovarian, 389
hemangioma, 447–448
Hodgkin's disease
dose, 224
energy, 224
factors that affect, 222
hypothyroidism, 475–476
refractory/relapse cases, 220–221
stage-based approaches, 217–218
therapy sequence, 224
total lymphoid irradiation, 218
volume, 222–224
infantile subglottic hemangioma, 411
for infants and young children, 59
juvenile nasopharyngeal angiofibroma,
402–403, 403t
juvenile pilocytic astrocytoma, 45–46
Langerhans' cell histiocytosis
clinical studies, 432–433

Radiotherapy, Langerhans' cell histiocytosis
(*contd.*)
   dose, 438–439, 439f–440f
   volume, 439
  late effects of
   bone growth. *See* Bone
   central nervous system. *See* Central
    nervous system, radiation-induced late
    effects of
   genitourinary system, 502t
   growth hormone production and release.
    See Growth hormone
   kidney. *See* Kidney, radiation-induced
    dysfunction
   lung. *See* Lung, radiation-induced late
    effects of
   ovary. *See* Ovary, radiation-induced effects
   prostate, 502t
   testes. *See* Testes, radiation-induced
    effects
   thyroid gland. *See* Thyroid gland, radiation-
    induced endocrine abnormalities
   tissue, 459–461
   uterus, 502t
  low-grade gliomas
   description of, 42–43
   dose, 46–47
   technique, 47
   volume, 45–46
  malignant gliomas
   description of, 52–53
   dose, 54–55
   technique, 54
   volume, 54
  malignant melanoma, 453–454
  medulloblastoma
   clinical studies, 88–89
   dose, 88–89
   efficacy of, 85–86
   technique, 89–93
   volume, 86–87
  nasopharyngeal carcinoma, 404–406
  non-Hodgkin's lymphoma
   description of, 239–240
   hypothyroidism, 475–476
  non-rhabdomyosarcoma soft-tissue sarcomas
   brachytherapy, 332–334
   clinical studies, 326–327
   dose, 332–333
   preoperative use, 331
   volume, 332
  optic pathway tumor, 49–50
  osteosarcoma
   charged particle therapy, 283
   dose, 280–281
   intraoperative use, 283–284
   neutron therapy, 282
   palliative use, 284

   prebiopsy, 271
   radioisotopes, 284
   technique, 281–282
   volume, 281
  pheochromocytoma, 397
  pineal region tumors, 69–71
  primary malignant liver tumors, 378–379,
   382
  retinoblastoma
   clinical studies, 147
   description of, 138
   dose, 144–147
   history of, 140
   secondary malignant neoplasms associated
    with, 547–548
   technique, 138–144
  rhabdomyosarcoma
   clinical studies, 302–305
   description of, 289
   secondary malignant neoplasms associated
    with, 549t
  salivary gland tumors, 410–411
  thyroid carcinoma, 399–400
  tolerance doses, 459t
  Wilms' tumor
   bilateral disease, 364–365
   bone growth effects, 464t
   clinical studies, 362
   dose, 363–364
   pulmonary metastasis, 366
   timing considerations, 363
   volume, 363
RAI. *See* Radioactive iodine
RB1 gene, 267, 539, 547
Reed-Sternberg cells
  characteristics of, 203–204
  history of, 203
  in Hodgkin's disease, 203–204, 206
  illustration of, 207f
  multilineage origin of, 204
Retinoblastoma
  age of onset, 126
  choroidal invasion, 133–134, 152
  composition of, 126
  diagnostic tests, 130–131, 131f–132f
  extraocular extension, 152
  genetics of, 126–129
  growth patterns of, 126, 127f
  heritable
   description of, 126–129, 130f
   secondary malignant neoplasms incidence
    associated with, 547–549
  histologic features of, 126, 127f
  incidence of, 2t–3t, 126
  metastases, 152
  in orbital cavity, 152–153
  prognostic factors, 133–134
  protein, 129

recurrent, 151–152
retreatment of, 151–152
sporadic, 127–128
staging of, 133–134, 134t
treatment of
  cataracts secondary to, 156
  chemotherapy, 147, 148t–149t, 150
  cryotherapy, 136
  enucleation, 134–135
  exenteration, 135
  goals, 134
  lacrimal gland abnormalities from,
    158–159
  laser hyperthermia, 136
  orbital development retardation secondary
    to, 156–158
  photocoagulation, 135–136
  radioactive plaque application, 136–138
  radiotherapy. *See* Radiotherapy,
    retinoblastoma
  secondary nonocular tumors associated
    with, 153–156
  survival rates after, 134
  vitreous seeding, 138
trilateral, 150–151
workup for, 130–131, 131f–132f
Rhabdoid tumor, of kidney, 347
Rhabdomyosarcoma
alveolar, 295
anatomic sites of, 293
biological factors
  cell cycle control, 292
  cytogenetics, 291–292
  overview, 291
  proto-oncogenes, 292–293
bladder, treatment approaches for, 305–309,
  306t–307t
botryoid, 294
of cervix, 311
characteristics of, 289–290
clinical presentation of, 293
clinical studies of, 289–290
diagnostic evaluation, 293–294
embryonal, 295
environmental factors that affect development
  of, 290
epidemiology of, 290–291
extremity, 311–312
future investigations, 315–316
grouping of, 295–297
of head and neck, 313
hepatobiliary tree, 314
histologic classification of, 294–295
incidence of, 2t–3t, 290
of larynx, 411
metastasis
  anatomic sites of, 294
  chemotherapy for, 315

incidence of, 315
  lymph nodes, 299t
nasopharyngeal, 312, 407
orbital, 293, 313–314
parameningeal, 293, 312–313
paratesticular, 310
perineal, 314
prognostic variables
  biology, 299–300
  clinical group, 297
  histology, 299
  lymphatic spread, 297–298
  primary site, 297–298
prostatic, treatment approaches for, 309
relapse, 304
retroperitoneal, 314
spindle cell, 294
staging of, 295–297
survival rates, 296
treatment of
  chemotherapy, 289, 301–302
  future investigations, 315
  general principles, 300
  radiotherapy. *See* Radiotherapy,
    rhabdomyosarcoma
  surgery, 300–301
  survival rates, 289, 290f
truncal, 314
undifferentiated, 295
of uterus, 311
of vagina, 310–311
of vulva, 310–311
RIS. *See* Radiation-induced sarcoma
Rosenthal's fibers, 40

S
Sacrococcygeal germ cell tumors, 391–392
Salivary gland
  radiation-induced late effects, 520t, 521
  tumors of, 410
Sarcoma. *See also* Fibrosarcoma;
    Leiomyosarcoma; Soft-tissue sarcomas
  alveolar soft part, 322
  bone, 549
  epithelioid, 322
  Ewing's. *See* Ewing's sarcoma
  fibromyxoid, 322
  neurogenic, 322
  osteogenic, 279
  radiation-induced, 557–558
  synovial, 332
Sarcoma botryoid, 293
Scoliosis, 463–464
Secondary malignant neoplasms
  chemotherapy and, 544–545
  in childhood survivors of primary malignancy
    clinical studies, 546, 546t–548t
    description of, 545–546

Secondary malignant neoplasms, in childhood
    survivors of primary malignancy
    (*contd.*)
  Ewing's sarcoma, 549
  Hodgkin's disease. *See* Hodgkin's disease,
    secondary malignant neoplasms
  incidence of, 538
  neuroblastoma, 557
  osteosarcoma, 557
  retinoblastomas, 153–156, 547–549
  soft-tissue sarcomas, 549
  Wilms' tumor, 549–550
  predisposing conditions, 558
  radiation-induced sarcoma and, comparison
    between, 557–558
SEER program. *See* Surveillance,
    Epidemiology, and End Results program
Sepsis, 569
Sevoflurane, 565–566
Skin cancer
  basal cell nevus syndrome, 450–451
  malignant melanoma. *See* Malignant
    melanoma
  squamous cell carcinoma, 450–451
Skull, osteosarcoma of, radiotherapeutic
    treatment approaches to, 283
Slipped femoral capital epiphysis, from
    radiotherapy, 464–465
Small bowel
  non-Hodgkin's lymphoma of, 414
  radiation-induced injuries to, 507–508
SMN. *See* Secondary malignant neoplasm
Soft-tissue sarcomas
  definition of, 320
  incidence of, 320
  non-rhabdomyosarcoma. *See* Non-
    rhabdomyosarcoma soft-tissue sarcoma
  rhabdomyosarcoma. *See* Rhabdomyosarcoma
  secondary malignant neoplasms after
    treatment for, 549, 549t
  survival rates, 4t
Solitary eosinophilic granuloma, 422
Somnolence syndrome, 497–498
Spermatogenesis
  description of, 484
  radiation-induced effects, 485, 486t, 490
Spinal cord
  neoplasms
    astrocytomas, 113–114
    ependymomas, 115
    extradural, 113
    intradural, 113
    magnetic resonance imaging evaluation of,
      115
    neuraxis dissemination, 118
    primary, 113
    radiotherapy for, 117–119
    signs and symptoms of, 115

  surgical therapy for, 115–117
  radiation-induced injuries to, 498, 499t,
    500
Spinal irradiation, 93. *See also* Craniospinal
    irradiation
Spitz nevi, 452
Splenectomy, leukemia and, 553–554
Squamous cell carcinoma
  description of, 450–451
  of head and neck region, 410
Stabilization devices. *See also* Immobilization
    devices
  bite block, 579–580
  ideal type, 577–578
  standard types of, 578f–579f, 578–579
Staging
  Burkitt's lymphoma, 235t
  germ cell tumor, 386–387, 391
  Hodgkin's disease
    Cotswold, 206t
    description of, 209
    surgical, 211–212
  juvenile nasopharyngeal angiofibroma, 401,
    402t
  laparotomy for, 211
  malignant melanoma, 452
  medulloblastoma, 83–84, 84t
  neuroblastoma, 173, 174t, 176t, 196t
  non-Hodgkin's lymphoma, 234–235, 235t
  non-rhabdomyosarcoma soft-tissue sarcomas,
    323, 325
  osteosarcoma, 268–269, 269t
  primary malignant liver tumors, 376–377
  retinoblastoma, 133–134, 134t
  rhabdomyosarcoma, 295–297
  Wilms' tumor, 349–351
Stomach, non-Hodgkin's lymphoma of, 412
Stromal tumors, 390–391
Sturge-Weber syndrome, 446
Suprasellar tumors, 40
Supratentorial compartment, 37, 39f
Supratentorial tumors
  astrocytomas. *See* Astrocytoma
  clinical presentation of, 40
  etiology of, 39–40
  incidence of, 38t
  in infants, 55
  malignant. *See* Malignant glioma
Surveillance, Epidemiology, and End Results
    program, 2–3
Swaddling, for patient immobilization, 585
Syngeneic transplantation, definition of, 25t
Synovial sarcoma, 332

T
TBI. *See* Total body irradiation
T cell leukemia
  anesthetic considerations, 573

cranial irradiation for, 16
description of, 11
Teeth
  development of, 518–519
  treatment-related late effects
    chemotherapy, 519, 520t
    radiation, 519–521, 520t
Tegmental tumors
  biopsy of, 100
  description of, 98
Teratomas
  description of, 67
  immature benign, 392
  malignant, 386
Testes
  germ cell tumors of, 391
  leukemia of
    in acute lymphoblastic leukemic patients,
      22–23, 29, 31
    description of, 22–23
    treatment of, 23
  radiation-induced effects
    infertility, 485–486
    overview, 484
    pathophysiology of, 484
    patient evaluation, 489t
    in prepubertal children, 487–488
    preventive measures, 490
  rhabdomyosarcoma of, 310
Testosterone, 484
Thiopental, 568
Thorotrast, 542–543
Thyroidectomy, 398
Thyroid gland
  anatomy of, 474–475
  carcinoma of
    gender predilection, 397
    incidence of, 397
    industrial causes of, 398
    metastases of, 398
    radiation-related, 543–544, 555–556
    radiotherapy for, 399–400
    signs and symptoms of, 398
    types of, 397–398
  radiation-induced endocrine abnormalities
    detection methods, 480
    hyperthyroidism, 478–480, 479t
    hypothyroidism, 475–478
    management of, 480
    pathophysiology, 474–475
    screening modalities, 480
    thyroid enlargement, 480
Thyrotoxicosis, 478
Thyrotropin-releasing hormone, treatment late
    effects related to, 472t
Tissue
  developmental patterns of, 460
  radiation-induced late effects

based on developmental stage of tissue,
    460–461
  description of, 459–460
TLI. *See* Total lymphoid irradiation
Total body irradiation
  administration techniques, 29, 30f
  brass plate use, 31f
  for Ewing's sarcoma, 262
  as preoperative regimen for bone marrow
    transplantation
    description of, 25, 28–29
    for neuroblastoma therapy, 189
    pneumonitis and, 504
  renal dysfunction and, 501
  veno-occlusive disease secondary to, 511
Total lymphoid irradiation, for Hodgkin's
    disease, 218
Transplantation
  bone marrow. *See* Bone marrow
    transplantation
  liver
    for Langerhans' cell histiocytosis, 438
    for primary malignant liver tumors, 378
  placental blood, 28
Treatment planning, 576
Trilateral retinoblastoma, 150–151
Tumor. *See* specific tumor
Tumor lysis syndrome, during Burkitt's
    lymphoma treatment, 239
Tumor suppressor genes
  function of, 128
  mutations in, 128
  in neoplastic transformation, 539, 539f
  p53. *See* p53
  radiation-induced effects, 540–541
  in rhabdomyosarcoma pathogenesis, 293
  Wilms' tumor and, 345

U

Ultrasonography, for retinoblastomas, 133f
Undifferentiated carcinoma, 397–398
Ureter, radiation-induced late effects on, 502t
Urethra, radiation-induced late effects on, 502t
Uterus
  radiation-induced late effects, 502t
  rhabdomyosarcoma of, 311

V

VACA regimen, 254
Vacuum bag, for patient immobilization, 585,
    585f
Vagina
  late effects of
    chemotherapy, 502t
    radiotherapy, 502t
  rhabdomyosarcoma of, 310–311
Valvular disease, secondary to radiotherapy,
    524, 527t

Vasoactive intestinal peptide, neuroblastomas
    and, 172, 178–179
Veno-occlusive disease, 508, 511
Ventriculoperitoneal shunts, 85, 99
Vertebrae
    Ewing's sarcoma metastasis to, 260–261
    hemangiomas of, 448
Vinca alkaloids, pulmonary toxicity associated
    with, 505t
Vincristine, for optic pathway tumors, 50
Vitreous Seeding, for retinoblastoma, 138
VOD. *See* Veno-occlusive disease
Vulva, rhabdomyosarcoma of, 310–311

W
WBC. *See* White blood cell count
White blood cell count, in acute lymphoblastic
    leukemia, 11–12
Whole-brain irradiation, 494
Whole-heart irradiation, 223
Whole-lung irradiation
    breast cancer and, 549
    for metastatic disease
        hepatoblastoma, 379
        osteosarcoma, 275–279, 276t–277t
        Wilms' tumor, 348, 363, 366
    for pulmonary involvement in Hodgkin's
        disease patients, 223
Wilms' tumor
    age of onset, 343
    anaplastic, 346–347
    bilateral, treatment approaches for,
        364–365
    biology of, 343, 345
    clinical presentation of, 347–348

    congenital anomalies associated with,
        344–345
    diagnostic workup, 348–349
    epidemiology of, 343
    history of, 343, 344f
    incidence of, 343
    metastasis of
        abdomen, 363–364
        pulmonary, 348, 507
        treatment of, 365–366
    NWTS studies of, 351–352, 354–360
    pathology of, 345–347
    progression genes, 345
    recurrent, 366–367
    renal function posttreatment, 500t
    SIOP studies of, 351–354
    staging of, 349–351
    syndromes associated with, 347
    treatment of
        brachytherapy, 364
        chemotherapy, 362
        complications associated with, 367–369
        inoperable states, 361–362
        intraoperative radiation, 364
        neoplasms secondary to, 368–369
        nephrectomy, 362
        radiotherapy. *See* Radiotherapy, Wilms'
          tumor
        surgery, 361–362
        survival rates, 4t, 8
WLI. *See* Whole-lung irradiation

X
Xeroderma pigmentosa, 451
Xerostomia, radiation-induced, 520t, 521